# Respiratory Infections

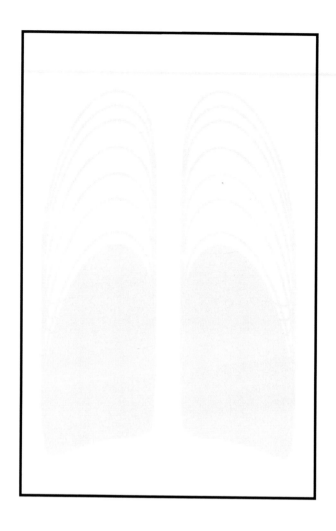

MICHAEL S. NIEDERMAN, MD

Associate Professor of Medicine
SUNY at Stony Brook
Stony Brook, New York
Director of the Medical and
Respiratory Care Unit
Director of the Critical Care Subsection
Winthrop University Hospital
Mineola, New York

GEORGE A. SAROSI, MD

Professor of Medicine
Stanford University Medical School
Stanford, California
Chairman, Department of Internal Medicine
Santa Clara Valley Medical Center
San Jose, California

JEFFREY GLASSROTH, MD

Gilbert H. Marquardt Professor of Medicine
Northwestern University School of Medicine
Chicago, Illinois

# Respiratory Infections

## A Scientific Basis for Management

W.B. SAUNDERS COMPANY
*A Division of Harcourt Brace & Company*
Philadelphia  London  Toronto  Montreal  Sydney  Tokyo

**W.B. SAUNDERS COMPANY**
*A Division of*
*Harcourt Brace & Company*

The Curtis Center
Independence Square West
Philadelphia, Pennsylvania 19106

**Library of Congress Cataloging-in-Publication Data**

Niederman, Michael S.
Respiratory infections / Michael S. Niederman, George Sarosi, Jeffrey
Glassroth.

     p.    cm.

ISBN 0–7216–4347–7

1. Respiratory infections.    I. Sarosi, George A.
   II. Glassroth, Jeffrey.    III. Title.

[DNLM: 1. Respiratory Tract Infections. WF 140 N666r 1994]

RC740.N54 1994

616.2—dc20

DNLM/DLC                              93-35615

Respiratory Infections

ISBN 0–7216–4347–7

Printed in the United States of America.

Last digit is the print number:    9   8   7   6   5   4   3   2   1

To Ronna, Alex, and Eric for their support and understanding
during the completion of this project

MICHAEL S. NIEDERMAN

To Grace for her understanding and support

GEORGE A. SAROSI

To Carol, Marley, and Drew

JEFFREY GLASSROTH

# CONTRIBUTORS

**Richard C. Ahrens, MD**
Associate Professor of Pediatrics at the
University of Iowa; Staff, University of
Iowa Hospitals and Clinics, Iowa City,
Iowa
*Cystic Fibrosis and Respiratory Infections*

**Robert L. Atmar, MD**
Assistant Professor, Department of
Medicine, Microbiology, and
Immunology, Baylor College of
Medicine; Assistant Attending, Ben
Taub General Hospital, Houston, Texas
*Atypical Pneumonia*

**David M. Bamberger, MD**
Associate Professor of Medicine,
University of Missouri–Kansas City
School of Medicine; Attending
Physician, Truman Medical Center;
Medical Education Affiliate Staff
Physician, St. Luke's Hospital, Kansas
City, Missouri
*Upper Respiratory Tract Infections:
Pharyngitis, Sinusitis, Otitis Media, and
Epiglottitis*

**John B. Bass, Jr., MD**
Professor and Vice-Chair, Department of
Medicine, and Director, Division of
Pulmonary and Critical Care Medicine,
University of South Alabama College of
Medicine; Staff, University of South
Alabama Medicine Center, Mobile,
Alabama
*Invasive Techniques for the Diagnosis of
Lower Respiratory Tract Infections*

**Steven L. Berk, MD**
Professor, Department of Internal
Medicine, East Tennessee State
University, James H. Quillen College of
Medicine; Staff, Veterans Affairs
Medical Center and Johnson City
Medical Center Hospital, Johnson City,
Tennessee
*Group B Streptococcal and Other
Nonpneumococcal Streptococcal
Pneumonia;* Moraxella (Branhamella)
catarrhalis *Pneumonia*

**Thomas R. Cate, MD**
Professor of Medicine and of
Microbiology and Immunology, Baylor
College of Medicine; Attending, Harris
County Hospital District (Ben Taub
General Hospital), Houston, Texas
*Viral Pneumonia in Immunocompetent
Adults*

**Richard E. Chaisson, MD**
Associate Professor of Medicine, Division
of Infectious Diseases, Department of
Medicine, Johns Hopkins University
School of Medicine; Associate
Professor of Epidemiology and
International Health, Johns Hopkins
University School of Hygiene and
Public Health, Staff, Johns Hopkins
Hospital and Francis Scott Key Medical
Center, Baltimore, Maryland
*Respiratory Infections in Persons Infected
With Human Immunodeficiency Virus*

**Wendy Colin, PharmD**
Clinical Preceptor, State University of
New York at Buffalo; Clinical
Specialist, Pediatrics, University of
Rochester, Strong Memorial Hospital,
Department of Pharmacy, Rochester,
New York
*Cystic Fibrosis and Respiratory Infections*

**Donald E. Craven, MD**
Professor of Medicine and Epidemiology,
Boston University Schools of Medicine
and Public Health; Director, Adult
Clinical AIDS Program, Boston City
Hospital, Boston, Massachusetts
*Nosocomial Pneumonia in Critically Ill
and Mechanically Ventilated Patients*

**Anthony R. Dal Nogare, MD**
Associate Professor of Internal Medicine,
University of Texas Southwestern
Medical Center; Attending Physician,
Parkland Memorial Hospital, Dallas,
Texas
*Nosocomial Pneumonia Outside the
Intensive Care Unit*

**Scott F. Davies, MD**
Associate Professor of Medicine,
University of Minnesota Medical
School; Director, Division of
Pulmonary and Critical Care Medicine,
Hennepin County Medical Center,
Minneapolis, Minnesota
*Pneumococcal Pneumonia; Fungal
Diseases of the Lung*

**Michael N. Dohn, MD**
Assistant Professor of Clinical Medicine,
University of Cincinnati College of
Medicine, Department of Internal
Medicine, Division of Pulmonary
Critical Care Medicine; Attending
Physician, University of Cincinnati
Medical Center, Cincinnati, Ohio
*Preventive Interventions for Persons
Infected With the Human Immuno-
deficiency Virus*

**Robert A. Duncan, MD, MPH**
Hospital Epidemiologist, Lahey Clinic,
Burlington, Massachusetts
*Nosocomial Pneumonia in Critically Ill
and Mechanically Ventilated Patients*

**Marc M. Dunn, MD**
Assistant Professor, Wayne State
University School of Medicine; Director
of Critical Care, Sinai Hospital of
Detroit, Detroit, Michigan
*Pseudomonal Infections of the Lung*

**Mariam Esat, MD, MBChB**
Assistant Professor of Medicine, College
of Physicians and Surgeons; Assistant
Attending, Harlem Hospital, New York,
New York
*Prevention of Pneumococcal and Influenza
Infections*

**Neil A. Ettinger, MD**
Assistant Professor of Medicine,
Washington University School of
Medicine; Attending, Barnes Hospital,
St. Louis, Missouri
*Immunocompromised Patients: Solid
Organ and Bone Marrow
Transplantation*

**Alan M. Fein, MD**
Professor of Medicine, Health Science
Center, State University of New York at
Stony Brook; Director, Pulmonary and
Critical Care Medicine Division, and
Co-Director, Pulmonary Research
Institute, Winthrop-University Hospital,
Mineola, New York
*Nonresolving, Slowly Resolving, and
Recurrent Pneumonia*

**Steven H. Feinsilver, MD**
Associate Professor of Medicine, Health
Sciences Center, State University of
New York at Stony Brook; Director,
Pulmonary Function Laboratory and
Sleep Disorder Center, Winthrop-
University Hospital, Mineola, New
York
*Nonresolving, Slowly Resolving, and
Recurrent Pneumonia*

**Robert B. Fick, Jr., MD**
Clinical Associate Professor of Medicine,
Stanford University School of
Medicine, Division of Pulmonary and
Critical Care, Stanford, California;
Associate Director, Genentech, Inc.,
S. San Francisco, California
*Cystic Fibrosis and Respiratory Infections*

**Gregory A. Filice, MD**
Associate Professor, Department of
Medicine, University of Minnesota;
Chief, Infectious Disease Section,
Veterans Affairs Medical Center,
Minneapolis; Minnesota
*Nocardiosis; Actinomycosis*

**Mitchell P. Fink, MD**
Associate Professor of Surgery, Harvard
Medical School; Director, Division of
Trauma and Surgical Critical Care, Beth
Israel Hospital, Boston, Massachusetts
*Nosocomial Pneumonia in Surgical
Patients*

**Peter T. Frame, MD**
Professor of Clinical Medicine, University
of Cincinnati; Director, AIDS
Treatment Center, University of
Cincinnati Medical Center, Cincinnati,
Ohio
*Preventive Interventions for Persons
Infected With the Human
Immunodeficiency Virus*

**Joel E. Gallant, MD, MPH**
Assistant Professor of Medicine, Division
of Infectious Diseases, Department of
Medicine, Johns Hopkins University
School of Medicine; Active Staff, Johns
Hopkins Hospital and Francis Scott Key
Medical Center, Baltimore, Maryland
*Respiratory Infections in Persons Infected
With Human Immunodeficiency Virus*

**Eugene F. Geppert, MD**
Professor of Clinical Medicine, University
of Chicago Pritzker School of Medicine,
Chicago, Illinois
*Lung Abscess and Other Subacute
Pulmonary Infections*

**Dale N. Gerding, MD**
Professor and Associate Chairman,
Department of Medicine, Northwestern
University; Chief, Medical Service,
Veterans Affairs Lakeside Medical
Center, Chicago, Illinois
*Antimicrobials for the Treatment of
Respiratory Infection*

**Jeffrey Glassroth, MD**
Gilbert H. Marquardt Professor of
Medicine, Northwestern University
School of Medicine, Chicago, Illinois
*Tuberculosis*

**Robert J. Glennon, MD**
Instructor of Medicine, Mount Sinai
School of Medicine; Co-Physician in
Charge, Intensive Care Units, Beth
Israel Medical Center, North Division,
New York, New York
*Adjunctive Measures in the Treatment of
Respiratory Infections*

**Stephen B. Greenberg, MD**
Vice-Chairman, Department of Medicine,
and Professor of Medicine, Micro-
biology and Immunology, Baylor
College of Medicine; Chief, Medical
Service, Ben Taub General Hospital,
Houston, Texas
*Atypical Pneumonia*

**David E. Griffith, MD**
Associate Professor of Medicine,
University of Texas Health Center at
Tyler, Tyler, Texas
*Bronchitis and Acute Febrile Tracheo-
bronchitis*

**Jeffrey K. Griffiths, MD, MPH&TM**
Assistant Professor of Medicine and
Comparative Medicine, Tufts University
Schools of Medicine and Veterinary
Medicine; Director of Clinical
Microbiology, and Division of
Infectious Diseases, St. Elizabeth's
Medical Center of Boston, Boston,
Massachusetts
*Anaerobic Pleuropulmonary Infections:
Aspiration, Pneumonia, Abscess, and
Empyema*

**John E. Heffner, MD**
Staff, St. Joseph's Hospital and Medical
Center, Phoenix, Arizona
*Pneumonia and Empyema*

**Hoi Ho, MD, MACP**
Associate Professor, Division of Infectious
Diseases, Texas Tech; Attending
Physician and Consultant, R.E.
Thomason Hospital, El Paso, Texas
*Community-Acquired Gram-Negative
Pneumonias*

**Jonathan S. Ilowite, MD**
Assistant Professor of Medicine, State
University of New York at Stony
Brook; Director, Pulmonary
Rehabilitation and Respiratory Therapy,
Winthrop-University Hospital, Mineola,
New York
*Inhaled Antibiotics*

**Carlos M. Isada, MD**
Staff, Department of Infectious Diseases,
Cleveland Clinic Foundation,
Cleveland, Ohio
*Chronic Bronchitis: Role of Antibiotics*

**Mary Anne Jackson, MD**
Associate Professor of Pediatrics,
University of Missouri–Kansas City
School of Medicine; Pediatrician in
Infectious Diseases, The Children's
Mercy Hospital, Kansas City, MO
*Upper Respiratory Tract Infections:
Pharyngitis, Sinusitis, Otitis Media, and
Epiglottitis*

**Richard F. Jacobs, MD**
Horace C. Cabe Professor of Pediatrics,
University of Arkansas for Medical
Sciences; Chief, Pediatric Infectious
Diseases, Arkansas Children's Hospital,
Little Rock, Arkansas
*Lower Respiratory Tract Infections of
Infants and Childen; Nosocomial
Pneumonia in Children*

**Philip C. Johnson, MD**
Associate Professor and Director, Division
of General Medicine, Baylor College of
Medicine; Attending, Hermann
Hospital, Houston, Texas
*Fungal Diseases of the Lung*

**Kethy M. Jules-Elysee, MD**
Resident, Department of Anesthesiology,
Cornell University Medical Center,
New York, New York
*Immunocompromised Patients:
Nontransplant Chemotherapy
Immunosuppression*

**Michael B. Kirkpatrick, MD**
Professor of Medicine, Division of
Pulmonary and Critical Care Medicine,
University of South Alabama College of
Medicine, and University of South
Alabama Medical Center, Mobile,
Alabama
*Invasive Techniques for the Diagnosis of
Lower Respiratory Tract Infections*

**Richard S. Kronenberg, MD**
Professor and Chairman of Medicine,
University of Texas Health Center at
Tyler, Tyler, Texas
*Bronchitis and Acute Febrile
Tracheobronchitis*

**Alexandro Liberati, MD**
Laboratory of Clinical Epidemiology,
Mario Negri Institute, Milan, Italy
*Prevention of Respiratory Tract Infections
in Intensive Care by Selective
Decontamination of the Digestive Tract*

**Thomas J. Marrie, MD, FRCP(C)**
Professor of Medicine, Dalhousie
University; Active Staff, Victoria
General Hospital; Consultant Staff,
Camp Hill Medical Center, Halifax,
Nova Scotia, Canada
*Community-Acquired Pneumonia*

**William J. Martin II, MD**
Floyd and Reba Smith Professor of
Medicine, Indiana University School of
Medicine; Director, Division of
Pulmonary and Critical Care, Indiana
University Medical Center,
Indianapolis, Indiana
Pneumocystis carinii

**William Merrill, MD**
Associate Professor, Yale University
School of Medicine; Chief, Pulmonary
Section, West Haven Division of
Veterans Affairs Medical Center, New
Haven, Connecticut
*Humoral Immunity in the Lung:
Expression and Therapeutic
Manipulation*

**Robert M. Middleton, MD**
Pulmonologist, Keesler Medical Center,
Keesler Air Force Base, Mississippi
*Invasive Techniques for the Diagnosis of
Lower Respiratory Tract Infections*

**Robert R. Muder, MD**
Assistant Professor of Medicine,
University of Pittsburgh; Chief,
Infection Control, Veterans Affairs
Medical Center, Pittsburgh,
Pennsylvania
Legionella

**Daniel M. Musher, MD**
Professor of Medicine, and of
Microbiology and Immunology, Baylor
College of Medicine; Chief, Infectious
Disease Section, Veterans Affairs

Medical Center, Houston, Texas
Haemophilus influenzae *as a Cause of
Acute Tracheobronchitis or Pneumonia*

**James Myers, MD**
Assistant Professor, University of
Tennessee College of Medicine–
Chattanooga; Attending, Erlanger
Medical Center, Chattanooga,
Tennessee
Moraxella (Branhamella) catarrhalis
*Pneumonia*

**Edward A. Nardell, MD**
Assistant Professor of Medicine, Harvard
Medical School; Chief, Pulmonary
Medicine, The Cambridge Hospital,
Cambridge, Massachusetts
*Respiratory Tract Infections Among the
Economically Disadvantaged*

**Steve Nelson, MD**
Associate Professor of Medicine and
Physiology (Pulmonary/Critical Care),
Louisiana State University Medical
Center; Director of Critical Care,
University Hospital, New Orleans,
Louisiana
*New Therapeutic Strategies for Sepsis and
Pneumonia*

**Michael S. Niederman, MD**
Associate Professor of Medicine, SUNY at
Stony Brook, Stony Brook, New York;
Director, Medical and Respiratory
Intensive Care Unit and Director,
Critical Care Subsection, Winthrop-
University Hospital, Mineola, New
York
*Nutrition and Infection; Approach to
Pneumonia in the Elderly Nursing
Home Patient; Nonresolving, Slowly
Resolving, and Recurrent Pneumonia*

**Gary A. Noskin, MD**
Assistant Professor of Clinical Medicine,
Northwestern University Medical
School; Attending, Northwestern
Memorial Hospital and VA Lakeside
Medical Center, Chicago, Illinois
*Host Impairments in Human
Immunodeficiency Virus Infection*

**John P. Phair, MD**
Samuel J. Sackett Professor of Medicine
and Chief, Division of Infectious
Diseases, Northwestern University
Medical School; Attending,
Northwestern Memorial Hospital and
VA Lakeside Medical Center, Chicago,
Illinois
*Host Impairments in Human
Immunodeficiency Virus Infection*

**Susan K. Pingleton, MD**
Professor of Medicine and Director,
  Division of Pulmonary and Critical
  Care Medicine, University of Kansas
  Medical School, Kansas City, Kansas
*Nutrition and Infection*

**Reuben Ramphal, MD**
Associate Professor of Medicine, Division
  of Infectious Diseases, Department of
  Medicine, University of Florida;
  Attending Physician, Shands Hospital,
  Gainesville, Florida
*Pathogenesis of Airway Colonization*

**M. Patricia Rivera, MD**
Clinical Assistant Physician, Memorial
  Sloan-Kettering Cancer Center, New
  York, New York
*Immunocompromised Patients:
  Nontransplant Chemotherapy
  Immunosuppression*

**Glenn D. Roberts, PhD**
Professor of Microbiology and of
  Laboratory Medicine, Mayo Medical
  School; Consultant, Division of Clinical
  Microbiology, Mayo Clinic and Mayo
  Foundation, Rochester, Minnesota
*An Approach to Diagnostic Methods*

**Richard M. Rose, MD**
Associate Professor of Medicine,
  University of California, San Diego;
  Vice President, Drug Development,
  Cytel Corporation, San Diego,
  California
*The Host Defense Network of the Lungs:
  An Overview*

**Mark J. Rosen, MD**
Associate Professor of Medicine, Mount
  Sinai School of Medicine; Chief,
  Division of Pulmonary and Critical
  Care Medicine, Beth Israel Medical
  Center, New York, New York
*Adjunctive Measures in the Treatment of
  Respiratory Infections*

**Matthias Salathe, MD**
Fellow, Pulmonary Division University of
  Miami, Miami, Florida
*Nonspecific Host Defenses: Mucociliary
  Clearance and Cough*

**George A. Sarosi, MD**
Clinical Professor of Medicine, University
  of Arizona, Tucson; Chairman,
  Department of Internal Medicine,
  Maricopa Medical Center, Phoenix,
  Arizona
*Fungal Diseases of the Lung*

**Gordon E. Schutze, MD**
Assistant Professor of Pediatrics and
  Pathology, University of Arkansas for
  Medical Sciences; Attending, Arkansas
  Children's Hospital, Little Rock,
  Arkansas
*Lower Respiratory Tract Infections of
  Infants and Children*

**Michael S. Simberkoff, MD**
Associate Professor of Medicine, New
  York University School of Medicine;
  Chief, Infectious Diseases Section, New
  York Veterans Affairs Medical Center;
  Associate Attending in Medicine, Tisch
  (NYU) Hospital; Associate Visiting
  Physician in Medicine, Bellevue
  Medical Center, New York, New York
*Prevention of Pneumococcal and Influenza
  Infections*

**David R. Snydman, MD**
Professor of Medicine and Pathology,
  Tufts University School of Medicine;
  Director, Clinical Microbiology, New
  England Medical Center, Boston,
  Massachusetts
*Anaerobic Pleuropulmonary Infections:
  Aspiration, Pneumonia, Abscess, and
  Empyema*

**Steven W. Sonnesyn, MD**
Assistant Clinical Professor, Department
  of Medicine, University of Minnesota;
  Staff Physician, Infectious Diseases,
  Abbott Northwestern Hospital,
  Minneapolis, Minnesota
*Antimicrobials for the Treatment of
  Respiratory Infection*

**Kathleen A. Steger, MPH, RN**
Assistant Professor of Public Health,
  Boston University School of Public
  Health; Associate Director, Adult
  Clinical AIDS Program, Boston City
  Hospital, Boston, Massachusetts
*Nosocomial Pneumonia in Critically Ill
  and Mechanically Ventilated Patients*

**James K. Stoller, MD**
Associate Professor of Medicine, Ohio
  State University School of Medicine,
  Columbus; Head, Section of Respiratory
  Therapy, Department of Pulmonary and
  Critical Care Medicine, Cleveland
  Clinic Foundation, Cleveland, Ohio
*Chronic Bronchitis: Role of Antibiotics*

**Christiaan P. Stoutenbeek, MD, PhD**
Director, Department of Intensive Care,
  Onze Lieve Vrouwe Gasthuis,
  Amsterdam, Holland

*Prevention of Respiratory Tract Infections in Intensive Care by Selective Decontamination of the Digestive Tract*

**Diane E. Stover, MD**
Professor of Clinical Medicine, Cornell University Medical Center; Chief, Pulmonary Service, and Head, Division of General Medicine, Memorial Sloan-Kettering Cancer Center, New York, New York
*Immunocompromised Patients: Nontransplant Chemotherapy Immunosuppression*

**Warren R. Summer, MD**
Professor of Medicine (Pulmonary/Critical Care), Louisiana State University Medical Center; Director of Respiratory Services, University Hospital, New Orleans, Louisiana
*New Therapeutic Strategies for Sepsis and Pneumonia*

**Gregory P. Thompson, MD**
Former Instructor of Medicine, Mayo Medical School, Rochester, Minnesota; Staff Physician, Gundersen Clinic and LaCrosse Lutheran Hospital, LaCrosse, Wisconsin
*An Approach to Diagnostic Methods*

**Hendrik K.F. van Saene, MD, PhD**
Senior Lecturer, Department of Medical Microbiology, University of Liverpool; Department of Medical Microbiology, Alderhey Childrens Hospital, Liverpool, United Kingdom
*Prevention of Respiratory Tract Infections in Intensive Care by Selective Decontamination of the Digestive Tract*

**Abraham Verghese, MD, FACP, FRCP(C)**
Professor of Medicine and Chief, Division of Infectious Diseases, Texas Tech; Consultant, R.E. Thomason Hospital, El Paso, Texas
*Community-Acquired Gram-Negative Pneumonias*

**Jeanne Marie Wallace, MD**
Associate Professor of Medicine, UCLA School of Medicine, Los Angeles; Attending, Olive View–UCLA Medical Center, Sylmar, California
*Mimics of Infectious Pneumonia in Persons Infected With Human Immunodeficiency Virus*

**Richard J. Wallace, Jr., MD**
Professor and Chairman, Department of Microbiology, University of Texas Health Science Center at Tyler, Tyler, Texas
*Pneumonic Forms of Bacterial Zoonosis: Plague, Anthrax, and Tularemia; Mycobacteria Other Than Mycobacterium tuberculosis*

**Adam Wanner, MD**
Professor of Medicine and Chief, Pulmonary Division, University of Miami School of Medicine; Staff, Mount Sinai Medical Center, Miami Beach, FL
*Nonspecific Host Defenses: Mucociliary Clearance and Cough*

**Robert A. Weinstein, MD**
Professor of Medicine, University of Illinois (Chicago) College of Medicine; Program Director, Joint University of Illinois/University of Chicago Infectious Disease Fellowship Training Program; Director, Infection Control, Michael Reese Hospital and Medical Center, Chicago, Illinois
*Infection Control Methods*

**Janis Wiener, MD**
Clinical Instructor of Medicine, The University of Illinois (Chicago); Clinical Instructor of Medicine, Northwestern University Medical School; Attending Physician, Michael Reese Hospital and Medical Center and Northwestern University Hospital, Chicago, Illinois
*Infection Control Methods*

**Victor L. Yu, MD**
Professor of Medicine, University of Pittsburgh; Chief, Infectious Disease Section, Veterans Administration Medical Center, Pittsburgh, Pennsylvania
*Legionella*

**Paul E. Zimmerman, MD**
Assistant Clinical Professor, University of Minnesota–Duluth School of Medicine; Attending, The Duluth Clinic Ltd, St. Mary's Medical Center, St. Luke's Medical Center and Miller-Dwan Medical Center, Duluth, Minnesota
*Pneumocystis carinii*

# PREFACE

There is currently a resurgence of interest in respiratory infections, for a number of compelling reasons. Pneumonia is the sixth leading cause of death in the United States, but it is the number one cause of death from infectious diseases. Also, certain types of infections are becoming increasingly common in the 1990s. Specific populations of patients, notably elderly persons, patients with human immunodeficiency virus infection, and those with other chronic medical illnesses, have a particularly high rate of acquiring lung infections. Among hospitalized individuals, nosocomial pneumonia is the second or third most common hospital-acquired infection, and the one most likely to lead to death.

There have also been multiple developments related to the epidemiology and biology of specific respiratory tract pathogens. For example, mycobacterial disease, including tuberculosis, has become an increasingly common problem. In addition, mycobacteria, as well as other pathogens such as *Streptococcus pneumoniae, Staphylococcus aureus, Haemophilus influenzae,* and a number of enteric gram-negative bacteria, have developed resistance to common antimicrobial agents, which adds to the difficulties in managing illness caused by these organisms. At the same time that the complexity of respiratory infections is increasing, the technologies available for diagnosis, treatment, and prevention are expanding. Molecular biology has given us new diagnostic and therapeutic approaches, new antimicrobial therapies are becoming available, and vaccines for common infections are being developed.

We have organized this text in order to summarize this expanding field and to provide a practical approach for clinicians to treat patients with respiratory infection. Unlike other similar texts, the focus of this effort is to provide a clinical approach to specific at-risk populations who present with respiratory infection. This approach, rather than an organism-directed organization, has been used because of our firm belief that one must consider the clinical and epidemiologic picture of the patient before one can consider a specific microbial cause for a suspected lung infection. This clinical approach must have a firm scientific foundation; therefore, we have summarized the current state of knowledge relevant to understanding the pathogenesis of pneumonia and other infections.

This text is intended to be a state-of-the art review of the field of respiratory infections, designed to meet the needs of both clinicians and scientists. It starts with a scientific review of infection pathogenesis and provides the principles on which clinical assessment, as well as diagnostic and therapeutic stragegies, are based. The next section is the "clinical core" of the book, in which respiratory infections are discussed from a unique and practical perspective. Specific risk groups are described, along with a review of the presentations and likely pathogens for lung infection in each group. This section can be consulted by a clinician at the time of initial evaluation of a patient suspected of having a respiratory infection. This part of the book is intended to focus on diagnosis and therapy for the specific patient and the set of clinical and epidemiologic circumstances at hand. After these efforts have led to the identification of a pathogen, the clinician can consult the next section, which reviews the specific features of individual respiratory pathogens.

Although each chapter in the clinical approach section is self-sufficient, issues are raised that are related to diagnosis, therapy, and prevention that apply to all patients, and these are reviewed in the later portions of the text. Practical reviews of the handling of laboratory samples, the use of new antimicrobial agents, and the benefits of available preventive approaches are presented.

This book is edited by three individuals with experience and interests in different aspects of lung infections. In this way, we believed that we could identify and recruit authoritative authors for each chapter. We are grateful to our contributing authors for all of their efforts and interest in this project. As with any multi-authored text, there is some repetition of information, but we have attempted to edit the chapters carefully to limit this to areas in which duplication might provide insight into various approaches to a particular problem.

We are grateful to Judy Fletcher at W.B. Saunders Company for her supervision of this project and for her encouragement. We also thank our families for indulging us the time required to complete this text.

MICHAEL S. NIEDERMAN, MD

GEORGE A. SAROSI, MD

JEFFREY GLASSROTH, MD

# CONTENTS

# Respiratory Infections

P A R T

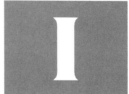

I

# Pathogenesis of Pneumonia

# The Host Defense Network of the Lungs: An Overview

RICHARD M. ROSE

The development of lung defense mechanisms capable of restricting the growth of infectious agents was an essential step in the evolution of air-breathing animals. To exchange oxygen and carbon dioxide with the environment, the lungs must avoid damage from a myriad of potentially injurious agents in the airstream. The agents include microorganisms shed from the skin and mucosal surfaces during routine activities such as coughing and sneezing. In the form of droplet nuclei, microbes can survive for extended periods in the environment and often have aerodynamic profiles that permit their penetration and deposition in the airways and gas exchange structures of the respiratory tract.

This presents a formidable challenge to the lungs. For a person with a minute ventilation of 6 L/min, it is necessary for the lungs to filter almost 9000 L of air daily. This task is daunting because the surface area of the lungs requiring protection is more than 75 times the external surface area of an average man! Host defenses must respond to this challenge and withstand the threat of infectious agents reaching the lungs through the bloodstream or by aspiration of oropharyngeal secretions, which may contain as many as $10^8$ bacteria per 1 mL of fluid.

Airways in the human lower respiratory tract normally contain few colonies of mostly commensal microorganisms.[1] The relative sterility of the lungs is the result of a complex network of antimicrobial defenses. The general properties of this host defense network are as follows.

1. It consists of immunologically specific and nonspecific components.
2. Its components are interactive and, under physiologic conditions, are carefully controlled.
3. It can be amplified by an influx of systemic antimicrobial factors.

In the first part of this chapter, the cellular basis of lung defenses is discussed. Other aspects of immunologically nonspecific defenses and humoral aspects of immune defenses are discussed in subsequent sections of this book. The second part of this chapter describes how lung defenses interact with specific respiratory pathogens.

## GENERAL MECHANISMS OF MICROBIAL CLEARANCE

The consequences of respiratory exposure to potentially infectious pathogens depend on factors that are specific for the organism and the host. Microbial attributes that may influence the outcome of the host-parasite interaction include inoculum size and virulence factors, such as the ability to produce toxins that adversely affect various components of the respiratory defense network (Table 1–1). For microorganisms in the airstream, the aerodynamic proper-

Table 1–1. **Microbial Virulence Factors That Affect Lung Defenses**

| Factor | Organism | Biologic Effects |
|---|---|---|
| Cilotoxin | *Haemophilus influenzae* | Retards ciliary beat frequency |
| IgA protease | *Pseudomonas aeruginosa* | Degrades secretory IgA |
| Inhibitors of oxidative metabolism | *Legionella pneumophila* | Suppresses generation of oxygen radicals by phagocytes |
| Components of cell wall | *Mycobacterium tuberculosis* | Inhibits phagolysosomal fusion in macrophages |

ties of infectious particles are critical determinants of respiratory deposition. Particles greater than 10 μm in diameter are filtered in the nasopharynx; decreasing particle size to the range of 1 to 2 μm results in a pattern of increasing deposition in small airways and alveoli. For droplet nuclei containing certain infectious agents, such as *Mycobacterium tuberculosis*, the mean aerodynamic diameter is estimated to be 1 to 5 μm, a range that favors retention in the distal lung.

A variety of host factors influence the efficiency of lung clearance mechanisms for infectious agents. Under normal circumstances, infectious particles impacting the mucosal surface of the airways are removed from the lungs by the mucociliary escalator (Fig. 1–1). Removal by this process can be accelerated if microbes stimulate neural receptors in the airways capable of mediating increased mucus production and cough. Airway clearance may also be aided by phagocytic cells and antimicrobial factors in the airway secretions, including lactoferrin, a protein with broad-spectrum antibacterial activity based on its capacity to bind iron, which is an essential element for microbial growth.[2, 3] Another potent antimicrobial factor in airway secretions is a cysteine-rich peptide related biochemically to the family of defensins, cationic antimicrobial peptides found in many mammalian phagocytic cells.[4] Like the defensins, this tracheal antimicrobial peptide has antimicrobial activity against gram-positive and gram-negative bacteria and against *Candida albicans*.

Infectious agents reaching the terminal airways and alveoli are cleared by cellular mechanisms. Alveolar macrophages are the predominant phagocytic cell in this region of the normal lung and are capable of ingesting and destroying many microorganisms. This process can be assisted by local factors such as fibronectin and surfactant protein A, which exhibit opsonic activity for some microbes.[5]

Complement components are found in the lower respiratory tract[6] and can be activated through the alternate pathway by structures on the microbial surface such as endotoxin and certain highly conserved carbohydrate domains. In immune hosts, binding of specific immunoglobulin G (IgG) or immunoglobulin M (IgM) molecules to the microbial surface initiates activation of the classic pathway. Both pathways of complement activation result in binding of C3b to the infectious agent, which can then be recognized by the type 1 complement receptors on neutrophils and macrophages. Enzymatic modification of the C3 complex yields C3bi, a factor that is more stable than C3b and acts as a ligand for the type 3 complement receptors on these phagocytic cells. The complement system has direct antimicrobial activity through cleavage of C5 into C5b, which is the foundation of the membrane attack complex consisting of highly bioreactive terminal complement components.[7]

Ingestion of infectious agents by pulmonary macrophages may lead to microbial killing. The mobile macrophage can also physically remove microbes from the lower respiratory tract (see Fig. 1–1). Pathways available for macrophage egress include the mucociliary escalator and interstitial and pleural lymphatics. If macrophage antimicrobial activities are inadequate for containing the growth of a microorganism, these normal pathways for microbial clearance can transport the infectious process to different anatomic regions of the lungs.

One method for evaluating the relative role of these immunologically nonspecific defense mechanisms in microbial clearance in the normal host is demonstrated in Figure 1–2. If these defenses are adequate for clearing an infectious challenge (eg, small microbial inoculum, avirulent organism), eradication of viable organisms from the lower respiratory tract is a highly efficient and rapid process in which microbial killing by phagocytes is usually of greater importance than actual physical clearance (see Fig. 1–2A). If normal protective mechanisms are inadequate to handle an infectious challenge (eg, large microbial inoculum, virulent organism), the failure is typically caused by the inability of lung phagocytic cells to restrict microbial replication (see Fig. 1–2B). Uncontrolled infection in the normal host induces an inflammatory response in which systemic defenses such as neutrophils are recruited. Such augmentation of local lung defenses is of value in limiting the extent of the infectious process (see Fig. 1–2C). These local and systemic defenses can be further amplified by activation of an immune response that characteristically develops in the later phases of the infectious process (see Fig. 1–2D).

## PHYSIOLOGIC CONTROL OF THE RESPIRATORY DEFENSE NETWORK

The factors controlling the complex interactions of the respiratory defense network are incompletely understood. Pulmonary macrophages are undoubtedly central to the orchestration of inflammatory and immune reactions in the lungs. Macrophages are found at the locus of microbial deposition at an early stage in infection and are capable of

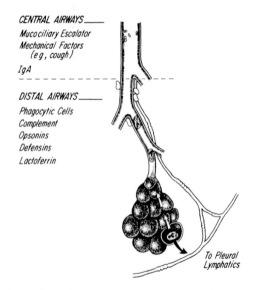

CENTRAL AIRWAYS
Mucociliary Escalator
Mechanical Factors
   (e g, cough)
IgA

DISTAL AIRWAYS
Phagocytic Cells
Complement
Opsonins
Defensins
Lactoferrin

To Pleural
Lymphatics

**Figure 1–1.** Schematic representation of the anatomic pathways for microbial clearance from the lungs. The major factors affecting microbial clearance from the airways and alveoli are listed on the left. At the alveolar level, phagocytic cells harboring microorganisms have two pathways of egress: centrifugal movement to pleural-based lymphatics and proximal movement up the mucociliary escalator in the distal and central airways. During the latter process, phagocytes can interact with lymphoid tissue associated with the airways, which are shown as ovoid structures at the airway bifurcations or in contiguity with the lymphatic system.

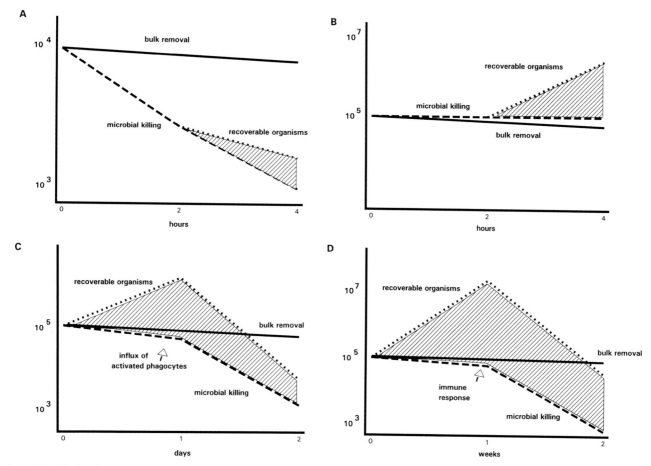

**Figure 1–2.** Idealized patterns of microbial clearance, showing the contribution of bulk physical removal by mucociliary clearance *(solid line)* and microbial killing by the pulmonary defense network *(dashed line)* at intervals after microbial challenge *(horizontal axis)*. Colony-forming units of a theoretical respiratory pathogen are displayed on the vertical axis. The number of viable organisms recoverable in the lungs is shown by the dotted line. The number of recoverable organisms at time ti is predicted by (microbial inoculum$_{t0}$ + microbial growth$_{t0-ti}$) − (bulk removal$_{t0-ti}$ + microbial killing$_{t0-ti}$). The line-filled area represents an estimate of net microbial growth: total microbial growth$_{t0-ti}$ − (bulk removal$_{t0-ti}$ + microbial killing$_{t0-ti}$).

*(A)* Short-term outcome of pulmonary challenge with a small inoculum of an avirulent organism. *(B)* Results of a challenge with a larger inoculum of a more virulent organism during the same period. If native pulmonary defenses are inadequate to restrict microbial replication, *(C)* augmentation of the lungs' defense network by recruitment of activated phagocytes and *(D)* the development of an immune response can be protective, although days or weeks may be required to elicit these responses.

secreting a variety of soluble factors important in the development of local inflammation. Macrophages are also a vehicle for the movement of antigenic particles to local lymphoid tissue as a first step in the generation of an immune response.[8] Although macrophages appear to be a key factor in the initiation and perpetuation of inflammatory and immune reactions during lung infection, it is not known if they play a role in the termination of these events after the infectious focus has been eradicated. A factor produced by human alveolar macrophages is capable of suppressing neutrophil migration in response to a variety of chemoattractants.[9] This factor is able to inhibit agonist-mediated oxidative burst activity by neutrophils. Prostagladin $E_2$ and transforming growth factor-β, both macrophage secretory products, may play a similar role in dampening T- and B-lymphocyte responses.[10, 11] This ability to limit certain responses may be one homeostatic mechanism for appropriately controlling the respiratory defense network after the active infectious process has been contained. This capability is important because persistent inflammatory and immune responses in the lower respiratory tract are commonly associated with end-organ injury.

## Lung Defense Cells

Studies employing the technique of bronchoalveolar lavage (BAL) to sample cellular constituents of the distal airways and alveoli indicate that approximately 85% of lavageable defense cells in normal adults are macrophages, 1% to 3% are neutrophils, and 10% are lymphocytes.[12] The number and functional agenda of these cells can be dramatically altered in response to an infectious challenge in a manner that is often characteristic for a specific class of microbial pathogen. For instance, the inflammatory response to lung infection with common bacterial pathogens such as *Streptococcus pneumoniae* typically increases the number and activation state of macrophages and neutrophils obtained by BAL. Mycobacterial infection is often associated with a pattern of mononuclear cell predominance.

Lung defense cells occur on the epithelial surface, in the pleural space, and within the interstitium and lymphoid structures of the lungs. There is mounting evidence to support an intravascular location for macrophages in many animal species.[13] What little is known about defense cells in these different anatomic locales suggests that their biology can be quite diverse and may differ in substantive ways from that of cells retrieved by BAL. The number of defense cells in nonalveolar regions of the lungs is large. Morphometric studies indicate that macrophages associated with lung connective tissue may be more numerous than in alveoli.[14] These interstitial cells differ antigenically[15] and functionally[16] from alveolar macrophages. The origin of this biologic diversity is partially related to the specialized microenvironments in which lung defense cells must operate. For instance, an alveolar macrophage must be adapted to residing on the oxygen-rich gas exchange surface of the lungs, but an interstitial macrophage is conditioned by direct contact with the biochemically complex connective tissue matrix. It is likely that recruitment of defense cells from various regions to the site of infection results in a population composed of cell types that are biologically and functionally heterogeneous.

## Macrophages

These "big eaters" have an established role as the primary defense of the lungs against a broad array of microorganisms (Table 1–2). Pulmonary macrophages are derived from precursors in the bone marrow that reach the lungs under steady-state and inflammatory conditions through the circulation in the form of blood monocytes.[17, 18] The limited proliferative capacity of macrophages provides a mechanism for local renewal of macrophage numbers. This process may be fostered by a lineage-specific growth factor for macrophages (ie, macrophage colony-stimulating factor) in the lower respiratory tract.[19] Because macrophages are relatively long-lived cells (ie, their life span can be on the order of months) and have several pathways of cell renewal, the population of macrophages in the lungs is

stable even under conditions (eg, chemotherapy) in which other myeloid cell lines are severely depleted.[20]

Ultrastructural studies of macrophages demonstrate a highly convoluted plasma membrane, which provides an expanded surface area for interaction with microorganisms (Fig. 1–3). The first step in macrophage recognition of microbes involves attachment of the organism to the membrane, a process that requires the binding of specific ligands on the organism to a receptor on the macrophage plasma membrane. Receptor occupation initiates the process of phagocytosis in which the infectious particle is engulfed by pseudopodal extensions arising from the macrophage surface. This process appears to be controlled by the availability of appropriate receptors along the surface of the pseudopod and the distribution of ligands on the microbe.[21] The energy-dependent process of phagocytosis is fueled by the abundant, energy-generating mitochondria in the macrophage cytoplasm.

Internalization of the plasma membrane-bound microorganism results in the formation of an intracytoplasmic vacuole (see Fig. 1–3). Movement of the vacuole centrally provides an opportunity for fusion with acid hydrolase-containing vesicles to form the secondary lysosome. Morphologically, this structure appears as an electron-dense granule by electron microscopy. The acidic environment and a variety of hydrolases in the secondary lysosome lead to the digestion of many macromolecules. Cell wall-containing microorganisms may resist digestion. Under these circumstances, macrophages can restrict microbial growth by their ability to generate highly toxic intermediates of oxygen[22] and nitrogen.[23] The contribution of oxidative products from L-arginine metabolism to produce nitrous oxide radicals is a well-developed property of rodent macrophages but appears to be of less importance to the antimicrobial arsenal of human phagocytes.[24]

Certain microorganisms have evolved mechanisms for evading macrophage killing and, as a result, can become chronic intracellular parasites of macrophages. In the case of *M. tuberculosis*, components of the bacterial cell wall are capable of preventing fusion of the primary phagosome

Table 1–2. **Lung Defense Cells**

| Cell Type | Pathogen Recognition | Antimicrobial Activity | Key Cellular Factors Involved in Containing Microbes |
|---|---|---|---|
| Macrophage | Receptor interaction with microbial ligand or opsonin | Endocytosis | Generation of toxic oxygen and nitrogen radicals; lysosomal digestive enzymes |
| | | Inhibition of microbial growth in other cells; inhibition of extracellular microbial growth | Direct and antibody-dependent cytotoxicity; secretion of interferon, TNF, transferrin |
| Neutrophil | Receptor interaction with microbial ligand or opsonin | Endocytosis | Generation of toxic oxygen radicals; defensins, lactoferrin, lysozyme |
| T lymphocytes | | | |
| CD4+ | MHC class II restricted | Production of macrophage-activating cytokines, stimulation of lymphocyte-mediated cytotoxicity | IFN-γ IL-2, IL-12 |
| CD8+ | MHC class I restricted | Direct cytotoxicity Cytokine production | Perforins, granzymes, TNF-β IFN-γ |
| γ-δ | Minor MHC requirements | May initiate early immune response | IL-2 |
| Natural killer cells | No MHC restriction | Direct cytotoxicity | Perforins, granzymes |
| B lymphocytes | Immunoglobulin receptor and microbial ligand interaction | Production of specific immunoglobulins | IgG, IgA, IgM |

Abbreviations: IFN, interferon; IL, interleukin; MHC, major histocompatibility complex; TNF, tumor necrosis factor.

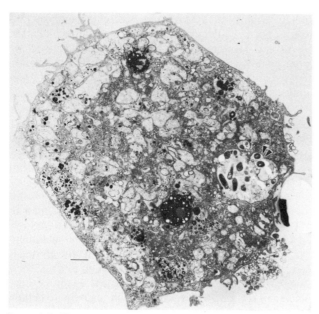

**Figure 1-3.** Ultrastructural view of a human alveolar macrophage with ingested *Mycobacterium avium* complex organisms *(arrows).* Notice the multiple intracytoplasmic vacuoles, some of which contain ingested organisms. (Courtesy of Angeline Warner, D.V.M., Ph.D., Respiratory Biology Program, Harvard School of Public Health, Cambridge, MA.)

with lysosomes.[25] The human immunodeficiency virus (HIV) is also able to persistently infect macrophages.[26] A variety of mechanisms appear to be active, including the ability of HIV to form stable extra- and intrachromosomal DNA precursors, restricted replication (and cell lysis) in cells of monocyte lineage, and the capacity of mature retrovirions to persist in intracytoplasmic vacuoles. Under these circumstances of intracellular parasitism, immune factors such as interferon-γ (IFN-γ) may be necessary to activate macrophages to a state in which they can resist microbial persistence.

In addition to microbial killing through the process of phagocytosis, mononuclear phagocytes may contribute to the control of infection by direct or antibody-dependent cytotoxicity for cells expressing microbial antigens. Although these activities are well described in vitro for peripheral blood-derived monocytes and to a lesser degree for alveolar macrophages,[27] it is unclear how important these mechanisms are in the actual host response to lung infection in situ.

### Neutrophils

Neutrophils occur in small numbers in the normal lung but can be quickly recruited from the circulation in response to infectious challenge (Fig. 1-4). Movement of neutrophils into the lower respiratory tract requires generation of signals mediating the adherence of cells to the pulmonary endothelium, translocation of cells across this membrane, and directed chemotaxis to the site of active infection. The process of leukocyte adherence is mediated in part by expression of neutrophil surface glycoproteins of the integrin superfamily: LFA-1, CR3, and p150,95.[28] The counter receptors on endothelial cells for the integrins are

intercellular adhesion molecules 1 and 2 (ICAM-1, ICAM-2) and possibly other factors. Vascular cells also express P-selectin and E-selectin, adhesion molecules that recognize carbohydrate ligands on the neutrophil surface. Diapedesis is fostered by attractants such as C5a and interleukin-8 (IL-8); in some cases, these factors stimulate directed cellular movement and activate neutrophils to secrete enzymes such as collagenase and elastase that facilitate the ability of cells to cross tissue planes.

Like macrophages, neutrophils interact with microorganisms by the process of receptor-mediated phagocytosis, resulting in the exposure of microbes to numerous antimicrobial substances within membrane-bound granules. Azurophilic primary granules contain small, positively charged proteins called defensins that possess broad antimicrobial activity.[29] Defensins probably bind to negatively charged regions on the microbial surface, a process that leads to altered membrane permeability and death. Neutrophils also contain numerous secondary granules in which antimicrobial factors such as lysozyme and the iron-binding protein lactoferrin are found.

Phagocytosis stimulates the generation of antimicrobial products of oxidative metabolism. Unlike macrophages, neutrophil respiratory burst activity depends on the actions of NADPH oxidase and myeloperoxidase. The presence of myeloperoxidase in primary granules greatly augments the range of antimicrobial products generated, because this enzyme is capable of forming several chlorine-containing tox-

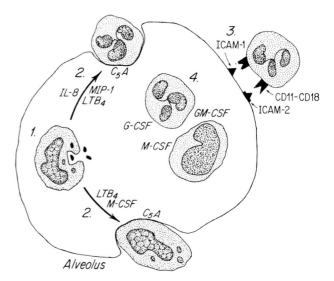

**Figure 1-4.** Schematic representation of inflammatory cell recruitment to the alveolus in response to microbial challenge. *(1)* Alveolar macrophage interaction with microorganisms leads to the secretion of a variety of proinflammatory signals such as interleukin-8 (IL-8), leukotriene B$_4$ (LTB$_4$), MIP-1, and macrophage colony-stimulating factor (M-CSF). *(2)* These signals help recruit and activate neutrophils and monocytes to the site of infection within the alveolus. *(3)* The process by which these inflammatory cells translocate from the circulation involves the binding of cell surface receptors of the integrin family (eg, CD11-CD18) to adhesion molecules on alveolar lining cells (ICAM-1 and ICAM-2). Expression of these adhesion molecules can be upregulated by local production of monokines such as IL-1β and tumor necrosis factor-α (TNF-α). *(4)* The number and activation state of inflammatory cells are maintained in the alveolus by exposure to myeloid colony-stimulating factors (eg, M-CSF, G-CSF, GM-CSF) produced in response to infection.

ins (eg, hypochlorous acid) in the presence of hydrogen peroxide.

### Lymphocytes

T and B lymphocytes and natural killer (NK) cells are normally present in the lungs and can participate as effector cells in the defense against infectious challenge in addition to their important role in the generation of immunologic responses to microbial antigens. In the normal lung, lymphocytes are found in lymphoid tissue and extranodal locations. In airways, aggregates of lymphocytes occur in regions of bronchus-associated lymphoid tissue (BALT).[30] In rodents and to a lesser degree, in humans, BALT is found at airway bifurcations, where a specialized epithelial surface facilitates exposure of antigens in the airstream to immunocompetent cells in BALT. Lymphocytes are also scattered throughout the interstitium and alveolar walls. As estimated by BAL, the distribution of lymphocyte subclasses is comparable to that found in blood. Unlike the T lymphocytes in blood, lung lymphocytes more frequently express activation markers such as HLA-DR and the IL-2 receptor,[31] and they exhibit a ''memory'' phenotype in that they exhibit substantial secretory and proliferative responses to activation of the T-cell receptor and express a variety of surface epitopes mediating adhesion and homing.[32] These alterations suggest that lung lymphocytes normally demonstrate various degrees of cellular activation, possibly in response to chronic antigen stimulation by factors in the airstream.

The CD4+ subclass of T lymphocytes recognizes antigens associated with class II molecules of the major histocompatibility complex (MHC) and can facilitate the development of cellular and humoral responses by secretion of cytokines (see Table 1–2). The CD8+ subclass of T lymphocytes recognizes antigens associated with class I MHC molecules and can modulate immune responses by directly suppressing T- and B-cell activities or through production of cytokines. In addition, CD8+ lymphocytes can be cytotoxic for cells expressing microbial antigens. Cytotoxicity results from the release of cytokines such as tumor necrosis factor-β (TNF-β) or IFN-γ or from toxic substances in preformed cytoplasmic granules. These toxins include a novel class of molecules capable of perforating cell membranes, the perforins,[33] and granzymes, which are proteases related to the serine esterase family.[34]

T lymphocytes expressing the γ-δ receptor are found on the epithelial surface of the lung and can be activated by certain microbial antigens (eg, mycobacterial proteins) in a manner that is restricted only by minor MHC determinants.[35] The precise host defense function of γ-δ T cells is still unclear, but their anatomic localization and MHC requirements suggest that they may be a rapid response element for initiating immune reactions at mucosal surfaces.

B lymphocytes compose a small fraction (<2%) of lung lymphocytes but play a central role in the development of local humoral immune responses in the lungs through secretion of immunoglobulins (see Chap. 3).

NK cells compose a small proportion of the lungs' lymphocyte population. NK cells do not express epitopes related to the T-cell receptor and are of unclear hematopoietic lineage. This cell type exhibits the capacity for direct cyto-

toxicity against cells expressing microbial antigens. The activity has been demonstrated against target cells harboring several respiratory viruses and intracellular bacterial pathogens such as *Mycobacterium avium*.[36] The mechanism of cytotoxicity appears to involve granular release of toxins similar to those found in cytotoxic CD8+ lymphocytes (eg, perforins, granzymes).[37]

### Recruitment of Lung Defense Cells

During active lung infection, lung defense cells are mobilized to the anatomic focus of infection. In response to infection at the alveolar level, phagocytes are rapidly recruited locally from the interstitium and airways and systemically from blood (see Fig. 1–4). Neutrophil and monocyte movement into the lung during the early phases of infection is mediated by the local production of a variety of chemotactic and proinflammatory signals. Many of these factors are secreted by macrophages in response to cellular interaction with microbial pathogens. After activation, lung macrophages produce two potent inflammatory mediators, leukotriene B$_4$ (LTB$_4$) and IL-8. LTB$_4$ is an arachidonic acid metabolite that is converted to a biologically active lipid by the lipoxygenase pathway. It exhibits chemoattractant activity comparable to C5a for neutrophils and monocytes, activates neutrophils functionally, and increases vascular permeability.[38] The action of IL-8 is restricted to chemoattraction and activation of neutrophils.[39] Macrophage inflammatory protein 1 (MIP-1), a heparin-binding protein, has properties similar to IL-8 but appears to be a less potent inflammatory stimulus.[40] Macrophages produce factors such as IL-1 and TNF-α that exhibit multiple proinflammatory activities on a variety of lung cell types.

The colony-stimulating factors (CSFs) are important in orchestrating the complex interactions of the lung defense network in response to microbial challenge.[41] These lineage-specific factors are produced by numerous cell types distributed on epithelial and endothelial surfaces, including macrophages, T lymphocytes, fibroblasts, and endothelial cells. CSF production from these sources can be rapidly stimulated by microorganisms and their component parts.[42] One of the CSFs, granulocyte colony-stimulating factor (G-CSF), is among the few cytokines demonstrated in the lungs of humans during active infection.[43] After they are produced at the locus of lung infection, the CSFs can have pleiotropic effects on lung defense cells, including enhanced motility,[44] increased membrane expression of phagocytic receptors and adhesion molecules, stimulation of macrophage monokine secretion,[45] and augmented antimicrobial function of macrophages[46] and neutrophils.[47]

### Generation of an Immune Response

If nonspecific lung defenses are inadequate to contain microbial invasion, the generation of an immune response specifically directed against the microbial antigen usually contains the infection (Fig. 1–5). The development of an immune response in the lungs can benefit host defenses by the production of specific immunoglobulin, which can opsonize the invading organism and promote its destruction

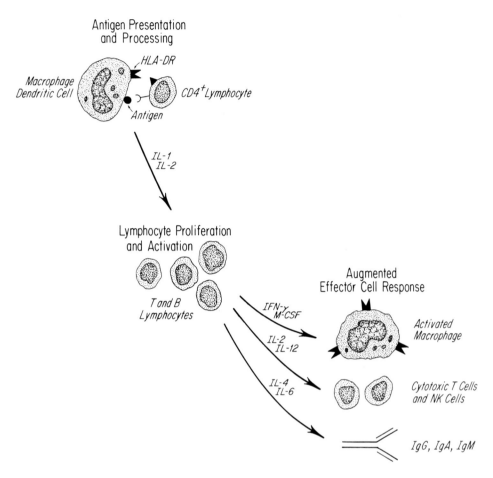

**Figure 1–5.** Development of immune responses in the lungs can be conceptualized as three distinct steps: antigen presenting and processing; lymphocyte proliferation and activation; and augmented effector cell response. Details are provided in the text.

through the process of receptor-mediated endocytosis, and by secretion of T-cell–derived cytokines, which are capable of activating antimicrobial activities of macrophages and cytolytic functions of CD8+ lymphocytes and NK cells.

The initiation of a new immune response requires presentation of antigen to T lymphocytes in conjunction with MHC class I and II molecules.[48] This process requires the antigen-presenting cell to be capable of metabolizing complex microbial antigens into smaller fragments recognizable by T cells and of displaying these molecules on its surface within the MHC locus. In the lower respiratory tract, macrophages and dendritic cells have this capacity. The latter cell type is frequently found in the walls of small airways, where its cytoplasmic extensions protruding toward the bronchial lumen provide a unique surface for antigen sampling.

After presenting cells have processed microbial antigen appropriately, they must physically interact with T lymphocytes. This interaction is orchestrated by the ability of the α-β T-cell receptor to recognize the antigen-MHC complex displayed on antigen-presenting cells. The interaction can take place in the lung interstitium, in airway lymphoid tissue (eg, BALT), and in intrapulmonary lymph nodes. Depending on the inoculum and physiochemical characteristics of a given antigen, there may be ''spillover'' into systemic lymphoid tissue as well.

Regardless of the anatomic localization of the process, the induction of an immune response in the lungs probably proceeds as in other organs. However, lung macrophages

may differ from other mononuclear phagocytes in their ability to function as accessory cells to promote lymphocyte proliferation in response to presented antigen. Compared with blood monocytes, alveolar macrophages appear to be inferior accessory cells; in some cases, human alveolar macrophages may suppress lymphocyte responses.[49] The dendritic cell population of the lungs functions competently in this regard.[50] Surfactant lipids and proteins may dampen lymphocyte blastogenic responses to antigen.[51] Factors that down-regulate immune responsiveness in the lungs may be desirable as a means of preventing inappropriate immune stimulation in the face of the antigen load chronically present in the airstream.

A critical step in the induction of an immune response is the secretion of IL-1 by antigen-presenting cells.[52] In response to IL-1, memory T cells produce IL-2, a potent inducer of T-cell proliferation and activation. IL-1 also fosters expansion of the B-cell pool. In addition, IL-1 is a well-established mediator of systemic responses to infection such as fever and increased synthesis of acute-phase reactants by the liver.

T lymphocytes activated by IL-2 elicit key host defense cytokines. Certain T-cell products such as IFN-γ have an established role as macrophage activators.[53] IFN-γ stimulates macrophage antimicrobial function by increasing membrane expression of MHC molecules and augmenting oxygen-dependent and -independent pathways of microbial killing. Several IFN-γ–stimulated oxygen-independent pathways have been described, including limitation of the availability of essential elements for microbial growth (eg, iron and tryptophan in the extracellular milieu) and exclusion of obligate intracellular parasites such as *Listeria monocytogenes* from the macrophage cytoplasm.[54] In addition to inducing an antiviral state in exposed cells, IFN-γ–activated macrophages are capable of restricting the growth of a wide spectrum of microbial pathogens that parasitize macrophages. Included in this group are important respiratory pathogens such as *Legionella pneumophila*, some mycobacterial species, the pathogenic fungi, *Pneumocystis carinii*, and *Chlamydia*.

Other cytokines produced by activated T cells play a potential role in the immune potentiation of lung defenses. IL-2 is a potent stimulant of cytotoxic CD8$^+$ lymphocytes and NK cells. IL-12, a recently discovered lymphokine, can directly activate NK cells.[55] Lymphotoxin, which shares structural and functional homology with TNF-β, may have a role in macrophage antimicrobial activation.[56] IL-4 and IL-6 can facilitate B-cell growth and immunoglobulin production.

Two essential features of host defense cytokines are that they frequently exhibit overlapping activities and that they are interactive. These interactions can stimulate and suppress host defense activities. For instance, exposure of human alveolar macrophages to macrophage colony-stimulating factor (M-CSF) or IFN-γ alone fails to substantially augment cellular killing of *M. avium*, even though the combination of these cytokines is remarkably effective in reducing mycobacterial growth.[57] In contrast, IL-4 and IFN-γ have antagonistic effects on certain elements of the host defense system. For example, IFN-γ stimulation of macrophage production of TNF-α is directly inhibited by IL-4.[58] IL-4 nullifies the ability of IFN-γ to augment macrophage killing of certain parasitic organisms (eg, *Leishmania* spp.). These complex cytokine interactions probably reflect a sophisticated mechanism for adjusting the scope of the immune responses necessary to defend the lungs against infectious challenge.

## INTERACTION OF LUNG DEFENSES WITH MICROBIAL PATHOGENS

How does the host defense network in the lungs meet the challenge posed by specific respiratory pathogens? Knowledge of the defense mechanisms required to contain a pathogen can be useful diagnostically, because defects in discrete defenses frequently predispose the patient to infection with specific classes of microorganisms (Table 1–3).

The process of identifying these host-specific defects in the lung defense network can be useful in guiding the choice of diagnostic procedures and in devising rational antiinfective therapy. The following sections discuss specific classes of respiratory pathogens from the perspective of host defense.

### Common Aerobic and Anaerobic Bacteria

Aerobic gram-positive and gram-negative bacteria such as *S. pneumoniae* and *Escherichia coli* are encapsulated in a polysaccharide-rich cell wall that resists phagocytosis by lung defense cells. Experimentally, ingestion and killing of these organisms by phagocytes require the fixation of complement to the bacterial surface, a process that is facilitated by the presence of specific immunoglobulin.[59] If complement and specific antibody are bound to the bacterial cell wall, ingestion and killing are mediated by the complement receptor of neutrophils and macrophages. The efficient defense against these pathogens requires the presence of appropriate opsonins in respiratory secretions, a normal number of functionally competent phagocytic cells, and the assistance of intact airway-clearance mechanisms such as the mucociliary escalator. As described in Figure 1–2A, resident macrophages may be capable of controlling challenge with small inocula of bacteria such as *Staphylococcus aureus*. However, other gram-positive organisms such as *L. monocytogenes* and gram-negative organisms characteristically require recruited neutrophils and monocytes for an adequate defense (see Fig. 1–2C).

Anaerobic bacteria such as *Bacteroides fragilis* possess a cell wall and may resist phagocytosis by lung defense cells. Under conditions of reduced oxygen tension in which anaerobic growth is favored, defense cells exhibit defective intracellular killing. As with aerobic bacteria, binding of C3bi and immunoglobulin to the surface of anaerobes is necessary for their efficient ingestion and killing by neutrophils. However, in experimental models of anaerobic abscess formation, protection is the result of cellular rather than humoral immune factors.[60] These cellular defenses include CD4$^+$ T lymphocytes, which are critical for the induction of abscess formation, and CD8$^+$ T cells, which secrete a low-molecular-weight factor that confers protection on challenge of immune animals with *Bacteroides* species.

### Legionella

*Legionella* organisms are able to persist and replicate within macrophages and neutrophils. Evasion of intracellu-

Table 1–3. **Lung Defenses That Protect Against Specific Respiratory Pathogens**

| | Nonimmune System | Immune System | | | | |
|---|---|---|---|---|---|---|
| **Pathogen** | *Mucociliary Clearance* | *Phagocytes* | *Complement* | *Activated Phagocytes* | *Cytotoxic T and Natural Killer Cells* | *Immunoglobulins* |
| Common bacteria | + + | + + | + + | + + | − | + + |
| *Legionella* | − | + | − | + + | + | − |
| Mycobacteria | − | − | − | + + | + + | − |
| Fungi | − | + | + | + + | + | − |
| *P. carinii* | − | + | − | + + | − | + |
| Viruses | + | + | + | + + | + + | + |

Symbols: + +, central defense, impairment of which predisposes the host to infection; +, plays a supportive role in defense; −, not known to be an important defense.

lar killing is associated with the capacity of *Legionella* to reside within membrane-bound vacuoles that resist lysosomal fusion and acidification.[61] The precise mechanisms accounting for this microbial persistence are unknown. Infectivity for macrophages requires a 24-kd membrane protein that appears to be linked to intracellular survival.[62] Moreover, *Legionella*-infected cells produce a low-molecular-weight peptide that inhibits neutrophil oxidative metabolism.[63]

An effective host defense against *Legionella* is mediated by the development of a cellular immune response. An essential step in this process is secretion of IFN-γ by sensitized T lymphocytes and possibly NK cells. IFN-γ–exposed macrophages resist the intracellular replication of *Legionella*.[64] IFN-γ activity against this pathogen is partly attributable to suppression of macrophage transferrin receptor expression and concomitant limitation of intracytoplasmic iron, an essential cofactor for bacterial growth.[65]

## Mycobacteria

The interactions of mycobacteria with the respiratory defense network are remarkably complex and incompletely understood. Like *Legionella*, mycobacteria reside and replicate within cells of monocyte lineage. The control of mycobacterial parasitism involves the participation of all classes of T lymphocytes and NK cells to develop a protective cellular immune response.

This response may not always be beneficial to the host. For instance, cytokines such as TNF appear to be essential for granuloma formation during mycobacterial disease but may also be central mediators of the lung injury associated with active infection.[66] In some experimental systems, certain cytokines may facilitate mycobacterial growth in macrophages.[67]

Mycobacteria can directly inhibit the development of an effective immune response. In human tuberculosis, circulating blood monocytes exhibit the ability to suppress lymphocyte proliferative responses to tuberculin; this effect appears to be mediated by increased production of IL-1.[68] Cell wall constituents of mycobacteria may exert immunosuppressive effects, such as the inhibition of macrophage activation.[69]

The generation of protective immunity against mycobacteria appears to depend on the carefully orchestrated interaction of different host defense mechanisms at each stage in the infectious process. In the early stages of the host response to *M. tuberculosis*, γ-δ T cells, which recognize mycobacterial antigens similar to or crossreactive with mammalian cell heat shock proteins,[70] proliferate and secrete IL-2.[71] At later stages, infection is controlled through the secretion of macrophage-activating cytokines by CD4+ and CD8+ lymphocytes and the destruction of cells displaying mycobacterial antigens by cytotoxic T cells and NK cells.[72, 73] The importance of cytokines in defense against mycobacteria was highlighted by a study of tuberculous pleurisy, which documented that cytokines such as IFN-γ and TNF are present at the site of infection during human disease.[74]

The precise nature of the protective cytokine response is unclear. The ability to activate antimycobacterial mechanisms in mononuclear phagocytes has been attributed to lymphokines like IFN-γ, IL-2, and IL-4; monokines such as TNF; and several of the CSFs.[75, 77] These cytokines may help potentiate the antimycobacterial activity of factors like 1,25-dihydroxyvitamin $D_3$, which can also stimulate macrophage killing of mycobacteria.[78] Because these cytokine effects depend on the specific mycobacterial strain and target cell under investigation, it has not been possible to characterize the precise pattern of cytokine response necessary for a protective host defense at various stages in the pathogenesis of mycobacterial disease. The manner in which the host orchestrates this complex network of antimycobacterial defenses into a protective response is an important issue for future research.

## Pathogenic Fungi and Yeasts

Inhalation of fungal spores with an aerodynamic profile favoring deposition in distal airways and alveoli is the first step in the development of infection with many of the pathogenic fungi. In experimental models, this process leads to an inflammatory response involving the appearance of neutrophils and mononuclear phagocytes at the site of deposition. Organisms are ingested by macrophages, and their intracellular growth fosters expansion of the infectious focus. The subsequent development of a cellular immune response leading to a granulomatous tissue reaction often contains the disease in a normal host.

Recognition of fungal elements by macrophages involves the interaction of carbohydrate-containing ligands on the microbial surface with lectin-like receptors on the cell membrane. In the case of *Aspergillus*, the mannose receptor appears to mediate binding,[79] and in the case of *Histoplasma capsulatum*, this role is served by integrin-binding domains.[80] Opsonization of fungal elements is frequently not a requirement for macrophage ingestion. After ingestion, fungi can be killed by toxic oxygen radicals[81] and reactive intermediates of L-arginine oxidation.[82]

Neutrophils play a role in the local control of certain fungal diseases in the lungs. In the case of *Aspergillus*, neutrophils appear to be more important than monocyte-macrophages in restricting the growth of extracellular hyphal forms of the fungus. In vitro neutrophils are capable of killing hyphae by a process involving their attachment and spreading along the surface of the fungal element.[83] In experimental models of fungal infection, NK cells can contribute to the pulmonary clearance of certain fungi like *Cryptococcus neoformans*.[84]

The fungistatic properties of lung defense cells are augmented by T-cell–derived cytokines through fostering phagolysosomal fusion and activating endogenous oxidative and nonoxidative pathways of fungal killing.[85, 86] IFN-γ can activate fungistatic mechanisms against a variety of pathogenic fungi.[53] CSFs, particularly M-CSF, are also active in stimulating mononuclear phagocyte killing of the pathogenic yeast *C. albicans*.[87]

Like mycobacteria, certain fungal pathogens have evolved the capacity to suppress an effective host response. *Aspergillus fumigatus* can produce factors that inhibit activation of the alternative complement pathway[88] and decrease the phagocytic capacity of macrophages.[89] The glycoprotein-rich surface of fungi is another important virulence factor that may be associated with resistance to phagocytosis. In the case of *C. neoformans*, mannan-containing carbohydrate moieties derived from the cell wall of the organism directly activate suppressor T cells.[90] Similarly, T-cell responses can be inhibited by certain antigens of *Coccidioides immitis*.

### *Pneumocystis carinii*

Although now classified phylogenetically as a yeast-like organism, *P. carinii* is contained by respiratory defenses in a manner distinct from that of the pathogenic fungi. Normal alveolar macrophages recognize mannose-rich ligands on *Pneumocystis* by means of the mannose receptor; this ligand-receptor interaction leads to ingestion.[91] *P. carinii* is then efficiently killed by macrophages[92] through a process involving oxidative burst activity[93] and possibly the generation of monokines such as TNF-α.[94] Unlike many other opportunistic pathogens, *P. carinii* is an obligate extracellular parasite that can be destroyed by normal macrophages.

In experimental models, humoral immunity[95] and cellular immunity[96] contribute to the defense against *Pneumocystis*. Protection against this pathogen can be passively transferred to immunodeficient mice by competent CD4+ but not CD8+ T lymphocytes. The specific role of CD4+ cells in the defense against *Pneumocystis* remains to be fully elucidated, but it is likely that their importance relates to the production of macrophage-activating cytokines such as IFN-γ, which are required for optimal macrophage handling of this organism in vivo.[97]

### Respiratory Viruses

For viruses deposited on the surface of the upper airways in the form of droplet nuclei, initial contact occurs with nonspecific defenses in the mucociliary escalator. The ability of viral agents to resist these defenses is associated with the elaboration of enzymes such as neuraminidase that facilitate the penetration of the mucous barrier and the attachment of virus to underlying epithelial cells, which can support viral replication. Viruses reaching the lower airways and gas exchange units by spread from an upper airway focus or by aerosol deposition must interact with cellular defenses, particularly alveolar macrophages. The macrophage-virus interaction is often a key determinant of the outcome of infection. In general, macrophages are a poorly permissive target cell for viral growth. This may reflect the

capacity of macrophages to produce interferons of various subclasses.[98] The reduced proliferative potential of macrophages can contribute to inhibition of viral expression for certain agents (eg, the human immunodeficiency virus type 1) for which efficient replication is linked to the process of cellular division.[99] Macrophages can also suppress viral growth in neighboring cells. This extrinsic antiviral activity is associated with a variety of mechanisms, including direct cytotoxicity for virally infected cells and macrophage secretion of certain factors (eg, interferon) capable of suppressing the virus replicative cycle in other cell targets.[100]

Interaction of macrophages with viral agents is modulated by immune factors. Specific immunoglobulins of the G, M, and A classes can neutralize viral infectivity. Binding of specific IgG to virally infected cells can lead to their lysis by complement. The cellular immune response involves cytolytic NK cells, T lymphocytes, and certain antiviral secretory products from these cells such as IFN-γ.

Several components of the immune response to respiratory viruses can have adverse effects on lung defenses. Bacterial superinfection during viral infection of the lower respiratory tract is associated with a diminished ability of epithelial cells to resist colonization and with impaired mucociliary clearance.[101, 102] However, the greatest impact of viruses on the lung defense network is on the functional integrity of phagocytes, which exhibit defects in motility, ingestion, and microbial killing.[103] Immune factors such as specific antibodies may foster certain of these abnormalities in cells expressing viral antigens.[104] Immune impairment of phagocytic cell function during viral respiratory infection is further supported by studies with Sendai virus pneumonia of rodents in which the risk of bacterial superinfection was diminished by the administration of an immunosuppressive agent.[105]

## FUTURE STUDIES OF THE LUNG DEFENSE NETWORK

As the roles of specific immunomodulatory factors of the lung defense network become clarified, the factors can perhaps be used to correct critical defects in lung defenses. This strategy may be of value in the treatment and prevention of serious respiratory infection. It is reasonable to believe that the lungs will be an early target organ for efforts to stimulate host defenses with exogenous factors because of their direct accessibility to aerosol therapy.[106] Many potentially useful immune modulators are available for human investigation and will begin to assume a clinical role in the

Table 1–4. **Strategies for Immunopotentiation of the Lung Defense Network**

| Strategy | Benefit | Potential Therapy |
|---|---|---|
| Expand lung phagocytic pool | Increases resistance to microbial challenge | M-CSF GM-CSF |
| Activate antimicrobial activity of lung phagocytes | Augments killing of intra- and extracellular organisms | IFN-γ |
| Activate and expand lung pool of natural killer and cytotoxic T cells | Stimulates cellular cytotoxicity against target cells displaying microbial antigens | IL-2 IL-12 |
| Enhance opsonic activity in respiratory secretions | Facilitates bacterial clearance by phagocytes | Type-specific monoclonal antibody |

Abbreviations: CSF, colony-stimulating factor; GM, granulocyte-macrophage; IFN, interferon; IL, interleukin; M, macrophage.

approach to respiratory infection in the near future (Table 1–4).

Lung defense mechanisms can be a double-edged sword, and physiologic control of the complex lung defense network is essential to the development of a response that protects the host. Failure to control certain components of this network can lead to lung injury. Activated phagocytic cells, for example, are a cornerstone of the lungs' defense network but are also key effector cells in common forms of lung injury such as pulmonary fibrosis and emphysema. Improved understanding of the factors controlling the lung defense network will be important in protecting lung health from the challenge posed by infectious agents and in preventing lung disease resulting from uncontrolled immunologic and inflammatory reactions in the lower respiratory tract.

## ACKNOWLEDGMENT

Supported in part by Public Health Service grants HL 41312 and HL 43510.

## REFERENCES

1. Halperin SA, Suratt PM, Gwaltney JM, et al: Bacterial cultures of the lower respiratory tract in normal volunteers with and without experimental rhinovirus infection using a plugged double catheter system. Am Rev Respir Dis 125:678–680, 1982.
2. Thompson AB, Bohling T, Payvandi R, et al: Lower respiratory tract lactoferrin and lysozyme arise primarily in the airways and are elevated in association with chronic bronchitis. J Lab Clin Med 115:148–158, 1990.
3. Arnold RR, Brewer M, Gauthier JJ: Bactericidal activity of human lactoferrin: sensitivity of a variety of microorganisms. Infect Immun 28:893–898, 1980.
4. Diamond G, Zasloff M, Eck H, et al: Tracheal antimicrobial peptide, a cysteine-rich peptide from mammalian tracheal mucosa: Peptide isolation and cloning of a cDNA. Proc Natl Acad Sci U S A 88:3952–3956, 1991.
5. Van Iwaarden JF, van Strijp JAG, Ebskamp MJM, et al: Surfactant protein A is an opsonin in phagocytosis of herpes simplex virus type 1 by rat alveolar macrophages. Am J Physiol 261:L204–L209, 1991.
6. Giclas PC, King TE, Baker SL, et al: Complement activity in normal rabbit bronchoalveolar fluid. Description of an inhibitor of C3 activation. Am Rev Respir Dis 135:403–411, 1987.
7. Muller-Eberhard HJ: The membrane attack complex of complement. Annu Rev Immunol 4:503–528, 1986.
8. Harmsen AG, Muggenburg BA, Snipes MB, et al: The role of macrophages in particle translocation from lungs to lymph nodes. Science 230:1277–1280, 1985.
9. Sibille Y, Merrill WW, Naegel GP, et al: Human alveolar macrophages release a factor that inhibits phagocyte function. Am J Respir Cell Mol Biol 1:407–416, 1989.
10. Kunkel SL, Fantone JC, Ward PA, et al: Modulation of inflammatory reactions by prostaglandins. Prog Lipid Res 20:633–640, 1981.
11. Yamauchi K, Martinet Y, Basset P, et al: High levels of transforming growth factor-β are present in the epithelial lining fluid of the normal human lower respiratory tract. Am Rev Respir Dis 137:1360–1363, 1988.
12. Reynolds HY: Bronchoalveolar lavage—state of the art. Am Rev Respir Dis 135:250–263, 1987.
13. Warner AE, Brain JD: The cell biology and pathogenic role of pulmonary intravascular macrophages. Am J Physiol 258:L1–L12, 1990.
14. Pinkerton KE, Barry BE, O'Neil JJ, et al: Morphologic changes in the lung during the lifespan of Fischer 344 rats. Am J Anat 164:155–174, 1982.
15. Kobzik L, Godleski J, Brain JD: Isolation and antigenic identification
16. Warren JS, Kunkel RG, Johnson KJ, et al: Comparative responses of lung macrophages and blood phagocytic cells in the rat. Possible relevance to IgA immune complex induced lung injury. Lab Invest 57:311–320, 1987.
17. Blusse van Oud Alblas A, van Furth R: Origin, kinetics and characteristics of pulmonary macrophages in the normal steady state. J Exp Med 149:1504–1518, 1979.
18. Blusse van Oud Alblas A, van der Linden-Schrever B, van Furth R: Origin and kinetics of pulmonary macrophages during an inflammatory reaction induced by intra-alveolar administration of aerosolized heat-killed BCG. Am Rev Respir Dis 128:276–281, 1983.
19. Rose RM, Kobzik L, Filderman AE, et al: Characterization of colony stimulating factor activity in the human respiratory tract: Comparison of healthy smokers and non-smokers. Am Rev Respir Dis 145:394–399, 1992.
20. Golde DW, Finley TN, Cline MJ: The pulmonary macrophage in acute leukemia. N Engl J Med 290:875–878, 1974.
21. Griffin FM, Griffin JA, Leider JE, et al: Studies on the mechanism of phagocytosis. I. Requirements for circumferential attachment of particle-bound ligands to specific receptors on the macrophage plasma membrane. J Exp Med 142:1263–1282, 1975.
22. Klebanoff, SJ: Oxygen metabolism and the toxic properties of phagocytes. Ann Intern Med 93:490–493, 1980.
23. Hibbs JB, Jr, Taintor RR, Vavrin Z: Macrophage cytotoxicity: Role for L-arginine deiminase and imino nitrogen oxidation to nitrate. Science 235:473–476, 1987.
24. Murray HW, Teitelbaum RF: L-Arginine-dependent reactive nitrogen intermediates and the antimicrobial effect of activated human mononuclear phagocytes. J Infect Dis 165:513–517, 1992.
25. Goren MB, D'Arcy Hart P, Young MR, et al: Prevention of phagosome–lysosome fusion in cultured macrophages by sulfatides of *Mycobacterium tuberculosis*. Proc Natl Acad Sci U S A 73:2510–2514, 1976.
26. Salahuddin SZ, Rose RM, Groopman JE, et al: Human T lymphotropic virus type III infection of human alveolar macrophages. Blood 68:281–284, 1986.
27. Stott EJ, Probert M, Thomas LH: Cytotoxicity of alveolar macrophages for virus-infected cells. Nature 255:710–712, 1975.
28. Zimmerman GA, Prescott SM, McIntyre TM: Endothelial cell interactions with granulocytes: Tethering and signaling molecules. Immunol Today 13:93–99, 1992.
29. Ganz T, Selsted ME, Lehrer RI: Defensins. Eur J Haematol 44:1–9, 1990.
30. Bienenstock J: Bronchus-associated lymphoid tissue. Int Arch Allergy Appl Immunol 76:62–69, 1985.
31. Saltini C, Hemler ME, Crystal RG: T lymphocytes compartmentalized on the epithelial surface of the lower respiratory tract express the very late activation antigen complex VLA-1. Clin Immunol Immunopathol 46:221–233, 1988.
32. Saltini C, Kirby M, Trapnell B, et al: Biased accumulation of T-lymphocytes with ''memory''-type CD45 leukocyte common antigen gene expression on the epithelial surface of the human lung. J Exp Med 171:1123–1140, 1990.
33. Lichtenheld MG, Olsen KJ, Lu P, et al: Structure and function of human perforin. Nature 335:448–451, 1988.
34. Jenne DE, Tschopp J: Granzymes, a family of serine proteases released from granules of cytolytic T lymphocytes upon T cell receptor stimulation. Immunol Rev 103:53–71, 1988.
35. Janis EM, Kaufmann SHE, Schwartz RH, et al: Activation of gamma delta T cells in the primary immune response to *Mycobacterium tuberculosis*. Science 244:713–715, 1989.
36. Bermudez LEM, Young LS: Natural killer cell-dependent mycobacteriostatic and mycobactericidal activity in human macrophages. J Immunol 146:265–270, 1991.
37. Herberman RB, Reynolds CW, Ortaldo JR: Mechanism of cytotoxicity by natural killer (NK) cells. Annu Rev Immunol 4:651–680, 1986.
38. Goetzl EJ, Pickett WC: The human PMN leukocyte chemotactic activity of complex hydroxyeicosatetraenoic acids (HETEs). J Immunol 132:828–832, 1984.
39. Baggiolini M, Walz A, Kunkel SL: Neutrophil-activating peptide-1/interleukin-8, a novel cytokine that activates neutrophils. J Clin Invest 84:1045–1049, 1989.
40. Wolpe SD, Davatelis G, Sherry B, et al: Macrophages secrete a

novel heparin-binding protein with inflammatory and neutrophil chemokinetic properties. J Exp Med 167:570–581, 1987.

41. Rose RM: The role of colony stimulating factors in infectious disease. Current status, future challenges. Semin Oncol. 19:415–421, 1992.

42. Bickel M, Amstad P, Tsuda H, et al: Induction of granulocyte-macrophage colony-stimulating factor by lipopolysaccharide and anti-immunoglobulin M-stimulated murine B cell lines. J Immunol 139:2984–2988, 1987.

43. Tazi A, Nioche S, Chastre J, et al: Spontaneous release of granulocyte colony-stimulating factor (G-CSF) by alveolar macrophages in the course of bacterial pneumonia and sarcoidosis: Endotoxin-dependent and endotoxin-independent G-CSF release by cells recovered by bronchoalveolar lavage. Am J Respir Cell Mol Biol 4:140–147, 1991.

44. Weisbart RH, Golde DW, Gasson DW: Biosynthetic human GM-CSF modulates the number and affinity of f-Met-Leu-Phe receptors. J Immunol 137:3584, 1986.

45. Warren MK, Ralph P: Macrophage growth factor CSF-1 stimulates human monocyte production of interferon, tumor necrosis factor, and colony stimulating activity. J Immunol 137:2281–2285, 1986.

46. Smith PD, Lamerson CL, Banks SM, et al: Granulocyte-macrophage colony-stimulating factor augments human monocyte fungicidal activity for *Candida albicans* by the colony-stimulating factors (CSF): IL-3, granulocyte-macrophage-CSF, and macrophage-CSF. J Immunol 143:671–677, 1989.

47. Weisbart RH, Golde DW, Clark SC, et al: Human granulocyte-macrophage colony-stimulating factor is a neutrophil activator. Nature 314:361–363, 1985.

48. Unanue ER, Allen PM: The basis for the immunoregulatory role of macrophages and other accessory cells. Science 236:551–557, 1987.

49. Toews GB, Vial WC, Dunn MM, et al: The accessory cell function of human alveolar macrophages in specific T cell proliferation. J Immunol 132:181–186, 1984.

50. Nicod LP, Lipscomb MF, Weissler JC, et al: Mononuclear cells in human lung parenchyma: Characterization of a potent accessory cell not obtained by bronchoalveolar lavage. Am Rev Respir Dis 136:818–823, 1987.

51. Sitrin RG, Ansfield MJ, Kaltreider HB: The effect of pulmonary surface-active material on the generation and expression of murine B and T lymphocyte effector functions in vitro. Exp Lung Res 9:85–97, 1985.

52. Mizel SB: Interleukin-1 and T cell activation. Immunol Rev 63:51–72, 1982.

53. Murray HW: Interferon-gamma, the activated macrophage, and host defense against microbial challenge. Ann Intern Med 108:595–608, 1988.

54. Portnoy DA, Schreiber RD, Connelly P, et al: Gamma interferon limits access of *Listeria monocytogenes* to the macrophage cytoplasm. J Exp Med 170:2141–2146, 1989.

55. Wolf SF, Temple PA, Kobayashi M, et al: Cloning of cDNA for natural killer cell stimulatory factor, a hetero dimeric cytokine with multiple biologic effects on T and natural killer cells. J Immunol 146:3074–3081, 1991.

56. Paul NL, Ruddle NH: Lymphotoxin. Annu Rev Immunol 6:407–438, 1988.

57. Rose RM, Fuglestad JM, Remington L: Growth inhibition of *Mycobacterium avium* complex in human alveolar macrophages by the combination of recombinant macrophage-colony stimulating factor and interferon-gamma. Am J Respir Cell Mol Biol 4:248–254, 1991.

58. Hart H, Vitti GF, Burgess DR, et al: Potential antiinflammatory effects of interleukin 4: suppression of human monocyte tumor necrosis factor alpha, interleukin 1, and prostaglandin $E_2$. Proc Natl Acad Sci U S A 86:3803–3807, 1989.

59. Horwitz MA, Silverstein SC: Influence of the *Escherichia coli* capsule on complement fixation and on phagocytosis and killing by human phagocytes. J Clin Invest 65:82–94, 1980.

60. Crabb JH, Finberg R, Onderdonk AB, et al: T cell regulation of *Bacteroides fragilis*-induced intraabdominal abscesses. Rev Infect Dis 12(Suppl 2):S178–S183, 1990.

61. Horwitz MA, Maxfield FR: *Legionella pneumophila* inhibits acidification of its phagosome in human monocytes. J Cell Biol 99:1936–1943, 1984.

62. Cianciotto NP, Eisenstein BI, Mody CH, et al: A *Legionella pneumophila* gene encoding a species-specific surface protein potentiates initiation of intracellular infection. Infect Immun 57:1255–1262, 1989.

63. Friedman RL, Lochner JE, Bigley RH, et al: The effects of *Legionella pneumophila* toxin on oxidative processes and bacterial killing of human polymorphonuclear leukocytes. J Infect Dis 146:328–334, 1982.

64. Bhardwaj N, Nash TW, Horwitz MA: Interferon gamma-activated human monocytes inhibit the intracellular multiplication of *Legionella pneumophila*. J Immunol 137:2662–2669, 1986.

65. Byrd TF, Horwitz MA: Interferon gamma-activated human monocytes downregulate transferrin receptors and inhibit the intracellular multiplication of *Legionella pneumophila* by limiting the availability of iron. J Clin Invest 83:1457–1465, 1989.

66. Kindler V, Sappino AP, Grau GE, et al: The inducing role of tumor necrosis factor in the development of bactericidal granulomas during BCG infection. Cell 56:731–740, 1989.

67. Shiratsuchi H, Johnson JL, Ellner JJ: Bidirectional effects of cytokines on the growth of *Mycobacterium avium* within human monocytes. J Immunol 146:3165–3170, 1991.

68. Fujiwara H, Kleinhenz ME, Wallis RS, et al: Increased interleukin-1 production and monocyte suppressor cell activity associated with human tuberculosis. Am Rev Respir Dis 133:73–77, 1986.

69. Pabst MJ, Gross JM, Brozna JP, et al: Inhibition of macrophage priming by sulfatide from *Mycobacterium tuberculosis*. J Immunol 140:634–640, 1988.

70. O'Brien RL, Happ MP, Dallas A, et al: Stimulation of a major subset of lymphocytes expressing T cell receptor gamma delta by an antigen derived from *Mycobacterium tuberculosis*. Cell 57:667–674, 1989.

71. Havlir DV, Ellner JJ, Chervenak KA, et al: Selective expansion of human gamma delta cells by monocytes infected with live *Mycobacterium tuberculosis*. J Clin Invest 87:729–733, 1991.

72. Kaufmann SHE, Flesch IEA: The role of T cell–macrophage interactions in tuberculosis. Springer Semin Immunopathol 10:337–358, 1988.

73. Kaufmann SHE: In vitro analysis of the cellular mechanisms involved in immunity to tuberculosis. Rev Infect Dis 2(suppl 2):S448–S454, 1989.

74. Barnes PF, Fong SJ, Brennan PJ, et al: Local production of tumor necrosis factor and IFN-gamma in tuberculosis pleuritis. J Immunol 145:149–154, 1990.

75. Flesch IEA, Kaufmann SHE: Activation of tuberculostatic macrophage functions by gamma interferon, interleukin-4, and tumor necrosis factor. Infect Immun 58:2675–2677, 1990.

76. Bermudez LEM, Young LS: Tumor necrosis factor, alone or in combination with IL-2, but not IFN-γ, is associated with macrophage killing of *Mycobacterium avium* complex. J Immunol 140:3006–3013, 1988.

77. Denis M, Gregg EO, Ghandirian E: Cytokine modulation of *Mycobacterium tuberculosis* growth in human macrophages. Int J Immunopharmacol 12:721–727, 1990.

78. Crowle AJ, Ross EJ, May MH: Inhibition by 1,25(OH)$_2$-vitamin D$_3$ of the multiplication of virulent tubercle bacilli in cultured human macrophages. Infect Immun 55:2945–2950, 1987.

79. Kan VL, Bennett JE: Lectin-like attachment sites on murine pulmonary alveolar macrophages bind aspergillus. J Clin Invest 69:617–631, 1982.

80. Bullock WE, Wright SD: Role of the adherence-promoting receptors, CR3, LFA-1, and p150,95, in binding of *Histoplasma capsulatum* by human macrophages. J Exp Med 165:195–210, 1987.

81. Washburn RG, Gallin JI, Bennett JE: Oxidative killing of *Aspergillus fumigatus* proceeds by parallel myeloperoxidase-dependent and independent pathways. J Immunol 55:2088–2092, 1987.

82. Granger DL, Hibbs JB Jr, Perfect JR, et al: Specific amino acid (L-arginine) requirement for the microbiostatic activity of murine macrophages. J Clin Invest 81:1129–1136, 1987.

83. Diamond RD, Krzesicki R, Epstein B, et al: Damage to hyphal forms of fungi by human leukocytes in vitro. Am J Pathol 91:313–323, 1978.

84. Hidore MR, Murphy JW: Natural cellular resistance of beige mice to *Cryptococcus neoformans*. J Immunol 137:3624–3631, 1986.

85. Weinberg PB, Becker S, Granger DL, et al: Growth inhibition of *Cryptococcus neoformans* by human alveolar macrophages. Am Rev Respir Dis 136:1242–1247, 1987.

86. Beaman L, Benjamini B, Pappagianis D: Activation of macrophages by lymphokines: Enhancement of phagosome–lysosome fusion and killing of *Coccidioides immitis*. Infect Immun 39:1201, 1983.

87. Wang M, Friedman H, Djeu JY: Enhancement of human monocyte

function against *Candida albicans* by the colony-stimulating factors (CSF): IL-3, granulocyte-macrophage-CSF, and macrophage-CSF. J Immunol 143:671–677, 1989.

88. Washburn RG, Hammer CH, Bennett JE: Inhibition of complement by culture supernatants of *Aspergillus fumigatus*. J Infect Dis 154:944–951, 1986.

89. Mullbacher A, Eichner RD: Immunosuppression in vitro by a metabolite of a human pathogenic fungus. Proc Natl Acad Sci U S A 81:3835–3837, 1984.

90. Mosley RL, Murphy JW, Cox RA: Immunoadsorption of *Cryptococcus*-specific suppressor T-cell factors. Infect Immun 51:844–850, 1986.

91. Ezekowitz RAB, Williams DJ, Koziel H, et al: Uptake of *Pneumocystis carinii* mediated by the macrophage mannose receptor. Nature 351:155–158, 1991.

92. Von Behren L, Pesanti EL: Uptake and degradation of *Pneumocystis carinii* by macrophages in vitro. Am Rev Respir Dis 118:1051–1059, 1978.

93. Hidalgo HA, Helmke RJ, German VF: *Pneumocystis carinii* induces an oxidative burst in alveolar macrophages. Infect Immun 60:1–7, 1992.

94. Pesanti EL: Interaction of cytokines and alveolar cells with *Pneumocystis carinii* in vitro. J Infect Dis 163:611–616, 1991.

95. Gigliotti F, Hughes WT: Passive immunoprophylaxis with specific monoclonal antibody confers partial protection against *Pneumocystis carinii* pneumonitis in animal models. J Clin Invest 81:1666–1668, 1988.

96. Harmsen AG, Stankiewicz M: Requirement for CD4+ cells in resistance to *Pneumocystis carinii* pneumonia in mice. J Exp Med 172:937–945, 1990.

97. Beck JM, Liggitt HD, Brunette EN, et al: Aerosolized interferon-gamma augments host defense against *Pneumocystis carinii* in mice. Am Rev Respir Dis 143:A399, 1991.

98. Roberts NJ Jr, Douglas RG Jr, Simons RM, et al: Virus-induced interferon production by human macrophages. J Immunol 123:365–369, 1979.

99. Meltzer MS, Nakamura M, Hansen BD, et al: Macrophages as susceptible targets for HIV infection, persistent viral reservoirs in tissue, and key immunoregulatory cells that control levels of virus replication and extent of disease. AIDS Res Human Retroviruses 6:967–971, 1990.

100. Morahan PS, Connor JR, Leary KR: Viruses and the versatile macrophage. Br Med Bull 41:15–21, 1985.

101. Davidson VE, Sanford BA: Factors influencing adherence of *Staphylococcus aureus* to influenza A virus-infected cell cultures. Infect Immunol 37:946–955, 1982.

102. Couch RB: The effects of influenza on host defense. J Infect Dis 144:284–291, 1981.

103. Abramson JS, Mills EL: Depression of neutrophil function induced by viruses and its role in secondary microbial infections. Rev Infect Dis 10:326–341, 1988.

104. Jakab GJ, Warr GA: Immune enhanced phagocytic dysfunction in pulmonary macrophages infected with parainfluenza 1 (Sendai) virus. Am Rev Respir Dis 124:575–581, 1981.

105. Jakab GJ, Warr GA: Lung defenses against viral and bacterial challenges during immunosuppression with cyclophosphamide in mice. Am Rev Respir Dis 123:524–528, 1981.

106. Jaffe HA, Buhl R, Mastrangeli A, et al: Organ specific cytokine therapy: Local activation of mononuclear phagocytes by delivery of an aerosol of recombinant interferon-gamma to the human lung. J Clin Invest 88:297–302, 1991.

# CHAPTER 2

# Nonspecific Host Defenses: Mucociliary Clearance and Cough

MATTHIAS SALATHE and ADAM WANNER

The lungs exchange up to 21,000 L of air in 24 hours. This exposes the epithelium of the conducting airways and the alveoli to large amounts of organic and inorganic particulate and gaseous matter, including pollutants, with potentially injurious actions. From the nose, where the air enters the body during quiet breathing, down to the alveoli, several nonspecific defense mechanisms lower the amount of potentially dangerous substances that can enter the body or remove them efficiently after they have entered. A mechanical barrier at the entrance of the nose, the nasal hairs, serves as a coarse filter. The turbulent flow in the upper airways causes larger particles to settle before they can enter the lower airways. Turbulent flow in the larger lower airways enhances the deposition of particles on the surface liquid covering the epithelium. At locations with extremely turbulent flow (eg, airway birfurcations), the particle deposition rate is about 100 times higher than elsewhere.[1] The particle size itself plays an important role in deposition.[2] Particles larger than 10 μm in diameter settle in the upper airways and rarely enter the lower airways; particles in the range of 5 to 10 μm deposit mainly between the trachea and bronchi with a diameter of about 2 mm; particles between 2 and 5 μm deposit by gravity in the alveoli; and those smaller than 2 μm behave like an insoluble gas during quiet breathing and may not deposit at all. Deposited particles are removed from the airways by the mucociliary transport system; the ones that enter the alveoli are phagocytosed by alveolar macrophages. The macrophages are removed from the alveoli by the mucociliary transport system or by lymphatic drainage.[3] Secretory immunoglobulin

A (IgA) forms an immunologic barrier in the respiratory system.

The mucociliary transport system consists of two major parts: cilia that beat in a periciliary fluid layer and an overlying sheet of mucus that is transported out of the airways by means of the ciliary beating. If this system fails, respiratory secretions accumulate in the airways. This leads to an increased susceptibility to bacterial colonization of the normally sterile airways, airflow obstruction by accumulated mucus, increased airway deposition of inhaled aerosols, and a greater possibility of injury by pollutants. Theoretically, accumulation of mucus can increase the risk for bronchogenic carcinoma, but increased amounts of mucus in the airways also protect the epithelium from some injurious agents (Fig. 2–1).[4]

This chapter focuses on the mucociliary transport system, including the regular function of this system and how it may be impaired in different diseases. We also discuss the role of cough as a backup system if mucociliary transport fails.

## MORPHOLOGY OF THE RESPIRATORY EPITHELIUM

The upper air passages are covered by a ciliated epithelium. Exceptions are the entrance of the nose, parts of the pharynx and larynx (ie, squamous epithelium), and the olfactory region (ie, special sensory epithelium). The lower airways are ciliated down to the nonalveolar parts of the

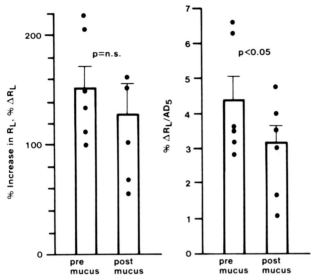

**Figure 2–1.** The injection of artificial mucus into both main bronchi of sheep decreases the bronchoconstrictor response to a standard dose of carbachol. The mean increase in pulmonary airflow resistance ($R_L$) after carbachol is only slightly less after the injection of mucus *(left panel)*. If allowance is made for the increased deposition of carbachol aerosol ($AD_5$) and the greater carbachol dose deposited in the airways because of the excessive mucus, the bronchoconstrictor response to carbachol is markedly reduced *(right panel)*. Excessive mucus increases aerosol deposition but also protects the airways from the effects of an inhaled aerosol. (From Kim CS, Eldridge MA, Wanner A: Airway responsiveness to inhaled and intravenous carbachol in sheep: Effect of airway mucus. J Appl Physiol 65:2744–2751, 1988.)

respiratory bronchioles. The normal ciliated epithelium consists of at least eight different cell types. Besides the columnar ciliated cells, there are mucus-producing goblet cells, serous cells, Clara cells, small mucous granule cells, brush cells, neuroendocrine cells, and basal cells.[5–7] Different forms of intermediate cells are found as well (Fig. 2–2).

Columnar ciliated cells, which are 5 to 10 μm long (measured from the basal membrane to the cell apex), carry about 200 cilia on an apical (luminal) cell surface diameter of about 5 μm. The ciliary length increases from 4 μm in the periphery of the lung to 6 μm in the central airways. The ciliary diameter is 0.1 to 0.2 μm. Short microvilli (1–3 μm long) are interspersed between the cilia; six microvilli surround each cilium. The ciliated cells are in physical contact with each other at belt-like desmosomes at the lateral cell surface (ie, tight junctions) and in chemical communication through gap junctions.[8, 9]

Three different epithelial cell types produce surface liquid: mucous (goblet) cells, serous cells, and Clara cells. The mucous cells are mainly found in large airways and are the principal source of mucus. The serous and Clara cells are found only in smaller airways; they produce watery secretions. Serous cells have been identified only in fetal tissues in humans. Small mucous granule cells are also found in human bronchi; their function is unknown.[10]

Brush cells form a small part of the luminal surface of the epithelium, but their presence in the human epithelium is in doubt. They have no cilia but do have microvilli as long as 2 μm and may serve an absorptive function,[11] sensory function,[12] or ciliogenesis.[11–13]

Basal cells probably help to attach the different columnar cells to the basal lamina.[14] They were long thought to be the only proliferative cells in the airway epithelium. However, some authors think that the secretory cells (especially Clara cells) are the primary stem cells for the renewal of the ciliated epithelium.[15]

Distinct differences exist between larger and smaller airways. The pseudostratified columnar ciliated epithelium of the trachea thins toward the peripheral airways to a ciliated cuboidal epithelium in the terminal bronchioles.[16] The distribution of cell types that form the epithelium changes as well. In the trachea, the ratio of ciliated cells to goblet cells is approximately 5:1,[17] only a few brush cells are found, and the cilia form an almost continuous carpet; small areas of about 1 mm² can be devoid of cilia,[18, 19] and small areas of squamous metaplasia may be found.[20] In the smaller airways, the ciliated and goblet cells are less dense, and intermediate cells are numerous.[21, 22] In the terminal bronchioles, the only secretory cells found are Clara cells.[23]

Submucosal glands are important for overall mucus production. They are chiefly located in the cartilaginous portion of the airways, with a density of one gland per 1 mm² of epithelium. Their total volume (4 mL) is approximately 40 times that of the goblet cells.[24, 25] The submucosal glands are branching tubular structures with serous cells at their distal ends and mucous cells at their proximal ends. They possess a ciliated duct opening into the airways with a diameter of 50 μm.

## Cilia

### Ciliary Structure

Mammalian cilia possess the well-known 9 + 2 microtubular structure, which is ubiquitous in animal cilia and flagella (Fig. 2–3).[26, 27] The microtubular axoneme can be separated from the ciliary membrane by detergent treatment. The major axonemal proteins are tubulin and dynein, but more than 200 other proteins have been identified in cilia and are associated with a variety of circumferential and radial linkage and spoke structures that maintain axonemal structure and may also play a role in ciliary beating.

The microtubules are constructed primarily from heterodimers of α- and β-tubulin. The outer nine doublet microtubules consist of a complete A subfiber (made of 13 protofilaments) on which a B subfiber (10–11 protofilaments) assembles. Some parts of the region in which the two subfibers come together are composed of tektin, which is related to intermediate-filament proteins.[28, 28a] At the tip of the cilium, the nine outer doublets simplify into only A fibers, which insert into a disk, the cytoplasmic part of a transmembrane complex: the ciliary crown.[29] The crown carries three to seven short "claws" (25–35 nm long), whose function is to engage mechanically or chemically with the overlying mucus sheet during the effective stroke of the cilium. Near the ciliary base, another transmembrane complex is found: the necklace, above which the cilium detaches from the cell after calcium shock treatment. At the base, the nine outer doublets end in the basal body, which is anchored to the cytoskeleton.[30] The basal body has a foot, which points with its narrow end in the direction of the

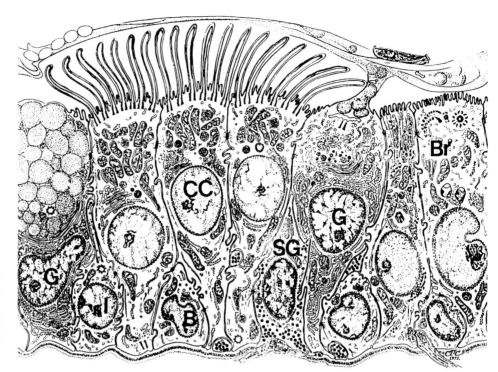

**Figure 2–2.** Morphology of the respiratory epithelium. Shown are different cell types of the ciliated epithelium. *CC,* ciliated cells; *G,* goblet cells; *Br,* brush cells; *SG,* small granule or neuroendocrine cells; *B,* basal cells; *I,* intermediate cells. Not shown are serous cells, Clara cells, and small mucous granule cells. (From Soroki SP: Respiratory system. *In* Weiss L, Greep RO (eds): Histology, ed 4. New York, McGraw-Hill, 1977:765–830.)

effective stroke of the cilium.[31] Because all basal feet of a cell point in nearly the same direction, the effective strokes of all cilia of a cell have a common orientation, but neither the orientation of the feet nor the orientation of the ciliary beats is absolutely identical in adjacent cells.[32–34]

The outer nine doublet microtubules of the axoneme are connected with each other by paired doublet links (made out of nexin) and with projections connected to the inner

singlet microtubules by radial spokes, which occur in groups of three along subfiber A with a 96-nm periodicity.[35] Bridges between the ciliary membrane and the outer nine doublet microtubules exist along the entire length of the cilium.[36]

Dynein is the site of energy usage in the cilium; it is an ATPase.[37] Outer and inner dynein arm molecules originate from each A subunit of the outer doublet microtubule and

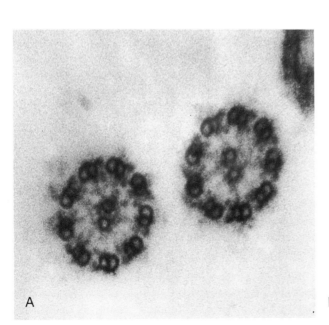

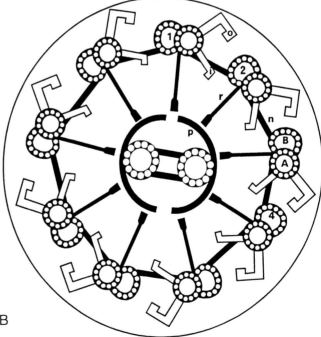

**Figure 2–3.** *(A)* Transmission electron microscopy reveals the structure of a normal cilium in cross section. *(B)* The schematic section is seen from the ciliary base toward the tip. Shown is the conventional numbering of the outer doublet microtubules made out of A and B subfibers and connected with each other by nexin *(n)*. The A subfibers carry outer *(o)* and inner *(i)* dynein arms, which project in a clockwise direction toward the B subfibers. Radial spokes *(r)* connect the outer doublet microtubules with projections *(p)* associated with the inner pair of microtubules.

project in a clockwise direction (as seen from the base) toward the B subunit of the next doublet. The outer arm dynein from tracheal cilia is a two-headed, bouquet-like molecule with a molecular mass of 1 to 2 Md.[38] Each head contains a heavy chain ATPase of 400 to 500 kd.

Along the entire axonemal length (except for the tip region with the ciliary crown and the base), the doublet is a repetitive structure. The repetitive unit is 96 nm long and consists of four outer dynein arms, three or four inner dynein arms, one spoke group (three radial spokes), and one pair of interdoublet links.[8]

### Normal Ciliary Function

During ciliary motion, the dynein arms projecting from the A subfiber interact transiently with the B subfiber of the adjacent outer doublet and, using the energy from ATP hydrolysis, undergo a conformational change that causes the latter doublet to slide tipward relative to the former.[39] The tipward movement has a maximal velocity of about 10 $\mu$m/s.[40, 41] The maximal sliding per half beat is in the region of 0.1 to 0.4 $\mu$m.[42] Different patterns of sliding on one side or the other side of the axoneme provide the different shape of the cilium during the effective and recovery strokes.[8] The power that the cilium produces is closely related to the number and rate of the dynein-microtubule interactions.[43]

Airway cilia have a special beating cycle that differs from that of water-propelling cilia (Fig. 2–4).[34, 44] From a resting state, the cilium swings through its recovery stroke almost 180° backward and to the right (compared with its effective stroke) close to the cell surface. After the completion of the recovery stroke, the cilium fully extends and goes directly through its effective stroke. The effective stroke takes place in a plane perpendicular to the cell surface; the extended cilium describes an arc of about 110°; and its tip has a maximal velocity of 1000 $\mu$m/s. During

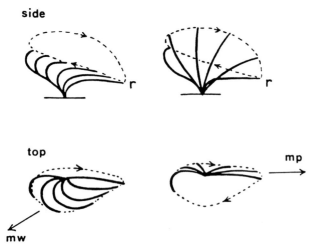

**Figure 2–4.** Beat cycle of a rabbit tracheal cilium seen from the side and from above. In the recovery stroke *(left)*, the cilium starts from a rest position *(r)* and unrolls clockwise *(top view)* to the right. During the effective stroke *(right)*, it remains fully extended and describes an arc of about 110° in a plane perpendicular to the cell surface. Mucus is propelled toward the right *(mp)*, and the metachronal wave is propagated toward the lower left *(mw)*. (From Sleigh MA, Blake JR, Liron N: The propulsion of mucus by cilia. Am Rev Respir Dis 137:726–741, 1988.)

the effective stroke the "claws" at the ciliary tip engage with the mucus and push it in the direction of the effective stroke. After completion of the effective stroke, the cilium rests for a short period and then goes again through its recovery and effective stroke. In the lower airways, the effective stroke has a cephalad orientation and is about three times faster than the recovery stroke.[45] When ciliary beat frequency increases, all three phases of the beat cycle are shortened, especially the rest period.[45]

Airway cilia beat in a coordinated fashion, (ie, as part of a metachronal wave). As the cilium swings backward from its resting state into the recovery stroke to the right (relative to its effective stroke), it pushes against other cilia that are resting, stimulating them to go into a recovery stroke.[46, 47] This mechanical recruitment is probably the most important factor in the propagation of a metachronal wave.[47] This limited coordination between cilia is the reason why metachronal waves are normally limited, restricting the field of metachrony.[34, 44]

Ciliary beat frequency is most often measured in vitro in a watery environment. Methods to measure it in vivo exist but are difficult to perform and to interpret.[48] Human cilia beat at 12 to 15 Hz at body temperature.[49] Except in the nose, the cilia beat slower if the temperature drops. Physiologically, this could play a role in mouth breathing during exercise. Unlike cilia in some animals, human cilia beat with the same frequency from the trachea through the bronchi when ciliary beat frequency is measured after tissue removal in vitro.[50] In the rat, the beat frequency decreases toward the periphery of the lung.[51]

### Control of Ciliary Beating

For more than 100 years, it has been known that the cilia of vertebrates are spontaneously active[52] (the frog palate is an exception). However, Sanderson and Dirksen showed that at room temperature the unstimulated beat frequency of rabbit cultured ciliated epithelial cells varied between 3 and 10 Hz.[53] When the cells were stimulated by mechanically touching the cell surface with a glass probe, their ciliary beat frequency increased.[53] This observation supports the hypothesis that physiologic regional loads to the airway epithelium (eg, increasing amounts of mucus) could mechanically and locally activate ciliary beating in vivo.[54, 55]

The same glass probe touch stimulus increased cytosolic calcium levels in ciliated cells.[56] It was concluded that the increased ciliary beat might be caused by the increase in cytoplasmic calcium. Other work confirms a coupling between the level of intracellular calcium and ciliary beat frequency: stimuli that increase cytosolic calcium levels (measured in cultured epithelial cells) also increase ciliary beat frequency (measured in the same kind of cell culture, but not in the identical cell); treatments that decrease calcium levels also inhibit beating.[57, 58] Work in our laboratory measuring intracellular calcium concentration and ciliary beat frequency in the same cell confirmed again the close link between the two.[58a] Additional work has shown that the increase in ciliary beat frequency in response to calcium elevation is mediated through a calcium/calmodulin-dependent kinase.[57, 59] The inhibition of this enzyme by trifluoperazine can blunt the effect of higher calcium concentrations

Table 2–1. **Mediators and Pharmaceuticals That Increase Ciliary Beat Frequency**

| Substance | Approximate $EC_{50}$ (M)* | Maximal Increase (%) | Epithelium | Reference |
|---|---|---|---|---|
| Acetylcholine | $1 \times 10^{-5}$ | 50 | Brushed human tracheal cells | 132 |
| | | | Cultured ciliated frog cells | 195 |
| Cyclic AMP | | 15 | Brushed human nasal cells | 63 |
| | $3 \times 10^{-7}$ | 30 | Cultured rabbit trachea | 62 |
| Angiotensin II | $5 \times 10^{-12}$ | 36 | Cultured rabbit trachea | 196 |
| Bradykinin | $1 \times 10^{-7}$ | 40 | Cultured rabbit trachea | 197 |
| CRF† | $3 \times 10^{-12}$ | 25 | Cultured rabbit trachea | 198 |
| ACTH‡ | $5 \times 10^{-14}$ | 34 | Cultured rabbit trachea | 198 |
| Endothelin I | $3 \times 10^{-9}$ | 36 | Cultured canine trachea | 199 |
| Isoproterenol | $3 \times 10^{-7}$ | 27–100 | Cultured rabbit trachea | 53, 200 |
| Leukotriene $C_4$ | | 33 | Brushed ovine tracheal cells | 72 |
| Leukotriene $D_4$ | $1 \times 10^{-6}$ | 16 | Brushed ovine tracheal cells | 70 |
| Neurokinin A | $5 \times 10^{-8}$ | 15 | Cultured rabbit trachea | 201 |
| Prostaglandin $E_1$ | $1 \times 10^{-7}$ | 26 | Brushed ovine tracheal cells | 72 |
| Prostaglandin $E_2$ | $1 \times 10^{-8}$ | 21 | Brushed ovine tracheal cells | 72 |
| Substance P§ | | 15 | Cultured rabbit trachea | 201 |
| Substance P | $1 \times 10^{-8}$ | 350 | In vivo (beagles) | 202 |
| U46619‖ | $3 \times 10^{-7}$ | 30 | Cultured rabbit trachea | 203 |
| VIP# | $6.1 \times 10^{-11}$ | 18 | Cultured rabbit trachea | 204 |

*Concentration required to produce a half-maximal increase in ciliary beat frequency.
†Corticotropin-releasing factor.
‡Adrenocorticotropic hormone.
§In the presence of thiorphan (enkephalinase inhibitor).
‖Thromboxane $A_2$ mimetic.
#Vasoactive intestinal peptide.

on ciliary beating.[57] The inhibition of the calcium/calmodulin-dependent kinase decreases ciliary beating at rest without changing cytosolic calcium levels.[57] The inhibition of protein kinase C by the amount of trifluoperazine used in these studies seems not to influence basal ciliary beat frequency.[57]

A cyclic AMP-dependent kinase is also involved in the control of ciliary beating. In *Paramecium*, a cyclic AMP-dependent protein kinase phosphorylates specific axonemal targets.[60] One with a molecular mass of 29 kd was extractable by procedures used for the isolation of dynein and may therefore be associated with dynein in the axoneme.[60] The phosphorylation of this protein has been linked to increased velocity of microtubule gliding across dynein-coated surfaces in vitro.[61] Other cyclic AMP-dependent protein kinase targets have been described in several species,[61a] and we have identified the first mammalian target in ovine axonemes with a molecular mass of 26 kd as estimated by sodium dodecyl sulfate–polyacrylamide gel electrophoresis.[61b] The phosphorylation of this protein may be responsible for the increase in ciliary beat frequency when cyclic AMP levels are elevated in mammalian cells.[62, 63]

Adrenergic drugs use the cyclic AMP-dependent protein kinase pathway to increase ciliary beat frequency. They bind to β-receptors that activate adenylate cyclase through G-proteins and increase intracellular cyclic AMP levels. Methylxanthines are also ciliostimulatory.[64, 65] They are weak phosphodiesterase inhibitors and could also increase cyclic AMP levels in the cell. Adenosine, which inhibits adenylate cyclase through a specific $A_1$-receptor, lowers cellular cyclic AMP levels and decreases ciliary beat frequency.[66] Another pathway to increase ciliary beat frequency, the stimulation of nitric oxide synthase, has been proposed for isoproterenol. In bovine bronchial epithelial cells, nitric oxide synthase inhibitors blunted the ciliostimulatory effect of isoproterenol.[66a] It is interesting to suggest

that a gas that easily crosses membranes transmits cell body signals to the cilium, because such a pathway is much faster than diffusion inside a cilium.

Ciliary beat frequency is exquisitely sensitive to temperature variations. Lower airway cilia beat optimally near body temperature, at a frequency between 12 and 15 Hz (measured in vitro).[67] Lowering the temperature to 25°C decreases the frequency to a range of 5 to 12 Hz, and supranormal temperatures increase ciliary beating to values between 26 and 30 Hz.[68]

A large body of literature has been published on mediator- and drug-induced changes of ciliary beating. Tables 2–1 and 2–2 summarize these data. It is still unclear whether a direct sympathomimetic and parasympathomimetic neural control of ciliary beat frequency exists; it is probably lacking in vertebrates. A clear proof of a direct cholinergic stimulation of mammalian ciliary beating has been absent until recently. It can be shown that acetylcholine directly stimulates ciliary beat in a mucus-free system, thus eliminating the possibility of a mechanical stimulation of cilia.[47, 58a]

Many inflammatory mediators stimulate ciliary beating in vitro, although mucociliary transport velocity is decreased during inflammation[69–73] (see later). Exceptions are the platelet-activating factor[74, 75] and the major basic protein of eosinophils that accumulates in the sputum of asthmatic patients.[76, 77] Serum proteins released into the airway lumen during inflammation, leukocyte elastase, and neutral protease are cilioinhibitory.[77–79]

### Influences of Soluble Bacterial Products on Ciliary Beating

In the mid-eighties, Wilson and coworkers described the cilioinhibitory effect of soluble products of *Haemophilus influenzae* and *Pseudomonas aeruginosa*.[80, 81] Pyocyanin

**Table 2–2. Mediators and Pharmaceuticals That Decrease Ciliary Beat Frequency**

| Substance | Approximate $IC_{50}$ (M)* | Maximal Inhibition (%) | Epithelium | Reference |
|---|---|---|---|---|
| Adenosine | $1 \times 10^{-4}$ | 32 | Cultured rabbit trachea | 66 |
| Atrial natriuretic factor | $3 \times 10^{-12}$ | 25 | Cultured rabbit trachea | 205 |
| Eosinophilic major basic protein | $1 \times 10^{-6}$ | 100 | Guinea pig tracheal cultures | 76 |
| Dextromethorphan | | 21 | Rat tracheal explants | 206 |
| Diphenhydramine | | 100 | Rat tracheal explants | 206 |
| Hydrogen peroxide | $1 \times 10^{-8}$ | 24 | Cultured ovine trachea | 84 |
| PMA† | $3 \times 10^{-10}$ | 21 | Cultured rabbit trachea | 207 |
| | $5 \times 10^{-8}$ | 20 | Cultured ovine trachea | 84 |
| PAF‡ | $1 \times 10^{-8}$ | | Ethmoid sinus tissue culture | 74 |
| | | | Brushed ovine tracheal cells | 75 |

*Concentration required to produce a half-maximal decrease in ciliary beat frequency.
†12-Phorbol-13-myristate acetate.
‡Platelet-activating factor.

and 1-hydroxyphenazine were the responsible agents of *P. aeruginosa* (mucoid strain).[82] Jackowski showed later that these two products do not act directly on epithelial cells or cilia, but stimulate luminal neutrophils to produce noncytotoxic amounts of hydrogen peroxide, which has a cilioinhibitory effect.[83] The effect of hydrogen peroxide could be mimicked by 12-phorbol-13-myristate acetate, a phorbol ester that strongly activates protein kinase C (Fig. 2–5).[84] Both cilioinhibitory effects can be blocked by a protein kinase inhibitor, suggesting that a protein kinase, probably protein kinase C, may be involved in mediating the cilioinhibition. The exact cellular pathway of this process is not clear. In vitro phosphorylation experiments suggest that a protein kinase C-like activity is present in isolated ovine cilia and that a specific 37-kd ciliary membrane protein is phosphorylated after protein kinase C activation. Therefore, protein kinase C, in addition to cyclic AMP-dependent and calcium/calmodulin-dependent kinase, may play a role in the regulation of ciliary beating.

Soluble products of *P. aeruginosa* act as cilioinhibitors and alter mucus production and transepithelial ion secretion.[85] They decrease overall mucociliary clearance. It has long been thought that bacterial colonization of the normally sterile airways[86] may predispose to infection without having a direct ill effect on the host. These results indicate, however, that bacterial colonization of the airways does have the deleterious effect of directly impairing mucociliary transport by inhibiting ciliary beating and by influencing other critical parts of the mucociliary transport system.

## Periciliary Fluid

The periciliary fluid is a watery secretion that, in the presence of mucus, is a little less deep than the extended cilium in length.[87] A small osmiophilic film covers the luminal surface of the periciliary fluid layer and is composed of phospholipids from alveoli or lipids secreted by the epithelial cells. The cilia beat throughout their entire cycle in this periciliary fluid. The fluid level is critical for regular mucociliary transport. If the fluid level is too high, the ciliary tips cannot interact with the mucus, and the mucus, which floats on top of the periciliary fluid, cannot be moved. If the fluid level is too low, the mucus itself impedes ciliary beating by interacting with the cilia during

the recovery stroke. The periciliary fluid near the cell surface oscillates (ie, it is not transported), because the cilia beat forward and backward in this fluid during their effective and recovery strokes. However, a small but unknown portion of this fluid is transported with the mucus, because the cilium moves through it only during its effective stroke.[47]

Besides its function as a proper environment for ciliary beating and mucus propulsion, the periciliary fluid has a role in mucus hydration after its secretion by mucus-producing cells[88] (see later). Most of the fluid is produced in the distal airways and absorbed as it passes up the bronchial tree.

The periciliary fluid level is probably regulated by an active ion transport across the epithelial cells with a concomitant passive fluid transfer.[89] Capillary action between the cilia may help in the production and maintenance of the periciliary fluid level. Particularly if there is no mucus, this action ensures a smooth water surface above the cilia to

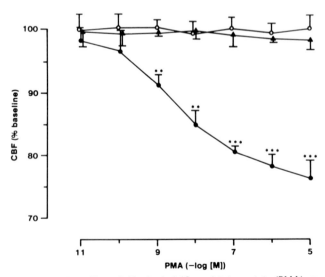

**Figure 2–5.** The effect of 12-phorbol-13-myristate acetate (PMA) on ciliary beat frequency (CBF) in sheep tracheal epithelium is shown *(closed circles)*. *Open circles*, buffer time control; *triangles*, pretreatment with H-7, a protein kinase inhibitor. The mean (n = 5) and SEM are represented by brackets. \*\*$P<.01$ and \*\*\*$P<.001$ are compared with time control and H-7. (From Kobayashi K, Salathe M, Pratt MM, et al: Mechanism of hydrogen peroxide induced inhibition of sheep airway cilia. Am J Respir Cell Mol Biol 6:667–673, 1992.)

prevent substantial negative pressures around ciliary tips.[90] The epithelial cells possess two major ion transport systems, which are both ATP dependent: one for chloride secretion and one for sodium absorption. There is a tendency to switch from chloride secretion to sodium absorption during development after birth. Sodium absorption predominates under basal conditions in larger airways in humans.[91] Chloride secretion is achieved through several different types of chloride channels.[92–94] Most research has focused on one that opens on phosphorylation by cyclic AMP-dependent kinase.[95, 96] Patients with cystic fibrosis exhibit defective function of this chloride channel. The channel fails to open because of a phosphorylation defect of the cyclic AMP-dependent kinase in the apical membrane.[96, 97] The failure of the chloride channel and probably the increase in sodium absorption result in thick, viscous secretions that contribute to airway obstruction in these patients.[98, 99]

## Mucus

Mucus is mandatory for mucociliary transport. If no mucus is present, the system fails.[100] Mucus is a mixture of glycoproteins, proteoglycans, lipids, other proteins, and sometimes DNA.[101] DNA is found in relevant concentrations only during colonization or inflammation of the airways. Large amounts of DNA increase the viscosity of mucus markedly, which is important in patients with cystic fibrosis (see later). The DNA originates from dead luminal leukocytes. Mucus also contains secretory IgA immunoglobulins that form an immunologic barrier against bacterial colonization; lysozyme, which is bactericidal; and lactoferrin, which scavenges oxygen radicals and traps iron ions. Iron ions are a growth requirement for many bacteria. The dry weight of mucus (measured as sputum) is about 20 to 40 mg/mL (nondialyzable solids, about 4–10 mg/mL). These values can increase dramatically during infection.[102]

Mucins form the main structure of mucus; they are glycoconjugates (ie, glycoproteins).[103] Mucins are polyionic at or near neutral pH. The glycoproteins are linked to each other in an end-to-end fashion by disulfide bonds and form very long molecules (0.5–6 μm).[104, 105] These long molecules are not covalently linked with each other but are entangled in the mucous matrix and have a random coil conformation in solution.[106]

Mucus is formed within the Golgi apparatus and secreted from vesicles in a concentrated form through exocytosis by a ''Jack-in-the-box'' mechanism (Fig. 2–6). To stay in a condensed form inside the cell, the charges of the polyions of the mucus must be rendered neutral by acidic pH or counterion shielding. This is achieved by high calcium concentrations inside the vesicles.[103] The shielding alone explains neither mucin condensation in secretory granules nor decondensation on secretion from the cell. The best physical paradigm for explaining condensation and decondensation events is Tanaka's theory of polymer gel phase transition.[107] Polymer gels (mucins are polymers) exist in only two phases: a condensed phase and an expanded hydrated phase. After the secretory granules fuse with the cell membrane, the calcium ions in the vesicles are probably exchanged with sodium ions from the extracellular space.

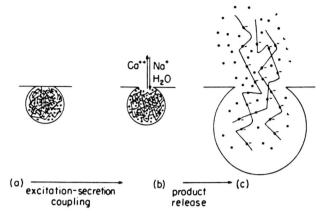

**Figure 2–6.** Mechanism of mucin exocytosis. The excitation-secretion coupling steps lead to docking of a secretory granule to the plasma membrane, formation of a secretory pore, and switching of the pore to high ionic conductance (a). After a high conductance is established, sodium and calcium exchange follows, triggering a phase transition that turns the mucus polymer from a condensed to a hydrated phase (b); the gel extends and is ''secreted'' into the airway lumen (c). (From Verdugo P: Mucin exocytosis. Am Rev Respir Dis 144(suppl):S33–S37, 1991.)

Because monovalent cations are weaker supporters of the condensed phase form,[107] this exchange results in a rapid mucus hydration, driven by a Donnan potential. The volume of the gel increases several hundredfold in only 3 seconds.[88] The periciliary fluid serves as a water and electrolyte donor in this event. The rheologic properties of mucus are mainly determined by the tangle density in the gel, which decreases during mucus hydration.[108] Critical factors regarding mucus rheology are mucus hydration and mucin molecule length.[103] Mucus hydration depends on the salt concentration and pH of the airway liquid. This is another reason why the disturbed transepithelial ion secretion in patients with cystic fibrosis results in thick mucus.[109]

Mucus appears in the smaller airways as droplets, rafts, or flakes and not as a continuous sheet.[110] It is possible that mucus is secreted only on stimulation by foreign particles to transport them out of the lung.[47, 54] The secreted mucus droplets coalesce and get larger as they migrate toward the trachea. In contrast to the periciliary fluid layer, which is continuous down to the smallest bronchi, the mucus does not form a continuous sheet (major bronchi and trachea may be exceptions).[111, 112] The thickness of the mucus increases toward the trachea, reaching a maximum of 10 μm. About 10 to 100 mL of mucus is transported through the trachea each day, as estimated in patients with tracheostomies.[113]

Mucus shows a non-Newtonian behavior. The viscosity decreases as the applied force increases. Airway mucus has a very long relaxation time (up to 30 seconds).[114] The long relaxation time enables the mucus to trap and retain foreign particles. On the other hand, the cilia apply their effective strokes to the mucus at much faster intervals than this relaxation time. The cilia encounter the mucus as a solid and are able to transport it. The transport rate of the mucus is indirectly proportional to viscosity and directly proportional to elasticity.[115] Other physical properties such as surface tension and spinability (ie, thread-forming ability)[116] are also important in particle and mucus interactions and mucus transportability but are less well defined.

Little is known about how alterations in the structure of mucus change its physical properties. Efforts to correlate qualitative changes in the physical properties of airway secretions in terms of elasticity and viscosity with mucociliary transportability in vivo have not been successful so far, primarily because expectorated sputum has been used for these measurements. Sputum does not necessarily represent lower airway secretions. A low water content, a high glycoconjugate content, a high serum protein content,[117] and a high DNA content (purulence)[118] have been associated with high viscosity and high elasticity. It is hard to predict how changes in mucus properties affect mucociliary interactions and mucus transportability. Some theoretical models predict certain behaviors of this system, but they are of limited use.

## MUCOCILIARY FUNCTION AND COORDINATION

### Assessment of Mucociliary Transport Rates and Mucociliary Clearance

Several different methods exist to assess mucociliary transport velocity and mucociliary clearance rates in vivo. The cinebronchofiberscopic technique measures the motion velocity of small Teflon discs insufflated through a catheter or through a bronchoscope into the trachea.[119] Tracheal transport rates of about 20 mm/min are measured with this method. With the radiographic technique, the transport rate of bismuth-coated Teflon discs is monitored by fluoroscopy.[120] Tracheal transport rates of 10 mm/min are typically measured. With the radioaerosol bolus technique, the movement of inhaled radiolabelled microspheres is monitored with a gamma camera.[121] The inhalation technique is designed to enhance central deposition of the microspheres. Tracheal transport rates of 4 to 5 mm/min are measured. This last method is the least invasive procedure and probably best approximates the real value of the mucociliary transport rate. The transport rates decrease toward the periphery of the lung, reaching the lowest value in the bronchioles with rates of less than 0.4 mm/min. In healthy adults, the transport rate in the nose is the same as or a little less than in the trachea, but there are wide individual variations in both. Transport rates decrease with age.

If radiolabelled particles are inhaled and the total radioactivity in both lungs is followed over time (without following individual particles), the overall mucociliary clearance of the lung can be assessed.[122] This clearance has two exponential phases. An initial fast phase, completed in less than 24 hours, with a half-life of about 4 hours, represents mucociliary clearance of the tracheobronchial tree. A later, slower phase with a half-life of several weeks or months represents the clearance of the alveoli by a nonmucociliary mechanism. Because of the differences between transport rates in the periphery of the lung and in the central airways, initial particle deposition influences the measured overall clearance rates. In older subjects, in smokers, and in patients with airflow obstruction, the central deposition of particles is enhanced.[123] It is therefore critical to alter the breathing pattern during particle inhalation to produce similar particle deposition in all subjects. Only if this is done can different subjects be compared. Lung clearance is significantly reduced in the elderly, in chronic smokers (even if they are asymptomatic), and in patients with chronic obstructive lung diseases such as chronic bronchitis, bronchiectasis, bronchial asthma, and cystic fibrosis.[123–125]

### Normal and Abnormal Function

Mucociliary function is coordinated throughout the airways. The mucus-fluid transport is very slow in the peripheral airways (see earlier) and increases progressively, up to 50 times from the bronchioles to the trachea.[110, 128] In the trachea, the transport direction describes a clockwise spiral (ie, when viewed from the larynx).[20] In sheep, mucociliary function already exists at birth. The ciliary beating is mature (ie, frequencies are comparable to frequencies of adults), but the overall transport rates are slower.[127] The maturation of the transport system takes a few weeks. In ferrets, the mucociliary transport system is not functional at birth and develops entirely after birth.

Mucociliary function can be disturbed by a change in any of its components: mucus secretion, ciliary activity, or the mucociliary interaction. It is extremely difficult to determine drug influences on cilia in vivo or in epithelial explants, because as soon as mucus secretion is stimulated, the cilia are indirectly influenced as well (see earlier). Changes in relative humidity between 10% and 70% do not affect the nasal mucociliary transport.[128] This is not surprising, because the nose serves as a major air conditioner. However, a relative humidity of less than 30% produces ciliostasis and transport stasis in the trachea.[129] Low temperature decreases ciliary beat frequency (see earlier) and transport rates. Both of these influences on mucus transport are critically important to patients who bypass the nose during breathing (eg, patients with tracheostomies); they should breathe warmed and humidified air.

Cigarette smoke, air pollutants (eg, $SO_2$, $NO_2$), anesthetic gases, high inspiratory oxygen concentrations, and inhalations of platelet-activating factor decrease transport rate.[20, 130] Cholinergic agonists increase mucus clearance, by increasing the amount of mucus secretion and increasing directly the ciliary beat frequency.[91] Atropine, a tertiary ammonium compound, decreases mucociliary clearance and transport rates.[131, 132] This could be the result of decreased mucus production or decreased ciliary beat frequency. Ipratropium bromide, a quaternary ammonium compound, has no effect on mucus clearance and transport rates; some studies even report an increase.[133] β-Adrenergic agonists increase intracellular cyclic AMP levels, which increase ciliary beating,[62, 63] ion-fluid secretion,[95] and mucus secretion.[89, 134] They lead to a general increase in transport and clearance rates in most healthy persons and patients (at least in the trachea).[135–137] Methylxanthines enhance mucociliary clearance, possibly by influencing the system through changes in cyclic AMP levels.[138] α-Adrenergic agonists have little or no influence on the mucociliary clearance rate in the lower airways, but they stimulate the nasal mucus transport rate by elevating mucus secretion or altering the physical properties of the mucus.

Soluble products of *P. aeruginosa* decrease ciliary beat frequency, increase periciliary fluid levels, and increase mucus secretion of guinea pig and human tracheal tissue pieces.[85] As a result, they decrease mucociliary transport rates.

## AIRWAY DISEASE AND MUCOCILIARY DYSFUNCTION

### Primary Ciliary Dysfunction as the Cause of Mucociliary Dysfunction

It is important to differentiate congenital from acquired primary ciliary dysfunction. Perhaps the best known primary congenital ciliary dysfunction is the primary dyskinesia syndrome.[139] In 50% of the patients, this syndrome is associated with a situs inversus and is then designated Kartagener's syndrome. The disease probably has an autosomal recessive inheritance pattern. The cilia of these patients have typical structural defects of their axonemes. The absence of the outer dynein arms is the most common defect; missing radial spokes and translocation of the outer doublet microtubules are also seen in this syndrome.[140–143] The lack of essential dynein arms is responsible for the ciliary immotility. Clinically these patients suffer from chronic sinusitis and chronic bronchitis that leads to bronchiectasis. Men are infertile because of the same axonemal defect in the sperm tail.

Other structural defects can impair mucociliary clearance. Abnormal lengths of cilia and disoriented cilia that cannot beat in a metachronal wave have been described in patients with bronchiectasis and chronic pulmonary infections.[144]

Acquired primary ciliary disorders are most often secondary to inflammation. In addition to misalignments of the central microtubules between adjacent cilia, compound cilia, supernumerary microtubules, and other malformations,[145–148] the destruction of the epithelial layer by inflammatory cell products or bacterial products, with apparent loss of cilia over a wide area, is important. The destruction must include more than 50% of the ciliated cells of a given area to decrease the mucociliary transport rate.[149] This extended destruction is seen commonly in infections with *Mycoplasma pneumoniae*,[150] and certain viruses,[151] and after aspiration of acid gastric content.[152] In viral diseases, the decrease of mucociliary clearance can persist as long as 6 weeks after the disappearance of the clinical symptoms.[151] The cilia of patients with cystic fibrosis show probably acquired deformations (eg, compound cilia, necklace dysmorphology) that may explain in part their depressed ciliary activity.[153]

### Abnormal Secretions as the Cause of Mucociliary Dysfunction

Abnormal secretions are the predominant cause of mucociliary dysfunction in most airway diseases. Quantitative and qualitative changes of the periciliary fluid and mucus are usually the result of an airway inflammation. Leukocyte products (eg, proteolytic enzymes, toxic oxygen metabolites), peptides released from afferent nerves, and inflammatory mediators (eg, bradykinin) are involved in this process. The airway epithelial layer typically changes in chronic

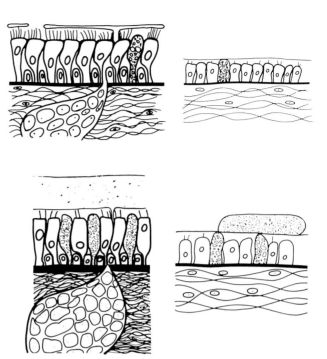

**Figure 2–7.** Schematic representation of mucociliary apparatus in large *(left)* and small *(right)* airways. The normal structure *(top)* is contrasted with the typical changes seen in airway disease *(bottom)*. In airway disease, decreased ciliation, goblet cell hyperplasia in the central airways, metaplasia in the smaller airways, submucosal gland hyperplasia and hypertrophy in the central airways, excessive mucus in the central airways, and luminal mucus in the peripheral bronchioles are typically seen. (From Wanner A: The role of mucociliary dysfunction in bronchial asthma. Am J Med 67:477–485, 1979.)

airway diseases (Fig. 2–7). Decreased ciliation, goblet cell hyperplasia in the central airways, metaplasia in peripheral bronchioles, and submucosal gland hyperplasia and hypertrophy in the central airways lead to excessive mucus production and accumulation of mucus in the airways. The machinery to propel the mucus cannot adequately function with this additional load.

The autonomic nervous system participates in airway inflammation. Local axonal reflexes seem to play a role through stimulation of afferent nerve fibers, which leads to the release of neuropeptides. In several species, including humans, the surface epithelium is in proximity to substance P and vasoactive intestinal peptide immunoreactive nerves; the submucosal glands are surrounded by them.[154] Vasoactive intestinal peptide is released from efferent nerve fibers and substance P from afferent nerve fibers.[155] The evidence that neuroinflammation in the airways can produce changes in airway secretion is based on the observations that capsaicin releases substance P in the lung;[156] exogenous substance P stimulates mucus secretions by stimulating serous cell secretion[157, 158] and goblet cell secretion[159] and by contracting the ducts of submucosal glands;[160–162] substance P stimulates chloride secretion of epithelial cells;[163] and inhibitors (eg, thiorphan) of enkephalinase, an enzyme found in membranes of airway epithelial cells[164] that degrades substance P,[165] potentiate substance P-induced secretion of glycoconjugates.[156, 160] Vasoactive intestinal peptide increases glycoconjugate secretion from mucous cells of submucosal glands in ferrets,[166] but in human tracheal explants, it has been found to inhibit secretion.[167] Vasoactive intestinal peptide is a potent stimulator of chloride secretion of tracheal epithelium,[168] and a high density of vasoactive intestinal peptide receptors is seen on human airway epithelial cells. It is unknown to what extent neuroinflammation participates in airway disease-associated mucociliary dysfunction.

## Asthma

The airway mucosa of asthmatic patients shows goblet cell hyperplasia and metaplasia and submucosal gland hypertrophy, which lead to excessive luminal secretions, and infiltration of the luminal wall by inflammatory cells.[16, 169–171] The mucociliary transport rates are reduced in these patients, even in the absence of symptoms (Fig. 2–8).[172–176]

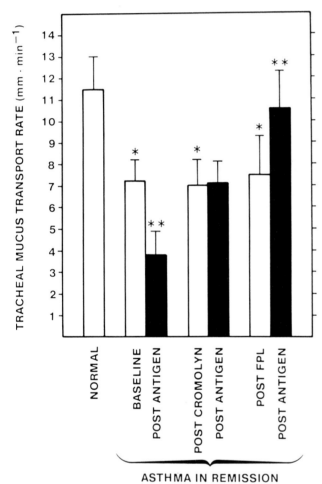

**Figure 2–8.** The velocity of tracheal mucus in asymptomatic, ragweed-hypersensitive asthmatics is compared with normal nonsmokers. Tracheal mucus velocity is already decreased at the baseline compared with normal subjects and is further reduced 1 hour after inhalation challenge with ragweed extract. Mean of 6 (SEM in brackets)*, significant difference from normals; **, significant difference from respective baseline. Cromolyn sodium prevents the ragweed effect, and the leukotriene antagonist FPL 55712 converts an expected decrease of tracheal mucus velocity after ragweed into an increase, which may be caused by the stimulating effects of other chemical mediators. (From Ahmed T, Greenblatt DW, Birch S, et al: Abnormal mucociliary transport in allergic patients with antigen-induced bronchospasm: Role of slow reactive substance of anaphylaxis. Am Rev Respir Dis 124:110–114, 1981.)

A further reduction in transport rates is seen after an allergen challenge.[173] This reduction can be blocked by pretreatment with cromolyn sodium or a leukotriene antagonist. Experimental allergen challenges of allergic dogs and sheep showed a regular decrease of mucociliary clearance even in the absence of bronchospasm.[177, 178] In contrast to the airway function, which showed an immediate and a late phase response, the decrease in mucociliary transport lasted several days.[179] Histamine or acetylcholine inhalation in concentrations known to produce bronchoconstriction comparable to the allergen challenge resulted in a transient increase in tracheal mucociliary transport rates in allergic dogs.[177] The bronchoconstriction seen on allergen challenge does not explain the mucociliary dysfunction. In vitro studies showed that ciliary activity was not depressed on allergen challenge.[69, 70] Hypersecretion of mucus and increased net transepithelial ion and water transport (ie, immediate fluid absorption, followed by fluid secretion), could be detected, reflecting a change in periciliary fluid production.[180–184] These changes may alter the luminal mucus layer and the thickness of the periciliary fluid level and impair mucociliary interaction. Leukotriene $D_4$ was identified as the responsible mediator. Histamine was important only in mediating active water transport toward the lumen, presumably by stimulation of $H_2$-receptors.[185–187] In vivo studies showed that leukotriene $D_4$ given to allergic sheep increased mucus production and changed transepithelial water transport. These changes were associated with a decrease in mucociliary transport comparable to that seen with allergen challenge.[188] The importance of leukotriene $D_4$ in mediating a mucociliary transport impairment was later confirmed in patients with ragweed asthma.[175]

## Cystic Fibrosis

The sputum of patients with cystic fibrosis is highly viscous. The failure of the chloride channel of epithelial cells in these patients has already been discussed. The incompetence to maintain an adequate periciliary fluid level results in an impairment of ciliary beating, and the failed hydration of the mucus leads to a high viscosity (see earlier). Sputum of these patients contains a large amount of DNA, which originates from luminal leukocytes that are present in large numbers because of the chronic colonization and infection of the airways. This high amount of DNA increases the viscosity of the mucus dramatically and impedes the normal clearance of the mucus by means of the mucociliary transport system, even if all the other parts were to function perfectly. DNase is effective in lowering in vitro the viscosity of sputum of these patients.[118] As early as the 1950s, bovine pancreatic DNase was tested as a therapeutic agent in these patients, but unacceptable allergic reactions to the nonhuman enzyme or "irritations" due to contaminating proteases occurred. Studies with recombinant human DNase are now under way to test its efficacy in lowering sputum viscosity, which could ease expectoration for these patients (see later). A phase II trial was published, which showed that recombinant DNase was safe and improved lung function in cystic fibrosis patients after a short-term application.[188a]

## COUGH AND FORCED EXPIRATION

When the mucociliary transport system is severely impaired or fails, mucus must be cleared from the airways by coughing. A forced expiration can help in mucus clearance, if certain criteria are met.

Gas-liquid interactions play a critical role in both of these clearing mechanisms. Energy derived from airflow is needed to move the mucus. The efficacy of these clearance mechanisms depends on the fluid dynamic interaction between the mucus layer and the airflow. Interacting with the mucus layer, the airflow develops a shear force on the interfacial surface of the mucus layer. The magnitude of the shear force is directly proportional to the kinetic energy of the airflow, which is defined as the product of the air density times the square of the mean airflow velocity.[189] To move the mucus in the direction of the proximal airways, the shear force created by the airflow has to overcome the mucus viscosity and gravitational forces.

Depending on the magnitude of airflow velocity and the physical characteristics of mucus, the mucus layer moves in different patterns (Fig. 2–9).[190] If mucus accumulates at a low airflow velocity and the airways are plugged with mucus, air may flow as bubbles through the plug and push the mucus very slowly. As the airflow velocity increases, the bubbles combine and form the slug flow. A further increase in airflow velocity eventually forms a channel of air through the mucous plug; this is called annular flow. At very high airflow velocities, mucus can be torn off the

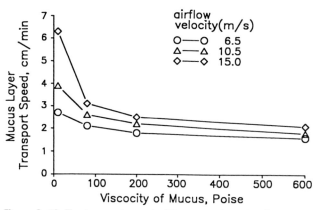

**Figure 2–10.** The transport speed of the mucus layer is a function of its viscosity at different levels of airflow velocity in an upward vertical tube (1.0-cm inside diameter) with a continuous supply of viscous artificial mucus at a rate of 0.5 mL/min. (Adapted from Kim CS, Rodriguez CR, Eldridge MA, et al: Criteria for mucus transport in the airways by two-phase gas-liquid flow mechanism. J Appl Physiol 60:901–907, 1986.)

surface as droplets (ie, mist flow) typically seen during expectoration of sputum from the trachea.

In small airways, particularly at high mucus viscosities, the bubble or slug flow pattern is unlikely to occur, because the airflow velocity is not high enough to penetrate the mucus. There, mucus is moved by a squeezing action as alveolar pressure distal to the mucous plug increases. The annular and mist flow patterns are therefore more important in vivo. The annular flow pattern requires about 1 m/s airflow velocity for a viscous mucus. Such airflow velocities can be reached even in the small airways during cough or forced expiration. If the airflow requirements are met, the effectiveness of mucus clearance depends on the depth of the mucus layer and its rheologic properties (Fig. 2–10).[191, 192]

For a given airflow velocity, a critical mucus depth is required for mucus to be moved (Fig. 2–11).[192] The critical depth increases with increasing mucus viscosity (the ideal viscosity for gas-liquid interaction being 10 to 100 poise), and with constant viscosity the critical depth tends to increase with elasticity.[193] The critical depth decreases with increasing airflow velocity (Fig. 2–12). For a steady-state clearance, a much thicker mucus layer than the critical depth is required to clear the airways. Normal persons cannot clear their airway mucus by coughing, because the normal mucus thickness is too thin for an effective gas-liquid interaction.[193]

Because the critical depth for viscous mucus is high, mucus builds up a thick layer before it moves. Lowering the viscosity is therefore an essential clinical goal. However, if the viscosity drops below 10 poise, gravitational forces dominate and produce mucous flooding of airways.

For a cough maneuver, the glottis is closed for approximately 0.2 second after a rapid inhalation of a volume of air greater than the normal tidal volume. The intrathoracic pressure then rises to 50 to 100 mm Hg, the glottis is opened, and a rapid exhalation follows. The airflow reaches a maximum of 10 L/s (supramaximal flow). Due to a dramatic airway narrowing during cough (up to 80% in the trachea), the airflow velocity reaches 160 to 280 m/s in the

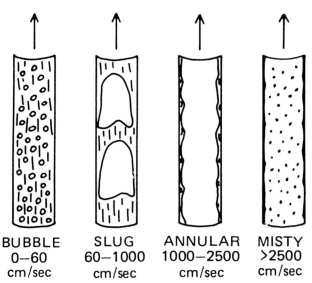

**Figure 2–9.** Typical patterns of two-phase gas-liquid flow in a vertically positioned circular tube: bubble, slug, annular, and mist flow. In an air-water two-phase flow system, the flow patterns change from the bubble to mist flow with increasing airflow velocities: 0–60 cm/s for the bubble, 60–1000 cm/s for the slug, 1000–2500 cm/s for the annular, and >2500 cm/s for the mist flow. With the high-viscosity mucus in the airways, the bubble and slug flow patterns are unlikely to occur. The annular flow pattern can occur at airflow velocities as low as 1 m/s and is the major mechanism for mucus clearance from the lower airways. The misty flow pattern can occur in the trachea and the major bronchi during cough. (Reprinted from Leith DE: Cough. In Brain JD, Proctor DF, Reid LM (eds): Respiratory Defense Mechanisms, part II. New York, Marcel Dekker, 1977:545–592, by courtesy of Marcel Dekker, Inc.)

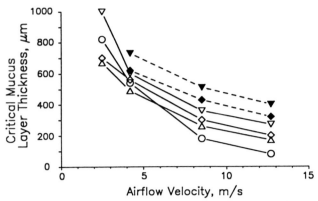

**Figure 2–11.** Minimal mucus layer thickness required for effective clearance by a two-phase flow mechanism in an upward tube flow (0.5-cm inside diameter) as a function of airflow velocity with artificial mucus with different rheologic properties: four viscous (*open symbols:* o 13; △, 79; ◇, 200; ▽, 600 poise) and two viscoelastic (*closed symbols:* ▼ 2.1% (wt/vol) and ◆ 1.5% (wt/vol) polyethylene oxide powder in water, 248 and 90 dynes/cm², respectively) mucus substances. The critical mucus layer thickness decreases with increasing airflow velocity and decreasing mucus viscosity. (Adapted from Kim CS, Rodriguez CR, Eldridge MA, et al: Criteria for mucus transport in the airways by two-phase gas-liquid flow mechanism. J Appl Physiol 60:901–907, 1986.)

trachea and approaches sonic velocity. This high airflow velocity explains the high efficiency of cough in the trachea.

Cough clearance is essentially a stepwise process mobilizing mucus toward larger airways by successive coughs.[190] It is a backup system for mucociliary transport, the regular clearance mechanism. Repetitive coughs can damage the airway epithelium.

Cough is deficient if maximal airflow velocity is below normal or if mucus viscosity is inappropriately high. The former occurs in patients with obstructive pulmonary dis-

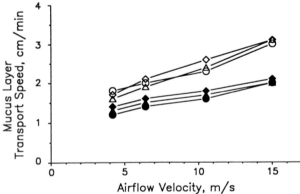

**Figure 2–12.** Relation between the mucus layer transport velocity and airflow velocity in an upward vertical tube flow (1.0-cm inside diameter) with a continuous supply of viscous artificial mucus at a rate of 0.5 mL/min. The mucus transport speed increases approximately in a linear fashion with increasing airflow velocity, and is higher with low viscosity (*open symbols*, 80 poise) than with high viscosity (*closed symbols*, 600 poise). Within the same viscosity range, the role of elasticity of mucus (o, high; △, medium; ◇, low value) appears to be insignificant. (Adapted from Kim CS, Rodriguez CR, Eldridge MA, et al: Criteria for mucus transport in the airways by two-phase gas-liquid flow mechanism. J Appl Physiol 60:901–907, 1986.)

ease, expiratory muscle weakness, or the inability to close the glottis (eg, tracheostomy, intubation). The latter is found in patients with asthma, chronic bronchitis, or cystic fibrosis.

A forced expiratory maneuver can also move mucus. This is an expiration from middle lung volume to a low lung volume. As with coughing, airway narrowing is essential to enhance airflow velocity in the smaller airways. However, the supramaximal flow rates are absent because the glottis closure does not occur. The forced expiratory maneuver acts on mucus for a longer time than cough and is less traumatic. Its effectiveness in mucus clearance has been shown clinically in patients with chronic bronchitis and cystic fibrosis.[194]

## REFERENCES

1. Schlesinger RB, Gurman JL, Lippmann M: Particle deposition within bronchial airways: Comparison using constant and cyclic inspiratory flow. Ann Occup Hyg 26:47, 1982.
2. Swift DL: Aerosols and humidity therapy. Generation and deposition of therapeutic aerosols. Am Rev Respir Dis 122(suppl):71, 1980.
3. Brain JD, Godlaski JJ, Sorokin SP: Quantification, origin, and fate of pulmonary macrophages. In Brain JD, Proctor DF, Reid LM (eds): Respiratory Defense Mechanisms, part II. New York, Marcel Dekker, 1977:849.
4. Kim CS, Eldridge MA, Wanner A: Airway responsiveness to inhaled and intravenous carbachol in sheep; effect of airway mucus. J Appl Physiol 65:2744, 1988.
5. Plopper CG: Comparative morphologic features of bronchiolar epithelial cells: The Clara cell. Am Rev Respir Dis 128(suppl):37, 1983.
6. Breeze R, Wheeldon EB: The cells of the pulmonary airways. Am Rev Respir Dis 116:705, 1977.
7. Jeffery PK, Reid LM: The respiratory mucous membrane. In Brain JD, Proctor DF, Reid LM (eds): Respiratory Defense Mechanisms, part I. New York, Marcel Dekker, 1977:193.
8. Satir P, Sleigh MA: The physiology of cilia and mucociliary interactions. Annu Rev Physiol 52:137, 1990.
9. Sanderson MJ, Dirksen ER: Intercellular communication between ciliated cells in culture. Am J Physiol 254:C63, 1988.
10. Mc Dowell EM, Barrett LA, Glavin F, et al: The respiratory epithelium. I. Human bronchus. J Natl Cancer Inst 61:539, 1978.
11. Jeffery PK: Structure and function of adult tracheobronchial epithelium. In McDowell EM (ed): Lung Carcinomas. Edinburgh, Churchill Livingstone, 1987:42.
12. Luciano L, Reale E, Ruska H: Über eine "chemo-rezeptive" Sinneszelle in der Trachea der Ratte. Zellforsch Mikrosk 85:350, 1968.
13. Rhodin JAG, Dalhamn T: Electron microscopy of the tracheal ciliated mucosa in rat. Z Zellforsch Mikrosk Anat 44:345, 1956.
14. Evans MJ, Cox RA, Shami SG, et al: The role of basal cells in attachment of columnar cells to the basal lamina of the trachea. Am J Respir Cell Mol Biol 1:463, 1989.
15. Johnson NF, Hubbs AF: Epithelial progenitor cells in the rat trachea. Am J Respir Cell Mol Biol 3:579, 1990.
16. Wanner A: The role of mucociliary dysfunction in bronchial asthma. Am J Med 67:477, 1979.
17. Rhodin JAG: Ultrastructure and function of the human tracheal mucosa. Am Rev Respir Dis 93:1, 1966.
18. Alexander I, Ritchie BC, Maloney JE, et al: Epithelial surfaces of the trachea and principal bronchi in the rat. Thorax 30:171, 1975.
19. Holma B: Scanning electron microscopic observation of particles deposited in the lung. Arch Environ Health 18:330, 1969.
20. Wanner A: Clinical aspects of mucociliary transport. Am Rev Respir Dis 116:73, 1977.
21. Leeson TS, Leeson CR: A light and electron microscope study of developing respiratory tissue in the rat. J Anat 98:183, 1964.
22. Serafini SM, Michaelson ED: Length and distribution of cilia in human and canine airways. Bull Eur Physiopathol Respir 13:551, 1977.
23. Widdicombe JG, Pack RJ: The Clara cell. Eur J Respir Dis 63:202, 1982.

24. Reid L: Natural history of mucus in the bronchial tree. Arch Environ Health 10:265, 1965.

25. Reid L: Measurement of the bronchial mucous gland layer: A diagnostic yardstick in chronic bronchitis. Thorax 15:132, 1960.

26. Fawcett DW, Porter KW: A study of the fine structure of ciliated epithelia. J Morphol 94:221, 1954.

27. Afzelius B: Electron microscopy of the sperm tail. Results obtained with a new fixative. J Biophys Biochem Cytol 5:269, 1959.

28. Linck RW, Amos LA, Amos WB: Localization of tektin filaments in microtubules of sea urchin sperm flagella by immunoelectron microscopy. J Cell Biol 100:126, 1985.

28a. Hastie A, Colizzo F, Evans L, et al: Initial characterization of tektins in cilia of respiratory epithelial cells. Chest 101(suppl):47S, 1992.

29. Foliguet B, Puchelle E: Apical structures of human respiratory cilia. Bull Eur Physiopathol Respir 22:43, 1986.

30. Sleigh MA, Silvester NR: Anchorage functions of the basal apparatus of cilia. J Submicrosc Cytol 15:101, 1983.

31. Gibbons IR: The relationship between the fine structure and direction of beat in gill cilia of a lamellibranch mollusc. J Biophys Biochem Cytol 11:179, 1961.

32. Holley MC, Afzelius BA: Alignment of cilia in immotile-cilia syndrome. Tissue Cell 18:521, 1986.

33. Iravani J: Physiologie und Pathophysiologie der Cilientätigkeit und des Schleimtransportes im Tracheobronchialbaum (Untersuchungen an Ratten). Pneumologie 144:93, 1971.

34. Sanderson MJ, Sleigh MA: Ciliary activity of cultured rabbit tracheal epithelium: Beat pattern and metachrony. J Cell Sci 47:331, 1981.

35. Luck DJL: Genetic and biochemical dissection of the eucaryotic flagellum. J Cell Biol 98:789, 1984.

36. Dentler WL: Microtubule–membrane interactions in cilia and flagella. Int Rev Cytol 72:1, 1981.

37. Gibbons IR: Chemical dissection of cilia. Arch Biol (Liege) 76:317, 1965.

38. Hastie AT, Marchese-Ragona SP, Johnson KA, et al: Structure and mass of mammalian respiratory ciliary outer arm 19S dynein. Cell Motil Cytoskeleton 11:157, 1988.

39. Satir P, Wais-Steider J, Lebduska S, et al: The mechanochemical cycle of the dynein arm. Cell Motil 1:303, 1981.

40. Paschal BM, King SM, Moss AG, et al: Isolated flagella outer arm dynein translocates brain microtubules in vitro. Nature 330:672, 1987.

41. Takahashi K, Shingyoji C, Kamimura S: Microtubule sliding in reactivated flagella. Soc Exp Biol Symp 35:159, 1982.

42. Satir P: Mechanisms and controls of microtubule sliding in cilia. Soc Exp Biol Symp 35:172, 1982.

43. Gibbons BH, Gibbons IR: Flagellar movement and adenosine triphosphatase activity in sea urchin sperm extracted with Triton X-100. J Cell Biol 54:75, 1972.

44. Marino MR, Aiello E: Cinemicrographic analysis of beat dynamics of human respiratory cilia. Cell Motil 1(suppl):35, 1982.

45. Sanderson MJ, Dirksen ER: A versatile and quantitative computer-assisted photoelectronic technique used for the analysis of ciliary beat cycles. Cell Motil 5:267, 1985.

46. Sleigh MA: The integrated activity of cilia; function and coordination. J Protozool 31:16, 1984.

47. Sleigh MA, Blake JR, Liron N: The propulsion of mucus by cilia. Am Rev Respir Dis 137:726, 1988.

48. Braga PC: In vivo observation and counting methods for ciliary motion. In Braga PC, Allegra L (eds): Methods in Bronchial Mucology. New York, Raven Press, 1988:269.

49. Low PM, Luk CK, Dulfano MJ, et al: Ciliary beat frequency of human respiratory tract by different sampling techniques. Am Rev Respir Dis 130:497, 1984.

50. Yager JA, Ellman H, Dulfano MJ: Human ciliary beat frequency at three levels of the tracheobronchial tree. Am Rev Respir Dis 121:661, 1980.

51. Iravani J: Flimmerbewegungen in den intrapulmonalen Luftwegen der Ratte. Pflugers Arch 297:221, 1967.

52. Englemann TW: Zur Anatomie und Physiologie der Flimmerzellen. Pflugers Arch 23:505, 1880.

53. Sanderson MJ, Dirksen ER: Mechanosensitive and beta-adrenergic control of the ciliary beat frequency of mammalian respiratory tract cells in culture. Am Rev Respir Dis 139:432, 1989.

54. Spungin B, Silberberg A: Stimulation of mucus secretion, ciliary activity, and transport in frog palate epithelium. Am J Physiol 247:C299, 1984.

55. Puchelle E, Zahm J-M, Sadoul P: Mucociliary frequency of frog palate epithelium. Am J Physiol 242:C31, 1982.

56. Sanderson MJ, Charles AC, Dirksen ER: Mechanical stimulation and intercellular communication increase intracellular calcium in epithelial cells. Cell Regulation 1:585, 1990.

57. Di Benedetto G, Magnus CJ, Gray PTA, et al: Calcium regulation of ciliary beat frequency in human respiratory epithelium in vitro. J Physiol (London) 439:103, 1991.

58. Girard PG, Kennedy JR: Calcium regulation of ciliary activity in rabbit tracheal explants and outgrowth. Eur J Cell Biol 40:203, 1986.

58a. Salathe M, Bookman R: Acetylcholine increases intracellular calcium and ciliary beat frequency: Measurement in single cultured tracheal epithelial cells. Am Rev Respir Dis 147:A48, 1993.

59. Verdugo P, Raess BV, Villalon M: The role of calmodulin in the regulation of ciliary movement in mammalian epithelial cilia. J Submicrosc Cytol 15:95, 1983.

60. Hamasaki T, Murtaugh TJ, Satir BH, et al: In vitro phosphorylation of Paramecium axonemes and permeabilized cells. Cell Motil Cytoskeleton 12:1, 1989.

61. Hamasaki T, Barkalow K, Richmond J, et al: cAMP-stimulated phosphorylation of an axonemal polypeptide that copurifies with the 22S dynein arm regulates microtubule translocation velocity and swimming speed in Paramecium. Proc Natl Acad Sci U S A 88:7918, 1991.

61a. Stephens RE, Prior G: Dynein from serotonin-activated cilia and flagella: Extraction characteristics and distinct sites for cAMP-dependent protein phosphorylation. J Cell Sci 103:999, 1992.

61b. Salathe M, Pratt MM, Wanner A: Cyclic AMP-dependent phosphorylation of a 26 kD axonemal protein in ovine cilia isolated from small tissue pieces. Am J Respir Cell Mol Biol 9:306, 1993.

62. Tamaoki J, Kondo M, Takizawa T: Effect of cyclic AMP on ciliary function in rabbit tracheal epithelial cells. J Appl Physiol 66:1035, 1989.

63. Di Benedetto G, Manara-Shediac FS, Mehta A: Effect of cyclic AMP on ciliary activity of human respiratory epithelium. Eur Respir J 4:789, 1991.

64. Iravani J, Melville GN: Wirkung von Pharmaka und Milieuveränderungen auf die Flimmertätigkeit der Atemwege. Respiration 32:157, 1975.

65. Wanner A: Effects of methylxanthines on airway mucociliary function. Am J Med 79:16, 1985.

66. Tamaoki J, Kondo M, Takizawa T: Adenosine-mediated cyclic AMP-dependent inhibition of ciliary activity in rabbit tracheal epithelium. Am Rev Respir Dis 139:441, 1989.

66a. Bharat J, Rubinstein I, Robbins RA, et al.: Modulation of airway epithelial cell ciliary beat frequency by nitric oxide. Biochem Biophys Res Commun 191:83, 1993.

67. Sleigh MA: The Biology of Cilia and Flagella. Oxford, Pergamon Press, 1974.

68. Mercke U: The influence of temperature on mucociliary activity: Temperature range 40°C to 50°C. Otorhinolaryngology 78:253, 1974.

69. Maurer DR, Sielczak M, Oliver W Jr, et al: Role of ciliary motility in allergic mucociliary dysfunction. J Appl Physiol 52:1018, 1982.

70. Wanner A, Sielczak M, Mella JF, et al: Ciliary responsiveness in allergic and non-allergic airways. J Appl Physiol 60:1967, 1986.

71. Maurer DR, Schor J, Sielczak M, et al: Ciliary motility in airway anaphylaxis. Prog Clin Biol Res 80:67, 1982.

72. Wanner A, Maurer DR, Abraham WM, et al: Effects of chemical mediators of anaphylaxis on ciliary function. J Allerg Clin Immunol 72:663, 1983.

73. Iravani J, Melville GN: Mucociliary activity in the respiratory tract as influenced by prostaglandin E$_1$. Respiration 32:305, 1975.

74. Ganbo T, Hisamatsu K, Nakazawa T, et al: Platelet activating factor (PAF) effects on ciliary activity of human paranasal sinus mucosa in vitro. Rhinology 29:231, 1991.

75. Seybold ZS, Mariassy AT, Stroh D, et al: Mucociliary interaction in vitro: Effects of physiological and inflammatory stimuli. J Appl Physiol 68:1421, 1990.

76. Frigas E, Loegering DA, Gleich GJ: Cytotoxic effects of the guinea pig eosinophil major basic protein on tracheal epithelium. Lab Invest 42:35, 1980.

77. Kennedy JR, Lin KD, Duckett KE: Serum complement (C3a and C5)-induced inhibition of rabbit tracheal cilia. Cell Motil 1(suppl):71, 1982.

78. Sanderson MJ, Sleigh MA: Serum proteins agglutinate cilia and modify ciliary coordination. Pediatr Res 15:219, 1981.

79. Tegner H, Ohlsson K, Toremalm NG, et al: Effect of human leukocyte enzymes on tracheal mucosa and its mucociliary activity. Rhinology 17:199, 1979.

80. Wilson R, Cole PJ: The effect of bacterial products on ciliary function. Am Rev Respir Dis 138(suppl):49, 1988.

81. Wilson R, Roberts D, Cole P: Effect of bacterial products on human ciliary function in vitro. Thorax 40:125, 1985.

82. Wilson R, Pitt T, Taylor G, et al: Pyocyanin and 1-hydroxyphenazine produced by *Pseudomonas aeruginosa* inhibit the beating of human respiratory cilia in vitro. J Clin Invest 79:221, 1987.

83. Jackowski JT, Szepfalusi ZS, Wanner DA, et al: Effects of *P. aeruginosa*-derived bacterial products on tracheal ciliary function: Role of $O_2$ radicals. Am J Physiol 260:L61, 1991.

84. Kobayashi K, Salathe M, Pratt MM, et al: Mechanism of hydrogen peroxide induced inhibition of sheep airway cilia. Am J Respir Cell Mol Biol 6:667, 1992.

85. Adler KB, Winn WC Jr, Alberghini TV, et al: Stimulatory effect of *Pseudomonas aeruginosa* on mucin secretion by the respiratory epithelium. JAMA 249:1615, 1983.

86. Wanner A, Amikam B, Robinson MJ, et al: Comparison between the bacteriologic flora of different segments of the airways. Respiration 30:561, 1973.

87. Hulbert WC, Forster BB, Laird W, et al: An improved method for fixation of the respiratory epithelial surface with the mucous and surfactant layers. Lab Invest 47:354, 1982.

88. Verdugo P: Hydration kinetics of exocytosed mucins in cultured secretory cells of the rabbit trachea: A new model. Ciba Found Symp 109:212, 1984.

89. Phipps RJ: Production of airway secretions. Semin Respir Med 5:314, 1984.

90. Meyer FA, Silberberg A: The rheology and molecular organization of epithelial mucus. Biorheology 17:163, 1980.

91. Knowles M, Murray G, Shallal J, et al: Bioelectrical properties and ion flow across excised human bronchi. J Appl Physiol 56:868, 1984.

92. Frizzell RA, Rechkemmer G, Shoemaker RL: Altered regulation of airway epithelial cell chloride channels in cystic fibrosis. Science 233:558, 1986.

93. Shoemaker R, Frizzell RA, Dwyer TM, et al: Single chloride channel currents from canine tracheal epithelial cells. Biochem Biophys Acta 858:235, 1986.

94. Welsh MJ: An apical-membrane chloride channel in human tracheal epithelium. Science 232:1648, 1986.

95. Al-Bazzaz FJ: Role of cyclic AMP in regulation of chloride secretion by canine tracheal mucosa. Am Rev Respir Dis 123:295, 1981.

96. Li M, Mc Cann J, Liedtke C, et al: Cyclic AMP-dependent protein kinase opens chloride channels in normal but not cystic fibrosis airway epithelium. Nature 331:358, 1988.

97. Schoumacher RA, Shoemaker RL, Halm DR, et al: Phosphorylation fails to activate chloride channels from cystic fibrosis airway cells. Nature 330:752, 1987.

98. Widdicombe JH, Welsh MJ, Finkbeiner WE: Cystic fibrosis decreases the apical membrane chloride permeability of monolayers cultured from cells of tracheal epithelium. Proc Natl Acad Sci U S A 82:6167, 1985.

99. Boucher RC, Stutts MF, Knowles RC, et al: Na transport in cystic fibrosis respiratory epithelia. Abnormal basal rate and response to adenylate cyclase activation. J Clin Invest 78:1245, 1986.

100. Sadé J, Eliezer N, Silberberg A, et al: The role of mucus in transport by cilia. Am Rev Respir Dis 102:48, 1970.

101. Coles SJ, Bhaskar KR, O'Sullivan DD, et al: Airway mucus: Composition and regulation of its secretion by neuropeptides in vitro. Ciba Found Symp 109:40, 1984.

102. Lopez-Vidriero MT, Das I, Reid LM: Airway secretion: Source, biochemical, and rheological properties. *In* Brain JD, Proctor DF, Reid LM (eds): Respiratory Defense Mechanisms, part I. New York, Marcel Dekker, 1977:289.

103. Verdugo P: Mucin exocytosis. Am Rev Respir Dis 144(suppl):S33, 1991.

104. Carlstedt I, Sheehan JK: Macromolecular properties and polymeric structure of mucus glycoproteins. Ciba Found Symp 109:121, 1984.

105. Sheehan JK, Oates K, Carlstedt I: Electron microscopy of cervical, gastric, and bronchial mucus glycoproteins. Biochem J 239:147, 1986.

106. Harding SE, Rowe AJ, Creeth JM: Further evidence for a flexible and highly expanded spheroidal model for mucus glycoproteins in solution. Biorheology 209:893, 1983.

107. Tanaka T: Gels. Sci Am 244(1):124, 1981.

108. Edwards SF: The theory of macromolecular networks. Biorheology 23:589, 1986.

109. Tam PY, Verdugo P: Control of mucus hydration as a Donnan equilibrium process. Nature 292:340, 1981.

110. Iravani J, van As A: Mucus transport of the tracheobronchial tree of normal and bronchitic rats. J Pathol 106:81, 1972.

111. Hilding AC: Ciliary streaming in the lower respiratory tract. Am J Physiol 191:404, 1957.

112. Sturgess JM: The mucus of major bronchi in the rabbit lung. Am Rev Respir Dis 115:19, 1977.

113. Toremalm MG: The daily amount of tracheobronchial secretion in man. A method for continuous tracheal aspiration in laryngectomised and tracheostomised patients. Acta Otolaryngol (suppl 158):43, 1960.

114. Gilboa A, Silberberg A: In situ rheological characterization of epithelial mucus. Biorheology 13:59, 1976.

115. Ross SM, Corrsin S: Results of an analytical model of mucociliary pumping. J Appl Physiol 37:333, 1974.

116. Puchelle E, Zahm JM, Duvivier C: Spinability of bronchial mucus. Relationship with viscoelasticity and mucous transport properties. Biorheology 20:239, 1983.

117. List SJ, Findlay BP, Forstner GG, et al: Enhancement of the viscosity of mucin by serum albumin. Biochem J 175:565, 1978.

118. Shak S, Capon DJ, Hellmiss R, et al: Recombinant human DNase I reduces the viscosity of cystic fibrosis sputum. Proc Natl Acad Sci U S A 87:9188, 1990.

119. Sackner MA, Rosen MJ, Wanner A: Estimation of tracheal mucus velocity by bronchofiberoscopy. J Appl Physiol 34:495, 1973.

120. Friedman MF, Scott D, Poole DO, et al: A new roentgenographic method for estimating mucous velocity in airways. Am Rev Respir Dis 115:67, 1977.

121. Yeates DB, Aspin N, Levison H, et al: Mucociliary tracheal transport rates in man. J Appl Physiol 30:487, 1975.

122. Albert RE, Arnett LC: Clearance of radioactive dust from the lung. AMA Arch Indust Health 12:99, 1955.

123. Del Donno M, Pavia D, Agnew JE, et al: Variability and reproducibility in the measurement of tracheobronchial clearance in healthy subjects and patients with different obstructive lung diseases. Eur Respir J 1:613, 1988.

124. Goodman RM, Yergin BM, Landa JF, et al: Relationship of smoking history and pulmonary function tests to tracheal mucous velocity in non-smokers, young smokers, ex-smokers, and patients with chronic bronchitis. Am Rev Respir Dis 117:205, 1978.

125. Puchelle E, Zahm J-M, Bertrand A: Influence of age on bronchial mucociliary transport. Scand J Respir Dis 60:307, 1979.

126. Serafini SM, Wanner A, Michaelson ED: Mucociliary transport in central and intermediate size airways: Effect of aminophylline. Bull Eur Physiopathol Respir 12:415, 1976.

127. Phipps RJ, Abraham WM, Mariassy AT, et al: Developmental changes in the tracheal mucociliary system in neonatal sheep. J Appl Physiol 67:824, 1989.

128. Anderson IB, Lundquist GR, Proctor DF: Human mucosal function under four controlled humidities. Am Rev Respir Dis 106:438, 1972.

129. Hirsch JA, Tokayer JL, Robinson MJ, et al: Effects of dry air and subsequent humidification on tracheal mucous velocity in dogs. J Appl Physiol 39:242, 1975.

130. Nieminen MM, Moilanen EK, Nyholm JEJ, et al: Platelet-activating factor impairs mucociliary transport and increases plasma leukotriene $B_4$ in man. Eur Respir J 4:551, 1991.

131. Gallagher JT, Kent PW, Passatore M, et al: The composition of tracheal mucus and the nervous control of its secretion in the cat. Proc R Soc Lond [Biol] 192:49, 1975.

132. Corrsen G, Allen CR: Acetylcholine: Its significance in controlling ciliary activity of human respiratory epithelium in vitro. J Appl Physiol 14:901, 1959.

133. Wanner A: Effect of ipratropium bromide on airway mucociliary function. Am J Med 81(suppl 5A):23, 1986.

134. Peatfield AC, Richardson PS: The control of mucin secretion into the lumen of the cat trachea by alpha- and beta-adrenoreceptors, and their relative involvement during sympathetic nerve stimulation. Eur J Pharmacol 81:617, 1982.

135. Foster WM, Bergofsky EH, Bohning DE, et al: Effect of adrenergic agents and their mode of action on mucociliary clearance in man. J Appl Physiol 41:146, 1976.

136. Mossberg B, Strandberg K, Philipson K, et al: Tracheobronchial

clearance in bronchial asthma: Response to beta-adrenoreceptor stimulation. Scand J Respir Dis 57:119, 1976.

137. Wood RE, Wanner A, Hirsch J, et al: Tracheal mucociliary transport in patients with cystic fibrosis and its stimulation by terbutaline. Am Rev Respir Dis 111:733, 1975.

138. Sutton PP, Pavia D, Bateman JRM, et al: The effect of oral aminophylline on lung mucociliary clearance in man. Chest 80:889, 1981.

139. Afzelius BA: The immotile-cilia syndrome and other ciliary diseases. Int Rev Exp Pathol 19:1, 1979.

140. Rossman CM, Forrest JB, Lee RM, et al: The dyskinetic cilia syndrome. Ciliary motility in immotile cilia syndrome. Chest 78:580, 1980.

141. Rossman CM, Forrest JB, Lee RM, et al: The dyskinetic cilia syndrome; abnormal ciliary motility in association with abnormal ciliary ultrastructure. Chest 80(suppl):860, 1981.

142. Sturgess JM, Chao J, Turner JAP: Transposition of ciliary microtubules: Another cause of impaired ciliary motility. N Engl J Med 303:318, 1980.

143. Sturgess JM, Chao J, Wong J, et al: Cilia with defective radial spokes: A cause of human respiratory disease. N Engl J Med 300:53, 1979.

144. Afzelius BA, Gargani G, Romano C: Abnormal length of cilia as a possible cause of defective mucociliary clearance. Eur J Respir Dis 66:173, 1985.

145. Laitinen LA, Heino M, Laitinen A, et al: Damage of the airway epithelium and bronchial reactivity in patients with asthma. Am Rev Respir Dis 131:599, 1985.

146. Lundgren R: Scanning electron microscopic studies of bronchial mucosa before and during treatment with beclomethasone dipropionate inhalations. Scand J Respir Dis 101(suppl):179, 1977.

147. Konradova V, Copova C, Sukova B, et al: Ultrastructure of the bronchial epithelium in three children with asthma. Pediatr Pulmonol 1:182, 1985.

148. Afzelius BA, Camner P, Mossberg B: Acquired ciliary defects compared to those seen in the immotile-cilia syndrome. Eur J Respir Dis 64(suppl 127):5, 1983.

149. Battista SP, Denine EP, Kensler CJ: Restoration of tracheal mucosa and ciliary particle transport activity after mechanical denudation in the chicken. J Toxicol Appl Pharmacol 22:56, 1972.

150. Biberfeld C, Biberfeld P: Ultrastructural features of *Mycoplasma pneumoniae*. J Bacteriol 102:855, 1970.

151. Camner P, Jarstrand C, Philipson K: Tracheobronchial clearance in patients with influenza. Am Rev Respir Dis 108:69, 1973.

152. Wynne JW, Ramphal R, Hood CI: Tracheal mucosal damage after aspiration. Am Rev Respir Dis 124:728, 1981.

153. Carson JL, Collier AM, Gambling TM, et al: Ultrastructure of airway epithelial cell membranes among patients with cystic fibrosis. Hum Pathol 21:640, 1990.

154. Uddman R, Sundler F: Vasoactive intestinal peptide nerves in the human upper respiratory tract. Otorhinolaryngology 41:221, 1979.

155. Barnes PJ: The third nervous system in the lung: Physiology and clinical perspectives. Thorax 39:561, 1984.

156. Saria A, Martling CR, Yan Z, et al: Release of multiple tachykinins from capsaicin-sensitive nerves in the lung by bradykinin, histamine, dimethylphenyl piperazinium, and vagal nerve stimulation. Am Rev Respir Dis 137:1330, 1988.

157. Gashi AA, Borson DB, Finbeiner WE, et al: Neuropeptides degranulate serous cells of ferret tracheal glands. Am J Physiol 251:C223, 1986.

158. Webber SE: Receptors mediating the effects of substance P and neurokinin A on mucous secretion and smooth muscle tone of the ferret trachea: Potentiation by enkephalinase inhibition. Br J Pharmacol 98:1197, 1989.

159. Kuo H-P, Rhode JAL, Tokuyama K, et al: Capsaicin and sensory neuropeptide stimulation of goblet cell secretion in guinea pig trachea. J Physiol (London) 431:629, 1990.

160. Borson DB, Corrales R, Varsano S, et al: Enkephalinase inhibitors potentiate substance P-induced secretion of $^{35}SO_4$ macromolecules from ferret trachea. Exp Lung Res 12:21, 1987.

161. Coles SJ, Neill KH, Reid LM: Potent stimulation of glycoprotein secretion in canine trachea by substance P. J Appl Physiol 57:1323, 1984.

162. Rogers DF, Aursudkij B, Barnes PJ: Effects of tachykinins on mucus secretion on human bronchi in vitro. Eur J Pharmacol 174:283, 1989.

163. Al-Bazzaz FJ, Kelsey JG, Kaage WD: Substance P stimulation of chloride secretion by canine tracheal mucosa. Am Rev Respir Dis 131:86, 1985.

164. Sekizawa K, Tamaoki J, Graf PD, et al: Enkephalinase inhibitor potentiates mammalian tachykinin-induced contraction in ferret trachea. J Pharmacol Exp Ther 243:1211, 1987.

165. Skidgel RA, Engelbrecht S, Johnson AR, et al: Hydrolysis of substance P and neurotensin by converting enzyme and neutral endopeptidase. Peptides (Fayetteville) 5:769, 1984.

166. Peatfield AC, Barnes PJ, Bratcher C, et al: Vasoactive intestinal peptide stimulates submucosal gland secretion in ferret. Am Rev Respir Dis 128:89, 1983.

167. Coles SJ, Said SI, Reid LM: Inhibition of vasoactive intestinal peptide of glycoconjugate and lysozyme secretion by human airways in vitro. Am Rev Respir Dis 124:531, 1981.

168. Nathanson I, Widdicombe JH, Barnes PJ: Effect of vasoactive intestinal peptide on ion transport across dog tracheal epithelium. J Appl Physiol 55:1844, 1983.

169. Dunnill MS, Massarella GR, Anderson JA: A comparison of the quantitative anatomy of the bronchi in normal subjects, in status asthmaticus, in chronic bronchitis, and in emphysema. Thorax 24:176, 1969.

170. Cutz E, Levison H, Cooper DM: Ultrastructure of airways in children with asthma. Histopathology 2:407, 1978.

171. Dunnill MS: The pathology of asthma with special reference to changes in the bronchial mucosa. J Clin Pathol 13:27, 1960.

172. Mitchell-Heggs P, Palfrey AJ, Reid L: The elasticity of sputum at low shear rates. Biorheology 11:418, 1974.

173. Mezey RJ, Cohn MA, Fernandez RJ, et al: Mucociliary transport in allergic patients with antigen-induced bronchospasm. Am Rev Respir Dis 118:677, 1978.

174. Santa Cruz R, Landa J, Hirsch J, et al: Tracheal mucous velocity in normal man and patients with obstructive lung disease: Effects of terbutaline. Am Rev Respir Dis 109:458, 1974.

175. Ahmed T, Greenblatt DW, Birch S, et al: Abnormal mucociliary transport in allergic patients with antigen-induced bronchospasm: Role of slow reactive substance of anaphylaxis. Am Rev Respir Dis 124:110, 1981.

176. Pavia D, Bateman JRM, Sheahan NF, et al: Tracheobronchial mucociliary clearance in asthma: Impairment during remission. Thorax 40:171, 1985.

177. Wanner A, Zarzecki S, Hirsch J, et al: Tracheal mucous transport in experimental canine asthma. J Appl Physiol 39:950, 1975.

178. Weissberger D, Oliver W Jr, Abraham WM, et al: Impaired tracheal mucus transport in allergic bronchoconstriction: Effect of terbutaline pretreatment. J Allergy Clin Immunol 67:357, 1981.

179. Allegra L, Abraham WM, Chapman GA, et al: Duration of mucociliary dysfunction following antigen challenge in allergic sheep. J Appl Physiol 55:726, 1983.

180. Phipps R, Denas SM, Wanner A: Antigen stimulates glycoprotein secretion and alters ion fluxes in sheep trachea. J Appl Physiol 55:1593, 1983.

181. Marom Z, Shelhamer JH, Kaliner M: Effects of arachidonic acid, monohydroxyeicosatetraenoic acid and prostaglandins on the release of mucous glycoproteins from human airways in vitro. J Clin Invest 67:1695, 1981.

182. Marom Z, Shelhamer JH, Bach MK, et al: Slow-reacting substances (LTC4 and LTD4) increase the release of mucus from human airways in vitro. Am Rev Respir Dis 126:449, 1982.

183. Coles SJ, Neill KH, Reid LM, et al: Effects of leukotrienes $C_4$ and $D_4$ on glycoprotein and lysozyme secretion by human bronchial mucosa. Prostaglandins 25:155, 1983.

184. Johnson HG, McNee ML: Secretagogue responses of leucotrienes $C_4$, $D_4$: Comparison of potency in canine trachea in vivo. Prostaglandins 25:237, 1983.

185. Marin MG, Davis B, Nadel JA: Effect of histamine on electrical and ion transport properties of tracheal epithelium. J Appl Physiol 42:735, 1977.

186. Olver RE, Davis B, Marin MG, et al: Active transport of Na and Cl across the canine tracheal epithelium in vitro. Am Rev Respir Dis 112:811, 1975.

187. Durand J, Durand-Arczynska W, Haab P: Volume flow, hydraulic conductive and electrical properties across bovine tracheal epithelium in vitro: Effect of histamine. Pflugers Arch 392:40, 1981.

188. Russi EW, Abraham WM, Chapman GA, et al: Effects of leukotriene $D_4$ on mucociliary and respiratory function in allergic and nonallergic sheep. J Appl Physiol 59:1416, 1985.

188a. Ramsey BW, Astley SJ, Aitken ML, et al: Efficacy and safety of short-term administration of aerosolized recombinant human deoxyribonuclease in patients with cystic fibrosis. Am Rev Respir Dis 148:145, 1993.

189. Wallis GB: One-Dimensional Two-Phase Flow. New York, Mc-Graw-Hill, 1969.

190. Leith DE: Cough. *In* Brain JD, Proctor DF, Reid LM (eds): Respiratory Defense Mechanisms, part II. New York, Marcel Dekker, 1977:545.

191. Kim CS, Greene MA, Sankaran S, et al: Mucus transport in the airways by two-phase gas-liquid flow mechanism: Continuous flow model. J Appl Physiol 60:908, 1986.

192. Kim CS, Rodriguez CR, Eldridge MA, et al: Criteria for mucus transport in the airways by two-phase gas-liquid flow mechanism. J Appl Physiol 60:901, 1986.

193. Kim CS, Iglesias AJ, Sackner MA: Mucus clearance by two-phase gas-liquid flow mechanism: Asymmetric periodic flow model. J Appl Physiol 62:959, 1987.

194. Pryor JA, Weller BA, Hodson ME, et al: Evaluation of the forced expiration technique as an adjunct to postural drainage in treatment of cystic fibrosis. Br Med J 2:417, 1979.

195. Aiello E, Kennedy J, Hernandez C: Stimulation of frog ciliated cells in culture by acetylcholine and substance P. Comp Biochem Physiol [C]99:497, 1991.

196. Kobayashi K, Tamaoki J, Sakai N, et al: Angiotensin II stimulates airway ciliary motility in rabbit cultured tracheal epithelium. Acta Physiol Scand 138:497, 1990.

197. Tamaoki J, Kobayashi K, Sakai N, et al: Effect of bradykinin on airway ciliary motility and its modulation by neutral endopeptidase. Am Rev Respir Dis 140:430, 1989.

198. Kobayashi K, Tamaoki J, Sakai N, et al: Corticotropin-releasing factor and adrenocorticotropin stimulate ciliary motility in rabbit tracheal epithelium. Life Sci 45:2043, 1989.

199. Tamaoki K, Kanemura T, Sakai N, et al: Endothelin stimulates ciliary beat frequency and chloride secretion in canine cultured tracheal epithelium. Am J Respir Cell Mol Biol 4:426, 1991.

200. Verdugo P, Johnson NT, Tam PY: Beta-adrenergic stimulation of respiratory ciliary activity. J Appl Physiol 48:868, 1980.

201. Kondo M, Tamaoki J, Takizawa T: Neutral endopeptidase inhibitor potentiates the tachykinin-induced increase in ciliary beat frequency in rabbit trachea. Am Rev Respir Dis 142:403, 1990.

202. Wong LB, Miller IF, Yeates DB: Pathways of substance P stimulation of canine tracheal ciliary beat frequency. J Appl Physiol 70:267, 1991.

203. Chiyotani A, Tamaoki J, Sakai N, et al: Thromboxane $A_2$ mimetic U46619 stimulates ciliary motility of rabbit tracheal epithelial cells. Prostaglandins 43:111, 1992.

204. Sakai N, Tamaoki J, Kobayashi K, et al: Vasoactive intestinal peptide stimulates ciliary motility in rabbit tracheal epithelium: Modulation by neutral endopeptidase. Regul Pept 34:33, 1991.

205. Tamaoki K, Kobayashi K, Sakai N, et al: Atrial natriuretic factor inhibits ciliary motility in cultured rabbit tracheal epithelium. Am J Physiol 260:C201, 1991.

206. Karttunen P, Silvasti M, Virta P, et al: The effects of vadocaine, dextromethorphan, diphenhydramine, and hydroxyzine on the ciliary beat frequency in rats in vitro. Pharmacol Toxicol 67:159, 1990.

207. Kobayashi K, Tamaoki J, Sakai N, et al: Inhibition of ciliary activity by phorbol esters in rabbit tracheal cells. Lung 167:277, 1989.

# CHAPTER 3

# Humoral Immunity in the Lung: Expression and Therapeutic Manipulation

WILLIAM MERRILL

The lung must be open to the outside world to perform its main function of gas exchange. This openness leaves the lung accessible to foreign substances, including infectious organisms. Fortunately, the lung is protected by a complex overlapping series of mechanisms called "host defenses."[1-3] This chapter considers elements of the host defense associated with immunoglobulins. It begins with a review of the B cell, because this cell is responsible for immunoglobulin synthesis. The mechanisms for immunoglobulin localization and function in the lung are considered with the roles of immunoglobulins and immunoglobulin replacement therapy in the modulation of pulmonary host defense.

## MECHANISMS OF B-CELL IMMUNITY

### B-Cell Ontogeny

The B cell is a product of the division of the hematopoietic stem cell. Cells destined for B-cell lineage appear first in the fetal liver and later populate the adult bone marrow.[4] As shown in Figure 3–1, the life cycle of the B cell is complex. The first step in B-cell differentiation appears to be the rearrangement of the genetic material on chromosome 14, which contains the genes coding for the immunoglobulin heavy chain molecule.[5] This genetic material occurs in every cell in the germline configuration, in which the variable or V region genes, the diversity or D region genes, and the joining or J region genes are separated from one another. The initial step in B-cell differentiation is a recombination of the genetic material in this chro-

mosome such that genetic material for one discrete V region is opposed to that of a single D region and a single J region. This recombined DNA contains the DNA message for the antibody-combining or variable region of the immunoglobulin molecules synthesized by this cell.

### Synthesis of Immunoglobulin Isotypes

Immunoglobulin synthesis after novel immunization requires an intricate and carefully coordinated series of events. Heavy and light chain regions must be synthesized to form the final molecule. Immunoglobulin molecules are classified by their isotype into one of five groups (ie, IgM, IgD, IgG, IgA, IgE) determined by the constant regions of the immunoglobulin heavy chain. Some isotypes contain several subclasses (Fig. 3–2). The genetic material coding for the Ig isotype is contained downstream from the variable region. The first constant region of the heavy chain located downstream from the variable region is that for the μ chain, the constant region of the heavy chain of the IgM molecule (see Fig. 3–2). Transcription of immunoglobulin heavy chain proceeds through this region, and the initial molecule transcribed by early B cells is the heavy chain of IgM. These cells are referred to as μ positive. Early in B-cell development, light chains are not transcribed, and the μ chains that are expressed accumulate in the cytoplasm. Subsequently, the light chain gene undergoes a similar rearrangement, light chains are synthesized, and the completed molecule, including two heavy chains and two light chains, is expressed. This early IgM protein expressed by

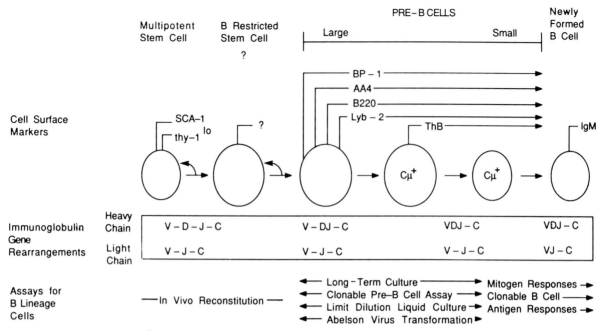

**Figure 3–1.** Schematic representation of some aspects of normal murine B-cell differentiation. The figure displays the multiple stages in the life cycle of the B cell (*top line*) and the evolution of cell surface markers (eg, SCA-1, THY-1, BP-1) as cells develop progressive ability to synthesize immunoglobulin molecules. (Adapted from Paige CJ and Wu GE: The B-cell repertoire. FASEB J 3:1818–1824, 1989.)

naive B cells contains a membrane-spanning region, and the IgM protein is a cell-surface molecule.[4,6]

The next bit of genomic data in the immunoglobulin chromosomal domain is that of the constant regions for the δ chain. This material is rapidly transcribed and is coupled to the antibody-combining region through alternative splicing. Naive B cells often express both IgM and IgD on their surface.[7] After stimulation by antigen and by growth factors released by other cells, the B cell may use constant region genetic material farther downstream from δ initially through alternative splicing. However, B cells appear to determine definitively their ultimate immunoglobulin isotype by opposing the variable region to a specific constant region through a deletion process called ''looping out'' that deletes the intervening constant region genetic material. Mature or memory B cells express a single population of immunoglobulin molecules on their surfaces.[8] The pattern of proteins secreted during the immune response (IgM followed by IgD, IgG3, and so on) follows the pattern of organization of genetic material on chromosome 14. During this process of rearrangement of the genetic material, the B cell expresses a variety of other surface molecules (see Fig. 3–1) that allow it to be identified definitively as having B-cell lineage.[9]

# IgH Isotypes

## Long arm chromosome 14

| VH | DH | JH | M | D | G3 | G1 | E | A1 | G2 | G4 | A2 |
|----|----|----|---|---|----|----|---|----|----|----|----|

| Cell Type | Ig Product |
|-----------|------------|
| Pre-B cell- | Cytoplasmic IgM |
| Naive B cell- | Surface IgM, IgD |
| Early response- | IgM, IgG3, IgG1 |
| Chronic response- | IgG2, IgG4 |

**Figure 3–2.** The relative position of genetic material on chromosome 14 is important in the synthesis of the immunoglobulin heavy chain (IgH). Shown in the figure is the pattern of immunoglobulin molecule expression during the immune response. The IgH constant regions proximal to the variable region genetic material are synthesized early in the immune response, and the immunoglobulin constant region material distal to the variable region tends to be used late in the immune response.

## Isotype Structure and Function

As depicted in Figure 3–2, the immunoglobulin genes can synthesize molecules with five different isotypes. Moreover, within IgG, there are four subclasses. Each isotype or subclass is characterized by a distinct constant heavy chain region.[10] This diversity of immunoglobulin isotypes and IgG and IgA subclasses suggests that there are important functional differences among immunoglobulin molecules. This idea is supported by analysis of the expression of immunoglobulins during various types of immune response and by assessment of immunoglobulin function in in vitro assays.[11,12] IgM is characterized by a high molecular mass (900 kd) and by early synthesis during a primary immune response. Because of its large molecular size, it is found chiefly in the circulating blood pool. It fixes complement well but is an ineffective opsonin. IgA is the primary immunoglobulin involved in mucosal immunity.[13] At the mucosal surface, dimeric IgA synthesized in submucosal sites is transported into external secretions by secretory component, a transport protein made by mucosal epithelial cells.[14] Some monomeric IgA is synthesized in the regional lymph nodes and circulates in blood. IgA can act as an opsonin. Its ability to fix complement is controversial. Its chief role may be "immune exclusion" whereby it binds an antigen or organism and prevents its attachment to the mucosa.

IgG is exclusively a monomer synthesized in lymph nodes and circulated in the blood pool. It enters the tissues by passive diffusion, although some local synthesis in tissue is possible. There are four subclasses of IgG.[10] IgG1 and IgG3 have much in common. IgG3 is the earliest IgG subclass molecule synthesized during the immune response.[15] It has potent complement-fixing properties. IgG1 is synthesized later in the immune response, but it also is potent in complement fixing and precipitation activity. IgG2 is the chief component of the immune response to polysaccharide antigens such as bacteria.[16] IgG4 is synthesized relatively late in the immune response, especially after recurrent antigenic challenge. Its role is uncertain. In some situations, it appears to be associated with antigenic tolerance,[17] but others have suggested that it may act as a weakly cytophilic analog of IgE, associated with allergic reactions. In some immunopathologic conditions such as bullous pemphigus, IgG4 can demonstrate significant toxic effects.[18] IgE has a powerful cytophilic attraction for mast cells and basophils and acts as the chief biologic trigger for mast cell and basophil degranulation. It exists in relatively low amounts in serum, but because it is tightly bound to tissue mast cells, the tissue concentration may be significantly higher.

## Lymphocyte Circulation

Naive B cells are made in the bone marrow and circulate throughout the body. There is some evidence that these cells are relatively freely passed into the pulmonary interstitium through postcapillary venules.[19] In the mouse, if these cells do not encounter antigen, they survive for only 2 weeks. However, if they encounter antigen and T-cell growth factors, the cells undergo the differentiation steps referred to earlier and become memory B cells with a much longer life span. These cells can gain access to lymph nodes and lymphatics and ultimately reenter the blood stream. The thoracic duct fluid of a rat provides transit for millions of lymphocytes daily, and many of these cells are memory B cells that return to the circulation.[19]

In the circulation, these cells have access to all the organs of the body, but their ability to migrate into an organ appears to depend on two factors. The first is the organ in which they originated. Cells that arise from an antigenic stimulation in the gut home to gut mucosal sites 8 to 10 times better than to peripheral lymph nodes. They also home somewhat better to the lung than to peripheral lymph nodes. Memory B cells that arise from intratracheal antigen priming appear to home to the lung much more strongly than they do to the gut. The second factor that determines distribution of memory B cells is the presence of inflammation. Some memory B cells appear to home to inflammatory sites in a non–organ-specific manner.[19] These memory B cells appear to express the cognate receptors for cell adhesion molecules expressed on endothelial cells exposed to inflammatory factors. For all of these cell adhesion molecules (eg, organ-specific homing factors, inflammation-specific adhesion molecules), the precise characterization of

the molecules is a topic of intense current research activity.[20, 21]

## Lung Lymphocyte Populations

Within the lung, lymphocytes are contained in several discrete locations. These include submucosal lymphocytes, loose parenchymal lymphocyte aggregates, and hilar lymph nodes.[22] Lymphocytes are also contained in special submucosal patches in larger airways. In some species, these patches are obvious and distinct, but in other species, including humans, they are more difficult to find. This submucosal collection of lymphocytes is covered with a specialized epithelium, and this unit is called bronchus-associated lymphoid tissue (BALT).[3]

Many experiments have demonstrated that antigen that enters the lung is processed locally in the lung, in hilar nodes, and subsequently in mediastinal lymph nodes.[1] However, the precise mechanisms of immunoglobulin responses have been difficult to observe. Because of the complexity of organization of pulmonary lymphocyte populations, gut analogies have been employed. The gut is more simply organized. Peyer patches (PP) are localized submucosal collections of lymphocytes, which are covered by a specialized epithelium. Antigen is processed locally in PP, and antigen-primed cells emigrate to mesenteric lymph nodes.[19] The response is amplified in mesenteric nodes, and lymphocytes emigrate to the circulation and subsequently home back to the gut. Many of the B cells in this traffic are destined to become IgA-secreting plasmocytes in the submucosa of the intestinal tract. As the IgA immune response is amplified, cells that can suppress synthesis of other immunoglobulin isotypes are also expanded and emigrate from the mesenteric nodes. Immunization of the gut results in an immune response that favors IgA synthesis and tends to suppress that of other isotypes.

Despite some similarities between the lung and the gut (eg, both are mucosal sites open freely to interaction with foreign antigen, both have relatively specialized collections of lymphocytes to interact with this foreign antigen), several investigators have demonstrated important differences between lung and gut immunization. For example, van der Brugge-Gamelkoorn and colleagues showed that after priming of the lung with tetanus toxoid, antibody-secreting cells tend to home much more specifically back to lung than to the intestinal tract.[23] Several investigators demonstrated that the immune response to sheep erythrocyte antigen deposited in the lung is of the IgG isotype.[24] PP appear to be an extremely important element of the intestinal tract response to foreign substances, and BALT, the lung PP analog, is not well developed in the human lung. It is difficult to draw simple analogies between the immunoglobulin immune responses in the lung and in the gut.

## Immunoglobulin Species on the Epithelial Surface of the Lung

Table 3–1 depicts the amounts of albumin, immunoglobulin classes, and IgG subclasses measured in serum and bronchoalveolar lavage (BAL) fluid of normal volunteers.

Table 3–1. **Absolute and Relative Concentrations of Immunoglobulin Species in Serum and Bronchoalveolar Lavage**

|         | Albumin | IgG1 | IgG2 | IgG3 | IgG4 | IgA  | IgE  |
| ------- | ------- | ---- | ---- | ---- | ---- | ---- | ---- |
| Serum*  | 49      | 4.5  | 2.1  | 0.03 | 0.09 | 1.98 | 199  |
| BAL     | 655     | 50   | 22   | 1.4  | 4.0  | 183  | 9.1  |
| Ratio   |         | 0.88 | 0.95 | 4.2  | 5†   | 7.9† | 3.8† |

*Values for serum are mg/mL and for bronchoalveolar lavage (BAL) are μg/mL, with the exception of IgE, which is in ng/mL for serum and BAL.

†The ratio is expressed as (BAL [Ig]/BAL [Albumin])/(Serum [Ig]/Serum [Albumin]) • 100; the BAL value is significantly greater than the serum value ($P < .05$).

Data from Merrill W, Naegel GP, Olchowski JJ, Reynolds HY: Immunoglobulin G subclass proteins in serum and lavage fluid of normal subjects. Am Rev Respir Dis 131:583, 1985.

These data demonstrate that significant quantities of all immunoglobulin classes and IgG subclasses can be detected in BAL fluid. The mechanism by which immunoglobulin gains access to the epithelial surface of the lung is uncertain, but some insight can be gained by assessment of ratios comparing immunoglobulin concentrations in serum and lavage fluid with simultaneously measured albumin concentrations in serum and lavage fluid. This type of assessment indicates that most IgG subclasses have similar relative concentrations in serum and lavage fluid, suggesting that passive diffusion from the serum onto the epithelial surface of the lung is the likely mode of access. Only IgG4 was significantly increased in BAL compared with serum. However, IgG has a larger molecular mass than albumin, and it is possible that some other IgG species are synthesized locally in the lung of normal subjects. The relative concentrations of IgA are considerably higher in the lung compared with serum. This increased relative concentration reflects the special excretory mechanism available for IgA transit from the submucosal region into the bronchial lumen.[19, 25] IgE is tightly bound to mast cell IgE surface receptors. The lung contains significant numbers of mast cells and therefore significant local concentrations of IgE.

In disease states, total concentrations of IgG recovered from the lower respiratory tract are significantly increased, as are amounts of albumin recovered. Often, the relative concentration of IgG is also increased.[26] This observation suggests that in the diseased lung a significant amount of IgG is produced locally. Studies by Hance and coworkers in patients with inflammatory lung disease support this,[27] and experiments involving chronic immunization of primate lung also indicate that chronically immunized lobes can have recruitment of immunoglobulin-secreting cells. Chronic inflammation probably enhances the migration of B cells into the lung through receptor-mediated mechanisms.

## THERAPEUTIC MANIPULATION OF HUMORAL IMMUNITY

### Immunization

The 1990s have ushered in a variety of exciting high-tech approaches for manipulation of the immune system. For example, the administration of cytokines forms an important part of our treatment of hematologic malignancies.[28]

Gene therapy is being explored as a method for treatment of immunodeficiencies associated with adenosine deaminase deficiency.[29] Despite this impressive array of high-tech approaches to therapy, it is likely that the single greatest advance in the manipulation of the immune response has been immunization. By an early age, most people in the United States have been immunized against a variety of diseases that previously caused severe childhood morbidity. Smallpox has been eradicated in the United States by an aggressive immunization policy. Debilitating illnesses such as polio and measles have been markedly curbed.[30] Moreover, this benefit to the health of the population accrues to the entire population and not just the small fraction that is likely to benefit from novel high-tech and expensive approaches to manipulation of the immune response.

The host defense in the lung can be significantly improved by immunization. Influenza is a common cause of respiratory illness. In the healthy adult or child, influenza causes a respiratory disease of variable severity that commonly results in significant loss of time from work or school. Patients who have chronic illnesses fare worse with influenza infections. A common method of following an influenza epidemic is to plot excess mortality. Excess mortality in the population tends to parallel influenza epidemics, because they cause mortality chiefly in persons who have other chronic medical illnesses. Immunization with the current vaccine affords significant protection against symptomatic influenza disease.[31–33] This protection can be achieved in anyone who has a normal immune system and who is given the influenza vaccine. Because the risk of vaccination complications is low, any adult willing to be vaccinated should receive the vaccine. It is especially important to immunize patients with known chronic medical illnesses, because this population suffers the greatest influenza-induced morbidity and death. Annual influenza immunization forms an important part of health maintenance for the average person with chronic illnesses, and it is a reasonable approach for healthy people with increased exposure to respiratory illnesses, such as health care workers.

Immunization provides effective prophylaxis for bacterial diseases.[34] Persons who have significant immune system diseases may not be protected[35] and may require more than one treatment with pneumococcal vaccine. Annual immunization should be considered. A trial using normal subjects and patients with a variety of human immunodeficiency virus (HIV)-related syndromes employed immunization with *Haemophilus influenzae* type B polysaccharide.[36] In this trial, patients with acquired immunodeficiency syndrome (AIDS) were shown to have significant responses to the antigen that were associated with rises in immunoglobulin concentration into the protective range (Fig. 3–3). More than 80% of AIDS patients achieved a protective response. Their titers were lower than those in the normal subjects and tended to wane more quickly over time. The trial was conducted with two different types of antigens, the polysaccharide antigen and the polysaccharide complexed to a carrier protein (PRP-CRM). Normal and HIV-infected persons in the trial with normal CD4 counts responded better to PRP-CRM. This is compatible with having normal immune systems and having T-cell–mediated help for B-cell immunoglobulin synthesis[37] available to them (Fig. 3–4, panel *B*). Patients with AIDS responded better to the simple polysaccharide antigen by itself (Fig.

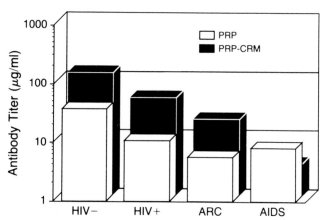

**Figure 3–3.** The geometric mean titer of antibody (*ordinate*) in four subject groups: HIV⁻ controls, HIV⁺ subjects without AIDS or AIDS-related complex (ARC), HIV⁺ subjects with ARC, and AIDS patients. The open bar depicts the response to polysaccharide antigen (PRP), and the closed bar represents response to polysaccharide antigen complexed to diphtheria toxoid (PRP-CRM). Although the immuno-globulin response to immunization was depressed with worsening stages of HIV infection, the response to polysaccharide antigen was preserved compared with that of PRP-CRM. (From Steinhoff MC, Auerbach BS, Nelson KE, et al: Antibody responses to *Haemophilus influenzae* type B vaccines in men with human immunodeficiency virus infection. Reprinted with permission from The New England Journal of Medicine, 325, 1837–1842, 1991.)

3–4, panel *A*), and there was no relation between CD4 counts and antibody response. This is compatible with the known immune defense lesion of AIDS, which affects chiefly the T cells. B cells are relatively unaffected and B cells can respond to polysaccharide antigens without T-cell help. Although this trial is preliminary, it suggests that the humoral response of patients with AIDS and other forms of immunocompromise can be manipulated by immunization against polysaccharide antigens. However, the trial also suggested that further research is necessary to determine optimal schedules for immunization.

Research in this important immunotherapy continues. Investigators are studying novel ways to stimulate the immune response. These methods include synthesis of peptide epitopes complexed to carrier proteins for immunization[38] and the use of lipophilic immune-stimulating complexes as immune adjuvants.[39] A group reported successful immunization of monkeys against simian immunodeficiency virus (SIV), the primate analog of HIV.[40] These investigators inserted the genes for SIV coat proteins into vaccinia virus and then immunized the monkeys with recombinant vaccinia viruses. The recombinant virus expressed SIV proteins in the immunized animals and effectively induced a significant immune response against SIV. One year after immunization, the animals were shown to be resistant to SIV infection. These results suggest that we may be getting closer to solving the paradox of HIV immunization.[41]

### Immunoglobulin Replacement Therapy

Several diseases compromise the host's ability to form immunoglobulin molecules specific for novel antigens. Among patients who have documented deficiencies in immunoglobulin synthesis, recurrent respiratory tract infec-

tions (eg, pneumonia, bronchitis, upper airway infection) are responsible for most significant symptomatic episodes (Table 3–2).[42] If a clinician is faced with a problem of recurrent symptomatic infections of the upper or lower respiratory tract, it is reasonable to consider the possibility of immunoglobulin deficiency. A quantitative assessment of serum immunoglobulins, including IgG subclasses, is a relatively common diagnostic step in the assessment of patients with recurrent infectious lung diseases. An important caveat in this assessment is that the clinician's actual concern is the patient's ability to make specific antibody. The patient's serum level of immunoglobulin is helpful information but may not be definitive by itself. For example, patients who have very low total levels of IgG (<4 g/L) almost always have significant abnormalities in synthesis of specific antibodies. For these patients, a decision to replace immunoglobulins can be made relatively simply, taking

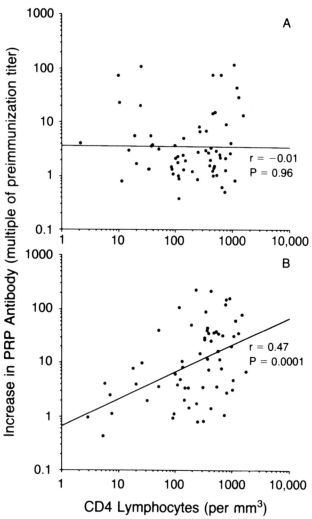

**Figure 3–4.** Relation between CD4⁺ lymphocyte count and antibody response in HIV-seropositive patients. The antibody response (*ordinate*) is plotted against the CD4⁺ lymphocyte count (*abscissa*). Patients receiving the complexed antigen (PRP-CRM, *panel B*) had a significant correlation between lymphocyte number and antibody titer. The responses of patients immunized with polysaccharide antigen (*panel A*) were not related to the number of CD4⁺ lymphocytes. (From Steinhoff MC, Auerbach BS, Nelson KE, et al: Antibody responses to *Haemophilus influenzae* type B vaccines in men with human immunodeficiency virus infection. Reprinted with permission from The New England Journal of Medicine, 325, 1837–1842, 1991.)

Table 3–2. **Infections in Hypoglobulinemic Patients**

| Infection | No. of Patients |
|---|---|
| Recurrent bronchitis, sinusitis, otitis | 103 |
| Conjunctivitis | 90 |
| Pneumonia | 80 |
| Hepatitis | 13 |
| Meningitis | 4 |
| History of severe herpes zoster | 2 |
| *Pneumocystis carinii* infection | 2 |
| Osteomyelitis | 1 |
| Suppurative parotitis | 1 |
| Recurrent parotitis | 1 |
| Septic arthritis | 1 |
| Pyoderma gangrenosum | 1 |

From Cunningham-Rundles C: Clinical and immunologic analyses of 103 patients with common variable immunodeficiency. J Clin Immunol 9:22–33, 1989.

into account the frequency of infections and the cost and inconvenience of treatment.

Patients with definitively abnormal levels of total IgG are relatively uncommon, and the physician can be faced with a patient with recurrent infections and low-normal total IgG levels or reductions in the concentration of specific IgG subclasses. In this situation, the ability to form specific antibodies is paramount, and serum level of immunoglobulin protein is less important. Some patients who have immunoglobulin subclass deficiency (ie, IgG2, IgG4) have significant problems with recurrent infections,[43] and others do not. The serum subclass level is more important as a marker of a *possible* immunodeficiency state than as definitive evidence of immunodeficiency. Such evidence can be determined by attempting to immunize the patient against a known antigen (eg, pneumovax, influenza vaccine) and quantifying the immune response to this antigen.[44] This service can be provided by many state laboratories and also by commercial labs. Although patients who have borderline or normal total IgG levels or isolated reductions in IgG subclasses may have significant deficiencies in immunoglobulin synthesis, it is important to demonstrate this definitively by immunization before embarking on therapy.

## Provision of Treatment

The past decade has seen a significant improvement in our ability to provide immunoglobulin replacement therapy. Before the 1980s, immunoglobulin preparations contained significant amounts of immunoglobulin aggregates. Intravenous infusion of these substances caused an unacceptable frequency of adverse effects. Improved purification strategies have managed to avoid this problem, and several commercial products are now available that allow for intermittent intravenous infusion (Table 3–3).[44]

These products are extremely safe. The purification method appears to inactivate HIV, and testing of immunoglobulin pools can exclude the hepatitis viruses. A significant potential complication of treatment is an anaphylactic or anaphylactoid reaction. Most patients with well-defined immunoglobulin deficiency diseases have some ability to form a humoral immune response. About a quarter of patients with common variable immunodeficiency were found to have clinical evidence of autoimmune diseases in one review of this illness.[42] Some patients with immunodeficiencies have no detectable IgA molecules. Some can make anti-IgA antibodies after receiving commercial immunoglobulin preparations that contain IgA. Subsequent challenge with these preparations can produce significant anaphylactic or anaphylactoid reactions. When receiving the infusion, the patient must have access to therapy for this potential complication. Some immunoglobulin preparations that have very low amounts of IgA can be substituted for patients who develop anti-IgA antibodies during treatment.[44] Another rare complication of immunoglobulin replacement therapy is aseptic meningitis syndrome. Only a few cases have been reported, and the causative mechanism is unknown.

The standard approach to treatment of these patients is to give a single infusion of approximately 400 mg/kg and to measure total IgG concentration 4 weeks later.[44–46] The goal of therapy is to maintain the serum level of IgG higher than 5.0 g/L with an interval between infusions of 4 weeks or more. The ability to achieve this depends on the immuno-

Table 3–3. **Characteristics of the Preparations of Intravenous Immune Globulin Available in the United States**

| Brand Name | Manufacturing Process | Additives | Approximate IgA Content* (μg/mL) | Form Supplied | Manufacturer |
|---|---|---|---|---|---|
| Gamimune N | pH 4.25, diafiltration | 10% maltose | 270 | 5% liquid, pH 4.25 | Cutter Biological, Miles Laboratories |
| Gammagard† | Polyethylene glycol, DEAE-Sephadex, ultrafiltration | 2% maltose, 0.2% polyethylene glycol, 0.3 M glycine, 0.15 M sodium chloride, 3% albumin | 0.4–1.9‡ | Lyophilized, 5%, pH 6.8 | Hyland Division, Baxter Healthcare |
| Gammar-IV | Low-ionic-strength ethanol | 5% sucrose, 2.5% albumin, 0.5% sodium chloride | 20‡ | Lyophilized, 5%, pH 7.0 | Armour Pharmaceutical |
| IVEEGAM | Immobilized trypsin, polyethylene glycol | 5% glucose, 0.3% sodium chloride, 0.5 polyethylene glycol | 5‡ | Lyophilized, 5%, pH 6.8 | Immuno-US |
| Sandoglobulin | pH 4.0, 1:10,000 trypsin | 5% or 10% sucrose (sodium chloride in diluent) | 720 | Lyophilized, 3% or 6%, pH 6.6 | Sandoz Pharmaceutical |
| Venoglobulin-I | Polyethylene glycol, DEAE-Sephadex | 2% D-mannitol, 1% albumin, 0.5% sodium chloride, <0.6% polyethylene glycol | 24‡ | Lyophilized, 5%, pH 6.8 | Alpha Therapeutics |

*Values are approximate; there is much lot-to-lot variability.

†Another preparation, marketed by the American Red Cross, is prepared by Baxter Hyland with plasma from Red Cross volunteer donors.

‡Data provided by manufacturer.

From Buckley R, Schiff RI: The use of intravenous immune globulin in immunodeficiency disease. Reprinted with permission from The New England Journal of Medicine, 325, 110–117, 1991.

globulin half-life. The immunoglobulin half-life in normal persons is 3 to 4 weeks, but the immunoglobulin half-life may be prolonged in patients with chronic immunodeficiency diseases. Because the treatment is expensive and the infusion is time consuming for the patient, it is important to optimize the amount of immunoglobulin infused and the infusion interval for each patient. This is an empiric process that requires provision of an initial dose, monitoring the effect of that dose, and adjustment of the dose or the interval between doses to achieve the desired effect.

### Effectiveness of Therapy

**Common Variable Immunodeficiency.** This is a heterogeneous disease. The onset of immunodeficiency is relatively late in life (Fig. 3–5), and it is a comparatively mild immunodeficiency. Patients are often treated by internists of diverse specialties. This patient population was one of the first to be treated with intravenous immunoglobulin therapy, and it was relatively simple to demonstrate a significant reduction in the frequency of infections with treatment.[47] Although controlled studies have not been performed, comparison of recently treated patients with historical controls suggests that the life spans of these patients may have been significantly increased by this treatment. A detailed analysis of the costs and benefits of this treatment has not been performed for this important but small patient population.

**Chronic Lymphocytic Leukemia.** Chronic lymphocytic leukemia (CLL) is a neoplasm of B cells, characterized by a monoclonal expansion of B cells with a reduction in total serum immunoglobulins. These patients have a significant frequency of respiratory infections, and bronchiectasis is not uncommon. A careful cost-effectiveness study of immunoglobulin replacement therapy in CLL was reported.[48] The investigators provided standard immunoglobulin re-

placement to patients who had CLL and immunoglobulin deficiency. They found a significant reduction in symptomatic infections with this treatment. However, their analysis of cost-effectiveness was sobering. The investigators found that most infections prevented were of relatively modest severity and that the impact on survival was small. Moreover, an attempt to assess the improvement in the quality of life afforded by immunoglobulin therapy (in quality-adjusted life-years) yielded a similarly small benefit. When gauged against this type of careful analysis, the cost of providing immunoglobulin replacement treatment to this patient population was prohibitively high (> $4,000,000/ quality-adjusted life-year of increased survival). These are important data for the entire field of chronic immunoglobulin replacement, because this represents the first attempt to assess carefully the cost effectiveness of this expensive (± $40,000/y) treatment.

**Acquired Immunodeficiency Syndrome.** Patients with AIDS have primarily a deficiency in helper T cell function. Although, hyperglobulinemia is common, these patients demonstrate poor responses to immunization with protein antigens; moreover, serious bacterial infections are not uncommon in patients with this syndrome.[49] Anecdotal reports have suggested some benefits from intravenous immunoglobulin replacement therapy.[50] A controlled trial demonstrated that patients with congenital HIV infections who received immunoglobulin replacement therapy had a significant reduction in the number of severe bacterial infections.[51] This benefit appeared to accrue only to patients with relatively mild immunocompromised (CD4+ cells > 200/ μL). Patients with lower CD4 counts appeared not to benefit from immunoglobulin infusion. Because this trial was done several years ago, only a few patients received standard antiretroviral therapy or *Pneumocystis carinii* prophylaxis; again, a careful assessment of cost effectiveness of this treatment was not performed. These results do suggest

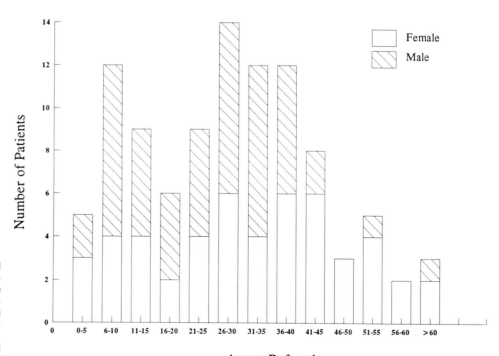

**Figure 3–5.** Histogram of age and sex of patients with common variable immunodeficiency at the time of first clinic visit. (From Cunningham-Rundles C: Clinical and immunologic analyses of 103 patients with common variable immunodeficiency. J Clin Immunol 9:22–33, 1989.)

some utility for immunoglobulin replacement therapy in congenitally HIV-infected patients. However, they also raise additional research questions. Preliminary data suggest that adult AIDS patients can mount significant IgG responses to T-cell–independent antigens (ie, polysaccharide antigens), and it seems unlikely that immunoglobulin replacement therapy will have a large role to play in the treatment of adults with AIDS. The role of immunization of children with AIDS also needs further exploration.

**Cytomegalovirus Infection.** In addition to the use of chronic immunoglobulin replacement therapy, immunoglobulins have been given acutely to treat viral infections. Most of these reports are anecdotal (eg, treatment of red cell aplasia secondary to parvovirus infection[52]). However, an extensive literature has developed concerning the use of immunoglobulin therapy in patients at risk for cytomegalovirus (CMV) infection. In these studies, patients who have received organ transplants and are immunosuppressed received immunoglobulin infusions in an effort to prevent or reduce the severity of CMV pneumonitis. These data were reviewed by Snydman.[53] For patients with renal transplants who are at risk for primary CMV infection (eg, CMV-negative recipients, CMV-positive donors), hyperimmune anti-CMV globulin provides significant protection against acute primary CMV disease (Table 3–4). His review of other solid organ transplantations suggested that anti-CMV immunoglobulin might have a similar effect; however, in most situations too few data were available for careful analysis.

There has been considerable interest in treating patients receiving bone marrow transplantations with immunoglobulin therapy. Preliminary results suggested that immunoglobulin therapy by itself did little to affect CMV syndromes in this patient population. However, several large, uncontrolled studies suggested that the combination of immunoglobulin administration plus antiviral therapy with ganciclovir may be useful. Several trials have been studied

patients with CMV pneumonia in the setting of bone marrow transplantation. These studies were all uncontrolled and involved combination therapy with immunoglobulin and ganciclovir. The outcome from the four studies demonstrated survival rates ranging from 52% to 87%, which is dramatically better than survival rates in historical controls (Table 3–5).

Despite this relatively exciting preliminary information, these results are not definitive. The period after bone marrow transplantation is complex. A variety of acute pulmonary syndromes can emerge, and a specific diagnosis of pulmonary infiltrates during this period is difficult. Graft-versus-host disease[54] and pulmonary drug and radiation reactions[55] can resemble CMV pneumonitis and cause diagnostic problems. The dose of immunoglobulins used in these studies is similar to that used for immunomodulation with immunoglobulin. It is not clear that the chief influence of the agent at this dose is an antibody-mediated antiviral effect. Conceivably, its main role is to down-regulate the host immune response. This effect could be useful in situations of viral infection and in graft-versus-host disease and pulmonary drug and radiation toxicity syndromes.[56]

Significant progress has been made in modulating CMV syndromes in the period after bone marrow transplantation. The fact that CMV infection in the posttransplant period may represent reactivation of a latent infection or a new infection in a previously uninfected host allows the development of additional strategies. Investigators have begun to explore the possibility of suppressing viral reactivation with ganciclovir during the period of greatest risk, approximately 30 days after transplantation.[57] A second strategy, to prevent new infection in previously uninfected recipients, is to employ blood products screened for the presence of CMV. Recipients who are uninfected with CMV should receive only CMV-negative blood products.[58] These recipients will have an extremely low rate of significant CMV infection. Despite these reservations, the reports of successful treatment of pneumonitis in the bone marrow transplant period are exciting and deserve further exploration.

**Other Passive Immunization.** Host immunity can also be altered by administering immunoglobulins with a more narrow spectrum of affinity. Several special-use immunoglobulin preparations are commercially available. High-titer human sera are available to treat patients with recent exposure to rabies or tetanus. The passively administered immunoglobulin is meant to act until the host can be actively immunized by giving appropriate intramuscular injections of antigen. By contrast, high-titer human anti-Rh serum is given to Rh-negative mothers at term or after abortion. This treatment is meant to block the host response to intravenous antigen (in this case, fetal Rh-positive erythrocytes). Other high-titer human immunoglobulin preparations have been employed in other specific situations, but the beneficial effects of these preparations have been difficult to prove. For example, high-titer anti-CMV immunoglobulins were thought to have a beneficial effect on CMV infection in transplant recipients. However, similar beneficial effects also accrue to the use of standard immunoglobulin preparations. In one trial, patients thought to be at high risk of bacterial infection were treated with a high-titer antilipopolysaccharide (anti-LPS) immunoglobulin preparation, with pooled immunoglobulins, or with albumin. The patient population receiving pooled immunoglobulins had a significantly im-

Table 3–4. **Interim Comparison of Outcome in Randomized Trial and Open-Label Trial of Intravenous Administration of CMV Immunoglobulin in Renal Transplant Recipients**

| Outcome | No. in Indicated Group With Outcome (%) | | |
|---|---|---|---|
| | *Randomized* | | *Open-Label* |
| | *Controls (n = 35)* | *Globulin (n = 24)* | *Globulin (n = 27)* |
| Clinical | | | |
| Virologically confirmed CMV syndrome | 21 (60)*† | 5 (21)* | 9 (33)† |
| Fungal or parasitic opportunistic infection | 7 (20)‡§ | 0‡ | 1 (4)§ |
| Death | 5 (14) | 1 (4) | 2 (7) |
| Graft loss | 10 (29) | 4 (17) | 5 (19) |
| Virologic | | | |
| CMV viremia | 15 (43) | 6 (25) | 6 (22) |
| Virus isolation (any size) | 20 (57) | 13 (54) | 15 (56) |
| Seroconversion | 27 (77) | 17 (71) | 16 (59) |

*$\chi^2 = 8.94$, $P < .01$.
†$\chi^2 = 4.34$, $P < .05$.
‡Fisher's exact test, $P = .02$.
§Fisher's exact test, $P = .06$ open-label vs. control group.

From Snydman DR: Cytomegalovirus immunoglobulins in the prevention and treatment of cytomegalovirus disease. Rev Infect Dis 12(suppl 7):S839–S848, 1990. © 1990 by the University of Chicago.

Table 3–5. **Controlled Trials of Immunoglobulin for CMV Prophylaxis in Bone Marrow Transplantation**

| Globulin (Manufacturer)* | Dose | CMV Serologic Status of Recipient | Conditioning Regimen† | Comparison | Outcome‡ |
|---|---|---|---|---|---|
| Hyperimmune plasma | 10 mL/kg IV on days −3, 3, 30, 45, 60, 75, 90, and 120 | Negative and positive | TBI, multiple | Randomized | Decreased CMV disease and CMV interstitial pneumonia, no granulocytes |
| Immunoglobulin (Miles/Cutter) | 20mL/kg IV once a week for 4 mo. | Negative and positive | Multiple, HLA identical sibling | Randomized | Decreased CMV disease, CMV pneumonia, and GVH |
| Hyperimmune (Condie) | 200 mg/kg IV on days 25, 50, and 75 | Negative and positive | TBI, cytoxan | With immunoglobulin lacking CMV antibody and matched untreated | Decreased CMV infection, interstitial pneumonia, and mortality |
| Hyperimmune (Massachusetts Biologic Laboratories) | 6 mL/m² IM on days −4, −2, and 0 and then every 7 d for 11 doses | Negative | TBI, cytoxan | Randomized | Decreased CMV infection for CMV-seronegative marrow donor, no granulocytes |
| Hyperimmune (Massachusetts Biologic Laboratories) | 150 mg/kg IV on days −5, −1, 6, 20, and 34 and 100 mg/kg on days 48 and 62 | Negative | Not stated | Randomized, factorial, screened blood | Decreased infection with screened blood |

*Miles/Cutter (West Haven, Connecticut), Condie (Minneapolis), and Massachusetts Biologic Public Health Laboratories (Jamaica Plain, Massachusetts).
†TBI, total body irradiation.
‡GVH, graft-versus-host disease.
Modified from Snydman DR: Cytomegalovirus immunoglobulins in the prevention and treatment of cytomegalovirus disease. Rev Infect Dis 12(suppl 7):S839–S848, 1990. © 1990 by the University of Chicago.

proved outcome compared with patients receiving albumin or the high-titer anti-LPS immunoglobulin preparation.[59]

Monoclonal antibodies can also be employed for passive immunization. Two preparations are commercially available. Antidigitalis monoclonal antibodies (Fab fraction) can significantly alter the risk of serious outcomes from digitalis intoxication in children.[60] Antibodies specific for CD3 are effective for the depletion of lymphocytes as part of a conditioning regimen for transplantation.[61] Many other monoclonal antibody preparations have been prepared for potential use in humans. A humanized IgM antibody preparation said to be specific for LPS was reported to improve the outcome in bacteremic septic patients.[62] Because of some concerns about the conduct of the trial, this agent has not been approved.[63, 64] Monoclonal antibodies specific for tumor necrosis factor, intracellular adhesion molecule-1, and tissue factor are in the early stages of investigation in humans. It is likely that these antibody preparations will have potent effects on the immune response and that these agents could offer significant benefits for treating some human diseases.

## Immunomodulation With Immunoglobulin

Immunoglobulins are considered to be important components of host defense that act by binding to antigen and destroying it through complement-mediated mechanisms or opsonizing the antigen and facilitating its ingestion by phagocytes. However, immunoglobulin molecules have other important effects on the immune system.[65, 66] Immunoglobulin molecules can bind to Fc receptors on several cell types. In general, this type of binding is facilitated by aggregates or immune complexes, and small amounts of these aggregates exist in commercial preparations. Large infusions of intravenous immunoglobulins, such as those given with the usual monthly dose of 400 mg/kg, could

have significant effects on IgG Fc receptors on immunocompetent cells. The second important mechanism of immunoglobulin alteration of the immune response is the anti-idiotype antibody. The immunoglobulin molecule has a constant region and a variable region. The variable or antigen-binding region represents a new protein epitope never previously synthesized by the host. It is possible for the host to form an antibody response against this "idiotypic" region of the immunoglobulin molecule. These anti-idiotype antibodies are thought to be important antiinflammatory components of the immune response. Anti-idiotype antibodies have been detected in commercial immunoglobulin preparations. Some of these anti-idiotypic antibodies are directed against the idiotypes of autoantibodies.[67, 68] Anti-idiotypic antibodies may modulate autoimmune reactions by an anti-idiotypic mechanism that is for some reason lacking in the host. A variety of other mechanisms have been demonstrated or proposed for immunomodulating effects of immunoglobulin infusion, and these are listed in Table 3–6.

This form of therapy has been tried in virtually every disease thought to have an immune mechanism.[66] This popularity results from the difficulty in controlling these diseases and the relatively low toxicity of this treatment compared with other attempts to manipulate the immune response. The best-studied diseases include idiopathic thrombocytopenic purpura and Guillain-Barré syndrome. In these diseases, large amounts of immunoglobulin are infused on successive days (eg, 400 mg/kg/d for 5 days), and the response to therapy is monitored. In general, some therapeutic response is seen within the first 3 to 5 days. In children, significant long-term responses are often seen. In adults, although improvement is frequently noted, it tends to be more transient.

Intravenous immunoglobulin has been tried in a variety of other illnesses, ranging from asthma[69] to Wegener's vasculitis.[70] In most of these reports, the agent has been admin-

Table 3–6. **Immunosuppressive Effects of Intravenous IgG**

| |
| --- |
| Fc receptor blockade |
| Anti-idiotype antibodies |
| Increased CD8$^+$ suppressor cells |
| Suppressed lymphocyte division |
| Suppressed B-cell differentiation |
| Reduced antibody-dependent cytotoxicity |
| Altered IgG subclass responses |
| Reduced natural killer cell activity |
| Reduced mixed lymphocyte reaction |

Abstracted from Woolf AD, Wenger T, Smith TW, Lovejoy FH: The use of digoxin-specific Fab fragments for severe digitalis intoxication in children. Reprinted with permission from The New England Journal of Medicine, 326, 1739–1744, 1992.

istered in an uncontrolled fashion and firm evidence of improvement has not been provided. However, when improvement does occur in immune disease, it usually occurs rapidly, within the first several doses of intravenous immunoglobulin. In these studies, investigators usually employed 400 mg/kg, administered daily for 3 to 5 days; such courses of treatment are generally nontoxic. Although immunoglobulin therapy is expensive, the cost accrues chiefly to the support of immunoglobulin concentrations over a long period. Short-term use of IgG preparations to regulate acute severe illnesses are less costly to the health care system in the long term.

## CONCLUSION

Humoral immunity and its investigation have formed the foundation for modern immunology. Humoral immune mechanisms were the first and are still the best-studied aspects of the immune system. Moreover, manipulation of humoral immunity by immunization has brought about major improvements in life expectancy and the quality of life. Progress in vaccine technology has raised our appreciation for the possibility of immunization, even against such daunting agents as HIV. Intravenous immunoglobulin infusions provide another mechanism for affecting humoral immunity and perhaps for providing antiinflammatory immunoregulation. Although this therapy is safe and can reduce infection in immunocompromised persons, the cost effectiveness of chronic immunoglobulin replacement therapy has been questioned. Future studies should address this important topic. Although preliminary data suggest that acute infusions of immunoglobulin may be useful as an immunoregulatory modality, most reports are essentially anecdotal. It is premature to recommend that this form of immunoregulation should be the primary therapy for any disease. However, experience with idiopathic thrombocytopenic purpura and Guillain-Barré syndrome indicates that it can play an important therapeutic role. Immunoglobulin infusion has a high therapeutic index compared with other immunomodulating agents, and it is appropriate that use of these agents continue so that a useful body of comparative data can be developed. For many appropriate diseases, the frequency of the illness is low, and controlled trials are difficult, but some illnesses treated with this therapy are common, and it would be inappropriate to continue the use of this agent without conducting appropriate controlled trials. The next decade should provide clinical information

indicating the appropriate role for immunomodulatory therapy with intravenous immunoglobulin.

## REFERENCES

1. Kaltreider HB: Local immunity. *In* Bienenstock J (ed): Immunology of the Lung and Upper Respiratory Tract. New York, McGraw-Hill, 1984:191–215.
2. Willoughby WF, Willoughby JB: Antigen handling. *In* Bienenstock J (ed): Immunology of the Lung and Upper Respiratory Tract. New York, McGraw-Hill, 1984:174–190.
3. Clancy R, Bienenstock J: A framework for immunization strategy. *In* Immunology of the Lung and Upper Respiratory Tract. 1984:216–231.
4. Paige CJ, Wu GE: The B cell repertoire. FASEB J 3:1818–1824, 1989.
5. Lieber MR: Site-specific recombination in the immune system. FASEB J 5:2934–2944, 1991.
6. Duperray C, Boiron JM, Boucheix C, et al: The CD24 antigen discriminates between pre-B and cells in human bone marrow. J Immunol 145:678–683, 1990.
7. Lees A, Morris SC, Thyphronitis G, Holmes JM, Inman JK, Finkelman FD: Rapid stimulation of large specific antibody responses with conjugates of antigen and anti-IgD antibody. J Immunol 145:3594–3600, 1990.
8. Snapper CM, Finkelman FD: Rapid loss of IgM expression by normal murine B cells undergoing IgG1 and IgE class switching after in vivo immunization. J Immunol 145:3654–3660, 1990.
9. Zola H: The surface antigens of human B lymphocytes. Immunol Today 8:308–315, 1987.
10. Schur PH: IgG subclasses: A review. Ann Allergy 58:89–99, 1989.
11. Bindon CI, Hale G, Bruggemann M, Waldmann H: Human monoclonal IgG isotypes differ in complement activating function at the level of C4 as well as C1q. J Exp Med 168:127–142, 1988.
12. Tao Mi-Hua, Canfield SM, Morrison SL: The differential ability of human IgG1 and IgG4 to activate complement is determined by the COOH-terminal sequence of the CH$_2$ domain. J Exp Med 173:1025–1028, 1991.
13. Kaetzel CS, Robinson JK, Chintalacharuvu KR, Vaerman JP, Lamm ME: The polymeric immunoglobulin receptor (secretory component) mediates transport of immune complexes across epithelial cells: A local defense function for IgA. Proc Natl Acad Sci U S A 88:796–800, 1991.
14. Merrill WW, Goodenberger D, Strober W, Matthay RA, Naegel GP, Reynolds HY: Free secretory component and other proteins in human lung lavage. Am Rev Respir Dis 122:156–161, 1980.
15. Rubin RL, Tang F, Lucas AH, Spiegelberg HL, Tan EM: IgG subclasses of anti-tetanus toxoid antibodies in adult and newborn normal subjects and in patients with systemic lupus erythematosus, Sjögren's syndrome, and drug-induced autoimmunity. J Immunol 137:2522–2527, 1988.
16. Shackelford P, Nelson SJ, Palma AT, Nahm MH: Human antibodies to group A streptococcal carbohydrate: Ontogeny, subclass restriction, and clonal diversity. J Immunol 140:3200–3205, 1988.
17. Kwan-Lim G-E, Forsyth KP, Maizels RM: Filarial-specific IgG4 response correlates with active *Wuchereria bancrofti* infection. J Immunol 145:4298–4305, 1990.
18. Rock B, Martins CR, Theofilopoulos AN, et al: The pathogenic effect of IgG4 autoantibodies in endemic pemphigus foliaceus (fogo selvagem). N Engl J Med 320:1463–1469, 1989.
19. Yednock TA, Rosen SD: Lymphocyte homing. Adv Immunol 44:313–379, 1989.
20. Chin Y-H, Cae J-P, Johnson K: Lymphocyte adhesion to cultured Peyer's patch high endothelial venule cells is mediated by organ-specific homing receptors and can be regulated by cytokines. J Immunol 145:3669–3677, 1990.
21. Shimizu Y, Shaw S: Lymphocyte interactions with extracellular matrix. FASEB J 5:2292–2299, 1991.
22. Lauweryns JM: The blood and lymphatic microcirculation of the lung. Pathol Annu 6:365–415, 1971.
23. Van Der Brugge-Gamelkoorn GJ, Claassen E, Sminia T: Anti-TNP-forming cells in bronchus-associated lymphoid tissue (BALT) and paratracheal lymph node (PTLN) of the rat after intratracheal priming and boosting with TNP-KLH. Immunology 57:405–409, 1986.

24. Mason MJ, Bice DE, Muggenburg BA: Local pulmonary immune responsiveness after multiple antigenic exposures in the cynomolgus monkey. Am Rev Respir Dis 132:657–660, 1985.
25. Merrill W, Naegel GP, Olchowski JJ, Reynolds HY: Immunoglobulin G subclass proteins in serum and lavage fluid of normal subjects. Am Rev Respir Dis 131:583–587, 1985.
26. Gerli R, Darwish S, Broccucci L, Spinozzi F, Rambotti P: Helper inducer T cells in the lungs of sarcoidosis patients. Chest 95:811–816, 1989.
27. Hance AJ, Saltini C, Crystal RG: Does de novo immunoglobulin synthesis occur on the epithelial surface of the human lower respiratory tract? Am Rev Respir Dis 137:17–24, 1988.
28. Harding AE: Treatment of a marrow stem-cell disorder with granulocyte colony-stimulating factor. N Engl J Med 320:1343–1344, 1989.
29. Blaese RM: Progress toward gene therapy. Clin Immunol Immunopathol 61:S47–S55, 1991.
30. General Recommendations on Immunization (Guidelines from the Immunization Practices Advisory Committee). Ann Intern Med 111:133–142, 1989.
31. Patriarca PA, Arden NH, Koplan JP, Goodman RA: Prevention and control of type A influenza infections in nursing homes. Ann Intern Med 107:732–740, 1987.
32. Gross PA, Quinnan GV, Rodstein M, et al: Association of influenza immunization with reduction in mortality in an elderly population. Arch Intern Med 148:562–565, 1988.
33. Oates JA, Wood AJ: Prophylaxis and treatment of influenza. N Engl J Med 322:433–450, 1990.
34. Research Committee of the British Thoracic Society: Community-acquired pneumonia in adults in British hospitals in 1982–1983: A survey of aetiology, mortality, prognostic factors and outcome. Q J Med 62:195–220, 1987.
35. Shapiro ED, Berg AT, Austrian R, et al: The protective efficacy of polyvalent pneumococcal polysaccharide vaccine. N Engl J Med 325:1453–1460, 1991.
36. Steinhoff MC, Auerbach BS, Nelson KE, et al: Antibody responses to *Haemophilus influenzae* type B vaccines in men with human immunodeficiency virus infection. N Engl J Med 325:1837–1842, 1991.
37. Noelle RJ, Snow CE: T-helper cell-dependent B cell activation. FASEB J 5:2770–2776, 1991.
38. Takahashi H, Nakagawa Y, Pendelton CD, et al: Induction of broadly cross-reactive cytotoxic T-cells recognizing an HIV-1 envelope determinant. Science 255:333–336, 1992.
39. Mowat AM, Donachie AM: ISCOMS—a novel strategy for mucosal immunization? Immunol Today 12:383–385, 1991.
40. Hu S-L, Abrams K, Barber GN, et al: Protection of macaques against SIV by subunit vaccines of SIV envelope glycoprotein gp160. Science 255:456–459, 1992.
41. Nara PL, Garrity RR, Goudsmit J: Neutralization of HIV-1: A paradox of humoral proportions. FASEB J 5:2437–2455, 1991.
42. Cunningham-Rundles C: Clinical and immunologic analyses of 103 patients with common variable immunodeficiency. J Clin Immunol 9:22–33, 1989.
43. Oxilius VA: Immunoglobulin G (IgG) subclasses and human disease. Am J Med 76(suppl 3A):7–18, 1984.
44. Buckley R, Schiff RI: The use of intravenous immune globulin in immunodeficiency diseases. N Engl J Med 325:110–117, 1991.
45. Stiehm RE, Ashida E, Kwang SK, Winston DJ, Haas A, Gale RP: Intravenous immunoglobulins as therapeutic agents. Ann Intern Med 107:367–382, 1987.
46. Berkman SA, Lee ML, Gale RP: Clinical uses of intravenous immunoglobulins. Ann Intern Med 112:278–292, 1990.
47. Cunningham-Rundles C, Siegal FP, Smithwick EM, et al: Efficacy of intravenous immunoglobulin in primary humoral immunodeficiency disease. Ann Intern Med 101:435–439, 1984.
48. Weeks JC, Tierney MR, Weinstein MC: Cost effectivelness of prophylactic intravenous immune globulin in chronic lymphocytic leukemia. N Engl J Med 325:81–86, 1991.
49. Schlamm HT, Yankovitz SR: *Haemophilus influenzae* pneumonia in young adults with AIDS, ARC or risk of AIDS. Am J Med 86:11–14, 1989.
50. Wood CC, McNamara JG, Schwarz DF, Merrill WW, Shapiro ED: Prevention of pneumococcal bacteremia in a child with acquired immunodeficiency syndrome-related complex. Pediatr Infect Dis J 6:564–566, 1987.
51. Willoughby A, Mofenson LM, Nugent R, et al: Intravenous immune globulin for the prevention of bacterial infections in children with symptomatic human immunodeficiency virus infection. N Engl J Med 325:73–80, 1991.
52. McGuire WA, Yang HH, Bruno E, et al: Treatment of antibody-mediated pure red-cell aplasia with high-dose intravenous immunoglobulin. N Engl J Med 317:1004–1008, 1987.
53. Snydman DR: Cytomegalovirus immunoglobulins in the prevention and treatment of cytomegalovirus disease. Rev Infect Dis 12(Suppl 7):S839–S848, 1990.
54. Ferrara JLM, Deeg HJ: Graft-versus-host disease. N Engl J Med 324:667–674, 1991.
55. Rosiello RA, Merrill WW: Radiation-induced lung injury. Clin Chest Med 11:65–71, 1990.
56. Sullivan KM, Kopecky KJ, Jocom J, et al: Immunomodulatory and antimicrobial efficacy of intravenous immunoglobulin in bone marrow transplantation. N Engl J Med 323:705–712, 1990.
57. Schmidt GM, Horak DA, Niland JC, Duncan SR, Forman SJ, Zaia JA: A randomized controlled trial of prophylactic ganciclovir for cytomegalovirus pulmonary infection in recipients of allogeneic bone marrow transplants. N Engl J Med 324:1005–1011, 1991.
58. Frank I, Friedman HM: Progress in the treatment of cytomegalovirus pneumonia. Ann Intern Med 109:769–771, 1988.
59. The Intravenous Immunoglobulin Collaborative Study Group: Prophylactic intravenous administration of standard immune globulin as compared with core-lipopolysaccharide immune globulin in patients with high risk of postsurgical infection. N Engl J Med 327:234–240, 1992.
60. Woolf AD, Wenger T, Smith TW, Lovejoy FH: The use of digoxin-specific Fab fragments for severe digitalis intoxication in children. N Engl J Med 326:1739–1744, 1992.
61. Ascher NL, Stock PG, Bumgardner GL, Payne WD, Najarian JS: Infection and rejection of primary hepatic transplant in 93 consecutive patients treated with triple immunosuppressive therapy. Surg Gynecol Obstet 167:474–484, 1988.
62. Ziegler EJ, Fisher CJ, Sprung CL, et al: Treatment of gram negative bacteremia and septic shock with HA-1A human monoclonal antibody against endotoxin. N Engl J Med 324:429–436, 1991.
63. Wenzel RP, Andriole VT, Bartlett JG, et al: Antiendotoxin antibodies for gram-negative sepsis: Guidelines from the IDSA. Clin Infect Dis 14:973–976, 1992.
64. Warren HS, Danner RL, Munford RS: Antiendotoxin monoclonal antibodies: A second look. N Engl J Med 326:1151–1157, 1992.
65. Hassner A, Adelman DC: Biologic response modifiers in primary immunodeficiency disorders. Ann Intern Med 115:294–307, 1991.
66. Dwyer, JM: Manipulating the immune system with immune globulin. N Engl J Med 326:107–116, 1992.
67. Dietrich G, Kazatchkine MD: Normal immunoglobulin G (IgG) for therapeutic use (intravenous Ig) contain antiidiotypic specificities against an immunodominant, disease-associated, cross-reactive idiotype of human anti-thyroglobulin autoantibodies. J Clin Invest 85:620–625, 1989.
68. Rossi F, Kazatchkine MD: Antiidiotypes against autoantibodies in pooled normal human polyspecific Ig1. J Immunol 143:4104–4109, 1989.
69. Larsen GL, Mazer BD, Gelfand EW: New concepts in the pathogenesis of allergies and asthma. *In* Imbach P (ed): Immunotherapy With Intravenous Immunoglobulins. London, Academic Press, 1991:319–331.
70. Jayne DRW, Davies MJ, Fox CJV, Black CM, Lockwood CM: Treatment of systemic vasculitis with pooled intravenous immunoglobulin. Lancet 337:1137–1139, 1991.

# CHAPTER 4

# Pathogenesis of Airway Colonization

REUBEN RAMPHAL

Colonization of the airways is recognized by the persistent growth of microorganisms from repeated cultures. At the microscopic level, this phenomenon is characterized by the adhesion of microorganisms to cells of the respiratory tract or to stagnant mucus secretions within the respiratory tract. The adhesion phenomenon is the microscopic basis of colonization, and in discussing the pathogenesis of airway colonization, it is essential to focus on the factors that allow the approximation of the microbe to the adhesive sites and on the biochemical nature of this interaction.[1] However, the mere approximation or attachment of a microbe to an adhesive site does not necessarily lead to colonization, because host factors ordinarily protect a normally sterile site. Failure of one or more of the host defenses of the lower respiratory tract is required for colonization to occur. In the respiratory tract, failure of host defenses may be genetic, acquired, or microbe mediated.

This chapter discusses the host-microbe interaction, highlighting what is known and not known about these aspects of the pathogenesis of airway colonization. Information about the mechanisms of colonization of the respiratory tract by most bacteria remains scarce. Because only *Pseudomonas aeruginosa* has been extensively studied, certain generalizations have been made that may not necessarily be true for other bacteria.

## ANATOMY

### Factors Influencing Colonization

The respiratory tract may be conveniently divided into the upper respiratory tract, consisting of the mucosal areas above the vocal cords, and the lower respiratory tract, con-

sisting of the conducting airways as far down as the bronchioles. Because the upper respiratory tract is in contact with the upper end of the gastrointestinal tract, the flora of the upper respiratory tract should be considered the same as oral flora. The endogenous flora of the mouth, which probably consists of several hundred species of bacteria, has been partially characterized, but its normal function has not been elucidated, except that it may prevent the implantation and colonization of pathogenic species of bacteria.[2]

The oral flora is generally stable from early childhood until death, but it is alterable by states of illness[3] and by the use of antimicrobial agents that eradicate or suppress the resident bacteria.[4] These alterations consist primarily of the acquisition and colonization of the upper respiratory tract by gram-negative bacteria and by some fungi. Convincing studies of several populations show the effects of illness. The severity of a systemic illness appears to have a direct bearing on colonization of the upper respiratory tract by gram-negative bacteria,[3] and in the elderly population, the greater the physical disability, the greater is the risk of gram-negative colonization.[5] It has also been shown that antibiotics change this normal flora,[4] and there is a body of data that suggests that intubated patients receiving antacids are also at higher risk for gram-negative colonization of the upper respiratory tract and pneumonia.[6]

The lower respiratory tract usually is considered to be sterile, but several studies have shown that a percentage of normal subjects do carry small numbers of upper respiratory tract bacteria in the lungs.[7, 8] It is thought that this is transient carriage and represents the aspiration of upper respiratory tract bacteria into the lungs, an event that is thought to occur frequently[9] and to be of little consequence in the majority of persons. However, this event may predispose the person to severe acute lung infections if large inocula, solid particles, or acid is aspirated with this normal flora.[10] Patients who have chronic colonization of the lower respiratory tract, whether by normal flora or potentially pathogenic microorganisms, are likely to be those who have some underlying structural or functional disease involving the defense mechanisms of the lower respiratory tract.

### Factors Influencing Sterility

To maintain sterility of the airways, air-breathing animals have developed powerful mechanisms to protect the lungs, the process of oxygen transport, and the bloodstream, which is separated from the air by a layer of cells only a few micrometers wide. Without such an efficient system, the evolution of the species might have been quite different. These defense mechanisms have been described in the previous chapters, and it is sufficient to reiterate that there are three main components—the mucociliary apparatus, which functions alone or in concert with some components of the immune system; a phagocytic system, which functions in a nonspecific, scavenging fashion or as part of an opsonophagocytic system; and a humoral immune system, which interacts with the other components to remove microorganisms. Patients with acquired or congenital abnormalities of any of these systems are predisposed to airway colonization.

Even in the face of an abnormality of host defense mechanisms, respiratory tract cells are remarkably resistant to colonization by bacteria. Deliberate colonization of animal tracheae (rather than acute pneumonitis) by direct inoculation of most of the bacteria known to chronically colonize the respiratory tract is difficult to achieve, unless these cells are injured in some way,[11–13] a theme that is developed later in this chapter. Thus, respiratory tract cells may possess a surface defense mechanism that prevents the attachment of bacteria which fails when there is some alteration of the cellular surface due to injury[11] or perhaps nutritional deprivation.[14] This aspect of individual cell defense has not been studied, but it is known that respiratory tract cell surfaces are covered by a layer of glycosaminoglycans that are generally acidic[15] and possess large amounts of sulfate, which imparts a strong negative charge to the surface. Charged substances such as glycosaminoglycans protect the bladder mucosa from bacterial colonization,[16, 17] and a similar mechanism could be the basis of the protection of a normal, healthy respiratory tract cell in vivo. Therefore in considering the failure of host defense mechanisms leading to airway colonization, a complex set of defenses from the cellular surface to systemic immunity must be dissected.

## CLINICAL STATES OF AIRWAY COLONIZATION

The clinical states of airway colonization can be defined as acute or chronic. Acute airway colonization can be defined as airway colonization occurring after an injury to the lower respiratory tract that is entirely reversible with removal of the exogenous factor. Chronic airway colonization can be defined as the establishment and maintenance of an endogenous bronchial flora secondary to a congenital or acquired defect of the host defense mechanisms that is permanent.

An examination of the microbial flora involved in acute and chronic colonization of the respiratory tract highlights some interesting tropisms (Table 4–1). Acute colonization of the respiratory tract most commonly involves *P. aeruginosa*, *Staphylococcus aureus*, and enteric gram-negative bacilli. Chronic colonization of the respiratory tract is most commonly due to *P. aeruginosa*, *S. aureus*, *Haemophilus influenzae*, and *Streptococcus pneumoniae*. The fact that these four species, among the hundreds of bacteria, are responsible for most cases of colonization indicates that these organisms are remarkably adapted to the respiratory tract. Further study of respiratory tract colonization may elucidate clear-cut adhesin-receptor systems and other virulence factors for these organisms that play roles in the colonization process.

### Acute Airway Colonization

The prototypic condition showing acute airway colonization is endotracheal intubation. As many as 75% of all patients who undergo endotracheal intubation eventually become colonized in the lower respiratory tract by one or another bacterium; the predominant species are gram negative, and the chief offender is *P. aeruginosa*.[18] Why this occurs could easily be explained by stating that the mechanisms responsible for clearance of the lower respiratory tract have been abrogated. However, there must be a much more complex scheme of events than this intuitive answer suggests. First, the bacteria must get to the upper respiratory tract in most cases before getting to the lower respiratory tract. This simple event involves the passage of microorganisms from the hands of caregivers or others to the oropharynx of the intubated patient. Second, biochemical alterations must occur on the cellular surfaces of the mouth of the sick patient to allow colonization. Third, the microorganisms must pass below the cuff of the endotracheal tube. Fourth, phagocytic mechanisms below the cuff of the endotracheal tube must fail. Fifth, the colonizing organism must find some receptor substrate in the lower respiratory tract. Sixth, there must be continued evasion of the host defenses as specific and nonspecific defense mechanisms come into play. Although this phenomenon of lower respiratory tract colonization in the intubated patient has been known for years and its medical significance is enormous, only a few steps in this complex process have been extensively studied.

Besides endotracheal intubation, it is difficult to demonstrate that other forms of injury lead to acute airway colo-

Table 4–1. **Major Colonizing Bacteria of the Respiratory Tract**

| Acute Colonization | Chronic Colonization |
|---|---|
| *Pseudomonas aeruginosa* | *Pseudomonas aeruginosa* |
| *Staphylococcus aureus* | *Staphylococcus aureus* |
| Enteric gram-negative bacilli | *Haemophilus influenzae* |
| | *Streptococcus pneumoniae* |
| | *Moraxella catarrhalis* |
| | *Pseudomonas cepacia* |

nization, because airway secretions are not frequently sampled in other illnesses. However, it is thought that acute lung injury, such as that caused by thermal burns or gastric acid aspiration, may injure the tracheobronchial tree and allow certain microorganisms to attach to and colonize these injured areas or at least to injure the mucociliary apparatus to such an extent that mucociliary clearance becomes abnormal. In such cases, the clinical importance of airway colonization is probably masked by concomitant lung injury and pneumonitis. The paucity of data concerning acute colonization in these areas does not allow much discussion.

## Chronic Airway Colonization

Chronic airway colonization is of enormous significance in chronic obstructive lung diseases. Exacerbations of many forms of chronic obstructive lung disease are often characterized by an inflammatory response to the resident bronchial flora of chronic colonization. In most cases, the stimulus for this response is not known, but viruses and mycoplasmas may be triggers.[19, 20] Alternatively, the microbial population may have increased to such an extent that it is the host response, consisting of mucus hypersecretion and inflammation, that produces clinical illness. Regardless of which is the stimulus, it is the host response to chronic colonization that is the main reason for illness.

### Chronic Bronchitis

The clinical condition known as chronic bronchitis is the classic example of a chronic state of colonization of the airways. Studies have shown that patients with the diagnosis of chronic bronchitis carry a lower respiratory tract flora that consists of organisms such as *S. pneumoniae, H. influenzae, Moraxella catarrhalis*, and even oral bacteria.[19, 21, 22] There is considerable debate about the role of these colonizers in exacerbation of chronic bronchitis,[19] but antibiotics are beneficial in some patients.[23] These patients usually do not have profound defects in mucociliary clearance, although a stable microbial flora, consisting primarily of a group of microorganisms known to be the common causes of acute bacterial pneumonia, is well established and is maintained in the face of a normal phagocytic host defense and a seemingly normal humoral immune system. However, the intriguing question about the bacteria found in chronic bronchitis concerns the nature of the host biochemical changes that select out these particular organisms as chronic colonizers, compared with those seen in other chronic lung diseases (eg, *P. aeruginosa*). The answer to this question could open avenues to novel forms of therapy.

### Ciliary Dyskinesia Syndrome

The ciliary dyskinesia syndrome has several characteristics. Chronic infection of the airways is a result of a variety of congenital abnormalities of the ciliary apparatus of the respiratory tract that result in motility disorders.[24] Typically, in early childhood, the microbial flora of a patient suffering from this syndrome, if it is severe enough, consists of the organisms that normally cause pneumonitis in children (ie,

*S. pneumoniae, H. influenzae, S. aureus*). These characteristic microorganisms persist in the lung despite of what appears to be normal phagocytic and humoral defense mechanisms, suggesting that these mechanisms have acquired a deficiency. As these patients survive into adulthood, there may be a gradual change of this flora, with the emergence of *P. aeruginosa* as a colonizing organism,[24] and even the peculiar mucoid form of *P. aeruginosa* has been seen in some of these patients (unpublished observations). Cardiorespiratory failure due to chronic lung infection is the most common cause of death.

### Cystic Fibrosis

Chronic airway colonization by *P. aeruginosa*, leading to continued lung injury, is the cause of death in most patients with cystic fibrosis.[25] As in the ciliary dyskinesia syndromes, a child with cystic fibrosis is colonized early in life by three common pathogens: *S. aureus, H. influenzae*, and *S. pneumoniae*. However, in cystic fibrosis *P. aeruginosa* begins to replace these microorganisms, and by early adulthood, it becomes the predominant organism in most of these patients and the one that ultimately leads to death. One peculiarity of the bacteriology of cystic fibrosis is that mucoid strains of *P. aeruginosa* are the rule later in the disease, rather than the exception, and colonization by mucoid strains heralds a decline in lung function.[26] The systemic phagocytic and humoral defense mechanisms of these patients are grossly normal. The abnormalities in the humoral immune system that have been described are secondary phenomena[27] that could worsen the state of colonization, but they do not explain the prominent role of *P. aeruginosa*. It is thought that, early in life, small bronchi become plugged with dehydrated mucus, leading to abnormal mucociliary clearance in the smaller airways.[25] However, because phagocytic host defenses also are unable to clear these areas, it can be concluded that mucus plugging in some way affects the local phagocytic and humoral defense mechanisms, resulting in chronic colonization. What differentiates cystic fibrosis from other diseases is the marked predilection for *S. aureus* and *P. aeruginosa* and the early age at which *P. aeruginosa* colonization occurs. These specificities raise questions about a possible relation between these organisms and the basic defect.

### Immunoglobulin Deficiency

Immunoglobulin G (IgG) deficiency has been associated with acute and recurrent sinopulmonary infections.[28] The most likely reason for this is the absence of effective opsonic activity against pulmonary pathogens. These deficiencies, which include congenital agammaglobulinemia and selective deficiencies of IgG subclasses, probably of themselves do not result in chronic colonization but rather in recurrent infection. However, repeated pulmonary infections eventually lead to airway injury and bronchiectasis in many of these patients. Patients are then left with two abnormalities of their host defense mechanism: lack of opsonic activity and an acquired abnormality of mucociliary clearance resulting from bronchiectasis. In the face of bronchiectasis and repeated antibiotic therapy, these patients suffer from colonization by the common respiratory pathogens, and eventually these pathogens may be replaced by *P. aeruginosa.*

### Bronchiectasis

Bronchiectasis is not described in detail here, but it is important to discuss it in the context of chronic colonization, because most patients who suffer from bronchiectasis eventually have chronic bacterial colonization of the airways. The causes of bronchiectasis are myriad, including childhood bronchopulmonary infections, bronchial obstruction, congenital anatomic defects of the trachea, and the genetic defects listed earlier.

The histologic and structural changes that occur in bronchiectasis result in markedly abnormal mucociliary clearance and the pooling of mucus secretions within segments or the entire tracheobronchial tree. The patterns of colonization in bronchiectasis, except when seen as a complication of cystic fibrosis, seem to be the same. Early in the patient's life, respiratory pathogens such as *H. influenzae* and *S. pneumoniae* are important, but they are subsequently replaced by *P. aeruginosa.* This change probably occurs as a result of antibiotic therapy, at least in the idiopathic forms of bronchiectasis. However, another group of microorganisms, the anaerobic bacteria, must also be considered in bronchiectasis. Most studies of the bacteriology of bronchiectasis were done before anaerobic bacteriology was available, but even at that time, the clinical association of putrid sputum with bronchiectasis was well known.[29] A complication of bronchiectasis was brain abscesses due to mixed aerobes and anaerobes. Autopsy specimens from bronchiectasis patients before the antimicrobial era showed anaerobic-like organisms in sections of the airways.[30] However, this group of organisms no longer features prominently in this complication, an observation that supports the idea that antibiotic therapy is an important factor in determining the final colonizing flora in bronchiectasis.

## SITES OF AIRWAY COLONIZATION

It is customary to consider that colonization of a site in or on the animal host occurs on a cellular surface, thus most studies on colonization of the respiratory tract used cells or tissues. Earlier studies focusing on the colonization of the upper respiratory tract showed that a variety of respiratory pathogens were capable of attaching to human buccal epithelial cells.[31–33] Similar studies were done with human tracheal cells and *P. aeruginosa*, and under certain conditions, there also was adhesion to these cells.[34, 35] However, the assumption cannot be made that cells are the sites of colonization in all infectious states. In chronic colonization of the respiratory tract by *P. aeruginosa* in cystic fibrosis, despite bacterial counts approaching $10^9$ organisms per 1 mL of sputum, bacteria were not present on the airway cells of patients whose lungs were examined at postmortem or after removal for lung transplantation.[36–38] When bacteria were seen in the respiratory tract, they were associated only with respiratory tract secretions. Unfortunately, only patients with cystic fibrosis and *P. aeruginosa* were studied. There are no comparable clinical data for chronic bronchitis. The observation that mucus could be an adhesive site

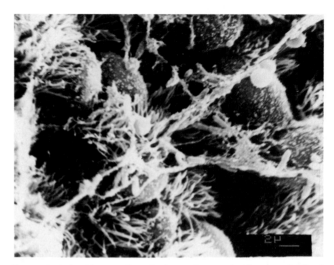

**Figure 4–1.** In this scanning electron micrograph of mouse tracheal epithelium inoculated with *Pseudomonas aeruginosa*, the bacteria are associated with mucus strands on the tracheal surfaces. (From Ramphal R, Pyle M: Adherence of mucoid and nonmucoid *Pseudomonas aeruginosa* to acid-injured epithelium. Infect Immun 41:345–351, 1983.)

for *P. aeruginosa* was also made for mice[11] (Fig. 4–1), hamsters,[39] and dogs in vivo[13] and with purified human mucins[40–43] in vitro. Therefore, both cells and mucins must be considered as adhesive sites for bacteria, although the receptor materials found on cellular surfaces may be different from those found in mucins, and the respective adhesins may differ. A reasonable hypothesis to explain the disparate binding studies is that cells may be the sites of adhesion in states of acute colonization after insult to the tracheobronchial tree and mucus the site of colonization in chronic obstructive lung diseases.

There is one important question concerning cells that needs to be answered. Is the normal, healthy tracheal cell surface susceptible to colonization in the living human or animal? Earlier studies of buccal cells indicated that they have a fibronectin coat that protects them from adhesion by gram-negative organisms.[44] Although it appears that cells have some sort of protection, the identity of this protection is now in question.[45] Studies with human tracheal cells removed at bronchoscopy showed that *P. aeruginosa* is capable of attaching to these cells,[34, 35] but it should be remembered that these cells have suffered trauma during removal from the tracheal epithelium. Studies of adhesion to healthy tissues with cultures of hamster tracheal epithelium indicated that there was minimal *Pseudomonas* adhesion to cells except over a long period of incubation.[39] Studies with mouse,[11] rat,[46] ferret,[47] and dog[13] tracheae do not show adhesion of *P. aeruginosa* except after injury to the tracheobronchial tree (Figs. 4–2 and 4–3). Most evidence indicates that the normal healthy tracheal cell in vivo may be quite resistant to bacterial adhesion because the receptors may be masked or there is some sort of surface protection. Similar but fewer observations have been made with *H. influenzae* and to some extent with *Klebsiella pneumoniae.* *H. influenzae* adheres to tracheal cells only after there has been tracheal cell injury,[48, 49] and *K. pneumoniae* attaches only to cryptic receptors on the basolateral tracheal cell surface and the submucosal surface of the trachea.[50]

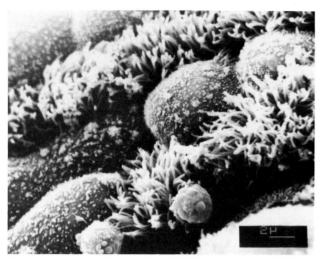

**Figure 4–2.** The scanning electron micrograph of intact tracheal epithelium without mucus shows a rare bacterium attached. (From Ramphal R, Pyle M: Adherence of mucoid and nonmucoid *Pseudomonas aeruginosa* to acid-injured epithelium. Infect Immun 41:345–351, 1983.)

Studies with cell lines, although capable of providing data on adhesins and receptors, may not answer the basic question, because these cellular surfaces do not necessarily represent what a microbe sees in vivo and probably do not have the normal repertoire of glycoconjugates that would be absorbed to the cellular surface after secretion from submucosal glands.

Two scenarios are hypothesized. First, if there is an acute tracheal injury, whether by viruses, chemical, or physical means or even metabolic disturbances, alterations in the tracheal surface allow adhesion of certain bacteria to the cellular surface,[11–14, 47] regenerating cells,[51] or submucosal surfaces.[46, 50] Secondly, in situations in which there is an abnormality of mucociliary clearance, there is stasis of mucus in the tracheobronchial tree, and colonizing microorganisms are able to remain there because of their ability to bind to mucus and mucins. After this initial encounter, their multiplication rate is faster than their rate of removal by residual mucociliary clearance and phagocytosis, or they resist removal by the phagocytic system. Whether bacteria can then move from high-affinity binding sites in mucus to low-affinity cellular receptors and colonize cells is unknown, but it is possible that if bacteria situated in mucus can injure cells, high-affinity receptors may be unmasked. Most studies have been done with *P. aeruginosa*; however, emerging data with *H. influenzae* suggest that similar mechanisms may also be operative.[48] It will be interesting to see whether studies with *S. pneumoniae* and *S. aureus* also show that there is a relative resistance of cells to adhesion by these organisms. A single study does suggest that *S. pneumoniae* may behave in this way, because it adheres to regenerating tracheal cells and not to healthy mature cells.[52]

## MICROBIOLOGIC PROPERTIES INFLUENCING COLONIZATION

Many of the microorganisms known to colonize the respiratory tract produce factors that have the potential to alter host defense mechanisms in the lower respiratory tract (Table 4–2). Theoretically, these factors may aid in the colonization process, but whether any of these factors play an actual role in vivo is still unproved. Most of these factors affect cell viability, ciliary function, or cell surfaces, and they could play a role by affecting mucociliary clearance. In experimental situations in which tracheal tissue is studied in culture, some of these factors may facilitate adhesion to cells[48, 53] and may produce other physiologic effects, such as excess mucus secretion,[54] which could modulate the colonization process.

### Pseudomonas aeruginosa

Compared with other gram-negative bacteria, *P. aeruginosa* is probably the most prolific organism in the production of exoproducts capable of affecting the tracheobronchial tree. Many of these exoproducts have pronounced effects on cellular function or cell surfaces that result in the loss of cell viability, impaired ciliary motility, or an alteration of cellular surfaces. Among those well characterized is *Pseudomonas* elastase, which has been shown to alter tracheal cellular surfaces.[55] Whether this protease occurs in sufficient quantity in vivo to affect airway function is debatable.[56] Other pseudomonal enzymes, such as exoenzyme A and exoenzyme S, which are ADP-ribosylating enzymes and which kill cells,[55, 57] could also be implicated in the adhesion process because cell viability is a pivotal aspect of the adhesion of *P. aeruginosa* to tracheal tissue; they may also alter mucociliary clearance. *Pseudomonas* produces a phospholipase C, which has profound effects on cellular surfaces and on surfactant, and it is possible that this substance may play a role in acute colonization and acute disease in the lower respiratory tract.[53, 58] The pigments produced by *P. aeruginosa* have been shown to inhibit ciliary beat frequency and mucociliary clearance.[59] Therefore, the colonization of mucus by *Pseudomonas* with the production of exoenzymes and pigments could worsen

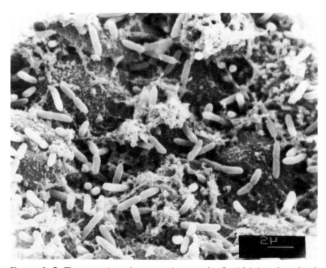

**Figure 4–3.** The scanning electron micrograph of acid-injured tracheal epithelium inoculated with *Pseudomonas aeruginosa* shows numerous organisms adhering to the injured epithelium. (From Ramphal R, Pyle M: Adherence of mucoid and nonmucoid *Pseudomonas aeruginosa* to acid-injured epithelium. Infect Immun 41:345–351, 1983.)

Table 4–2. **Microbial Products That Influence Colonization**

| Bacteria | Product | Action | Possible Consequence |
|---|---|---|---|
| *Pseudomonas aeruginosa* | Exoenzyme A | Cell injury | Mucociliary clearance and adhesion |
| | Exoenzyme S | Cell injury | |
| | Elastase | Cell injury | |
| | Elastase | Cleavage of IgG and C1 | Defective phagocytosis adhesion |
| | Phospholipase C | Cell injury | Mucociliary clearance and adhesion |
| | | Surfactant breakdown | ? |
| | Pigments | Ciliostasis | Mucociliary clearance |
| | IgA protease | Cleavage of IgA | ? |
| *Haemophilus influenzae* | Ciliostatic factor | Ciliostasis | Mucociliary clearance |
| | Toxin (?) | Cell injury | Adhesion |
| | IgA protease | Cleavage of IgA | ? |
| *Streptococcus pneumoniae* | Pneumolysin | Ciliostasis | Mucociliary clearance |
| | | Cell injury | Defective phagocytic killing |
| | Neuraminidase | Cleaves sialic acid off glycolipids, glycoproteins | Adhesion (?) |

mucociliary function, enhancing the cycle of chronic colonization. It has also been suggested that *P. aeruginosa* products may have effects on the immune system; for example, *P. aeruginosa* elastase is capable of degrading immunoglobulins and complement.[60] If this occurs in vivo, it would produce opsonophagocytic defects that would allow colonization. *P. aeruginosa* has been reported to produce an immunoglobulin A (IgA) protease[61] that cleaves IgA, but it is not known how this functions in vivo. If all these factors do play a role in the process of colonization by *P. aeruginosa*, it should not be surprising that in the final race for microbial dominance within the milieu of the respiratory tract, *P. aeruginosa* would be among the most successful of organisms.

### Haemophilus influenzae

*H. influenzae* produces a ciliostatic factor.[62] Its nature is unknown, but in respiratory tissue culture systems, this substance leads to a loss of ciliary activity and possibly a loss of respiratory tract cell viability, resulting in the adhesion of *H. influenzae* to injured respiratory tract cells.[48] Whether this factor plays a role in vivo in the chronic colonization of the respiratory tract by *H. influenzae* is unknown. In diseases such as chronic bronchitis, in which the defect in mucociliary clearance is not quite so profound as that seen in other diseases, such a substance could play a role in colonization by further slowing mucociliary clearance. *H. influenzae* has also been reported to produce an IgA protease.[63] Chronic colonization could occur if antiadhesive IgA is destroyed by this protease; however, there is no evidence to support this hypothesis. It is still not proved that secretory IgA plays a role in protecting the lungs against bacterial infection.

### Streptococcus pneumoniae

*S. pneumoniae* is seen as a chronic colonizer in the early stages of most of the diseases discussed earlier. Like the other chronic colonizers, this microorganism produces some virulence factors, which theoretically could allow it to persist in the respiratory tract for prolonged periods.

Pneumococcal neuraminidase could degrade mucus and assist in the persistence of this organism in the airways.[64, 65] This is a plausible scenario if this organism were adherent to mucins by means of a sialic acid molecule, but data are lacking. If, on the other hand, this organism were capable of binding to nonsialylated receptor molecules,[66] the neuraminidase could expose these receptors allowing adhesion to mucins or cells. It remains to be shown that *S. pneumoniae* is capable of binding to intact mature respiratory epithelial cells. The pneumococcus also secretes an enzyme, pneumolysin,[67] which is thiol activated. This enzyme has attracted much attention, and the evidence indicates that in high doses it is toxic for ciliated epithelium[68] and it is ciliostatic in lower doses. This enzyme also inhibits the bactericidal activity of phagocytic cells.[67] Such an enzyme could affect mucociliary clearance and phagocytosis, allowing pneumococci to stay for prolonged periods within the respiratory tract. It will require the appropriate animal models and isogenic bacterial mutants to test these theories.

## HOST FACTORS AND COLONIZATION

Some host factors that play a role in chronic colonization of the airways are primarily structural and related to a genetic disorder or an acquired defect of mucociliary clearance. During the interaction between microbe and host, certain host responses may also play a role in prolonging colonization. For example, leukocyte protease is found in excess in the mucus of patients with cystic fibrosis and other diseases during exacerbations[69] and could affect mucociliary clearance by virtue of its ability to injure the epithelium. Leukocyte protease can alter a mucosal surface so that bacterial receptors are exposed.[70] Whether this latter action plays a role in colonization is unknown. Another prominent host response to colonizing microbes is the release of mucus from submucosal glands and surface cells. Almost all important respiratory pathogens or their exoproducts trigger this response.[54] If mucociliary clearance is already abnormal, excess mucus secretion could result in obstruction of the airways, worsening the predisposition to colonization.

Table 4–3. **Bacterial Receptors in the Respiratory Tract**

| Bacteria | Cells | Mucus or Mucins |
|---|---|---|
| *Pseudomonas aeruginosa* | GalNAc($\beta$1→4)Gal | Gal($\beta$1–3/4)GlcNAc |
| | Gal($\beta$1→4)Glc | Sialylated oligosaccharides |
| | Sialylated glycolipids | Mucin peptide |
| *Haemophilus influenzae* | GalNAc($\beta$1→4)Gal | Mucus component unknown |
| | Neu$\alpha$(2→3)Gal($\beta$1→4)Glu | |
| | Anton blood group substance | |
| *Streptococcus pneumoniae* | GalNAc($\beta$1→4)Gal | |
| | GlcNAc($\beta$1→4)Gal | GlcNAc($\beta$1–4)Gal on mucins |
| *Staphylococcus aureus* | GalNAc($\beta$1→4)Gal | Mucus and mucins |
| *Pseudomonas cepacia* | GalNAc($\beta$1→4)Gal | Mucins |

## MECHANISMS OF AIRWAY COLONIZATION

### Adhesin-Receptor Systems

Adhesin-receptor systems have been described for a variety of bacteria. These systems are thought to be the explanation for the tropism shown by certain bacteria for colonization or infection of certain sites. It was envisaged that this specificity between bacterial adhesin and the epithelial surface receptor would eventually provide a clear understanding of the first step in the pathogenic process. However, this thesis appears to be only partially true, because many nonrespiratory bacteria attach to substances that have been described as receptors for respiratory tract bacteria but do not frequently colonize the lung.[66, 71, 72] It is possible that adhesin-receptor systems will eventually explain tropism, but the current data are insufficient.

Most of the adhesin-receptor systems that have been described involve a lectin-like interaction between a microbial protein and a host carbohydrate.[1] Alternatively, it is possible that microbial polysaccharides could interact with host proteins.[1] In the lower respiratory tract, the first host receptors that colonizing microorganisms are likely to encounter are the carbohydrate chains of the mucin molecules. These molecules are large glycoproteins with molecular masses between $2 \times 10^5$ and $20 \times 10^6$ d and are composed of a polypeptide core to which are attached hundreds of carbohydrate chains by O-glycosidic linkages.[73] The molecules are in the form of flexible threads when examined under the electron microscope. The typical molecule has many long, hydrophilic regions, containing one carbohydrate chain for about every three amino acids, and intervening hydrophobic regions relatively devoid of carbohydrate chains, often called the nude regions. There are also intramolecular disulfide bonds. Much work has been done to elucidate the structure of these carbohydrate chains, and about 100 different chains have been sequenced.[73] It is estimated that there may be hundreds of different chains in any mucin sample, based on the various linkage possibilities between the sugars found in mucins. The carbohydrate chains are made of the following five sugars, in chains of lengths from two to more than 20 sugar residues: D-galactose, *N*-acetylgalactosamine, L-fucose, *N*-acetylglucosamine, and *N*-acetylneuraminic acid. In addition to these sugars, human respiratory mucins contain significant amounts of sulfate, which is thought to be increased in the mucins of cystic fibrosis patients.[74] Some mucins probably undergo age-related changes in structure, leading to the expression of carbohydrate chains with different receptor properties; this has been shown for gastrointestinal mucins.[75] If the same holds for respiratory mucins, this may be an important determinant of colonization in different disease states and at different ages.

The other possible targets for microbial adhesion are the cell surface glycoconjugates. The cell surface glycoconjugates that could be important in binding are probably the glycolipids, gangliosides, and other neutral glycolipids.[76] Receptor glycolipids for many bacteria that infect the respiratory tract have been found in the lungs.[58, 76] Mucin-like substances on the surface of cells have been described,[77] but their role in adhesion to cells has not been studied. The other major class of cell surface glycoconjugates, the glycosaminoglycans, have not been implicated in bacterial adhesion until recently, when it was shown that *S. aureus* was capable of binding to them,[78] but it is not known whether this occurs in the respiratory tract (Table 4–3).

### Pseudomonas aeruginosa *Adhesins and Receptors*

The fact that the adhesion of *P. aeruginosa* has attracted the most attention and study underscores its role as the major colonizer in acute and chronic colonization of the respiratory tract. Besides the accumulated clinical experience, there is ample evidence that it is better adapted for adhesion to the respiratory tract than are other gram-negative bacteria.[40, 79] Several adhesins and receptors have been described for this organism, but the information is by no means complete. *P. aeruginosa* uses pili,[80–82] the mucoid exopolysaccharide,[82, 83] and even exoenzyme S as adhesins.[84] It also has nonpilus mucin-binding surface proteins,[85] which are being characterized. Pili, which are made up of subunits of about 14 to 15 kd, mediate the adhesion of this organism to cells[86] and, to lesser degree, to mucins.[82] The binding site on the pilin subunit is located at the carboxy-terminal end of the subunit.[87] Unfortunately, pilins are structurally heterogeneous, and antibody against one pilin type would not necessarily prevent adhesion of heterologous strains. *Pseudomonas* mucoid exopolysaccharide, the characteristic substance found on mucoid strains from cystic fibrosis patients and some bronchiectasis patients, has also been shown to bind to cells and mucins,[82, 84, 88] but it is not known whether they are specific binding epitopes on this exopolysaccharide. A substance fitting some of the characteristics of *Pseudomonas* exoenzyme S also mediates binding of *P. aeruginosa* to buccal cells and glycolipids,[84] and it has been suggested that its binding site and its receptors are similar to those of pilin.[89] The true role of this substance requires clarification, because it is in part a secreted substance and could block adhesion by occupying receptor sites rather than mediate adhesion. The presence of nonpilus adhesins on the surface of *P. aeruginosa* has been demonstrated. This substance or group of substances does bind to tracheal cells, pneumocytes, or respiratory mucins, even in the absence of other adhesins.[53, 85, 90]

Several receptors for *P. aeruginosa* have been described on glycolipids and on mucins. It is assumed that the glycolipid receptors that have been described are actually the receptors recognized in vivo on cells. These receptors are very short chains and are probably buried deep in the cell membrane. They include asialo $GM_1$ and asialo $GM_2$, both of which contain GalNAc($\beta1\rightarrow4$)Gal linked to ceramide[66] and lactosylceramide[91] (Gal($\beta1\rightarrow4$)Glc-ceramide) substances commonly found on cell membranes. In addition to these cellular receptors, sialylated cellular receptors have also been postulated.[91, 92] These have not been characterized, and they seem to contradict studies showing that sialylation hinders adhesion of *P. aeruginosa* to the GalNAc($\beta1\rightarrow4$)Gal disaccharide.[66] At least two classes of *P. aeruginosa* mucin receptors have been described. The type I and type II disaccharide units (ie, Gal$\beta1\rightarrow3$/4GlcNAc), which are found in mucins,[73] have been shown to be receptors for this organism,[93] and 2-3-sialylated forms of these chains, Neu$\alpha2\rightarrow3$Gal($\beta1\rightarrow3$/4)GlcNAc, also show receptor activity.[93] Desialylation of mucins reduces binding, implicating sialic acid as part of the receptors in mucins.[94] Although much data have been gathered on this system, the *P. aeruginosa* adhesion-receptor system is still not fully characterized (see Table 4–3).

### Haemophilus influenzae

The *H. influenzae* organisms that are found in the lower respiratory tract are generally unencapsulated. These unencapsulated organisms adhere more avidly to buccal and tracheal cells than do their capsulated counterparts.[95] These organisms attach to tracheal cells and to respiratory mucus.[48] Although piliated *H. influenzae* organisms do attach to buccal cells,[96] nonpilus adhesins may be the more important structures mediating adherence in the lower respiratory tract.[48] These nonpilus adhesins have recently been characterized.[97] They appear to be high molecular weight surface antigens which are structurally related to *Bordetella pertussis* filamentous hemagglutinin, an adhesin. At least three receptors for *H. influenzae* have been described on cells. The first one to be described is known as the Anton blood group substance, but its structure has not been elucidated.[98] A second receptor, identical in structure to the *Pseudomonas* cellular receptor GalNAc($\beta1\rightarrow4$)Gal, has also been suggested.[66] The third receptor, sialyl lactosylceramide,[99] adds greater complexity and contradiction to this system, because sialylation of the second receptor results in inhibition of adhesion. *H. influenzae* pili recognize the sialyl lactosylceramide receptor,[99] but it is not known which receptor is recognized by the nonpilus adhesin(s). The *H. influenzae* receptor, which is present in respiratory mucins or at least on some component of respiratory mucus, has not been characterized, but it may be similar to the last receptor described, because it has some similarities to the structures found in respiratory mucins (see Table 4–3).

These data together mean that *H. influenzae* could have three or more receptors and corresponding adhesins.

### Streptococcus pneumoniae

*S. pneumoniae* attaches to cells and mucus, but there are few data on these associations. This organism binds to oropharyngeal cells[100] and to the immature respiratory mucosa after an influenza virus infection.[52] It can attach to strands of mucus in the mouse respiratory tree (Fig. 4–4) and to the mucus of the frog's palate.[101] The nature of the *S. pneumoniae* adhesin is unknown, but at least two receptors have been described. One of these receptors is the GalNAc($\beta1\rightarrow4$)Gal disaccharide[66] found on asialo $GM_1$; this is a cellular receptor. The other receptor described for *S. pneumoniae* is the disaccharide GlcNAc($\beta1\rightarrow3$)Gal,[100] which occurs in respiratory mucins[73] and on cells.[100]

### Staphylococcus aureus

Much work has been done on the adhesion of *S. aureus* to nonrespiratory tract tissue. This organism binds to squamous cells, fibronectin, collagen, and vascular endothelial cells. Only recently has there been work on staphylococcal binding to respiratory tract targets. These studies have shown that *S. aureus* binds to human respiratory tract mucins[102] and to animal mucus,[103] and it is possible that there may be some adhesion to respiratory mucosal cells.[103] A staphylococcal lipotechoic acid adhesin for cells has been described,[104] but it has been speculated that a different adhesin, which may be proteinaceous, is responsible for staphylococcal binding to mucins.[103] Some data on a staphylococcal cellular receptor have been presented in preliminary form. These data suggest that *S. aureus* also binds to the same GalNAc($\beta1\rightarrow4$)Gal asialo $GM_1$ receptor described for many other bacteria.[66] Staphylococcal binding to the glycosaminoglycan heparan sulfate has been described.[78] It is not known whether this substance serves as a respiratory tract receptor, but it occurs on the surface of lower respiratory tract cells.[15]

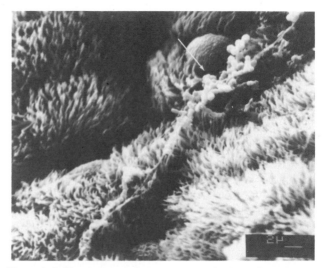

**Figure 4–4.** The scanning electron micrograph shows *Streptococcus pneumoniae* adhering to a mucus strand on the tracheal surface. (Unpublished observations, Ramphal R., 1981.)

## Binding to a Common Cellular Receptor

A variety of pulmonary pathogens bind to the same GalNAc($\beta$1→4)Gal cellular receptor (see Table 4–3). In addition to the four bacteria listed previously, other pulmonary pathogens, such as *Pseudomonas cepacia*, *Chlamydia pneumoniae*, *K. pneumoniae*, *Haemophilus parainfluenzae*, and *Xanthomonas maltophilia*, adhere to this same receptor.[66, 71] In addition to these bacteria, some nonpulmonary pathogens have been reported to adhere to this disaccharide.[71, 72] These include *Neisseria gonorrhoeae*, some strains of *Escherichia coli* that cause urinary tract infection, and a variety of other microorganisms. If this receptor provides a common binding site for all these bacteria, there may be a common or similar adhesin epitope mediating the adhesion of all these bacteria. This would be a fascinating evolutionary adaptation and would provide an unusual opportunity for vaccine development, but it does not provide us with an explanation for the specificity of certain bacteria for the respiratory tract in states of acute or chronic colonization. Similar data have been presented for the lactosylceramide receptor.[76] This receptor also mediates the adhesion of many other bacteria, most of which are not adapted to the respiratory tract. The significance of these receptors is not understood, and a synthesis of these disparate findings awaits future work.

## Mucin Receptors

Respiratory mucins contain receptors for viruses and mycoplasma.[73] However, the number of receptors described appears to be surprisingly limited. Although mucins should possess many specific receptors to trap the wide variety of bacteria the host may encounter, among the large unbiquitous class of enteric bacilli, none has been consistently shown to bind to respiratory mucins.[40, 41] Nevertheless, it is clear from animal studies that these bacteria and particulate material are trapped by mucus and removed by mucociliary clearance; evidently, this is done by nonspecific mechanisms. The presence of specific receptors in mucins for organisms that coincidentally are the major chronic colonizers of lung suggests that adaptation of these organisms, allowing them to recognize specific structures in mucins played a role in their evolution as respiratory pathogens. These aspiring pathogens should have possessed or evolved additional mechanisms that would aid them in achieving this successful state of parasitism (see Table 4–2). Most of these organisms recognize structures that are derived from the type 1 and 2 oligosaccharide units commonly found in mucins (Table 4–4). This probably evolved because of the abundance of these structures in mucins or because of some stereospecific exposure of these groups that allowed recognition. These units are the scaffolding for the blood group substances, another well-characterized recognition system.[73]

## Mucins and Bacterial Virulence

Why should certain bacteria bind to mucins, when binding puts them at a disadvantage in the face of normal mucociliary clearance? Why would they synthesize adhe-

**Table 4–4. Structurally Similar Receptors in Mucins and Glycolipids for Specific Organisms**

| Receptors | Organisms |
|---|---|
| Gal($\beta$1→3/4)GlcNAc($\beta$1→4)Gal | *Pseudomonas aeruginosa* |
| Neu($\alpha$2→3)Gal($\beta$1→4)GlcNAc($\beta$1→4)Gal | *Pseudomonas aeruginosa* |
| Neu($\alpha$2→3)Gal($\beta$1→4)GlcNAc-Gal | *Mycoplasma pneumoniae* |
| Gal($\beta$1→3/4)GlcNAc($\beta$1→4)Gal | *Streptococcus pneumoniae* |
| Neu($\alpha$2→3/6)Gal($\beta$1→4)GlcNAc ($\beta$1→4) Gal | Influenza virus |
| Neu($\alpha$2→3)Gal($\beta$1→4)Glc | *Haemophilus influenzae* |

sins for a substance that is not fixed and does not provide a firm basis of adherence? They could easily survive in the liquid milieu of stagnant mucus in the absence of mucociliary clearance, except perhaps for the possibility that they would be eradicated by phagocytes. These organisms would not expend energy to bind to mucus unless it were advantageous. This suggests that binding provides bacteria with some survival advantage, perhaps to evade host defenses, making them more virulent. Experimentally, this has been shown to be the case. Crude mucus protects a variety of microorganisms from host defenses or enhances their virulence, as demonstrated by the lowering of the lethal dose of bacteria required to kill 50% of a population of mice when mucus is injected together with the bacteria.[105] This observation was made with *S. pneumoniae*, and it was the method of choice in producing pneumonia in experimental animals. *S. pneumoniae* mixed with crude mucins reproducibly produced pneumonia, but the organism given alone required massive inocula to do the same.[106] However, these observations were clouded by the fact that crude mucus (ie, mixture of mucin, cells, DNA, lipid, and protein) enhanced the virulence of a variety of bacteria.[105] A clinical role for this phenomenon was not accepted.[107] However, it has been shown that pure respiratory mucins protect mucin-adhesive *P. aeruginosa*, but not other nonadhesive bacteria from phagocytic clearance.[108] This phenomenon may in part explain why certain bacteria, notably *P. aeruginosa*, have chosen mucins as an adhesive site. It could be argued that organisms capable of binding to mucins were the ones that became pulmonary pathogens, because they would be protected from phagocytosis. More work needs to be done with other mucin-adhesive bacteria for this to be considered a phenomenon of general importance.

## CONSEQUENCES OF AIRWAY COLONIZATION

Acute colonization of the airways by bacteria leads to disease. Prospective studies of colonized patients in intensive care units reinforce the point; 20% of patients who are colonized show clear-cut evidence of bacterial pneumonias rather than other causes of chest radiographic abnormalities.[109] In patients with pneumonia, most often gram-negative disease, the mortality rate may be quite high, depending on the microorganism. *P. aeruginosa* carries the greatest mortality rate. Most other patients pose a problem of considerable significance: the differentiation of tracheal colonization and tracheobronchitis from pneumonia when chest radiographic abnormalities are seen. Although the physician may use the familiar laboratory parameters, such as the presence of polymorphonuclear leukocytes in tracheal aspirates to assess the significance of a positive culture, he or she is still faced with the fact that patients who carry bacteria within the trachea, whether or not there is a host inflammatory response, are at risk for developing life-threatening nosocomial pneumonia. Newer diagnostic methods, such as the protected brush catheter, appear to offer some hope in making these distinctions,[110] but it is unlikely that this procedure will be used commonly outside of the academic situation. Because tracheobronchial colonization often leads to nosocomial pneumonia, the clinician is faced with the question of whether routine antibiotic therapy prevents the development of nosocomial pneumonias in the patient with acute airway colonization. In the past, attempted sterilization of the respiratory tract with aerosolized antibiotics led to the development of resistance,[111] and even parenteral administration resulted in an unacceptable rate of resistance. This question is still unanswered.

Chronic colonization of the airways has different consequences, perhaps based on the type of colonizing organism and the underlying lung disease. Chronic colonization by *H. influenzae* in chronic bronchitis does not have the same consequences as chronic colonization by *P. aeruginosa* in cystic fibrosis. Most patients with cystic fibrosis develop bronchiectasis, but this is not the case in those with chronic bronchitis. It is difficult to separate the contribution of the microorganism from that of the host, but a fair assumption may be that organisms that evoke a stronger host inflammatory response (eg, higher levels of proteases or immune complexes) may be associated with more destructive lung processes.

The ultimate consequence of chronic colonization is bronchiectasis, probably caused by the inflammatory response to colonizing bacteria:

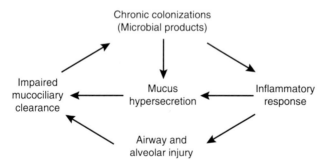

Chronic colonization may lead to acute pneumonias if the delicate balance between colonizing microbes and host defenses that prevent frank alveolar extension of this process is broken. Antecedent viral infections may be one cause.

## PREVENTION OF COLONIZATION

The prevention of airway colonization is a daunting but desirable goal because nosocomial pneumonia carries one of the highest mortality rates among nosocomial infections.[112] This has been attempted largely from the infection control point of view, using classic methods. The use of antibiotics is discussed in another chapter, but this is not the solution because of the plasticity of the bacterial ge-

nome in generating resistant mutants. Whether vaccines capable of preventing colonization are feasible is a difficult question, because most patients who become acutely or chronically colonized are capable of mounting an immune response to the colonizing pathogens yet remain colonized until reversible host factors are corrected. Nevertheless, this work needs to be done after the microbial determinants of colonization have been elucidated.

There are two possible mechanisms that require exploration: the generation of antiadhesive antibodies, presumably IgA, against the microbial adhesin in question and the generation of opsonophagocytic antibodies, presumably IgG, against a surface component of the bacterium. Many questions and hurdles must be dealt with before realizing these approaches. Does IgA function as an antiadhesin against bacteria in the lung? If so, what role do the IgA proteases play? Because most acute lower airway colonization occurs in the face of endotracheal intubation, will the defense systems function normally? Perhaps preventing oral colonization by vaccines is more feasible. The prospects for preventing chronic colonization seem even more difficult. There is always a coexistent abnormality of lung defense mechanisms. Even if IgA does prevent adhesion to cells, it would not prevent colonization of mucus, because this molecule may be mucinophilic.[113] This leaves the phagocytic defenses to prevent colonization, but there is the question of whether phagocytes function optimally against mucus-bound bacteria. Despite these obstacles, the medical consequences of acute and chronic colonization of the airways are important, and attempts should be made to elucidate the factors that influence colonization.

## REFERENCES

1. Beachey EH: Bacterial adherence: Adhesin-receptor interactions mediating attachment of bacteria to mucosal surfaces. J Infect Dis 143:325–345, 1981.
2. Sprunt K, Redman W: Evidence suggesting the importance of role of interbacterial inhibition in maintaining the balance of normal flora. Ann Intern Med 68:579–590, 1968.
3. Johanson WG Jr, Pierce AK, Sanford JP: Changing pharyngeal bacterial flora of hospitalized patients: Emergence of gram-negative bacilli. N Engl J Med 281:1137–1140, 1969.
4. Tillotson JR, Finland M: Bacterial colonization of the respiratory tract complicating antibiotic therapy of pneumonia. J Infect Dis 119:597–624, 1969.
5. Valenti WM, Trudell RG, Bentley DW: Factors predisposing to oropharyngeal colonization with gram-negative bacilli in the aged. N Engl J Med 298:1108–1111, 1978.
6. Driks MR, Craven DE, Bartolome R, et al: Nosocomial pneumonia in intubated patients given sucralfate as compared with antacids or histamine type 2 blockers. N Engl J Med 317:1376–1382, 1987.
7. Lees AW, McNaught W: Bacteriology of lower respiratory tract secretions, sputum, and upper respiratory tract secretions in "normals" and chronic bronchitics. Lancet 2:1112–1115, 1959.
8. Laurenzi GA, Potter RT, Kass EH: Bacteriologic flora of the lower respiratory tract. N Engl J Med 265:1273–1278, 1961.
9. Huxley EJ, Viroslav J, Gray WR: Pharyngeal aspiration in normal adults and patients with depressed consciousness. Am J Med 64:564–568, 1978.
10. Wynn JW, Modell JH: Respiratory aspiration of stomach contents. Ann Intern Med 87:466–474, 1977.
11. Ramphal R, Pyle M: Adherence of mucoid and nonmucoid *Pseudomonas aeruginosa* to acid-injured tracheal epithelium. Infect Immun 41:345–351, 1983.
12. Boyd RL, Ramphal R, Rice R, Mangos JA: Chronic colonization of

rat airways with *Pseudomonas aeruginosa*. Infect Immun 39:1403–1410, 1983.

13. Zoutman DE, Hulbert WC, Pasloske BL, et al: The role of polar pili in the adherence of *Pseudomonas aeruginosa* to injured canine tracheal cells. A semiquantitative morphologic study. Scanning Microsc 5:109–124, 1991.

14. Niederman MS, Merrill WW, Ferranti RD, et al: Nutritional status and bacterial binding in the lower respiratory tract in patients with chronic tracheostomy. Ann Intern Med 100:795–800, 1984.

15. Spicer SS, Chakrin LW, Wardell JR Jr: Effect of chronic sulfur dioxide inhalation on the carbohydrate histochemistry and histology of the canine respiratory tract. Am Rev Respir Dis 110:13–24, 1974.

16. Parsons CL, Mulholland SG: Bladder surface mucin: Its antibacterial effect against various species. Am J Pathol 93:423–432, 1978.

17. Parsons CL, Stauffer C, Schmidt JD: Bladder surface glycosaminoglycans: An efficient mechanism of environmental adaptation. Science 208:605–607, 1980.

18. Niederman MS: Gram-negative colonization of the respiratory tract: Pathogenesis and clinical consequences. Semin Respir Infect 5:173–184, 1990.

19. Sachs FL: Chronic bronchitis. *In* Pennington JE (ed): Respiratory Infection: Diagnosis and Management, ed 2. New York, Raven Press, 1988:142–158.

20. Marks MI: Respiratory viruses in cystic fibrosis. N Engl J Med 311:1695–1696, 1984.

21. Fagon JY, Chastre J, Trouillet JL, et al: Characterization of distal bronchial microflora during acute exacerbation of chronic bronchitis. Am Rev Respir Dis 142:1004–1008, 1990.

22. Wallace RJ, Musher DM: In honor of Dr. Sarah Branham. A star is born: The realization of *Branhamella catarrhalis* as a respiratory pathogen. Chest 90:447–450, 1986.

23. Anthonisen NR, Manfreda J, Warren CP, et al: Antibiotic therapy in exacerbations of chronic obstructive pulmonary disease. Ann Intern Med 106:196–204, 1987.

24. Pedersen M, Stafanger G: Bronchopulmonary symptoms in primary ciliary dyskinesia. Eur J Respir Dis 64(Suppl 127):118–128, 1983.

25. Woods RE, Boat TF, Doershuk C: Cystic fibrosis: State of the art. Am Rev Respir Dis 113:833–878, 1976.

26. Hoiby N: Microbiology of lung infections in cystic fibrosis patients. Acta Paediatr Scand 301(Suppl):33–54, 1982.

27. Fick RB Jr, Naegel GP, Squier RE, et al: Proteins of the cystic fibrosis respiratory tract: Fragmented immunoglobulin G opsonic antibody causing defective opsonophagocytosis. J Clin Invest 74:236–248, 1984.

28. Beck BS, Heiner DC: Selective immunoglobulin G$_4$ deficiency and recurrent infections of the respiratory tract. Am Rev Respir Dis 124:94–96, 1981.

29. Perry KMA, King DS: Bronchiectasis. A study of prognosis based on a follow-up of 400 patients. Am Rev Tuberc 41:531–548, 1940.

30. Ogilvie AG: The natural history of bronchiectasis. A clinical roentgenologic and pathologic study. Arch Intern Med 68:395–465, 1941.

31. Johanson WG Jr, Woods DE, Chaudhuri T: Association of respiratory tract colonization with adherence of gram-negative bacilli to epithelial cells. J Infect Dis 139:667–673, 1979.

32. Lampe RM, Mason EO, Kaplan SL et al: Adherence of *Hemophilus influenzae* to buccal epithelial cells. Infect Immun 35:166–172, 1982.

33. Andersson B, Ericksson B, Falsen E, et al: Adhesion of *Streptococcus pneumoniae* to human pharyngeal epithelial cells in vitro, differences in adhesive capacity among strains isolated from subjects with otitis media, septicemia or meningitis or from healthy carriers. Infect Immun 32:311–317, 1981.

34. Niederman MS, Rafferty TD, Sasaki CT, et al: Comparison of bacterial adherence to ciliated and squamous epithelial cells obtained from the human respiratory tract. Am Rev Respir Dis 127:85–90, 1983.

35. Franklin AC, Todd T, Gurman G, et al: Adherence of *Pseudomonas aeruginosa* to cilia of human tracheal epithelial cells. Infect Immun 55:593–597, 1987.

36. Simel DL, Mastin BS, Pratt PC, et al: Scanning electron microscopy of the airways in normal children and in patients with cystic fibrosis and other lung diseases. Pediatr Pathol 2:47–64, 1984.

37. Jeffrey PK, Brain APR: Surface morphology of human airway mucosa: Normal, carcinoma or cystic fibrosis. Scanning Microsc 2:345–351, 1988.

38. Baltimore RS, Christie CDC, Smith GJ: Immunohistopathologic localization of *Pseudomonas aeruginosa* in lungs from patients with cystic fibrosis. Am Rev Respir Dis 140:1650–1661, 1989.

39. Marcus H, Baker NR: Quantitation of adherence of mucoid and nonmucoid *Pseudomonas aeruginosa* to hamster tracheal epithelium. Infect Immun 47:723–729, 1985.

40. Vishwanath S, Ramphal R: Adherence of *Pseudomonas aeruginosa* to human tracheobronchial mucin. Infect Immun 85:197–202, 1984.

41. Nelson JW, Tredgett MW, Sheehan DJ, et al: Mucinophilic and chemotactic properties of *Pseudomonas aeruginosa* in relation to pulmonary colonization in cystic fibrosis. Infect Immun 58:1489–1495, 1990.

42. Sajjan U, Reismann J, Doig P, et al: Binding of nonmucoid *Pseudomonas aeruginosa* to normal human intestinal mucin and respiratory mucin from patients with cystic fibrosis. J Clin Invest 89:657–665, 1992.

43. Reddy MS: Human tracheobronchial mucin: Purification and binding to *Pseudomonas aeruginosa*. Infect Immun 60:1530–1535, 1992.

44. Woods DE, Straus DC, Johanson WG Jr, Bass JA: Role of salivary protease activity in adherence of gram-negative bacilli to mammalian buccal epithelial cells in vivo. J Clin Invest 68:1425–1440, 1981.

45. Mason CM, Bawdon RE, Pierce AK, DalNogare AR: Fibronectin is not on the intact buccal epithelial surface of normal rats or humans. Am J Respir Cell Mol Biol 3:563–570, 1990.

46. Yamaguchi T, Yamada H: Role of mechanical injury on airway surface in the pathogenesis of *Pseudomonas aeruginosa*. Am Rev Respir Dis 144:1147–1152, 1991.

47. Ramphal R, Small PM, Shands JW Jr, et al: Adherence of *Pseudomonas aeruginosa* to tracheal cells injured by influenza infection or by endotracheal intubation. Infect Immun 27:614–619, 1980.

48. Read RC, Wilson R, Rutman A, et al: Interaction of nontypable *Hemophilus influenzae* with human respiratory mucosa in vitro. J Infect Dis 163:549–558, 1991.

49. Johnson AP, Clark JB, Osborn MF: Scanning electron microscopy of the interaction between *Hemophilus influenzae* and organ cultures of rat trachea. J Med Microbiol 16:477–482, 1983.

50. Hornick DB, Allen BL, Horn MA, Clegg S: Adherence to respiratory epithelia by recombinant *Escherichia coli* expressing *Klebsiella* type 3 fimbrial gene products. Infect Immun 60:1577–1588, 1992.

51. Plotkowski MC, Chevillard M, Pierrot D, et al: Differential adhesion of *Pseudomonas aeruginosa* to human respiratory epithelial cells in primary culture. J Clin Invest 87:2018–2028, 1991.

52. Plotkowski MC, Puchelle CE, Beck G, et al: Adherence of type 1 *Streptococcus pneumoniae* to tracheal epithelium of mice infected with influenza A/PR8 virus. Am Res Respir Dis 134:1040–1044, 1986.

53. Saiman L, Ishimoto K, Lory S, Prince A: The effect of piliation and exoproduct expression on the adherence of *Pseudomonas aeruginosa* to respiratory epithelial monolayers. J Infect Dis 161:541–548, 1990.

54. Adler KB, Hendley D, Davis GS: Bacteria associated with obstructive pulmonary disease elaborate extracellular products that stimulate mucin secretion by explants of guinea pig airway. Am J Pathol 125:501–514, 1986.

55. Baker NR: Role of exotoxin A and proteases of *Pseudomonas aeruginosa* in respiratory tract infections. Can J Microbiol 28:248–255, 1982.

56. Döring G, Goldstein W, Roll A, et al: Role of *Pseudomonas* exoenzymes in lung infections of patients with cystic fibrosis. Infect Immun 49:557–562, 1985.

57. Woods DE, To M, Sokol PA: *Pseudomonas aeruginosa* exoenzyme S as a pathogenic determinant in respiratory tract infections. Antibiot Chemother 42:27–35, 1989.

58. Vasil ML: *Pseudomonas aeruginosa*: Biology, mechanisms of virulence, epidemiology. J Pediatr 108:800–805, 1986.

59. Wilson R, Pitt T, Taylor GW, et al: Pyocyanin and 1-hydroxy phenazine produced by *Pseudomonas aeruginosa* inhibit the beating of human respiratory cilia in vitro. J Clin Invest 79:221–229, 1987.

60. Fick RB, Hata JS: Pathogenetic mechanisms in lung disease caused by *Pseudomonas aeruginosa*. Chest 95(Suppl):206S–213S, 1989.

61. Milazzo FH, Delisle GJ: Immunoglobulin A proteases in gram-negative bacteria isolated from human urinary tract infections. Infect Immun 43:11–13, 1984.

62. Denny FW: Effect of a toxin produced by *Hemophilus influenzae* on ciliated respiratory epithelium. J Infect Dis 129:93–100, 1974.

63. Cole MF, Hale CA: Cleavage of chimpanzee secretory immunoglobulin A by *Hemophilus influenzae* IgA1 protease. Microb Pathog 11:39–46, 1991.

64. Hughes RC, Jeanloz RW: The extracellular glycosidases of *Diplococcus pneumoniae* 1. Purification and properties of a neuraminidase

and β-galactosidase: Action on α-1-acid glycoprotein of human plasma. Biochemistry 3:1535–1543, 1964.

65. Drzeniek R: Viral and bacterial neuraminidases. Curr Top Microbiol Immunol 59:35–75, 1972.

66. Krivan HC, Roberts DD, Ginsburg V: Many pulmonary bacteria bind specifically to the carbohydrate sequence GalNAc(β1→4)Gal in some glycolipids. Proc Natl Acad Sci U S A 85:6157–6161, 1988.

67. Paton JC, Lock RA, Hansman D: Inhibition of human polymorphonuclear leukocyte respiratory burst, bactericidal activity and migration by pneumolysin. Infect Immun 41:548–552, 1983.

68. Feldman C, Mitchell TJ, Andrew PW, et al: The effect of *Streptococcus pneumoniae* pneumolysin on human respiratory epithelium in vitro. Microb Pathog 9:275–284, 1990.

69. Suter S, Schaad UB, Tegner H, et al: Granulocyte neutral proteases and *Pseudomonas* elastase as possible causes of airway damage in patients with cystic fibrosis. J Infect Dis 149:523–531, 1984.

70. Plotkowski MC, Beck G, Tournier JM, et al: Adherence of *Pseudomonas aeruginosa* to respiratory epithelium and the effect of leukocyte elastase. J Med Microbiol 30:285–293, 1989.

71. Krivan HC, Nilsson B, Lingwood CA, Ryu H: *Chlamydia trachomatis* and *Chlamydia pneumoniae* bind specifically to phosphatidylethanol-amine in HeLa cells and to GalNAcβ1-4Galβ-4Glc sequences found in asialo-GM1 and asialo-GM2. Biochem Biophys Res Commun 175:1082–1089, 1991.

72. Deal CD, Krivan HC: Lacto and ganglio series glycolipids are adhesion receptors for *Neisseria gonorrhoeae*. J Biol Chem 265:12774–12777, 1990.

73. Lamblin G, Lhermitte M, Klein A, et al: The carbohydrate diversity of human respiratory mucins: A protection of the underlying mucosa. Am Rev Respir Dis 144:S19–S24, 1991.

74. Lamblin G, Lafitte JJ, Lhermitte M, et al: Mucins from cystic fibrosis sputum. Mod Probl Paediatr 19:153–164, 1978.

75. Conway PL, Welin A, Cohen PS: Presence of K-88 specific receptors in porcine ileal mucus is age dependent. Infect Immun 58:3178–3182, 1990.

76. Karlsson KA: Animal glycosphingolipids as membrane attachment sites for bacteria. Annu Rev Biochem 58:309–350, 1989.

77. Kim KC, Wasano K, Niles RM, et al: Human neutrophil elastase releases cell surface mucins from primary cultures of hamster tracheal epithelial cells. Proc Natl Acad Sci U S A 84:9304–9308, 1987.

78. Liang OD, Ascencio F, Fransson LA, Wadstrom T: Binding of heparan sulfate to *Staphylococcus aureus*. Infect Immun 60:899–906, 1992.

79. Grant MM, Niederman MS, Poehlman MA, Fein AM: Characterization of *Pseudomonas aeruginosa* adherence to cultured hamster tracheal epithelial cells. Am J Respir Cell Mol Biol 5:563–570, 1991.

80. Woods DE, Straus DC, Johanson WG Jr, et al: Role of pili in adherence of *Pseudomonas aeruginosa* to mammalian buccal epithelial cells. Infect Immun 29:1146–1151, 1980.

81. Ramphal R, Sadoff JC, Pyle M, Silipigni JD: Role of pili in adherence of *Pseudomonas aeruginosa* to injured tracheal epithelium. Infect Immun 44:38–40, 1984.

82. Ramphal R, Guay C, Pier GB: *Pseudomonas* adhesins for tracheobronchial mucins. Infect Immun 55:600–603, 1987.

83. Ramphal R, Pier GB: Role of *Pseudomonas aeruginosa* mucoid exopolysaccharide in adherence to tracheal cells. Infect Immun 47:1–4, 1985.

84. Baker NR, Minor V, Deal C, et al: *Pseudomonas* exoenzyme S is an adhesin. Infect Immun 59:2859–2683, 1991.

85. Ramphal R, Koo L, Ishimoto KS, et al: Adhesion of *Pseudomonas aeruginosa* pilin deficient mutants to mucin. Infect Immun 59:1307–1311, 1991.

86. Doig P, Todd T, Sastry PA, et al: Role of pili in adhesion of *Pseudomonas aeruginosa* to human respiratory epithelial cells. Infect Immun 56:1641–1646, 1988.

87. Doig P, Todd T, Hodges RS, et al: Inhibition of adhesion of *Pseudomonas aeruginosa* to human buccal epithelial cells by monoclonal antibodies directed against pili. Infect Immun 58:124–132, 1990.

88. Hata JS, Fick RB: Airway adherence of *Pseudomonas aeruginosa*: Mucoexopolysaccharide binding to human and bovine airway proteins. J Lab Clin Med 117:410–422, 1991.

89. Paranchych W, Irvin RT, Hodges RS, Woods DE: Functional analy-

sis of synthetic analogues of bacterial adhesins specific for mammalian glycoconjugate receptors. Pediatr Pulmonol S6-1:134–135, 1991.

90. Chi E, Mehl T, Nunn D, Lory S: Interaction of *Pseudomonas aeruginosa* with A549 pneumocyte cells. Infect Immun 59:949–954, 1991.

91. Baker N, Hansson GC, Leffler H, et al: Glycosphingolipid receptors for *Pseudomonas aeruginosa*. Infect Immun 58:2361–2366, 1990.

92. Ramphal R, Pyle M: Evidence for mucins and sialic acid as receptors for *Pseudomonas aeruginosa* in the lower respiratory tract. Infect Immun 41:339–344, 1983.

93. Ramphal R, Carnoy C, Fievre S, et al: *Pseudomonas aeruginosa* recognizes carbohydrate chains containing type 1 (Galβ1-3GlcNAc) and type 2 (Galβ1-4GlcNAc) disaccharide units. Infect Immun 59:700–704, 1991.

94. Vishwanath S, Ramphal R: Tracheobronchial mucin receptor for *Pseudomonas aeruginosa*: Predominance of amino sugars in binding sites. Infect Immun 48:331–335, 1985.

95. Lampe RM, Mason EO, Kaplan SH, et al: Adherence of *Hemophilus influenzae* to buccal epithelial cells. Infect Immun 35:166–172, 1982.

96. Guerina NG, Langermann S, Clegg HW, et al: Adherence of piliated *Hemophilus influenzae* to human oropharyngeal cells. J Infect Dis 146:564, 1982.

97. St Geme JW, Falkow S, Barencamp SJ: High molecular weight proteins of nontypable *Haemophilus influenzae* mediate attachment to human epithelial cells. Proc Natl Acad Sci USA 90:2875–2879, 1993.

98. Van Alphen L, Poole J, Overbeeke M. The Anton blood group antigen is the erythrocyte receptor for *Hemophilus influenzae*. FEMS Microbiol Lett 37:69–71, 1986.

99. Van Alphen L, van den Broek LG, Blaas L, et al: Blocking of fimbria mediated adherence of *Haemophilus influenzae* by sialyl gangliosides. Infect Immun 59:4473–4477, 1991.

100. Andersson B, Dahmen J, Frejd T, et al: Identification of an active disaccharide unit of a glycoconjugate receptor for pneumococci attaching to human pharyngeal epithelial cells. J Exp Med 158:559–570, 1983.

101. Plotkowski MC, Beck G, Jacquot J, Puchelle E: The frog palate mucosa as a model for studying bacterial adhesion to mucus coated respiratory epithelium. J Comp Pathol 100:37–46, 1989.

102. Ramphal R: The role of bacterial adhesion in cystic fibrosis including the staphylococcal aspect. Infection 18:61–64, 1990.

103. Sanford BA, Thomas VL, Ramsay MA: Binding of *Staphylococci* to mucus in vivo and in vitro. Infect Immun 57:3735–3742, 1989.

104. Carruthers MM, Kabat WJ: Mediation of staphylococcal adherence to mucosal cells by lipotechoic acid. Infect Immun 40:444–446, 1983.

105. Olitzki L: Mucin as a resistance lowering substance. Bacteriol Rev 12:149–172, 1948.

106. Nungester WJ, Jourdonais LF: Mucin as an aid in the experimental production of lobar pneumonia. J Infect Dis 59:258–265, 1936.

107. Smith H: The virulence enhancing actions of mucins: A survey of human mucins and mucosal enhancing extracts. J Infect Dis 88:207–211, 1951.

108. Vishwanath S, Ramphal R, Guay C, Desjardin D, Pier GB: Respiratory mucin inhibition of the opsonophagocytic killing of *Pseudomonas aeruginosa*. Infect Immun 56:2218–2222, 1988.

109. Johanson WG Jr, Pierce AK, Sanford JP, Thomas GD: Nosocomial respiratory infections with gram-negative bacilli. Ann Intern Med 77:701–706, 1972.

110. Fagon YJ, Chastre J, Dosnart Y, et al: Nosocomial pneumonia in patients receiving continuous mechanical ventilation. A prospective analysis of 52 episodes with use of a protected specimen brush and quantitative culture techniques. Am Rev Respir Dis 139:877–886, 1989.

111. Feely TW, DuMoulin GC, Hedley-Whyte J, et al: Aerosol polymyxin and pneumonia in seriously ill patients. N Engl J Med 293:471–475, 1975.

112. Stevens RM, Teres D, Skillman JJ, Feingold DS: Pneumonia in an intensive care unit. Arch Intern Med 134:106–111, 1974.

113. Magnusson KE, Stjernstrom I: Mucosal barrier mechanisms. Interplay between secretory IgA (SIgA), IgG and mucins on the surface properties and association of salmonellae with intestines and granulocytes. Immunology 45:239–248, 1982.

# Host Impairments in Human Immunodeficiency Virus Infection

GARY A. NOSKIN and JOHN P. PHAIR

Acquired immunodeficiency syndrome (AIDS) is the consequence of infection with the human immunodeficiency virus type-1 (HIV-1), HIV-2, and possibly others.[1] These agents are lentiviruses and are related to similar retroviruses that infect nonhuman primates and produce immunosuppression in other species. Infection in humans ultimately results in development of opportunistic infections and malignancies secondary to the primary pathologic process, impairment of normal cellular and humoral immunity.[2] The target of the virus is the surface molecule of the helper T (CD4+) lymphocyte. Binding of the viral envelope protein gp120 to the CD4 receptor results in entry of viral RNA into the cytoplasm of the lymphocyte, followed by transcription of proviral DNA mediated by the viral enzyme, reverse transcriptase. Proviral DNA is integrated into cellular DNA on appropriate stimulation of the infected cell followed by viral replication.[2, 3]

With time, infection with HIV leads to suppression of T-cell function, infection of monocyte-macrophages, B-cell dysfunction, and alteration in cytokine production. This complex process, which has not been completely elucidated, ultimately results in quantitative and functional abnormalities in immunity.[4–10a] A hallmark of the increasing immune dysfunction is the progressive depletion of CD4+ lymphocytes in the circulating blood. Initially, it was postulated that this loss of helper T cells was related primarily to the cytopathic effect associated with HIV replication. It is now recognized that there are many potential mechanisms leading to CD4+ lymphocyte depletion. This chapter reviews these immunologic abnormalities and characterizes the clinical consequences of HIV infection.

## T-LYMPHOCYTE ABNORMALITIES

### Quantitative Defects

T lymphocytes are primarily subdivided by expression of the surface molecules, CD4 and CD8, which identify cells of differing function. The CD4+ lymphocyte (ie, helper T cell) serves to augment the immune response by production of lymphokines. One of the functions of CD8+ cells (ie, suppressor or cytotoxic T cells) is to down-regulate this response. An early observation in patients with AIDS was the recognition of severe depletion of CD4+ lymphocytes in homosexual men with *Pneumocystis carinii* pneumonia (PCP).[11] This fall in CD4+ lymphocytes and depression of the CD4:CD8 ratio correlates with progressive HIV infection (Table 5–1). Asymptomatic HIV-infected persons often have a relatively normal CD4+ lymphocyte count (normal, $1000 \pm 250$ cells/mm$^3$). There is a gradual and progressive decline in the number of CD4+ lymphocytes in the circulating blood. After the CD4+ lymphocyte count approaches 200 cells/mm$^3$, persons are at increased risk of developing opportunistic infections.[12, 13] There is, however, a marked variation in the rate of CD4+ lymphocyte decline among HIV-infected patients. Some have an initial fall in CD4+ cells followed by a relatively stable period, others demonstrate a gradual decline, and a few have a rapid progressive drop in the level of these lymphocytes.[14]

The mechanism of CD4+ lymphocyte depletion in HIV infection is not completely understood, but virulence of the infecting HIV strain may play a role in this process.[15] HIV-1 replication can cause cell death but is unlikely to

Table 5–1. **Immunologic Abnormalities in Human Immunodeficiency Virus Infection**

| Cell | Asymptomatic Infection | Acquired Immunodeficiency Syndrome |
|---|---|---|
| T lymphocytes | | |
|   CD4+ | ↓ | ↓ ↓ |
|   CD8+ | ↑ ↑ | ↑ |
|   CD4+:CD8+ | ↓ | ↓ ↓ |
| B lymphocytes | 0 | ↓ ↓ |
| Monocytes | ↑ | ↓ |
| Natural killer cells | ↓ | ↓ ↓ |
| Interleukin-1 | ↑ | ↑ |
| Interleukin-2 | ↓ | ↓ ↓ |
| Interferon-α | ↑ | ↑ ↑ |
| Interferon-γ | 0 | ↓ |
| Immunoglobulins (IgG, IgA, IgD) | ↑ | ↑ ↑ |
| Neopterin | 0 | ↑ |
| β$_2$-Microglobulin | 0 | ↑ ↑ |

Key: ↑, increased; ↓, decreased; 0, normal.

account for the total CD4+ lymphocyte depletion in vivo, because in early infection, few circulating CD4+ lymphocytes contain virus.[16] Other mechanisms have been hypothesized, including hyperactivation of CD4+ cells, autoimmune responses, destruction of memory CD4+ cells, and inappropriate cell death of uninfected cells.[17] It has been postulated that programmed cell death (ie, apoptosis) in mature helper T lymphocytes is a consequence of the immune response to HIV-1.[17] There is evidence that the viral load in nodal lymphocytes may be much greater than in peripheral blood cells.

It appears that CD8+ lymphocytes may not be susceptible to HIV-1[18] and are capable of suppressing viral replication in vitro. CD8+ lymphocyte counts generally increase after seroconversion, as in many other viral infections,[19] and may remain elevated independent of changes in the number of CD4+ lymphocytes. As patients develop symptomatic HIV disease, the number of CD8+ lymphocytes falls in parallel with the decreases in absolute lymphocyte count.[2] Disease progression and the development of opportunistic infections are associated with decreased numbers of CD8+ cells (see Table 5–1).[2, 20] The ratio of CD4+ to CD8+ lymphocytes has been evaluated in HIV infection, and although clinical decisions usually are based on CD4+ lymphocyte counts, a low CD4:CD8 ratio (<0.2) also is indicative of disease progression.[2, 21]

### Functional Defects

The opportunistic infections such as *P. carinii* pneumonia, cryptococcal meningitis, central nervous system toxoplasmosis, disseminated histoplasmosis, disseminated *Mycobacterium avium* complex, and cytomegalovirus retinitis are a result of dysfunctional cell-mediated immunity. Delayed-type hypersensitivity to common antigens is usually absent in patients with advanced HIV infection and AIDS.[22] There is in vitro evidence that CD4+ lymphocytes obtained from patients with AIDS do not respond appropriately to various antigens.[23] In one study, a large percentage of asymptomatic HIV-infected men failed to demonstrate a proliferative response to soluble antigens despite normal CD4+ cell counts.[24] This observation is consistent with clinical experience in which HIV-infected persons develop an increased susceptibility to a variety of pathogens early in the course of their HIV infection. Other functional defects of T cells have been documented in vitro, including decreased proliferative responses to mitogens, abnormal lymphokine production, and defective cytotoxic function.[25]

Several mechanisms may account for the impaired function of CD4+ lymphocytes after HIV infection. Antigen presentation by mononuclear phagocytes to CD4+ lymphocytes requires the interaction of the major histocompatibility complex (MHC) class II receptor complex with the CD4 receptor. When the HIV-1 gp120 envelope protein binds to the CD4 receptor of lymphocytes, the normal interaction is impaired.[26, 27] Another possibility is that infection of CD4+ lymphocytes with HIV-1 may lead to a deficiency in postreceptor signal transduction. This is manifested by defects in calcium metabolism, which is required for T-cell activation.[28] Production of interleukin-2 (IL-2), necessary for lymphocyte proliferation, is diminished in HIV-infected patients.[29, 30] A second lymphokine, interferon-γ (IFN-γ), is produced less well by CD4+ cells from HIV-infected persons. After recombinant IL-2 administration, CD4+ lymphocytes from AIDS patients still produce almost 15 times less IFN-γ.[31] IL-2 deficiency alone does not account for abnormal INF-γ production.

### NATURAL KILLER CELL ACTIVITY

Natural killer (NK) cells are lymphocytes that are CD4 and CD8 negative and are responsible for immunologic surveillance against tumors and viral infections. The mechanism of this process has not been completely elucidated. NK cells are quantitatively normal in AIDS but have impaired function.[7] NK cells from patients with AIDS have an impaired ability to lyse tumor cells such as the K562 line.[32] The most significant defects in NK cells of AIDS patients occur at the level of the cytoskeletal microtubule,[6] which regulates the transport of lytic substances to a target. The release of natural killer cytotoxic factor is also impaired in HIV infection.[33] The decreased production of IL-2 by lymphocytes may contribute to the NK cell defects seen in AIDS. When IL-2 is added to HIV-1 infected lymphocytes in vitro, NK cell function is only partially restored.[33]

It is known that gp120 has significant immunomodulatory effects. Recombinant gp120 can inhibit microtubule polarization and lytic properties of NK cells;[6] gp120 may play a role in the cascade of events that ultimately leads to NK cell dysfunction, supporting the hypothesis that HIV-1 envelope glycoproteins are critical in many of the immunologic impairments in AIDS. The mechanism by which NK cell deficiency occurs in AIDS may be related to a direct interaction between HIV-1 and NK cells and an indirect process mediated by decreased IL-2 production.[6]

### MONOCYTE-MACROPHAGE FUNCTION

The monocyte-macrophage system is partially responsible for clearing the circulating blood of foreign antigens, antigen presentation, and the killing of intracellular pathogens. Monocytes and macrophages that express CD4 antigens can be infected by HIV-1.[34–39] Monocytes and macrophages present antigens to CD4[+] lymphocytes, and monocyte surface CD4 plays an important role in the interaction between HIV gp120 and T cells.[40] The effect of HIV infection on antigen presentation is an impaired proliferative response to soluble antigens such as tetanus toxoid.[41] Moreover, monocyte chemotaxis, phagocytosis, and intracellular killing have been reported as normal[42] and as dysfunctional.[25, 43] Chemotaxis, the monocyte function most frequently reported to be defective, is particularly important in the pathogenesis of *Candida* and *Toxoplasma* infections. It is unclear whether this impairment is directly related to infection with HIV-1 or is a result of immune suppression from other viral or malignant conditions. Because infection of this cell line often is not associated with cell death, monocytes may represent a reservoir for HIV-1 that contributes to the pathogenesis of HIV-1 infection of the central nervous system.[44, 45]

CD4[+] monocyte counts, which are increased early in HIV infection, decrease with disease progression (see Table 5–1). The role of depletion of CD4[+] monocytes in the pathogenesis of AIDS is unclear. However, monocytic infection may be related to the augmented production of tumor necrosis factor (TNF), IL-1 and IL-6 that has been documented in HIV-infected persons. IL-6 is believed to be partially responsible for the hypergammaglobulinemia that occurs in AIDS and correlates with serum IgG levels.[46]

## B-LYMPHOCYTE FUNCTION

There is conflicting data on absolute B-lymphocyte numbers in HIV infection. Investigators have reported quantitative increases and decreases and have demonstrated no abnormalities.[9, 47] Although less is known about effects of HIV on B-cell function than on T-cell function, HIV infection is clearly a B-cell disease. Striking evidence supporting B-lymphocyte dysfunction is the high incidence of B-cell lymphomas in adults with AIDS,[48] the hypergammaglobulinemia (especially IgA) occurring with disease progression,[49, 50] and the failure of AIDS patients to produce antibody after antigenic stimulation. The clinical significance of this defect is a poor response to immunizations[51] and the inability to use serologic tests to accurately diagnose infections, such as those due to toxoplasmosis or cytomegalovirus. The most severe consequences of impaired antibody production are seen in children infected with HIV-1, which accounts for the increased frequency and severity of infections with *Streptococcus pneumoniae* and *Haemophilus influenzae*.[52] B-cell dysregulation has been implicated in autoimmune phenomena, such as immune thrombocytopenia.[53, 54]

Several mechanisms have been postulated to explain the polyclonal B-cell activation seen in HIV disease. One suggested mechanism is activation of B lymphocytes by Epstein-Barr virus (EBV).[55] Alternatively, direct activation by HIV-1 may account for the hypergammaglobulinemia seen in AIDS, or B-cell dysregulation may reflect altered cytokine production by T cells and mononuclear phagocytes. B

cells that have been incubated with HIV-1 show increased immunoglobulin production.[56]

$\beta_2$-Microglobulin is a low-molecular-weight immunoglobulin that forms the light chain of the class I MHC. Levels of this compound are normal in asymptomatic patients but increase with disease progression. In one study, persons with a $\beta_2$-microglobulin level greater than 5 $\mu g/mL$ had a 17 times greater risk of developing AIDS than those with normal levels.[57]

## NEUTROPHIL FUNCTION

The neutrophil is the primary defense against pathogens such as *Staphylococcus aureus* and *Candida albicans*. Relatively few investigations have evaluated neutrophil function in patients with HIV infection, but one report demonstrated that neutrophils from patients with symptomatic infection or AIDS had defects in chemotaxis, bacterial killing, and binding of *Candida*.[58] Neutrophils from patients with AIDS also have an impaired ability to kill *S. aureus* compared with normal controls.[59] Another study evaluated patients with lymphadenopathy and found normal neutrophil migration but impaired chemotaxis.[60] Impaired chemotaxis is more severe during the early stage of HIV infection than in advanced disease.[42, 58] Neutropenia is not an uncommon finding in late-stage HIV-1 infection.

It is estimated that 18% to 35% of HIV-infected persons develop a serious bacterial infection.[42] An incompletely resolved issue is the role played by neutrophil defects unrelated to HIV infection in the predisposition to suppurative complications. For instance, HIV-seronegative intravenous drug users have abnormal neutrophil function. This raises the question of whether neutrophil defects are related to drug use alone or are the consequence of HIV-1 infection. Similar poylmorphonuclear leukocyte abnormalities have been reported in homosexual men and in hemophiliacs, independent of HIV infection.[60] Each risk group requires matched controls to accurately assess neutrophil function. Regardless of the mechanism, neutrophil abnormalities are found in HIV-infected persons and may enhance the development of bacterial and fungal infections.

## INTERFERONS AND INTERLEUKINS

Interferons are cytokines that have antiviral, antineoplastic, and immunomodulating properties. In normal persons, interferon levels usually are not measurable in serum, but in HIV-infected patients, interferons can be detected.[61] The interactions between HIV-1 and interferons are complex and not completely understood. In HIV-infected patients with disease progressing to AIDS, high levels of an interferon inhibitor substance have been measured in sera, especially in patients with Kaposi sarcoma (KS) or lymphoma.[61] Increasing levels of IFN-$\alpha$ (acid-labile) can be seen with disease progression (see Table 5–1).[62–64] IFN-$\gamma$ increases production of neopterin, a product of guanosine triphosphate biosynthesis, by macrophages. Consequently, serum neopterin levels serve as an indirect estimate of INF-$\gamma$ activity. Serum and urine neopterin levels increase with advancing HIV disease, and cerebrospinal fluid levels are elevated if neurologic manifestations are present, especially with opportunistic infections and lymphoma.[64, 65]

The interleukins, like interferons, are regulatory cytokines. IL-1 is produced by many cell types, but mononuclear phagocytes are the major source of this cytokine. IL-1 has many biologic effects, including induction of fever, T-cell activation, B-cell proliferation, enhancement of TNF, interferon and colony-stimulating factor production, and induction of polymorphonuclear release from the bone marrow. HIV-1 has been reported to stimulate the production of IL-1 from mononuclear cells,[66] and increased levels of IL-1 have been found in the sera of HIV-infected persons (see Table 5–1).[67, 68] The clinical significance of increased IL-1 production is unclear, although it may help explain the activation of T and B cells, fever, and wasting that occur with advanced disease. One investigation found that in the absence of endotoxin, HIV-1 did not induce production of IL-1.[69]

IL-2, IL-4, and IL-5 are all produced by T cells and serve as mediators of T-cell and B-cell function. IL-2 is the predominant mediator of T-lymphocyte proliferation and serves as a cofactor for B-cell development and immunoglobulin secretion. IL-4 stimulates production of IgE and plays an important role in the allergic response. IL-5 mediates IgA and IgM synthesis and eosinophil maturation. IL-2 production by peripheral blood mononuclear cells (PBMC) after exposure to HIV-1 peptides was documented at least 1 year before identification of HIV-1 DNA by polymerase chain reaction.[70] Such T-cell responses may serve as early markers of infection, before antibody production.[71] IL-2 production has also been examined as a marker of disease progression. Another longitudinal study demonstrated that prognosis and survival of HIV-infected patients depended on the ability of their PBMC to produce IL-2 after antigenic stimulation.[72] Based on the known immunologic effects of IL-2, several investigators have used it therapeutically for patients with HIV infection. Although IL-2 therapy in conjunction with conventional antiviral therapy is investigational, preliminary reports suggest it may have a role as an immunomodulating agent,[73] and it has been used successfully in the treatment of HIV-related lymphomas.[74]

The roles of IL-4 and IL-5 in the pathogenesis of HIV infection have not been fully elucidated. Because IL-4 is a potent stimulator of IgE synthesis, it may have a role in the pathophysiology of the increased prevalence of adverse drug reactions in these patients. In our HIV-infected patients, we have observed an increased incidence of eosinophilia, independent of opportunistic infections or malignancies, which may be related to the increased production of IL-5, although this requires confirmation.

IL-6, like IL-1, is derived from mononuclear phagocytes, T cells, and KS cells. Its major role in immunoregulation is the induction of immunoglobulin synthesis in activated B cells. HIV-1 stimulates IL-6 production in the absence of T cells.[75] IL-6 can enhance HIV-1 replication and the proliferation of KS cells. The reverse transcriptase inhibitors zidovudine and dideoxyinosine do not inhibit in vitro production of IL-6, but in vivo, they do result in decreases in serum concentrations of IL-6 and TNF, which may augment the antiviral effects.[76]

The immunopathogenic interaction of the interferons and interleukins in HIV infection is complex and not completely understood. A greater appreciation for the interactions of these cytokines, TNF, and the colony-stimulating factors will aid our understanding of the pathogenesis of AIDS. Through recombinant DNA technology, many of these substances are now available, and they soon may play important roles therapeutically.

## HUMAN IMMUNODEFICIENCY VIRUS-1 INFECTION

### Immunopathology

HIV-1 has three gene regions that code for structural proteins. The *gag* region codes for the viral core; the *pol* region transcribes reverse transcriptase; and the *env* region codes for envelope proteins.[77] Two major envelope glycoproteins, gp41 and gp120, appear to be responsible for initiation of HIV-1 infection. The gp120 molecule binds to the CD4 receptor on helper T lymphocytes, and gp41 attaches to a fusion site, also on the cell surface.[77, 78] After penetration into the cell, viral RNA transcribes viral DNA through the action of reverse transcriptase. The virus then circularizes and enters the host cell genome after stimulation of the cell. In the nucleus, proviral DNA can exist in a latent form or enter into the replicative phase. In the latter case, proviral DNA makes RNA, which transcribes viral proteins and genomic RNA.[79] After reassembly of the structural proteins, infectious virions bud from the cell.

Although CD4$^+$ cells are most frequently infected, CD4$^-$ cells, such as human glial cell fibroblasts and dendritic cells, can be infected.[80, 81] Fibroblasts and dendritic cells may serve as reservoirs for HIV-1 throughout the body. Many other cell lines have demonstrated HIV-1 infection, including macrophages of the central nervous system, colorectal cells, and cells in the duodenal lamina.[37, 39, 82]

The immunopathology of HIV-1 is not understood. One unexplained finding is the long clinical latency that occurs in some persons and the rapid development of immunosuppression in others. It has been shown in vitro that HIV-1 isolates from the same patient demonstrate more virulent characteristics as the immunosuppression progresses.[77] One investigation documented that HIV-1 facilitated endonuclease activation in T cells, which may regulate the growth and death of these lymphocytes.[83] This alteration in programmed cell death may be partially responsible for the cytopathology associated with HIV infection. Another report confirmed that quiescent T lymphocytes serve as a source of extrachromosomal HIV-1 DNA and that these cells are a reservoir for HIV-1.[84] In an epidemiologic study of gay and bisexual men, those with more than 500 sexual partners had an increased incidence of sexually transmitted diseases, and continued high-risk sexual activity after establishment of HIV infection produced a more rapid progression to AIDS.[85] These findings raise the issue of the roles of reinfection with HIV-1, exposure to a more pathogenic strain of HIV-1, and the presence of one or more cofactors that facilitate disease progression.

### Altered Pulmonary Host Defenses

There are many important defense mechanisms that protect the lower respiratory tract against invading organisms.

Table 5–2. **Immunologic Defects in Acquired Immunodeficiency Syndrome**

| Defect | Pathogen | Infection |
|---|---|---|
| T lymphocytes | Bacteria | |
| | *Legionella* | Pneumonia |
| | *Nocardia* | Pneumonia |
| | *Listeria* | Meningitis, disseminated infection |
| | *Salmonella* | Gastroenteritis, disseminated infection |
| | Fungi | |
| | *Candida albicans* | Mucosal, esophagitis, vaginitis |
| | *Cryptococcus neoformans* | Meningitis, disseminated infection, pulmonary |
| | *Histoplasma capsulatum* | Disseminated infection, pulmonary |
| | *Coccidioides immitis* | Disseminated infection, pulmonary |
| | *Aspergillus* | Invasive pneumonia |
| | *Pneumocystis carinii* | Pneumonia, disseminated infection |
| | Protozoa | |
| | *Toxoplasma gondii* | Brain abscess, rarely lung |
| | *Cryptosporidium* | Gastroenteritis, rarely pneumonitis |
| | *Isospora belli* | Gastroenteritis |
| | Mycobacteria | |
| | *Mycobacterium avium* complex | Disseminated infection |
| | *Mycobacterium tuberculosis* | Tuberculosis; disseminated infection |
| | Viruses | |
| | Cytomegalovirus | Retinitis, disseminated infection |
| | Epstein-Barr virus | Oral hairy leukoplakia, Burkitt lymphoma, lymphoid interstitial pneumonitis(?) |
| | Herpes simplex virus | Recurrent mucocutaneous ulcers, pneumonia |
| | Varicella-zoster virus | Dermatomal or disseminated infection |
| | Human papillomavirus | Rectal and cervical carcinoma |
| | Papovavirus | Progressive multifocal leukoencephalopathy |
| B lymphocytes | Bacteria | |
| | *Streptococcus pneumoniae* | Pneumonia, bacteremia |
| | *Haemophilus influenzae* | Pneumonia, disseminated infection |
| | Neoplasms | |
| | Non-Hodgkin lymphoma | |
| Granulocytes | Gram-negative bacteria | Disseminated infection, pneumonia |
| | *Staphylococcus aureus* | Abscess, bacteremia, pneumonia |

Adapted from Rubin RH: Acquired immunodeficiency syndrome. Scientific American Medicine, Rubenstein E, Federman DF, Eds. Section 7, Subsection XI. © 1993 Scientific American, Inc. All rights reserved.

Nasal cilia, cough reflexes, and the mucociliary blanket are the first lines of defense and play little role in the pulmonary immunopathology associated with HIV-1. However, additional host defenses in the respiratory tract, such as humoral and cellular immune responses, are altered in HIV-infected persons. In normal bronchoalveolar lavage (BAL) fluid, almost 90% of the cells are macrophages.[86] Lymphocytes account for as many as 10% of the cells; neutrophils, eosinophils, and basophils compose less than 1%. Most lymphocytes are T cells, and approximately one half of them are $CD4^+$.[87] The ratio of $CD4^+$ to $CD8^+$ cells in BAL fluid is similar to that in the serum.

In patients with AIDS, the percentage of $CD4^+$ cells in BAL fluid usually is decreased,[88, 89] although the total number is frequently normal.[90] The absolute $CD8^+$ number and the $CD8^+$ percentage are increased, resulting in a decreased CD4:CD8 ratio.[88–90] One question that has not been completely addressed is whether $CD4^+$ lymphocytes are recruited to the respiratory tract during acute infection. Lymphocytic alveolitis was found to consist of primarily $CD8^+$ lymphocytes, but these cells were not cytotoxic in vitro.[91]

Alveolar macrophages from patients with AIDS are structurally similar to those in normal hosts. The major defect appears to be in the functioning of these cells. Most likely, abnormalities in cytokine production in PBMC prob-ably are also present in alveolar macrophages.[86] This local immunologic deficiency may help explain ineffective macrophage killing of opportunistic pathogens. The numbers of pulmonary NK cells are increased in patients with AIDS, but have impaired release of cytotoxic substances.[91] In vitro stimulation of these cells with IL-2 improves their cytotoxic function.

## Clinical Aspects of Infection

The clinical consequence of HIV-1 infection is the deterioration of immune function, resulting in the development of "opportunistic" infections and neoplasms (Table 5–2). The opportunistic infections occur primarily because of defects in cell-mediated immunity. The most frequent is PCP, which is diagnosed in 60% to 70% of AIDS patients in the United States. The risk can be diminished by prophylaxis. Patients are at highest risk for PCP when their $CD4^+$ lymphocyte counts approach 200 cells/mm$^3$.[92] Based on data from the Multicenter AIDS Cohort Study, almost one third of HIV-infected patients not receiving prophylaxis and with $CD4^+$ lymphocyte counts less than 200 cells/mm$^3$ developed PCP within 36 months.[92]

Among the most common infections seen in HIV infection are oral candidiasis (thrush) and severe infections caused by herpes simplex virus and varicella-zoster virus. These infections usually do not occur in immunocompetent persons and should increase the clinical suspicion for HIV-1 infection. Mucosal candidiasis occurs as a result of defects in cell-mediated immunity and serves as an early marker of immune suppression (200–500 $CD4^+$ cells/mm$^3$). Widely disseminated *Candida* infections result from prolonged neutropenia and are unusual in HIV infection. In patients with these conditions, if no evidence of other immunosuppressive states exists, an inquiry into risk factors for HIV-1 is warranted. Another important viral infection is caused by the cytomegalovirus (CMV). Most AIDS patients develop active CMV infections at an extremely advanced stage ($CD4^+$ lymphocyte counts < 50/mm$^3$), and viremia often occurs during this end-stage disease. Although CMV can often be identified in the BAL fluid obtained from AIDS patients with pneumonia, its role in the production of pulmonary infection is difficult to ascertain. In AIDS patients, cytotoxic T-cell activity against CMV-infected cells is absent.[78] Infections with *Listeria monocytogenes,* an intracellular bacteria, are unusual in AIDS patients.

Although *C. albicans* is the most common fungal infection occurring in HIV-infected patients, other fungi are frequently seen in AIDS. *Cryptococcus neoformans* causes meningitis and disseminated infection. This infection is most commonly detected when a patient's $CD4^+$ cell count falls below 100 cells/mm$^3$.[93] HIV-infected persons living in the Mississippi and Ohio River valleys and the southwestern United States are at increased risk for disseminated histoplasmosis and coccidioidomycosis, respectively. Invasive and disseminated *Aspergillus* infection is reported in AIDS patients, although much less commonly than the endemic mycoses.

The inability of the monocyte-macrophage system to function effectively results in disseminated infections due to *Mycobacterium tuberculosis* and the nontypical *Mycobacteria* such as *M. avium* complex and *M. kansasii.* Infected macrophages from AIDS patients are frequently loaded with these acid-fast bacilli. *M. avium* complex tends to occur as immune function deteriorates. Pulmonary tuberculosis (TB) is an important infection, because it is transmissible to other persons from HIV-infected patients. TB can occur regardless of the patient's immune status. Multidrug-resistant tuberculosis has been reported in HIV-infected patients primarily in New York, Florida, and California.[93a]

Bacterial infections occur with increased frequency in HIV-infected patients. In adults and children, B-cell dysfunction is manifested by more frequent infections with encapsulated organisms such as the pneumococcus and *H. influenzae,* which are more commonly bacteremic.[51, 52, 94] Adults infected with HIV-1 should be vaccinated against the pneumococcus and receive annual influenza vaccines. The pneumococcal vaccine should be given early in the course of HIV-1 infection, when antibody response to the vaccine is most likely to occur.

Lymphoid interstitial pneumonitis (LIP) is a pulmonary process that occurs predominantly in HIV-infected children. LIP may be confused with PCP but is usually distinguishable based on clinical and radiographic manifestations. LIP typically is insidious in onset and leads gradually to hy-poxia and respiratory failure. The pathogenesis of LIP may be related to EBV or immunologic response to HIV-1.[95]

## CONCLUSION

HIV infection is best viewed as a continuum from seroconversion to profound immunosuppression, manifested as opportunistic infections, neoplasms, wasting syndrome, and encephalopathy.[96] The immunopathogenesis of this process is complex, and although our understanding has advanced tremendously in recent years, much is still not understood. Data describing this process may conflict because different populations are examined at various stages of the disease. To further complicate matters, viruses such as CMV and EBV can suppress the immune system independently of HIV-1 and may contribute to the pathogenesis of AIDS.

We know that HIV-1 infects $CD4^+$ lymphocytes and alters the function of monocyte-macrophages, B cells, neutrophils, NK cells, and cells in the central nervous system (see Table 5–1). Regulatory cytokines such as interleukins, interferons, colony-stimulating factors, and TNF apparently play a significant role in the pathogenesis of this infection. The development of therapeutic agents through recombinant DNA technology is already having an impact on the management of HIV disease and will undoubtedly play a larger role in the future. Advances in the management of HIV disease will depend on a greater understanding of the immunopathogenesis. Although we are unable to reverse the process of HIV infection and the inevitable deterioration in immune function, our goal is to stabilize immune function while attempting to prevent opportunistic infections. The challenge is to modify the pathogenesis of HIV-1 infection through pharmacotherapy or immunomodulation.

## REFERENCES

1. Fauci AS: The human immunodeficiency virus: Infectivity and mechanisms of pathogenesis. Science 239:617–622, 1988.
2. Zolla-Pazner S: Immunologic abnormalities in infections with the human immunodeficiency virus. Lab Med 17:685–689, 1986.
3. Shearer GM, Bernstein DC, Tung KSK, et al: A model for the selective loss of major histocompatibility complex self-restricted T cell immune responses during the development of acquired immune deficiency syndrome (AIDS). J Immunol 137:2514–2521, 1986.
4. Sodroski J, Goh WC, Rosen C, Campbell K, Haseltine WA: Role of the HTLV-III/LAV envelope in syncytium formation and cytopathicity. Nature 322:470–474, 1986.
5. Gartner S, Markovits P, Markovitz DM, Gallo RC, Popovic M: The role of mononuclear phagocytes in HTLV-III/LAV infection. Science 233:215–219, 1986.
6. Sirianni MC, Tagliaferri F, Aiuti F: Pathogenesis of the natural killer cell deficiency in AIDS. Immunol Today 11:81–82, 1990.
7. Poli G, Introna M, Zanaboni F, et al: Natural killer cells in intravenous drug abusers with lymphadenopathy syndrome. Clin Exp Immunol 62:128–134, 1985.
8. Montagnier L, Gruest J, Chamaret S, et al: Adaptation of lymphadenopathy associated virus (LAV) to replication in EBV-transformed B lymphoblastoid cell lines. Science 225:63–66, 1984.
9. Lane HC, Masur H, Edgar LC, Whalen G, Rook AH, Fauci AS: Abnormalities of B-cell activation and immunoregulation in patients with acquired immunodeficiency syndrome. N Engl J Med 309:453–458, 1983.
10. Rieckmann P, Poli G, Kehrl JH, Fauci AS: Activated B-lymphocytes from human immunodeficiency virus infected individuals induce virus expression in infected T cells and monocytes. J Exp Med 173:1–5, 1991.

10a. Levy JA: The transmission of HIV and factors influencing progression to AIDS. Am J Med 95:86–100, 1993.

11. Gottlieb MS, Schroff R, Schanker HM, et al: *Pneumocystis carinii* pneumonia and mucosal candidiasis in previously healthy homosexual men: Evidence of a new acquired cellular immunodeficiency. N Engl J Med 305:1425–1431, 1981.

12. Polk BF, Fox R, Bookmeyer R, et al: Predictors of the acquired immunodeficiency syndrome developing in a cohort of seropositive homosexual men. N Engl J Med 316:61–66, 1987.

13. Goedert JJ, Bigga RJ, Melbye M, et al: Effect of T4 count and cofactors on the incidence of AIDS in homosexual men infected with human immunodeficiency virus. JAMA 257:331–334, 1987.

14. Kaplan JA, Spira TJ, Fishbein DB, et al: Lymphadenopathy syndrome in homosexual men: Evidence for continuing risk of developing the acquired immunodeficiency syndrome. JAMA 257:335–337, 1987.

15. Cheng-Mayer C, Seto D, Tateno M, et al: Biologic features of HIV-1 that correlate with virulence in the host. Science 240:80–82, 1988.

16. Harper ME, Marselle LM, Gallo RC, Wong-Staal F: Detection of lymphocytes expressing human T-lymphotrophic virus type III in lymph nodes and peripheral blood from infected individuals by in situ hybridization. Proc Natl Acad Sci USA 83:772–776, 1986.

17. Ameisen JC, Capron A: Cell dysfunction and depletion in AIDS: The programmed cell death hypothesis. Immunol Today 12:102–105, 1991.

18. Zagury D, Bernard J, Leonard R, et al: Long-term cultures of HTLV-III infected T cells: A model of cytopathology of T-cell depletion in AIDS. Science 231:850–853, 1986.

19. Cooper DA, Maclean P, Finlayson R, et al: Acute AIDS retrovirus infection: Definition of clinical illness associated with seroconversion. Lancet 1:537–540, 1985.

20. Dobozin BS, Judson FN, Cohn DL, et al: The relationship of abnormalities of cellular immunity to antibodies to HTLV-III in homosexual men. Cell Immunol 98:156–171, 1986.

21. De Martini RM, Turner RR, Formenti SC, et al: Peripheral blood mononuclear cell abnormalities and their relationship to clinical course in homosexual men with HIV infection. Clin Immunol Immunopathol 46:258–271, 1988.

22. Lane HC, Depper JM, Green WC, et al: Qualitative analysis of immune function in patients with acquired immunodeficiency syndrome. N Engl J Med 313:79–84, 1985.

23. Shearer GM, Salahuddin SZ, Markham PD, et al: Prospective study of cytotoxic T lymphocyte responses to influenza and antibodies to human T lymphotropic virus-III in homosexual men. J Clin Invest 76:1699–1704, 1985.

24. Fauci AS: AIDS: Immunopathogenic mechanisms and research strategies. Clin Res 35:503–510, 1987.

25. Bowen DL, Lane HC, Fauci AS: Immunopathogenesis of the acquired immunodeficiency syndrome. Ann Intern Med 103:704–709, 1985.

26. Gay D, Maddon P, Sekaly R, et al: Functional interaction between human T-cell protein CD4 and the major histocompatibility complex HLA-DR antigen. Nature 328:626–629, 1987.

27. Doyle C, Strominger JL: Interaction between CD4 and class II MHC molecules mediates cell adhesion. Nature 330:256–259, 1987.

28. Linette GP, Hartzman RJ, Ledbetter JA, June CH: HIV-1 infected T cells show a selective signaling defect after perturbation of CD3/antigen receptor. Science 241:573–576, 1988.

29. Murray HW, Rubin BY, Masur H, Roberts RB: Impaired production of lymphokines and immune (gamma) interferon in the acquired immunodeficiency syndrome. N Engl J Med 310:883–889, 1984.

30. Goldsmith JM, Huprikar J, Wu SJY, Phair JP: Interleukin 1 and 2 production in homosexual men: A controlled trial of therafectin (SM-1213), a possible immunomodulator. J Immunopharmacol 8:1–14, 1986.

31. Murray HW, Welte K, Jacobs JL, Rubin BY, Mertelsmann R, Roberts RB: Production of and in vitro response to interleukin 2 in the acquired immunodeficiency syndrome. J Clin Invest 76:1959–1964, 1985.

32. Creemers PC, Stark DF, Boyko WJ: Evaluation of natural killer cell activity in patients with persistent generalized lymphadenopathy and acquired immunodeficiency syndrome. Clin Immunol Immunopathol 36:141–150, 1985.

33. Bonavida B, Katz J, Gottlieb M: Mechanism of defective NK cell activity in patients with acquired immunodeficiency syndrome (AIDS) and AIDS-related complex. Defective trigger on NK cells for NKCF production by target cells, and partial restoration by IL2. J Immunol 137:1157–1163, 1986.

34. De Martini RM, Parker JW: Immunologic alterations in human immunodeficiency infection: A review. J Clin Lab Anal 3:56–70, 1989.

35. Belsito DV, Sanchez MR, Baer RL, et al: Reduced Langerhans cell Ia antigen and ATPase activity in patients with the acquired immunodeficiency syndrome. N Engl J Med 310:1279–1282, 1984.

36. Tschachler E, Groh V, Popovic M, et al: Epidermal Langerhans cells—a target for HTLV-III/LAV infection. J Invest Dermatol 88:233–237, 1989.

37. Adachi A, Koenig S, Gendelman HE, et al: Productive, persistent infection of human colorectal cell lines with human immunodeficiency virus. J Virol 61:209–213, 1987.

38. Pomerantz RJ, De La Monte SM, Donegan SP, et al: Human immunodeficiency virus (HIV) infection of the uterine cervix. Ann Intern Med 108:321–327, 1988.

39. Pomerantz RJ, Kurizkes DR, De La Monte SM, et al: Infection of the retina by human immunodeficiency virus type 1. N Engl J Med 317:1643–1647, 1987.

40. Siliciano RF, Knall C, Lawton T, Berman P, Gregory T, Reinholz EL: Recognition of HIV glycoprotein gp 120 by T cells. Role of monocyte CD4 in the presentation of gp 120. J Immunol 142:1506–1511, 1989.

41. Wood GS, Burns BF, Dorfman RF, Warnke RA: The immunohistology of non-T cells in the acquired immunodeficiency syndrome. Am J Pathol 120:371–378, 1985.

42. Nielsen H, Kharazmi A, Faber V: Blood monocyte and neutrophil functions in the acquired immune deficiency syndrome. Scand J Immunol 24:291–296, 1986.

43. Smith PD, Ohura K, Masur H, Lane HC, Fauci AS, Wahl SM: Monocyte function in the acquired immune deficiency syndrome. J Clin Invest 74:2121–2128, 1984.

44. Koenig S, Gendelman HE, Orenstein JM, et al: Detection of AIDS virus in macrophages in brain tissue from AIDS patients with encephalopathy. Science 233:1089–1093, 1986.

45. Gendelman HE, Orenstein JM, Baca LM, et al: The macrophage in the persistence and pathogenesis of HIV infection. AIDS 3:475–497, 1989.

46. Breen EC, Rezai AR, Nakajima K, et al: Infection with HIV is associated with elevated IL-6 levels and production. J Immunol 144:480–484, 1990.

47. Stites DP, Casavant CH, McHugh TM, et al: Flow cytometric analysis of lymphocyte phenotypes in AIDS using monoclonal antibodies and simultaneous dual immunofluorescence. Clin Immunol Immunopathol 36:161–177, 1985.

48. Levine AM, Meyer PR, Begandy MK, et al: Development of B-cell lymphoma in homosexual men: Clinical and immunologic findings. Ann Intern Med 100:7–13, 1984.

49. Chess Q, Daniels J, North E, Macris NT: Serum immunoglobulin elevations in the acquired immunodeficiency syndrome (AIDS): IgG, IgA, IgM, and IgD. Diagn Immunol 2:148–153, 1984.

50. Pahwa SG, Quilop MTJ, Lange M, et al: Defective B-lymphocyte function in homosexual men in relation to the acquired immunodeficiency syndrome. Ann Intern Med 101:757–763, 1984.

51. Ammann AJ, Schiffman G, Abrams D, Volberding P, Ziegler J, Conant M: B-cell immunodeficiency in acquired immunodeficiency syndrome. JAMA 251:1447–1449, 1984.

52. Rubinstein A, Morecki R, Goldman H: Pulmonary disease in infants and children. Clin Chest Med 9:507–517, 1988.

53. Morris L, Distenfeld A, Amorosi E, Karpatkin S. Autoimmune thrombocytopenic purpura in homosexual men. Ann Intern Med 96:714–717, 1982.

54. Walsh CM, Nardi MA, Karpatkin S: On the mechanism of thrombocytopenic purpura in sexually active homosexual men. N Engl J Med 311:635–639, 1984.

55. Yarchoan R, Redfield RR, Broder S: Mechanisms of B cell activation in patients with acquired immunodeficiency syndrome and related disorders. J Clin Invest 78:439–447, 1986.

56. Schnittman SM, Lane HC, Higgins SE, Folks T, Fauci AS: Direct polyclonal activation of human B lymphocytes by the acquired immune deficiency syndrome virus. Science 233:1084–1086, 1986.

57. Moss AR, Bacchetti P, Osmond D, et al: Seropositivity for HIV and the development of AIDS or ARC: Three year follow-up of the San Francisco General Hospital cohort. Br Med J 296:745–750, 1988.

58. Ellis M, Gupta S, Galant S, et al: Impaired neutrophil function in patients with AIDS or AIDS-related complex: A comprehensive evaluation. J Infect Dis 158:1268–1275, 1988.

59. Murphy PM, Lane HC, Fauci AS, Gallin JI: Impairment of neutrophil bactericidal activity in patients with AIDS. J Infect Dis 158:627–630, 1988.

60. Valone FH, Payan DG, Abrams DI, Goetzl EJ: Defective polymorphonuclear leukocyte chemotaxis in homosexual men with persistent lymph node syndrome. J Infect Dis 150:267–271, 1984.

61. Ambrus JL, Poiesz BJ, Lillie MA, Stadler I, DiBeradino LA, Chadha KC: Interferon and interferon inhibitor levels in patients infected with varicella-zoster virus, acquired immunodeficiency syndrome, acquired immunodeficiency syndrome-related complex, or Kaposi's sarcoma, and in normal individuals. Am J Med 87:405–407, 1989.

62. Lane HC, Fauci AS: Immunologic abnormalities in the acquired immunodeficiency syndrome. Annu Rev Immunol 3:477–500, 1985.

63. Akao M, Yorifuji H, Hada M, Ikematsu S, Fujimaki M: Immune abnormalities of hemophiliacs in relation to HIV-1 infection (abstract 2184). Program and Abstracts of the 6th International Conference on AIDS. San Francisco, CA, 1990:400.

64. Griffin DE, McArthur JC, Cornblath DR: Neopterin and interferon-gamma in serum and cerebrospinal fluid of patients with HIV-associated neurologic disease. Neurology 41:69–74, 1991.

65. Fahey JL, Taylor JMG, Detels R, et al: The prognostic value of cellular and serologic markers in infection with human immunodeficiency virus type 1. N Engl J Med 322:166–172, 1990.

66. Merrill JE, Koyanagi Y, Chen ISY: Interleukin-1 and tumor necrosis factor α can be induced from mononuclear phagocytes by human immunodeficiency virus type 1 binding to the CD4 receptor. J Virol 63:4404–4408, 1989.

67. Berman MA, Sandborg CI, Calabia BS, Andrews BS, Friou GJ: Interleukin 1 inhibitor masks high interleukin 1 production in acquired immunodeficiency syndrome (AIDS). Clin Immunol Immunopathol 42:133–140, 1987.

68. Lepe-Zuniga JL, Mansell PWA, Hersh EM: Idiopathic production of interleukin-1 in the acquired immunodeficiency syndrome. J Clin Microbiol 25:1695–1700, 1987.

69. Molina JM, Scadden DT, Amirault C, et al: Human immunodeficiency virus does not induce interleukin-1, interleukin-6, or tumor necrosis factor in mononuclear cells. J Virol 64:2901–2906, 1990.

70. Clerici M, Berzofsky JA, Shearer GM, Tacket CO: Exposure to human immunodeficiency virus type 1-specific T helper cell responses before detection of infection by polymerase chain reaction and serum antibodies. J Infect Dis 164:178–182, 1991.

71. Giorgi JV, Clerici M, Berzofsky JA, Shearer GM: HIV-specific cellular immunity in high-risk HIV-1 seronegative homosexual men (abstract WA 1209). Program and Abstracts of the 7th International Conference on AIDS. Florence, Italy, 1991:44.

72. Morland P, Leclercq P, Giroux C, Brion JP, Benson C, Micoud M: Longitudinal follow-up of in vitro interleukin-2 (IL-2) production by HIV patients' lymphocytes (abstract WA 1277). Program and Abstracts of the 7th International Conference on AIDS. Florence, Italy, 1991:160.

73. Bartlett JA, Blakenship K, Waskin H, Sebastian H, Austin A, Weinhold K: The therapeutic uses of interleukin-2 in patients with HIV infection (abstract WB 2154). Program and Abstracts of the 7th International Conference on AIDS. Florence, Italy, 1991:220.

74. Mazza P, Bocchia M, Tumietto F, et al: rIL-2 in the treatment of lymphomas associated with HIV infection. Preliminary report (abstract WB 2369). Program and Abstracts of the 7th International Conference on AIDS. Florence, Italy, 1991:274.

75. Nakajima K, Martinez-Maza O, Hirano T, et al: Induction of IL-6 (B cell stimulatory factor-2/IFN-β₂) production by HIV. J Immunol 142:531–536, 1989.

76. Goujard C, Delfralssy JF, Wallon C, Boué F, Galanaud P: Effects of AZT and ddI on TNF alpha and IL6 production (abstract WB 2135). Program and Abstracts of the 7th International Conference on AIDS. Florence, Italy, 1991:215.

77. Levy JA: Human immunodeficiency viruses and the pathogenesis of AIDS. JAMA 261:2997–3006, 1989.

78. Fauci AS: Immunopathogenic mechanisms in human immunodeficiency virus (HIV) infection. Ann Intern Med 114:678–693, 1991.

79. Levy JA: The human immunodeficiency virus and its pathogenesis. Infect Dis Clin North Am 2:285–297, 1988.

80. Cheng-Mayer C, Rutka JT, Rosenblum ML, McHugh T, Stites DP, Levy JA: The human immunodeficiency virus (HIV) can productively infect cultured glial cells. Proc Natl Acad Sci U S A 84:3526–3530, 1987.

81. Tateno M, Gonzalez-Scarano F, Levy JA: The human immunodeficiency virus can infect CD4 negative human fibroblastoid cells. Proc Natl Acad Sci U S A 86:4287–4290, 1989.

82. Nelson JA, Wiley CA, Reynolds-Kohler C, Reese CE, Margaretten W, Levy JA: Human immunodeficiency virus detected in bowel epithelium of patients with gastrointestinal symptoms. Lancet 1:259–262, 1988.

83. Terai C, Kornbluth RS, Pauza CD, Richman DD, Carson DA: Apoptosis as a mechanism of cell death in cultured T lymphoblasts acutely infected with HIV-1. J Clin Invest 87:1710–1715, 1991.

84. Burkinsky MI, Stanwick TL, Dempsey MP, Stevenson M: Quiescent T lympocytes as an inducible virus reservoir in HIV-1 infection. Science 254:423–427, 1991.

85. Phair J, Detels R, Jacobson L, Rinaldo C, Saah A, Muñoz A: AIDS within five years of seroconversion. J AIDS 5:490–496, 1992.

86. Rankin JA: Pulmonary immunology. Clin Chest Med 9:387–393, 1988.

87. Shaw S: Characterization of human leukocyte differentiation antigens. Immunol Today 81:1–3, 1987.

88. Venet A, Clavel F, Israel-Biet D, et al: Lung in acquired immunodeficiency syndrome: Infections and immunological status assessed by bronchoalveolar lavage. Bull Eur Physiopathol Respir 21:535–543, 1985.

89. Wallace JM, Barbers RG, Oishi JS, et al: Cellular and T-lymphocyte subpopulation profiles in bronchoalveolar lavage fluid from patients with acquired immunodeficiency syndrome and pneumonitis. Am Rev Respir Dis 130:786–790, 1984.

90. Young KR Jr, Rankin JA, Naegel GP, et al: An immunologic analysis of bronchoalveolar lavage cells and proteins in patients with the acquired immunodeficiency syndrome. Ann Intern Med 103:522–533, 1985.

91. Semenzato G: Immunology of interstitial lung diseases: Cellular events taking place in the lung of sarcoidosis, hypersensitivity pneumonitis and HIV infection. Eur Respir J 4:95–102, 1991.

92. Phair JP, Muñoz A, Detels R, et al: The risk of *Pneumocystis carinii* pneumonia among men infected with human immunodeficiency virus type 1. N Engl J Med 322:161–165, 1990.

93. Larsen RA, Leal MAE, Chan LS: Fluconazole compared with amphotericin B plus flucytosine for cryptococcal meningitis in AIDS. Ann Inter Med 113:183–187, 1990.

93a. Frieden TR, Sterling T, Pablos-Mendez A, Kilburn JO, Cauthen GM, Dooley SW: The emergence of drug-resistant tuberculosis in New York City. N Engl J Med 328:521–526, 1993.

94. Polsky B, Gold JWM, Whimbey E, et al: Bacterial pneumonia in patients with the acquired immunodeficiency syndrome. Ann Intern Med 104:38–41, 1986.

95. Teirstein AS, Rosen MJ: Lymphocytic interstitial pneumonitis. Clin Chest Med 9:467–471, 1988.

96. Chaisson RE, Volberding PA: Clinical manifestations of HIV infections. *In* Mandell GL (ed): Principles and Practice of Infectious Diseases, ed 3. New York, Churchill Livingstone, 1990:1059–1092.

# Nutrition and Infection

SUSAN K. PINGLETON and MICHAEL S. NIEDERMAN

The role of nutritional impairment in promoting respiratory infection has been recognized for many years, but only recently have some of the mechanisms of malnutrition-induced respiratory host defense failures been clarified. Malnutrition has multiple influences on the lung's ability to resist invading pathogens, and these alterations in lung defenses lead to three clinical consequences: an increased incidence of lung infections, a more virulent and prolonged bout of infection than is usually seen, and a more subtle clinical presentation of pneumonia than is typical of well-nourished persons.[1, 1a]

In this chapter, the role of nutrition in respiratory infection is discussed, beginning with the effect of malnutrition on thoracopulmonary function. Malnutrition decreases respiratory muscle strength and impairs ventilatory drive. Special attention is focused on lung defense mechanisms and changes in host defenses seen in malnutrition. The effects of refeeding on infection are discussed. Nutritional support, especially enteral nutrition, may decrease infection complications of malnutrition by decreasing a process known as bacterial translocation in the gut. Nutritional support also can increase infectious complications, especially respiratory infection, by promoting gastric colonization with resultant tracheal colonization and nosocomial pneumonia.

Improved management includes strategies to decrease tracheal aspiration and respiratory infection, which are complications of nutritional support. Management strategies may include use of amino acids such as glutamine.

## MALNUTRITION AND LUNG DISEASE

### Epidemiology

Although malnutrition can adversely affect previously normal persons, the effects of nutritional deficiency on pa-

tients with acute and chronic lung disease have been especially studied. Investigators in the late 1960s first noticed the association between weight loss and increased mortality in chronic obstructive pulmonary disease (COPD).[2, 3] Weight loss has been found in 70% of patients hospitalized with COPD, and anthropomorphic measurements were abnormal in half of these patients.[4] Data from the recent large COPD population enrolled in the Intermittent Partial Pressure Breathing Trial evaluated the frequency of protein-calorie malnutrition in patients with COPD.[5] Approximately 25% of the patients enrolled in the study were malnourished (<90% ideal body weight). The frequency of malnutrition increased to 35% in patients with severe airflow obstruction (FEV$_1$, <30% predicted). The study confirmed an independent effect of weight loss on mortality, although the precise cause of increased mortality was not defined.

The frequency of malnutrition has been examined in patients with respiratory failure. Driver and colleagues assessed nutritional status of patients with COPD in respiratory failure.[6] Ideal body weight anthropomorphic measurements and visceral measurements of nutritional status were lower in respiratory failure patients than in those from a control group of 18 patients without respiratory failure. In a preliminary study, nutritional status of 80 consecutive respiratory intensive care unit (ICU) patients was evaluated.[7] Weight loss (<80% ideal body weight) was found in 24%. Anthropomorphic measurements of triceps skin-fold thickness and mid-arm muscle circumference were abnormal in almost one half of the patients. Although poor nutritional status did not appear to predispose the need for mechanical ventilation, malnourished patients who required mechanical ventilation had a significantly higher mortality than well-nourished patients requiring mechanical ventilation. Malnutrition is a common problem in patients with chronic lung disease and acute respiratory failure.

Hospitalized patients may experience a deterioration in nutritional status during their stay. In a retrospective study of 26 patients, Driver and LeBrun found inadequate nutri-

Portions of this chapter have been reproduced from Niederman MS: Malnutrition and host lung defenses: Implications for the pathogenesis and prevention of pneumonia. *In* Ferranti RD, Rampulla C, Fracchia C, Ambrosino N (eds): Nutrition and Ventilatory Function. Verona, Italy, Bi & Gi Publishers s.r.l., 1992:87–98.

tional support in 23.[8] They suggested that inadequate nutrition, on an iatrogenic basis, occurs in ventilated patients. Similar results were found in a retrospective assessment of nutritional therapy in respiratory ICU patients over a 1-year period.[9] Calorie, protein, and carbohydrate requirements were met on only 70%, 26%, and 51%, respectively, of ICU days. Patients with acute respiratory failure are at risk for worsening nutritional status without appropriate nutritional support. These data suggest that hospitalized patients and outpatients, with or without chronic lung disease, are at risk for malnutrition with its attendant adverse effects.

## Effect of Malnutrition on Thoracopulmonary Function

Poor nutritional status can adversely affect thoracopulmonary function by impairing respiratory muscle function, ventilatory drive, and pulmonary defense mechanisms (Table 6–1).[10] The adverse effects of malnutrition occur independently of those of primary lung disease. However, malnutrition's adverse effects on lung disease may be additive, especially in some patients with acute respiratory failure, such as those with respiratory failure caused by COPD. In COPD, primary abnormalities of decreased inspiratory pressure and increased work of breathing are found. Inspiratory muscle weakness, as assessed by maximal inspiratory pressure, results from mechanical disadvantage to inspiratory muscles after hyperinflation and from generalized muscle weakness.[11, 12] In COPD, inspiratory muscle weakness must be severe for hypercapnia to occur. In patients with myopathy, hypercapnia occurs when inspiratory pressures are less than one third of normal.[13] However, hypercapnia was found in 13 of 18 patients with COPD whose inspiratory pressures were less than half normal.[14] Hypercapnia occurs with much less respiratory muscle weakness if other mechanical abnormalities, such as those of COPD, increase the work of breathing.

Although none of these studies has addressed the patient critically ill with COPD, they do suggest that malnutrition may further compromise an already impaired lung function. Hypercapnic respiratory failure or difficulty in weaning from mechanical ventilation may be more easily precipitated in the malnourished patient with COPD than in the normally nourished patient with COPD.

In simple starvation or undernutrition, fat and protein are lost, but the loss of protein is minimized by reducing the need to use it as a source of energy.[15] Nitrogen loss is modified by mobilization of fat, and enhanced fat oxidation is the principal source of energy in the starving person. Some protein wasting does occur despite the availability of fat as a source of energy, and it becomes markedly accelerated after the fat stores are used up. In critical illness, protein catabolism occurs to provide energy. With inade-

quate caloric intake in critically ill patients, energy sources are derived from protein breakdown and gluconeogenesis. Of the various protein "pools" available, the muscle protein pool is susceptible to catabolism to provide fuel.[16] Inspiratory and expiratory respiratory muscles, primarily the diaphragm and intercostals, are skeletal muscles and therefore susceptible to this catabolic effect. Because the diaphragm is the critical respiratory muscle, the following discussion focuses on it, although these considerations are valid for all respiratory muscles.

Malnutrition reduces diaphragmatic muscle mass in health and disease.[17, 18] Thurlbeck[17] correlated low diaphragmatic mass with low body weight in patients with emphysema. The diaphragmatic weight was lower than predicted from body weight, suggesting that additional factors are operative. In a necropsy study, Arora and Rochester[18] evaluated diaphragmatic muscle mass, thickness, and area in normal-weight patients dying suddenly and underweight patients dying of a variety of diseases. Body weight and diaphragmatic muscle mass were reduced to 70% and 60%, respectively, of normal in poorly nourished patients. Another study measured the contribution of reduced diaphragmatic muscle mass to transdiaphragmatic pressures, an index of diaphragmatic muscle strength.[19] Compared with values in normal subjects, transdiaphragmatic pressures were reduced by 66%, and diaphragmatic muscle thickness was reduced by 25%. This suggests that transdiaphragmatic pressure is reduced not only because there is less muscle but also because the remaining muscle is weaker.

Animal studies confirm the loss of diaphragmatic strength in prolonged nutritional deprivation. In an in vivo hamster model in which food was reduced by 33.3% for 4 weeks, body weight was reduced to 75% of the control values.[20] Diaphragm weight and muscle thickness were similarly reduced to 73% and 70% of controls, respectively. Caloric restriction produced changes in diaphragm muscle fiber composition and muscle fiber size. The percentage of fast twitch glycolytic and oxidative fibers decreased ($-4\%$ and $-2\%$, respectively) slightly. More dramatic changes were found in the muscle fiber size. The cross-sectional area of fast twitch fibers (type II) was reduced to 76% of normal. The cross-sectional area of slow oxidative (type I) fibers was unchanged. Maximal isometric tension was reduced 73% in undernourished control subjects. Using isolated diaphragmatic strips from rats, Lewis evaluated the contractile and fatigue properties of the diaphragm when food was restricted until the body weight of the nutritionally deprived animals were 50% of that of the control group.[21] The diaphragmatic strength as assessed by peak twitch tension was reduced by almost 50%. After these were corrected for diaphragmatic weight, no difference between malnourished and normally nourished animals was found. The shape of the force-frequency curve was similar between the two groups except at 5 and 10 pulse/sec, where greater relative tension was produced in diaphragms from the nutritionally deprived animals.

Respiratory muscle function is also impaired in poorly nourished humans. In malnourished adult patients without lung disease, respiratory muscle strength, maximum voluntary ventilation, and vital capacity were reduced by 37%, 41%, and 63%, respectively, compared with the values in the well-nourished patients.[22] The data interpretation is clouded by the fact that the patients' malnutrition was

Table 6–1. **Effect of Malnutrition on Thoracopulmonary Function**

| |
|---|
| Impairment of respiratory muscle function |
| Decreased ventilatory drive |
| Alteration of pulmonary defense mechanisms |

caused by malignancy. Given the nature of this systemic disease, the researchers could not rule out catabolic factors other than malnutrition contributing to respiratory muscle weakness.

The status of respiratory muscles in poorly nourished children and young adults with cystic fibrosis (CF) is controversial. Normal or even greater than normal inspiratory pressures, despite severe malnutrition, have been found in CF patients.[23] In contrast, the inspiratory pressures were decreased in a homogeneous group of malnourished CF patients.[24] CF is characterized by malnutrition and chronic hyperinflation. Hyperinflation places the diaphragm at a mechanical disadvantage so it can no longer operate according to its optimal force-length relation. Conflicting data in the CF studies may arise over the appropriate correction factor for hyperinflation.[12] Lands and colleagues found that the decreased respiratory muscle strength in CF was caused by the mechanical disadvantage placed on the diaphragm by the marked hyperinflation. Respiratory muscle strength was mildly influenced by nutritional status, but not to any degree of clinical significance. Further impairment of respiratory function, even mild, may jeopardize respiratory muscle strength during periods of infectious exacerbation.

Respiratory muscle strength in patients without a systemic disease or hyperinflation is decreased. Kelly and associates studied respiratory muscle strength and body composition in adult patients hospitalized on a surgical service.[25] Maximal inspiratory pressures were lower (33 ± 3 cm $H_2O$) in malnourished patients than in those who were normal (45 ± 5 cm $H_2O$). Transdiaphragmatic pressures were decreased (stimulated transdiaphragmatic pressure (Pdi) 16 ± 5 cm $H_2O$) in 10 patients with anorexia nervosa, a relatively pure model of malnutrition without systemic disease.[26] The human data suggest malnutrition alone decreases respiratory muscle strength.

Malnutrition also affects ventilatory drive. Zwillich and colleagues suggested that the interaction of nutrition and ventilatory drive seems to be a direct function of the influence of nutrition on the metabolic rate.[27] Conditions that reduce the metabolic rate reduce the ventilatory drive. A decrease in the metabolic rate occurs with starvation.[28] Doekel and coworkers demonstrated a parallel fall in the metabolic rate and hypoxic ventilatory response, which returned toward normal with refeeding.[29] Studies of hospitalized patients receiving total parenteral nutrition demonstrated that an increased protein intake decreased the ventilatory response to $CO_2$.[30] This effect could be detrimental in patients with limited pulmonary reserve, leading to an unnecessary increase in respiratory effort. The consequences of decreased respiratory strength and ventilatory drive could include decreased cough and the increased likelihood of atelectasis and subsequent pneumonia in nonventilated patients. Decreased respiratory muscle strength and drive have the potential to prolong the duration of mechanical ventilation in patients who are otherwise candidates for weaning.

## MALNUTRITION AND RESPIRATORY HOST DEFENSES

### Normal Host Defenses[1]

To recognize the effects of malnutrition on lung defense mechanisms, the normal host defenses should be understood. After microorganisms are in the respiratory tract, they encounter a host defense system that has the capacity to repel them at every anatomic site. Whether pneumonia develops is a function of the size of the bacterial inoculum, the virulence of the specific organism, and the ability of the host to resist infection by means of an intact defense system.[1]

The normal oropharynx is usually free of gram-negative bacilli because of the cleansing action of secretions, salivary proteases (eg, lysozyme, lactoferrin, lactoperoxidase), and local IgA antibody.[31] The oropharyngeal epithelium resists gram-negative colonization by cellular desquamation and by the intrinsically poor ability of oral mucosal cells to adhere to this type of bacteria. With illness, mucosal cells of the upper and lower airways can bind more gram-negative bacteria than normal, and the airway can become colonized. For this to occur, cells expose more ''receptors'' that bind to adhesins on appropriately equipped bacteria.[1]

The lower respiratory tract has an even more complex host defense system that keeps this site sterile in normal persons.[31] To colonize and infect the lower airway, bacteria must first navigate the epiglottis and vocal cords and then pass through the physical barriers of the tracheobronchial tree. These physical defenses include cough, bronchoconstriction, airway angulation, and the mucociliary escalator. Beyond these barriers are the immunologic defenses, which can be organism specific or nonspecific. These include bronchus-associated lymphoid tissue, phagocytic cells (eg, polymorphonuclear leukocytes, alveolar macrophages), humoral immunity (eg, IgA antibody, IgG antibody, complement), and cell-mediated immunity with T lymphocytes. In the lower airway, as in the oropharynx, bacterial adherence is necessary for gram-negative bacteria to colonize the mucosa.[1a, 32]

Certain bacteria are handled by the lower airway host defense system in specific ways. For example, *Staphylococcus aureus* is primarily eliminated by resident alveolar macrophages, although certain gram-negative bacteria require the recruitment of neutrophils to be eliminated.[1a] Another organism, *Listeria monocytogenes,* which has been the subject of some studies of the effects of malnutrition, requires alveolar macrophages to be recruited to the lung in large numbers, because resident macrophages alone cannot effectively remove this organism.[1, 1a, 33]

### Host Defense Abnormalities

Many investigators have examined the cellular basis of impairment in respiratory host defenses that result from malnutrition, but there is little uniformity in the types of nutritional deficits that have been evaluated (Table 6–2). Some studies have involved animals, and others have involved human adults and children. Human studies have focused primarily on hospitalized patients with protein-calorie deficiency or global nutritional depletion. Animal studies have evaluated neonates and adults and have looked at acute starvation, chronic protein-calorie malnutrition, or combined food and water deprivation. The defects in humans and animals that have been documented by these methods are summarized in the following sections.

Table 6–2. **Host Defense Abnormalities With Malnutrition**

Airway colonization
Bacterial adherence
Alveolar macrophage function
Neutrophil function
Cell-mediated immunity lymphocyte function
Respiratory tract IgA

## Airway Colonization and Bacterial Adherence

In patients with chronic tracheostomy and in those treated with mechanical ventilation, malnutrition has promoted colonization by *Pseudomonas* species.[34] Some studies have used a multifactorial index of nutrition, the Prognostic Nutritional Index (PNI), which incorporates measurements of serum albumin, triceps skin-fold thickness, serum transferrin, and total lymphocyte count and becomes numerically higher with increasing degrees of global nutritional impairment. Among the tracheostomy patients, those colonized by *Pseudomonas* species had a higher PNI than noncolonized patients.[34] In a study of 14 mechanically ventilated patients, multiple tracheal cultures were collected for at least 1 week, with each patient having a minimum of three cultures. Among the 6 patients with the highest PNI, *Pseudomonas* species were found in 60% of their tracheal cultures, and among the 8 patients with the lowest PNI values, these bacteria occurred in only 25% of their lower airway cultures.[35] Among patients with community-acquired pneumonia, respiratory tract colonization by gram-negative bacteria was associated with malnutrition, as measured by serum albumin.[36]

It is likely that malnutrition leads to gram-negative colonization of the airway by making epithelial cells more receptive for the binding of bacteria. Tracheotomized patients colonized by *Pseudomonas* species had a higher mean tracheal cell adherence (measured in vitro, with isolated tracheal cells and *P. aeruginosa*) than noncolonized patients.[34] There was a linear correlation between the absolute tracheal cell adherence value and the PNI among 15 patients with chronic tracheostomy.[34] Similar data have been found in animal studies, with rats exposed to food and water deprivation developing an increase in buccal cell-binding capacity for *P. aeruginosa* that paralleled their loss in body weight.[11] In rats, this abnormality developed after only 3 days of starvation and disappeared after 2 days of refeeding. In the human studies, vigorous enteral nutrition was given, and in 1 patient studied for 10 weeks, this therapy led to a decline in the PNI, a fall in tracheal cell-binding capacity for bacteria, and an elimination of sputum colonization by *P. aeruginosa*.[34]

## Alveolar Macrophage Function

Green and Kass[38] first implied that malnutrition could interfere with macrophage function when they showed that mice, starved for 24 to 48 hours, had reduced clearance of aerosolized *S. aureus* and the reduction in clearance was directly related to how much weight each animal lost. The type of challenge used implied that resident alveolar macrophage dysfunction was responsible for the observed abnormalities. Shennib and colleagues studied rats exposed to acute food (but not water) deprivation and found that lung

macrophages from these animals had a reduced ability to phagocytose *P. aeruginosa,* although their bactericidal function was intact.[39] With refeeding, the deficit could be reversed, but only after 3 weeks, indicating that the abnormality was permanent and that new cells had to be produced for normal function to return.

When chronic protein-calorie malnutrition was studied in neonatal rats, different findings emerged. In this model, meant to simulate kwashiorkor, animals could clear aerosolized *S. aureus* and *P. aeruginosa* but could not remove *L. monocytogenes.*[40] The investigators concluded that chronic malnutrition did not interfere with resident phagocyte function, neutrophil recruitment, or macrophage bactericidal function. However, there was a deficit in the ability of macrophages to be recruited to the lung. In subsequent studies, alveolar macrophages from chronically malnourished rats, when stimulated by *L. monocytogenes,* did not have abnormalities in phagocytosis, bacterial killing, release of superoxide anion, or production of interleukin-1 or tumor necrosis factor.[41] However, the macrophages from malnourished animals did have a change in arachidonic acid metabolism compared with controls, with reduced production of leukotriene $B_4$ and an increased release of thromboxane $B_2$ and prostaglandin $E_2$ after stimulation by *L. monocytogenes.* This shift in metabolism appeared after 4 weeks of dietary restriction and reversed after 1 week of normal feeding.

## Neutrophil Function

Protein deficiency usually does not interfere with the microbicidal or phagocytic function of neutrophils, but one study of children observed an abnormal early-phase migration of blood neutrophils as a result of protein-calorie malnutrition.[42] The defects in neutrophil migration correlated with serum prealbumin levels and reversed after 3 to 4 weeks of normal feeding.

## Cell-Mediated Immunity and Lymphocyte Function

Skin test anergy and reductions in total lymphocyte count are common accompaniments of nutritional deficiency and are incorporated into clinical measurements of nutritional status. Lymphocyte differentiation may be abnormal with malnutrition, as shown by the finding that malnourished children can have reduced numbers of T lymphocytes, normal numbers of B lymphocytes, and increased numbers of null cells.[43]

## Respiratory Tract IgA

This major antibody of the lower respiratory tract can be reduced with nutritional deficiency, and sputum levels of IgA have been inversely related to the PNI in patients with chronic tracheostomy.[44]

# MALNUTRITION AND PNEUMONIA

## Incidence of Lung Infection

### Children[1]

In developing countries, the incidence of bronchopneumonia and viral lung infections is increased in children who are malnourished. In a study of 75 malnourished infants in Kampala, Uganda, many types of infection were common, with 12 infants developing pneumonia, including tuberculosis and possibly gram-negative infection.[45] In Bangladesh, similar findings have been reported, with almost half of severely malnourished children having pneumonia, including tuberculosis in more than 10%.[46] Viral infections, including measles and viral bronchitis, may also be more common among malnourished children.[1a]

### Adults[1]

In studies of survivors of ghetto conditions and prisoner of war camps in World War II, the incidence of pneumonia was increased among adults who were severely malnourished. In the Warsaw ghetto, tuberculosis was common, and in prisoners of war who were poorly fed, tuberculosis was seen with a higher than expected frequency.[1a] In the latter population, the incidence of common respiratory infections was not increased.

Most of the current interest in adult pneumonia and nutritional status centers on hospitalized patients. In a variety of medical and surgical patients, abnormal measurements of nutritional parameters are a common occurrence. Driver and coworkers found that patients with respiratory failure and chronic obstructive lung disease often had abnormalities in triceps skin-fold thickness, serum transferrin, and total lymphocyte count.[6] In the study, 56% of respiratory failure patients were below 80% of ideal body weight. This situation may be compounded by medical therapy, because patients treated with mechanical ventilation are often underfed. One study observed that, on average, among 26 patients receiving mechanical ventilation, daily caloric intake was 390 calories below basal metabolic need, even though 71% of these patients had a serum albumin below 3.2 g/dL.[8]

In a surgical population, Mullen and associates observed that nutritional impairment was common and related to an increased risk of postoperative infection.[47] For a group of 64 elective surgical patients, 16 nutritional and immunologic parameters were measured; 97% of the patients had at least one abnormality, and 35% had three or more abnormal findings.[47] Of the 64 patients, 15 developed serious postoperative complications, including 9 infections, 3 of which were pneumonia. These complications were more common in patients with the lowest serum albumin, transferrin, and delayed hypersensitivity testing.[47]

### Course of Pneumonia

In adults and children, malnutrition may portend a more serious course or even a fatal outcome of respiratory infection. In the Warsaw ghetto experience, tuberculosis was more severe in malnourished children, and pneumonia often presented almost asymptomatically.[1a] Both of these observations reflect an impairment in host defense function, which must be intact to ensure the best outcome from infection and the most appropriate inflammatory (ie, symptomatic) response to invading pathogens. In children in Bangladesh, mortality rates from pneumonia were higher among those with malnutrition.[1, 1a, 46]

In a study of 80 patients with suppurative lung disease requiring surgical therapy, nutritional status was found to be an important determinant of outcome.[48] In this group, 64 patients had empyema, 11 had tuberculous empyema or pleural effusion, 2 had lung abscess, and 3 had other infections. A fatal outcome best correlated with a low serum level of albumin, but mortality was also affected by reduced delayed hypersensitivity testing.[48] Studies such as these demonstrate the increased frequency and poor outcome of respiratory infection in those with malnutrition, but they do not tell us whether nutritional therapy can be employed to reverse this trend.

## NUTRITIONAL SUPPORT AND INFECTION

The primary cause of death in critically ill patients is infection, specifically sepsis and nosocomial pneumonia. Nutrition is used in part to counteract the adverse effects of malnutrition on lung defense mechanisms that are thought to be operative in the development of pneumonia. Enteral nutrition is often the method of choice for nutrient administration because it is generally perceived to be less invasive, more physiologic, and less expensive than total parenteral nutrition. As with all therapeutic modalities, complications of enteral nutrition exist.[49] Mechanical, metabolic, gastrointestinal, and infectious complications occur (Table 6–3). Mechanical problems include inappropriate location of feeding tubes, frequent obstruction, and inadvertent dislodgement of nasoenteral feeding tubes. Metabolic complications comprise various electrolyte disorders and nutrition-related hypercapnia. Gastrointestinal complications include nausea, vomiting, and diarrhea. The relation of enteral nutrition to infection is less well defined. Infectious complications occur, notably gastric and tracheal colonization with resultant nosocomial pneumonia. On the other hand, new data suggest that abnormalities of gut function play a primary role in initiating and promoting infection in critical illness. Malnutrition may worsen gut function and enteral nutrition improve it, potentially decreasing the risk of infection in critically ill patients.

### The Gut and Infection

The gut has not been thought of as having importance in functions other than digestion. If ileus occurs, the gut is thought to be inactive or quiescent. There are no "gut function" tests with which to monitor or determine normal function. Little attention is paid to the gut in ICU patients unless vomiting or diarrhea occurs. Recent data suggest that the gut is active in nondigestive functions, and that it may play a pivotal role in promoting or defending against infection.[50, 51] The gut may represent the "final frontier" of organ system study in the ICU.

Table 6–3. **Infectious Complications of Enteral Nutrition**

| |
|---|
| Gastric colonization of enteral nutrition |
| Tracheal colonization |
| Nosocomial lung infection |
| Nosocomial sepsis |

Gut function is more extensive than originally thought. In addition to the accepted primary role of digestion and absorption of nutrients, the gastrointestinal (GI) tract has important defense mechanisms. The intestinal mucosa functions as a major local defense barrier to prevent bacteria colonizing the gut. The normal intestine protects the host from intraluminal bacteria and their toxins, primarily because the structural maintenance of normal intestinal epithelial cells prevents transepithelial migration. A variety of immunologic mechanisms complement this barrier function. The intestinal wall contains immunologically active cells, such as lymphocytes and macrophages, and the mesentery is filled with regional lymph nodes. Secretory IgA intraluminally prevents adherence of bacteria to mucosal cells and is the principal component of the gut mucosal defense system. Kupffer cells of the liver and spleen provide a backup barrier to trap and detoxify bacteria and their toxic products, if penetration of the epithelium and regional lymph nodes has occurred. The gut can be described as a metabolically active, immunologically important, and bacteriologically decisive organ in critical illness.

After insult to the intestinal epithelium, indigenous bacteria colonizing the gastrointestinal tract pass through the epithelial mucosa to infect the mesenteric lymph nodes and systemic organs. This microbial migration has been called bacterial translocation.[3] Three major mechanisms promote bacterial translocation: altered permeability of the intestinal mucosa caused by hemorrhagic shock, sepsis, or endotoxemia; decreased host defense mechanisms such as immunosuppression; and increased bacterial numbers within the intestine, caused by bacterial overgrowth or intestinal stasis. Because many of the factors that facilitate bacterial translocation occur in critically ill patients, these patients may be vulnerable to the invasion of enteral bacteria. The data for evaluating bacterial translocation have been developed largely in animal experiments. The clinical significance of these observations remains uncertain, although it is recognized that infection in critically ill patients involves organs (eg, lung) that are not a part of the GI tract but are invaded by microflora usually only identified within the gut lumen. The available human data has accumulated from studies of patients with inflammatory bowel disease or surgical patients. Ambrose cultured intestinal serosa and mesenteric lymph nodes from patients undergoing abdominal operation.[52] The results of serosal and nodal cultures were positive for 15% and 5%, respectively, of patients with noninflammatory bowel disease; patients undergoing surgery for complications of Crohn disease had a 30% incidence of positive serosal cultures. More indirect human data from retrospective and epidemiologic studies have associated infection in certain patient populations with bacterial invasion from the gut. These data suggest bacterial invasion and translocation occur in patients with injury, multiorgan failure, or severe burns.[53–55]

Protein malnutrition affects intestinal cell structure and may increase the susceptibility for bacterial translocation in certain disease states. Li and associates studied the effects of acute 3-day starvation, prolonged protein malnutrition, and endotoxemia in mice, and severe mucosal atrophy was found.[56] Despite markedly diminished villus height and crypt depth, bacterial translocation did not occur. After endotoxin administration in normal mice, bacterial translocation to the mesenteric lymph nodes occurred in 80%.

However, the combination of malnutrition plus endotoxin was associated with an even higher incidence (100%) of translocation to systemic organs and a higher number of bacteria per organ than endotoxemia alone. The mortality rate was related directly to the degree of malnutrition, with increased mortality only among malnourished endotoxic animals. It appears that protein malnutrition in endotoxemia is synergistic with increased mortality. Additional studies from the same group evaluated the mechanism of increased mortality in this animal model.[57] Protein malnutrition in combination with endotoxemia resulted in the highest incidence of bacterial translocation to mesenteric lymph nodes, liver, and spleen (80%, 50%, 60%) compared with malnutrition alone (6%, 0%, 0%) or endotoxemia alone (70%, 5%, 0%), despite the finding that the intestinal barrier to luminal bacteria remained intact after protein malnutrition and was less severely injured after a combination of malnutrition and endotoxin compared with endotoxin alone. These data suggest the very high bacterial translocation rate found in malnutrition and endotoxemia probably is not caused primarily by altered epithelial permeability but may be caused by defects in cell-mediated and reticuloendothelial activity. These data suggest confirmation of a generally held concept of malnutrition's effect of increasing susceptibility to infection.

Enteral nutrition preserves the integrity of intestinal structure and promotes immunocompetence. Administered immediately in stress states, enteral nutrition preserves intestinal structure or returns it toward normal in starvation or after the administration of total parenteral nutrition (TPN).[58] Data suggest early enteral feeding decreases translocation across the gut. Inque and associates studied *Candida albicans* translocation after burn injury in guinea pigs.[59] Enteral nutrition given 3 hours after injury resulted in a 33% decrease in positive *Candida* cultures compared with animals given no nutrition. Data also indicate that some chemically defined liquid diets result in increased intestinal microflora and increased bacterial translocation from the gut. Alverdy and colleagues studied cecal cultures and bacterial translocation rates in normal rats fed usual rat chow, Vivonex, Ensure, Enrich, or Ensure plus ground corn cobs, a crude fiber source.[60] A 66% rate of bacterial translocation to mesenteric lymph nodes was found with Ensure and Enrich, compared with 21% with Vivonex, 20% with Ensure plus ground corn cobs, and 0% in animals fed normal rat chow. Cecal cultures were significantly increased in all feedings except rat chow, suggesting alterations in intestinal flora occur with chemically defined liquid diets in normal animals.

Most authorities agree that nutritional support is important in critically ill patients. Enteral administration of nutritional support is generally preferred as the route of substance delivery compared with TPN, because it is cheaper. Data provide substantial support for this practice and suggest enteral nutrition may affect the development of infection.

A stress-induced rise in catabolic hormones, such as cortisone and glucagon, occurs after injury. The injury stress response is characterized by a hypercatabolic hypermetabolic state. Enteral nutrition initiated as early as 2 hours after injury in an animal model of burn injury suppressed the expected rise in the level of stress hormones.[61] Fong and associates reevaluated the metabolic response to *Esch-*

*erichia coli* in human volunteers receiving TPN or enteral feeding for 7 days before the septic challenge.[62] Counterregulatory hormones and cytokinins (eg, glucagon, epinephrine, tumor necrosis factor) were significantly higher in the TPN group than in the enteral feeding group. In addition to the magnitude of acute phase response, peripheral amino acid mobilization and lactate production were increased with TPN compared with enteral feeding. These data suggest that bowel rest associated with TPN administration produces alterations in host resistance to injury independent of the nutritional status. TPN is also associated with bacterial translocation in the gut. In an animal study, Alverdy and coworkers gave TPN formula intravenously or intragastrically.[63] Fewer animals enterally fed with TPN solution had culture-positive mesenteric lymph nodes (9/27) compared with animals parenterally fed (18/27). Cecal bacterial counts were increased in enterally and parenterally fed groups compared with controlled rats.

Addition of special fuels to enteral nutrition or TPN may be useful in attenuating the catabolic response of critical illness. Amino acids such as glutamine and arginine and omega-3 fatty acids are additions to the diet of critically ill patients that may decrease infectious complications. Glutamine is an abundant free amino acid that was previously considered a nonessential amino acid. Nutritional requirements for the glutamine may increase during critical illness.[64] Glutamine functions as a primary fuel source for intestinal cells.[65] In animal studies, glutamine-enriched TPN is associated with decreased bacterial translocation compared with standard, non–glutamine-containing formulas.[66] In various stress states (eg, shock, sepsis, trauma) associated with decreased bacterial translocation, glutamine-supplemented diets may reduce the incidence of bacterial translocation, promote ''bowel rescue,'' and improve overall survival.[67] Human studies suggest that the addition of glutamine to TPN decreases infection.[68] Arginine may also be useful. In animals, arginine has enhanced wound healing and improved immunologic responses.[69] Few human data in critical illness are available. Omega-3 fatty acids in the diet may modify immune responses. Administration of these fatty acids has diminished the cytokine synthesis in vitro,[70] but the usefulness of this approach in seriously ill patients is unknown.

The preferred route of substance delivery and its effect on infection have been evaluated in a large group of surgical patients with abdominal trauma. Moore and colleagues compared early enteral nutrition, administered by jejunal feeding, with TPN in critically ill injury patients.[71] Nutritional intake (eg, total calories, nitrogen intake, and nitrogen balance) were similar during most periods with TPN or enteral feeding. Traditional nutritional protein makers were better restored in the enteral nutrition group. Infection developed in only 5 (17%) of the enterally fed patients but in 11 (37%) of the TPN group. A significant difference existed in major infections between the two groups. The incidence of major septic morbidity was 3% in patients receiving enteral nutrition compared with 20% receiving TPN. This study suggests early enteral feeding through the gut in a critically injured surgical patient reduces septic complications. The mechanism for the observed decrease in infection may be related to decreased bacterial translocation with enteral nutrition.

## Infectious Complications of Enteral Nutrition

Although early enteral nutrition may be helpful in decreasing the acute injury hypermetabolic response and may decrease the major infectious complications in trauma patients compared with TPN, infectious complications with its use also exist. Microbial growth occurs in the stomach of patients treated prophylactically for stress ulceration with antacids or $H_2$-antagonists. Atherton and White[72] found gastric microbial growth in 9 of 10 mechanically ventilated patients with paralytic ileus. Du Moulin and colleagues[73] later described gastric colonization in ventilated patients receiving antacids or cimetidine and suggested gastric to tracheal transmission had occurred in 17 of 52 patients. Gastric organism growth occurs as a result of gastric pH alteration. Stress ulcer prophylaxis alkalizes the potent antibacterial activity of hydrochloric acid. Microbial growth is virtually nonexistent at a gastric pH of 1 and increases exponentially with increases in gastric pH. Hillman and colleagues found the gastric contents of critically ill patients were acidic and sterile on admission to the intensive care unit.[74] Within 24 to 48 hours after alkalization, multiple organisms including gram-negative bacteria were cultured from the gastric aspirate. Daschner and associates[75] found that 85% of gastric aspirates in 142 critically ill patients developed gastric colonization, with an average of 2.1 bacterial species cultured. Microbial counts of gastric fluid increased significantly with an increase in gastric pH. The sequela of gastric colonization by microbial agents can be nosocomial pneumonia. Du Moulin and colleagues[73] suggested a gastric source of tracheal colonization and resultant nosocomial pneumonia in patients in the ICU, but cultures from the oropharynx, the primary source of tracheal colonization, were not reported in his study.

The frequency with which gastric colonization contributes to tracheal colonization may depend in part on the patient population. Although two thirds of 153 gastric aspirates were found to contain microorganisms in 40 young neurosurgical patients on mechanical ventilation, the stomach was thought to be the source of subsequent tracheal colonization and nosocomial pneumonia in only 1 patient.[76] Approximately one half of these patients were receiving stress ulcer prophylaxis with antacids or ranitidine, and the other half received no prophylactic therapy.

Enteral feeding appears to have a risk of infectious complications, including nosocomial sepsis from contaminated enteral feeding solutions. Bacterial contamination of enteral feeding was found to be responsible for *E. cloacae* sepsis in 10 of 40 patients studied by plasmid profile over a 7-year period.[77] Contamination appeared to result largely from in-hospital preparation of feeding formulas or administration through an open system. Sterile, commercially prepared solutions represent less infectious risk.[78]

A potentially more significant infectious risk of enteral nutrition results from gastric colonization and resultant transmission of gastric organisms to the trachea, with the development of nosocomial pneumonia. Pingleton and associates[79] evaluated simultaneous daily gastric, tracheal, and oropharyngeal cultures in 18 mechanically ventilated patients. Antacids and $H_2$-antagonists were not given. Gastric cultures demonstrated microbial growth in 75% of patients before enteral feeding began. Initial gastric cultures showed a high number of gram-negative and gram-positive organisms. After enteral feeding began, the number of gram-negative isolates increased significantly. Virtually all ventilated patients developed tracheal colonization by day 4. Sources of tracheal colonization included the oropharynx and stomach. Five patients (36%) had gram-negative rods recovered first in the stomach, which were subsequently identified in the trachea. Definite or probable nosocomial pneumonia occurred in 11 (62%) of 18 patients. Of three infections identified during the 5-day study period, 1 patient had nosocomial pneumonia due to a gram-negative rod first recovered in the stomach.

The mechanism of transfer of organisms from the stomach to the trachea is clearly aspiration, with esophageal reflux being the initial mechanism. The incidence of pulmonary aspiration reported with gastric intubation by feeding tubes varies widely, ranging from 0.8% to 77%.[80–85] In a review of 253 hospitalized patients treated with enteral nutritional support, only 2 patients (0.8%) were diagnosed with aspiration pneumonia.[82] Metheny and associates found physician-documented clinical aspiration occurred in only 5.7% (6/150) of patients.[82] If aspiration was detected by glucose-positive endotracheal secretions, aspiration was diagnosed in 21% of mechanically ventilated patients.[83] Likewise, 77% (24/31) of tracheally intubated patients were found to aspirate, as determined by the presence of methylene blue in tracheal secretions.[84] It is difficult to draw general conclusions about the effect of feeding tubes from these studies, because all differ in the population studied, study design, method of diagnosing aspiration, and size of enteral feeding tube.

Multiple factors can affect the frequency and severity of aspiration. The presence of an endotracheal tube and the type of endotracheal tube influence the incidence of aspiration. With high-volume, low-pressure endotracheal cuffs, aspiration decreased by 20% from that with low-volume, high-pressure cuffs.[86] Other risk factors for aspiration include a reduced level of consciousness, with consequential compromise in glottic closure, the presence of an artificial airway, and ileus or gastroparesis.

One of the most important factors in aspiration in patients receiving enteral nutrition is patient position. Nagler and Spiro studied acid reflux in normal volunteers with nasogastric tubes in the supine and 10°, 30°, and 45° positions and sitting upright. After a large volume of acid was instilled into the stomach, aspiration as detected by a fall in esophageal pH occurred only in the supine position.[87] Torres and colleagues found similar results when they studied pulmonary aspiration by scintiscanning tracheal secretions after isotopic labeling of enteral nutrition.[88] All patients received nutrition through a 5-mm nasogastric tube. Radioactive counts were four times higher in the supine position than in the semirecumbent positions. These data suggest that body position is a more important determinant of reflux and aspiration than the presence of a nasogastric tube.

Another important variable in gastroesophageal reflux is the duration of the supine position. Prolongation of time spent in the supine position can cause reflux. Torres and associates found time-dependent aspiration: increasing aspiration, as determined by scintiscanning of tracheal secretions in ventilated patients, with longer time in the supine position.[88] Counts per minute of radioisotope increased 650% from the first to the sixth hour of study when the patients were supine. Vinnik and Kern found esophageal pH decreased in 1 of 6 volunteers only after 68 hours of gastric intubation.[89]

The route of nutrient delivery is thought to be important in decreasing aspiration. Intragastric feeding has been suggested as resulting in less aspiration than intrajejunal feeding. Strong and associates found no difference in physician-diagnosed aspiration when hospitalized patients were fed in the stomach or by the jejunal route.[90]

The size of the feeding tube has been thought to affect aspiration. Small-bore feeding tubes are recommended to decrease gastroesophageal reflux and pulmonary aspiration, but data supporting this recommendation are controversial. No aspiration of methylene blue-dyed tube feedings was found in 30 ventilated patients with small-bore (8Fr) feeding tubes.[81] In contrast, bore size of feeding tubes was not a significant variable in witnessed aspiration or aspiration pneumonia in hospitalized patients.[85] Similar results were reported by Metheny and coworkers, who found small-bore feeding tubes had been used in 3 of 5 patients with physician-reported aspiration.[82] Many study differences make these data difficult to interpret. One study found no difference in radionuclide-detected aspiration with large (14Fr) nasogastric tubes compared with small (8Fr) tubes in 10 normal volunteers.[91]

Even if small-bore tubes are used, aspiration can easily occur if the tube is malpositioned. A retrospective study of adult patients showed a 40% incidence of inadvertent dislodgement of the feeding tube.[92] This was not a critically ill patient population, but all patients with displaced tubes were confused, disoriented, or obtunded periodically. These data agree with a prospective evaluation of a similar patient population, in which a 62% incidence of inadvertent dislodgement was observed.[93] Dislodgement increases the risk of aspiration, although the precise incidence of this complication has not been evaluated in an ICU population. Boscoe and Rosin described two cases of pulmonary aspiration in patients with fine-bore nasogastric tubes.[94] Aspiration occurred after the tubes were inadvertently displaced.

Enteral feeding tubes are not the sole culprit in aspiration. Cole and colleagues described significant aspiration detected by radionuclide studies in a patient with percutaneous gastroscopy.[95]

## CONCLUSIONS

Malnutrition has multiple effects on lung function, including diminished respiratory strength and ventilatory drive, which may increase the likelihood of pneumonia. More specifically, malnutrition alters lung defense mechanisms. Nutritional support in sick patients can replenish nutritional deficits. Enteral nutrition can offer the advantage of decreased bacterial translocation in the gut, theoretically decreasing the risk of infection. Complications of nutritional support also occur, especially aspiration resulting in nosocomial pneumonia. Specific management strategies decrease the risk of aspiration.

## REFERENCES

1. Niederman MS: Malnutrition and host lung defenses: Implications for the pathogenesis and prevention of pneumonia. *In* Ferranti RD,

Rampulla C, Fracchia C, Ambrosino N (eds): Nutrition and Ventilatory Function. Verona, Italy, Bi & Gi Publishers s.r.l., 1992:87–98.

1a. Martin TR: The relationship between malnutrition and lung infections. Clin Chest Med 8:359–372, 1987.

2. Vandenburgh E, Van de Woestigne K, Gyselen A: Weight changes in the terminal stages of chronic obstructive lung disease. Am Rev Respir Dis 96:556–565, 1967.

3. Renzetti AD, McClement JH, Litt BD: The Veterans Administration Cooperative Study of Pulmonary Function. Mortality in relation to respiratory function in chronic obstructive pulmonary disease. Am J Med 41:115–129, 1966.

4. Hunter AMB, Carey MA, Larsh HU: The nutritional status of patients with chronic obstructive pulmonary disease. Am Rev Respir Dis 124:376–381, 1981.

5. Wilson D, Wright E, Rodgers R, et al: Body weight in COPD. Am Rev Respir Dis 135:A144, 1987.

6. Driver AG, McAlvey MT, Smith JL: Nutritional assessment of patients with chronic obstructive pulmonary disease and acute respiratory failure. Chest 82A:568–571, 1982.

7. Pingleton SK, Eulberg M: Nutritional analysis of acute respiratory failure (abstract). Chest 84:A343, 1983.

8. Driver AG, LeBrun M: Iatrogenic malnutrition in patients receiving ventilatory support. JAMA 244:2195–2196, 1980.

9. Harmon G, Pingleton SK, Hanson FN, et al: Computer-assisted nutritional therapy (CANT) in the intensive care unit. Am Rev Respir Dis 131:A152, 1985.

10. Rochester DF, Esau SA: Malnutrition and respiratory system. Chest 85:411–415, 1984.

11. Weiner P, Suo J, Fernandez E, et al: The effect of hyperinflation on respiratory muscle strength and efficiency in healthy subjects and patients with asthma. Am Rev Respir Dis 141:1501–1505, 1990.

12. Lands L, Desmond KJ, Demizio D, et al: The effects of nutritional status and hyperinflation on respiratory muscle strength in children and young adults. Am Rev Respir Dis 141:1506–1509, 1990.

13. Braun NMT, Arora NS, Rochester DF: Respiratory muscle and pulmonary function in proximal myopathies. Thorax 38:616–623, 1983.

14. Rochester DF, Braun NMT: Determinants of maximal inspiratory pressure in chronic obstructive pulmonary disease. Am Rev Respir Dis 132:42–47, 1985.

15. Cahil G: Starvation in man. N Engl J Med 282:668–675, 1970.

16. Long CL, Birkham RH, Geiger JW: Contribution of skeletal muscle protein in elevated rates of whole body protein catabolism in trauma patients. Am J Clin Nutr 34:1087–1093, 1981.

17. Thurlbeck WM: Diaphragm and body weight in emphysema. Thorax 33:483–487, 1978.

18. Arora NS, Rochester DF: Effect of body weight and muscularity on human diaphragm muscle mass, thickness and area. J Appl Physiol 52:64–70, 1982.

19. Rochester DF, Arora NS, Braun NMT: Maximum contractile force of human diaphragm muscle, determined in vitro. Trans Am Clin Climatol Assoc 82:200–208, 1981.

20. Kelsen SG, Ference M, Kapoor S: Effects of prolonged undernutrition on structure and function of the diaphragm. J Appl Physiol 58:1354–1359, 1985.

21. Lewis MI, Sieck GV, Fournier M, et al: Effect of nutritional deprivation on diaphragm contractility and muscle fiber size. J Appl Physiol 68:1938–1944, 1986.

22. Arora NS, Rochester DF: Respiratory muscle strength and maximal voluntary ventilation in undernourished patients. Am Rev Respir Dis 126:5–8, 1982.

23. O'Neill S, Leahy F, Pasterkamp H, Tal A: The effects of chronic hyperinflation, nutritional status and posture on respiratory muscle strength in cystic fibrosis. Am Rev Respir Dis 128:1051–1054, 1983.

24. Szeinbers A, England S, Mindorff C, et al: Maximal inspiratory and expiratory pressures are reduced in hyperinflated, malnourished, young adult males with cystic fibrosis. Am Rev Respir Dis 132:766–769, 1985.

25. Kelly SM, Rosa A, Field S, et al: Inspiratory muscle strength and body composition in patients receiving total parenteral nutrition therapy. Am Rev Respir Dis 130:33–37, 1984.

26. Murciano D, Armengauk MH, Rigaurd D, et al: Effect of renutrition on respiratory and diaphragmatic function in patients with severe mental anorexia. Am Rev Respir Dis 141:A547, 1990.

27. Zwillich CW, Sahn SA, Weil JV: Effects of hypermetabolism on ventilation and chemosensitivity. J Clin Invest 60:900–906, 1977.

28. Keys A, Brozek J, Henschel A, et al: Biology of Human Starvation. Minneapolis, University of Minnesota Press, 1950.

29. Doekel RC Jr, Zwillich CW, Scoggin CH: Clinical semi-starvation: Depression of hypoxic ventilatory response. N Engl J Med 295:358–361, 1976.

30. Askanazi J, Rosenbaum SH, Hyman AI, et al: Effects of parenteral nutrition on ventilatory drive. Anesthesiology 53(Suppl 1):185, 1980.

31. Niederman MS, Fein AM: The interaction of infection and the adult respiratory distress syndrome. Crit Care Clin 2:471–495, 1986.

32. Niederman MS: Bacterial adherence as a mechanism of airway colonization. Eur J Clin Microbiol Infect Dis 8:15–20, 1986.

33. Skerrett SJ, Niederman MS, Fein AN: Respiratory infections and acute lung injury in systemic illness. Clin Chest Med 10:469–502, 1989.

34. Niederman MS, Merrill WW, Ferranti RD, et al: Nutritional status and bacterial binding in the lower respiratory tract in chronic tracheostomy. Ann Intern Med 100:795–800, 1984.

35. Niederman MS, Mantovani R, Schoch P, et al: Patterns and routes of tracheobronchial colonization in mechanically ventilated patients: The role of nutritional status in colonization of the lower airway by *Pseudomonas* species. Chest 95:155–161, 1989.

36. Ortqvist A, Hammers-Berggren S, Kalin M: Respiratory tract colonization and incidence of secondary infection during hospital treatment of community-acquired pneumonia. Eur J Clin Microbiol Infect Dis 9:725–731, 1990.

37. Higuchi JH, Johanson WG: The relationship between adherence of *Pseudomonas aeruginosa* to upper respiratory cells in vitro and susceptibility to colonization in vivo. J Lab Clin Med 95:698–705, 1980.

38. Green GM, Kass EH: Factors influencing the clearance of bacteria by the lung. J Clin Invest 43:769–776, 1964.

39. Shennib H, Chiu RCJ, Mulder DS, et al: Depression and delayed recovery of alveolar macrophage function during starvation and refeeding. Surg Gynecol Obstet 158:535–540, 1984.

40. Martin TR, Altman LC, Alvares OF: The effects of severe protein-calorie malnutrition on antibacterial defense mechanisms in the rat lung. Am Rev Respir Dis 128:1013–1019, 1983.

41. Skerrett SJ, Henderson WR, Martin TR: Alveolar macrophage function in rats with severe protein calorie malnutrition: Arachidonic acid metabolism, cytokine release, and antimicrobial activity. J Immunol 144:1052–1061, 1990.

42. Anderson DC, Krishna GS, Hughes BJ, et al: Impaired polymorphonuclear leukocyte motility in malnourished infants: Relationship to functional abnormalities of cell adherence. J Lab Clin Med 101:881–895, 1983.

43. Chandra RK: Cell-mediated immunity in nutritional imbalance. Fed Proc 39:3088–3092, 1980.

44. Niederman MS, Merrill WW, Polomski S, et al: Influence of sputum IgA and elastase on tracheal cell bacterial adherence. Am Rev Respir Dis 133:255–260, 1986.

45. Phillips I, Wharton F: Acute bacterial infection in kwashiorkor and marasmus. Br Med J 1:407–409, 1968.

46. Brown KH, Gilman RH, Gaffar A, et al: Infections associated with severe protein-calorie malnutrition in hospitalized infants and children. Nutr Res 1:33–46, 1981.

47. Mullen JL, Gertner MH, Buzby GP, et al: Implications of malnutrition in the surgical patient. Arch Surg 114:121–125, 1979.

48. Nwiloh J, Freeman H, McCord C: Malnutrition: An important determinant of fatal outcome in surgically treated pulmonary suppurative disease. J Natl Med Assoc 81:525–529, 1989.

49. Pingleton SK: Complication of acute respiratory failure. Am Rev Respir Dis 137:1463–1493, 1988.

50. Wilmore DW, Smith RJ, O'Dwyer SY, et al: The Gut: A central organ after surgical stress. Surgery 104:917–923, 1988.

51. Berg RD: Bacterial translocation from the gastrointestinal tracts of mice receiving immunosuppressive chemotherapeutic agent. Curr Top Microbiol Immunol 8:285–292, 1983.

52. Ambrose NS, Johnson M, Burden DW, et al: Incidence of pathogenic bacteria from mesenteric lymph nodes and ileal serosa during Crohns' disease surgery. Br J Surg 71:623–625, 1984.

53. Border JR, Hassett J, LaDuca J, et al: The gut origin septic state in blunt multiple trauma (ISS + 40) in the ICU. Ann Surg 206:425–427, 1987.

54. Carrico CJ, Meakins JL, Marshall JC, et al: Multiple-organ failure syndrome. Arch Surg 121:196–208, 1986.

55. Jarrett F, Balish E, Moylan JA, et al: Clinical experience with prophylactic antibiotic bowel suppression in burn patients. Surgery 83:523–527, 1978.

56. Li M, Specian RD, Berg RD, et al: Effects of protein malnutrition and

endotoxin on the intestinal mucosal barrier to the translocation of indigenous flora in mice. JPEN 13:572–578, 1989.

57. Dietch EA, Winterton J, Berg R: The gut as a portal of entry for bacteremia: Role of protein malnutrition. Ann Surg 205:681–692, 1987.

58. Lo CW, Walker WA: Changes in the gastrointestinal tract during enteral or parenteral feeding. Nutr Rev 47:193–198, 1989.

59. Inque S, Epstein MD, Alexander JW, et al: Prevention of yeast translocation across the gut by a single enteral feeding after burn injury. JPEN 13:565–571, 1989.

60. Alverdy JC, Aoys E, Moss GS: Effect of commercially available chemically defined liquid diets on the intestinal microflora and bacterial translocation from the gut. JPEN 14:1–6, 1990.

61. Saito H, Trocki O, Alexander JU, et al: The effect of nutrient administration on the nutritional state, catabolic hormone secretion and gut mucosal integrity after burn injury. JPEN 11:1–7, 1987.

62. Fong Y, Marano MA, Barber A, et al: Total parenteral nutrition and bowel rest modify the metabolic response to endotoxin in humans. Ann Surg 210:449–455, 1989.

63. Alverdy JC, Aoys E, Moss GS: Total parenteral nutrition promotes bacterial translocation from the gut. Surgery 104:185–190, 1988.

64. Wilmore DW, Black PR, Muhlbacher F: Injured man: Trauma and sepsis. *In* Winters RW, Greene HL (eds): Nutritional Support of the Seriously Ill Patient. New York, Academic Press, 1983:33–52.

65. Windmueller HG: Glutamine utilization by the small intestine. Adv Enzymol Relat Areas Mol Biol 53:201–237, 1982.

66. Salloum RM, Souba WW, Klimbers VS, et al: Glutamine is superior to glutamate in supporting gut metabolism, stimulating intestinal glutaminase activity and preventing bacterial translocation. Surg Forum 40:6, 1989.

67. Souba WW, Herskowitz K, Austgen TR, et al: Glutamine nutrition: Theoretical considerations and therapeutic impact. JPEN 14(suppl 1):237S–243S, 1990.

68. Scheltinga MR, Young LS, Benfell K, et al: Glutamine enriched intravenous feedings attenuate extracellular fluids expansion after a standard stress. Ann Surg 214:385–395, 1991.

69. Barbul A: Arginine: Biochemistry, physiology, and therapeutic implications. JPEN 10:227–238, 1986.

70. Endres S, Ghorbani R, Kelley VE, et al: The effect of dietary supplementation with n-3 polyunsaturated fatty acids on the synthesis of interleukin-1 and tumor necrosis factor by mononuclear cells. N Engl J Med 320:265–271, 1989.

71. Moore FA, Moore EE, Jones TN, et al: TEN versus TPN following major abdominal trauma–reduced septic morbidity. J Trauma 29:916–923, 1989.

72. Atherton ST, White DJ: Stomach as source of bacteria colonizing respiratory tract during artificial ventilation. Lancet 2:968–969, 1978.

73. DuMoulin GC, Paterson DB, et al: Aspiration of gastric bacteria in antacid-treated patients. Lancet 1:242, 1982.

74. Hillman KM, Riodan T, O'Farrell SM, et al: Colonization of the gastric contents in critically ill patients. Crit Care Med 109:444–447, 1982.

75. Daschner F, Kappstein I, Reuschenbach K, et al: Stress ulcer prophylaxis and ventilation pneumonia: Prevention by antibacterial cytoprotective agents. Infect Control Hosp Epidemiol 9:59–65, 1988.

76. Reusser P, Scheidegger D, Marbet GA, et al: Role of gastric colonization in nosocomial infections and endotoxemia: A prospective study in neurosurgical patients on mechanical ventilation. J Infect Dis 160:414–420, 1989.

77. Levy J, Van Laethem Y, Verhaegen G, et al: Contaminated enteral nutrition solutions as a cause of nosocomial bloodstream infection: A study using plasmid fingerprinting. JPEN 13:228–234, 1989.

78. Freedland CP, Roller RD, Wolfe BM, et al: Microbial contamination of continuous drip feedings. JPEN 13:18–22, 1989.

79. Pingleton SK, Hinthorn D, Lui C: Enteral nutrition in patients receiving mechanical ventilation. Am J Med 80:827–832, 1986.

80. Treloar DM, Stechmiller J: Pulmonary aspiration in tube fed patients with artificial airways. Heart Lung 15:256–261, 1986.

81. Cataldi-Betcher EL, Seltzer MH, et al: Complications occurring during enteral nutrition support: A prospective study. JPEN 7:546–552, 1983.

82. Metheny NA, Eisenberg P, Spies M: Aspiration pneumonia in patients fed through nasoenteral tubes. Heart Lung 15:256–261, 1986.

83. Kingston GW, Phang PT, Leathley MJ: Increased incidence of nosocomial pneumonia in mechanically ventilated patients with subclinical aspiration. Am J Surg 161:589–592, 1991.

84. Elpern EH, Jacobs ER, Bone RC: Incidence of aspiration in tracheally intubated adults. Heart Lung 16:527–531, 1987.

85. Mullan H, Roubenoff RA, Roubenoff R: Risk of pulmonary aspiration among patients receiving enteral nutrition support. JPEN 16:160–164, 1992.

86. Andrews MJ, Pearson FG: Incidence and pathogenesis of tracheal injury following cuffed tube tracheostomy with assisted ventilation. Ann Surg 173:249–263, 1971.

87. Nagler R, Spiro HM: Persistent gastroesophageal reflux induced during prolonged gastric intubation. N Engl J Med 269:495–500, 1963.

88. Torres A, Serra-Batlles J, Ros E, et al: Pulmonary aspiration of gastric contents in patients receiving mechanical ventilation: The effect of body position. Ann Intern Med 116:540–543, 1992.

89. Vinnik IE, Kern F: The effect of gastric intubation on esophageal pH. Gastroenterology 47:388–394, 1964.

90. Strong RM, Condon SC, Solinger MR, et al: Equal aspiration rates from post-pylorus and intra-gastric placed small-bore nasoenteral feeding tubes. JPEN 16:59–63, 1992.

91. Dotson R, Robinson R, Pingleton SK: The effect of nasogastric tube size on gastroesophageal reflux. Am Rev Respir Dis 143:A683, 1991.

92. Meer JA: Inadvertent dislodgment of nasoenteral feeding tubes: Incidence and prevention. JPEN 11:187–189, 1987.

93. Silk DBA, Rees RG, Keohane PP, et al: Clinical efficacy and design changes of "fine bore" nasogastric feeding tubes: A seven-year experience involving 809 intubations in 403 patients. JPEN 11:378–383, 1987.

94. Boscoe MJ, Rosin MD: Fine bore enteral feeding and pulmonary aspiration. Br Med J 289:1421–1422, 1984.

95. Cole MJ, Smith JT, Molnar C, et al: Aspiration after percutaneous gastrostomy: Assessment by Tc-99m labeling of the enteral feed. J Clin Gastroenterol 9:90–95, 1987.

# Clinical Approach to Upper and Lower Respiratory Tract Infections in Specific Populations

# CHAPTER 7

# Upper Respiratory Tract Infections: Pharyngitis, Sinusitis, Otitis Media, and Epiglottitis

DAVID M. BAMBERGER and MARY ANNE JACKSON

## PHARYNGITIS

Pharyngitis is one of the most common diseases treated in clinical practice, accounting for 40 million physician visits annually in the United States.[1] Despite its high incidence, many practical questions concerning the causes, diagnosis, and treatment of pharyngitis remain unanswered.

### Etiology

The causes of pharyngitis are listed in Table 7–1. The most common causes of pharyngitis are group A β-hemolytic streptococci and the respiratory viruses: rhinoviruses, coronaviruses, adenonviruses, influenza, and parainfluenza viruses. Studies have suggested that *Chlamydia pneumoniae* also may be a common cause of pharyngitis.[2] In approximately one third of patients, no pathogen can be identified despite extensive evaluation.[2] *Corynebacterium diphtheriae*, once a common infection in North America, is now exceedingly rare. In the last decade, no more than five cases were reported annually in the United States.[3]

The role of non-group A β-hemolytic streptococci, such as group C or G, as pathogens in pharyngitis remains controversial. Non-group A streptococci have been associated with outbreaks of pharyngitis, but in endemic settings, most studies have suggested that non-group A β-hemolytic streptococci are isolated from healthy persons as often as they are isolated from patients with pharyngitis.[4] However, two studies of young adults in an endemic setting demonstrated a higher rate of isolation of group C β-hemolytic streptococci from patients with pharyngitis than from controls.[5, 6] A community-wide outbreak of group G β-hemolytic streptococci in children also was reported.[7] Foodborne outbreaks of pharyngitis have been attributed to group C and G streptococci.[8]

*C. pneumoniae* has emerged as a potentially important common pathogen causing pharyngitis in young adults.[2, 9] Previous reports suggesting an important role of *Chlamydia trachomatis* based on serologic evidence of infection were probably influenced by crossreactivity with *C. pneumoniae*.[9] *C. trachomatis* was reported as a cause of pharyngitis in a sexually active young adult with a concomitant genital infection,[10] but the agent is isolated from the pharynx from a small percentage of sexually active adults without pharyngeal symptoms.[11]

*Mycoplasma pneumoniae*, a common cause of bronchitis and pneumonia, can cause pharyngitis.[12] *M. pneumoniae* is commonly cultured from the pharynxes of patients with pharyngitis,[2] and in a study based on serologic evidence of infection in adults, it was found to cause 10.6% of pharyngeal infections.[1] In several controlled studies, *M. pneumoniae* was not found more frequently in patients with pharyngitis than in healthy controls,[8] and the role of *M. pneumoniae* as an etiologic agent in patients presenting with a primary complaint of pharyngitis is probably minor.

Table 7–1. **Causes of Pharyngitis**

Bacteria
    Group A streptococci
    Group C streptococci*
    Group G streptococci*
    *Corynebacterium diphtheriae*
    *Corynebacterium ulcerans*
    *Arcanobacterium hemolyticum*
    *Yersinia enterocolitica*
    *Francisella tularensis*
    *Treponema pallidum*
    Mixed anaerobes
    *Chlamydia pneumoniae*
    *Chlamydia trachomatis**
    *Mycoplasma pneumoniae*
    *Mycoplasma hominis*
    *Legionella pneumophila**
    *Haemophilus influenzae**
    *Staphylococcus aureus* (eg, toxic shock syndrome)
Viruses
    Rhinoviruses†
    Respiratory syncytial virus†
    Coronaviruses†
    Enteroviruses
    Influenza A and B
    Epstein-Barr virus
    Parainfluenza virus
    Herpes simplex virus
    Cytomegalovirus
    Human immunodeficiency virus
    Rubella
    Rubeola
Fungi
    *Candida albicans* (eg, thrush)
Noninfectious causes
    Bullous pemphigoid
    Systemic lupus erythematosus
    Behçet syndrome
    Syndrome of periodic fever, pharyngitis, and stomatitis
    Kawasaki syndrome
    Paraquat ingestion
    Tracheal intubation
    Mucositis of chemotherapy
    Stevens-Johnson syndrome

*Its role as a true pathogen is controversial.
†It more commonly causes rhinitis or nasopharyngitis than pharyngitis alone.

## Epidemiology

Group A streptococci are most commonly observed in school-aged children from November to April. The incidence is lower among adults and children younger than 2 years of age than in school-aged children.[4, 13] Conversely, *C. pneumoniae* and *Arcanobacterium hemolyticum*[14] infections are more likely in young adults than in children. Influenza and coronaviruses are typically the causes of infections during the winter months, enteroviruses in the summer and fall, and rhinoviruses and parainfluenza viruses in the fall and spring. Humans provide a reservoir for the most common pathogens. Outbreaks of *Yersinia enterocolitica* pharyngitis have been attributed to contaminated pasteurized milk,[15] *Corynebacterium ulcerans* infections to raw milk, and tonsillopharyngeal tularemia to ingestion of improperly cooked rabbit meat or hand-to-mouth contact after handling infected animals.[16]

## Pathophysiology

The M protein of the cell wall of the structurally complex group A streptococcus is a crucial marker for virulence because of the protein's capacity to impede phagocytosis by polymorphonuclear leukocytes. There are more than 80 antigenically distinct M proteins. Infection is usually acquired by person-to-person contact through droplets of saliva or nasal secretions. During the acute phase of infection, there are a large number of M-typable organisms in the nose and the pharynx. If the patient is left untreated, the organisms disappear from the nose but persist in the tonsillar pharynx for long periods, although the patient has the acute symptoms of pharyngitis for a few days. Over several weeks, the colony counts in the pharynx decrease, infectivity decreases, and the M-protein content and virulence diminish.[17] If rheumatic fever occurs, it usually develops 3 to 5 weeks after an acute infection.[12] The persistence of the organism (ie, carriage) in the pharynx often makes defining an acute infection in a patient with clinical pharyngitis confusing.

*C. diphtheriae* is spread through respiratory droplets or direct contact with respiratory secretions or exudate from infected skin. The organism is not invasive; its main pathogenic mechanism is the production of a polypeptide exotoxin, which is encoded on a gene of a lysogenic β-phage. The polypeptide has two segments: B, which binds to specific receptors, and A, which enters the host cell and inactivates elongation factor 2, a necessary step in polypeptide formation in eukaryotic ribosomes. As a result of local toxin production, a dense coagulum of fibrin, leukocytes, respiratory cells, and organisms forms a pseudomembrane over the tonsils, pharynx, and nasal epithelium. Suffocation may result from membrane aspiration. The diffuse effects of toxin production include myocarditis, demyelination of nerves with resultant cranial and peripheral neuropathy, and acute tubular necrosis of the kidneys.

## Clinical Manifestations

The manifestations of the usual causes of pharyngitis are shown in Table 7–2. No clinical features are diagnostic of a specific cause, but fever, tonsillar exudate, and tender cervical lympadenopathy increases the likelihood of a group A streptococcal infection, and a cough, itchy eyes, or coryza decreases the likelihood.[18] Abdominal pain, nausea, and vomiting occur with streptococcal pharyngitis, especially in children, and infants may have excoriated nares. A history of sexual practices is important in the diagnosis of gonorrhea, syphilis, *C. trachomatis*, herpes simplex virus, and the pharyngitis associated with acute human immunodeficiency virus (HIV) infection. Particularly severe or life-threatening pharyngitis may be secondary to *Y. enterocolitica*[19] or anaerobic pharyngitis associated with jugular vein septic thrombophlebitis caused by *Fusobacterium necrophorum* (Lemierre disease).

The complications of group A streptococcal pharyngitis are suppurative and nonsuppurative. The suppurative complications include peritonsillar abscesses, retropharyngeal abscesses, otitis media, acute sinusitis, cervical adenitis, and pneumonia. Rarely, patients may develop meningitis, brain abscess, thrombosis of intracranial venous sinuses, or metastatic foci of infection due to bacteremia. The nonsuppurative complications of group A streptococcal pharyngitis are rheumatic fever and acute glomerulonephritis. *Streptococ-*

Table 7–2. **Clinical Features of Pharyngitis**

| Organism | Fever | Exudate | Cervical Adenopathy | Oral Findings | Other Findings |
|---|---|---|---|---|---|
| Group A streptococci | Common | Common | Common | Palatal petechiae, strawberry tongue | Scarlet fever |
| Rhinoviruses, respiratory syncytial virus, coronaviruses | Mild | Uncommon | Minimal | | Coryza |
| Adenovirus | Moderate | Common | Moderate | | Conjunctivitis, cough |
| Influenza | Common | | | | Coryza, myalgia, cough |
| Parainfluenza | Moderate | | Occasional | | Croup |
| Herpes simplex | Moderate | Occasional | Occasional | Vesicles, ulcers | |
| Enteroviruses | Moderate | Occasional | Occasional | Small vesicles | Rash |
| Epstein-Barr virus | Common | Common | Comon (posterior) | Petechiae | Splenomegaly |
| Chlamydia pneumoniae | Moderate | | | | Bronchitis, pneumonia |
| Arcanobacterium hemolyticum | Moderate | Moderate | Moderate | | Scarlatiniform rash |
| Corynebacterium diphtheriae | Common | Membranous | Moderate | | Neuritis, carditis |
| Mycoplasma pneumoniae | Common | | Occasional | | Bronchitis, pneumonia |
| Mixed anaerobes | Mild | Purulent membrane, foul odor | Mild | | Lemierre disease |

*cus zooepidemicus*, a group C streptococcus, has also been associated with glomerulonephritis,[5] but only group A streptococci cause rheumatic fever. A group A streptococcal toxic shock syndrome has been described in adults and children.

**Diagnosis**

The major decision in evaluating a patient is whether to administer antimicrobials to treat group A streptococcal pharyngitis. The prevalence of group A streptococci in patients with pharyngitis is usually between 5% and 40%, depending on the age of the patient, the clinical findings, the season, the prevalence in the community, and the setting (ie, a higher prevalence is observed in emergency centers than in office practice). Approximately half of children with pharyngitis and positive throat culture for group A streptococci do not have serologic evidence of infection. Patients with positive throat cultures without serologic evidence of infection respond to antimicrobials to a greater degree than those without positive cultures, a result that diminishes the utility of streptococcal antibody testing in differentiating the streptococcal carrier state from true streptococcal infection.[20] Because there is an inherent delay in the use of antibody detection, a patient with pharyngitis and a positive culture for group A streptococci is assumed to have a streptococcal infection.

Assuming an adequate technique for obtaining the pharyngeal culture, which requires a vigorous scrub of the tonsillar pillars and posterior pharynx under direct visualization, the sensitivity of a positive culture in detecting group A streptococci in most microbiology laboratories is in the range of 80% to 90%.[18] Over the past decade, many rapid tests that detect group A streptococcal antigen have been developed. Most have a very high specificity (95%–99%) but only moderate sensitivity (70%–90%) compared with throat culture.

Decisions regarding initial treatment without culturing, treatment on the basis of a rapid test or culture, or no treatment are made on the basis of the severity of the disease, the likelihood of a positive culture, the compliance of the patient, the likelihood of suppurative and nonsuppur-

ative complications, and cost. The relatively ill adult patient may be treated for streptococcal pharyngitis without the need for culture documentation if four of the following criteria are found: high fever, tender cervical lympadenopathy, exudate, absence of cough, and presentation to an emergency center.[18] If the illness is moderate, treatment can be initiated on the basis of a positive antigen test, with a culture performed if the antigen test is negative. If the illness is mild or the likelihood of group A streptococcal infection is low, treatment decisions can be made on the basis of a culture without antigen testing, assuming the physician has the ability to contact the patient regarding the results. The American Academy of Pediatrics has recommended that children with suggestive or classic findings of streptococcal pharyngitis should have a throat culture.[21] The throat culture helps to establish the presence of streptococcal disease and is helpful in the management of contacts who subsequently become ill. Adults or children younger than 2 years of age who are without fever, exudate, or tender cervical lymphadenopathy and who have symptoms more compatible with a viral upper respiratory tract infection need not be cultured.

**Treatment**

The goals of treatment of group A streptococcal pharyngitis include decreasing disease morbidity, lessening the chance of suppurative and nonsuppurative complications, and decreasing the contagiousness of the patient. Several studies have provided evidence that early initiation of penicillin alleviates the symptoms of streptococcal pharyngitis.[22] However, streptococcal pharyngitis is usually a self-limited disease, and treatment with penicillin shortens the duration of the clinical illness by approximately 24 hours.[18] Early treatment does not increase the likelihood of disease recurrence.[23] Treatment with penicillin lessens the incidences of suppurative complications and rheumatic fever by at least 10-fold. There is not convincing evidence that penicillin reduces the incidence of glomerulonephritis. Virtually all patients are no longer contagious 24 hours after the initiation of penicillin.

The American Heart Association recommends penicillin

for the treatment of streptococcal pharyngitis except in patients with a history of penicillin allergy.[24] Therapy can be a single administration of intramuscular benzathine penicillin (600,000 U if < 27 kg; 1,200,000 U if > 27 kg) or penicillin V (250 mg orally three times a day for 10 days). Although not contained within current American Heart Association recommendations, Gerber and associates[25] found that 250 mg of penicillin V twice daily is effective. Oral erythromycin estolate or ethylsuccinate should be used for the penicillin-allergic patient. Strains of group A streptococci resistant to erythromycin have been reported, including a large-scale outbreak in Finland.[26] Sulfonamides, trimethoprim, tetracyclines, and chloramphenicol are not recommended.

Bacteriologically defined treatment failures after penicillin therapy occur in 5% to 35% of patients, with higher rates reported in the last 15 years than in the 1950s and 1960s.[22, 27] Many mechanisms have been postulated to explain the high failure rate, including antimicrobial tolerance; the presence of β-lactamase-producing bacteria such as *Staphylococcus aureus, Haemophilus* spp., *Moraxella* spp., and anaerobes in the upper respiratory tract; a high proportion of streptococcal carriers among treatment failures; a lack of compliance; and reinfection from household contacts. None of these mechanisms, however, fully explains the problem with treatment failures. Several studies found no evidence that failures were caused by penicillin tolerance[27, 28] or the presence of β-lactamase-producing staphylococci in the pharynx.[22]

Some studies have suggested that alternative regimens may be more effective than penicillin, including the addition of rifampin to the last 4 days of penicillin V for treatment of acute disease,[29] the use of dicloxacillin for treatment failures,[28] or the use of clindamycin for treatment of group A streptococcal carriage.[30] Several studies utilizing a variety of oral cephalosporins have resulted in small but statistically significant higher bacteriologic cure rates and fewer clinical failures when compared with oral penicillin.[30a] Penicillin should remain the treatment of choice for acute disease. If symptomatic relapses occur, one of the alternative regimens should be considered. Pichichero has suggested that in communities with high rates of penicillin failures, cephalosporins should be considered as first-line therapy.[30a] Daily administration of cefadroxil for 10 days, or azithromycin for 5 days in adults only , may improve patient compliance.[31] Cultures of family members should be considered in cases of symptomatic recurrence.

Tonsillectomy was previously commonly performed to prevent recurrent streptococcal pharyngitis. Paradise and colleagues found that tonsillectomy did reduce infection rates for 2 years, but by the third year, the differences were no longer significant. In the nonsurgical group, infection rates declined over time, and by year 3, only 5% had more than one moderate or severe episode of pharyngitis per year.[32]

Diphtheria is usually treated with erythromycin, gonococcal pharyngitis with ceftriaxone, and yersinial pharyngitis with aminoglycosides, trimethoprim-sulfamethoxazole, or third-generation cephalosporins. *A. hemolyticum* responds to benzathine penicillin or erythromycin.[14] Although *C. pneumoniae* and *M. pneumoniae* are susceptible to tetracyclines and erythromycin in vitro, no clinical trials for the treatment of pharyngitis due to these pathogens have

been performed. In a trial of treatment of pharyngitis due to organisms other than group A streptococci, erythromycin had minimal efficacy and was associated with a high incidence of side effects.[33]

## SINUSITIS

Sinusitis is a common disease with significant morbidity. There were almost 16 million physician visits for sinusitis in 1989 in the United States.[34] Newer forms of sinusitis, including nosocomial sinusitis and allergic fungal sinusitis, have been recognized in the last decade. Improved diagnostic and therapeutic techniques (eg, newer antibiotics, high-resolution imaging, endoscopic techniques) have enhanced our capacity to manage difficult cases.

### Microbial Etiology

Table 7–3 lists the microbial causes of cases of maxillary sinusitis reported since 1981 for which cultures were obtained from sinus aspiration. The predominant pathogens in adults and children are *Streptococcus pneumoniae* and *Haemophilus influenzae*. In children, *Moraxella catarrhalis* is a common pathogen. Despite extensive microbiologic analysis, no pathogen could be recovered from a high percentage of patients in whom sinusitis was diagnosed on the basis of clinical or radiographic criteria.

Anaerobic pathogens are common in chronic sinusitis in adults, but in children, the role of anaerobes is less well understood.[42] In younger children or children with subacute sinusitis (ie, symptoms persisting 3 weeks to 2 months), anaerobes are infrequently found.[42] However, in older children with more complicated chronic sinusitis that requires surgical drainage, anaerobes predominate.[43]

Sphenoid or frontal sinusitis differs from acute maxillary sinusitis in that *S. aureus* is a frequent pathogen. Pneumococci, *H. influenzae*, and anaerobic streptococci are also found in acute sphenoid sinusitis, but gram-negative pathogens and *Aspergillus* species predominate in chronic sphenoid sinusitis.[44]

The microbes associated with nosocomial sinusitis are the usual nosocomial pathogens: *Pseudomonas aeruginosa*, enteric gram-negative bacilli, *S. aureus* and *S. epidermidis*, and enterococci. Less commonly, β-hemolytic streptococci, anaerobes, and *Candida albicans* are found.

### Pathogenesis

Occlusion of the sinus ostia, usually from mucosal swelling or mechanical obstruction, is the most important predisposing cause of sinusitis. Dental infections extending into the sinus are the cause of about 10% of cases of acute maxillary sinusitis. Mucosal swelling is most often caused by viral upper respiratory tract infections or allergic rhinitis. Chronic sinusitis develops if the obstruction persists, usually because of diseases of the anterior ethmoid and middle meatal (ie, ostiomeatal) complex. Important local factors predisposing to sinusitis include a deviated nasal septum, nasal polyps, tumors, overuse of nasal decongestants, and

**Table 7–3. Microorganisms Causing Acute Maxillary Sinusitis in Adults and Children**

| Microorganism | Studies of Adults* | | | | Sydnor[39] | Studies of Children* | |
| --- | --- | --- | --- | --- | --- | --- | --- |
| | Gwaltney[35] | Jousimies-Somer[36] | Berg[37] | Nord[38] | | Wald[40] | Wald[41] |
| *Streptococcus pneumoniae* | 25 | 21 | 57 | 18 | 17 | 36 | 28 |
| *Haemophilus influenzae* | 18 | 52 | 24 | 23 | 18 | 23 | 19 |
| *Moraxella catarrhalis* | 3 | 2 | 1 | 3 | 2 | 19 | 19 |
| *Streptococcus pyogenes* | 1 | 6 | 6 | 2 | 3 | 1 | 1 |
| Non-group A streptococci | 3 | 1 | | 3 | 2 | 1 | 2 |
| *Staphylococcus aureus* | 2 | 1 | 1 | 1 | | | |
| Coagulase-negative staphylococci | | 6 | | | | | |
| *Haemophilus parainfluenzae* | | | | | 4 | | |
| Other gram-negative bacilli | 2 | | | | 1 | | 1 |
| Anaerobic bacteria | 5 | 5 | 7 | 2 | 1 | | 1 |
| Viruses | | ND | ND | ND | ND | | |
| Rhinovirus | 5 | | | | | | |
| Influenza A | 2 | | | | | | |
| Parainfluenza | 1 | | | | | 1 | 1 |
| Adenovirus | | | | | | 1 | 1 |
| No pathogen isolated | 42 | 22 | 7 | 32 | 53 | 28 | 35 |

*The results of studies performed since 1981 are listed as a percentage of total cases. ND, not done.
Adapted from Bamberger DM: Antimicrobial treatment of sinusitis. Semin Respir Infect 6:77–84, 1991.

barotrauma due to flying, swimming, or diving. In children, adenoid hypertrophy may cause chronic sinusitis. Risk factors for nosocomial sinusitis include nasogastric tubes, nasoendotracheal tubes, facial and cranial trauma, and mechanical ventilation.[45]

Local and systemic immunodeficiencies predispose patients to sinusitis. Sinusitis, often caused by *P. aeruginosa* or *S. aureus*, is common in patients with cystic fibrosis or the immotile cilia syndrome. Important systemic immune abnormalities include hypogammaglobulinemia, a subclass deficiency of IgG2 or IgG3, and poor antibody responsiveness to a polysaccharide pneumococcal vaccine.[46] Sinusitis is common among HIV-infected patients, with a reported incidence as high as 68%,[47] and may be due to *P. aeruginosa*.[47a] Sinusitis due to *Aspergillus* spp., zygomycetes, or *Pseudallescheria boydii* usually occurs during periods of granulocytopenia due to cancer chemotherapy. Rhinocerebral zygomycosis is also observed as a complication of the acidosis and dehydration associated with diabetes mellitus.

Fungal sinusitis in the immunocompetent host may be invasive[48] or noninvasive. A newly described form of noninvasive fungal sinusitis is allergic fungal disease, which is similar to allergic bronchopulmonary *Aspergillus* infection. Patients present with a history of asthma, recurrent nasal polyposis, and pansinusitis.[49] The sinus mucin contains eosinophils, fungal hyphae, and Charcot-Leyden crystals. Total serum IgE levels and serum precipitins to *Aspergillus* spp. are common. Many cases may be caused by dematiaceous fungi, especially *Bipolaris* spp.[50]

## Clinical Manifestations

The most common symptoms of sinusitis are pain over the affected sinus and nasal congestion with purulent nasal discharge. There may be an associated postnasal drip, productive cough, or hyposmia. The discharge may be malodorous, especially if anaerobes are present, and associated with halitosis and pharyngeal discomfort. Patients are often afebrile. The pain of maxillary sinusitis is accentuated by straining, coughing, or bending at the waist to a head-down

position. This pain is often not relieved by decongestants and may be associated with a maxillary toothache.[50a] Patients with maxillary, ethmoid, or frontal sinusitis exhibit tenderness to palpation over the sinus area. The headache associated with sphenoid sinusitis is more deep-seated and may be occipital, frontal, temporal, periorbital, or retroorbital.[44]

The ostium of the maxillary sinus, frontal sinus, and anterior ethmoid cells opens into the middle meatus. The sphenoid sinus and posterior ethmoid cells open into the superior meatus. A purulent discharge at these sites is usually observed in patients with sinusitis.

In children, it is often difficult to differentiate acute bacterial sinusitis from a viral upper respiratory tract infection (URI). Facial pain and headache occur less frequently and are difficult to recognize in younger children. Viral URIs usually resolve in 5 to 10 days, but symptoms of sinusitis persist longer. Six percent to 13% of children 1 to 3 years of age with URIs have symptoms that last at least 15 days and are likely to have sinusitis.[51] The frequency of prolonged URI symptoms is higher in 2- to 3-year-old children in day care than in home care settings. The cough associated with sinusitis often occurs during the day and night, unlike a nocturnal cough alone, which may be a residual from a recent viral URI. Fever is more common in children than in adults, occurring in 19 of 30 patients in one series.[40] Younger children may have malodorous breath. In chronic sinusitis, cough or worsening asthma may be the primary complaint without symptoms of nasal congestion.

Nosocomial sinusitis usually manifests as fever or sepsis syndrome in a patient with an underlying altered mental status. Most do not have obvious findings of mucopurulent discharge on physical examination. The disease usually occurs during the second week after admission to the intensive care unit.[45]

Complications of sinusitis include meningitis, periorbital infections, subdural empyema, epidural abscess, brain abscess, cavernous sinus thrombosis, osteomyelitis, chronic sinusitis with nasal polyposis, or development of mucoceles. Because of the location of sinuses and the vascular supply, complication rates are higher in sinusitis of the frontal, ethmoid, or sphenoid sinuses than in maxillary sinusitis. Disease of the frontal sinus can extend into the dural veins, causing epidural, subdural, or intracranial abscesses or sagittal sinus thrombosis. Anterior extension can cause a subperiosteal abscess with edema (ie, Pott's puffy tumor). Frontal or ethmoid sinusitis can extend into the orbit, with resultant cellulitis or abscess formation. Common complications of sphenoid sinusitis are meningitis and cavernous sinus thrombosis.[43] The association between asthma and sinusitis is commonly reported, especially in children, but the mechanisms of this process are not well understood.[52] Although *S. aureus* is not a common cause of acute maxillary sinusitis, there are reports of toxic shock syndrome due to staphylococcal sinusitis.[53]

## Diagnosis

The diagnosis of sinusitis is difficult, because the signs and symptoms are nonspecific and the conclusive tests are expensive or invasive. It is often difficult to differentiate sinusitis from viral URI, allergic rhinitis, or vasomotor rhinitis.

Transillumination of the sinuses has been useful in the diagnosis of maxillary sinusitis in adults[54] but of little help in children.[52] The technique involves placing the transilluminator over the orbital rim in a completely darkened room. The hard palate is observed as normal, dull, or completely opaque. Normal findings help to exclude maxillary sinusitis. Opaque antrums highly correlate with sinusitis, although the fluid obtained at the time of sinus puncture may be purulent or nonpurulent. The finding of dullness is neither sensitive nor specific in the diagnosis of sinusitis.

Plain film radiographs, including Water's view, are helpful in the diagnosis of frontal or maxillary sinusitis but of little help in ethmoid or sphenoid disease. The finding of complete opacification of the maxillary sinus, an air-fluid level, or mucosal thickening greater than 8 mm suggests sinusitis. Mucosal thickening without opacification or air-fluid levels is often associated with allergic or nonallergic rhinitis.[52, 55] Plain film radiographs are of little help for children younger than 2 years of age, and the frontal sinuses are not observed until the age of 6. Computed tomographic scans provide excellent detail of all the sinuses, including the posterior ethmoid and sphenoid sinuses, and are useful in the evaluation of deep ostiomeatal air passages. Magnetic resonance scans are less useful because the appearance of normal nasal mucosa during the edematous phase of the nasal cycle on $T_2$-weighted images may resemble pathologic findings.[56]

The finding of pus on rhinologic examination may be more specific for the diagnosis of bacterial sinusitis than the plain film radiograph, because many patients with mucosal thickening, and a third of patients with sinus opacification or air-fluid levels, have nonpurulent sinusitis.[57] The use of fiberoptic rhinoscopy may be more sensitive than plain radiographs. Castellanos and Axelrod studied 246 patients with headache.[58] Ninety-eight patients had rhinoscopic evidence of sinusitis, based on the presence of purulent material emanating from the sinus orifice, but normal radiographs. Ninety-four percent of these patients re-

sponded to antimicrobial therapy, compared with 75% of the 84 patients who had rhinoscopic and radiographic evidence of infection and 5% of the 64 patients with no evidence of sinusitis. The low sensitivity for radiographs may be an artifact of the high frequency of sphenoethmoidal disease in their study. Patients with chronic sinusitis or recurrent episodes of acute sinusitis should be referred for functional nasal endoscopy to better define potential pathology of the ostiomeatal complex.[59]

Cultures of nasal secretions are less accurate than sinus aspiration in defining the microbiologic causes of sinusitis.[42] Sinus puncture for the purpose of microbiologic diagnosis is important in patients in whom the likelihood of disease from other than the usual sinus pathogens (eg, *S. pneumoniae, H. influenzae, M. catarrhalis*) is high and in patients who have a high likelihood of developing severe or life-threatening sinusitis, including those failing appropriate therapy, the immunocompromised, patients with nosocomial sinusitis, and patients with invasive disease or concurrent complications.

## Treatment

Empiric antimicrobial treatment is directed against the usual sinus pathogens (eg, *S. pneumoniae, H. influenzae, M. catarrhalis*). There is an increasing problem with antimicrobial resistance. In the United States from 1979 through 1987, 5% of pneumococci were relatively resistant to penicillin (MIC $\geq 0.1$ $\mu$g/mL) and 2.9% were resistant to tetracycline.[60] The relative resistance to penicillin and resistance to trimethoprim-sulfamethoxasole may be even higher in children with chronic sinusitis.[61] U.S. studies of adults showed that 42% of strains of *H. influenzae* in patients with acute sinusitis[39] and 44% of strains of *Bacteroides* with chronic sinusitis produced β-lactamases.[62] In children, 20% of *H. influenzae* and 27% of *M. catarrhalis* strains produced β-lactamases.[41] Several hospitals have reported strains of pneumococci resistant to penicillin, and erythromycin has poor activity against most strains of *H. influenzae*.

The efficacy of antimicrobials in the treatment of purulent sinusitis has been demonstrated in adults and children. In children, 43% of those given placebo were cured, compared with 66% of those given antimicrobials.[63] In adults, the difference in the cure rates between those given antimicrobials and those given decongestants alone is small.[64] It is difficult to perform clinical trials large enough to show a statistically significant difference between two active agents. In comparative studies, many antimicrobials have been demonstrated to be effective (Table 7–4). Most studies used 10-day treatment regimens. In only two studies was one regimen demonstrated to be superior to another. In one of these, all the patients were not randomized,[39] and in the other, cefixime and cefaclor had similar clinical efficacy, but the bacteriologic efficacy based on reaspiration at the end of therapy was greater for cefixime.[73] Based on the results of trials, the effective antimicrobials for the treatment of sinusitis include ampicillin, amoxicillin, amoxicillin-clavulanate, cefaclor, cefixime, cefuroxime axetil, trimethoprim-sulfamethoxasole, phenoxymethylpenicillin, minocycline, tetracycline, doxycycline, erythromycin,

Table 7–4. **Comparative Treatment Studies of Antimicrobial Agents Commonly Used in the United States for Acute Maxillary Sinusitis**

| Investigation | Results |
| --- | --- |
| **Adults** | |
| Carenfelt[66] | penicillin V = tetracycline = doxycycline |
| Eneroth[65] | penicillin V = tetracycline |
| Gwaltney[35] | amoxicillin = trimethoprim–sulfamethoxasole = ampicillin = cefaclor |
| von Sydow[67] | erythromycin base = penicillin V |
| Mattucci[68] | minocycline = amoxicillin |
| Brodie[69] | amoxicillin = cefuroxime axetil |
| Karma,[70] Marchi[71] | amoxicillin = clarithromycin |
| Casiano[72] | amoxicillin = azithromycin |
| Carenfelt[73] | cefixime > cefaclor |
| Sydnor[39] | cefuroxime axetil > cefaclor |
| **Children** | |
| Wald[41] | amoxicillin = cefaclor |
| Wald[63] | amoxicillin = amoxicillin-clavulanate |

Adapted from Bamberger DM: Antimicrobial treatment of sinusitis. Semin Respir Infect 6:77–84, 1991.

azithromycin, and clarithromycin. Despite the presence of β-lactamase-producing organisms, no clinical trial has reported superior results for agents that are β-lactamase stable,[41, 63] perhaps because a very large study would be needed to exclude a type II statistical error.

Based on in vitro susceptibility data, trimethoprim-sulfamethoxasole, cefuroxime, cefixime, amoxicillin-clavulanate, erythromycin-sulfisoxasole, azithromycin, clarithromycin, and the tetracyclines have activity against the usual sinus pathogens of *S. pneumoniae*, *H. influenzae*, and *M. catarrhalis*, including β-lactamase-producing strains. Trimethoprim-sulfamethoxasole, ampicillin, amoxicillin, and the tetracyclines have the advantage of low cost. Cefixime and azithromycin have the advantage of once-daily dosage.

No controlled trials have been performed for the treatment of chronic sinusitis. Based on in vitro susceptibility data, amoxicillin-clavulanate has activity against the usual pathogens. Some clinicians treat chronic sinusitis with a 3- to 4-week course.[74] Endoscopy to delineate a cause for obstruction and for sinus drainage are often required for chronic sinusitis. Most children with subacute sinusitis respond to antimicrobials.[75]

Nasal decongestants should be used to reduce edema and facilitate drainage. Effective topical agents include phenylephrine HCl and oxymetazoline HCl. Use of topical agents for more than several days should be discouraged to prevent rebound vasodilation. If decongestants are needed for more than 3 to 4 days, oral phenylpropanolamine or pseudoephedrine should be used. Antihistamines with anticholinergic effects may dry mucous membranes and interfere with the clearance of secretions. Antihistamines should be used only if there is evidence of allergic manifestations.

Antimicrobial therapy for nosocomial sinusitis should be based on the results of the sinus aspiration with knowledge of the antimicrobial susceptibility pattern of nosocomial isolates within the intensive care unit. If gram-negative bacilli are observed on the initial Gram stain, a broad-spectrum antipseudomonal penicillin plus an aminoglycoside should be initiated; if clusters of gram-positive cocci are found, vancomycin should be started if methicillin-resistant staphylococci are prevalent within the hospital; if

mixed flora are observed, vancomycin, metronidazole, and an aminoglycoside can be used.

Chronic noninvasive fungal sinusitis should be treated with debridement and drainage of the involved sinus without the need for systemic therapy. Sites affected with allergic fungal sinusitis should be debrided and drained and then treated with systemic corticosteroids but no antifungal therapy.[49] Invasive fungal sinusitis is usually treated with a prolonged course of amphotericin B. If *P. boydii* is isolated, miconazole should be considered, because most strains are resistant to amphotericin B. Fungal sinusitis in patients with granulocytopenia due to cancer chemotherapy often recurs, coinciding with the relapse of their leukemia and the need for additional cancer chemotherapy.[76]

## OTITIS MEDIA

### Epidemiology

Otitis media is one of the most common conditions encountered by the clinician caring for young children. The peak incidence is in children between 6 and 15 months of age.[77] The cumulative incidences during the first 6 months, first year, and second year are 35%, 53%, and 61%, respectively.[78] By 7 years of age, more than 90% of children will have had at least one episode of otitis media, and approximately 75% will have had three episodes or more.[79]

Children in day care experience otitis media more often than children in home care.[80] In one study, more than 40% of respiratory tract infections incurred by infants younger than 1 year of age who attended day care were complicated by otitis media.[81] The role of other factors, including male sex, Native American or Alaskan Eskimo race, parental smoking, bottle feeding while supine, familial predisposition, and crowded living conditions, in determining an increased risk of otitis media is still somewhat controversial; however, these factors may play a role in persistent effusion and chronic disease.[82, 83] The risk of otitis media increases from December through March, paralleling the peak of respiratory virus season.[84]

Serous otitis media, known as nonsuppurative otitis media, otitis media with effusion, or chronic otitis media with effusion, is defined as the presence of middle ear effusion behind an intact tympanic membrane without acute signs or symptoms. Chronic suppurative otitis media is diagnosed if a chronic discharge through a perforation of the tympanic membrane is observed.

### Microbial Etiology

Although there are differences in the microbiology of otitis media in children and adults, *S. pneumoniae* and *H. influenzae* are the most frequently isolated pathogens in all groups.[85–88] Many pneumococcal serotypes are implicated in cases of otitis media; however, serotypes 1, 3, 4, 6, 7, 9, 14, 15, 18, 19, and 23 account for 85% of those causing pediatric disease.[89–91]

Nontypable strains of *H. influenzae* that exist as normal flora in the upper respiratory tract are commonly isolated in otitis media cases. Biotypes II and III predominate in the pharynx and are the commonly found biotypes in the middle ear fluid of children with otitis media.[92, 93] Only 10% of middle ear isolates of *H. influenzae* are type b strains.

*M. catarrhalis* has become an increasingly important cause of otitis media, accounting for 10% of cases in one study.[94] Gram-negative enteric pathogens, *S. aureus*, and group B β-hemolytic streptococci are found in neonates but rarely encountered in older infants, children, or adults.[95–97]

Fewer than 1% of cases of chronic suppurative otitis media are caused by infection with *Mycobacterium tuberculosis*.[98] Tuberculous otitis media is often bilateral and characterized by profuse chronic otorrhea, excessive growth of granulation tissue, and severe conductive hearing loss. Underlying pulmonary tuberculosis is found in 67% of patients but is usually not considered the source of infection.

Eustachian tube dysfunction induced by viral upper respiratory tract infections allows nasopharyngeal organisms to proliferate in the middle ear. In some cases, viruses alone have been isolated in cases of otitis media, including respiratory syncytial virus, adenovirus, parainfluenza, and influenza A.[99] Mycoplasma otitis occurs in school-aged children and *Chlamydia* in young infants with afebrile pneumonia, but both are less commonly observed pathogens in otitis media.

*P. aeruginosa* has been implicated in 67% of cases of chronic suppurative otitis media.[100] Chronic otorrhea and tympanic membrane perforation may be associated with mastoiditis, and it is difficult to treat with oral antimicrobial agents in the pediatric population because oral quinolones are not recommended. Parenteral therapy using an agent effective against *P. aeruginosa* is indicated in cases of chronic suppurative otitis media.

In cases of nonsuppurative otitis media or otitis media with effusion, bacteria can be isolated from middle ear fluid in 30% to 50% of cases, usually *H. influenzae* or *S. pneumoniae*.[101]

## Clinical Manifestations

Otitis media is a spectrum of diseases involving inflammation of the mucoperiosteal lining of the middle ear. The diagnosis is straightforward if the clinician views a bulging, erythematous, opaque tympanic membrane otoscopically. Pneumatic otoscopy is used to evaluate the mobility of the tympanic membrane and may be the most sensitive measure of middle ear effusion other than tympanocenthesis. Ear pain, otorrhea, and the degree of tympanic membrane redness and bulging are used to differentiate acute suppurative from nonsuppurative otitis media. Fever may occur in the child with acute otitis media but is usually less than 39.4°C.

## Treatment

Spontaneous cure occurs in approximately one third of cases of acute otitis media. Few clinicians withhold drug treatment, because clinical improvement occurs within 48 to 72 hours with the use of an appropriate antimicrobial agent.

Antimicrobial treatment of acute otitis media also is used to prevent suppurative sequelae, shorten the time spent with middle ear effusion, and prevent recurrent disease.[102] Choosing an antimicrobial agent for treatment of acute otitis media involves decision making based on several factors and should be individualized (Table 7–5).

Serious bacterial infection, including sepsis and meningitis, are considered in the evaluation of the febrile neonate. The finding of acute otitis media does not exclude the former diagnostic considerations. Most neonates are treated with parenteral antibiotics (eg, ampicillin and cefotaxime) while awaiting culture results. Infants who have been intubated nasotracheally for a long period have a greater incidence of staphylococcal and gram-negative enteric infections, and antimicrobial therapy for these infants should be based on suspicion of infection with these pathogens and take into account the current nursery antimicrobial susceptibility patterns.

Most practitioners continue to use 10 to 14 days of amoxicillin for first-line treatment of acute suppurative otitis media in older infants and children. In cases of persistent or recurrent otitis media, a second-line drug that is stable against β-lactamase, such as trimethoprim-sulfamethoxasole, is effective. Amoxicillin-clavulanate and erythromycin-sulfisoxasole are alternatives. We prefer amoxicillin-clavulanate if acute otitis media occurs with conjunctivitis, cervical adenitis, sinusitis, or pneumonia. Cefixime is second-line agent that has the advantage of single daily dosing, but it has reduced bacteriologic efficacy against pneumococci (and *S. aureus*) and does not penetrate well into middle ear fluid. Newer agents include cefpodoxime and cefprozil, whereas formulations of cefuroxime axitel and clarithromycin are still investigational.

In areas of the country where 30% or more of *H. influenzae* infections are resistant to amoxicillin, β-lactamase-resistant antibiotics may be preferred initially. In these geographic locales, any of the second-line drugs may be used, but we prefer amoxicillin-clavulanate. The side effects of each antibiotic must be considered. Stevens-Johnson syndrome has been more commonly associated with trimethoprim-sulfamethoxasole than with other agents used to treat otitis media. Serum sickness-like illness occurs most frequently with cefaclor. Although rash and diarrhea can occur with any regimen, amoxicillin-clavulanate is most frequently associated with this adverse effect. In cases for which *Mycoplasma* or *Chlamydia* are considered, erythromycin-sulfamethoxasole is appropriate.

Table 7–5. **Choosing an Antimicrobial Agent for Treatment of Otitis Media**

Antimicrobial factors
    Penetration into the middle ear
    Documented therapeutic efficacy
    Cost
    Palatability
    Adverse effects
Patient factors
    Age
    Underlying disease
    History after otitis media
    Concomitant disease
    History of response to prior antimicrobial regimen
    Drug hypersensitivity
    Likelihood of compliance
Pathogen factors
    Prevailing bacterial susceptibility patterns

Approximately one third of patients treated for acute otitis media experience recurrence within 1 month of the initial diagnosis. In most cases, a new bacterium is recovered, or more often, the middle ear effusion is sterile. If relapse with the same pathogen initially isolated occurs, it is often caused by β-lactamase-producing strains.[103] Cefixime, which may have more activity than amoxicillin against *H. influenzae* and is β-lactamase resistant, is a useful agent for cases of amoxicillin-failed, recurrent disease.

Treatment of nonsuppurative otitis media (ie, serous otitis media) remains controversial. Antimicrobial therapy with amoxicillin may be effective in the 25% of cases caused by bacterial pathogens. We prefer to use amoxicillin in a dosage of 40 mg/kg/d for 10 days and then reduce to 10 mg/kg/d (single bedtime dose) for 4 weeks. Patients with middle ear effusion that persists more than 3 months and with documented hearing loss are candidates for referral to an otolaryngologist.

## Complications

Hearing loss and its effect on language development is the most important complication of acute otitis media and persistent middle ear effusion.[104] As many as 20% of patients with otitis media before the antibiotic era developed intracranial or intratemporal complications, including mastoiditis, meningitis, and epidural abscess.[105] If an intratemporal or intracranial complication is suspected, parenteral antimicrobial therapy is indicated, and surgical exploration or drainage is usually necessary.

## Prevention

Prevention of otitis media in the child with frequent recurrences should include a trial of antimicrobial prophylaxis. Amoxicillin and sulfasoxasole have been shown to be effective.[106] We use chemoprophylaxis for 3 to 6 months, usually continuing therapy through the respiratory virus season. Continued assessment of the child's auditory acuity and tympanometry may be used to select the patient in whom surgical management may be warranted.

Insertion of a tympanostomy tube alone or with adenoidectomy is effective in managing the child with frequently recurring otitis media and persistent middle ear effusion with conductive hearing loss.[107] Sequelae, including atrophy, tympanosclerosis, and poorer hearing in ears in which tubes were inserted, were found in one study, but concerns about the methodology of this study have been raised.[108] Adenoidectomy with or without tonsillectomy is effective but should be reserved for the select group of patients who have failed medical management and in whom adenoidal hypertrophy is clinically significant.

## EPIGLOTTITIS

Epiglottitis, which is also called supraglottitis, refers to infection of the epiglottis, aryepiglottic folds, and arytenoid soft tissues. Early intubation must be performed to avoid the most common life-threatening complication, acute airway obstruction.

## Epidemiology

Epiglottitis has been described in newborns and the elderly, but most cases occur in children 2 to 7 years of age.[109] Annual attack rates of 2 to 13 per 100,000 children younger than 5 years of age have been reported.[110] However, epiglottitis is rare in populations in whom early invasive *H. influenzae* type b disease occurs frequently, such as Alaskan Eskimos, other Native Americans, and Australian aboriginals.[111–113] Epiglottitis is reported to occur equally in males and females, although studies in children have demonstrated a 65% or greater male predominance.[114, 115]

Spring and winter seasonal peaks have been reported,[116] but cases occur in all months. Data suggest a preponderance of epiglottitis cases in the fall,[117] and in our institution, 46% of epiglottitis cases occurred from September through November.

## Clinical Manifestations

The diagnosis of epiglottitis should be suggested by the sudden onset of high fever, severe sore throat with dysphagia, and drooling in a previously well child.[118, 119] Cough is not a common presenting symptom. Although early symptoms may be mild, children with epiglottitis may progress rapidly and without warning to airway obstruction.[120]

On examination, the child is anxious and often appears toxic. The patient usually insists on the sitting position and leans forward with the neck hyperextended and chin protruding. The voice may be muffled but is usually not hoarse. Stridor and retractions are observed, and rapid progression to airway obstruction may occur.[121]

## Microbial Etiology

Acute epiglottitis is caused by *H. influenzae* type b in most cases. In two series, 142 of 144 positive blood cultures grew *H. influenzae* type b.[122, 123] Disease caused by pneumococci,[116] streptococci including groups A, B, and C,[125–127] *S. aureus*,[115] and *Haemophilus parainfluenzae*[128] has been described. Unusual pathogens such as *Klebsiella pneumoniae, Aspergillus flavus*,[129] and *Pasteurella multocida*[130] have been reported in immunocompromised hosts.

Nasopharyngeal cultures cannot differentiate asymptomatic colonization from infection. However, direct culture of the epiglottis or trachea has been successful in isolating *H. influenzae* type b among children in as many as 94% of cases.[131]

## Diagnosis

If a patient presents with characteristic manifestations of epiglottitis, no diagnostic procedures are necessary, and the physician should proceed directly to ensuring maintenance of the patient's airway. Oropharyngeal examination should not be performed, nor should any attempt be made to lay the child down, because both may precipitate sudden airway obstruction.[132] Although leukocyte counts of 20,000 with an increased number of bands are often found, veni-

Table 7–6. **Guidelines for Management of Suspected Epiglottitis**

1. Intubation and resuscitation equipment is prepared, and a physician skilled in intubation, preferably an anesthesiologist, otolaryngologist, or intensivist, is notified. An endotracheal tube one size smaller than usual should be used.
2. Do not transport patient unless the airway is secure. If the patient is sent from an outlying clinic or physician's office, personnel skilled in airway management and intubation must accompany the patient.
3. No invasive procedures should be performed. A blood culture may be performed after the airway is protected.
4. Do not lay the patient down or examine the oropharynx.
5. Oxygen may be administered by blow-by if tolerated by the patient.
6. If a lateral neck x-ray film is deemed necessary, do not transport the patient to the radiology department. A portable film can be obtained with the patient remaining upright.
7. Sudden airway obstruction can occur without warning. Be prepared to intubate at any time. Use bag and mask ventilation to stabilize the patient while preparing to intubate.

puncture should be avoided until the patient's airway is secured.

When a child with epiglottitis presents early in the course of illness, findings may be subtle and the diagnosis may not be considered. If the diagnosis of epiglottitis is in question, radiography may be used if personnel experienced in intubation and full resuscitation equipment are available (Table 7–6). The radiographs of the lateral neck should always be performed with the child sitting up, and preferably the patient should not leave the emergency room or intensive care unit. Transport of the patient to the radiology department is discouraged; if it is necessary, the patient should be accompanied by a physician skilled in intubation, resuscitation equipment should be accessible, and no delays should be encountered. Abnormalities found on lateral soft tissue neck roentgenograms include enlargement of the epiglottis and aryepiglottic folds, narrowing and possible obliteration of the valleculae, and an increased ratio of the hypopharynx to tracheal air columns (Fig. 7–1).[133]

If the diagnosis of epiglottitis is seriously considered, direct visualization of the epiglottis by laryngoscopy should be performed at the time of intubation. Demonstration of the enlarged, swollen, erythematous epiglottis, usually with involvement of the arytenoids and aryepiglottic folds, is diagnostic.

## Differential Diagnosis

Epiglottitis must be differentiated from viral laryngotracheitis, bacterial tracheitis, isolated uvulitis, and a foreign body lodged in the valleculae larynx.[134–137] Penetrating pharyngeal injury and parapharyngeal or paravertebral abscess that dissects pus anteriorly may mimic epiglottitis. Thermal epiglottitis has occurred after ingestion of very hot beverages. Nasopharyngeal diphtheria is rare, but the clinical manifestations may suggest the diagnosis of epiglottitis.

Differentiating epiglottitis from viral laryngotracheitis or bacterial tracheitis usually is not difficult. Children with viral laryngotracheitis tend to be younger than 3 years of age, have symptoms that begin gradually, have less fever, and have a more prominent cough, which typically has a barking quality. Children with bacterial tracheitis tend to

have a clinical picture suggesting croup but with more fever and progression to airway obstruction in some cases. Bacterial cultures commonly reveal *S. aureus, H. influenzae, M. catarrahalis,* and *S. pneumoniae.* Radiography reveals subglottic narrowing in viral and membranous croup, but the epiglottis appears normal. Appropriate airway management may include intubation in 1% to 3% of those with viral croup and as many as 85% of children with bacterial tracheitis (ie, membranous croup).[138] Most children with laryngotracheal foreign bodies present with cough and stridor. Dyspnea, which is uncommon in patients with epiglottitis, occurred in 74.3% of children with laryngotracheal foreign bodies in one series.[139]

Isolated uvulitis has been associated with infection due to *H. influenzae* type b and group A β-hemolytic streptococci and has occurred concomitantly with epiglottitis with *H. influenzae* type b bacteremia.[139]

## Treatment

Airway protection is mandatory in cases of epiglottitis. In a review by Cantrell of 740 cases of epiglottitis, mortal-

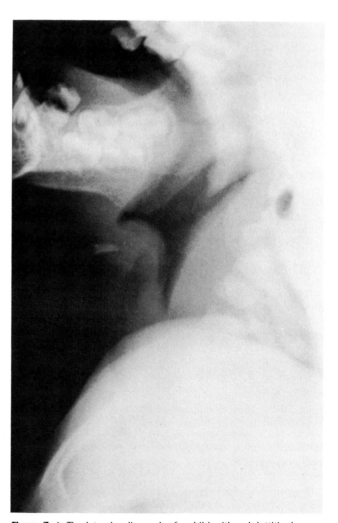

**Figure 7–1.** The lateral radiograph of a child with epiglottitis demonstrates an enlarged, rounded epiglottis and distention of the pharynx with air.

ity rates were 6.1%, 0.86%, and 0.92%, respectively, for patients managed with close observation, routine tracheotomy, or routine intubation.[140] Prompt elective nasotracheal intubation at the time of diagnosis has proved safer than tracheotomy in successfully managing the airways of patients with epiglottitis.[141] Most investigators recommend using a nasotracheal tube that is 1 mm smaller than that predicted by the patient's age. Supportive care should include the addition of humidified oxygen, hydration, and adequate sedation. Direct observation of the epiglottis should determine when extubation can be carried out successfully, which usually is possible in 36 to 48 hours.[142] Decreased swelling of the epiglottis does not correlate with the duration of fever, nor does it follow an arbitrary timetable.

We recommend parenteral cefotaxime, ceftriaxone, or cefuroxime for 5 to 7 days for treatment of acute epiglottis. As many as 40% of *H. influenzae* type b cases are resistant to ampicillin; since 1985, 26% of all *H. influenzae* type b isolates in our institution have produced β-lactamase. For other pathogens, modification of the antimicrobial agent should be based on antimicrobial susceptibility testing of the isolate.

## Complications

Airway obstruction can be avoided with improved recognition and proper airway management. Accidental extubation must be avoided, and the use of sedation and analgesia is advised, especially in the first 24 hours of intubation.

Extraepiglottic foci of *H. influenzae* type b disease are unusual. Meningitis and septic arthritis rarely have been encountered.[143]

Pulmonary edema rarely has been associated with upper airway obstruction before or after endotracheal intubation.[144] Some clinicians think that the provision of continuous positive airway pressure in intubated patients with epiglottitis can prevent this complication.

## Epiglottitis in Adults

Clinical manifestations of epiglottitis in adults are similar to those seen in children. Severe sore throat with increasing dysphagia and drooling occurs. The degree of pain is often disproportionate to the oropharyngeal findings on examination, and rapid progression to airway obstruction may occur without warning. Radiographic diagnosis using lateral neck x-ray films of the soft tissues of the neck may be useful; an epiglottis width greater than 8 mm and an aryepiglottic fold width greater than 7 mm suggest epiglottitis in adults.[145] However, in one study, only 80% of the lateral neck films were diagnostic. Indirect laryngoscopy performed with the adult patients upright and awake proved to be safe and more reliable than radiography.[146] Less aggressive airway management has been advocated for adults with epiglottitis, because the development of airway obstruction is less likely, especially in those presenting with a gradual onset of disease. However, a recent large series of adults with epiglottitis reported a mortality rate of 7%, prompting the

recommendation that early protection of the airway be considered mandatory in adults with epiglottitis. Antimicrobial therapy for epiglottitis in adults is similar to that in children. *H. influenzae* type b is the most commonly isolated pathogen; the blood cultures are positive for 20% to 30% of adults and 60% to 80% of children. Epiglottic abscesses were reported in 26% of patients in one series.[146]

## Prevention

The risk of invasive *H. influenzae* type b disease among household contacts of index patients is increased, particularly for those younger than 4 years of age. Asymptomatic colonization is more frequent among household contacts than in the general population. Thirty-nine percent of siblings of patients with epiglottitis are nasopharyngeal carriers of *H. influenzae* type b. Concurrent epiglottitis has been described in siblings.[147] Adults residing with a child with epiglottitis have an increased risk of developing epiglottitis; simultaneous disease has been described in a parent and child.[148] Rifampin eradicates *H. influenzae* type b from the nasopharynxes of most carriers. Prophylaxis is recommended for all household contacts with any affected child younger than 48 months of age. Children who have been immunized with *H. influenzae* b vaccine and unvaccinated children should be given rifampin prophylaxis.

Purified *H. influenzae* type b capsular polysaccharide vaccine has been used in the United States since 1985 for children 24 months of age or older. Vaccines that employ capsular polysaccharide or oligosaccharide covalently linked to a carrier protein have proven to be safe and effective in preventing *H. influenzae* disease in younger children. The first conjugate vaccine that uses a diphtheria toxoid carrier protein was licensed for use in 1987 and is recommended for children 15 months of age or older. Two subsequent conjugate vaccines, one using an oligosaccharide CRM197 and the other an outer membrane *Neisseria meningitidis* protein, were approved in 1990 and 1991, respectively, for use in infants at least 2 months of age. Universal *H. influenzae* type b immunization of all infants beginning at 2 months of age has already resulted in a decrease in the incidence of epiglottitis. In our institution, there has only been one case of epiglottitis diagnosed in the last 2 years, compared with the prevaccine experience of 3.5 cases per year.

## REFERENCES

1. Komaroff AL, Aronson MD, Pass TM, Ervin CT, Branch WT Jr: Serologic evidence of chlamydial and mycoplasmal pharyngitis in adults. Science 222:927–929, 1983.
2. Kuovinen P, Lahtonen R, Ziegler T, Meurman O, et al: Pharyngitis in adults: The presence and coexistence of viruses and bacterial organisms. Ann Intern Med 110:612–616, 1989.
3. Summary of notifiable diseases, United States, 1990. MMWR 39:1–61, 1990.
4. Todd JK: The sore throat: Pharyngitis and epiglotitis. Infect Dis Clin North Am 2:149–162, 1988.
5. Meier FA, Centor RM, Graham L, Dalton HP: Clinical and microbiological evidence for endemic pharyngitis among adults due to group C streptococci. Arch Intern Med 150:825–829, 1990.
6. Turner JC, Hayden GF, Kiselica D, Lohr J, Fishburne CF, Murren

D: Association of group C β-hemolytic streptococci with endemic pharyngitis among college students. JAMA 264:2644–2647, 1990.

7. Gerber MA, Randolph MF, Martin NH, Rizkallah MF, Cleary PP, Kaplan EL, Ayoub EM: Community-wide outbreak of group G streptococcal pharyngitis. Pediatrics 87:598–603, 1991.

8. Gwaltney JM Jr: Acute pharyngitis. In Mandel GL, Douglas RG, Bennett JE (eds): Principles and Practices of Infectious Diseases. New York, Churchill Livingstone, 1990:493–499.

9. Komaroff AL, Branch WT, Aronson MD, Schachter J: Chlamydial pharyngitis. Ann Intern Med 111:537–538, 1989.

10. Watanakunakorn C, Levy DH: Pharyngitis and urethritis due to Chlamydia trachomatis. J Infect Dis 147:364, 1983.

11. Jones RB, Rabinovitch RA, Katz BP, Batteiger BE, Quinn S, Terho P, Lapworth MA: Chlamydia trachomatis in the pharynx and rectum of heterosexual patients at risk for genital infection. Ann Intern Med 102:757–762, 1985.

12. Denny FW: Current problems in managing streptococcal pharyngitis. J Pediatr 111:797–806, 1987.

13. Hall CB, McBride JT: Upper respiratory tract infections: The common cold, pharyngitis, croup, bacterial tracheitis and epiglottis. In Respiratory Infections: Diagnosis and Management, ed 2. New York, Raven Press, 1988:97–118.

14. Miller RA, Brancato F, Holmes KK: Corynebacterium hemolyticum as a cause of pharyngitis and scarlatiniform rash in young adults. Ann Intern Med 105:867–872, 1986.

15. Tacket CO, Davis BR, Carter GP, Randolph JF, et al: Yersinia enterocolitica pharyngitis. Ann Intern Med 99:40–42, 1983.

16. Parkhurst JB, San Joaquin VH: Tonsillopharyngeal tularemia: A reminder. Am J Dis Child 144:1070–1071, 1990.

17. Bisno AL: Streptococcus pyogenes. In Mandel GL, Douglas RG, Bennett JE (eds). Principles and Practices of Infectious Disease. New York, Churchill Livingstone, 1990:49–499.

18. Centor RM, Meier RA, Dalton HP: Throat cultures and rapid tests for diagnosis of group A streptococcal pharyngitis in adults. In Sox, JC Jr (ed): Common Diagnostic Tests: Use and Interpretation, ed 2. Philadelphia, American College of Physicians, 1990:245–264.

19. Rose FB, Camp CJ, Antes EJ: Family outbreak of fatal Yersinia enterocolitica pharyngitis. Am J Med 82:636–637, 1987.

20. Gerber MA, Randolph MF, Mayo DR: The group A streptococal carrier state: A reexamination. Am J Dis Child 142:562–565, 1988.

21. Georges P (ed) and Committee on Infectious Diseases, American Academy of Pediatrics: Report of the Committee on Infectious Diseases, ed 22. Elk Grove Village, IL, American Academy of Pediatrics, 1991:438–447.

22. Pichichero ME: Controversies in the treatment of streptococcal pharyngitis. Am Fam Physician 42:1567–1576, 1990.

23. Gerber MA, Randolph MF, DeMeo KK, Kaplan EL: Lack of impact of early antibiotic therapy for streptococcal pharyngitis on recurrence rates. J Pediatr 117:853–858, 1990.

24. Dajani AS, Bisno AL, Chung KJ, Durack DT, et al: Prevention of rheumatic fever: A statement for health professionals by the Committee on Rheumatic Fever, Endocarditis, and Kawasaki Disease of the Council on Cardiovascular Disease in the Young, the American Heart Association. Circulation 78:1082–1086, 1988.

25. Gerber MA, Spadaccini LJ, Wright LL, Deutsch L, et al: Twice-daily penicillin in the treatment of streptococcal pharyngitis. Am J Dis Child 139:1145–1148, 1985.

26. Seppala H, Nissinen A, Jarvinen H, et al: Resistance to erythromycin in group A streptococci. N Engl J Med 326:292–297, 1992.

27. Feldman S, Bisno AL, Lott L, Dodge R, Jackson RE: Efficacy of benzathine penicillin G in group A streptococcal pharyngitis: Reevaluation. J Pediatr 110:783–787, 1987.

28. Smith TD, Huskins WC, Kim KS, Kaplan EL: Efficacy of β-lactamase-resistant penicillin and influence of penicillin tolerance in eradicating streptococci from the pharynx after failure of penicillin therapy for group A streptococcal pharyngitis. J Pediatr 110:777–782, 1989.

29. Chaudhary S, Bilinsky SA, Hennessy JL, et al: Penicillin V and rifampin for the treatment of group A streptococcal pharyngitis: A randomized trial of 10 days penicillin vs 10 days penicillin with rifampin during the final 4 days of therapy. J Pediatr 106:481–485, 1985.

30. Tanz RR, Poncher JR, Coydon KE, et al: Clindamycin treatment of chronic pharyngeal carriage of group A streptococci. J Pediatr 119:123–128, 1991.

30a. Pichichero ME: Cephalosporins are superior to penicillin for treat-

ment of streptococcal pharyngitis: Is the difference worth it? Pediatr Infect Dis J 12:268–274, 1993.

31. Gerber MA, Randolph MF, Chanatry J, et al: Once daily therapy for streptococcal pharyngitis with cefadroxil. Pediatr 109:531–537, 1991.

32. Paradise JL, Bluestone CD, Bachman RZ, et al: Efficacy of tonsillectomy for recurrent throat infection in severely affected children. N Engl J Med 310:674–83, 1984.

33. McDonald CJ, Tierney WM, Hui SL, et al: A controlled trial or erythromycin in adults with nonstreptococcal pharyngitis. J Infect Dis 152:1092–1094, 1985.

34. Kennedy DW: Overview. Otolaryngol Head Neck Surg 103:847–854, 1990.

35. Gwaltney JM, Sydnor A, Sande MA: Etiology and antimicrobial treatment of acute sinusitis. Ann Otol Rhinol Laryngol 90(suppl 84):6871, 1981.

36. Jousimies-Somer HR, Savolainen S, Ylikoski JS: Bacteriological findings of acute maxillary sinusitis in young adults. J Clin Microbiol 26:1919–1925, 1988.

37. Berg O, Carenfelt C, Kronvall G: Bacteriology of maxillary sinusitis in relation to character of inflammation and prior treatment. Scand J Infect Dis 20:511–516, 1988.

38. Nord CE: Efficacy of penicillin treatment in purulent maxillary sinusitis. A European multicenter trial. Infection 16:209–217, 1988.

39. Sydnor A, Gwaltney JM, Cocchetto DM, Scheld WM: Comparative evaluation of cefuroxime axetil and cefaclor for treatment of acute bacterial maxillary sinusitis. Arch Otolaryngol Head Neck Surg 115:1430–1433, 1989.

40. Wald ER, Milmoe GJ, Bowen A, et al: Acute maxillary sinusitis in children. N Engl J Med 304:749–754, 1981.

41. Wald ER, Reilly JS, Casselbrant M, et al: Treatment of acute maxillary sinusitis in childhood: A comparative study of amoxicillin and cefaclor. J Pediatr 104:297–302, 1984.

42. Bamberger DM: Antimicrobial treatment of sinusitis. Semin Respir Infect 6:77–84, 1991.

43. Brook I: Bacteriologic features of chronic sinusitis in children. JAMA 246:967–969, 1981.

44. Lew D, Southwick FS, Montgomery WW, et al: Sphenoid sinusitis: A review of 30 cases. N Engl J Med 309:1149–1154, 1983.

45. Caplan ES, Hoyt NJ: Nososcomial sinusitis. JAMA 247:639–641, 1982.

46. Shapiro GG, Virant FS, Furukawa CT, Pierson WE, Bierman CW: Immunologic defects in patients with refractory sinusitis. Pediatrics 87:311–316, 1991.

47. Rubin JS, Honigberg R: Sinusitis in patients with the acquired immunodeficiency syndrome. Ear Nose Throat J 69:460–463, 1990.

47a. O'Donnell JG, Sorbello AF, Condoluci DV, Barnish MJ: Sinusitis due to Pseudomonas aeruginosa in patients with human immunodeficiency virus infection. Clin Infect Dis 16:404–406, 1993.

48. Washburn RG, Kennedy DW, Begley MG, et al: Chronic fungal sinusitis in apparently normal hosts. Medicine (Baltimore) 67:231–247, 1988.

49. Waxman JE, Spector JF, Sale SR, Katzenstein AA: Allergic Aspergillus sinusitis: Concepts in diagnosis and treatment of a new clinical entity. Laryngoscope 97:261–266, 1987.

50. Manning SC, Schaefer SD, Close LG, Vuitch F: Culture-positive allergic fungal sinusitis. Arch Otolaryngol Head Neck Surg 117:174–8, 1991.

50a. Williams JW, Simel DL, Roberts L, Samsa GP: Clinical evaluation for sinusitis: Making the diagnosis by history and physical exam. Ann Intern Med 117:705–710, 1992.

51. Wald ER, Guerra N, Byers C: Upper respiratory tract infections in young children: Duration of and frequency of complications. Pediatrics 87:129–133, 1991.

52. Ott NL, O'Connell EJ, Hoffman AD, Beatty CW, Sachs MI: Childhood sinusitis. Mayo Clin Proc 66:1238–1247, 1991.

53. Ferguson MA, Todd JK: Toxic shock syndrome associated with Staphylococcus aureus sinusitis in children. J Infect Dis 161:953–954, 1990.

54. Evans FO, Sydnor JB, Moore WEC, et al: Sinusitis of the maxillary antrum. N Engl J Med 293:735–739, 1975.

55. Kurien M, Raman R, Job A: Roentgen examination of maxillary sinus, antral puncture and irrigation: A comparative study. Singapore Med J 30:565–567, 1989.

56. Zinreich SJ: Paranasal sinus imaging. Otolaryngol Head Neck Surg 103:863–869, 1990.

57. Berg O, Bergstedt H, Carenfelt C, et al: Discrimination of purulent from nonpurulent maxillary sinusitis. Ann Otol Rhinol Laryngol 90:272–275, 1981.
58. Castellanos J, Axelrod D: Flexible fiberoptic rhinoscopy in the diagnosis of sinusitis. J Allergy Clin Immunol 83:91–94, 1989.
59. Kennedy DW: Surgical update. Otolaryngol Head Neck Surg 103:884–886, 1990.
60. Spika JS, Facklam RR, Plikaytis BD, et al: Antimicrobial resistance of *Streptococcus pneumoniae* in the United States, 1979–1987. J Infect Dis 163:1273–1278, 1991.
61. Tinkelman DG, Silk J: Clinical and bacteriologic features of chronic sinusitis in children. Am J Dis Child 143:938–941, 1989.
62. Brook I: Bacteriology of chronic maxillary sinusitis in adults. Ann Otol Rhinol Laryngol 98:426–428, 1989.
63. Wald ER, Ciponis D, Ledesma-Medina J: Comparative effectiveness of amoxicillin and amoxicillin-clavulanate potassium in acute paranasal sinus infection in children: A double-blind, placebo-controlled trial. Pediatrics 77:795–800, 1986.
64. Axelsson A, Jensen C, Melin O, et al: Treatment of acute maxillary sinusitis. V. Amoxicillin, azidocillin, phenylpropanolamine and pivampicillin. Acta Otolaryngol (Stockh) 91:313–318, 1981.
65. Eneroth CM, Lundberg C: The antibacterial effect of antibiotics in treatment of maxillary sinusitis. Acta Otolaryngol (Stockh) 81:475–483, 1976.
66. Carenfelt C, Eneroth CM, Lundberg C, Wretlind B: Evaluation of the antibiotic effect of treatment of maxillary sinusitis. Scand J Infect Dis 7:259–264, 1975.
67. Von Sydow C, Axelsson A, Jensen C: Treatment of acute maxillary sinusitis: Erythromycin base and phenoxymethyl-penicillin (penicillin V). Rhinology 22:247–254, 1984.
68. Mattucci KF, Levin WJ, Habib MA: Acute bacterial sinusitis: Minocycline vs amoxicillin. Arch Otolaryngol Head Neck Surg 112:73–76, 1986.
69. Brodie DP, Knight S, Cunningham K: Comparative study of cefuroxime axetil and amoxycillin in the treatment of acute sinusitis in general practice. J Int Med Res 17:547–551, 1989.
70. Karma P, Pukander J, Pentilla M: The comparative efficacy and safety of clarithromycin and amoxycillin in the treatment of outpatients with acute maxillary sinusitis. J Antimicrob Chemother 27(suppl A):83–90, 1991.
71. Marchi E: The comparative efficacy and tolerability of clarithromycin and amoxicillin in the treatment of outpatients with acute maxillary sinusitis. Curr Med Res Opin 12:19–24, 1990.
72. Casiano RR: Azithromycin and amoxicillin in the treatment of acute maxillary sinusitis. Am J Med 91(suppl 3A):27S–30S, 1991.
73. Carenfelt, C, Melen I, Odkvist L: Treatment of sinus empyema in adults. Acta Otolaryngol (Stockh) 110:128–135, 1990.
74. Stafford CT: The clinician's view of sinusitis. Otolaryngol Head Neck Surg 103:870–875, 1990.
75. Wald ER, Byers C, Guerra N, et al: Subacute sinusitis in children. J Pediatr 115:28–32, 1989.
76. Viollier A, Peterson DE, DeJongh CA, et al: *Aspergillus* sinusitis in cancer patients. Cancer 58:366–371, 1986.
77. Klein JO: Epidemiology of otitis media. Pediatr Infect Dis 8(suppl 1):S9, 1989.
78. Casselbrandt ML: Epidemiology of otitis media in infants and preschool children. Pediatr Infect Dis 8(suppl 1):S10–S11, 1989.
79. Teele DW, Klein JO, Rosner B and the Greater Boston Otitis Media Study Group: Epidemiology of otitis media during the first seven years of life in children in Greater Boston: A prospective, cohort study. J Infect Dis 160:83–94, 1989.
80. Strangert K: Otitis media in young children in different types of day care. Scand J Infect Dis 9:119–123, 1977.
81. Wald ER, Dashefsky B, Byers C, et al: Frequency and severity of infections in day care. J Pediatr 112:540–546, 1988.
82. Kraemer MJ, Richardson MA, Weiss NS, et al: Risk factors for persistent middle-ear effusions. JAMA 249:1022–1025, 1983.
83. Stewart IA, Kirkland C, Simpson A, et al: Some developmental characteristics associated with otitis media with effusion. *In* Lim DJ, Bluestone DC, Klein JO, Nelson JD (eds). Recent Advances in Otitis Media With Effusion. Proceedings of the Third International Symposium. Toronto, BC Decker, 1984:25–27.
84. Medical Research Council Working Party Report: Acute otitis media in general practice. Lancet 2:510–514, 1957.
85. Howie VM, Ploussard JH, Lester R: Otitis media: A clinical and bacteriologic correlation. Pediatrics 45:29–35, 1970.
86. Brook I: Otitis media in children: A prospective study of aerobic and anaerobic bacteriology. Laryngoscope 89:992–997, 1979.
87. Schwartz AR: Bacteriology of otitis media: A review. Otolaryngol Head Neck Surg 89:444–450, 1981.
88. Celin SE, Bluestone CD, Stephenson J, et al: Bacteriology of acute otitis media in adults. JAMA 266:2249–2252, 1991.
89. Luotonen J, Herva E, Karma P, et al: The bacteriology of acute otitis media in children with special reference to *Streptococcus pneumoniae* as studied by bacteriological and antigen detection methods. Scand J Infect Dis 113:788–183, 1981.
90. Gray BM, Converse GM III, Dillon HC Jr: Serotypes of *Streptococcus pneumoniae* causing disease. J Infect Dis 140:979–983, 1979.
91. Kamme C, Ageberg M, Lundgren K: Distribution of *Diptococcus pneumoniae* types in acute otitis media in children and influence of the types on the clinical course in penicillin V therapy. Scand J Infect Dis 2:183–190, 1970.
92. Barenkamp SJ, Munson RS, Granoff DM: Outer membrane protein and biotype analysis of pathogenic nontypable *Haemophilus influenzae*. Infect Immunol 36:535–540, 1982.
93. Hendrickse WA, Shelton S, Kusmiesz H, et al: Biotypes of *Haemophilus influenzae* isolated from middle ear fluid of children with acute otitis media with effusion. *In* Lim DJ, Bluestone CD, Klein JO, Nelson JD (eds): Recent Advances in Otitis Media. Philadelphia, BC Decker, 1988:328–330.
94. Shurin PA, Marchant CD, Kim CH, et al: Emergence of beta-lactamase–producing strains of *Branhamella catarrhalis* as important agents of acute otitis media. Pediatr Infect Dis J 2:34–38, 1983.
95. Bland RD: Otitis media in the first six weeks of life: Diagnosis, bacteriology and management. Pediatrics 49:187–197, 1972.
96. Shurin PA, Howie VM, Pelton SI, et al: Bacterial etiology of otitis media during the first 6 weeks of life. J Pediatr 92:893–896, 1978.
97. Tetzlaff TR, Ashworth C, Nelson JD: Otitis media in children less than 12 weeks of age. Pediatrics 59:827–832, 1977.
98. Jeang MK, Fletcher EC: Tuberculous otitis media. JAMA 249:2231–2232, 1983.
99. Chonmaitree T, Howie VM, Truant AL: Presence of respiratory viruses in middle ear fluids and nasal wash specimens from children with acute otitis media. Pediatrics 77:698–702, 1986.
100. Kenna MA, Bluestone CD: Microbiology of chronic suppurative otitis media in children. Pediatr Infect Dis J 5:223–225, 1986.
101. Brook I, Yocum P, Shah K, Feldman B, et al: Aerobic and anaerobic bacteriologic features of serous otitis media in children. Am J Otolaryngol 4:389–392, 1983.
102. Giebink GS, Canafax DM, Kempthorne J: Antimicrobial treatment of acute otitis media. J Pediatr 119:495–500 1991.
103. Carlin SA, Marchant CD, Shurin PA, et al: Early recurrence of otitis media. Re-infection or relapse? J Pediatr 110:20–25, 1987.
104. Teele DW, Klein JO, Rosner BA: Otitis media with effusion during the first three years of life and development of speech and language. Pediatrics 74:282, 1984.
105. Hawkins DB: Acute mastoiditis in children: A review of 54 cases. Laryngoscope 93:568, 1983.
106. Perrin JM, Charney E, MacWhinney JD: Sulfisoxazole as chemoprophylaxis for recurrent otitis media: A double-blind crossover study in pediatric practice. N Engl J Med 291:664, 1974.
107. Gates GA, Avery CA, Prihoda TJ: Effectiveness of adenoidectomy and tympanostomy tubes in the treatment of chronic otitis media. N Engl J Med 317:1444, 1987.
108. Pichichero ME, Berghash LR, Hengeser AS. Anatomic and audiologic sequelae after tympanostomy tube insertion or prolonged antibiotic therapy for otitis media. Pediatr Infect Dis J 8:780–787, 1989.
109. Johnson GK, Sullivan JL, Bishop LA: Acute epiglottitis: Review of 55 cases and suggested protocol. Arch Otolaryngol 100:333–337, 1974.
110. Peltola H, Kayhty H, Virtanen M, et al: Prevention of *Haemophilus influenzae* type b bacteremia infections with capsular polysaccharide vaccine. N Engl J Med 310:1561–1566, 1984.
111. Ward JI, Lum MKW, Hall DV, et al: Invasive *Haemophilus influenzae* type b disease in Alaska: Background epidemiology for a vaccine efficacy trial. J Infect Dis 153:17–26, 1986.
112. Losonsky GA, Santosham M, Sehgal VM, et al: *Haemophilus influenzae* disease in the White Mountain Apaches: Molecular epidemiology of a high risk population. Pediatr Infect Dis J 3:539–547, 1984.
113. Harrsmarr D, Harma J, Morey F: High prevalence of invasive *Haemophilus influenzae* disease in Central Australia. Lancet 2:927–929, 1986.

114. Baxter J: Acute epiglottitis in children. Laryngoscope 77:1358–1368, 1967.
115. Bass JW, Steele RW, Wiebe RA: Acute epiglottitis: A surgical emergency. JAMA 229:671–675, 1974.
116. Vetto RR: Epiglottitis: Report of 37 cases. JAMA 17:990–994, 1960.
117. Briggs WH, Altenau MM: Acute epiglottitis in children. Otolaryngol Head Neck Surg 88:665–669, 1980.
118. Lewis JK, Gastner JC, Galvis AG: A protocol for management of acute epiglottitis. Clin Pediatr 17:494–496, 1978.
119. Diaz JH, Lockhart CH: Early diagnosis and airway management of acute epiglottitis in children. South Med J 75:399–403, 1982.
120. Bates JR: Epiglottitis: Diagnosis and treatment. Pediatr Rev 1:173, 1979.
121. Bass JW, Fajardo E, Brien JH: Sudden death due to acute epiglottitis. Pediatr Infect Dis J 4:447–449, 1985.
122. Faden HS: Treatment of *Haemophilus influenzae* type b epiglottitis. Pediatrics 63:402–407, 1979.
123. Barrier DB, Wark H, Overtin JR: Acute epiglottitis in children. Anaesth Intensive Care 13:25–28, 1984.
124. Berenberg W, Kevy S: Acute epiglottitis in childhood: A serious emergency, readily recognized at the bedside. N Engl J Med 258:870–874, 1958.
125. Lacroix J, Ahronheim G, Arcand P, et al: Group A streptococcal supraglottitis. J Pediatr 109:21–24, 1986.
126. Mills E: Group B streptococcal supraglottitis in a three month old infant. Am J Dis Child 140:411–412, 1986.
127. Schwartz RH, Kuen RJ, Hermansen K: Acute epiglottitis caused by β-hemolytic group C streptococci. Am J Dis Child 136:558–559, 1982.
128. Warner JA, Finlay WEI: Fulminating epiglottitis in adults. Report of 3 cases and review of the literature. Anaesthesia 40:348–352, 1985.
129. Bolivar R, Gomez LG, Luna M, et al: *Aspergillus* epiglottitis. Cancer 51:367–370, 1983.
130. Johnson RH, Rumans LW: Unusual infections caused by *Pasturella multicoda*. JAMA 237:146–147, 1977.
131. Margolis CZ, Colletti RB, Grundy G: *Hemophilus influenzae* type b: The etiologic agent of epiglottitis. J Pediatr 87:322–323, 1975.
132. Barker GA: Current management of croup and epiglottitis. Pediatr Clin North Am 26:565–579, 1979.
133. Rapskin RH: The diagnosis of epiglottitis: Simplicity and reliability of radiographs of the neck in the differentiation of croup syndrome. Pediatrics 80:96–98, 1972.
134. Denny FW, Murphy TF, Clyde WA, et al: Croup: An 11-year study in a pediatric practice. Pediatrics 71:871–876, 1983.
135. Jones R, Santus JI, Overall JC: Bacterial tracheitis. JAMA 242:721–726, 1979.
136. Li KI, Dieman S, Wald ER: Isolated uvulitis due to *Haemophilus influenzae* type b. Pediatrics 74:1054–1057, 1984.
137. Blazer S, Naveh Y, Friedman A: Foreign body in the airway: A review of 200 cases. Am J Dis Child 134:68–71, 1980.
138. Han BK, Dunbar JS, Stuher TW: Membranous laryngotracheobronchitis (membranous croup). AJR 113:53–58, 1979.
139. Kotloff KL, Wald ER: Uvulitis in children. Pediatr Infect Dis J 2:392–393, 1983.
140. Cantrell RW, Bell RA, Morioka WT: Acute epiglottitis: Intubation versus tracheostomy. Laryngoscope 88:994–1005, 1978.
141. Schuller DE, Birch HG: The safety of intubation in croup and epiglottitis. An eight year follow-up. Laryngoscope 85:33–46, 1975.
142. Rothstein P, Lister G: Epiglottitis: Duration of intubation, fever. Anesth Analg 62:785–787, 1983.
143. Molteni RA: Epiglottitis: Incidence of extra epiglottic infection. Report of 72 cases and review of the literature. Pediatrics 58:526–531, 1976.
144. Travis KW, Todres ID, Shannon DC: Pulmonary edema associated with croup and epiglottitis. Pediatrics 59:695–599, 1977.
145. Schumaker HM, Doris PE, Birnbaum G: Radiographic parameters in adult epiglottitis. Am J Emerg Med 13:588–590, 1984.
146. Mayosmith MF, Hirsh PJ, Wodzinski SF, et al: Acute epiglottitis in adults: An 8-year experience in the state of Rhode Island. N Engl J Med 314:1133–1139, 1986.
147. Handler SD, Plotkin SA, Potsic WP, et al: *Haemophilus influenzae* epiglottitis occurring concurrently in two siblings. Clin Pediatr 21:634–635, 1982.
148. Glode MP, Halsey NA, Murray M, et al: Epiglottitis in adults: Association with *Haemophilus influenzae* type b colonization and disease in children. Pediatr Infect Dis J 3:548–551, 1984.

# CHAPTER 8

# Bronchitis and Acute Febrile Tracheobronchitis

RICHARD S. KRONENBERG and DAVID E. GRIFFITH

Chronic bronchitis is probably the most common infection of the lower respiratory tract (Table 8–1). Prevalence data on chronic bronchitis in the United States are difficult to obtain because chronic bronchitis and emphysema are often lumped together under the umbrella of chronic obstructive pulmonary disease (COPD). Data from the National Health Interview Survey of 1980 estimate a total economic cost for chronic bronchitis in 1979 of over 1.5 billion dollars.[1] In this chapter, we discuss various aspects of this disease, focusing primarily on its role as a respiratory infection. We also discuss acute febrile tracheobronchitis, an entity with altogether different epidemiologic features.

## CHRONIC BRONCHITIS

Chronic bronchitis is a clinical disorder. It was defined in 1959 as the presence of productive cough for 3 months of the year for 2 consecutive years.[2] Other causes for sputum production, such as tuberculosis and bronchiectasis, should be ruled out. At the time this definition was adopted, a main focus of controversy was separating chronic bronchitis from emphysema, which was defined at the same

Table 8–1. **Impact of Chronic Obstructive Pulmonary Disease***

|  |  |  |
|---|---|---|
| Total affected |  |  |
| Chronic bronchitis | 11.4 | million |
| Emphysema | 2 | million |
| Office visits | 17 | million |
| Hospitalizations | 2 | million |

*Data from United States in 1976.

symposium on the basis of pathologic changes in the lung parenchyma. Although proposed more than 30 years ago, these definitions of bronchitis and emphysema are still used. The controversy in terms of defining the various entities that make up COPD has shifted from separating patients with emphysema from patients with chronic bronchitis to defining asthma and dealing with patients who fit the definition of chronic bronchitis but who also have significant bronchospasm. Although there have been several attempts to define asthma, any separation of asthma from chronic bronchitis is likely to be artificial.[3] Patients meeting the definition of productive cough for 3 months of the year in 2 consecutive years should be considered to have chronic bronchitis, even if they also have reversible airway obstruction that meets most definitions of asthma. Whether these patients constitute a subset of patients with chronic bronchitis or comprise a distinct group is discussed later in the chapter.

### Epidemiology and Pathogenesis

#### Structure and Function Correlations

Because chronic bronchitis was defined on clinical grounds, subsequent attempts at structure and function correlations have not been very successful. Initial efforts focused on enlargement of the mucous glands in the large airways (Fig. 8–1A). One of the more popular methods for determining mucous gland enlargement was the Reid index.[4] In this technique, the thickness of the mucous gland layer is compared with the overall thickness of the bronchial wall from the epithelial basal lamina to the inner perichondrium. Normally, the mucous gland layer should

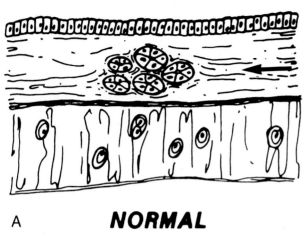

A **NORMAL**

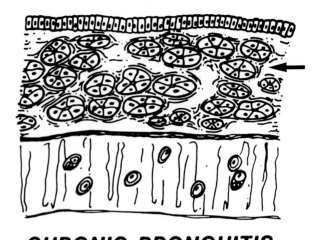

B **CHRONIC BRONCHITIS**

**Figure 8–1.** *A,* Diagram of mucous glands in a normal bronchus. *B,* Diagram of mucous gland hypertrophy in chronic bronchitis. In the normal bronchus, the mucous glands *(arrow)* comprise less than one third of the wall thickness.

be one third or less of the wall thickness. A Reid index of greater than 0.3 indicates mucous gland hypertrophy (Fig. 8–1*B*).

Although there is a general correlation between the Reid index and other measures of tracheobronchial mucous gland enlargement and the presence of clinical chronic bronchitis, there is a significant problem with this concept. There is considerable overlap in measurements of mucous gland size between patients with chronic bronchitis and those without.[5] The distribution curve of the Reid index and other measures of mucous gland size is unimodal.[5] This implies a gradual transition from normal to abnormal mucous gland size and, as a consequence, a poor ability of mucous gland size to predict who has chronic bronchitis and who does not. The lack of sensitivity and specificity of mucous gland size as an indicator of chronic bronchitis may be an artifact of the way chronic bronchitis is defined. The clinical definition of chronic bronchitis sharply separates patients with the disease from those without it, but it is unlikely that the actual disease process is so sharply separated. If mucous gland size and excess sputum production are related to the same disease process, perhaps the unimodal distribution of mucous gland size is more truly related to the gradual transition from normal to abnormal that is typical of most disease processes.

### Cigarette Smoke

Although exposure to environmental pollutants, particularly those encountered in certain occupations, can cause chronic bronchitis,[6, 7] the major causative agent in the United States is cigarette smoke. The evidence for this association is compelling. The 1984 Surgeon General's report, which focused on COPD, concluded, "Cigarette smoking is the major cause of chronic obstructive lung disease in the United States for both men and women. The contribution of cigarette smoking to chronic obstructive lung disease morbidity and mortality far outweighs all other factors."[8] The principal agent causing chronic bronchitis is known; there is considerably less knowledge about how cigarette smoke and environmental and occupational pollutants cause chronic sputum production. Most of the epide-

miologic and mechanistic research on COPD has focused on emphysema and the mechanisms of lung tissue destruction rather than on hypersecretion of mucus.

The sequence of morphologic changes occurring in the airways of cigarette smokers appears to start in the peripheral airways, with mucous gland hyperplasia in more central airways being a relatively late change (Fig. 8–2).[9, 10] The small airways of the lung that contain these inflammatory changes constitute the major site of airways obstruction in advanced symptomatic COPD.[11] These morphologic observations in small airways are of considerable importance to our understanding of the causes of airways obstruction, but their relation to chronic bronchitis is not obvious. Changes have been observed in other airway structures in patients with chronic bronchitis. Smokers show a loss of ciliary structures compared with nonsmokers.[12] This may account for the delay in mucociliary clearance observed in smokers.[13] Bronchi in surgical specimens obtained from heavy cigarette smokers demonstrate a significant decrease in the number of Clara cells. Although the exact function of the Clara cell is unknown, it is thought to be a secretory cell that may contribute to maintaining a normal viscosity in the bronchial mucous.[14]

Models of chronic bronchitis have been helpful in determining the role of cigarette smoke in the pathogenesis of this disease.[15] Organ cultures of tracheal explants demonstrate extensive damage to the epithelial layer and cilia after 1 to 12 hours of exposure to tobacco smoke.[16] Several investigators have examined the effects of cigarette smoke on the airways of animals exposed to smoke in chambers. Kilburn and colleagues exposed hamsters to 4 hours of whole cigarette smoke, followed by the particulate or gaseous phase of cigarette smoke.[17] Airway histology was examined at 2, 8, or 20 hours after smoke exposure. Whole cigarette smoke but not the gaseous or the particulate phases recruited polymorphonuclear leukocytes (PMNs) to the airways. The gaseous phase of cigarette smoke produced loss of cilia, epithelial exfoliation, and vacuoles in the cytoplasm and nuclei. Hoidal and Niewoehner examined the histology of hamster lungs after 2 to 6 weeks of smoke exposure.[18] They found an inflammatory cell infiltrate of predominately monocytes and macrophages and

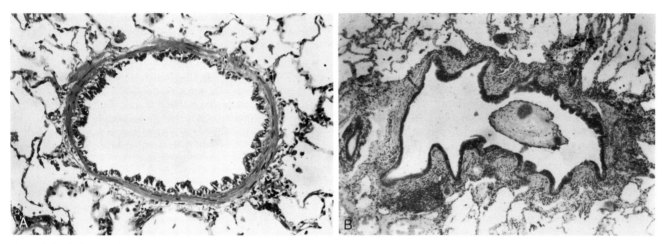

**Figure 8–2.** *A*, A normal human bronchiole (original magnification × 100). Notice the thin-walled epithelial layer and the absence of mucous glands. *B*, A bronchiole from a cigarette smoker shows the early changes of chronic obstructive pulmonary disease. There is a lymphocytic infiltrate, increased smooth muscle and goblet cells, and a mucous plug in the lumen (original magnification × 100). (*A* and *B* from Niewoehner DE: The role of chronic bronchitis in the pathogenesis of chronic obstructive pulmonary disease. Semin Respir Infect 3:14–26, 1988.)

relatively few PMNs, a response similar to that seen in asymptomatic human smokers. Filtration of the particulates from the smoke abolished this response.

The studies on the morphology and histology of human airways obtained from cigarette smokers and of animal airways after exposure to experimental smoke enable the development of a hypothesis on how cigarette smoke causes chronic bronchitis and COPD (Fig. 8–3). Cigarette smoke itself contains several constituents that are capable of injuring the airway epithelium directly. These include aldehydes, phenols, acrolein, and semiquinone contained in the tars and more than $10^{17}$ reactive oxygen species (ROS) per puff contained in the gas phase.[19] ROS are of major importance in the pathogenesis of chronic bronchitis and COPD. ROS may directly degrade lung matrix proteins, polysaccharides, tissue glycosaminoglycans, including hyaluronate,

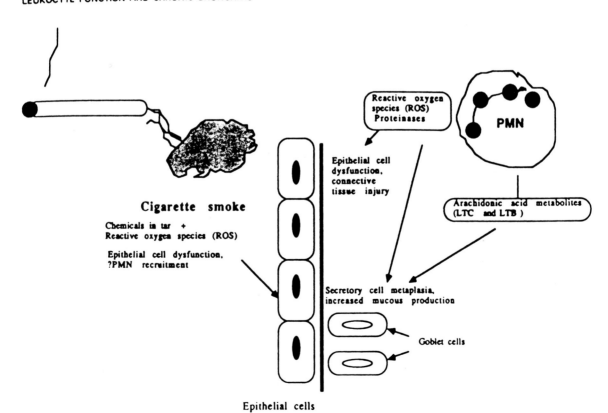

**Figure 8–3.** Mechanisms of airway injury from cigarette smoke. (From McCusker KT, Hoidal J: Leukocyte function in chronic bronchitis. Semin Respir Infect 3:5–13, 1988.)

type I collagen, desmosine, and isodesmosine.[20–23] ROS promote the protease-mediated destruction of lung matrix. ROS increase the protease burden in the lung by recruiting PMNs to the lung tissue. Under oxidant stress, the alveolar macrophage produces PMN chemotactic factors.[24] PMN numbers are increased in the bronchoalveolar lavage (BAL) fluid of cigarette smokers and are more metabolically active, further increasing the burden of ROS in the lung tissue.[18] PMNs are also an important source of proteases that, if unchecked, can degrade lung matrix proteins.[25]

Ordinarily, the proteases released by PMNs into the lung tissue are neutralized by antiproteases found in the lower respiratory tract.[26] The major inhibitor of serine proteases in the lower respiratory tract is $\alpha_1$-protease inhibitor ($\alpha$-PI).[27] $\alpha$-PI can be inactivated by ROS.[28] This effect may be particularly important in the pathogenesis of chronic bronchitis. The major antiprotease in airway mucus is bronchial mucous protease inhibitor (BMPi).[29] BMPi is inactivated by ROS contained in cigarette smoke or released by PMNs.[30] This effect can be prevented with antioxidants. The functional activity of BMPi is reduced in smokers compared with nonsmokers.[30] Intratracheal instillation of leukocyte proteases into the hamster causes chronic bronchial injury.[31] This suggests roles for proteases and ROS in the pathogenesis of chronic bronchitis.

PMNs secrete other substances that can damage the lung structurally and functionally. Arachidonic acid metabolites, including leukotrienes, cause bronchoconstriction, cellular infiltration, and increased vascular permeability.[32, 33] The increased permeability of the alveolar epithelium may allow proteases into the lung interstitium, where they have access to the lung matrix proteins. Leukotrienes $C_4$ and $D_4$ increase the secretion of mucus from human lung explants.[34] This implies a role for these substances in the mucus hypersecretion seen in chronic bronchitis.

The current hypothesis for the role of cigarette smoke in the pathogenesis of chronic bronchitis and COPD involves a complex interaction between proteases and ROS. The initial triggering event is probably direct injury to the airway and alveolar epithelium caused by ROS and other chemicals present in large amounts in cigarette smoke. These substances initiate the production of chemoattractants, primarily in the alveolar macrophages, which recruit large numbers of PMNs to lung tissue, including the airways. The PMNs add to the oxidant burden in the lung tissue by producing their own ROS, and they release serine proteases capable of destroying the lung matrix proteins. Ordinarily, the presence of antiproteases in the lung tissue, particularly $\alpha$-PI, is sufficient to neutralize the effect of proteases, but the increased protease burden produced by the large numbers of activated PMNs found in the lungs of cigarette smokers may overwhelm this protective mechanism. ROS may inactivate $\alpha$-PI, further altering the protease-antiprotease balance in the lung in favor of tissue destruction. PMNs also secrete leukotrienes, which can increase epithelial permeability, allowing the proteases and ROS access to the lung interstitium. Leukotrienes can induce bronchoconstriction, compromising the functional integrity of the lung.

The hypothesis outlined is supported by a large body of evidence developed over the last 30 years by numerous investigators; however, it remains a hypothesis. The ability of ROS to inactivate $\alpha$-PI within the lung interstitium re-

mains controversial.[35] There are also several observations not explained by the hypothesis. The biochemical effects of cigarette smoke on the lung and the cellular constituents of the lung appear to be universal, but only a minority of cigarette smokers develop significant airways obstruction.[36] It is not known why most smokers are protected from the effects of cigarette smoke, but genetic factors play a role in the epidemiology of COPD.[37] Some people exposed to cigarette smoke develop primarily airways disease, and others have much more significant destruction of their lung parenchyma. The factors that allow these two pathways remain unknown.

## Infections

It is difficult to establish the importance of infection as a cause of chronic bronchitis. Unlike normal people, patients with chronic bronchitis do not have a sterile tracheobronchial tree. Bacteria can be found in regions of damaged airways.[38] It is unknown whether these bacteria are a proximate cause of the airway damage and the mucus hypersecretion defines the disease or they are merely colonizing an already damaged airway. Perhaps a more fruitful approach is to examine the role of infection in acute exacerbations of chronic bronchitis, but there is not universal agreement about what constitutes an exacerbation of this disease. Some researchers have included in the definition features, such as changes in the chest radiograph, which would be more consistent with pneumonia.[39] Others have included significantly ill patients with fever and leukocytosis.[40] Many investigators include temperature elevation in their definition.[39, 40] In our experience, this degree of illness is not typical of an exacerbation of chronic bronchitis. The definition we favor is an increase in productive cough with a worsening of the patient's respiratory status.

Because the tracheobronchial tree of patients with chronic bronchitis is not sterile, the role of bacteria in exacerbations of chronic bronchitis can be inferred but not proven. Potentially pathogenic bacteria can be cultured from medically stable patients, and cultures obtained from the tracheobronchial tree grow the same bacteria from stable patients as from those suffering acute exacerbations.[41] If a patient who meets the clinical criteria for an acute exacerbation has a heavy growth of a pathogenic organism in relatively pure culture obtained from a good specimen of expectorated sputum or by direct aspiration of airway secretions, it seems reasonable to attribute the cause to the pathogen. Other techniques used to determine a bacterial cause for an exacerbation of chronic bronchitis include a rise in serum antibody titer and response to specific antibiotic therapy.

Respiratory bronchiolitis resembling the disease seen in postmortem human lungs occurs frequently in experimental animals as a consequence of bacterial or viral infection. In the rat, murine bronchiectasis is caused by *Mycoplasma pulmonis* and perhaps by other bacteria or viruses.[42, 43] Peripheral airways disease can be induced experimentally. Mice infected with A/PR8/34 influenza virus develop alveolitis and bronchiolitis.[44] Syrian hamsters develop a chronic bronchiolitis after intratracheal inoculation with *Legionella* but not after inoculation with *Streptococcus pneumoniae* or *Pseudomonas aeruginosa*.[45]

Table 8–2. **Common Causes of Chronic Bronchitis**

Bacteria
    *Haemophilus influenzae*
    *Streptococcus pneumoniae*
    *Moraxella catarrhalis*
    *Chlamydia psittaci*
Viruses
    Rhinovirus
    Influenza A virus
    Influenza B virus
    Coronavirus
    Herpes simplex virus
    Respiratory syncytial virus
    Adenovirus
*Mycoplasma pneumoniae*

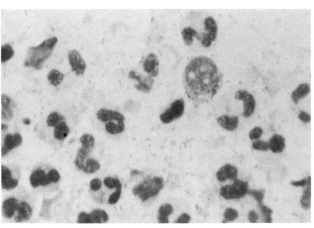

**Figure 8–5.** The Gram stain of sputum shows the gram-negative cocci of *Moraxella catarrhalis.* (Courtesy of Richard Wallace, M.D., University of Texas Health Center, Tyler, TX.)

*Haemophilus influenzae* is the most common bacterial organism associated with exacerbations of chronic bronchitis in humans, and *S. pneumoniae* is the next most common (Table 8–2).[41, 46, 47] Foremost among the agents more recently examined has been *Moraxella catarrhalis.*[47] *M. catarrhalis* is a gram-negative diplococcus that is indistinguishable from *Neisseriae* species by Gram stain, a fact that probably contributed to its neglect as a true respiratory pathogen for many years (Figs. 8–4, 8–5, and 8–6).[48] *M. catarrhalis* has acquired an ability to produce β-lactamase. Most isolates of *M. catarrhalis* from the human respiratory tract now produce this enzyme.[49] The recovery of *M. catarrhalis* from patients with clinical exacerbations of chronic bronchitis is seasonal, with more than 50% of the isolates occurring in the winter months.[48] The signs and symptoms of exacerbations caused by *M. catarrhalis* are indistinguishable from those caused by other agents such as *H. influenzae.* Another agent associated with exacerbations of chronic bronchitis is *Chlamydia pneumoniae* or the TWAR agent.[48] Infections with this organism appear quite similar to those associated with *Mycoplasma pneumoniae.*

Viruses account for a significant percentage of the exacerbations of chronic bronchitis. Estimates of their incidence vary between 18% and 41% of the total number of exacerbations within a given cohort.[41, 46, 50] Rhinovirus is the most frequently isolated, followed by influenza A, influenza B, coronavirus, herpes simplex, respiratory syncytial virus,

and adenovirus.[41, 46, 50–52] *M. pneumoniae* is also reported as a cause of exacerbations of chronic bronchitis, accounting for between 2% and 9% of cases.[53] Viruses and *M. pneumoniae* are much more important causes of acute febrile tracheobronchitis.

## Treatment

Many physicians are faced with the prospect of treating patients with bronchitis. Although some aspects are controversial, there is general agreement that smoking cessation is beneficial, even if the patients have far advanced disease. In their study of London postal workers, Fletcher and associates demonstrated this benefit.[36] Perhaps smoking cessation stops the accelerated loss of pulmonary function in those persons who are sensitive to the effects of cigarette smoke and restores it to the normal age-dependent decline, although it does not restore lung function already lost. Smoking cessation also reduces the mucus hypersecretion and productive cough that are the hallmarks of the disease. The benefits of smoking cessation occur over months and years, although the reduction in productive cough occurs within a shorter time.[54] Beyond smoking cessation, treat-

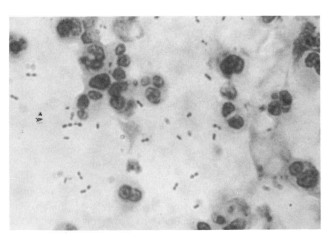

**Figure 8–4.** The Gram stain of sputum shows gram-positive diplococci that are characteristic of *Streptococcus pneumoniae.* (Courtesy of Richard Wallace, M.D., University of Texas Health Center, Tyler, TX.)

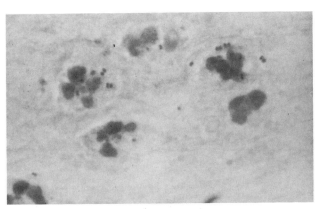

**Figure 8–6.** The sputum Gram stain demonstrates the gram-negative coccobacilli of *Haemophilus influenzae.* (Courtesy of Richard Wallace, M.D., University of Texas Health Center, Tyler, TX.)

ment of chronic bronchitis can be divided into two broad categories: treatments that can be applied to chronic obstructive lung disease in general, such as bronchodilators, physiotherapy, expectorants, oxygen, steroids, and rehabilitation, and antibiotics used to treat infectious exacerbations of chronic bronchitis.

A detailed examination of the possible role of bronchodilators in slowing the progression of COPD is beyond the scope of this chapter. Similarly, a discussion of the use of steroids, oxygen, and pulmonary rehabilitation would be more appropriate in a text on COPD than in one on respiratory infections. It is worthwhile, however, to consider some of the therapies for improving clearance of bronchial mucus, because it is the increased production of this mucus, resulting in chronic productive cough, that defines chronic bronchitis as a clinical entity (Table 8–3). Attempts to mobilize mucus have improved vital capacity in patients with chronic bronchitis.[55] Several studies have demonstrated an adverse effect of high-viscosity mucus on pulmonary function in patients with asthma, chronic bronchitis, and cystic fibrosis.[55–57] It is easy to demonstrate a reduction in mucous viscosity in vitro using a number of agents.[58] Unfortunately, it is much harder to show efficacy for these agents in clinical trials with chronic bronchitis patients.

Acetylcysteine is the best studied of the mucolytics. In a double-blind study involving 500 patients, acetylcysteine reduced the number of acute exacerbations and the quantity, thickness, and purulence of sputum production.[59] The forced expiratory volume in 1 second and the forced vital capacity increased only 100 mL. Although this was a statistically significant increase, it could not have had much clinical importance. A second study also documented a decrease in acute exacerbations in patients with chronic bronchitis receiving acetylcysteine for 6 months, but, there was no change in pulmonary function.[60] Studies of other types of expectorants have yielded similar results.[61, 62] Most of the evidence supporting the use of mucolytics appears to be subjective. Moreover, acetylcysteine may cause bronchospasm in asthmatics.[63] These agents may be useful if mucus is particularly thick and tenacious, but they should be used with caution in patients with reactive airways.

Chest physiotherapy includes postural drainage, percussion, and forceful coughing. These techniques may be useful in improving the clearance of secretions in patients with large volumes of mucus, such as those with bronchiectasis.[64] They do not seem to be as effective in patients with chronic bronchitis who do not have this problem.[65] The cutoff for excessive production of mucus, at least for COPD patients, is 30 mL per day.[66] Pulmonary function changes after chest physiotherapy are variable, with some studies showing no change[65] and others showing improvement.[67] Hypoxemia may occur during administration of chest

physiotherapy.[68] Patients undergoing chest physiotherapy may require supplemental oxygen.

Antibiotics have been used in the treatment of acute exacerbations of chronic bronchitis for years. As early as 1960, a large, controlled study reported less time lost from work by patients with chronic bronchitis treated prophylactically with tetracycline, although the frequency of exacerbations was not affected.[69] Other studies of the efficacy of antibiotics in acute exacerbations of chronic bronchitis produced different results. Many of these studies were small and not controlled. In 1975, Tager and Spizer reviewed the controlled studies available on the usefulness of short-term antibiotics in acute exacerbations of chronic bronchitis.[70] They were able to identify six placebo-controlled studies with adequate statistical data and outcome criteria to allow a conclusion. Two of the six studies showed a definite advantage for antibiotic therapy, one was indeterminate, and three showed no benefit. Tager and Spizer concluded that no definite decision on the efficacy of antibiotics in the treatment of acute exacerbations could be made on the basis of the data in the literature.

Since the publication of that review, Nicotra, Rivera, and Awe conducted a double-blind, randomized, placebo-controlled trial of the efficacy of tetracycline (500 mg every 6 hours for 1 week) in 40 patients hospitalized with an acute exacerbation of chronic bronchitis.[71] The patients were sick enough to require hospitalization but not severely ill. The placebo- and tetracycline-treated patients had significant improvements in $PaO_2$. The tetracycline-treated group also had small, statistically significant improvements in the differences between alveolar and arterial oxygen tension and in peak expiratory flow rates. The placebo-treated patients had similar improvements in these variables that did not reach statistical significance. The clinical utility of tetracycline as judged by the outcome of this study was doubtful.

In 1987, Anthonisen and colleagues published another study of the efficacy of antibiotics in the treatment of acute exacerbations of chronic bronchitis.[72] This study was a double-blind, placebo-controlled, randomized, crossover trial. Acute exacerbations were analyzed in 173 outpatients who suffered a total of 362 exacerbations. Treatment success was defined on the basis of improvement in symptoms. Treatment failure was defined as a patient who had no improvement in symptoms or who got worse during the 21-day study period. The antibiotics used were doxycycline, amoxicillin, and trimethoprim-sulfamethoxazole. Patients treated with antibiotics had a significantly higher incidence of treatment success (68% versus 55%) and lower rate of treatment failure (10% versus 19%) than did the placebo group. The antibiotic-treated group also had a more rapid recovery peak flow rate. The conclusion from this study was that antibiotics are beneficial.

Although there are some obvious differences in the studies by Nicotra, Rivera, and Awe and by Anthonisen and coworkers, there still does not seem to be sufficient data available to allow a solid conclusion about the efficacy of antibiotics in treating acute exacerbations of chronic bronchitis. The antibiotics used in both these studies were inexpensive, and no adverse side effects were seen; there seems some potential benefit in their use to treat exacerbations. Newer antibiotics developed to treat β-lactamase-producing bacteria such as *M. catarrhalis* are much more costly. It would be reasonable not to treat routinely with these agents

**Table 8–3. Nonantibiotic Treatment of Chronic Bronchitis**

Smoking cessation
Bronchodilators
Steroids
Oxygen
Pulmonary rehabilitation
Mucolytics
Chest physiotherapy

Table 8–4. **Antibiotic Therapy of Chronic Bronchitis**

| Antibiotic | Effective Against | Cost of Therapy ($)* |
|---|---|---|
| Tetracycline | β-Lact. neg. *Haemophilus influenzae* | 5.08–7.20 |
| Amoxicillin | *Streptococcus pneumoniae* β-Lact. neg. *H. influenzae* | 7.55–17.40 |
| Ciprofloxacin | *S. pneumoniae*† β-Lact. pos. *H. influenzae* β-Lact. pos. *Moraxella catarrhalis* *Pseudomonas* species | 55.89–66.50 |
| Cefixime | *S. pneumoniae* β-Lact. pos. *H. influenzae* β-Lact. pos. *M. catarrhalis* *Pseudomonas* species | 47.72–61.90 |

*Approximate cost of a 10-day course (as of spring/summer 1992).
†Not effective against all strains. Bacteremic pneumococcal pneumoniae has developed in patients during treatment with ciprofloxacin.

unless there is significant infection with fever or respiratory failure (Table 8–4).

Because of the frequency of exacerbations in patients with chronic bronchitis, several investigators have proposed the use of prophylactic antibiotics. This topic was reviewed by Rubin.[73] Studies of the efficacy of prophylactic antibiotics are difficult to evaluate because of the unpredictability and irregular timing of acute exacerbations. The success rates varied, and success was largely confined to patients with copious sputum production or frequent exacerbations, such as those with bronchiectasis or cystic fibrosis.

Tetracycline seems to be the most effective drug, especially considering its low cost and lack of side effects. A one-time dose of pneumococcal vaccine and annual influenza vaccination is recommended and seems reasonable. During influenza epidemics, amantadine should be used for unvaccinated persons.

## ACUTE FEBRILE TRACHEOBRONCHITIS

Acute febrile tracheobronchitis is a common clinical syndrome with multiple causes (Table 8–5) that is especially familiar to primary care physicians. The hallmark of acute febrile tracheobronchitis is cough, often accompanied by the production of sputum, which may be clear, discolored, thin, or tenacious. Coryza, pharyngitis, and headache are familiar prodromal symptoms. Other possible findings include fever, sweats, fatigue, wheezing, and chest pain secondary to cough. As with chronic bronchitis, the definition of acute febrile tracheobronchitis is descriptive, somewhat arbitrary, and often determined by what is excluded. The original American Thoracic Society definition stressed that in acute bronchitis there could be no physical or radiographic findings compatible with pneumonia.[76] In that context, acute febrile tracheobronchitis is part of a continuum that includes nasopharyngeal infection, bronchitis, bronchiolitis, and pneumonitis. Symptomatically, these processes may be indistinguishable.

Acute febrile tracheobronchitis also implies site-specific airway pathology, between the glottis and the bronchioles. This implication is artificial, because most episodes of infectious or irritative febrile tracheobronchitis are preceded by nasopharyngitis, although not all nasopharyngitis is followed by febrile tracheobronchitis. Similarly, the inflammatory process may not be limited to large airways but may also involve small airways (ie, bronchiolitis). The degree of penetration of the infectious or inflammatory process in the lung varies, because febrile tracheobronchitis probably coexists to some degree with bronchiolitis and alveolitis.

The mean annual attack rate in the United States for acute bronchitis is approximately 87 cases per 100,000 persons per week, peaking in winter at approximately 150 cases per 100,000 persons per week.[77] An estimated 12 million physician visits per year are made because of this disease, with an annual cost of 200 million to 300 million dollars for physician visits and prescription costs.[78] Hospitalizations for acute febrile tracheobronchitis are unusual.

## Pathogenesis

Determining the pathogenesis of acute febrile tracheobronchitis is complicated by several factors. Studies examining an infectious cause frequently fail to isolate a specific pathogen, similar to series of community-acquired pneumonia. Because most cases of acute febrile tracheobronchitis are considered to be viral in origin, one explanation may be the inevitable delay in seeking medical care after onset of symptoms, which may bring the patient to medical attention beyond the period of viral shedding.

Determination of a causative agent is further complicated in subjects with chronic lung disease who may have tracheobronchial colonization by potentially pathogenic bacteria, including nontypable *H. influenzae, S. pneumoniae,* and *M. catarrhalis*. These bacteria can be isolated from the sputum of patients at baseline and with acute bronchitic symptoms. It is frequently difficult to differentiate whether these organisms are responsible for acute febrile tracheobronchitis, cofactors with viruses, or colonizing organisms unrelated to acute bronchitic symptoms. A rise in serum antibody titers to bacteria associated with acute bronchitic symptoms suggests that bacteria may play a causative role,[79] although analysis of antibody coating of bacteria in sputum is not helpful.[80] Subjects with suspected bacterial acute febrile tracheobronchitis appear to respond to antibiotics directed at a specific bacterial pathogen. The supposition that bacteria produce acute febrile tracheobronchitis is therefore based on two major lines of evidence: serum

Table 8–5. **Causes of Acute Febrile Tracheobronchitis**

| Infectious Causes | Noninfectious Causes |
|---|---|
| Respiratory syncytial virus | Industrial gases |
| Parainfluenza virus | Ozone |
| Influenza virus | |
| Coronavirus | |
| Rhinovirus | |
| Adenovirus | |
| Herpes simplex virus | |
| *Mycoplasma* | |
| *Chlamydia* (TWAR strain) | |
| *Legionella* | |
| *Haemophilus influenzae* | |
| *Streptococcus pneumoniae* | |
| *Moraxella catarrhalis* | |

antibody response to a bacterial pathogen and an apparently favorable response to antibiotic therapy.

In children and otherwise healthy adults, viruses are the most common pathogens identified in acute febrile tracheobronchitis.[81–84] Important viruses in this syndrome include respiratory syncytial virus (RSV), parainfluenza virus, influenza virus, coronavirus, rhinovirus, adenovirus, and herpes simplex virus. Most viral acute febrile tracheobronchitis runs a benign, self-limited course; but herpes simplex type 1 has been described as causing severe febrile tracheobronchitis and respiratory failure in normal adults.[83]

*M. pneumoniae* and *C. pneumoniae* (TWAR strain) can cause acute febrile tracheobronchitis. Characteristically, the onset of disease with *C. pneumoniae* (TWAR strain) is subacute, often preceded or accompanied by pharyngitis. The protracted course resembles disease caused by *M. pneumoniae*. The identity of this agent is difficult to establish without specialized laboratory testing. One study suggested an association between respiratory infection with *C. pneumoniae* (TWAR strain) and adult-onset asthma.[85]

The incidence of *Legionella* infection in the setting of acute bronchitis is unknown. It is unlikely that the prevalence of nonpneumonic disease caused by *Legionella* species will ever be known because of the difficulty and expense in identifying these agents. In Pontiac fever, a self-limited endemic form of bronchitis caused by *Legionella* species, patients experience acute onset of headache, chills, myalgia, and sore throat.

Bacteria (eg, *H. influenzae*, *S. pneumoniae*, *M. catarrhalis*) can also cause tracheobronchitis in the setting of chronic lung diseases, such as chronic bronchitis, bronchiectasis, and cystic fibrosis. It is difficult or impossible to differentiate viral from bacterial bronchitis on the basis of symptoms.

Acute febrile tracheobronchitis may be a consequence of the inhalation of irritating, toxic substances as a result of air pollution or occupational exposures.[86] Agents causing this syndrome include ammonia, chlorine, sulfur dioxide, nitrogen dioxide, and ozone. In these circumstances, tracheobronchial irritation and inflammation probably alert a person to the dangerous environment. The inflammatory response induced by these exposures can be demonstrated by BAL. Large or overwhelming exposures are associated with persistent bronchitis and airflow obstruction.[87]

Acute febrile tracheobronchitis usually is not associated with severe or long-term medical consequences, but there are three potentially significant sequelae of acute febrile tracheobronchitis that are of justifiable concern (Fig. 8–7). First is the relation between viral bronchitis and acute bronchial hyperreactivity. Viral infections alone are associated with increases in airway hyperreactivity and airway resistance that may persist for 6 to 8 weeks after a respiratory infection.[88–92] The elevated airway resistance observed after a bronchial infection is largely reversible with β-sympathomimetic and anticholinergic bronchodilators. This enhanced bronchial hyperreactivity persisting after a viral infection may produce a bothersome cough, called a postviral or postinfluenza cough. Respiratory viruses may affect bronchial smooth muscle function by several mechanisms,[92] including stimulation of specific IgE antibody, respiratory epithelial damage, PMN-dependent inflammation, and enhanced mediator release. Respiratory viral infections also directly affect the anatomy and function of airways, including increase in submucosal gland size, increase in goblet

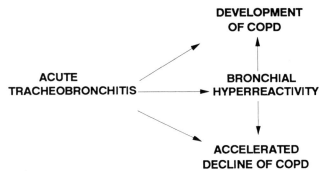

**Figure 8–7.** Possible long-term consequences of acute febrile tracheobronchitis.

cell number, muscle hypertrophy, and defects in cilia of respiratory epithelium.[93, 94] Epidemiologic studies demonstrate that children infected with RSV with bronchiolitis are more likely to have subsequent bronchial hyperreactivity and episodes of wheezing.[92] Although a history of RSV infection may be associated with enhanced bronchial hyperreactivity, there is a less well defined relation between this infection and persistent symptomatic asthma. In contrast to viral illness, there is no firm relation between bacterial infections and enhanced bronchial hyperreactivity, although bronchial inflammation can be a common mediating event.

A second major issue concerns the effect of bronchitic exacerbation on the long-term course of COPD. Do exacerbations of bronchitis accelerate lung function decline in patients with COPD? One potentially significant consequence of acute febrile tracheobronchitis in the setting of chronic tracheobronchial inflammation is exacerbation or temporary worsening of the chronic inflammatory response. The influx of neutrophils associated with an acute infection may produce an increase in the activity of proteinases, including elastase and cathepsin G, which overwhelms native inhibitory capacity. Whether these periodic proteolytic assaults impact the long-term course of chronic bronchitis is unknown. Although the severity of airway neutrophilia in chronic bronchitis correlates with the degree of airflow obstruction,[95] there is no firm or well-established relation between large airway inflammation and the development of significant airflow obstruction. Overall, pulmonary function in COPD patients may fall transiently with acute febrile tracheobronchitis, but there is no evidence of long-term accelerated decline in pulmonary function.[96]

## Chronic Airflow Obstruction

What relation exists between respiratory infections in childhood and later problems with chronic airflow obstruction. Several retrospective and prospective epidemiologic studies suggest a possible connection[97–100] but do not confirm a causal role for respiratory infection in childhood and later development of chronic airflow obstruction for several reasons. First, "Lower respiratory infection" in childhood encompasses much more than acute febrile tracheobronchitis (eg, bronchiolitis, pneumonitis), and it is difficult to assess the isolated effect of febrile tracheobronchitis. Second, information about respiratory infections is usually obtained by means of a questionnaire that relies on patient recall and may introduce significant bias into the analysis. Third, the nature of the early respiratory insult is obscure, and the cause is completely conjectural. Fourth, it may be impossible to know with certainty what is cause and what is effect in this setting. Are children who are more likely to develop chronic airflow obstruction also more susceptible to respiratory illness, or do respiratory illnesses enhance the development of chronic airflow obstruction?

In 1983, Samet and coworkers published an exhaustive review of the available literature evaluating the relation between respiratory illness in childhood and chronic airflow obstruction in adulthood.[101] They concluded that the data reviewed were consistent with a causal or a noncausal association between lower respiratory infection and impaired ventilatory function in children. The data, however, did not establish respiratory illness in childhood as a risk factor for chronic airflow obstruction in adulthood. This conclusion still appears reasonable. As Samet and coworkers suggested, a complete analysis of this important question would require prospective evaluation of a large number of study subjects from birth to adulthood, with close monitoring of respiratory infections and pulmonary function.[101]

## Diagnosis and Treatment

The evaluation of patients with acute febrile tracheobronchitis is usually uncomplicated and can be accomplished on the basis of history and a physical examination. Knowledge of viruses endemic in the community or the pattern of respiratory illness within a family is useful. Without a strong clinical suspicion or physical findings of pneumonia, there is little to be gained by obtaining a chest radiograph unless a noninfectious pulmonary process is suspected. For most patients with acute febrile tracheobronchitis, symptomatic therapy for this self-limited process is all that is necessary. Factors that may prompt the use of antibiotics include a patient's age, significant underlying medical problems, and persistent or severe symptoms. For children, antibiotic therapy has no benefit.[102]

Although we have stressed a conservative approach to antibiotic administration, some uses are appropriate. Viral infections of the upper airways lead to bacterial colonization of the nasopharynx and tracheobronchial tree, with the increased risk of bacterial infection.[103] The syndrome of acute febrile tracheobronchitis may be confused with other respiratory syndromes characterized by cough and sputum production that do require specific therapy, including purulent sinusitis and pneumonitis. Although the examining physician must not overuse antibiotics, it is also important to recognize situations in which antibiotics are necessary. An antibiotic may be effective if other specific treatable causes are suspected, such as *M. pneumoniae* or *C. pneumoniae* (TWAR strain).

Nonspecific therapy such as immunization to influenza is important in preventing or ameliorating bronchitic symptoms. Amantadine is effective for minimizing symptoms of influenza, as prophylaxis during an epidemic in nonimmunized subjects or in those who have contracted influenza. Smoking cessation is important for the patient with acute bronchitic symptoms and for the parent of a child with bronchitic symptoms.

## REFERENCES

1. Tenth Report of the Director, National Heart, Lung, and Blood Institute. Lung diseases, vol 30, publication no. 84–2358. Bethesda, National Institutes of Health, 1982.
2. Ciba guest symposium report: Terminology, definitions, and classification of chronic pulmonary emphysema and related conditions. Thorax 14:286–299, 1959.
3. American Thoracic Society: Standards for the diagnosis and care of patients with chronic obstructive pulmonary disease (COPD) and asthma. Am Rev Respir Dis 136:225–244, 1987.
4. Reid L: Measurement of the bronchial mucous gland layer: A diagnostic yardstick in chronic bronchitis. Thorax 15:132–141, 1960.
5. Thurlbeck WM: Chronic Airflow Obstruction in Lung Disease. Major Problems in Pathology, vol. 5. Philadelphia, WB Saunders, 1976.
6. Detels R, Tahkin DP, Sayre JW, et al: The UCLA population studies of chronic obstructive respiratory disease. Nine lung function changes associated with chronic exposure to photochemical oxidants; a cohort study among neversmokers. Chest 92:594–603, 1987.
7. Morgan WKC, Reger RB: Chronic airflow limitation and occupation. In Cherniack NS (ed): Chronic Obstructive Pulmonary Disease. Philadelphia, WB Saunders, 1991:270–285.
8. United States Public Health Service: The health consequences of smoking. Chronic obstructive lung disease: A report of the Surgeon General. DHHS Publ (PHS) 84–50205. Rockville, MD: US Government Printing Office, 1984.
9. Niewoehner DE, Kleinerman J, Rice DB: Pathologic changes in the peripheral airways of young cigarette smokers. N Engl J Med 291:755–758, 1974.
10. Megahed GE, Senna GA, Eissa, MH, et al: Smoking versus infection as the aetiology of bronchial mucous gland hypertrophy in chronic bronchitis. Thorax 22:271–287, 1967.
11. Hogg JC, Macklem PT, Thurlbeck WM: Site and nature of airway obstruction in chronic obstructive lung disease. N Engl J Med 278:1355–1360, 1968.
12. Regland B, Cajander S, Wiman LG, et al: Scanning electron microscopy of the bronchial mucosa in some lung diseases using bronchoscopy specimens. Scand J Respir Dis 57:171–182, 1976.
13. Foster WM, Langenback EG, Bergofsky EH: Dissociation in the mucociliary function of central and peripheral airways of asymptomatic smokers. Am Rev Respir Dis 132:633–639, 1985.
14. Murray JF: The Normal Lung. Philadelphia, WB Saunders, 1986:28.
15. Reid L, Jones, R: Experimental chronic bronchitis. Int Rev Exp Pathol 24:335–382, 1983.
16. Kennedy JR, Allen PL: Effects of cigarette smoke residue on rabbit tracheal epithelium in organ culture. Arch Environ Health 34:5–11, 1979.
17. Kilburn KH, McKenzie W: Leukocyte recruitment of airways by cigarette smoke and particle phase in contrast to cytotoxicity of vapor. Science 189:634–637, 1975.
18. Hoidal JR, Niewoehner DE: Lung phagocyte recruitment and metabolic alterations induced by cigarette smoke in humans and in hamsters. Am Rev Respir Dis 126:548–552, 1982.
19. Pryor WA, Prier DG, Church DF: An electron-spin resonance study of mainstream and sidestream cigarette smoke: The nature of the free radicals in gas-phase smoke and in cigarette tar. Environ Health Perspect 47:345–355, 1983.
20. Harris MJ, Herp A, Pigman W: Depolymerization of polysaccharides through the generation of free radicals at a platinum surface: A novel procedure for the controlled production of free-radical oxidation. Arch Biochem Biophys 142:615–622, 1971.
21. Moore JS, Phillips GO, Davis JV, et al: Reactions of connective tissue and related polyanions with hydrated electrons and hydroxyl radicals. Carbohydr Res 12:253–260, 1970.
22. Curran SF, Amoruso MA, Goldstein BD, et al: Degradation of soluble collagen by ozone or hydroxyl radicals. FEBS Lett 176:155–160, 1984.
23. Baurain R, Larochelle SF, Lamy F: Photolysis of desmosine and isodesmosine by ultraviolet light. Eur J Biochem 67:155–164, 1976.
24. Hunninghake GW, Crystal RG: Accumulation of neutrophils in the lungs of cigarette smokers. Am Rev Respir Dis 128:833–838, 1983.

25. Bruce MC: The extracellular matrix of the lung: Implications in COPD. *In* Cherniack NS (ed): Chronic Obstructive Pulmonary Disease. Philadelphia, WB Saunders, 1991:31.

26. Idell S, Cohen AB: The protease-inhibitor hypothesis of emphysema. *In* Flenley DC, Petty TL (eds): Recent Advances in Respiratory Medicine. Edinburgh, Churchill Livingstone, 1983:159–171.

27. Gadek JE, Fells GA, Zimmerman RL, et al: Antielastases of the human alveolar structure. Implications for the protease-antiprotease theory of emphysema. J Clin Invest 68:889–898, 1981.

28. Tsan M, Chen JW: Oxidation of methionine by human polymorphonuclear leukocytes. J Clin Invest 65:1041–1050, 1980.

29. Hoidal JR, McCusker KT, Marshall BC, et al: Oxidative damage and COPD. *In* Cherniack NS (ed): Chronic Obstructive Pulmonary Disease. Philadelphia, WB Saunders, 1991:46.

30. Carp H, Janoff A: Inactivation of bronchial mucous proteinase inhibitor by cigarette smoke and phagocyte derived oxidants. Exp Lung Res 1:225–237, 1980.

31. Snider GL, Lucey EC, Christensen TG, et al: Emphysema and bronchial secretory cell metaplasia induced in hamsters by human neutrophil products. Am Rev Respir Dis 129:155–160, 1984.

32. Samuelsson B: Leukotrienes: Mediators of immediate hypersensitivity reactions and inflammation. Science 220:568–575, 1983.

33. Martin T: Arachadonic acid metabolism in lung phagocytes. Semin Respir Infect 1:89–98, 1986.

34. Marom Z, Shelhamer JH, Bach MK, et al: Slow-reacting substances, leukotrienes C$_4$ and D$_4$, increase the release of mucous from human airways in vitro. Am Rev Respir Dis 126:449–451, 1982.

35. Stone PJ, Calore JD, McGowan SE, et al: Functional alpha$_1$-proteinase inhibitor in the lower respiratory tract is not decreased. Science 221:1187–1189, 1983.

36. Fletcher C, Peto R, Tinker C, et al: The Natural History of Chronic Bronchitis and Emphysema: An Eight-Year Study of Early Chronic Obstructive Lung Disease in Working Men in London. Oxford, England, Oxford University Press, 1976.

37. Redline S, Tishler PV, Lewitter FI, et al: Assessment of genetic and nongenetic influences on pulmonary function. A twin study. Am Rev Respir Dis 135:217–222, 1987.

38. Hers JFP, Mulder J: The mucosal epithelium of the respiratory tract in mucopurulent bronchitis caused by *H. influenzae*. J Path Bact 66:103–104, 1953.

39. Davis AL, Growbow EJ, Tompsett R, et al: Bacterial infection and some effects of chemoprophylaxis in chronic pulmonary emphysema. I. Chemoprophylaxis with intermittent tetracycline. Am J Med 31:365–381, 1961.

40. Pines A, Raafatt H, Greenfield JSB, et al: Antibiotic regimens in moderately ill patients with purulent exacerbations of chronic bronchitis. Br J Dis Chest 66:107–115, 1972.

41. Gump DW, Phillips CA, Forsyth BR, et al: Role of infection in chronic bronchitis. Am Rev Respir Dis 113:465–474, 1976.

42. Lamb D: Rat lung pathology and quality of laboratory animals. The user's view. Lab Anim 9:1–8, 1975.

43. Greaves P, Faccini JM: Rat Histopathology. A Glossary for Use in Toxicity and Carcinogenicity Studies. Amsterdam, Elsevier, 1984.

44. Jakab GJ, Astry CL, Warr GA: Alveolitis induced by influenza virus. Am Rev Respir Dis 128:730–739, 1983.

45. Niewoehner DE: The role of chronic bronchitis in the pathogenesis of chronic obstructive pulmonary disease. Semin Respir Infect 3:14–26, 1988.

46. Smith CB, Golden CA, Kanner RE, et al: Association of viral and *Mycoplasma pneumoniae* infections with acute respiratory illness in patients with chronic obstructive pulmonary diseases. Am Rev Respir Dis 121:225–232, 1980.

47. Nicotra MB, Rivera M, Luman JI, et al: *Branhamella catarrhalis* as a lower respiratory tract pathogen in patients with chronic lung disease. Arch Intern Med 146:890–893, 1986.

48. Wallace RJ Jr: Newer oral antimicrobials and newer etiologic agents of acute bronchitis and acute exacerbations of chronic bronchitis. Semin Respir Infect 3:49–54, 1988.

49. Alvarez S, Jones M, Holtsclaw-Berk S, et al: In vitro susceptibilities and β-lactamase production of 53 clinical isolates of *Branhamella catarrhalis*. Antimicrob Agents Chemother 27:646–647, 1985.

50. Carilli AD, Gohd RS, Gordon W: A virological study of chronic bronchitis. N Engl J Med 270:123–127, 1964.

51. McNamara MJ, Phillips IA, Williams OB: Viral and *Mycoplasma pneumoniae* infections in exacerbations of chronic lung disease. Am Rev Respir Dis 100:19–24, 1969.

52. Stenhouse AC: Rhinovirus infection in acute exacerbations of chronic bronchitis: A controlled prospective study. Br Med J 3:461–463, 1967.

53. Nicotra MB, Rivera M: Chronic bronchitis: When and how to treat. Semin Respir Infect 3:61–71, 1988.

54. Tobin MJ, Suffredini AF, Grenvik A: Short-term effects of smoking cessation. Respir Care 29:641–651, 1984.

55. Pham QT, Peslin R, Puchelle E, et al: Respiratory function and the rheological status of bronchial secretions collected by spontaneous expectorations and after chest physiotherapy. Bull Physiopathol Respir 9:293–314, 1973.

56. Polgar G, Denton R: Cystic fibrosis in adults. Studies of pulmonary function and some physical properties of bronchial mucus. Am Rev Respir Dis 85:319–327, 1972.

57. Chodosh S, Medici TC, Ishikawa S, et al: Relationship of physical sputum characteristics and ventilatory capacity in chronic bronchial disease. Chest 63(suppl):56–58, 1973.

58. Sheffner A: The reduction in vitro in viscosity of mucoprotein solutions by a new mucolytic agent, *N*-acetylcysteine. Ann N Y Acad Sci 106:298–310, 1963.

59. Multicenter Study Group: Long-term oral acetylcysteine in chronic bronchitis, a double-blind controlled study. Eur J Respir Dis 61(suppl 111):93–108, 1980.

60. Boman G, Backer U, Larsson S, et al: Oral acetylcysteine reduces exacerbation rate in chronic bronchitis: Report of a trial organized by the Swedish Society for Pulmonary Diseases. Eur J Respir Dis 64:405–415, 1983.

61. Hamilton WFD, Palmer KNV, Gent M: Expectorant action of bromhexine in chronic obstructive bronchitis. Br Med J 3:260–261, 1970.

62. Lieberman J, Kurnick NB: Proteolytic enzyme activity and the role of deoxyribonucleic acid content on the proteolysis of sputum and pus. Nature 196:988–990, 1962.

63. Rao S, Wilson DB, Brooks RC, et al: Acute effect of nebulization of *N*-acetylcysteine on pulmonary mechanics and gas exchange. Am Rev Respir Dis 102:17–22, 1970.

64. Bateman JR, Newman SP, Daunt KM, et al: Is cough as effective as chest physiotherapy in the removal of excessive tracheobronchial secretions? Thorax 36:683–687, 1981.

65. Anthonisen P, Riis P, Sogaard-Anderson T: The value of lung physiotherapy in the treatment of acute exacerbations in chronic bronchitis. Acta Med Scand 175:715–719, 1964.

66. Mohsenifar Z, Rosenberg N, Goldberg HS, et al: Mechanical vibration and conventional chest physiotherapy in outpatients with stable chronic obstructive lung disease. Chest 87:483–485, 1985.

67. Cochrane GM, Webber BA, Hodson ME, et al: Effects of sputum on pulmonary function. Br Med J 2:1181–1183, 1977.

68. Connors AF, Hammon WE, Martin RJ, et al: Chest physical therapy: The immediate effect on oxygenation in acutely ill patients. Chest 78:559–564, 1980.

69. Medical Research Council of Great Britain: Value of chemoprophylaxis and chemotherapy in early chronic bronchitis. Br Med J 1:1317–1322, 1966.

70. Tager I, Speizer FE: Role of infection in chronic bronchitis. N Engl J Med 292:563–571, 1975.

71. Nicotra MB, Rivera M, Awe RJ: Antibiotic therapy of acute exacerbations of chronic bronchitis—A controlled study using tetracycline. Ann Intern Med 97:18–21, 1982.

72. Anthonisen NR, Manfreda J, Warren CPW, et al: Antibiotic therapy in exacerbations of chronic obstructive pulmonary disease. Ann Intern Med 106:196–204, 1987.

73. Ruben FL: Prophylactic therapy of chronic bronchitis. Semin Respir Infect 3:72–80, 1988.

74. National Center for Health Statistics: Current estimates from the National Health Interview Survey, United States, 1986. Vital and Health Statistics, Series 10, No 164. DHHS (PHS) 897–1592.

75. Higgins MW, Thorn T: Incidence, prevalence, and mortality: Intra- and intercountry differences. *In* Hensley MJ, Saunders NA (eds): Clinical Epidemiology of Chronic Obstructive Pulmonary Disease. New York, Marcel Dekker, 1989:23–29.

76. American Thoracic Society: Definitions and classifications of infectious reactions of the lung. Am Rev Respir Dis 101:119, 1970.

77. Ayres JG: Seasonal pattern of acute bronchitis in general practice in the United Kingdom. Thorax 41:106–110, 1986.

78. Rodnick JE, Gude JK: The use of antibiotics in acute bronchitis and acute exacerbations of chronic bronchitis. West J Med 149:347–351, 1988.

79. Musher DM, Kubitschek KR, Crennan J, Baughn RE: Pneumonia and acute febrile tracheobronchitis due to *Haemophilus*. Ann Intern Med 99:444–450, 1983.
80. Yoo O, Donath J, Desmond E, et al: The problem of diagnosing bacterial pneumonia in patients with chronic bronchitis: Bacteria in sputum and bronchial washings from patients with chronic bronchitis are antibody coated. Mt Sinai J Med 55:5, 1988.
81. Boldy DAR, Skidmore SJ, Ayres JG: Acute bronchitis in the community: Clinical features, infective factors, changes in pulmonary function and bronchial reactivity to histamine. Respir Med 84:377–385, 1990.
82. Smith CB, Golden CA, Kanner RE, Renzetti AD Jr: Association of viral and *Mycoplasma pneumoniae* infections with acute respiratory illness in patients with chronic obstructive pulmonary diseases. Am Rev Respir Dis 121:225–232, 1980.
83. Sherry MK, Klainer AS, Wolff M, Gerhard H: Herpetic febrile tracheobronchitis. Ann Intern Med 1:229–233, 1988.
84. Pennington JE: Community-acquired pneumonia and acute bronchitis. *In* Pennington JE: Respiratory Infections: Diagnosis and Management, ed 2. New York, Raven Press, 1988.
85. Hahn DL, Dodge RW, Golubjatnikov R: Association of *Chlamydia pneumoniae* (strain TWAR) infection with wheezing, asthmatic bronchitis, and adult-onset asthma. JAMA 266:225, 1991.
86. Griffith DE, Levin JL: Occupational bronchitis. *In* Bardana E, Montanaro A, O'Hallaren M (eds): Occupational Asthma. Philadelphia, Hanley & Belfus, 1992.
87. Schwartz DA: Acute inhalational injury. Occup Med State Art Rev 2:297–318, 1987.
88. Empey DW, Laitinen LA, Jacobs L, et al: Mechanisms of bronchial hyperreactivity in normal subjects after upper respiratory tract infection. Am Rev Respir Dis 113:131–138, 1976.
89. Hall WJ, Douglas RG Jr, Hyde RW, et al: Pulmonary mechanics after uncomplicated influenza A infection. Am Rev Respir Dis 113:141–146, 1976.
90. Little JW, Hall WJ, Douglas RG Jr, et al: Airway hyperreactivity and peripheral airway dysfunction in influenza A infection. Am Rev Respir Dis 118:295–303, 1978.
91. Hall WJ, Hall CB, Speers DM: Respiratory syncytial virus infection in adults. Ann Intern Med 88:203–205, 1978.
92. Schroeckenstein DC, Busse WW: Viral ''bronchitis'' in childhood: Relationship to asthma and obstructive lung disease. Semin Respir Infect 3:40–48, 1988.
93. Reid L: Influence of the pattern of structural growth of lung on susceptibility to specific infectious diseases in infants and children. Pediatr Res 11:210–215, 1977.
94. Carson JL, Collier AL, Hu SS. Acquired ciliary defects in nasal epithelium of children with acute viral upper respiratory infections. N Engl J Med 312:463–468, 1985.
95. Thompson, AB, Daughton D, Robbins RA, Ghafouri MA, Oehlerking M, Rennard SI: Intraluminal airway inflammation in chronic bronchitis. Am Rev Respir Dis 140:1527–1537, 1989.
96. Smith CB, Kanner RE, Golden CA, Klauber MR, Renzetti AD Jr: Effect of viral infections on pulmonary function in patients with chronic obstructive pulmonary diseases. J Infect Dis 141:271–280, 1980.
97. Burrows B, Knudson RJ, Lebowitz MD: The relationship of childhood respiratory illness to adult obstructive airway disease. Am Rev Respir Dis 115:751–760, 1977.
98. Britten N, Davies JMC, Colley JRT: Early respiratory experience and subsequent cough and peak expiratory flow rate in 36 year old men and women. Br Med J 294:1317–1320, 1987.
99. Gold, DR, Tager, IB, Weiss ST, Tosteson TD, Speizer FE: Acute lower respiratory illness in childhood as a predictor of lung function and chronic respiratory symptoms. Am Rev Respir Dis 140:877–884, 1989.
100. Barker DJP, Osmond C: Childhood respiratory infection and adult chronic bronchitis in England and Wales. Br Med J 293:1271–1275, 1986.
101. Samet JM, Tager IB, Speizer FE: The relationship between respiratory illness in childhood and chronic air-flow obstruction in adulthood. Am Rev Respir Dis 127:508–523, 1983.
102. Sutrisna B, Frerints R, Reingold A, et al: Randomized, controlled trial of effectiveness of ampicillin in mild acute respiratory infections in Indonesian children. Lancet 338:471–474, 1991.
103. Smith CB, Golden C, Klauber MR, Kanner R, Renzetti A: Interactions between viruses and bacteria in patients with chronic bronchitis. J Infect Dis 134:552–560, 1976.

# Lower Respiratory Tract Infections of Infants and Children

GORDON E. SCHUTZE and RICHARD F. JACOBS

The overall incidence and significance of acute lower respiratory tract infections (LRTI) in infants and preschool-aged children has not been fully appreciated until recently. It is estimated that 4.5 million children die each year as a consequence of LRTI,[1] accounting for approximately one third of childhood deaths worldwide. Children in developed countries usually experience six to eight respiratory infections per year, with many involving the lower respiratory tract.[2–5] In 1989, preschool-aged children in the United States experienced 45 million episodes of acute respiratory illnesses, with approximately 30% involving the lower respiratory tract.[6] The illnesses were of sufficient severity that 73% of patients were medically attended. Most LRTI present as bronchiolitis or pneumonia. Infections of the lower respiratory tract may be difficult to differentiate from simple upper respiratory infections because many of the presenting symptoms vary according to the age of the patient and the extent of pulmonary involvement. It is therefore prudent for the clinician to be familiar with the common presenting symptoms and causes of LRTI in infants and preschool-aged children.

## PATHOGENESIS

Children are born with an anatomic design that protects against LRTI. The nares filter particulate matter, and the epiglottal and cough reflexes prevent aspiration. Organisms that do pass into the lower respiratory tract become entrapped by mucus-secreting cells and are expelled by the ciliated cells of the airways or are ingested and killed by alveolar macrophages and polymorphonuclear cells. Local and systemic immune modulators (eg, complement, immunoglobulins, cytokines) and the lymphatic system also aid in pulmonary defense.[7] Each child may also have factors that increase susceptibility to LRTI (Table 9–1). Extraneous factors, such as lower socioeconomic class, parental smoking, and day care, place children at greater risk for LRTI.[8, 9] For pulmonary infections to occur, one or more of the protective defenses usually becomes impaired (eg, cleft palate), or an underlying condition (eg, congenital immunodeficiency) exists that predisposes the child to infection.

The pathogenesis of acute viral LRTI usually begins with inoculation of the upper respiratory tract by large droplet contact (eg, respiratory syncytial virus [RSV]) or through aerosolization (eg, influenza, measles). The virus proliferates and spreads to involve the lower respiratory tract. As the virus replicates, it destroys the ciliated epithelium, causing accumulation of mucus and cellular debris. Normal ciliary function can be directly compromised by the virus

Table 9–1. **Risk Factors for Lower Respiratory Tract Infections**

| | |
|---|---|
| Anatomic defects: | cleft palate, pulmonary sequestration, tracheoesophageal fistula |
| Immune defects: | severe combined immunodeficiency, Bruton disease, selective IgA deficiency, common variable immunodeficiency, chronic granulomatous disease, acquired immunodeficiency, sickle cell anemia |

Cystic fibrosis
Gastroesophageal reflux
Swallowing dysfunction with chronic aspiration
Congenital heart disease

without destruction of the epithelium. As the destruction continues, there is loss of surfactant production, an increase in hyaline membrane deposition, and development of pulmonary edema. Acute inflammatory cells are attracted to the area, contributing further to occlusion of the airways and leading to complete or partial obstruction. Partial obstruction results in poor expiration and causes air trapping with hyperinflation; complete obstruction may result in lobular atelectasis, especially in the young infant with RSV infection. The atelectasis is caused by the lack of collateral ventilation between alveolar spaces (ie, pores of Kohn) that normally exists in older children and adults.[7, 10]

Unlike viruses, bacteria that cause LRTI often colonize the oropharynx of healthy children. For instance, *Streptococcus pneumoniae* can be isolated from the nasopharynxes of approximately 45% of healthy children, compared with a 5% isolation rate for *Haemophilus influenzae* type b.[11, 12] Most bacterial infections of the lower respiratory tract begin by aspiration of colonizing flora. This is especially true for the newborn infant. LRTI at this age may be acquired before, during, or after birth. Intrauterine pneumonia may develop as a consequence of aspiration of infected amniotic fluid after prolonged rupture of the membranes. A second, less common route of infection is transplacental acquisition. This type of infection is usually passed hematogenously and involves multiple fetal tissues, including the lungs. The most common route of infection in the newborn is acquisition during labor and delivery. The infants become colonized from the maternal vaginal flora with potentially pathogenic organisms, and some aspirate these bacteria and develop infections.[13]

In older children, aspiration of the colonizing flora reaches the lower airways and, in some cases, causes an outpouring of edema fluid and leukocytes within the alveoli. As the process continues, the infection can spread to contiguous sections of the lung or into blood through the lymphatic system. Less commonly, infection may occur through hematogenous spread to the lungs from an infected focus elsewhere in the body. A third mechanism for developing infection is a preceding viral illness. The viral destruction of the airways contributes to bacterial infections of the respiratory tract. This is especially true with LRTI caused by influenza viruses, which are often followed by a secondary infection with *Staphylococcus aureus*.[7] Viral destruction of the ciliated cells of the airways and altered mucus production greatly reduce the ability to clear infected secretions. Bacterial adherence to influenza-infected cells is enhanced through unknown mechanisms. The combination of the inability to clear infected secretions and enhanced bacterial adherence may increase the likelihood of secondary bacterial infections.[14]

## EPIDEMIOLOGY

The epidemiologic patterns of LRTI vary according to the age and sex of the patient, the time of year, and the geographic location. Most LRTI occur in children less than five years of age, with a slight male predominance. The incidence of disease is inversely proportional to the age of the patient. The rates of LRTI in children younger than 1 year of age range from 46 to 300 cases per 1000 children

per year. As age increases above 1 year, these rates decline.[5, 10, 15] Although LRTI are encountered throughout the year, they are more common during the winter months. The seasonal variations and endemic pathogens unique to each domain make geographic location important.[16] For instance, RSV infection tends to produce disease for a shorter period in warmer climates than in colder ones.

Improvement in diagnostic techniques makes determination of a causative agent possible in approximately 75% of cases of LRTI in preschool-aged children.[17, 18] Most pathogens isolated are nonbacterial (Table 9–2). The most common pathogens at all ages are the respiratory viruses. RSV is the most common cause of LRTI in young children, especially those younger than 2 years of age. The remaining respiratory viruses—parainfluenza types 1, 2, and 3, influenza virus A or B, and adenovirus—also are commonly encountered. Rhinovirus, although a major pathogen in adults, has a relatively minor role in causing infections in young children.[10, 17–19]

Bacterial infections of the lower respiratory tract tend to be more common in the older child. The most common community-acquired bacterial pathogens outside the newborn age group are *S. pneumoniae*, *H. influenzae* type b, and *S. aureus*. Because these organisms may colonize the oropharyngeal areas in many children, differentiation of colonized children from those who will develop invasive disease is not possible. Colonization may persist for several months, and the pathogenetic explanation for children who do develop disease is unknown.[20, 21] There is evidence that concomitant infections with bacteria and viruses may contribute to LRTI.[17, 18] Pathogens usually associated with school-aged children and adults, *Mycoplasma pneumoniae* and *Chlamydia pneumoniae*, are not major pathogens of preschool-aged children.

Bacteria are the most common cause of LRTI in newborns (Table 9–3). The pathogens usually encountered are those colonizing the mother's genital tract. Group B *Streptococcus* is the most common bacteria isolated in this age group. Other pathogens, including the enteric gram-negative bacilli and *Listeria monocytogens*, are encountered in this age group but to a lesser degree.[14]

Day care centers have added a new dimension to the epidemiology of LRTI. More than one half of preschool-aged children attend some sort of day care facility. These children have a larger number of respiratory infections (6–

**Table 9–2. Causes of Lower Respiratory Tract Infections in Preschool-Aged Children**

| Bacteria | Viruses |
|---|---|
| *Streptococcus pneumoniae* | Respiratory syncytial virus |
| *Haemophilus influenzae* type b | Parainfluenza types 1,2,3 |
| *Staphylococcus aureus* | Influenza A and B |
| Group A *Streptococcus* | Adenovirus |
| *Moraxella catarrhalis* | Measles |
| *Neisseria meningitidis* | |
| *Bordetella pertussis* | |
| *Mycoplasma pneumoniae* | |
| *Chlamydia pneumoniae* | |
| *Coxiella burnetti* | |
| *Francisella tularensis* | |
| *Ehrlichia chaffeensis* | |
| *Mycobacterium tuberculosis* | |

Table 9–3. **Causes of Lower Respiratory Tract Infections in Newborns**

| Bacteria | Viruses |
|---|---|
| Group B *Streptococcus* | Herpes simplex |
| *Escherichia coli* | Adenovirus |
| *Klebsiella* species | Enterovirus |
| Other gram-negative bacilli | |
| *Staphylococcus aureus* | |
| Nontypable *Haemophilus influenzae* | |
| Other *Streptococcus* | |
| *Enterococcus* | |
| *Listeria monocytogenes* | |
| Anaerobes | |

8/y) than children in home care (3–4/y)[3, 22] Transmission of the respiratory viruses occurs readily in the day care setting and can be difficult to control. Efforts to prevent spread should include hand washing and good hygiene. It may be prudent for infants younger than 6 months of age not to enter day care during the respiratory infection season.[23] Children attending day care are at the greatest risk of developing invasive *H. influenzae* type b infections acquired through respiratory spread from another child. This is potentially the most serious infection associated with day care centers.[24, 25]

## CLINICAL MANIFESTATIONS

As in many infections of the newborn, the presentation of LRTI is nonspecific. Newborns who become ill at birth or shortly thereafter often have mothers with problems that place them at increased risk for infections. Infants born to mothers with prolonged rupture of membranes, prolonged labor or excessive obstetric manipulations, poor prenatal care, foul-smelling amniotic fluid, or chorioamnionitis are at risk for LRTI. The initial symptoms may be hypothermia, hyperthermia, poor feeding, lethargy, cough, or congestion.[14] These symptoms may progress with time to include apnea, shock, and respiratory failure.[26] Symptoms related to the respiratory tract, such as tachypnea, tachycardia, nasal flaring, grunting, retractions, and cyanosis, do not always develop. Infant respiratory distress syndrome, congenital heart disease, transient tachypnea of the newborn, infections of the central nervous system, and meconium aspiration may mimic LRTI in this age group.[27]

The clinical manifestations of LRTI depend on the etiologic agent and the severity of the disease in the older infant and child. Nonspecific indicators of infection include fever, rigors, headache, malaise, restlessness, and irritability. Gastrointestinal complaints of abdominal pain, vomiting, abdominal distention, and diarrhea are not uncommon. Pulmonary symptoms may include nasal flaring, tachypnea, dyspnea, apnea, grunting, and retractions. Cough is often nonproductive. Percussion may not be helpful in a young infant or child if the infection is diffuse and patchy. Dullness in response to percussion is more likely to represent the presence of pleural fluid. Auscultatory changes, such as decreased breath sounds or rales, that occur in the older patients may be absent in young children. Pleural irritation is not an uncommon finding and is associated with chest pain, usually at the site of inflammation. This pain may

mimic other disorders. If the irritation includes the diaphragm, the pain may be referred to the posterior or lateral neck or produce abdominal pain not unlike appendicitis. Irritation of the right upper lobe may produce meningism. Extrapulmonary findings such as abscesses of the skin and soft tissues, otitis media, sinusitis, conjunctivitis, meningitis, pericarditis, and epiglottitis can also be encountered.[10, 20, 21]

## INFECTION IN YOUNG CHILDREN

### Infections of Newborns

Newborns may present with an LRTI that was acquired in utero. Organisms that produce infection in utero include cytomegalovirus, herpes simplex, rubella, enterovirus, tuberculosis, *Toxoplasma gondii*, syphilis (pneumonia alba) and *L. monocytogenes*. These congenitally acquired respiratory infections are not common.[28]

Perinatally acquired bacterial infections are the most common cause of LRTI in the newborn (see Table 9–3). Group B *Streptococcus* (eg, *Streptococcus agalactiae*) is the predominant pathogen isolated.[29] The onset of this illness is characteristically within the first hours of life, but it may occur at any time. Group B streptococcal disease within the first 5 days of life is referred to as early-onset disease. Pulmonary involvement is common in early-onset disease and is demonstrated in approximately 40% of the patients. Infections that begin after 7 days are referred to as late-onset disease and are usually meningitis or osteomyelitis.[30] Almost all patients with early-onset pulmonary involvement demonstrate signs and symptoms of respiratory difficulty, such as grunting, tachypnea, and apnea. These newborns have a generalized septicemia that can lead to apnea and shock. Although a chest roentgenogram may demonstrate a discrete infiltrate, changes indistinguishable from hyaline membrane disease may occur (Fig. 9–1).[27] These infections predominantly affect low-birth-weight infants whose mothers have a history of obstetric complications (eg, prolonged rupture of membranes, maternal fever) that predispose the newborn to infection.[30] Early-onset disease may be seen in full-term newborns with no known predisposing risk factors. Not uncommonly, a history of group B streptococcal colonization can be obtained from the mother.

Second to group B streptococcal organisms as a cause of newborn pulmonary infections are the gram-negative enteric bacilli. *Escherichia coli* K1 and, to a lesser extent, the *Klebsiella* species and others from the Enterobacteriaceae group are commonly isolated. These infections tend to be necrotizing and produce extensive tissue destruction, resulting in pneumatocele formation that is detected on chest roentgenogram.[31, 32]

Other bacteria isolated in this age group include *S. aureus*, nontypable *H. influenzae*, other streptococci (eg, group A and α-hemolytic species), *Enterococcus*, *Listeria*, and anaerobic bacteria.[28]

The most common virus associated with LRTI of newborn infants is herpes simplex. These patients present in respiratory distress from the third to tenth day of life. Rapidly progressing interstitial infiltrates on chest roentgeno-

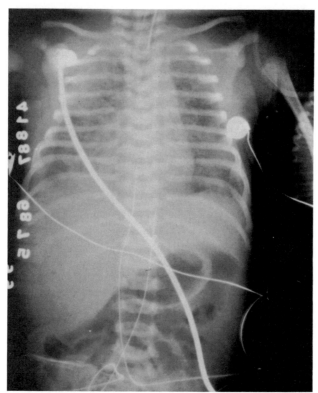

**Figure 9–1.** Chest roentgenogram of a newborn with group B streptococcal pneumonia.

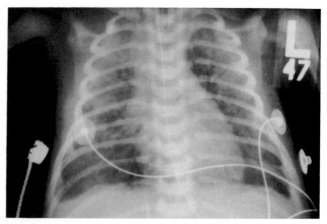

**Figure 9–2.** Herpes simplex pneumonia in a newborn, demonstrating interstitial infiltrates.

gram despite appropriate antimicrobial therapy aids the clinician in the diagnosis (Fig. 9–2). The mortality of patients with this type of herpes infection approaches 75%. Other clues to the diagnosis are thrombocytopenia, evidence of disseminated intravascular coagulopathy, elevated liver function tests, and development of skin vesicles.[33, 34] There usually is no maternal or paternal history of herpetic infection. The mode of transmission is thought to be through aspiration of infected secretions during birth or as an extension of a viremia.

Other viral infections that present in a similar fashion include adenovirus and enterovirus. Newborns infected with adenovirus usually have interstitial infiltrates on chest roentgenogram along with respiratory distress, fever, apnea, and hepatomegaly.[35] After an acute presentation, some infants appear to improve but soon have a rapid decline in their respiratory and neurologic status, and approximately 85% of these infants die. Enteroviral infections localized only to the respiratory tract are rare.[36] This is usually present as part of a severe disseminated illness in newborns that has a mortality rate exceeding 75%. In adenoviral and enteroviral diseases of the newborn, there is usually a maternal history of illness in the perinatal period.

Newborns who develop respiratory distress should always be evaluated for possible bacterial sepsis. This process involves evaluating and culturing blood, urine, and cerebrospinal fluid. A complete blood count may aid the clinician in identifying the infected newborn. In early-onset bacterial infections, leukopenia or neutropenia correlates well with infection.[37] A chest roentgenogram and arterial blood gas analysis should be included in the evaluation of the newborn with respiratory distress. Routine cultures of skin and

mucous membranes may only reveal colonizing microorganisms. The bacteria that are isolated from such cultures may not accurately reflect the causative agent of the illness and should not be collected. Gram stain and the culture of a fresh tracheal aspirate in a recently intubated newborn younger than 12 hours of age have proven useful in the diagnosis of LRTI.[38, 39] If cultures are obtained later, the Gram stain and culture become difficult to interpret because of the rapid colonization of the respiratory tract. Rapid antigen tests are available for group B *Streptococcus* and *E. coli* K1. These rapid tests may be run on serum, cerebrospinal fluid, pleural fluid, or urine. The results of these rapid antigen tests should be used cautiously because of possible contamination of specimens from newborns who are simply colonized.[40]

Empiric antimicrobial therapy should be started in newborn infants with respiratory compromise. This empiric therapy should be directed at the most common neonatal pathogens (Table 9–4). Newborns with LRTI should not be evaluated and treated as outpatients. Ampicillin (150–300 mg/k/d divided every 6–8 h) and an aminoglycoside (eg, gentamicin, 2.5 mg/kg dose every 8–12 h) are the preferential choices. Antimicrobial therapy can be altered based on the culture and sensitivity results. For instance, after sensitivities are determined, group B *Streptococcus* can be treated with penicillin G at a dose of 200,000 to 300,000 U/kg/d divided every 6 to 8 h (Table 9–5). The total length of therapy should be specified based on associated problems such as bacteremia or meningitis. For most cases of bacterial pneumonia, the length of therapy should be 10 to 14 days of parenteral antimicrobial treatment.

Newborns who present with thrombocytopenia, disseminated intravascular coagulopathy, elevated liver function tests, or skin lesions after the first 5 to 7 days of life should always have herpes simplex or another natally acquired

Table 9–4. **Empiric Antimicrobial Therapy**

| Infants 0 to 3 Months | Preschool-Aged Children |
| --- | --- |
| Ampicillin + gentamicin | Ampicillin + chloramphenicol |
| or | or |
| Ampicillin + cefotaxime | Cephalosporin (e.g., cefuroxime, cefotaxime, ceftriaxone, ceftazidime) |

Table 9–5. **Treatment of Lower Respiratory Tract Infections**

| Organism | Antibiotic |
| --- | --- |
| Group B *Streptococcus* | Penicillin, ampicillin |
| *Escherichia coli* | Ampicillin, aminoglycoside |
| *Klebsiella* species | Aminoglycosides, cephalosporin |
| *Staphylococcus aureus* | Methicillin,* nafcillin |
| Nontypable *Haemophilus influenzae* | Cephalosporin |
| Enterococcus | Penicillin, ampicillin |
| *Listeria monocytogenes* | Penicillin, ampicillin |
| *Streptococcus pneumoniae* | Penicillin, ampicillin |
| *Haemophilus influenzae* type b | Ampicillin, cephalosporin |
| Group A *Streptococcus* | Penicillin, ampicillin |
| *Moraxella catarrhalis* | Ampicillin, cephalosporin |
| *Neisseria meningitidis* | Penicillin, ampicillin |
| *Mycoplasma pneumoniae* | Erythromycin, tetracycline |
| *Chlamydia pneumoniae* | Erythromycin, tetracycline |
| *Legionella pneumophila* | Erythromycin |
| *Coxiella burnetti* | Tetracycline, chloramphenicol |
| *Francisella tularensis* | Streptomycin,† gentamicin |
| *Ehrlichia chaffeensis* | Tetracycline, chloramphenicol |

*For methicillin-resistant *S. aureus,* use vancomycin.
†Use if available.

viral infection considered in the differential diagnosis. The evaluation of the newborn should include blood, urine, and cerebrospinal fluid cultures for bacterial pathogens and nasopharyngeal and rectal cultures for viruses. Empiric antiviral therapy should be initiated until culture results are available. Acyclovir and vidarabine are the two medications used for herpetic infections. Acyclovir is as effective as vidarabine in the treatment of neonates with herpetic infections.[41] The ease of administration in the neonate has probably made acyclovir the drug of choice. The desired dose should be 10 to 15 mg/kg every 8 hours. The dosage and schedule should be modified in young prematures or extremely ill newborns who have renal or hepatic compromise caused by the accumulation of acyclovir.[42] No specific antiviral medications are available for enteroviral or adenoviral infections. If the LRTI is part of an overwhelming infection, the use of specific neutralizing antibody in the form of intravenous γ-globulin has been proposed. Although there is no evidence that this mode of therapy is beneficial for treating acute infections, proponents use it based on results with treatment of chronic enteroviral meningoencephalitis infections in agammaglobulenemic patients.[43] Antibodies to the common enteroviral serotypes usually are well represented in the commercially available preparations of intravenous γ-globulin. There are no recommendations for its use.

## Afebrile Pneumonitis of the Young Infant

*C. trachomatis* is a gram-negative bacteria that exists in the female genital tract. Approximately 50% of infants born to infected mothers acquire infection through their conjunctiva or respiratory tract.[44] Of the infected infants, approximately 60% suffer from conjunctivitis, with 20% having pneumonia and another 15% judged to be asymptomatically infected.[45] This illness represents the most common form of lower respiratory infection encountered in the 3-week to 3-month age group.[46]

This clinical syndrome usually presents in a gradual fashion with symptoms increasing over several weeks. This infection is not severe, and the infants are rarely febrile. Febrile infants should be suspected of having a different illness. Afebrile pneumonitis is characterized by a short staccato cough with diffuse crackles audible on auscultation. Approximately one half of affected infants have a history of conjunctivitis. Fifty percent of the infants also have abnormal-appearing tympanic membranes. These abnormalities consist of opaque, pearly white tympanic membranes with a diffuse light reflex and poorly differentiated landmarks.[45–48] Chest roentgenograms reveal hyperexpansion and diffuse interstitial or alveolar infiltrates (Fig. 9–3).[49] On a complete blood count, about 50% to 60% of infants have peripheral eosinophilia. Other abnormalities include an increase in serum IgM levels and a possible IgG and IgA elevation in levels.[47, 48]

Other organisms implicated with the afebrile pneumonitis syndrome are cytomegalovirus, *Pneumocystis carinii,* and *Ureaplasma urealyticum,* alone or in combination with *Chlamydia.*[50, 51] These agents can produce clinical syndromes indistinguishable from *C. trachomatis.*

The diagnosis of chlamydial pneumonia requires proof that the infant is infected with *C. trachomatis* and that this infection is related to the infant's problems. Culture of this organism from nasopharyngeal secretions is the most sensitive and specific method available. Direct immunofluorescence assay of nasopharyngeal and conjunctival secretions can be used in place of culture. This test is easy to perform, easy to interpret, and has levels of sensitivity and specificity that exceed 90%.[52] Serologic confirmation requires a fourfold rise in antibody titer to *C. trachomatis* or the demonstration of specific IgA or IgM antibody.

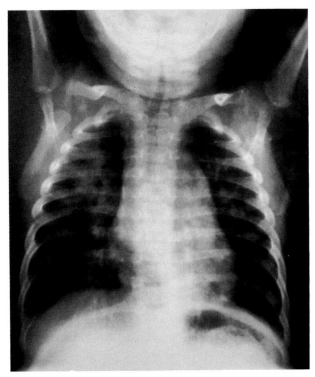

**Figure 9–3.** The chest roentgenogram of afebrile pneumonitis syndrome reveals hyperinflation and diffuse interstitial infiltrates.

The therapy of choice for *C. trachomatis* is erythromycin (40–50 mg/kg/d) or sulfisoxazole (150 mg/kg/d) for 14 days. Improvement should be seen between the third and the fifth days of therapy. Infants tend to be completely asymptomatic and have a normal physical examination at the end of therapy.

## Infections of Infants and Preschool-Aged Children

Except for newborns, most LRTI in young children can be attributed to viral infections (see Table 9–2). Understanding the seasonal predominance of the different viruses can be important in determining the common causes of illness in preschool-aged children.

RSV is the most common cause of LRTI of infants and small children.[15, 17, 53] These infections usually present in the form of pneumonia or bronchiolitis. Specific neutralizing antibody is passed from the mother to the child and is thought to offer full-term newborns some initial protection until 6 to 8 weeks of age.[54] The peak incidence of hospitalizations for RSV is 2 to 5 months of age, with most LRTI confined to children of younger than 2 years of age.[55] Epidemics occur each winter and tend to be abrupt in onset, lasting from 2 to 5 months. The severity of these outbreaks varies from year to year.[15] Approximately 40% of the primary infections result in LRTI, and at least 1% of children younger than 1 year of age have an illness severe enough for hospitalization. In chronically ill patients with bronchopulmonary dysplasia or congenital heart disease, the admission rate to the hospital usually exceeds 50%, with a mortality rate that approaches 70% for hospitalized infants.[56, 57] Therapy with ribavirin may be indicated in selected patients with RSV.

The usual illness begins with fever (37.7°C–39°C) and signs of upper respiratory tract infection. Coughing increases over a 3-day period, and wheezing ensues. The patients with severe illness may demonstrate intercostal retractions, hyperpnea, and mild to moderate hypoxia with or without cyanosis.[10] Hypoxemia is a clear indication for hospitalization of the infant. Chest roentgenograms of infants hospitalized with RSV demonstrate a wide array of abnormalities (Fig. 9–4). The most common findings are hyperexpansion, peribronchial, perihilar, or interstitial infiltrates and segmental atelectasis.[58, 59] Illness caused by RSV is usually mild and may last a few days to 3 weeks. Hospitalized infants usually improve after 3 to 4 days, with total hospitalization lasting 5 to 7 days.[60, 61]

Although parainfluenza virus infections can occur throughout the year, there are distinct seasonal trends. Parainfluenza type 1 tends to occur in the autumn of odd numbered years. Type 2 infections are much less predictable but also tend to occur in the autumn. Type 3 infections are more common in the spring.[15, 62] Most parainfluenza infections are asymptomatic. Of the primary infections that are symptomatic, the disease usually localizes in the larynx and trachea, leading to croup or acute laryngotracheobronchitis. If parainfluenza does involve the lower respiratory tract, the clinical course and radiograph findings are similar to those seen with RSV infection.[10]

A third important group of viral pathogens in children

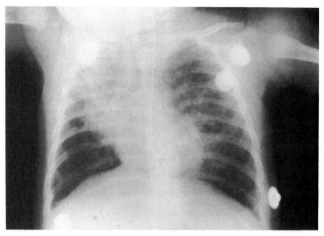

**Figure 9–4.** Respiratory syncytial virus infection with hyperinflation and atelectasis.

are the influenza viruses. Influenza usually presents during the winter months in epidemic forms. The two subtypes of influenza virus are classified as influenza A and B. The clinical presentation and course of influenza infections in infants and young children are not unlike those for other respiratory viral infections, except that these patients are febrile, appear ill, and may have neurologic involvement.[63] These viruses can be very destructive to the respiratory epithelium and often lead to a secondary bacterial infection involving *S. aureus, S. pneumoniae, H. influenzae,* and occasionally, *K. pneumoniae, Streptococcus pyogenes,* and *Neisseria meningitidis.*[13, 64]

Effective vaccines are available for the prevention of influenza infection and should be offered to children who are at high risk. The targeted high-risk group who should be vaccinated are children older than 6 months of age who have chronic pulmonary diseases (eg, severe asthma, bronchopulmonary dysplasia, cystic fibrosis), hemodynamically significant cardiac disease, immunosuppressive therapy, sickle cell anemia, and other hemoglobinopathies. Children with chronic illnesses such as diabetes mellitus, symptomatic human immunodeficiency virus infection, or chronic renal disease may benefit from the vaccine. Patients receiving long-term aspirin therapy for rheumatoid arthritis or Kawasaki disease should also be considered for vaccination because of the risk of development of Reye syndrome. Household contacts and primary caretakers of high-risk children should also be immunized.[65] High-risk patients may benefit from chemoprophylaxis with amantidine after exposure if they failed to receive the vaccine.

Adenoviral infections are an exceedingly common problem in young children, and the spectrum of disease is quite broad. These infections have a predilection for children younger than 5 years of age who spend a great amount of time in day care or other closed environments.[66] Sporadic infections can be seen throughout the year, with epidemics usually occurring in the winter, spring, and early summer. LRTI can be severe or fatal, especially in the child younger than 18 months of age.[67] The onset of illness is usually abrupt. Patients may demonstrate cough, fever, lethargy, vomiting, diarrhea, pharyngitis, or conjunctivitis and moderate to severe dyspnea and tachypnea. Extrapulmonary signs may be present in the form of meningitis, encephalitis, seizures, hepatosplenomegaly, hepatitis, myocarditis, nephritis, and exanthems.[68] Chest roentgenograms may reveal diffuse bilateral infiltrates, which may be bronchial, peribronchial, or interstitial. Atelectasis and hilar adenopathy may also be demonstrated.[58, 59] Serious complications resulting from adenoviral respiratory infections include bronchiectasis, bronchiolitis obliterans, and unilateral hyperlucent lung (ie, increased translucency of all or part of one lung with reduction in size).[69–72]

Outside of the industrialized nations, measles is a major cause of morbidity and mortality related to LRTI. The infection of the respiratory tract may result from the virus itself or from a secondary bacterial or viral infection. These infections are responsible for the largest percentage of deaths associated with measles and may represent as many as 20% of deaths attributable to LRTI.[73] New recommendations for measles vaccine suggest that a child should have received two vaccinations by 12 years of age. The first is suggested at 15 months, with a second immunization at the start of school (5–6 years) or on entry into middle school (11–12 years).[74]

The bacterial causes of lower respiratory tract infections are much less common than viral causes among preschool-aged children. The most common bacterial pathogen continues to be *S. pneumoniae*. There are more than 80 stereotypes of this bacteria, and in children, types 1, 3, 6, 7, 14, 18, 19, and 23 cause most of the disease.[21] The pneumococci are normal inhabitants of the pharynx in healthy children and are usually spread form child to child through the aerosolization of respiratory secretions. The incidence of LRTI with pneumococci is more common in the winter and spring.

The spectrum of pneumococcal disease can be mild to life threatening. Patients who are congenitally or acquired immunosuppressed or who have splenic dysfunction, sickle cell anemia, Hodgkin disease, nephrotic syndrome, splenectomy, or organ transplantation have a greater risk of acquiring disease from this organism.[75] The most common presentation is a sudden onset of symptomatic illness with hyperpyrexia, chills, and diaphoresis. An equally characteristic feature is the abrupt improvement when appropriate antimicrobial agents are instituted. Children usually present with an elevated temperature, a leukocytosis, and a lobar or segmental consolidation on chest roentgenogram (Fig. 9–5).[76] Cases can be complicated by empyema formation or by extrapulmonary disease such as meningitis.

Preventive measures can be initiated for high-risk patients by using the 23-valent pneumococcal vaccine. This vaccine is recommended for high-risk children 2 years of age and older. Revaccination should be considered after 3 to 5 years for children less than 10 years of age or those who demonstrate a rapidly declining antibody titer.[77]

*H. influenzae* is the second most common cause of bacterial LRTI in the pre-school-aged child. The most prevalent serotype is type b, but occasionally other strains have been reported. This disease is usually seen in children less than 5 years of age, with the greatest incidence being between 4 and 7 months of age.[20] The clinical presentation is similar to that of pneumococcal pneumonia. Children present with fever, cough, and a leukocytosis. The chest roentgenogram findings with this pathogen demonstrate no characteristic or consistent pattern. Approximately one half of patients have additional foci of infection. These extrapul-

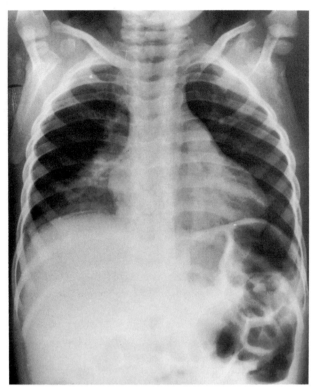

**Figure 9–5.** *Streptococcus pneumoniae* pneumonia.

monary infections include otitis media, meningitis, epiglottitis, and pericarditis.[12]

*H. influenzae* type b conjugate vaccines are recommended to begin at 2 months of age.[78] With widespread use of this vaccine, the number of infections caused by this organism should decrease. Other preventive measures include chemoprophylaxis of household contacts of children who have invasive disease such as bacteremia, meningitis, septic arthritis, or epiglottitis. There is an increased risk of transmission to household contacts younger than 48 months of age.[25] It is recommended that any members of the household where a case has been identified, who live with other members younger than 48 months of age, should receive rifampin prophylaxis. If the exposed child has received all of his or her *Haemophilus* vaccines, then prophyaxis is not required.[79] Children younger than 2 years of age who spend more than 25 hours each week in contact with the source case in day care facilities should also receive prophylaxis. If two or more cases have occurred within 60 days in the same institution, all children and personnel in the day care center should receive prophylaxis. The index case should also receive a course of rifampin before discharge to prevent the carrier state. Pregnant women should be excluded from treatment. The dose is 20 mg/kg, with a maximum of 600 mg given once daily for 4 days.[79a]

LRTI caused by *S. aureus* is a rapidly progressive disease. The patient's presenting symptoms usually include fever, lethargy, and severe respiratory distress. Characteristically, there is rapid progression on chest roentgenograms from normal to consolidated lesion with empyema (Fig. 9–6). Repeated chest roentgenograms are often helpful. Although a large percentage of patients develop pneumatoceles during their illness, a combination of pneumothorax

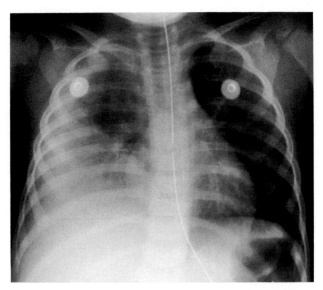

**Figure 9–6.** *Staphylococcus aureus* pneumonia with empyema.

and empyema is highly suggestive of staphylococcal disease.[80]

Other bacteria cause LRTI less frequently (see Table 9–2). Anaerobes (eg, *Fusobacterium, Bacteriodes),* group A *Streptococcus, Moraxella catarrhalis, N. meningitidis,* and *P. aeruginosa* are all potential pathogens.[81–84] *Bordetella pertussis* continues to cause many LRTI, especially in children younger than 6 months of age. As a result of vaccine strategies in the industrialized nations, this disorder is mostly seen in developing countries.[85]

*M. pneumoniae* and *C. pneumoniae,* although predominant organisms in the school-aged child, rarely cause infection in preschool-aged children.[86, 87] Infection caused by *Legionella pneumophila* (eg, legionnaires disease), *Chlamydia psittaci* (eg, bird fancier's disease), *Francisella tularensis* (eg, tularemia), *Coxiella burnetti* (eg, Q fever), *Ehrlichia chaffeensis,* and *Rickettsia* are also rare.[88, 89]

*Mycobacterium tuberculosis* infections may present in this age group. Because of the increasing prevalence of this infection, careful histories should be obtained from patients with LRTI to discover any exposure to active cases of tuberculosis. Children with a significant exposure history should be considered to be at risk for infections with *M. tuberculosis.* Exposure to adults in the household with acquired immunodeficiency syndrome (AIDS) also places children at an increased risk for developing tuberculosis. Mycobacterial infections in these patients are common and can be difficult to treat. The effect this will have on childhood tuberculosis is unknown. Patients with mycobacterial infections usually demonstrate hilar adenopathy or atelectasis on chest roentgenograms and demonstrate a positive tuberculosis skin test.[90]

Patients with AIDS may have their case-defining illness in the form of a LRTI. Infections with *Pneumocystis carinii,* cytomegalovirus, or histoplasmosis are among the most common opportunistic pathogens in this patient group. A history of intravenous drug abuse, prostitution, blood transfusion, or other high-risk behavior may help to identify these patients early so that appropriate steps to diagnosis and therapy can be taken.

Foreign-body aspiration should always be considered. Hyperinflation limited to one side of a chest roentgenogram can be diagnostic.

## DIAGNOSIS

A chest roentgenogram should be obtained for confirmation and characterization of any infiltrate before antimicrobial therapy in patients with LRTI. Chest roentgenograms are indicated if children with fever display any of the following pulmonary findings: nasal flaring, grunting, intercostal retractions, tachypnea, crackles, or decreased breath sounds. With the use of these criteria, the number of unnecessary roentgenograms is greatly reduced.[91, 92] The results of roentgenograms must be interpreted with caution. Although there are certain characteristic abnormalities unique to bacterial (ie, lobar infiltrates) and viral (ie, interstitial infiltrates) pulmonary infections, it is not practical to differentiate the two based on roentgenograms alone.[93, 94]

Peripheral blood examinations obtained in the evaluation of LRTI rarely enable the clinician to differentiate between bacterial and viral illnesses. Although more common in patients with presumed bacterial pathogens, leukocyte counts elevated above 15,000 cells/mm[3] and elevated erythrocyte sedimentation rates are not specific enough to dismiss viral causes.[95] One infection for which a peripheral blood examination is helpful is *B. pertussis.* These children usually have a severe leukocytosis (20,000–50,000 cells/mm[3]) with an absolute lymphocytosis.

A positive culture can provide a specific bacteriologic diagnosis, but this can be a problem in the preschool-aged child. Blood cultures are positive only 5% to 10% of the time, depending on the etiologic agent and the number of samples obtained.[18, 94, 96] Because younger children usually do not expectorate their secretions, sputum cultures for bacterial pathogens are not helpful. Nasopharyngeal and throat cultures are not of value because results may only represent colonization by bacterial organisms. Cultures that are obtained through an endotracheal tube from a recently intubated patient, lung puncture, bronchoalveolar lavage, or open biopsy can be diagnostic in selected patients. Patients who are candidates for such procedures include those who are severely ill, have progressive or unresponsive disease, or are immunosuppressed (see Chap. 10). Because bacterial pathogens are difficult to isolate, antigen detection can be attempted as a means of diagnosing bacterial LRTI. Although bacterial antigen detection systems have a higher yield than blood cultures, specific bacteria are detected only 20% of the time with these techniques.[94, 97] Because most LRTI are not the result of bacteremia, positive bacterial antigen tests may reflect other conditions, such as otitis media or recent vaccination, and not the cause of the LRTI.[97–99] If bacterial antigens are employed, the highest yield is obtained from concentrated urine specimens. Antigen tests are available for *H. influenzae* type b, *S. pneumoniae,* and *N. meningitidis,* but their role in a diagnostic evaluation should be limited.

Viral pathogens may be isolated by culturing secretions obtained from the nasopharynx. Because of the length of time necessary for the growth of these cultures, the clinician often does not benefit from the results. Rapid diagnostic techniques are available for the detection of respiratory syncytial virus.[100] These immunofluorescence or enzyme-linked immunosorbent assays are commercially available and help the diagnosis. The sensitivity and specificity of these tests exceed 80% to 90% when compared with culture, and when compared with each other, they are in agreement more than 86% of the time.[101]

## MANAGEMENT

Most children with LRTI are treated as outpatients, but some children benefit from inpatient therapy. Children should be considered for inpatient therapy if they are younger than 6 months of age, are hypoxemic, have significant respiratory distress, are unable to eat or drink, have a toxic appearance, are unresponsive to oral medications, have an underlying disease state, have recurrent pneumonias, or have a family that is unable to care for the patient.

When patients with LRTI are admitted to the hospital, isolation techniques should be observed. These techniques should prevent both aerosol and large droplet transmission so that other patients in the hospital do not become infected.[102, 103]

Antiviral therapy was impeded for many years by the lack of reliable and rapid diagnostic techniques. With the ability to establish a diagnosis quickly, many of the respiratory viral pathogens can be treated. Ribavirin is a broad-spectrum antiviral agent that inhibits replication of respiratory syncytial virus, influenza, and other respiratory viruses.[104, 105] The mechanism of action is not entirely understood. Because of the cost of the medication, the cumbersome administration techniques, and the self-limited nature of the disease, ribavirin is recommended by the American Academy of Pediatrics only for high-risk infants who have RSV infections. High-risk children are those with congenital heart disease or bronchopulmonary dysplasia, premature infants, transplant patients, and other immunodeficient patients. These infants are at an increased risk of having severe complications associated with their RSV infection. Infants who have a $PaO_2$ of less than 65 mm Hg and a rising $PaCO_2$ are also candidates for therapy.[106] Ill infants requiring mechanical ventilation may also be treated with ribavirin, but only if proper precautions are followed to avoid ventilator dysfunction caused by the delivery of the medication.[107] Six grams of ribavirin are mixed into a solution and given by aerosolization for 18 hours over 5 to 7 days. Keeping infants under the aerosol for most of the day can be difficult. Incidental exposure of hospital personnel and visitors to ribavirin is to be expected. Ribavirin is teratogenic in rodents, but has not been proven to have similar effects in primates. However, concern still exists about exposure of pregnant women to this medication. Until further studies are available, it would be prudent for personnel who are pregnant to avoid working directly with aerosolized ribavirin.[104]

Amantadine is available for the treatment and prophylaxis of influenza A. This medication is recommended for patients with severe disease or with chronic underlying conditions that place them at risk for complications caused by influenza infections. Little information is available on the use of this medication in children younger than 1 year of age. Therapy should begin soon after the onset of symptoms and be continued from 2 to 7 days, depending on clinical improvement.[108] The recommended dose of amantadine is 4.4 mg/kg (150 mg/d maximum) in two divided doses each day for children 1 to 9 years of age. If the child is older than 9 years of age, the dose is 200 mg in two divided doses each day. Amantadine is contraindicated in patients with seizure disorders, and it has been associated with other central nervous system side effects such as insomnia, lightheadedness, and difficulty in concentrating. These complaints resolve after the medication is discontinued.[104] Rimantadine, a close relative of amantadine, has been proven effective for use in children with influenza A infection, but it is investigational in the United States.[109] Children with influenza infections should not receive salicylate therapy because of the risk of developing Reye syndrome.

Children who are ambulatory and have a presumed bacterial LRTI can be placed on a broad-spectrum antimicrobial agent. These antibiotics should have good activity against the two most common pathogens, *S. pneumoniae* and *H. influenzae*. Amoxicillin is the drug of choice. Some of the *Haemophilus* species may be resistant to aminopenicillins and, if previous experience has demonstrated this to be a problem, a change of antimicrobial agents may be indicated if there is no improvement after 24 to 48 hours. Available preparations include amoxicillin-clavulanate potassium, erythromycin ethylsuccinate-sulfisoxazole, trimethoprim-sulfamethoxazole, cefuroxime axetil, cefixime, and cefaclor. These preparations vary in preparation availability, spectrum of efficacy, dosing schedule, and cost to the patient.[110] An intramuscular injection of ampicillin or ceftriaxone is often administered before starting oral medications. These intramuscular medications should be seen only as adjuncts to oral therapy and not as substitutes for hospital admission with severely ill children. There is currently no role for quinolones in this age group. The total length of therapy should be between 10 and 14 days.

For the hospitalized child older than 3 months of age, empiric antimicrobial therapy may be initiated with ampicillin and chloramphenicol, cefotaxime, cefuroxime, ceftriaxone, or ceftazidime (see Table 9–4). These antimicrobial agents ensure a broad range of coverage. In patients in whom *S. aureus* is a major concern, nafcillin should be added to the regimen or substituted for ampicillin. The total length of intravenous therapy depends on the organism isolated and the patient's clinical course. In uncomplicated cases, intravenous administration of antimicrobial agents can be continued until the patient has been afebrile for 24 to 48 hours, and then an oral preparation may be given to complete 10 to 14 days of therapy. In patients with pulmonary or extrapulmonary complications, the length of intravenous therapy may be extended.

## REFERENCES

1. Gwatkin DR: How many die? A set of demographic estimates of the annual number of infant and child deaths in the world. Am J Public Health 70:1286, 1980.
2. Dingle JH, Badger GF, Jordan WS Jr: Illness in the Home: A Study of 25,000 Illnesses in a Group of Cleveland Families. Cleveland, Press of Case Western Reserve University, 1964.

3. Wald ER, Dashefsky B, Byers C, et al: Frequency and severity of infections in day care. J Pediatr 112:540, 1988.
4. Loda FA, Glezen WP, Clyde WA Jr: Respiratory disease in group day care. Pediatrics 49:428, 1972.
5. Glezen WP, Loda FA, Clyde WA Jr, et al: Epidemiologic patterns of acute lower respiratory disease of children in a pediatric group practice. Pediatrics 78:397, 1971.
6. Glezen WP: Viral respiratory infections. Pediatr Ann 20:407, 1991.
7. Busse WW: Pathogenesis and sequelae of respiratory infections. Rev Infect Dis 13:S477, 1991.
8. Schenker MB, Samet JM, Speizer FE: Risk factors for childhood respiratory disease: The effect of host factors and home environmental exposures. Am Rev Respir Dis 128:1038, 1983.
9. Vedal S, Schenker MB, Samet JM, et al: Risk factors for childhood respiratory disease: Analysis of pulmonary function. Am Rev Respir Dis 130:187, 1984.
10. Glezen WP: Viral pneumonia. In Chernick V, Kendig EL Jr (eds): Disorders of the Respiratory Tract in Children, ed 5 . Philadelphia, WB Saunders, 1990:394.
11. Loda FA, Collier AM, Glezen WP, et al: Occurrence of *Diplococcus pneumoniae* in the upper respiratory tract of children. J Pediatr 87:1087, 1975.
12. Mendelman PM, Smith AL: *Haemophilus influenzae*. In Feigin RD, Cherry JD (eds): Textbook of Pediatric Infectious Diseases, ed 2. Philadelphia, WB Saunders, 1987:1142.
13. Dennehy PH: Respiratory infections in the newborn. Clin Perinatol 14:667, 1987.
14. Leigh MW, Carson JL, Denny FW: Pathogenesis of respiratory infections due to influenza virus: Implications for developing countries. Rev Infect Dis 13:S501, 1991.
15. Glezen WP, Denny FW: Epidemiology of acute lower respiratory disease in children. N Engl J Med 288:498, 1973.
16. Maletzky AJ, Cooney MK, Luce R, et al: Epidemiology of viral and mycoplasmal agents associated with childhood lower respiratory illness in a civilian population. J Pediatr 78:407, 1971.
17. Paisley JW, Lauer BA, McIntosh K, et al: Pathogens associated with acute lower respiratory tract infection in young children. Pediatr Infect Dis 3:14, 1984.
18. Nohynek H, Eskola J, Laine E, et al: The causes of hospital-treated acute lower respiratory tract infection in children. Am J Dis Child 145:618, 1991.
19. Zollar LM, Krause HE, Mufson MA: Microbiologic studies on young infants with lower respiratory tract disease. Am J Dis Child 126:56, 1973.
20. Arguedas AG, Stutman HR, Marks MI: Bacterial pneumonias. In Chernick V, Kendig EL Jr (eds): Disorders of the Respiratory Tract in Children, ed 5. Philadelphia, WB Saunders, 1990:371.
21. Klein JO: Bacterial pneumonias. In Feigin RD, Cherry JD (eds): Textbook of Pediatric Infectious Diseases, ed 2. Philadelphia, WB Saunders, 1987:329.
22. Wald ER, Guerra N, Byers C: Frequency and severity of infections in day care: Three-year follow-up. J Pediatr 118:509, 1991.
23. Glezen WP: Viral respiratory infections. Pediatr Ann 20:407, 1991.
24. Shapiro ED: Bacterial respiratory infections and otitis media. Pediatr Ann 20:413, 1991.
25. Istre GR, Conner JS, Broome CV, et al: Risk factors for primary invasive *Haemophilus influenzae* disease: Increased risk from day care attendance and school-aged household members. J Pediatr 106:190, 1985.
26. Bruhn FW, Mokrohisky ST, McIntosh K: Apnea associated with respiratory syncytial virus infection in young infants. J Pediatr 90:382, 1977.
27. Ablow RC, Driscoll SG, Effmann EL, et al: A comparison of early-onset group B streptococcal neonatal infection and the respiratory-distress syndrome of the newborn. N Engl J Med 294:65, 1976.
28. Teele D: Pneumonia: Antimicrobial therapy for infants and children. Pediatr Infect Dis 4:330, 1985.
29. Baker CJ: Group B streptococcal infections in neonates. Pediatr Rev 1:5, 1979.
30. Baker CJ, Edwards MS: Group B streptococcal infections. In Remington JS, Klein JO (eds): Infectious Diseases of the Fetus and Newborn Infant, ed 3. Philadelphia, WB Saunders, 1990:742.
31. Papageorgiou A, Bauer CR, Fletcher BD, et al: *Klebsiella* pneumonia with pneumatocele formation in a newborn infant. Can Med Assoc J 109:1217, 1973.
32. Kuhn JD, Lee SB: Pneumatoceles associated with *Escherichia coli* pneumonias in the newborn. Pediatrics 51:1008, 1973.
33. Barker JA, McLean SD, Jordan GD, et al: Primary neonatal herpes simplex virus pneumonia. Pediatr Infect Dis J 9:285, 1990.
34. Hubbell C, Dominguez R, Kohl S: Neonatal herpes simplex pneumonitis. Rev Infect Dis 10:431, 1988.
35. Abzug MJ, Levin MJ: Neonatal adenovirus infection: Four patients and review of the literature. Pediatrics 87:890, 1991.
36. Morens DM: Enteroviral disease in early infancy. J Pediatr 92:374, 1978.
37. Boyle RJ, Chandler BD, Stonestreet BS, et al: Early identification of sepsis in infants with respiratory distress. Pediatrics 62:744, 1978.
38. Sherman MP, Chance KH, Goetzman BW: Gram's stains of tracheal secretions predict neonatal bacteremia. Am J Dis Child 138:848, 1984.
39. Sherman MP, Goetzman BW, Ahlfors CE, et al: Tracheal aspiration and its clinical correlates in the diagnosis of congenital pneumonia. Pediatrics 65:258, 1980.
40. Sanchez PJ, Siegel JD, Cushion NB, et al: Significance of a positive urine group B streptococcal latex agglutination test in neonates. J Pediatr 116:601, 1990.
41. Whitley R, Arvin A, Prober C, et al: A controlled trial comparing vidarabine with acyclovir in neonatal herpes simplex virus infection. N Engl J Med 324:444, 1991.
42. Englund JA, Fletcher CV, Balfour HH: Acyclovir therapy in neonates. J Pediatr 119:129, 1991.
43. McKinney RE, Katz SL, Wilfert CM: Chronic enteroviral meningoencephalitis in agammaglobulinemic patients. Rev Infect Dis 9:334, 1987.
44. Schachter J: Chlamydial infections. N Engl J Med 298:540, 1978.
45. Beem MO, Saxon EM, Tipple MA: Chlamydial infections of infants. In Chernick V, Kendig EL Jr (eds): Disorders of the Respiratory Tract in Children, ed 5. Philadelphia, WB Saunders, 1990:807.
46. Stagno S, Brasfield DM, Brown MB, et al: Infant pneumonia associated with cytomegalovirus, *Chlamydia, Pneumocystis* and *Ureaplasma*: A prospective study. Pediatrics 68:322, 1981.
47. Rettig PJ: Infections due to *Chlamydia trachomatis* from infancy to adolescence. Pediatr Infect Dis 5:449, 1986.
48. Tipple MA, Beem MO, Saxon EM: Clinical characteristics of the afebrile pneumonia associated with *Chlamydia trachomatis* infection in infants less than six months of age. Pediatrics 63:192, 1979.
49. Radkowski MA, Kranzler JK, Beem MO, et al: *Chlamydia pneumonia* in infants: Radiography in 125 cases. Am J Radiol 137:703, 1981.
50. Dworsky ME, Stagno S: Newer agents causing pneumonitis in early infancy. Pediatr Infect Dis 1:188, 1982.
51. Rudd PT, Waites KB, Duffy LB, et al: *Ureaplasma urealyticum* and its possible role in pneumonia during the neonatal period and infancy. Pediatr Infect Dis 5:S288, 1986.
52. Paisley JW, Lauer BA, Melinkovich P, et al: Rapid diagnosis of *Chlamydia trachomatis* pneumonia in infants by direct immunofluorescence microscopy of nasopharyngeal secretions. J Pediatr 109:653, 1986.
53. Berman S: Epidemiology of acute respiratory infections in children of developing countries. Rev Infect Dis 13:S454, 1991.
54. Glezen WP, Paredes A, Allison JE, et al: Risk of respiratory syncytial virus infection for infants from low-income families in relationship to age, sex, ethnic group and maternal antibody level. J Pediatr 98:708, 1981.
55. Gardner PS: Respiratory syncytial virus infections: Postgrad Med J 49:788, 1973.
56. Groothuis JR, Gutierrez KM, Lauer BA: Respiratory syncytial virus infection in children with bronchopulmonary dysplasia. Pediatrics 82:199, 1988.
57. MacDonald NE, Hall CB, Suffin SC, et al: Respiratory syncytial viral infection in infants with congenital heart disease. N Engl J Med 307:397, 1982.
58. Rice RP, Loda FA: A roentgenographic analysis of respiratory syncytial virus pneumonia in infants. Radiology 87:1021, 1966.
59. Wildin SR, Chonmaitree T, Swischuk L: Roentgenographic features of common pediatric viral respiratory tract infections. Am J Dis Child 142:43, 1988.
60. Hall CB, Douglas RG, Geiman JM: Quantitative shedding patterns of respiratory syncytial virus in infants. J Infect Dis 132:151, 1975.
61. Hall CB, Hall WJ, Speers DM: Clinical and physiological manifestations of bronchiolitis and pneumonia: Outcome of respiratory syncytial virus. Am J Dis Child 133:798, 1979.
62. Glezen WP, Frank AL, Taber LH, et al: Parainfluenza virus type 3:

Seasonality and risk of infection and re-infection in young children. J Infect Dis 150:851, 1984.

63. Glezen WP, Paredes A, Taber LH: Influenza in children: Relationship to other respiratory agents. JAMA 243:1345, 1980.

64. Schwarzmann SW, Adler JL, Sullivan RL Jr, et al: Bacterial pneumonia during the Hong Kong influenza epidemic of 1968–69. Arch Intern Med 127:1037, 1971.

65. Committee on Infectious Diseases, American Academy of Pediatrics: Report of the Committee on Infectious Diseases, ed 22. Elk Grove Village, IL: American Academy of Pediatrics, 1991:274.

66. Cesario TC, Kriel RL, Caldwell GG, et al: Epidemiologic observations of virus infection in a closed population of young children. Am J Epidemiol 94:457, 1971.

67. Becroft DMO: Histopathology of fatal adenovirus infection of the respiratory tract in young children. J Clin Pathol 20:561, 1967.

68. Spencer MJ, Cherry JD: Adenoviral infections. In Feigin RD, Cherry JD (eds): Textbook of Pediatric Infectious Diseases, ed 2. Philadelphia, WB Saunders, 1987:1688.

69. MacPherson RI, Cumming GR, Chernick V: Unilateral hyperlucent lung: A complication of viral pneumonia. J Can Assoc Radiol 20:225, 1969.

70. Lang WR, Howden CW, Laws J, et al: Bronchopneumonia with serious sequelae in children with evidence of adenovirus type 21 infection. Br Med J 1:73, 1969.

71. Gold R, Wilt JC, Adhikari PK, et al: Adenoviral pneumonia and its complications in infancy and childhood. J Can Assoc Radiol 20:218, 1969.

72. Simila S, Linna O, Lanning P, et al: Chronic lung damage caused by adenovirus type 7: A ten-year follow-up study. Chest 80:127, 1981.

73. Markowitz LE, Nieburg P: The burden of acute respiratory infection due to measles in developing countries and the potential impact of measles vaccine. Rev Infect Dis 13:S555, 1991.

74. Committee on Infectious Diseases, American Academy of Pediatrics: Report of the Committee on Infectious Diseases, ed 22. Elk Grove Village, IL: American Academy of Pediatrics, 1991:308.

75. Krasinski K, Borkowsky W, Bonk S, et al: Bacterial infections in human immunodeficiency virus-infected children. Pediatr Infect Dis J 7:323, 1988.

76. Teele DW: Pneumococcal infections. In Feigin RD, Cherry JD (eds): Textbook of Pediatric Infectious Diseases, ed 2. Philadelphia, WB Saunders, 1987:1243.

77. Committee on Infectious Diseases, American Academy of Pediatrics: Report of the Committee on Infectious Diseases, ed 22. Elk Grove Village, IL: American Academy of Pediatrics, 1991:373.

78. Peter G, Easton JG, Halsey NA, et al: Haemophilus influenzae type b conjugated vaccines: Recommendations for immunization of infants and children 2 months of age and older: Update. Pediatrics 88:169, 1991.

79. Murphy TV, Pastor P, Medley F, et al: Decreased Haemophilus colonization in children vaccinated with Haemophilus influenzae type B conjugate vaccine. J Pediatr 122:517, 1993.

79a. Committee on Infectious Disease, American Academy of Pediatrics: Report of the Committee on Infectious Diseases, ed 22. Elk Grove Village, IL: American Academy of Pediatrics, 1991:220.

80. Hendren WH, Haggerty RJ: Staphylococcal pneumonia in infancy and childhood: Analysis of 75 cases. JAMA 168:6, 1958.

81. Brook I: Anaerobic infections in childhood. Rev Infect Dis 6:S187, 1984.

82. Wheeler MC, Roe MH, Kaplan EL, et al: Outbreak of group A Streptococcus septicemia in children: Clinical, epidemiologic, and microbiological correlates. JAMA 266:533, 1991.

83. Molteni RA: Group A β-hemolytic streptococcal pneumonia: Clinical course and complications of management. Am J Dis Child 131:1366, 1977.

84. Berg RA, Bartley DL: Pneumonia associated with Branhamella catarrhalis in infants. Pediatr Infect Dis J 6:569, 1987.

85. Wright PF: Pertussis in developing countries: Definitions of the problem and prospects for control. Rev Infect Dis 13:S528, 1991.

86. Broughton RA: Infections due to Mycoplasma pneumoniae in childhood. Pediatr Infect Dis 5:71, 1986.

87. Grayston JT, Wang SP, Kuo CC, et al: Current knowledge on Chlamydia pneumoniae, strain TWAR, an important cause of pneumonia and other acute respiratory diseases. Eur J Clin Microbiol Infect Dis 8:191, 1989.

88. Carlson NC, Kuskie MR, Dobyns EL, et al: Legionellosis in children: An expanding spectrum. Pediatr Infect Dis J 9:133, 1990.

89. Tuazon CU: Atypical pneumonias: When symptoms just don't add up. J Respir Dis 7:91, 1986.

90. Snider DE, Rieder HL, Coombs D, et al: Tuberculosis in children, Pediatr Infect Dis 7:271, 1988.

91. Leventhal JM: Clinical predictors of pneumonia as a guide to ordering chest roentgenograms. Clin Pediatr 21:730, 1982.

92. Zukin DD, Hoffman JR, Cleveland RH, et al: Correlation of pulmonary signs and symptoms with chest radiographs in the pediatric age group. Ann Emerg Med 15:792, 1986.

93. McCarthy PL, Spiesel SZ, Stashwick CA, et al: Radiographic findings and etiologic diagnosis in ambulatory childhood pneumonias. Clin Pediatr 20:686, 1981.

94. Turner RB, Lande AE, Chase P, et al: Pneumonia in pediatric outpatients: Cause and clinical manifestations. J Pediatr 111:194, 1987.

95. McCarthy PL, Jekel JF, Dolan TF: Comparison of acute-phase reactants in pediatric patients with fever. Pediatrics 62:716, 1978.

96. Gooch WM: Bronchitis and pneumonia in ambulatory patients. Pediatr Infect Dis J 6:137, 1987.

97. Ramsey BW, Marcuse EK, Foy HM, et al: Use of bacterial antigen detection in the diagnosis of pediatric lower respiratory tract infections. Pediatrics 78:1, 1986.

98. Martin SJ, Hoganson DA, Thomas ET. Detection of Streptococcus pneumoniae and Haemophilus influenzae type b antigens in acute nonbacteremic pneumonia. J Clin Microbiol 25:248, 1987.

99. Rothstein EP, Madore DV, Girone JAC, et al: Comparison of antigenuria after immunization with three Haemophilus influenzae type b conjugate vaccines. Pediatr Infect Dis J 10:311, 1991.

100. McIntosh K: Respiratory syncytial virus infections in infants and children: Diagnosis and treatment. Pediatr Rev 9:191, 1987.

101. Krilov LR, Marcoux L, Isenberg HD: Comparison of three enzyme-linked immunosorbent assays and a direct fluorescent-antibody test for detection of respiratory syncytial virus antigen. J Clin Microbiol 26:377, 1988.

102. Serwint JR, Miller RM, Korsch BM: Influenza type A and B infections in hospitalized pediatric patients: Who should be immunized? Am J Dis Child 145:623, 1991.

103. Avendano LF, Larranaga C, Palomino MA, et al: Community- and hospital-acquired respiratory syncytial virus infections in Chile. Pediatr Infect Dis J 10:564, 1991.

104. Balfour HH, Englund JA: Antiviral drugs in pediatrics. Am J Dis Child 143:1307, 1989.

105. Steele RW: Antiviral agents for respiratory infections. Pediatr Infect Dis J 7:457, 1988.

106. Committee on Infectious Diseases, American Academy of Pediatrics: Report of the Committee on Infectious Diseases, ed 22. Elk Grove Village, IL: American Academy of Pediatrics, 1991:581.

107. Smith DW, Frankel LR, Mathers LH, et al: A controlled trial of aerosolized ribavirin in infants receiving mechanical ventilation for severe respiratory syncytial virus infection. N Engl J Med 325:24, 1991.

108. Committee on Infectious Diseases, American Academy of Pediatrics: Report of the Committee on Infectious Diseases, ed 22. Elk Grove Village, IL: American Academy of Pediatrics, 1991:274.

109. Hall CB, Dolin R, Gala CL, et al: Children with influenza A infection: Treatment with rimantadine. Pediatrics 80:275, 1987.

110. Grossman M, Klein JO, McCarthy PL, et al: Consensus: Management of presumed bacterial pneumonia in ambulatory children. Pediatr Infect Dis 3:497, 1984.

# CHAPTER 10

# Nosocomial Pneumonia in Children

## RICHARD F. JACOBS

Acute respiratory infections are a major worldwide public health problem because of the associated high morbidity and mortality rates in neonates, infants, and children. The incidence and severity of nosocomial pneumonia in children is equally impressive. Viruses are the most common cause of lower respiratory tract infections in children, and nosocomial pneumonia due to common respiratory viruses constitutes one of the largest groups of nosocomial infections in children. During viral respiratory seasons, nosocomial respiratory syncytial virus (RSV) accounts for as many as 15% of all hospitalized patients with RSV infections.[1] Older children are usually not prone to lower respiratory tract RSV disease. However as many as 60% of all hospitalized RSV infections are acquired nosocomially, with as many as 100% of immunocompromised older children manifesting serious lower respiratory tract disease.[2] Nosocomial influenza infection has been confirmed in 4% to 14% of low- to high-risk children.[3]

Nosocomial bacterial pneumonia is a common and potentially life-threatening complication of hospitalization in children. With the recognition that nosocomial bacterial pneumonia is an important cause of morbidity came the understanding that aerobic gram-negative bacilli predominate as the major bacterial agents in older children and adolescents.[4–6] The emergence of gram-negative bacilli as the predominant cause of nosocomial bacterial pneumonia in this group is related to the increased use of broad-spectrum antibiotics, the use of prolonged ventilatory assistance for critically ill patients, and newly developed respiratory equipment using mainstream reservoir nebulizers.[7–10] These risk factors have been described in retrospective analyses that suggested a fourfold increase in the incidence of nosocomial gram-negative pneumonia among hospitalized patients.[5] The demonstration that nosocomial bacterial infec-

tions due to *Staphylococcus epidermidis* and *Candida* species have increased in neonatal intensive care units (NICU) has also affected treatment algorithms.[11]

Nosocomial pneumonia in all ages is the third most common type of hospital-acquired infection, accounting for approximately 15% of all nosocomial infections.[4, 5, 8] The lung ranks third in frequency behind the urinary tract and skin as a site of hospital-acquired infection in children. Although the mortality rates for infection in the latter two organ systems range from 1% to 4%, the estimated mortality rate associated with nosocomial pneumonia is 20% to 50%. As many as 15% of all deaths occurring in hospitalized patients of all ages are directly related to nosocomial pneumonia, and nosocomial pneumonia is the most common fatal nosocomial infection for all ages in the United States.[8]

During the past two decades, more information has been published about the epidemiology and pathogenesis of this disease process, but controversy continues concerning the proper diagnostic tests and treatment regimens.[10] This controversy is amplified for the pediatric age group because of the high-risk patient populations, the increased risk of viral nosocomial pneumonia, the absence of safe invasive diagnostic testing, the increasing number of new antibacterial and antiviral drugs, and the advent of new vaccines.[4, 11] The risk of nosocomial pneumonia with a poor outcome has been increased by the use of modern intensive care facilities with the ability to maintain critically ill neonates and older children for prolonged periods with invasive life support techniques.[12–16] The ability of modern pediatricians to maintain life in very low-birth-weight premature newborns and in immunocompromised patients has also exposed more of these high-risk patients to nosocomial pneumonia with its subsequent complications, morbidity, and mortality.[11]

The incidence of nosocomial pneumonia depends on the

patient group, the patient environment, and the immunologic and nutritional status of the patient. The National Nosocomial Infections Study (NNIS) has recorded an annual incidence of nosocomial lower respiratory tract infection of approximately 0.55% (5.5 cases per 1000 discharges) for all ages.[8] In the NNIS report, the highest incidence (0.5%–1%) of nosocomial pneumonia occurred in the medical-surgical services. Pediatric services registered one of the lowest risks at 0.03% to 0.3% incidence. Increased patient risk groups in certain patient settings were evident. Respiratory intensive care units accounted for 20% of all nosocomial pneumonias, compared with a 17.5% rate for postoperative patients. NICU accounted for 7% of nosocomial pneumonias under similar circumstances.[8]

The postoperative patient has an increased risk of developing nosocomial pneumonia, the rate may approach 15 per 100 operations.[9, 15] Within this group, persons undergoing thoracic, thoracoabdominal, and upper abdominal surgical procedures are at the greatest risk because of postoperative pain that can result in an inability to clear secretions adequately, sedation and analgesia, and the use of chest tubes that can provide a direct conduit for bacterial entrance into the lower respiratory tract.

## PATHOGENESIS OF NOSOCOMIAL PNEUMONIA

In hospitalized patients, the pathophysiology of nosocomial pneumonia is related to altered or circumvented pulmonary antimicrobial defenses in the upper and lower respiratory tract.[16–18] Most cases of nosocomial pneumonia result from subclinical aspiration of oropharyngeal secretions that have become colonized by the resident hospital flora, including aerobic gram-positive and gram-negative organisms.[13, 16] In the pediatric hospital, it also includes viral agents because of patients hospitalized with contagious and seasonal respiratory viral illnesses.[19–23] The normal flora of most patients on admission to the hospital consists of gram-positive and gram-negative organisms, with species of *Neisseria*, α-streptococci, and staphylococci predominating. In colder months, many healthy persons are routinely colonized with *Haemophilus influenzae* and *Streptococcus pneumoniae*. Children, in particular, may be asymptomatically colonized with *Streptococcus pyogenes*.[13] Respiratory viruses are not common flora of the upper respiratory tract. This normal flora routinely protects against colonization with aerobic gram-negative bacilli and gram-positive organisms. Only 3% of healthy persons are colonized with gram-negative bacilli on admission to the hospital.

Although most animal and human research on bacterial pathogenesis in nosocomial pneumonia has been done in adults, the principles are important in the pathophysiology in children. Studies in healthy adult volunteers have shown that radioactively labeled concentrations of $10^8$ colony-forming units (CFU) per 1 mL of *Escherichia coli*, *Klebsiella pneumoniae*, and *Proteus mirabilis* have regularly failed to result in oropharyngeal colonization over a period of hours. Colonization, which is defined as the presence without the clinical consequences of these organisms, not considered part of normal flora, occurs regularly in hospitalized patients. The role of gram-negative bacterial coloni-

zation increases with the severity of the patient's illness, and the organisms occur in as many as 45% of patients hospitalized in an adult medical-surgical intensive care unit after 96 hours. As many as 25% of these patients become colonized within the first 24 hours. The risk factors for colonization include acidosis, endotracheal intubation, hypotension, and broad-spectrum antibiotic therapy.[14, 16, 18] Turbulence in the nasal passageways normally results in the impaction of large particles, preventing deposition in the lower respiratory tract. Nasotracheal, orotracheal, or tracheostomy tubes bypass this initial host defense mechanism for preventing colonization of the upper respiratory tract. Twenty-three percent of patients with gram-negative oropharyngeal colonization develop nosocomial pneumonia, but only 3% of noncolonized hospitalized patients do so.[15]

Defining the source of colonizing flora in these patient populations is important for developing schemes for prevention of upper airway colonization. A fecal-oral route for bacterial contamination of respiratory airways has historically been suspected for bedridden patients.[14, 16] This route does not readily explain the frequency of colonization by organisms such as *Pseudomonas aeruginosa* and *Acinetobacter* species that are not usual inhabitants of the human gastrointestinal tract. Patients having daily cultures monitored from rectal, hypopharyngeal, and tracheal sites after prolonged intubation commonly have Enterobacteriaceae in the hypopharynx and rectum before their appearance in tracheal cultures.[13, 16] In contrast, non-Enterobacteriaceae and colonizing Enterobacteriaceae originate primarily from changes in the patient's endogenous flora.[13–16] Investigators have suggested that the most important factor for transmission of this environmental flora is the hands of health care personnel and the respiratory therapy equipment. Other factors in the intensive care unit that can enhance bacterial colonization of critically ill patients include the use of nebulized or aerosolized respiratory therapy medications and the use of gastric alkalization to prevent stress gastritis, ulcers, and bleeding. These procedures increase the number of patients with extensive bacterial overgrowth in the upper gastrointestinal and respiratory tract. This appears to lead to airway colonization secondary to aspiration of gastric microflora. Many of these same factors are vital in the spread of respiratory viral pathogens in the hospital.[14–18]

Nosocomial pneumonia occurs when these organisms evade the mucociliary and cellular defenses of the lower respiratory tract. This may result from a direct effect on the mucociliary apparatus (eg, RSV infection) or on the cellular host defenses in the lower respiratory tract (eg, influenza) or from a primary or secondary immunodeficiency state (eg, neutropenic chemotherapy patients). The most important factor predisposing a patient to nosocomial pneumonia is endotracheal intubation. Short-term intubation for surgery or airway maintenance and longer periods of intubation for respiratory failure are associated with the highest rates (15%–20%) of nosocomial pneumonia. The incidence of nosocomial pneumonia for intubated patients is fourfold higher than for nonintubated patients; tracheostomy tube placement has an even higher risk of nosocomial pneumonia. The fact that these are critically ill patients requiring prolonged hospitalization in intensive care units is an obvious explanation for this increased risk.[15, 19] However, the endotracheal tube eliminates the effective natural host defense mechanisms of the upper airway. The filtration system of the upper airway and the mucociliary clearance system of the larger airways are bypassed during intubation. Accentuating this loss of mucociliary transport is the mechanical irritation and damage to the respiratory epithelium, which can predispose the patient to local colonization with potential bacterial and viral pathogens. In a prospective surveillance in the NICU environment, low birth weight and patent ductus arteriosus were variables strongly associated with nosocomial infection. Nosocomial pneumonia occurred in 33.3% of patients because of the risk factors of prolonged hospitalization, endotracheal intubation, nasogastric tubes, and broad-spectrum antibiotics.[19]

Nosocomial pneumonia may occur as a result of metastatic infection secondary to bacteremia or primary infection at a distant site. Distant infections, such as peritonitis, may contribute to the establishment of nosocomial pneumonia. The infrequent association of nosocomial pneumonia with bacteremia suggests that primary respiratory infection is the most common route.[4, 9, 11] This may not be valid in neonates because umbilical catheters for vascular access predispose these patients to bacteremia from a variety of organisms such as *S. epidermidis* and *Candida albicans*. Distant infection may selectively sequester polymorphonuclear leukocytes away from the lung and potentially explain the increased mortality from gram-negative pneumonia in these cases.

The factors predisposing to nosocomial pneumonia include age (eg, premature and low-birth-weight newborns), poor nutritional status, underlying pulmonary immune status, length of time in the hospital, season (ie, predominantly viral pathogens), general anesthesia, endotracheal intubation, tracheostomy, inhalation therapy, antibiotic therapy, and respiratory tract colonization with gram-negative bacilli.[4, 11, 19]

## Patient Groups

The prognosis for children with nosocomial pneumonia is determined by the major risk factors for acquisition of this disease, and those with the highest risk also have the worst outcome. Any hospitalized patient is considered to have an added risk for nosocomial pneumonia. However, patients who manifest acidosis, hypotension, hypoperfusion, or an altered state of consciousness or who require nasotracheal or orotracheal intubation or nasogastric tube placement have an increased risk for a poor outcome.[5, 15] A special pediatric category comprises patients at risk for symptomatic or asymptomatic aspiration, including children with tracheoesophageal fistulas, swallowing dyscoordination, or gastroesophageal reflux and surgery patients with unprotected airways. These patients are at increased risk for aspiration of resident flora the hypopharynx.

The circumstances in which these children have been hospitalized for diagnostic workup or treatment of the underlying diseases increase the risk for nosocomial pneumonia with hospital-acquired pathogens. Included in this group are patients with primary and secondary myopathies with altered swallowing mechanisms and children with facial burns and smoke inhalation requiring prolonged hospitalization. Children with underlying pulmonary disease, cardiac disease (especially shunt lesions with pulmonary hypertension), and primary immunodeficiencies (severe combined immune deficiency) have a marked risk for fatal nosocomial pneumonia caused by common viral pathogens.[4, 20–23] The special circumstances involving pediatric patients include the spread of highly contagious viral pathogens such as measles, varicella-zoster virus (VZV), and influenza. The ease of spread of RSV as fomites on human or inanimate contacts and the transmission of cytomegalovirus (CMV) through blood products to CMV-seronegative newborns are added risks for nosocomial infections in children.[20–23]

Malnutrition increases the incidence of nosocomial pneumonia in pediatric patients. Included in this group of high-risk patients are immunocompromised children with a failure to thrive. The risk for bacterial and viral pneumonia with a fatal outcome in children with primary immunodeficiencies has been well documented.[20, 21] Secondary immunodeficiency states such as those of children receiving cancer chemotherapy, transplanted organ recipients, and AIDS patients place these patients at high risk for nosocomial pneumonia.[22, 24] Included in this group of high-risk children are premature newborns. A premature newborn requires prolonged hospitalization, frequently with extended endotracheal intubation, a major risk factor for nosocomial pneumonia.[11] These predisposing factors, coupled with an underlying immune system that is not the equivalent of that of older children and adults, and the continued problem of poor nutrition, make premature newborns one of the highest-risk pediatric patient groups for nosocomial pneumonia.[11, 19] In addition to having predisposing factors for upper respiratory tract colonization, altered local or systemic host defense parameters, and underlying disease states, these patients are at increased risk for nosocomial pneumonia and excessive mortality.[4]

## Etiologic Agents

Viral nosocomial pneumonias, although not fatal in most circumstances, are particularly dangerous in children with secondary immunodeficiency states caused by cancer chemotherapy and organ transplantation.[2, 23] RSV nosocomial pneumonia in patients with congenital heart disease, especially those with shunt lesions, and patients with pulmonary hypertension has an excessive mortality rate, ranging from 40% to 80%.[4, 5, 8]

The relation between etiologic agents and mortality from nosocomial pneumonia has been of great clinical interest. Most cases are caused by gram-negative bacillary organisms, and gram-positive organisms make up the second largest group. The mortality rate associated with gram-negative bacillary pneumonias is frequently estimated to be about 50%, but the mortality rate from gram-positive pneumonias is between 5% and 24%. Among gram-negative bacillary deaths, those infections associated with *P. aeruginosa* have demonstrated the highest mortality rate, between 70% and 80%.[5, 8, 15]

Significant viral agents, spread by aerosol droplets or fomites, include influenza A and B, parainfluenza 1, 2, and 3, adenovirus, and RSV during the fall and winter months. Enteroviruses are predominant pathogens in the spring and summer months, although pulmonary involvement is uncommon. During outbreaks, or throughout the year, other pathogens include VZV and measles. In immunocompromised neonates and children, herpes simplex virus (HSV), CMV, and VZV are predominant pathogens.

The specific etiologic organisms for nosocomial pneumonia vary form institution to institution. Clinicians must be aware of the organisms and the antibiotic susceptibility data of these organisms at their own institutions. Among the gram-negative bacilli, *E. coli, K. pneumoniae,* and *P. aeruginosa* are the most common and comprise as many as 73% of all isolates described in nosocomial pneumonia studies. *Staphylococcus aureus* and *S. epidermidis* are found in as many as 20% of cases. Other gram-negative bacilli, including *Acinetobacter* species and *Proteus* species, make up most of the remainder. In most cases, single pathogens have been identified, but in 10% to 25% of cases, polymicrobial gram-negative pneumonias have been reported.[4, 5, 7, 9, 11] The NNIS data[8] indicate that the two most common bacterial agents causing nosocomial pneumonia in children are gram-negative rods (Table 10–1). The predominance of gram-negative bacillary pathogens as etiologic agents for nosocomial pneumonia has been observed in community hospitals and teaching centers. Among the gram-positive bacteria, *S. aureus* is by far the most common. *S. pneumoniae,* the most frequent bacteria in community-acquired pneumonias for patients older than 6 years of age, accounts for fewer than 3% of all bacterial nosocomial pneumonias. *Legionella pneumophila* and *Legionella micdadei* have also been implicated in outbreaks of nosocomial pneumonia. The true incidence of nosocomial pneumonia for the *Legionella* species is not known for children and probably varies among hospitals. In pediatric hospitals, the possibility of nonpneumococcal streptococci and *H. influenzae* type b exists. Although these organisms are much more common as etiologic agents in community-acquired pneumonias, nosocomial acquisition of these bacterial pathogens secondary to a distant infection with bacteremia or direct respiratory tract spread should be considered.

In the NICU, *S. epidermidis* is a potentially important cause of nosocomial infections, including pneumonia (see Table 10–1). In the NICU, gram-negative bacilli and gram-positive aerobic infections including *S. epidermidis* must be considered as potential causes of nosocomial pneumonia.[11, 19] Although *S. epidermidis* is the most common isolate described in the literature, other coagulase-negative staphylococci may be equally important and warrant therapy until the microbiology laboratory verifies the specific species and antibiotic susceptibilities.

Nosocomial pneumonia caused by fungi has been an increasing part of the clinician's dilemma during the past two decades. Fungal infections have become special problems in immunocompromised children. The lung remains one of the most commonly identified sites of infection among immunocompromised patients. Neutropenic patients are at particular risk for acquiring aerobic gram-negative bacillary pneumonias, even in the absence of endotracheal intubation.[24]

With the use of broad-spectrum antibiotic therapy in immunocompromised patients for suspected bacterial infections, the fungal causes of pulmonary infections have become increasingly important (see Table 10–1). *Aspergillus* pneumonia has been associated with neutropenia. Construction with contaminated fireproofing materials and air-conditioning equipment have been associated with nosocomial pulmonary aspergillosis. *Candida* species, including *C. albicans, C. tropicalis,* and *C. parapsilosis,* and *Torulopsis glabrata* have become increasingly frequent causes of nosocomial infection, including pneumonia in neutropenic chemotherapy patients.[24] The potential importance of fungal infections in these patient groups is recognized by the current use of empiric antifungal therapy in febrile neutropenic patients who are unresponsive to initial antibacterial therapy.

## DIAGNOSIS

Although radiographic patterns of interstitial or alveolar (lobar) infiltrates do not correlate with specific viral and bacterial infections, respectively, to a degree high enough to be diagnostic,[25] the chest roentgenograph is considered an optimal initial test. The appearance of a lobar infiltrate in a young infant during RSV season (Fig. 10–1) is a significant finding. In an infant with documented influenza A, the radiographic appearance of a consolidated lobar infiltrate suggests a nosocomial pneumonia secondary to *S. aureus* (Fig. 10–2). A diffuse parenchymal infiltrate in an immunocompromised child (Fig. 10–3) indicates a nosocomial pneumonia with a possible bacterial cause, such as gram-negative bacillary organisms.

In viral nosocomial pneumonia, the culture of a respiratory virus from a nasopharyngeal swab is diagnostic, but it is usually not helpful in the acute situation because of the 7- to 14-day incubation period that may be required for final identification. Rapid diagnostic techniques that include immunofluorescent staining of nasopharyngeal lavages (ie, cellular debris) with monoclonal antibodies or enzyme immunoassays have reduced the time for identification to hours and have proven useful in the acute situation. The reported sensitivity and specificity of these tests range from 80% to 95%.[26, 27] The development of even more rapid assays for RSV can make the diagnosis quick enough for infection control policies to be undertaken at the time of admission.[27] One concern about the rapid diagnosis of RSV is the possibility of false-negative results[28] in patients who would qualify for consideration of antiviral therapy with ribavirin. Proper collection of cellular debris is vital for any of the rapid diagnostic tests. Identification of other viral nosocomial pneumonias depends on recognition of characteristic viral exanthems (eg, measles, VZV) or oropharyn-

Table 10–1. **Etiologic Agents Causing Nosocomial Pneumonia in Children**

| Bacteria | Fungi | Viruses |
|---|---|---|
| *Escherichia coli* | *Candida* | Respiratory syncytial virus |
| *Klebsiella pneumoniae* | *Aspergillus* | Influenza A and B |
| *Pseudomonas aeruginosa* | | Parainfluenza virus |
| *Staphylococcus aureus* | | Cytomegalovirus |
| *Staphylococcus epidermidis* | | Varicella-zoster virus |
| Enterococci | | Herpes simplex virus |
| Other gram-negative bacilli | | Measles |
| *Streptococcus pneumoniae* | | |
| *Haemophilus influenzae* | | |

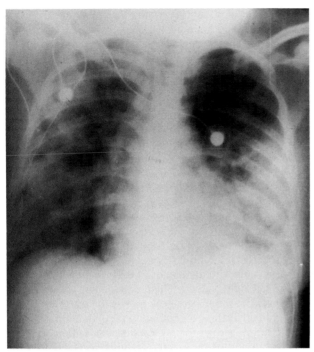

**Figure 10–1.** A posteroanterior chest roentgenograph of a 5-month-old boy with respiratory syncytial virus nosocomial pneumonia that required ribavirin therapy because of underlying immunodeficiency disease.

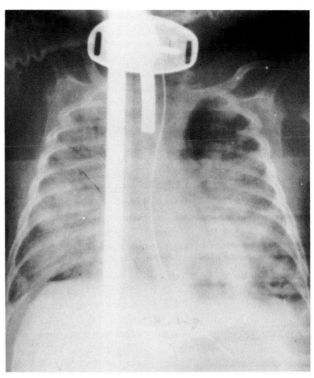

**Figure 10–3.** A posteroanterior chest roentgenograph of a 22-month-old boy with underlying laryngotracheomalacia and hypogammaglobulinemia and a diffuse infiltrate involving all five lobes of the lung. The blood cultures were positive for *Klebsiella pneumoniae*, which was responsible for a nosocomial pneumonia with sepsis.

geal lesions (eg, HSV) and subsequent cultures or rapid fluorescent assays for viral antigens.

The optimal method for diagnosis of nosocomial bacterial pneumonia remains undefined and controversial.[29–34]

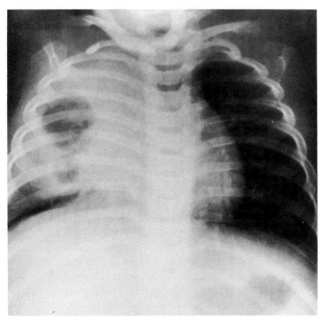

**Figure 10–2.** A posteroanterior chest roentgenograph of a 3-month-old girl with culture-proved influenza A virus infection who subsequently developed a right middle and upper lobe infiltrate with pneumatocele formation. The blood cultures were positive for *Staphylococcus aureus*, which was responsible for a nosocomial pneumonia with bacteremia.

Diagnosis has historically been made on clinical grounds with an appropriate chest roentgenogram, Gram stain, and culture of lower respiratory tract secretions. This definition has probably overestimated the true incidence of nosocomial pneumonia because many other entities can be easily misdiagnosed in the critically ill patient. The recognition that chest roentgenographic changes seen in adult respiratory distress syndrome are not necessarily associated with an infectious process has also made the diagnosis of nosocomial pneumonia difficult in some pediatric patients. The confusing underlying diseases seen in adults are not as commonly encountered in children. However, high-risk patient groups, including children with congenital heart disease or bronchopulmonary dysplasia, cancer chemotherapy patients receiving irradiation or antimetabolite chemotherapy, and patients receiving granulocyte-monocyte colony-stimulating factor (GM-CSF) therapy, have clinical pictures with similar radiographic presentations. These situations have been further confused by the finding that fever can be associated with the pulmonary infiltrates caused by several of these nonbacterial entities.

Data suggest a poor correlation between culture results obtained from endotracheal suction specimens and those from otherwise sterile sites, such as the lung, blood, and pleural fluid. As many as 75% of upper airway cultures represent colonization rather than invasive infections, but as many as 30% of the infections are mistaken for colonization.[10, 14, 30–33] The difficulty in interpreting upper airway bacterial cultures is accentuated by the fact that patients in the intensive care environment usually have abnormal chest roentgenograms with or without lung infection, and fever and leukocytosis are common in patients with or without pneumonia. Cough and sputum production have little relevance in the intubated patient and are infrequent diagnostic indicators in children. Even if the tracheobronchial secretions are purulent, differentiation between tracheobronchitis and pneumonia may be difficult. Clinical suspicion is the first step in the proper diagnosis of nosocomial bacterial pneumonia.

Nosocomial pneumonia may be indicated by a change in the clinical status of the patient that is unexplained by other events. These changes may include a drop in oxygenation, an increased requirement for supplemental oxygen therapy, metabolic acidosis, or increasing ventilator requirements. A change in the fever pattern with a concomitant increase in the quantity and purulence of respiratory secretions should be a clue to the possibility of an infectious process. These factors in combination with a sudden increase in a previously diagnosed lung infiltrate or a new infiltrate should make the clinician suspect nosocomial pneumonia. Although such criteria may lack sensitivity and specificity, they may be the only available parameters for the clinician. Included in the diagnostic considerations are the likely causes of nosocomial pneumonia and the epidemiology of the intensive care and patient environment. Close contact, with adjacent patients sharing nursing or respiratory therapy personnel, should be considered as a potential source for the spread of infection. Recent patient exposure to RSV or influenza virus implicates these organisms, and recent transfusions of unscreened blood products in newborns or organ transplantation recipients suggest CMV as a possible cause. The bacteriologic flora of the intensive care or patient care facility also should be considered.

After deciding that a potential nosocomial pneumonia exists, the clinician must determine which samples should be obtained to identify the specific etiologic organism. In patients with prolonged intubation and respiratory therapy, serial respiratory tract secretion Gram stains may assist the clinician in ascertaining whether an inflammatory and potentially infectious process exists. Microscopic examination of upper respiratory tract secretions by gram stain can reveal an influx of polymorphonuclear leukocytes (PMNs) and the presence of a predominant bacterial organism. Unfortunately, these specimens are often contaminated with upper airway flora, and cultures of such specimens may or may not reflect the microbiology of infected lung tissue. Isolation of a single organism, bacterial or fungal, from blood cultures can help differentiate contaminating from infecting bacterial isolates in the respiratory secretions of these patients, but data suggest that only 2% to 5% of blood cultures are positive for bacterial organisms from patients with nosocomial pneumonia.[4, 11, 19, 24] Blood cultures in a patient with suspected nosocomial pneumonia are justified, but a high-percentage yield should not be expected. Pleural fluid should always be investigated. Because microbiologic evaluation of contaminated respiratory specimens can be misleading, several invasive methods have been developed to obtain uncontaminated specimens for diagnostic evaluation.[35–38] The use of quantitative sputum cultures, washed sputum cultures, and microscopic screening of sputa for the presence of upper airway cells suggesting contamination have been evaluated, but the usefulness of these methods is controversial.[4, 38] Unfortunately, these are the major sources of specimens available to clinicians treating critically ill

intubated children for nosocomial pneumonia. Transtracheal aspiration in nonintubated patients, percutaneous thin needle lung aspiration in ventilated patients, and protected shielded-tip bronchoscopic sampling of lower airway secretions are not advisable or available for children.

Although an excellent microbiologic correlation between lung tissue and bronchoscopic specimens has been observed for patients with histologic evidence of pneumonia, a high incidence of false-positive results has been reported for bronchoscopic specimens obtained from patients without pneumonia. In immunocompromised patients, the demonstration that bronchoalveolar lavage (BAL) yields results similar to open lung biopsy for the diagnosis of CMV, *Pneumocystis carinii*, and atypical mycobacteria was important. Flexible bronchoscopy is a relatively new avenue for obtaining these specimens from intubated patients with nosocomial pneumonia or adult respiratory distress syndrome. Methods to allow sensitive and specific differentiation of patients with these entities from those without pneumonia are being evaluated. These procedures are less well investigated for the pediatric population because of the small-caliber flexible bronchoscope required for use with only a single access for suctioning and sampling of the lower respiratory tract. In smaller children unable to safely receive an adult flexible bronchoscope, the use of BAL alone has been investigated.[35]

Although the concern about contamination with upper airway microorganisms still exists, semiquantitative cultures looking for organisms forming more than $10^4$ CFU/mL of a predominant bacteria have proven useful.[36] Urinary bacterial antigen detection systems are somewhat useful in identifying common community-acquired etiologic agents of pneumonia in children.[37, 38] Bacterial antigen detection systems for *H. influenzae* type b, *S. pneumonia*, group B streptococci, and *E. coli* (eg, newborn) have added to the diagnostic capabilities of blood culture isolation for children with community-acquired pneumonia. However, because these organisms are not common causes of nosocomial pneumonia in children, their utility in this setting is minimal. Identification of some bacterial organisms by direct fluorescent antibody microscopy has added to the diagnostic capabilities for nosocomial acquisition of *L. pneumophila* and *Bordetella pertussis*. Specimens taken from the nasopharynx or endotracheal tube are examined by using fluoresceinated monoclonal antibody-stained specimens. A few pediatric patients can tolerate thin needle direct lung aspiration for the diagnosis of bacterial nosocomial pneumonia.

The existence of an influx of PMNs with a predominant organism in the endotracheal tube culture, although suggesting a nosocomial infectious process, has not been proven to be diagnostic. The use of a double-lumen plugged catheter by blind passage has been proposed for critically ill children, but the procedure awaits further study to determine its usefulness and safety.

In immunocompromised children with nosocomial pneumonia unresponsive to broad-spectrum antibiotic therapy regimens, the alternative of open lung biopsy with histologic special stains and cultures has been used. The diagnosis of nosocomial pneumonia due to *Aspergillus* and *Candida* species may be suspected by examination of wet preps of BAL samples, and confirmation may be obtained by histologic examination and culture of the open lung biopsy material. The culture of bacterial isolates is important because of the need for antibiotic susceptibility data. In the era of widespread use and abuse of antibiotics, susceptibility testing enables the clinician to select the appropriate drugs for empiric and specific therapy regimens.

## TREATMENT

With the availability of new antiviral compounds, clinicians must investigate all nosocomial pneumonias with the same diligence they apply to bacterial infections. Ribavirin (Virazole), an aerosolized synthetic nucleoside, has activity against many respiratory viruses. The expense, potential toxicity to health care workers, and requirements for prolonged aerosol exposure have made the use of ribavirin less attractive. However, treatment of high-risk patients has improved clinical severity scores,[39-44] decreased days of hospitalization, and decreased time on oxygen and mechanical ventilation[45] for patients with RSV nosocomial pneumonia. High-risk patient groups, including those with cyanotic congenital heart disease, pulmonary hypertension, prematurity, underlying pulmonary disease (eg, bronchopulmonary dysplasia), immunodeficiency disorders, human immunodeficiency infection, and severe infection in infancy are considered candidates for treatment under the American Academy of Pediatrics guidelines.[46] Acyclovir therapy for HSV or VZV nosocomial pneumonia in immunocompromised children or VZV nosocomial pneumonia in otherwise normal children is considered standard therapy.

Treatment of nosocomial bacterial pneumonia may be empiric or specific. Empiric treatment is employed for patients with clinically suspected pneumonia in whom an identified etiologic agent is not available to guide specific therapy. If a specific bacterial agent is identified and antibiotic susceptibility data are available, specific therapy should be used. Intravenous antibiotics remain the conventional form of treatment for nosocomial bacterial pneumonia, although investigations with inhaled endobronchial antibiotics and passive immunization have been reported.[47-49]

Several factors must be considered in the selection of an appropriate empiric antibiotic therapy regimen. Patient records must be reviewed to identify recently administered antibiotics and possibly indicate resistant organisms as the cause of this nosocomial infection. The parents must be interviewed for the possibility of underlying disease states (eg, cystic fibrosis) that could predispose the patient to *Pseudomonas* infections. Special circumstances include the premature newborn with an increased risk for *S. epidermidis* infections and the consideration of immunocompromised patients for empiric antifungal therapy.[4, 11, 24] The demonstration that recent BAL results and surveillance cultures in the intensive care unit have identified a particular organism should guide broad-spectrum antibiotic empiric therapy.[35, 36] It is important to review recent antibiotic susceptibility patterns of nosocomial pathogens in the specific hospital or intensive care unit. If the environment has had a particularly high incidence of pneumonia or other nosocomial infections caused by multiple antibiotic-resistant *Pseudomonas* species, *Xanthamonas* species, or *Acinetobacter antitratus* during the past several months, empiric antibiotic therapy should include antibiotics that cover those isolates.

Another important consideration is the presence of *Legionella* species in the proven cases of nosocomial pneumonia at that institution. Relevant to pediatric units is the consideration of recent hospitalized patients with *B. pertussis* respiratory infections.

Empiric treatment of nosocomial bacterial pneumonias should include coverage of aerobic gram-negative bacilli. In high-risk patients, coverage should also include highly resistant organisms such as *Pseudomonas* and *Acinetobacter*. Empiric therapy should cover gram-positive organisms such as *S. aureus*. The identification in the specific institution of a high frequency of methicillin-resistant *S. aureus* or the consideration of *S. epidermidis* in the premature newborn should guide the clinician in selecting a specific antistaphylococcal regimen that includes vancomycin. Based on these considerations, several regimens have been employed for the empiric treatment of nosocomial pneumonia (Table 10–2). These regimens provide broad-spectrum antibacterial activity for nosocomial pneumonia in pediatrics. If a specific etiologic agent is identified, the specific antibacterial therapeutic regimens of single or multiple drugs should be selected based on the antibiotic susceptibility data for that pathogen.

Some investigations have questioned the usefulness of aminoglycosides in treating gram-negative pneumonia. The narrow therapeutic ratios for achievable levels in serum of aminoglycosides and the difficulty in penetration from blood into the respiratory secretions and tissues may result in local drug concentrations insufficient for treating the infecting organisms. However, aminoglycosides may be more active than β-lactam antibiotics against certain resistant gram-negative bacilli. In one report, patients receiving parenteral antibiotics plus aerosol aminoglycoside therapy in saline suspension instilled into the respiratory tract every

Table 10–2. **Empiric Treatment of Nosocomial Pneumonia**

| Patient Group | Treatment | | |
|---|---|---|---|
| Immunocompetent | | | |
| Noninstrumented | | | Cefotaxime |
| Intubated or instrumented | Nafcillin* or clindamycin | plus | aminoglycoside† or cefotaxime |
| Methicillin-resistant organisms prevalent | Vancomycin‡ | plus | aminoglycoside or cefotaxime |
| Nonintubated, patient younger than 6 years§ | | | Cefotaxime |
| Immunocompromised | | | |
| No prior antibiotics | Nafcillin or clindamycin | plus | aminoglycoside or ceftazidime |
| Prior antibiotics ± indwelling catheter | Vancomycin | plus | aminoglycoside‖ or ceftazidime |
| Unresponsive to antibiotics | Erythromycin# and amphotericin B | | |

*Substitute methicillin in the neonate.

†The use of gentamicin, tobramycin, amikacin depends on susceptibility data for the institution.

‡Vancomycin is also indicated in the neonatal intensive care unit if *S. epidermidis* is prevalent.

§Includes *H. influenzae* type b found in a secondary site.

‖Change of aminoglycoside or cephalosporin or the addition of a ticarcillin, ticarcillin-clavulanate, piperacillin, azlocillin, or imipenem to cover resident *Pseudomonas* species.

#Added to existing regimen to cover *Legionella* species, if endemic.

8 hours had an increased treatment success rate compared with those treated with saline aerosol instillations.[47–49] An equal superinfection rate with resistant flora occurred in the two groups. The use of aerosolized or directly instilled aminoglycosides should be limited to patients who have multiple antibiotic-resistant gram-negative bacilli and in whom parenteral therapy produces only borderline achievable serum concentrations compared with the minimal inhibitory concentration of the organism.

A prospective study of 51 patients with culture-proven bacterial nosocomial pneumonia compared the broad-spectrum antibiotics cefotaxime and ceftriaxone.[50] The age, Apache II scores, and BAL results were similar, but 19 of 26 cefotaxime-treated patients had improvement in their global scores, compared with 12 of 25 ceftriaxone-treated patients ($P = .04$). The effectiveness of cefotaxime or ceftriaxone yielded ratings of clinical effectiveness, (73% versus 48%, $P = .01$), premature clinical failure (4% versus 29%, $P = .01$), microbiological response or cure (57% versus 36%), and clearance of organisms (79% versus 50%). This study demonstrated an overall superior outcome for nosocomial pneumonia patients treated with cefotaxime than those receiving ceftriaxone therapy.[50]

The treatment of nosocomial pneumonia still relies on intravenous antibiotics as the mainstay of therapy. Empiric treatment with amphotericin B in high-risk patients, with or without 5-flucytosine, should be considered for certain *Candida* species. There are no prospective studies evaluating the imidazoles (eg, ketoconazole, itraconazole, fluconazole) versus amphotericin B for the treatment of fungal infections frequently involved in nosocomial pneumonia. Although the imidazoles are effective against certain dimorphic fungal pulmonary infections such as cryptococcosis, blastomycosis, and histoplasmosis, their usefulness in invasive nosocomial fungal infections caused by *Aspergillus* and *Candida* species has not been verified.

## PREVENTION

The most obvious preventive method for some nosocomial pneumonias is immunization. Current vaccine schedules prevent pertussis, measles, and *H. influenzae* type b infections. Routine influenza vaccine administration to high-risk children and health care professionals can dramatically reduce influenza rates.

The other prevention schemes for nosocomial pneumonia depend on the environment, patient, and personnel. The fundamental objective in preventing nosocomial pneumonia is to reduce the acquisition of potential pathogens in the upper airways, reducing the potential for the aspiration of these organisms into the lower respiratory tract. Compulsive care of the ventilator apparatus is always indicated. Ventilated patients should be suctioned regularly to decrease intrabronchial secretions, and those without support instrumentation should be routinely forced to cough and deep breathe with respiratory therapy. Care should be taken to ensure that medications and other materials used for respiratory support are sterile. Disposable substances should be used if feasible. Patients should be treated on the ventilator for the shortest possible time, with extubation a constant consideration to be weighed against the risk of

nosocomial pneumonia. If resistant strains of organisms exist within an intensive care area, appropriate isolation precautions must be maintained. Patients who are infected or colonized should be selectively grouped or isolated (ie, cohorted). Aerosolized antibiotics for prophylaxis against bacterial colonization should not be considered a routine procedure, but in outbreaks of pneumonia caused by a single pathogen such as *Acinetobacter*, the use of this modality for short periods may prove beneficial. The appropriate design and staffing of critical care areas is an important environmental consideration for the prevention of nosocomial pneumonia. Attention to environmental factors such as hand washing between patient contacts, compliance with hospital infection control policy, adherence to isolation procedures, and reporting of communicable diseases, along with a multidisciplined approach among infection control personnel, infectious disease specialists, and primary care clinicians, helps to prevent or diminish the incidence of nosocomial pneumonia.

Although most attention has been focused on preventing nosocomial gram-negative pneumonia, effective methods for reducing endemic nosocomial bacterial and viral infections have also been reported. Measures employing hyperchlorination of contaminated potable water within the hospital have been shown to reduce the incidence of nosocomial infection by *Legionella*. Limited success has been achieved in controlling nosocomial viral respiratory infections. RSV is spread primarily by direct inoculation of large droplets or by direct contact.[23] Secretion precautions have been advocated for known cases. In some centers, isolation cohorting of staff to infected infants has reduced the spread of RSV among patients but not among hospital personnel.

It is the opinion of most infection control personnel that many of the causes of nosocomial pneumonia are not preventable. The best chance to decrease morbidity and mortality lies in early diagnosis and treatment with appropriate antiinfectives. Supportive therapy should be aggressive, and attempts to decrease or reverse organ failure should be vigorous.

## CONCLUSION

Nosocomial pneumonia continues to be a leading cause of fatal nosocomial infection in children in the United States. Although there are differences in the pathogens isolated in various age groups, the importance of nosocomial pneumonia is apparent in all pediatric patient groups. The ability to diagnose these infections using clinical suspicion and microbiologic and rapid diagnostic tests allows the clinician to treat effectively nosocomial pneumonia in critically ill patients. Unfortunately, the treatment modalities and preventive measures have not kept pace with our understanding of the pathogenesis of this disease. Pediatric patients present several unique infection control, diagnostic, and treatment problems for the practicing clinician. The appropriate infection control and isolation policies for specific viral and multiple antibiotic–resistant bacterial isolates remain a cornerstone in the prevention of nosocomial pneumonia. The judicious use of empiric antibacterial chemotherapy remains important in the treatment of patients with nosocomial pneumonia. However, in the pediatric patient population, the recognition that viruses and fungi are important causes of nosocomial pneumonia challenges the clinician to apply appropriate diagnostic and effective treatment regimens. For any institution, the causes of nosocomial pneumonia, drug susceptibility patterns, and the seasonal and patient distribution of these infections are critical. Rapid diagnostic testing, improved treatment modalities, and better prevention measures will be aided by the advent of immunologic therapy for these diseases. Although these modalities show great promise, it will be up to the clinician to stay current in the field of nosocomial pneumonia because it will continue to be a significant cause of morbidity, mortality, and hospital cost.

## REFERENCES

1. Avendano LF, Larranaga C, Palomino MA, et al: Community- and hospital-acquired respiratory syncytial virus infection in Chile. Pediatr Infect Dis J 10:564, 1991.
2. Hall CB, Powell KR, MacDonald NE, et al: Respiratory syncytial viral infection in children with compromised immune function. N Engl J Med 315:77, 1986.
3. Serwint JR, Miller RM, Korsch BM: Influenza type A and B infections in hospitalized pediatric patients. Who should be immunized? Am J Dis Child 145:623, 1991.
4. Jacobs RF: Nosocomial pneumonia in children. Infection 19:64, 1991.
5. Graybill JR, Marshall LW, Charache P, et al: Nosocomial pneumonia: A continuing major problem. Am Rev Respir Dis 108:1130, 1973.
6. Johanson WG Jr, Pierce AK, Sanford JP: Changing pharyngeal bacterial flora of hospitalized patients: Emergence of gram-negative bacilli. N Engl J Med 281:1137, 1969.
7. Bartlett JG, O'Keefe P, Tally FP, et al: Bacteriology of hospital-acquired pneumonia. Arch Intern Med 146:868, 1986.
8. Centers for Disease Control: National Nosocomial Infections Study Report. Annual Summary, 1983. Atlanta, Centers for Disease Control. MMWR 33:955, 2155, 1985.
9. Bryan CS, Reynolds KL: Bacteremic nosocomial pneumonia. Am Rev Respir Dis 129:668, 1984.
10. Bartlett JG: Invasive diagnostic techniques in respiratory infections. *In* Pennington JE (ed): Respiratory Infections: Diagnosis and Management. New York, Raven Press, 1983:55.
11. Hemming VG, Overall JC Jr, Britt MR: Nosocomial infections in a newborn intensive care unit. N Engl J Med 294:1310, 1976.
12. LaForce FM, Hopkins J, Trow R, et al: Human oral defenses against gram-negative rods. Am Rev Respir Dis 114:929, 1976.
13. Brook I: Bacterial colonization, tracheobronchitis, and pneumonia following tracheostomy and long-term intubation in pediatric patients. Chest 76:420, 1979.
14. Johanson WG, Pierce AK, Sanford JP, et al: Nosocomial respiratory infections with gram-negative bacilli. Ann Intern Med 77:701, 1972.
15. Craven DE, Kunches LM, Kilinsky V, et al: Risk factors for pneumonia and fatality in patients receiving continuous mechanical ventilation. Am Rev Respir Dis 133:792, 1986.
16. Schwartz SN, Dowling JN, Benkovic C, et al: Sources of gram-negative bacilli colonizing the trachea of intubated patients. J Infect Dis 138:227, 1978.
17. Louria DB, Kaminski T: The effects of four antimicrobial drug regimens on sputum superinfection in hospitalized patients. Am Rev Respir Dis 85:649, 1962.
18. Johanson WG Jr: Pathogenesis and prevention of nosocomial pneumonia in a nonhuman primate model of acute respiratory failure. Am Rev Respir Dis 130:502, 1984.
19. Goldmann DA, Freeman J, Durbin WA Jr: Nosocomial infection and death in a neonatal intensive care unit. J Infect Dis 147:635, 1983.
20. Jarvis WR, Middleton PJ, Gelfand EW: Significance of viral infections in severe combined immunodeficiency syndrome. Pediatr Infect Dis 2:187, 1983.
21. Karp D, Willis J, Wilfert CM: Parainfluenza virus II and the immunocompromised host. Am J Dis Child 127:592, 1974.
22. Hall CB, McBride JT, Walsh EE: Aerosolized ribavirin treatment of

infants with respiratory syncytial virus infection: A randomized, double-blind study. N Engl J Med 308:1443, 1983.
23. Hall CB, Douglas RG Jr, Geiman JM, Messner MK: Nosocomial respiratory syncytial virus infection. N Engl J Med 293:1343, 1975.
24. Pizzo PA, Robichaud KJ, Gill FA, et al: Empiric antibiotic and antifungal therapy for cancer patients with prolonged fever and granulocytopenia. Am J Med 72:101, 1982.
25. Sunakorn P, Chunchit L, Niltawat S, et al: Epidemiology of acute respiratory infections in young children from Thailand. Pediatr Infect Dis J 9:873, 1990.
26. Halstead DC, Todd S, Fritch G: Evaluation of five methods for respiratory syncytial virus detection. J Clin Microbiol 28:1021, 1990.
27. Swierkosz EA, Flanders R, Melvin L, et al: Evaluation of the Abbott TESTPACK RSV enzyme immunoassay for detection of respiratory syncytial virus in nasopharyngeal swab specimens. J Clin Microbiol 27:1151, 1989.
28. Arandien M, Pettersson CA, Gardner B, et al: Rapid viral diagnosis of acute respiratory infections: Comparison of ELISA and IF techniques for the detection of viral antigens in nasopharyngeal secretions. J Clin Microbiol 22:757, 1985.
29. Bartlett JG, Rosenblatt JE, Finegold SM: Percutaneous transtracheal aspiration in the diagnosis of anaerobic pulmonary infection. Ann Intern Med 79:535, 1973.
30. Fossieck B, Parker R, Cohen M, et al: Fiberoptic bronchoscopy and culture of bacteria from the lower respiratory tract. Chest 72:5, 1977.
31. Hayes D, McCarthy L, Friedman M: Evaluation of two bronchofiberscopic methods of culturing the lower respiratory tract. Am Rev Respir Dis 122:319, 1980.
32. Higuchi JH, Coalson JJ, Johanson WG Jr: Bacteriologic diagnosis of nosocomial pneumonia in primates: Usefulness of the protected specimen brush. Am Rev Respir Dis 125:53, 1982.
33. Chastre J, Viau F, Brun P, et al: Prospective evaluation of the protected specimen brush for the diagnosis of pulmonary infections in ventilated patients. Am Rev Respir Dis 130:924, 1984.
34. Coleman DL, Dodek PM, Luce JM, et al: Diagnostic utility of fiberoptic bronchoscopy in patients with *Pneumocystis carinii* pneumonia and the acquired immune deficiency syndrome. Am Rev Respir Dis 128:795, 1983.
35. Stokes DC, Shenep JL, Parham D, et al: Role of flexible bronchoscopy in the diagnosis of pulmonary infiltrates in pediatric patients with cancer. J Pediatr 115:561, 1989.
36. Frankel LR, Smith DW, Lewiston NJ: Bronchoalveolar lavage for diagnosis of pneumonia in the immunocompromised child. Pediatrics 81:785, 1988.
37. Ramsey BW, Marcuse EK, Foy HM, et al: Use of bacterial antigen detection in the diagnosis of pediatric lower respiratory tract infections. Pediatrics 78:1, 1986.
38. Jacobs RF: Rapid diagnosis of infection in pulmonary disease. Am Rev Respir Dis 134:829, 1986.
39. Hall CB, Powell KR, MacDonald NE: Respiratory syncytial virus infection in children with compromised immune function. N Engl J Med 315:77, 1986.
40. MacDonald NE, Hall CB, Suffin SC, et al: Respiratory syncytial virus infection in infants with congenital heart disease. N Engl J Med 307:397, 1982.
41. Hall CB, Walsh EE, Hruska JF: Ribavirin treatment of experimental respiratory syncytial virus infection: A controlled double-blind study in young adults. J Am Med Assoc 249:2666, 1983.
42. Hall CB, McBride JT, Walsh EE: Aerosolized ribavirin treatment of infants with respiratory syncytial virus infection. A randomized double-blind study. N Engl J Med 308:1443, 1983.
43. Taber LH, Knight V, Gilbert BE: Ribavirin aerosol treatment of bronchiolitis associated with respiratory syncytial virus infection in infants. Pediatrics 72:613, 1983.
44. Hall CB, McBride JT, Gala CL: Ribavirin treatment of respiratory syncytial virus infection in infants with underlying cardiopulmonary disease. JAMA 254:3047, 1985.
45. Smith DW, Frankel LR, Mathers LH, et al: A controlled trial of ribavirin in infants receiving mechanical ventilation for severe respiratory syncytial virus infection. N Engl J Med 325:24, 1991.
46. Committee on Infectious Diseases, American Academy of Pediatrics: Ribavirin Therapy of Respiratory Syncytial Virus. Report of the Committee on Infectious Diseases, ed 22. Elk Grove, IL, American Academy of Pediatrics, 1991:581.
47. Gough PA, Jordan NS: A review of the therapeutic efficacy of aerosolized and endotracheally instilled antibiotics. Pharmacotherapy 2:367, 1982.

48. Pennington JE, Reynolds HY: Pharmacokinetics of gentamicin sulfate in bronchial secretions. J Infect Dis 131:158, 1975.

49. Klastersky J, Juysmans E, Weerts D, et al: Endotracheally administered gentamicin for the prevention of infections of the respiratory tract in patients with tracheostomy: A double-blind study. Chest 65:650, 1974.

50. Reeves JH, Russell GM, Cade JF, et al: Comparison of ceftriaxone with cefotaxime in serious chest infections. Chest 96:1292, 1989.

# CHAPTER 11

# Community-Acquired Pneumonia

THOMAS J. MARRIE

Community-acquired pneumonia (CAP) is pneumonia in outpatients rather than nosocomial pneumonia or hospital-acquired pneumonia. Pneumonia used to be easy to diagnose but difficult to treat. In 1938, *Streptococcus pneumoniae* accounted for almost all cases of CAP.[1] Unfortunately, there was no specific therapy. In the 1990s the situation is reversed; we have specific therapy for almost every microbial cause of pneumonia, but our problem is making a specific diagnosis. Although many causes of CAP have been identified, in 30% to 40% of cases, the cause remains unknown.[2, 3] To further complicate matters, the population at risk for CAP has changed. The segment of the population 65 years of age or older is the fastest growing one.[4] This has led to a new nosologic entity—nursing home-acquired pneumonia (NHAP). The explosion of infection caused by human immunodeficiency virus[5] and the success of organ transplantation with its attendant need for ongoing immunosuppression have produced a large number of immunocompromised persons. These factors dictate that the physician have an organized approach to the diagnosis and therapy of CAP.

## INCIDENCE

The attack rates for CAP are highest at the extremes of age. Foy and colleagues,[6] in a study of 180,000 persons in the 1960s and 1970s, found that the overall annual rate of pneumonia was 12 per 1000. For those between the ages of 0 and 4 years, it was 12 to 18 per 1000, and it was 1 to 5 per 1000 for those between 5 and 60 years of age. MacFarlane and coworkers,[7] in a study carried out in England,

found that for adults the annual incidence of pneumonia was 1 to 3 cases per 1000. Jokinen and associates carried out a 1-year study of the incidence of pneumonia in Kuopio province in Eastern Finland.[7a] The overall incidence was 11.6 per 1000. For persons 2 to 5 years of age it was 36 per 1000; for those 5 to 14 years of age, 16.2 per 1000; for those 15 to 19 years of age, 6 per 1000; for those 60 to 74 years of age, 15.4 per 1000; and for those aged 75 years and older, the rate was 34.2 per 1000. Studies focusing on pneumonia caused by specific microbial agents suggest that the rate for pneumococcal pneumonia is 37.5 cases per 100,000 persons per year.[8] Among Alaskan Natives, pneumococcal disease rates are 6 to 34 times higher than rates reported for other U.S. populations.[9] The annual rate for *Mycoplasma pneumoniae* pneumonia in Seattle was 1 per 1000, but in some years it was as high as 3 per 1000.[10]

The hospitalization rate for pneumonia ranges from 17%[11] to 35% (Marrie TJ, unpublished observations) for patients seen in their physicians' offices and to 50% for those seen in emergency rooms.[12] In the Finnish study, 42% of the patients were admitted to the hospital.[7a]

## ETIOLOGY

Patients with CAP requiring admission to the hospital have been studied most extensively.[2, 3, 8, 12–28] Some studies did not state their criteria for the diagnosis of pneumonia, valid cases of pneumonia were excluded in some studies, and the diagnostic workup varied considerably.[3] Table 11–1 summarizes data from two studies of CAP requiring hospitalization. These two studies used similar criteria for the

Table 11–1. **Causes of Community-Acquired Pneumonia Requiring Hospitalization**

| Cause of Pneumonia | Investigation | |
|---|---|---|
| | Fang et al[2] (359 patients)* | Marrie et al[3] (719 patients)† |
| Unknown | 118 (32.9)‡ | 340 (47)‡ |
| More than one cause | | 74 (10.3) |
| *Streptococcus pneumoniae* | 39 (10.9) | 61 (8.5) |
| Aspiration | 12 (3.3) | 52 (7.2) |
| *Mycoplasma pneumoniae* | 7 (2) | 40 (5.6) |
| Influenza A | Not tested | 40 (5.6) |
| *Staphylococcus aureus* | 12 (3.3) | 29 (4.0) |
| *Haemophilus influenzae* | 39 (10.9) | 27 (3.7) |
| *Coxiella burnetii* | Not tested | 22 (3.1) |
| Aerobic gram-negative bacteria | 21 (5.9) | 22 (3.1) |
| Influenza B | Not tested | 17 (2.4) |
| *Pneumocystitis carinii* | 9 (2.5) | 14 (1.9) |
| *Legionella* species | 24 (6.7) | 16 (2.2) |
| *Mycobacterium tuberculosis* | 4 (1.1) | 10 (1.4) |
| *Chlamydia pneumoniae* | 22 (6.1) | 18/301 (6)§ |
| Postobstructive disease | 19 (5.3) | 13 (1.8) |

*Study conducted between July 1, 1986, and June 30, 1987.
†Study conducted between November 1, 1981, and March 18, 1987.
‡Percentage of the total patient number is given in parentheses.
§Only 301 patients had serum samples tested for antibodies to *C. pneumoniae*.

diagnosis of pneumonia, and patients in both studies had extensive serologic workups. Pneumonia is said to exist if there is acute onset of respiratory symptoms with cackles, rhonchi, or consolidation. In addition, an opacity that does not have a noninfectious cause, such as congestive heart failure, malignancy, or pulmonary infarction, must be seen on the chest radiograph.[3]

The cause of pneumonia should be classified as definite, presumptive, or unknown.[2] Blood cultures yielding a pathogen, pleural fluid positive for a pathogen, *Pneumocystis carinii* on bronchoalveolar lavage, open lung biopsy diagnosis, isolation of *M. pneumoniae* from respiratory secretions or a fourfold rise in antibody titer to this agent, or fourfold rise in antibody to *Chlamydia pneumoniae* or to *Legionella pneumophila* constitutes evidence that the indicated pathogen is the *definite* cause of pneumonia. Heavy or moderate growth of a predominant bacterial pathogen on sputum culture, light growth of a pathogen if the sputum Gram stain reveals a bacterium compatible with the culture results, bacterium isolated on multiple sputum cultures within 3 days of admission, or multiple potential pathogens growing on sputum culture indicates that the *presumptive* cause is the predominant organism seen on Gram stain that is compatible with one of these isolates or multiple pathogens if the Gram stain is compatible with multiple isolates. Cases showing normal flora on respiratory tract culture, producing light growth of multiple organisms on tract culture, or not fulfilling any of the above conditions are attributed to *unknown* agents.[2]

The results of two studies[2, 3] were remarkably similar. One third to almost one half of the cases were of unknown origin. From its dominant position six decades ago, *S. pneumoniae* now causes 8% to 10% of CAP requiring hospitalization. However, it is still the dominant cause of bacteremic pneumonia, accounting for 58% of such bacteremias (Table 11–2). The major finding from these two studies is the diversity of causes of CAP requiring hospitalization. It

is evident that there are local variations in the causes of pneumonia; *Legionella* was more common in Pittsburgh than in Halifax, and *Coxiella burnetii*, which caused 3.3% of the pneumonias in Halifax, was not sought in the Pittsburgh study. *P. carinii* and *C. pneumoniae* represent relatively new causes of CAP.

Although many cases are attributed to unknown causes because of inadequate diagnostic studies (eg, respiratory secretions not available for culture), it is likely that there are agents causing pneumonia that we have not discovered or agents that will emerge as changes occur in the populations at risk. This thesis is substantiated by the findings of Ortqvist and colleagues,[29] who were unable to make an etiologic diagnosis in 5 (20%) of 24 patients with CAP despite bronchoscopy and serologic studies in all the patients.

There have been few studies of pneumonia as it presents in a physician's office.[30] This is a much different patient population from those who are hospitalized, and there is a high diagnostic yield (54%) from serologic studies.[30] In a study of 75 such patients, we were able to identify an etiologic agent by serologic means in 45% (Marrie TJ, unpublished observations). *M. pneumoniae* accounted for 65% of these cases and 29% of the cases overall. *C. pneumoniae* caused 5%, and *L. pneumophila* caused 3% of these cases of pneumonia. Other agents identified included influenza A (7%), *C. burnetti* (3%), and adenovirus (3%). Thirty-five percent of the 75 patients were hospitalized. The mortality rate was 4%. Similar results were obtained in a practitioner-based study in Switzerland[116]: 14 (8.7%) of 161 patients required hospitalization, and the overall mortality rate was 1.2%. The agents implicated included *S. pneumoniae* (17 cases), *Haemophilus* sp. (2 cases), *Moraxella catarrhalis* (1 case), *Streptococcus* sp. (1 case), *Legionella* sp. (3 cases), *Chlamydia* sp. (9 cases), *M. pneumoniae* (28 cases), *C. burnetii* (3 cases), influenza (19 cases), and other respiratory viruses (7 cases). No etiologic diagnosis was made in 47% of the cases.

Table 11–2. **Causes of Pneumonia Cultured From Blood Samples**

| Pathogen | Investigation | |
|---|---|---|
| | Fang et al[2] (314 patients)* | Marrie et al[3] (539 patients)† |
| *Streptococcus pneumoniae* | 16 (57)‡ | 28 (58)‡ |
| *Staphylococcus aureus* | 4 | 1 (2) |
| *Haemophilus influenzae* | 1 | 2 (4) |
| *Streptococcus* species | 2 | 8 (16) |
| *Legionella pneumophila* | 1 | 0 |
| *Actinomyces israelii* | 1 | 0 |
| *Pseudomonas aeruginosa* | 1 | 1 (2) |
| *Serratia marcescens* and *Acinetobacter calcoaceticus* | 1 | 0 |
| *Bacteroides fragilis* | 1 | 1 (1) |
| *Escherichia coli* | 0 | 3 (6) |
| *Klebsiella pneumoniae* | 0 | 2 (4) |
| *Neisseria meningitidis* W135 | 0 | 1 (1) |
| *Salmonella montevideo* | 0 | 1 (1) |
| *Bifidobacterium* species | 0 | 1 (1) |
| Polymicrobial | 1 | 4 (8) |

*Of 314 patients who had blood cultures, 28 (8.9%) had positive results.
†Of 539 patients who had blood cultures, 48 (8.9%) had positive results.
‡Percentage of the total patient number is given in parentheses.

## EPIDEMIOLOGY

### Comorbidity

Most patients with pneumonia have one or more comorbidities. Such comorbidities are often age dependent (Table 11–3). The mean number of comorbidities increased from 0.73 for those 30 years of age or older to 2.75 for those between the ages of 71 and 80 years.[31] Alcoholism, chronic obstructive pulmonary disease (COPD), ischemic heart disease, malignancy, diabetes mellitus, and neurologic disease are important in predisposing the patient to pneumonia (eg, neurologic disease resulting in aspiration) or influencing recovery from pneumonia (eg, COPD, ischemic heart disease, malignancy).

### Mortality Rates

Pneumonia is a serious illness; the overall mortality rate is 1% to 3%. For patients requiring hospitalization, the mortality varies considerably depending on the exclusion criteria used in the study, ranging from 6% to 24%.[2, 3, 12–31] However, for subpopulations within this group mortality rates are much higher—40% for patients with nursing home-acquired pneumonia requiring hospitalization,[40] and 22% to 57% for those with CAP requiring intensive care unit treatment.[32–37] In our study, patients who required ventilator therapy had the highest mortality rate, reaching a high of 56% for those between the ages of 71 and 80 years.[31] The percentage of patients with CAP who need admission to an intensive care unit (ICU) depends greatly on the criteria used for admission. Alkhayer and coworkers[35] from Norwich, England, estimate that as many as 5% of patients admitted with CAP require ICU treatment. At our center, 17% of patients admitted with CAP required assisted ventilation as part of the management of their pneumonic illness.[31]

Several studies have tried to determine the factors that predict mortality. The results of three such studies that used multivariate analysis are shown in Table 11–4. More recently, Farr and colleagues studied 245 patients and found three factors to be predictive of mortality using a stepwise logistic regression analysis.[40a] These were respiratory rate $\geq$30/min, diastolic blood pressure $\leq$60mm Hg, and blood urea nitrogen $>$19.6 mg/dL. Mortality increased from 9- to

Table 11–3. **Major Comorbidities of 1118 Patients With Community-Acquired Pneumonia Requiring Hospitalization**

| Comorbidity | No. of Patients (%) |
|---|---|
| Neurologic disease | 305 (27.2) |
| Chronic obstructive pulmonary disease | 222 (19.8) |
| Ischemic heart disease | 179 (16) |
| Hypertension | 153 (13.6) |
| Malignancy | 137 (12.3) |
| Diabetes mellitus | 80 (7.1) |
| Renal disease | 68 (6.1) |
| Acquired immunodeficiency syndrome | 40 (3.5) |

From Marrie TJ: Epidemiology of community-acquired pneumonia in the elderly. Semin Respir Infect 5:260, 1990.

Table 11–4. **Predictors of Mortality From Studies of Community-Acquired Pneumonia That Used Multivariate Analysis**

| Investigation | No. of Patients | Predictors of Mortality |
|---|---|---|
| Marrie et al[3] | 719 | Number of lobes involved on chest radiograph, number of antibiotics, age, ventilatory support, number of complications, admission from a nursing home |
| British Thoracic Society[23] | 453* | Age, absence of chest pain or vomiting, tachypnea, diastolic hypotension, confusion, elevated blood urea nitrogen, leukocytosis or leukopenia, digitalis toxicity |
| Zweig et al[38] | 133† | Impaired level of consciousness, tachypnea, temperature lower than normal, leukocyte count $>$20 $\times$ 10$^9$/L, cyanosis |

*This study excluded patients 75 years of age or older and those with a terminal course, tuberculosis, or postobstructive disease.
†This retrospective study only included patients older than 60 years of age.

21-fold if two of these factors were present, compared with when two factors were not present. Fine and colleagues[39] studied 170 patients with CAP to determine who could safely be treated in an ambulatory care setting. They found that five factors predisposed to a complicated course:

1. Age older than 65 years (odds ratio 2.7)
2. Comorbid illness (odds ratio 3.2)
3. Temperature greater than 38 °C (odds ratio 4.1)
4. Immunosuppresion (odds ratio 12)
5. High-risk cause (odds ratio 23.3), such as staphylococcal, gram-negative rod, aspiration, or postobstructive pneumonia

These findings are reflected in the criteria for admission of patients with CAP to the hospital. Seriously ill patients with respiratory distress or central cyanosis should be admitted. Patients who are at high risk for a complicated course (eg, those 70 years of age or older with comorbid illness such as COPD or ischemic heart disease), those of any age who have severe comorbidity that is likely to be adversely affected by the pneumonia, and immunocompromised patients should be admitted.

Several investigators have used various laboratory measurements to try and predict the outcome of patients with CAP. $\alpha_1$-Proteinase inhibitor in serum was found to be functionally inactivated in patients with fulminating CAP.[40] This low functional level of $\alpha_1$-proteinase inhibitor may result in proteolytic lung damage and an unfavorable outcome. In a population of AIDS patients with *P. carinii* pneumonia, the single best prognostic indicator of acute mortality was a total serum triiodothyronine ($T_3$) of less than 0.7 nmol/L.[41] Profound alterations in serum thyroid hormone indices occur in severely ill patients.[42, 43] In severe illness, an acquired defect in thyroid hormone binding to serum proteins develops.[43] Depression in serum $T_3$ levels reflects an impaired conversion of thyroxine to $T_3$ by the peripheral tissues.[44]

In pneumococcal pneumonia, low levels of unsaturated

Table 11–5. **Settings in Which Outbreaks of Pneumonia Have Occurred and the Infecting Microorganisms**

| Microorganism | Setting | Reference |
|---|---|---|
| *Legionella pneumophila* | Contaminated water source: air conditioning, cooling tower, grocery store mist machine | 50, 52 |
| | | 51 |
| *Streptococcus pneumoniae* | Shelter for homeless men, jails, South African mines, Army barracks | 53 |
| | | 54 |
| *Mycoplasma pneumoniae* | Family outbreak (intrafamilial spread) | 55 |
| *Coxiella burnetii* | Exposure to infected parturient cats, sheep, cattle, goats | 56 |
| | | 57 |
| | | 58 |
| *Mycobacterium tuberculosis* | Exposure to an infected person, especially one with cavitary disease in a closed setting, such as a nursing home, shelters for the homeless | 59 |
| *Histoplasma capsulatum* | Exposure to contaminated bat caves; excavation in endemic areas; fallen trees in endemic areas | 60 |
| | | 61 |
| *Blastomyces dermatitidis* | Exposure to disturbed contaminated soil; exposure to a contaminated beaver lodge | 62, 63 |
| *Coccidioides immitis* | After a windstorm in an endemic area | 64 |

transferrin have been associated with a fatal outcome,[45] and high levels of antibodies to phosphorylcholine in patients 70 years of age predicts subsequent fatal pneumonia.[46]

## Other Epidemiologic Factors

In the northern hemisphere, pneumonia is more common during the winter months. Cases of *M. pneumoniae* pneumonia seem to peak every 7 years.

Pneumonia usually occurs as sporadic cases, but outbreaks are not uncommon if there is exposure to a point source of contamination or in an enclosed environment.[47–59] Some of the most dramatic outbreaks of pneumonia have been caused by *L. pneumophila*. The event that drew this form of pneumonia to our attention was the 1976 convention of the American Legion at the Bellevue-Stratford Hotel in Philadelphia, after which 221 of the conventioneers developed pneumonia.[49] Table 11–5 summarizes the circumstances that have led to outbreaks of pneumonia.

## CLINICAL FEATURES

Respiratory tract symptoms such as cough usually predominate in pneumonia; however, only about 80% of patients with pneumonia complain of cough.[3] In patients with NHAP, only 60% have a cough.[3] Even in patients who were bacteremic as a result of pneumococcal pneumonia, only 81% complained of cough, and it was productive in 66% (Marrie TJ, unpublished observations). Fever, anorexia, and chills are other common complaints. A variety of nonspecific symptoms are reported by 10% to 30% of patients with pneumonia. These include headache, nausea, vomiting, sore throat, myalgia, arthralgia, rigors, abdominal pain, and diarrhea.[3] Pleuritic chest pain occurs in as many as 40% of patients with pneumonia.

The most frequent physical finding on examination of the chest is cackles (78%), followed by rhonchi (34%), and consolidation (29%).[3]

The clinical diagnosis of pneumonia is fraught with difficulty, and a chest radiograph must be part of the evaluation of a febrile patient. Singal and colleagues,[65] using decision analysis, ''were unable to derive or validate useful low-yield criteria to improve on the seasoned clinician's

probable estimate of pneumonia.'' However, Heckerling and coworkers,[66] found that a prediction rule based on the findings of temperature greater than 37.8°C, pulse greater than 100 beats per minute, rales, decreased breath sounds, and the absence of asthma accurately predicted which patients would have pneumonia. Others[67] have used variables predictive of various etiologic agents in a discriminant function analysis to predict the microbial origin of pneumonia. Using this technique, they were able to correctly predict the cause of the pneumonia in 42% of cases.[67] Pneumonia may present with minimal or no symptoms referable to the respiratory system, and clinical and radiographic features usually do not allow the physician to make an accurate etiologic diagnosis.

There are hazards in the recognition of pneumonia, and there are certain aspects of the diagnosis and treatment of pneumonia that commonly cause problems. In 1965, Shulman, Phillips, and Petersdorf[68] reviewed records of patients with pneumonia in a geriatric teaching hospital and detailed seven errors and hazards in the diagnosis and treatment of bacterial pneumonias. These are listed with annotations indicating the current status of these considerations:

1. The frequency with which the etiologic agent is missed on Gram smears of sputum. This is largely caused by inexperience, such as missing pleomorphic, small, gram-negative coccobacilli (eg, *H. influenzae*) or overdiagnosing *S. pneumoniae* although only normal flora is present. The Gram stain, however, remains an important tool in the presumptive etiologic diagnosis of pneumonia and for providing guidance for initial antimicrobial therapy.

2. Failure to suspect the appropriate organism in certain clinical situations. Late diagnosis of reactivated pulmonary tuberculosis, especially among the residents of nursing homes, is the most frequent error in this category.

3. Delay in recognition of superinfections. This remains a major problem. The real difficulty is differentiating colonization from infection. Bronchoscopy using a protected specimen brush is often the only reliable means, and even this technique is not 100% sensitive or 100% specific.

4. Tardy appreciation of the systemic complications of bacterial pneumonia, particularly meningitis. In the elderly, confusion due to meningitis is likely to be attributed to

Alzheimer disease. Endocarditis complicating pneumonia, especially among the elderly, is a problem.

5. Inappropriate use of antibiotics, particularly because mechanical factors interfering with bronchial drainage remained undetected.

6. Failure to appreciate the alterations in flora of the sputum in patients receiving antibiotics. In the 1990s, this is more appropriately stated as a failure to appreciate the effects of broad-spectrum antibiotics in altering the patient's flora of the respiratory tract and of the gastrointestinal tract. The latter is important because microaspiration and macroaspiration are common in seriously ill patients with pneumonia, especially those who have nasogastric or endotracheal tubes in place.

7. The propensity of nonbacterial complications of pneumonia, such as sterile pleural effusion or atelectasis, to produce fever. Although rare, it should be considered in the patient with pneumonia who remains febrile.

## APPROACH TO THE PATIENT WITH PNEUMONIA

A decision tree for approaching the patient with pneumonia is given in Figure 11–1.

The first consideration should be whether the patient has pneumonia or one of the noninfectious entities that mimic pneumonia (Table 11–6).

If the physician decides the patient has pneumonia, but there is no sputum available for Gram stain and culture, he or she should categorize the patient according to one of the pneumonia syndromes shown in Table 11–7. This concept, first popularized by Donowitz and Mandell,[69] is useful for guiding initial empiric antimicrobial therapy. We have added several categories to the original ones, including pneumonia complicating human immunodeficiency virus infection as a new category of agents predisposing to CAP.[70] Given the increasing number of organ transplant recipients who are leading healthy, productive lives in the community but nevertheless are immunosuppressed, it is appropriate to create a new category for this group. Many of these syndromes are discussed in later chapters, but an overview is provided here. For the purposes of this discussion, the causes of pneumonia occurring 3 months or longer after transplantation are considered.[71–77] Empiric antibiotic therapy for each syndrome is given in Table 11–7. The syndrome approach to the diagnosis and therapy of pneumonia is only a guide, it has not been tested in a prospective study. There may be overlap among the syndromes. For example, *L. pneumophila* and *M. pneumoniae*, both agents that cause atypical pneumonia, may result in a productive cough in some patients and could therefore be classified as typical pneumonia and perhaps treated inappropriately. For these reasons, guidelines for the initial empiric antimicrobial treatment of CAP now emphasize the severity of the pneumonia, site of acquisition (home or nursing home), and site of treatment (home or hospital) rather than clinical syndromes (Table 11–8).[77a] Tables 11–7 and 11–8 supplement each other.

### History and Physical Examination

A careful history is critical and frequently is the only way an etiologic diagnosis can be made. Table 11–5 lists the settings in which various outbreaks of pneumonia have occurred. Table 11–9 shows clues to the cause of pneumonia that may be gleaned from the history, and Table 11–10 shows physical findings that may be associated with specific causes of pneumonia.

### Radiographic Evaluation

The chest radiograph (Table 11–11) represents a key element in the diagnosis of pneumonia. An opacity must be seen on the chest radiograph to substantiate a diagnosis of pneumonia. If the clinical findings indicate a diagnosis of pneumonia but the chest radiograph is negative, repeat radiographs should be obtained in 24 to 48 hours. The world of chest radiology is one of shadows. Pneumonia is infected pulmonary edema, and many infectious and noninfectious conditions can give rise to opacities that mimic pneumonia. Radiologists use a variety of terms when reporting chest radiographic findings. The terms pneumonia and pneumonitis are used interchangeably, although most radiologists prefer the term pneumonia.[91] Opacity or density should be used in preference to consolidation as a radiologic term.

There often is a poor correlation between the findings on

Table 11–6. **Noninfectious Causes of Cough, Fever, and Pulmonary Opacities**

Congestive heart failure
Pulmonary infarction
Atelectasis
Collagen vascular diseases
   Lupus erythematosus
   Wegner granulomatosis
   Churg-Strauss vasculitis
   Rheumatoid vasculitis, especially in coal miners (Caplan syndrome)
Sarcoidosis
Hypersensitivity pneumonitis
Lymphangitic carcinomatosis
Lymphoma
Eosinophilic pneumonia
Drug-induced pulmonary disease
   Reticulonodular disease that may lead to pulmonary fibrosis[78]
      Cytosine arabinoside
      Busulfan
      Bleomycin
      Cyclophosphamide
      Methotrexate
      Procarbazine
      Mitomycin
      Vinblastine
      Amiodarone
      Hydrochlorthiazide
      Nitrofurantoin
      Penicillamine
      Sulfasalazine
      Tocainamide
      Gold salts
Pulmonary edema (noncardiogenic)[79–86]
   Salicylates
   Narcotics (eg, heroin, cocaine)
   Ethchlorvynol (Placidyl)
   Chlordiazepoxide (Librium)
   Propoxyphene
Septic pulmonary emboli[87]
   Intravenous drug abuse resulting in right-sided endocarditis
Hypersensitivity pneumonitis[88]
   Nonsteroidal antiinflammatory drugs

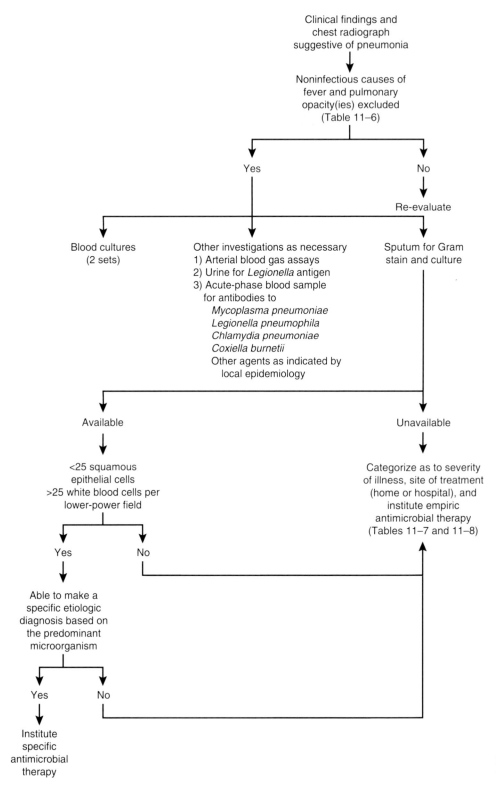

**Figure 11–1.** Approach to the patient with pneumonia.

Table 11–7. **Cause and Treatment of Pneumonia Syndromes**

| Pneumonia Syndrome | Agent | Therapy |
|---|---|---|
| Atypical | *Mycoplasma pneumoniae* <br> *Chlamydia pneumoniae* <br> *Legionella pneumophila* <br> *Chlamydia psittaci* <br> *Coxiella burnetii* <br> *Pneumocystis carinii* | Erythromycin or tetracycline (if *Pneumocystis carinii* suspected, trimethoprim-sulfamethoxazole) |
| Typical <br>   Age <60, no comorbidity <br>   Comorbidity <br>   Chronic obstructive lung disease <br><br>    Alcoholism | <br> *Streptococcus pneumoniae* <br> *Streptococcus pneumoniae* <br> *Haemophilus influenzae* <br> *Moraxella catarrhalis* <br> *Streptococcus pneumoniae* <br> *Klebsiella pneumoniae* <br> *Staphylococcus aureus* <br> *Mycobacterium tuberculosis*† | <br> Penicillin* <br> Second-generation cephalosporin (eg, cefuroxime) <br> Tetracycline or trimethoprim-sulfamethoxazole <br> Second-generation cephalosporin (eg, cephamandole or cefuroxime) |
| Aspiration <br>   No H$_2$-blockers <br>   H$_2$-blockers | <br> Acid <br> Polymicrobial oral flora and aerobic gram-negative bacteria in elderly patients | <br> No antibiotics <br> Penicillin plus third-generation cephalosporin |
| Nursing home acquired | *Streptococcus pneumoniae* <br> *Staphylococcus aureus* <br> *Haemophilus influenzae* <br> Aerobic gram-negative rods <br> *Mycobacterium tuberculosis*† | Second-generation cephalosporin or penicillin plus ciprofloxacin |
| Rapidly progressive pneumonia | All the agents that cause pneumonia, but most commonly: <br>   *Legionella pneumophila* <br>   *Mycoplasma pneumoniae* <br>   *Staphylococcus aureus* <br>   Aerobic gram-negative rods <br>   *Coxiella burnetii* | Erythromycin plus rifampin plus ceftazidime |
| Acquired immunodeficiency syndrome with pneumonia | *Pneumocystis carinii* <br> Pyogenic bacteria (*Streptococcus pneumoniae* most common) <br> *Cryptococcus neoformans* <br> *Mycobacterium avium-intracellulare* <br> *Mycobacterium tuberculosis*† <br> Cytomegalovirus <br> *Legionella* | Necessary to make an etiologic diagnosis |
| Organ transplant recipient (>3 mo after transplant) | *Streptococcus pneumoniae* <br> *Haemophilus influenzae* <br> *Legionella* spp. <br> *Pneumocystis carinii* <br> Cytomegalovirus <br> *Strongyloides* <br> *Mycobacterium tuberculosis*† <br> *Nocardia asteroides* | Aggressive approach to diagnosis necessary |

*Consider local epidemiology and resistance patterns.
†Specific antituberculous therapy if this disease is diagnosed or suspected.

Table 11–8. **Initial Empiric Treatment of Community-Acquired Pneumonia***

A. Age ≤60 years; no comorbidity; outpatient therapy (oral): Macrolide or tetracycline
B. Age >60 years; comorbidity; outpatient therapy (oral): Second-generation cephalosporin, trimethoprim-sulfamethoxazole, or β-lactam/β-lactamase inhibitor; add macrolide if infection with *Legionella* is a concern
C. Therapy in hospital (parenteral): Second-generation cephalosporin or β-lactam/β-lactamase inhibitor; add macrolide if infection with *Legionella* is a concern
D. Therapy in hospital—severe pneumonia (parenteral): Macrolide plus antibiotic with antipseudomonal activity such as ceftazidime; ciprofloxacin or imipenem/cilastatin; add rifampin PO if *Legionella* is diagnosed

*Patients with HIV infection excluded.
Modified from Mandell LA, Niederman MS, The Canadian Community-Acquired Pneumonia Consensus Group: Antimicrobial treatment of community-acquired pneumonia in adults: A conference report. Reproduced with permission of Canadian Journal of Infectious Diseases. 1993; 4:25.

Table 11–9. **Indications of the Cause of Pneumonia From the Patient's History**

| History | Agent |
|---|---|
| Animal exposure[89, 90] | |
| Cats (parturient) | *Coxiella burnetii* (Q fever) |
| | *Pasteurella multocida* |
| Cattle, sheep, goats | *C. burnetii* |
| Rabbits, squirrels, coyotes, skunks, rodents, foxes, dogs, cats | *Francisella tularensis* (tularemia) |
| Turkeys, chickens, ducks, psittacine birds (eg, parrots, parakeets, macaws, cockatiels) | *Chlamydia psittaci* (psittacosis) |
| Rats, squirrels, rabbits, prairie dogs | *Yersinia pestis* (plague) |
| Rats, mice | *Leptospira* spp. (leptospirosis) |
| Horses | *Pseudomonas mallei* (glanders) |
| Travel | |
| Thailand; other countries in Southeast Asia | *Pseudomonas pseudomallei* (melioidosis) |
| Asia, Africa, Central and South America | *Paragonimus westermani* (paragonimiasis) |
| Anywhere with exposure to contaminated air conditioning (eg, cooling towers, evaporative condensers) | *Legionella pneumophila* (legionnaires disease) |
| Occupational exposure | |
| Irritant gas exposure: ammonia, sulfur dioxide, nitrogen dioxide, chlorine, phosgene | Pulmonary edema |
| Demographics | |
| Alcoholism | *Klebsiella pneumoniae* |
| | *Streptococcus pneumoniae* |
| | *Staphylococcus aureus* |
| Chronic obstructive pulmonary disease | *Streptococcus pneumoniae* |
| | *Haemophilus influenzae* |
| | *Moraxella catarrhalis* |
| Corticosteroid therapy | *Staphylococcus aureus* |
| | *Mycobacterium tuberculosis* |
| | *Pneumocystis carinii* |

Table 11–10. **Physical Findings That Suggest an Etiologic Diagnosis of Pneumonia**

| Finding | Agent |
|---|---|
| Cutaneous findings | |
| Erythema multiforme | *Mycoplasma pneumoniae* |
| Maculopapular rash | Measles |
| Erythema nodosum | *Chlamydia pneumoniae,* |
| Ecythema gangrenosum | *Mycobacterium tuberculosis* |
| | *Pseudomonas aeruginosa* |
| | *Serratia marcescens* |
| Oral findings | |
| Periodontal disease | Anaerobic pneumonia |
| Foul smelling sputum | |
| Ears | |
| Bullous myringitis | *M. pneumoniae* |
| Neurologic disease | |
| Absent gag reflex, altered level of consciousness, recent seizure, | Aspiration |
| Cerebellar ataxia | *M. pneumoniae* |
| | *Legionella pneumophila* |
| Encephalitis | *M. pneumoniae* |
| | *Coxiella burnetii* |
| Toxic encephalopathy | Nonspecific, all agents that can cause pneumonia |

Table 11–11. **Differential Diagnosis of Common Radiographic Patterns in Patients With Pneumonia**

| Infective Cause | Noninfective Cause |
|---|---|
| **Focal opacity** | |
| *Streptococcus pneumoniae* | Bronchial obstruction |
| *Mycoplasma pneumoniae* | Pulmonary infarction |
| *Legionella pneumophila* | Sarcoidosis |
| *Staphylococcus aureus* | Collagen vascular disease |
| *Chlamydia pneumoniae* | Bronchoalveolar carcinoma |
| *Mycobacterium tuberculosis* | |
| Aspiration | |
| *Blastomyces dermatitidis* | |
| **Multifocal opacities** | |
| *S. aureus* | Hypersensitivity pneumonitis |
| *Coxiella burnetii* | Pulmonary infiltrates with eosinophilia (eg, PIE syndrome) |
| *L. pneumophila* | Sarcoidosis |
| *S. pneumoniae* | Allergic bronchopulmonary aspergillosis |
| | Bronchiolitis obliterans organizing pneumonia (BOOP) |
| **Interstitial pattern** | |
| Viral causes | Pulmonary edema |
| *M. pneumoniae* | Sarcoidosis |
| *Pneumocystis carinii* | Drug reactions |
| *Chlamydia psittaci* | Pulmonary fibrosis |
| | Hypersensitivity pneumonitis |
| **Miliary pattern** | |
| *M. tuberculosis* | Sarcoidosis |
| *Histoplasma capsulatum* | Lymphoma |
| *Coccidioides immitis* | Histiocytosis |
| *B. dermatitidis* | Hypersensitivity pneumonia |
| Varicella zoster | |
| **Interstitial pneumonia with lymphadenopathy** | |
| Epstein-Barr virus | Metastatic carcinoma |
| *Francisella tularensis* | Sarcoidosis |
| *C. psittaci* | Lymphoma |
| **Segmental or lobar pneumonia with lymphadenopathy** | |
| *M. tuberculosis* (primary infection) | Carcinoma with bronchial obstruction |
| Fungal infection | |
| Atypical measles | |
| **Cavitation** | |
| Anaerobic lung abscess | Bronchogenic carcinoma |
| *S. aureus* | Metastatic carcinoma |
| Aerobic gram-negative bacilli | Pulmonary infarction |
| *(Escherichia coli; Klebsiella; Pseudomonas aeruginosa)* | Vasculitis |
| *L. pneumophila* | |
| *M. tuberculosis* | |
| *Cryptococcus neoformans* | |
| *C. immitis* | |
| *Nocardia asteroides* | |
| *Actinomyces israelii* | |

Some data from Lynch DA, Armstrong JD II: A pattern-oriented approach to chest radiographs in atypical pneumonia syndromes. Clin Chest Med 12:203, 1991, and from Reed JC: Chest Radiography. Patterns and Differential Diagnosis. Chicago, Year Book Medical Publishers, 1981:107–250.

clinical examination and the radiograph. As many as 25% of young adults with pneumonia have no abnormal auscultatory findings.[92] It is likely that most of these patients have atypical pneumonia.

The clinician should have a logical approach to evaluating the chest radiograph of a patient with suspected pneumonia. The first principle is to examine the radiograph and use the radiologist as a consultant whenever necessary. In adults, a posteroanterior (PA) and a lateral chest radiograph should be performed. In children, there may be little value

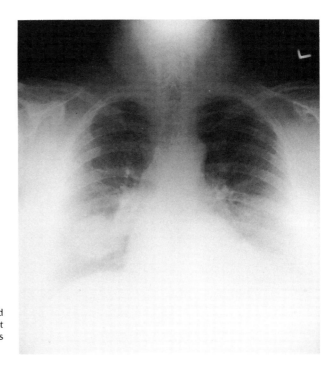

**Figure 11–2.** Bacteremic pneumococcal pneumonia. This 67-year-old woman has a rounded opacity, "round pneumonia," involving the right lower lobe. This is a mass lesion, and the differential diagnosis includes malignancy.

in obtaining a lateral chest radiograph in suspected pneumonia; in one study, in only 9 of 414 children with suspected pneumonia did the lateral radiograph add any information to the PA film.[93] The technical quality of the film can influence the interpretation. Films that are underpenetrated make it difficult to assess the interstitium of the lung and may result in overdiagnosis of interstitial pneumonia. With portable chest radiographs, 10° to 15° of lordosis can result in various degrees of loss of definition of the left hemidiaphragm and can create a false impression of disease in the left lower lobe, pleural space, or both.[94]

In most instances, it is impossible to make an etiologic diagnosis from the appearance of the pneumonia on the

chest radiograph. Several studies have shown that radiologists cannot differentiate bacterial from nonbacterial pneumonia on the basis of the chest radiograph.[95–97] The etiologic agent may be suggested from the appearance on chest radiograph, such as upper lobe cavitation due to tuberculosis or multiple pneumatocoeles due to *Staphylococcus aureus* infection.

There is a considerable variation in the radiographic features of pneumonia due to any one microorganism (Figs. 11–2 through 11–7).[98] The preexisting state of the lung can influence greatly the radiographic appearance of pneumonia. For example, incomplete consolidation is common if pneumonia complicates emphysema,[99] and atypical distri-

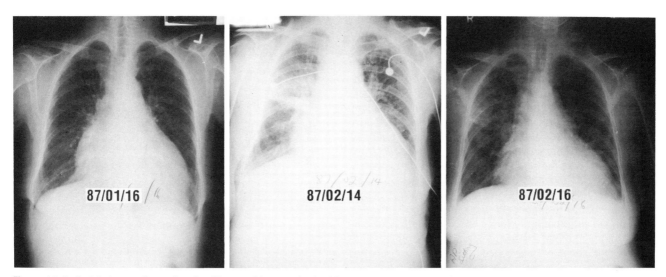

**Figure 11–3.** Serial chest radiographs of a 70-year-old man who had bacteremic pneumococcal pneumonia and coexisting congestive heart failure. The radiograph obtained on January 16, 1987, before his pneumonia, shows cardiomegaly and vascular redistribution. At the time of admission to the hospital on February 14, 1987, there was a pulmonary edema and a right upper lobe opacity. Two days later, after treatment with diuretics, there was considerable clearing of the pulmonary edema and the right upper lobe opacity. However, the opacity remained distinct, suggesting that this patient had pneumonia and pulmonary edema.

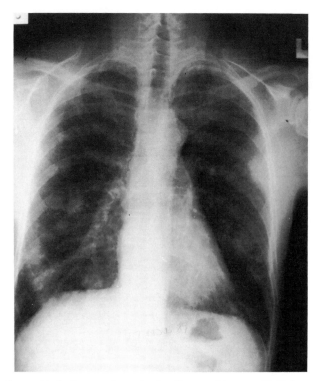

**Figure 11–4.** Chest radiograph of a 56-year-old man with Q fever pneumonia. This man who had a 60 pack-year smoking history has multiple, rounded opacities (ie, nodules) scattered throughout both lung fields. The radiologist reported that this was probably metastatic carcinoma.

bution of bacterial pneumonia may occur after radiation therapy to the thorax.[100]

Febrile dehydrated patients may have pneumonia despite a normal chest radiograph. Although one study demonstrated that rehydration in dogs with pneumococcal pneumonia does produce a heavier pneumonic lobe than develops in control dogs who are not hydrated,[101] there is little clinical evidence other than a few case reports to support this concept.[102]

In reviewing the chest film, it is useful to calculate the amount of the pulmonary parenchyma that is involved by the pneumonic process. In general, a bronchopulmonary segment represents 10% of the lung volume. The extent of pneumonic involvement correlates with outcome.[3]

The frequency with which follow-up radiographs should be obtained is dictated by the clinical status of the patient. Patients who are responding to antibiotic therapy need have only one follow-up film to ensure that the pneumonia has resolved. The timing of this radiograph is related to the patient's age and the underlying state of the lung parenchyma. Patients older than 50 years of age with chronic obstructive lung disease may require as long as 10 weeks for radiographic resolution of the pneumonia.[103] Patients who are not improving or whose condition is deteriorating may require multiple chest radiographs, and other radiologic techniques may be necessary. The thoracic computed tomographic scan has proven extremely helpful in evaluating critically ill patients with pneumonia. It is especially useful for detecting empyema.[104]

Chest radiographs probably are overused in the management of pneumonia. In our hospital, the mean number of chest radiographs per episode of pneumonia was 4.2.[31] Dans and coworkers,[105] in a study at the Johns Hopkins Hospital in Baltimore, Maryland, found that the mean number of chest radiographs per episode of pneumonia was 3.68, but if thoracentesis was necessary, 10.5 chest radiographs were obtained per episode of pneumonia.

Figures 11–2 through 11–7 illustrate the spectrum of radiographic findings in pneumococcal pneumonia,[106–109] pneumonia due to *C. burnetti*,[110–113] *M. pneumoniae*, *L. pneumophila*, *Chlamydia psittaci*, and *P. carinii*.

For the nonradiologist, pattern recognition is extremely useful in interpreting the chest radiograph. The common causes of the various patterns seen are given in Table 11–10.

### Diagnostic Workup

All patients should have Gram stain and culture of sputum. Decisions regarding transtracheal aspiration, bronchoscopy with bronchoalveolar lavage, or protected specimen brush depend on the clinical setting. All patients seen in a hospital should have two sets of blood cultures performed.

All patients with pneumonia serious enough to require hospitalization should have a blood gas determination. All patients with pneumonia complicated by cyanosis, severe

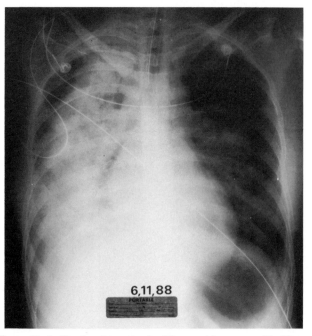

**Figure 11–5.** Chest radiograph of a 26-year-old woman with *Mycoplasma pneumoniae* pneumonia. This young woman, who had insulin-dependent diabetes mellitus, was 2 weeks postpartum when she developed fever, nonproductive cough, and progressive dyspnea, resulting in respiratory failure. She required assisted ventilation for 5 days. There is extensive opacification involving the right lung, and similar although less pronounced changes are evident in the left lung.

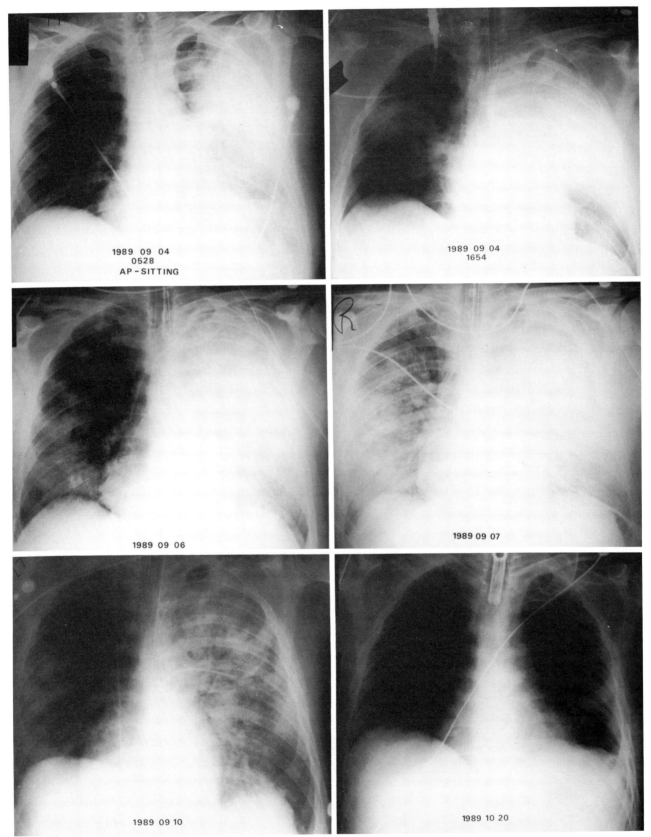

**Figure 11–6.** Serial chest radiographs of a 40-year-old man with rapidly progressive pneumonia due to *Legionella pneumophila* serogroup 1. There is dense opacification of the left lung, which quickly spread to the right lung. Such spread may represent development of adult respiratory distress syndrome. Almost complete radiographic resolution of the pneumonia occurred 46 days after admission to the hospital.

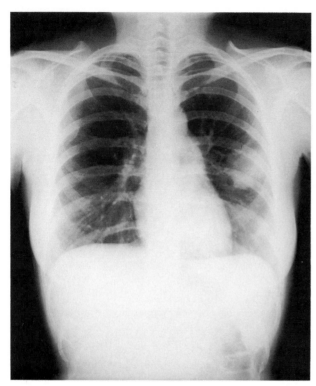

**Figure 11–7.** Rounded opacity in the left lower lobe of an 18-year-old female store worker with psittacosis.

dyspnea, hypotension, COPD, or an unconscious state must have blood gas analysis.[116]

## Therapeutic Decisions Other Than Antimicrobial Therapy

An early therapeutic decision must be made about whether to intubate and provide assisted ventilation. In some instances, this poses an ethical dilemma; however, there are clear-cut medical indications for intubation and for assisted ventilation (Table 11–12). Comorbid illnesses are common in patients with pneumonia requiring hospitalization, and these require management as well.

The problem of pneumonia is a challenging one. The greatest need is for sensitive and specific tests that can rapidly detect antigens in the serum of the agents that cause pneumonia. The results of these tests can be used to guide specific therapy.

**Table 11–12. Indications for Intubation and Mechanical Ventilation of Patients With Pneumonia**

Inability to maintain an adequate arterial $Po_2$ (50–60 mm Hg) despite administration of maximal supplemental oxygen
Respiratory acidosis
Respiratory muscle fatigue (gradually increasing $Paco_2$ with acidosis, paradoxic breathing pattern, and increasing respiratory rate)
Occasionally to protect the airway to prevent aspiration in an unconscious patient
Inability to clear secretions, with likelihood of impending respiratory failure

## REFERENCES

1. Heffron R: Pneumonia: With Special Reference to Pneumococcus Lobar Pneumonia. Cambridge, MA, Harvard University Press, 1939 (second printing, 1979).
2. Fang G-D, Fine M, Orloff J, et al: New and emerging etiologies for community-acquired pneumonia with implications for therapy. A prospective multicenter study of 359 cases. Medicine (Baltimore) 69:307, 1990.
3. Marrie TJ, Durant H, Yates L: Community-acquired pneumonia requiring hospitalization: 5-year prospective study. Rev Infect Dis 11:586, 1989.
4. Fredman L, Haynes SG: An epidemiologic profile of the elderly. In Phillips HT, Gayland SA (eds): Aging and Public Health. New York, Springer Verlag, 1985.
5. Update: Acquired immunodeficiency syndrome—United States, 1981–1990. MMWR 40:358, 1991.
6. Foy HM, Cooney MK, Allan I, et al: Rates of pneumonia during influenza epidemics in Seattle, 1964 to 1975. JAMA 241:253, 1979.
7. MacFarlane J: Community-acquired pneumonia. Br J Dis Chest 81:116, 1987.
7a. Jokinen C, Heiskanen L, Juvonen H, et al: Incidence of community-acquired pneumonia in the population of four municipalities in eastern Finland. Am J Epidemiol 137:977, 1993.
8. Mufson MA, Oley G, Hughey D: Pneumococcal disease in a medium-sized community in the United States. JAMA 248:1486, 1982.
9. Davidson M, Schraer CD, Parkinson AJ, et al: Invasive pneumococcal disease in an Alaska Native population 1980 through 1986. JAMA 261:715, 1989.
10. Foy HM, Cooney MK, McMahan R, et al: Viral and mycoplasmal pneumonia in a prepaid medical care group during an eight-year period. Am J Epidemiol 97:93, 1973.
11. Foy HM, Wentworth B, Kenny GE, et al: Pneumococcal isolations from patients with pneumonia and control subjects in a prepaid medical care group. Am Rev Respir Dis 111:595, 1975.
12. Fekety FR Jr, Caldwell J, Gump D, et al: Bacteria, viruses and mycoplasmas in acute pneumonia in adults. Am Rev Respir Dis 104:499, 1971.
13. Sullivan RJ Jr, Dowdle WR, Marine WM, et al: Adult pneumonia in a general hospital: Etiology and host risk factors. Arch Intern Med 129:935, 1972.
14. Dorff GJ, Rytel MW, Farmer SG, et al: Etiologies and characteristic features of pneumonia in a municipal hospital. Am J Med Sci 266:349, 1973.
15. Garb JL, Brown RB, Garb JR, et al: Differences in etiology of pneumonias in nursing home and community patients. JAMA 240:2169, 1978.
16. White RJ, Blainey AD, Harrison KJ, et al: Causes of pneumonia presenting to a district general hospital. Thorax 36:566, 1981.
17. McNabb WR, Shanson DC, Williams TDM, et al: Adult community-acquired pneumonia in central London. J R Soc Med 77:550, 1984.
18. MacFarlane JT, Finch RG, Ward MJ, et al: Hospital study of adult community-acquired pneumonia. Lancet 2:255, 1982.
19. Kerttula Y, Leinonen M, Koskela M, et al: The etiology of pneumonia. Application of bacterial serology and basic laboratory methods. J Infect Dis 14:21, 1987.
20. Holmberg H, Badin L, Jonsson I, Krook A: Rapid aetiological diagnosis of pneumonia based on routine laboratory features. Scand J Infect Dis 22:537, 1990.
21. Bath JCJL, Boissard GPB, Calder MA, et al: Pneumonia in hospital practice in Edinburgh 1960–1962. Br J Dis Chest 58:1, 1964.
22. Larsen RA, Jacobson JA: Diagnosis of community-acquired pneumonia: Experience at a community hospital. Compr Ther 10:20, 1984.
23. Research Committee of the British Thoracic Society and the Public Health Laboratory Service: Community-acquired pneumonia in adults in British hospitals in 1982–1983: A survey of aetiology, mortality, prognostic factors and outcome. Q J Med 62:195, 1989.
24. Mohamed ARE, Price Evans DA: The spectrum of pneumonia in 1983 at the Riyadh Armed Forces Hospital. J Infect Dis 14:31, 1987.
25. Holmberg H: Aetiology of community-acquired pneumonia in hospital treated patients. Scand J Infect Dis 19:491, 1987.
26. Levy M, Dromer F, Brion N, et al: Community-acquired pneumonia. Importance of initial noninvasive bacteriologic and radiographic investigations. Chest 92:43, 1988.

27. Lim I, Shaw DR, Stanley DP, et al: A prospective study of the aetiology of community-acquired pneumonia. Med J Aust 151:87, 1989.

28. Ausina V, Coll P, Sambeat M, et al: Prospective study on the etiology of community-acquired pneumonia in children and adults in Spain. Eur J Clin Microbiol Infect Dis 7:343, 1988.

29. Ortqvist A, Kalin M, Lejdeborn L, et al: Diagnostic fiberoptic bronchoscopy and protected brush culture in patients with community-acquired pneumonia. Chest 97:576, 1990.

30. Berntsson E, Lagergard T, Strannegard O, et al: Etiology of community-acquired pneumonia in outpatients. Eur J Clin Microbiol Infect Dis 5: 446, 1986.

31. Marrie TJ: Epidemiology of community-acquired pneumonia in the elderly. Semin Respir Infect 5:260, 1990.

32. Sorenson J, Forsberg P, Hakanson E, et al: A new diagnostic approach to the patient with severe pneumonia. Scand J Infect Dis 21:33, 1989.

33. Ortqvist A, Sterner G, Nilsson JA: Severe community-acquired pneumonia: Factors influencing need of intensive care treatment and prognosis. Scan J Infect Dis 17:377, 1985.

34. Sorensen J, Cederholm I, Carlsson C: Pneumonia: A deadly disease despite intensive care treatment. Scand J Infect Dis 18:329, 1986.

35. Alkhayer M, Jenkins PF, Harrison BDW: The outcome of community-acquired pneumonia treated on the intensive care unit. Respir Med 84:13, 1990.

36. Feldman C, Kallenbach JM, Levy H, et al: Community-acquired pneumonia of diverse etiology: Prognostic features in patients admitted to an intensive care unit and "severity of illness score." Intensive Care Med 15:302, 1989.

37. Woodhead MA, MacFarlane JT, Rodgers FG, et al: Aetiology and outcome of severe community-acquired pneumonia. J Infect 10:204, 1985.

38. Zweig S, Lawhorne L, Post R: Factors predicting mortality in rural elderly hospitalized for pneumonia. J Fam Pract 30:153, 1990.

39. Fine MJ, Smith DN, Singer DE: Hospitalization decision in patients with community-acquired pneumonia. A prospective cohort study. Am J Med 89:713, 1990.

40. Van Eeden SF, deBeer P: Community-acquired pneumonia: Evidence of functional inactivation of alpha 1 proteinase inhibitor. Crit Care Med 18:1204, 1990.

40a. Farr BM, Sloman AJ, Fisch MJ: Predicting death in patients hospitalized for community-acquired pneumonia. Ann Intern Med 115:428, 1991.

41. Fried JC, LoPresti JS, Micon M, et al: Serum triodothyroxine values. Prognostic indicator of acute mortality due to *Pneumocystis carinii* pneumonia associated with the acquired immunodeficiency syndrome. Arch Intern Med 150:406, 1990.

42. Chopra IJ, Hershman JM, Pardridge WM, et al: Thyroid function in non-thyroidal illnesses. Ann Intern Med 98:946, 1983.

43. Kaptein EM, Grieb DA, Spencer EM, et al: Thyroxine metabolism in the low thyroxine state of critical non-thyroidal illness. J Clin Endocrinol Metab 53:764, 1981.

44. Chopra IJ, Huang TS, Bereda A et al: Evidence for an inhibitor of extrathyroidal conversion of thyroxine to 3,5,3'-triodothyronine in sera of patients with non-thyroidal illnesses. J Clin Endocrinol Metab 60:666, 1985.

45. Lambert CC, Hunter RL: Low levels of unsaturated transferin as a predictor of survival in pneumococcal pneumonia. Ann Clin Lab Sci 20:140, 1990.

46. Nordenstam G, Andersson B, Briles D, et al: High anti-phosphorylcholine antibody levels and mortality associated with pneumonia. Scan J Infect Dis 22:187, 1990.

47. Pneumonia and influenza mortality—United States, 1988–89 season. MMWR 38:97, 1989.

48. Foy HM, Kenny GE, Cooney MK, et al: Long term epidemiology of infections with *Mycoplasma pneumoniae*. J Infect Dis 139:681, 1979.

49. Fraser DW, Tsai TR, Orenstein W, et al: Legionnaires' disease: Description of an epidemic pneumonia. N Engl J Med 297:1189, 1977.

50. Dondero TJ, Rendtorff RC, Mallison GF, et al: An outbreak of Legionnaires' disease associated with a contaminated air-conditioning cooling tower. N Engl J Med 302:365, 1980.

51. LaMaire W, Jackson H, McFarland L: Legionnaires' disease associated with a grocery store mist machine—Louisiana, 1989. MMWR 39:108, 1990.

52. Muder RR, Yu VL, Fang G-D: Community-acquired legionnaires' disease. Semin Respir Med 4:32, 1989.

53. Mercat A, Nguyen J, Dautzenberg B: An outbreak of pneumococcal pneumonia in two men's shelters. Chest 99:147, 1991.

54. Hoge C, Reichler M, Mastro T, et al: Outbreak of invasive pneumococcal disease in a jail. [Abstract no. 510] Interscience Conference on Antimicrobial Agents and Chemotherapy, Atlanta, GA, October 21–24, 1990: 171. American Society of Microbiologists, Washington, DC, 1990.

55. Hanukoglu A, Hebroni S, Fried D: Pulmonary involvement in *Mycoplasma pneumoniae* infection in families. Infection 14:1, 1986.

56. Marrie TJ, Durant H, Williams JC, et al: Exposure to parturient cats is a risk factor for acquisition of Q fever in maritime Canada. J Infect Dis 158:108, 1988.

57. Dupuis G, Petite J, Peter O, et al: An important outbreak of human Q fever in a Swiss alpine valley. Int J Epidemiol 16:282, 1987.

58. Marrie TJ: Q fever pneumonia. Semin Respir Infect 4:47, 1989.

59. Morris CDW, Nell H: Epidemic of pulmonary tuberculosis in geriatric homes. S Afr Med J 74:117, 1988.

60. Goodwin RA Jr, Des Prez RM: Histoplasmosis. State of the art. Am Rev Respir Dis 117:929, 1978.

61. Ward JI, Weeks M, Allen D, et al: Acute histoplasmosis: Clinical epidemiologic and serological findings of an outbreak associated with exposure to a fallen tree. Am J Med 65:587, 1979.

62. Tosh FE, Hammerman KJ, Weeks RJ, et al: A common source epidemic of North American blastomycosis. Am Rev Respir Dis 109:525, 1974.

63. Sarosi GA, Davies SF: Blastomycosis. State of the art. Am Rev Respir Dis 120:911, 1979.

64. Drutz DJ, Catanzaro A: Coccidiodomycosis. State of the art. Am Rev Respir Dis 117:559;727, 1978.

65. Singal BM, Hedges JR, Radack KL: Decision rules and clinical prediction of pneumonia: Evaluation of low-yield criteria. Ann Emerg Med 18:13, 1989.

66. Heckerling PS, Tape TG, Wigton RS, et al: Clinical prediction rule for pulmonary infiltrates. Ann Intern Med 113:664, 1990.

67. Farr BM, Kaiser DL, Harrison BDW, et al: Prediction of microbial aetiology at admission to hospital for pneumonia from the presenting clinical features. Thorax 44:1031, 1989.

68. Shulman JA, Phillips LA, Petersdorf RG: Errors and hazards in the diagnosis and treatment of bacterial pneumonias. Ann Intern Med 62:41, 1965.

69. Donowitz GR, Mandell GL: Empiric therapy for pneumonia. Rev Infect Dis 5:540, 1983.

70. Murray JF, Felton CP, Garay SW, et al: Pulmonary complications of the acquired immunodeficiency syndrome: Report of a National Heart, Lung, and Blood Institute workshop. N Engl J Med 310:1682, 1984.

71. Mermel LA, Maki DG: Bacterial pneumonia in solid organ transplantation. Semin Respir Infect 5:10, 1990.

72. Amysel NM, Wing EJ: *Legionella* infection in transplant patients. Semin Respir Infect 5:30, 1990.

73. Anderson DJ, Jordon MC: Viral pneumonia in recipients of solid organ transplants. Semin Respir Infect 5:38, 1990.

74. Dummer JA: *Pneumocystis carinii* infections in transplant recipients. Semin Respir Infect 5:50, 1990.

75. Stone WJ, Schaffner W: *Strongyloides* infections in transplant recipients. Semin Respir Infect 5:58, 1990.

76. Sinnott JT IV, Emmanual PJ: Mycobacterial infections in the transplant patient. Semin Respir Infect 5:65, 1990.

77. Chapman SW, Wilson JP: Nocardiosis in transplant recipients. Semin Respir Infect 5:74, 1990.

77a. Mandell LA, Niederman MS, The Canadian Community-acquired Pneumonia Consensus Group: Antimicrobial treatment of community-acquired pneumonia in adults: A conference report. Can J Infect Dis 4:25, 1993.

78. Taylor CR: Diagnostic imaging techniques in the evaluation of drug-induced pulmonary disease. Clin Chest Med 11:87, 1990.

79. Anderson RJ, Potts DE, Gabour PA, et al: Unrecognized adult salicyclate intoxication. Ann Intern Med 85:745, 1976.

80. Heffner JE, Sahn SA: Salicyclate-induced pulmonary disease. Clinical features and prognosis. Ann Intern Med 95:405, 1981.

81. Louria DB, Hensle T, Rose J: The major medical complications of heroin addiction. Ann Intern Med 67:1, 1967.

82. Saba GP, James AE, Johnson BA, et al: Pulmonary complications of narcotic abuse. AJR 122:733, 1974.

83. Cucco RA, Yoo OH, Cregler L, et al: Nonfatal pulmonary edema after "freebase" cocaine smoking. Am Rev Respir Dis 136:179, 1987.

84. Burton WN, Vender J, Shapiro BA: Adult respiratory distress syndrome after Placidyl abuse. Crit Care Med 8:48, 1980.

85. Richman SR, Harris RD: Acute pulmonary edema associated with Librium abuse. Radiology 103:57, 1972.

86. Bogartz LJ, Miller WC: Pulmonary edema associated with propoxyphene intoxication. JAMA 215:259, 1971.

87. O'Donnell AE, Pappas LA: Pulmonary complications of intravenous drug use. Chest 94:251, 1988.

88. Weber JCP, Essigmen WK: Pulmonary alveolitis and NSAID—Fact or fiction? [Letter] Br J Rheumatol 25:5, 1986.

89. Casey KR: Atypical pneumonia and environmental factors. Where have you been and what have you done? Clin Chest Med 12:285, 1991.

90. Winer-Muram T, Rubin SA: Pet-associated lung diseases. J Thorac Imaging 6:6, 1991.

91. Heitzman RE: The radiological diagnosis of pneumonia in the adult: A commentary. Semin Roentgenol 24:212, 1989.

92. Osmer JC, Cole BK: The stethoscope and roentgenogram in acute pneumonia. South Med J 59:75, 1966.

93. Kennedy J, Dawson KP, Abbott GD: Should a lateral chest radiograph be routine in suspected pneumonia? Aust Paediatr J 22:299, 1986.

94. Zylak CJ, Littleton JT, Durizch ML: Illusory consolidation of the left lower lobe: A pitfall of portable radiography. Radiology 167:653, 1988.

95. Friis B, Eiken M, Hornsleth A, et al: Chest x-ray appearances in pneumonia and bronchoilitis. Correlation to virological diagnosis and secretory bacterial findings. Acta Paediatr Scand 79:219, 1990.

96. Courtoy I, Lande AE, Turner RB: Accuracy of radiographic differentiation of bacterial from non-bacterial pneumonia. Clin Pediatr 28:261, 1989.

97. Ponka A, Sarna S: Differential diagnosis of viral, mycoplasmal and bacteremic pneumococcal pneumonia on admission to hospital. Eur J Respir Dis 64:360, 1983.

98. Scanlon GT, Unger JD: The radiology of bacterial and viral pneumonias. Radiol Clin North Am 11:317, 1973.

99. Ziskind MM, Schwarz MI, George RB, et al: Incomplete consolidation in pneumococcal lobar pneumonia complicating pulmonary emphysema. Ann Intern Med 72:835, 1970.

100. Fujita J, Bungo M, Nakamura H, et al: Atypical distribution of bacterial pneumonia after thoracic radiation therapy. AJR 155:1135, 1990.

101. Colligan TG, Light R, Duke K, et al: The effect of volume infusion in canine lobar pneumonia. Am Rev Respir Dis 121:122, 1990.

102. Hall FM, Simon M: Occult pneumonia associated with dehydration: Myth or reality? AJR 148:853, 1987.

103. Jay SJ, Johnson WG Jr, Pierce AK: The radiographic resolution of *Streptococcus pneumoniae* pneumonia. N Engl J Med 293:791, 1975.

104. Mirvis SE, Tobin KD, Kostrubiak I, et al: Thoracic CT in detecting occult disease in critically ill patients. AJR 148:685, 1987.

105. Dans PE, Charache P, Fahey M, et al: Management of pneumonia in the prospective payment era. A need for more clinician and support service interaction. Ann Intern Med 144:1392, 1984.

106. Taryle DA, Potts DE, Sahn SA: The incidence and clinical correlates of parapneumonic efusions in pneumococcal pneumonia. Chest 74:170, 1978.

107. Ort S, Ryan J, Barden G, et al: Pneumococcal pneumonia in hospitalized patients. Clinical and radiological presentations. JAMA 249:214, 1983.

108. Fraser RG, Wortzman G: Acute pneumococcal lobar pneumonia: The significance of non-segmental distribution. J Can Assoc Radiol 10:37, 1959.

109. Rose RW, Ward DH: Spherical pneumonias in children simulating pulmonary and mediastinal masses. Radiology 106:179, 1973.

110. Gordan JD, MacKeen AD, Marrie TJ, et al: The radiographic features of epidemic and sporadic Q fever pneumonia. J Can Assoc Radiol 35:293, 1984.

111. Millar JK: The chest findings in Q fever—a series of thirty-five cases. Clin Radiol 29:317, 1978.

112. Seggev JS, Levin S, Schey G: Unusual radiological manifestations of Q fever. Eur J Respir Dis 69:120, 1986.

113. Janigan DT, Marrie TJ: An inflammatory pseudotumor of the lung in Q fever pneumonia. N Engl J Med 30:86, 1983.

114. Lynch DA, Armstrong JD II: A pattern-oriented approach to chest radiographs in atypical pneumonia syndromes. Clin Chest Med 12:203, 1991.

115. Reed JC: Chest Radiology. Patterns and Differential Diagnosis. Chicago, Year Book Medical Publishers, 1981:107–250.

116. Marrie TJ: Community-acquired pneumonia. Clin North Med Am 4:1064, 1990.

117. Erard PH, Moser F, Wenger A, Saghafi L, Bille J, Francioli P: Prospective study on community-acquired pneumonia diagnosed and followed up by private practitioners. Interscience Conference on Antimicrobial Agents and Chemotherapy, Chicago, IL, September 29 to October 2, 1991. [Abstract no. 56] Washington, DC, American Society of Microbiologists, 1991:108.

# CHAPTER 12

# Nosocomial Pneumonia Outside the Intensive Care Unit

ANTHONY R. DAL NOGARE

Nosocomial pneumonia is a major problem in the United States and other Western countries, as illustrated by data obtained from two large epidemiologic studies. The Study on the Efficacy of Nosocomial Infection Control (SENIC) retrospectively reviewed infections in patients hospitalized at 338 U.S. institutions between 1975 and 1976. Nosocomial pneumonia occurred in 1.1% of patients and was the third most common hospital-acquired infection, after urinary tract and surgical wound infections. The National Nosocomial Infections Study (NNIS) prospectively investigated infections at 58 U.S. hospitals between 1980 and 1982 and found a pneumonia rate of 0.6 per 100 discharges. The lower rate in the NNIS study probably reflects the more rigorous NNIS diagnostic criteria (ie, 85% of the NNIS pneumonias were culture-positive; fewer than 50% of the SENIC cases were) and the exclusion of fatal cases from the NNIS database.[1, 2] Assuming there are about 38 million hospital discharges per year, nosocomial pneumonias affect approximately 300,000 patients annually. Because of the aging American population and the ability of modern medicine to keep severely ill patients alive, it is likely that the prevalence of nosocomial pneumonias will increase.

The morbidity, cost, and mortality of nosocomial pneumonias are high. In 1976, it was estimated that nosocomial pneumonias added an average of 5 hospital days and $1194 (in 1976 dollars) to each affected patient's case.[3] A review of 200 consecutive deaths occurring in one university and one community hospital determined that nosocomial pneumonia directly caused 16% of the deaths.[4] Other investigations have reported nosocomial pneumonia mortality rates between 28% and 37%.[5] Because new antibiotics and other advances in medical care have not appreciably affected mortality, one goal of this chapter is to provide clinicians with the information required to recognize high-risk patients and minimize their risk factors. The primary focus is on aerobic bacterial pneumonias in immunocompetent patients outside of the intensive care unit; about 50% of all nosocomial pneumonias occur in this population.[6] Nosocomial pneumonia in the intensive care unit is discussed in Chapter 13.

## DIAGNOSTIC CRITERIA

The criteria used for establishing a diagnosis of pneumonia vary widely among studies. Because there is no readily available, noninvasive standard test to establish the diagnosis, the specificity of a clinical diagnosis of pneumonia is often questionable.[7] The Centers for Disease Control (CDC) has published a list of criteria for nosocomial pneumonia that are based on the criteria used in the NNIS studies.[8] The CDC diagnostic criteria for nosocomial pneumonia are as follows:

1. Onset of pneumonia more than 72 hours after hospital admission.
2. A physical examination showing rales, dullness to percussion, or an infiltrate on the chest radiograph and one or more of the following:
   A. Purulent sputum
   B. Isolation of a pathogen from blood, transtracheal aspirate, biopsy specimen, or bronchial brushing
   C. Isolation of a virus in respiratory secretions

D. Diagnostic antibody titers for a pathogen

E. Histopathologic evidence of pneumonia

Most of the studies reviewed in this chapter used similar criteria to diagnose nosocomial pneumonia.

## EPIDEMIOLOGY

The SENIC and NNIS investigations found that nosocomial pneumonia occurred primarily in patients hospitalized with medical problems or recovering from abdominal or thoracic surgery; few pneumonias occurred in obstetric, surgical specialty, orthopedic, or pediatric patients. Infection rates were highest in large teaching hospitals: 0.7 per 100 discharges, compared with a rate of 0.36 per 100 for private, nonteaching hospitals. The patient's sex was not a factor, but pneumonia prevalence varied directly with age, increasing from a low of 0.5 cases per 100 patients younger than 35 years of age to 1.5 per 100 for those older than 65 years of age.[1, 2]

## PATHOGENESIS

Pneumonia occurs when microbes are introduced into the lower respiratory tract by one of four routes: aspiration, inhalation, transport by blood, or spread from a contiguous site. Most nosocomial pneumonias occur by aspiration of pathogen-laden oropharyngeal secretions into the lung. Nosocomial pneumonia caused by inhalation of aerosolized gram-negative bacteria (eg, contaminated respiratory therapy equipment) has been described, as have cases of hematogenously acquired *Escherichia coli* pneumonia,[9, 10] but such cases are uncommon. Aspiration of upper respiratory tract secretions occurs even in healthy subjects during sleep, and 70% of subjects with depressed consciousness have been observed to aspirate secretions.[11] Patients at risk for nosocomial pneumonia commonly have some predisposition to aspirate. When a large dose of bacteria enters the normally sterile lower respiratory tract, host defense mechanisms may fail to clear the inoculum, resulting in bacterial proliferation, inflammation, and pneumonia.

An overview of pneumonia pathogenesis is shown on Figure 12–1. If the appropriate host and exogenous factors coexist, pathogenic bacteria can colonize the upper respiratory or gastrointestinal tract. Anaerobic bacteria and streptococcal species compose the normal oral flora but rarely cause nosocomial pneumonia, and the major nosocomial pneumonia pathogens, gram-negative bacteria and *Staphylococcus aureus*, are present in less than 5% of healthy persons' respiratory tracts.[12] Colonization of the respiratory tract by these pathogens is a cardinal event, usually preceding the development of pneumonia and defining patients at high risk for pneumonia.[13]

Hospitals are favorable environments for the growth of gram-negative bacteria and *S. aureus*. Many of the gram-negative bacteria that cause nosocomial pneumonia are colonic flora, and patients commonly become orally colonized with species from their gastrointestinal tracts. In one study of 145 patients, 23% of those receiving no antibiotics and 40% of the patients receiving antibiotics developed oropha-

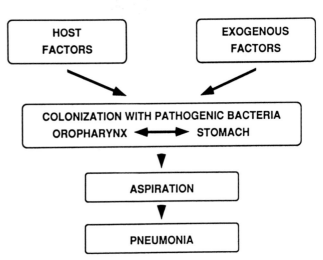

# PATHOGENESIS

**Figure 12–1.** Pathogenesis of nosocomial pneumonia.

ryngeal gram-negative bacterial colonization, almost always with the same species previously isolated from their rectums.[14] How bacteria get to the oropharynx from the perineum is not clear, although transmission by the hands of health care workers is a likely route; by using careful culturing techniques, it has been shown that most medical personnel carry gram-negative bacteria on their hands.[15] Gram-negative bacteria, especially *Pseudomonas aeruginosa*, proliferate in wet areas, which are common in hospitals. Transmission of *S. aureus* occurs when carriers, whose nasopharynxes are colonized with *Staphylococcus*, contact patients.[16]

## RISK FACTORS

The endogenous and exogenous risk factors for colonization and pneumonia are reviewed here, with an emphasis on clinical factors; a discussion of the cellular and biochemical events is presented in the first section of this book. Although risk factors are analyzed separately, it is important to realize that patients commonly present with multiple risk factors. Investigations that associate single risk factors with pneumonia, without using multivariant analysis to determine the effect of other dependent variables, are of questionable significance. For example, if an elderly, debilitated nursing home patient develops a nosocomial infection, it may be difficult to determine the separate roles of debility, age, prior antibiotic administration, the nasogastric feeding tube, and sedative drugs in contributing to the pneumonia.

### Host Risk Factors

Three endogenous factors associated with increased risk are debility, underlying illness, and age. In a sample of 407 persons older than 65 years of age living in institutions, none of whom had received antibiotics in the preceding 4 weeks, the major factor associated with oropharyngeal gram-negative bacterial colonization was debility. Nineteen percent of the patients living independently were colonized, but 37% of the bedridden elderly were colonized. Underlying cardiac, pulmonary, and neoplastic diseases were also associated with colonization but only insofar as they affected the subjects' ability to ambulate and care for themselves.[17] A strong independent association between debility and pneumonia was found in another study, in which deteriorating health status was associated with a 24-fold increased risk of pneumonia for nursing home patients and elderly patients admitted from the community.[18]

One prospective study examined the effect of underlying illnesses in 3315 patients admitted to the medical service of a Veterans Administration hospital. The results of a univariant analysis showed that 1.2% of patients hospitalized with nonfatal conditions, 5.8% of those with ultimately fatal conditions, and 11.6% of patients with rapidly fatal illnesses developed pneumonia.[19] Severity of illness correlates directly with the prevalence of gram-negative bacterial colonization, rising from 2% for hospitalized psychiatric patients to 16% for moderately ill patients and 57% for moribund subjects. The different colonization rates were not explicable in terms of antibiotic use.[12] The presence of one disease, chronic obstructive pulmonary disease (COPD), was independently associated with a 3.7 times greater risk of nosocomial pneumonia.[20]

Demographic surveys indicate that there will be 30 million elderly people in the United States by the year 2000, and it is likely that nosocomial pneumonia in elderly patients will become increasingly common. The diagnosis of pneumonia is difficult in older people, because the usual signs and symptoms are often absent.[21] Multiple epidemiologic studies conducted in the United States and Europe have confirmed that age per se is associated with a two to three times greater risk.[22] In elderly patients, the presence of nasogastric tubes, difficulty in handling secretions, and aspiration of oropharyngeal contents further increase the degree of risk. Nursing home patients constitute a special group because the bacteriology of nursing home-acquired pneumonia closely resembles that of nosocomial pneumonia. In one case-control study of 35 nursing home-acquired pneumonias, 40% of sputum cultures grew *Klebsiella pneumoniae*, compared with 9% of the age-matched controls presenting with community-acquired pneumonia, and 26% grew *S. aureus*, compared with 14% of the control cases. Almost half of the nursing home patients had received antibiotics in the 7 days before admission, and the investigators postulated that antibiotic use explained the high rate of gram-negative and staphylococcal colonization.[23] Another study of 63 nursing home-acquired pneumonias used transtracheal aspiration, bronchoscopy with protected specimen brush, and tracheal suctioning to obtain culture material and found that 49% of the patients had samples that grew gram-negative bacteria and 25% had samples that grew *S. aureus*.[24] These data indicate that nursing home patients are colonized and infected with bacterial species usually associated with nosocomial pneumonias.

## Exogenous Factors

### Surgery

Pneumonia in postoperative patients is common; in the SENIC survey, postoperative pneumonias accounted for 74% of all nosocomial pneumonias,[1] and other investigators have found most pneumonias to be postoperative.[25]

One prospective study of 520 surgical patients determined by univariant analysis that a serum albumin level of less than 3.0 mg/dL, an American Association of Anesthesiologists score of 4, obesity, a history of smoking or COPD, a preoperative stay of more than 7 days, and prolonged (>4 hours) surgery were associated with a significantly increased pneumonia risk. The site of surgery was also important; pneumonia complicated the postoperative course of 40% of thoracotomy patients, 17% of those with upper abdominal surgery, and only 5% of those recovering from lower abdominal operations.[26] The SENIC study also found a risk gradient by surgical site; the risk of pneumonia was 14 times greater after thoracic surgery, 7 times greater after upper abdominal operations, and 1.6 times greater after lower abdominal procedures.[1] The high risk of thoracic surgery may not apply to patients undergoing coronary artery bypass surgery; a review of 498 cases found only 3.8% developed pneumonia.[27]

### Antibiotic Use

Many antibiotics, especially those of the penicillin group, affect the normal oral and bowel flora. Streptococcal species in normal mouth flora release bacteriocins that inhibit the growth of gram-negative bacteria. Sprunt and Redman showed that patients treated with large doses of penicillin had decreased numbers of oral gram-positive bacteria and developed oral gram-negative bacterial colonization. After penicillin administration was stopped, the number of gram-positive bacteria returned to normal, and the gram-negative bacteria disappeared.[28] Although some investigators have found that antibiotic administration increases the prevalence of gram-negative bacterial colonization,[14] others have not found such an association.[12] Two investigations documented frequent oral gram-negative colonization during antibiotic therapy of community-acquired pneumonia. A review of 149 consecutive patients admitted with pneumonia found that 59% became colonized with gram-negative bacteria or *S. aureus*. Twelve percent developed nosocomial pneumonia, usually from the same pathogen with which they were colonized.[29] A study of 245 community-acquired pneumonias found that 24% developed gram-negative colonization.[30] These data indicate that, although colonization and nosocomial pneumonia may occur without prior antibiotic exposure, antibiotics can facilitate colonization in some patients. Antibiotics that are active against oral streptococci and bowel anaerobes may be especially effective in promoting colonization.

### Respiratory Therapy Equipment

The reservoir nebulizers used for aerosolized drug delivery provide a favorable environment for the growth of gram-negative bacteria, especially *P. aeruginosa*, and are capable of aerosolizing bacteria and sending them deep into the lungs. Outbreaks of gram-negative pneumonia have been associated with contaminated nebulizers.[9, 10] However, the widespread use of effective sterilization procedures has made nebulizers uncommon vectors for pneumonia.

### Nasogastric Tubes, Antacids, and Enteral Alimentation

Nasogastric tubes, antacids, and enteral alimentation are considered together because they commonly act in concert to promote gastric colonization. Normal subjects rarely have gastric gram-negative bacteria, maintain a fasting gastric pH of less than 3.0, and are able to rapidly clear any ingested bacteria.[31] Achlorhydric persons have large numbers of gastric gram-negative bacteria.[32] Antacids and $H_2$-blockers are commonly given to hospitalized patients as prophylaxis against stress ulcers and are usually titrated to maintain a gastric pH greater than 4.0.[33] Coincident with the widespread use of stress ulcer prophylaxis during the past 20 years, gastric gram-negative bacterial colonization has become recognized as a serious problem. Large numbers ($10^6$–$10^8$ CFU/mL) of aerobic gram-negative bacteria exist in the stomachs of iatrogenically achlorhydric patients, and the same gram-negative species in the stomach are often isolated from the oropharynx and trachea.[34] Studies using serial cultures have shown that initial gastric colonization is frequently (22%–36%) followed by the appearance of the same bacterial species in the respiratory tract, raising the possibility that patients' stomachs act as reservoirs for airway colonization.[35] Sucralfate is a cytoprotective agent that does not affect gastric pH and, when compared with antacid therapy, sucralfate use was associated with significantly less gastric, oral, and tracheal gram-negative colonization and fewer episodes of nosocomial pneumonia.[36] Nasogastric tubes, commonly used to administer antacids and enteral feedings, disrupt the lower esophageal sphincter and may facilitate movement of gastric contents to the respiratory tract.[37] Enteral feeding solutions have a neutral pH of 6.4 to 7.0 and have been implicated as a factor promoting gram-negative gastric and airway colonization.[38, 39]

### Hospital Environment

The hospital milieu is favorable for propagating gram-negative bacteria and *S. aureus*. Pneumonia outbreaks caused by other, more unusual microbes have been associated with the hospital environment. Nosocomial *Legionella* pneumonia has been attributed to contaminated hospital water supplies.[40] Outbreaks of nosocomial *Aspergillus fumigatus* and *Histoplasma capsulatum* pneumonia have been associated with construction work at or near hospitals.[41] The influenza A virus is spread person to person by coughing, and the spread of aerosolized virus is enhanced by crowded hospital wards. Nosocomial outbreaks of influenza A, during which the virus was spread between patients and hospital personnel, have been described.[42]

## BACTERIOLOGY

Accurate identification of the microbes causing a nosocomial pneumonia may be difficult. The same bacteria that cause nosocomial pneumonia also commonly colonize the airways, and samples obtained through the airways, such as expectorated sputum, transtracheal aspirates, or bronchoscopically obtained samples, may be contaminated by airway flora. Few investigations reporting bacteriologic data have included a "gold standard" test, such as open or needle biopsy of the involved lung, to confirm the results

of sputum cultures. A positive blood culture is usually taken as evidence that the blood isolate caused the pneumonia, but only 5% of all nosocomial pneumonias have positive blood cultures, and it is uncertain whether this small number of bacteremic patients is representative of most patients with nonbacteremic pneumonias.[43] Expectorated sputum or transtracheal aspirates frequently grow two or more potential pathogens, and choosing one as the causal organism may be somewhat arbitrary. All of these caveats must be kept in mind when interpreting microbiologic results.

Bacteriologic data from three large nosocomial pneumonia studies are shown on Table 12–1. In the NNIS study most bacteria were identified by sputum culture and 85% of all pneumonias had a pathogen isolated (ie, 65% grew a single pathogen; 20% grew more than one). The predominant isolates were aerobic gram-negative organisms from the Enterobacteriaceae group, followed by *P. aeruginosa* and *S. aureus*. Samples from few patients grew *Streptococcus pneumoniae*, and the number of anaerobic and viral isolates was small, which is not surprising because anaerobic and viral cultures were not routinely done. Culture material in the Bartlett study[44] was obtained mainly (80%) from transtracheal aspirates, with the remainder from blood and pleural fluid samples. Fifty-four percent of the samples grew more than one pathogen. Anaerobic cultures were routinely done, and anaerobes were grown from 35%, although most of the anaerobe-containing specimens also grew aerobic bacteria.[44]

The study by Bryan and colleagues[45] reported data from 168 bacteremic nosocomial pneumonias, and the predominant species (aerobic gram-negative bacteria and *S. aureus*) isolated by blood culture were similar to those isolated from sputum or transtracheal aspirates in the NNIS and Bartlett studies. In the Bryan study, there were 202 potential pathogens isolated from sputum, and in only 51% of cases was the blood culture isolated also grown from sputum. In fully half of the cases, the bacteria species in the bloodstream could not have been predicted from sputum culture. Polymicrobial bacteremic pneumonia, usually involving *S. aureus*, *P. aeruginosa*, or *K. pneumoniae*, occurred in 12%, suggesting that nosocomial pneumonia may be caused by more than one pathogen.[45]

**Table 12–1. Bacteriologic Findings From Three Nosocomial Pneumonia Studies**

| Feature Assessed | Study | | |
| --- | --- | --- | --- |
| | NNIS[2] | Bartlett et al.[44] | Bryan and Reynolds[45] |
| Culture material | Sputum | TTA* | Blood |
| *Pseudomonas aeruginosa* | 17% | 9 | 15 |
| *Staphylococcus aureus* | 13 | 26 | 27 |
| Enterobacteriaceae† | 37 | 48 | 42 |
| Fungi | 6 | ND‡ | ND |
| Anaerobic bacteria | 2 | 35 | 2 |
| *Streptococcus pneumoniae* | <3 | 31 | 12 |
| *Haemophilus influenzae* | <3 | 17 | <4 |
| Viruses | <3 | ND | ND |

*TTA, transtracheal aspirate.
†Includes *Klebsiella pneumoniae*, *Enterobacter* species, *Escherichia coli*, *Serratia*, and proteins.
‡ND, not done.

Table 12–2. **Unusual Causes of Nosocomial Pneumonia**

Viruses, especially influenza A
*Haemophilus influenzae*
*Legionella* species
*Chlamydia* strain TWAR
*Branhamella catarrhalis*

In summary, sputum from nosocomial pneumonia patients usually grows aerobic gram-negative bacteria or *S. aureus*, and the same species are isolated from blood samples. Sputum and transtracheal aspirates often grow multiple pathogens, which may differ from the bacteria species isolated from blood, and in many patients, bacteria cultured from sputum may not identify bacteria infecting the lung.

## UNUSUAL PATHOGENS

Uncommon causes of nosocomial pneumonia are listed in Table 12–2. The exact prevalence of viral nosocomial pneumonia is difficult to discern, because few epidemiologic studies have used appropriate culture and serologic techniques to detect viral disease. It is thought that viruses rarely cause pneumonia in immunocompetent adults. A 2-year study in one hospital, in which comprehensive viral cultures and serologies were performed, revealed that 10% of all adult nosocomial pneumonias were caused by viruses; influenza A virus, parainfluenza virus, and adenovirus were common isolates.[46] Nosocomial outbreaks of influenza A virus pneumonia have been well documented, usually in the fall and winter of pandemic years. Attack rates for patients and hospital staff of 48% have been reported, with severe pneumonias occurring mainly in patients with rheumatic heart disease.[42]

Nontypable *Haemophilus influenzae* strains commonly colonize the airway of COPD patients. One review of 100 consecutive *H. influenzae* sputum cultures revealed 25 pneumonias attributed to *H. influenzae*. Pneumonia occurred almost exclusively (90%) in males, 40% of whom had COPD. In 30% of the cases, the *Haemophilus* pneumonia was nosocomial.[47] *H. influenzae* always should be considered when COPD patients develop nosocomial pneumonia.

The largest described outbreak of nosocomial *Legionella* pneumonia occurred at the Wadsworth Veterans Administration Hospital. Sixty-five cases, all confirmed by antibody tests or culture, were observed over a 19-month period. Ninety-four percent of the patients had one of the known risk factors for *Legionella* infection, such as immunosuppression or cardiac, pulmonary, malignant, or renal disease. The clinical presentation of high fever with relative bradycardia, scant sputum, chest radiographic progression from a patchy infiltrate to lobar consolidation, and rapid response to erythromycin was typical for *Legionella* pneumonia.[40] Another cluster of 16 cases, 65% of whom had received kidney transplants, has been described.[48]

A novel *Chlamydia* species known as *Chlamydia* TWAR was originally described as causing community-acquired pneumonia. A retrospective study of serum from 198 pneumonia patients from two Seattle hospitals found 20 serologically confirmed cases of TWAR pneumonia. Forty-five

percent of the TWAR pneumonias were nosocomial, and the patients recovered without specific antibiotic therapy effective against TWAR.[49]

*Branhamella catarrhalis* colonizes the airways of COPD patients and may cause pneumonia. Two small series of nosocomial *B. catarrhalis* pneumonia have been described. In both, COPD and postoperative patients were primarily affected.[50, 51]

## APPROACH TO THE PATIENT WITH NOSOCOMIAL PNEUMONIA

### Prevention

Because of the high mortality of nosocomial pneumonia, clinicians caring for hospitalized patients should attempt to reduce the controllable risk factors (Table 12–3). Influenza A and pneumococcal vaccines are of proven efficacy in immunocompetent patients and should be given before hospitalization, especially to elderly patients with chronic disease.[52] Spread of bacteria between patients can be prevented if consistent hand-washing practices are followed by medical personnel. The institution of careful hand-washing practices with antiseptic soap solutions has been associated with fewer nosocomial pneumonias.[15] Unfortunately, few health care personnel routinely wash their hands after patient contact.[53] Careful disinfection practices reduce the risk of aerosol transmission of bacteria by respiratory therapy equipment.[10] To avoid aspiration, physicians should assess patients' ability to swallow; this can be done at the bedside and is especially important for patients with neuromuscular disorders (eg, myasthenia gravis, polymyositis, Guillain-Barré syndrome), elderly patients with multiple strokes, and patients with depressed or fluctuating consciousness. Sedative drugs should be given judiciously, nasogastric tubes should be removed whenever possible, and enteral feedings should be started cautiously to avoid gastric distention and massive aspiration of gastric bacteria. Because they decrease normal oral and bowel flora and may contribute to colonization by pathogenic bacteria, antibiotics should be used sparingly and for clearly defined indications. If prophylactic therapy for acid-induced gastric bleeding is indicated, a cytoprotective agent such as sucralfate, which does not raise gastric pH, should be used in lieu of antacids or $H_2$-blockers. Patients undergoing elective upper abdominal or thoracic surgery should be told to stop smoking at least 2 weeks before surgery and should be informed of the importance of postoperative incentive spirometry and coughing, measures which may decrease the risk of pulmonary complications and pneumonia.[54]

Table 12–3. **Measures to Prevent Nosocomial Pneumonia**

Vaccination
Prevent transmission of pathogens
Avoid aspiration
Avoid unnecessary antibiotic use
Maintain gastric acidity
Preoperative and postoperative respiratory care

## Diagnosis

The usual constellation of symptoms, signs, and laboratory abnormalities that are useful for diagnosing community-acquired pneumonia may be less helpful for diagnosing nosocomial pneumonia. Not uncommonly, the patient's underlying condition obscures the diagnosis. For example, sedation or an altered mental status affect symptoms. Fever, chest pain, or shortness of breath may be wrongly attributed to the patient's primary illness. Weak, debilitated patients are often unable to expectorate sputum samples for examination. Diagnosis may be extremely difficult in elderly patients, in whom an altered mental status may be the only clue.[21] There are no particular symptoms, signs, or laboratory abnormalities that allow the physician to confidently diagnose a specific bacterial pathogen, although the combination of a high (>103°F) fever and a relative bradycardia is said to be characteristic of *Legionella* pneumonia.[40]

Pneumonia is indicated by an infiltrate on the chest radiograph. A minimum requirement for a pneumonia diagnosis is a chest radiographic infiltrate, which is usually a focal, patchy bronchopneumonia pattern or a dense lobar infiltrate caused by lobar consolidation. The pattern of the radiographic infiltrate is not specific for particular microbes. Many noninfectious conditions commonly affect hospitalized patients and cause roentgenographic infiltrates; these include atelectasis, aspiration of gastric contents, and pulmonary emboli. The possibility of a noninfectious process should always be considered in the differential diagnosis of nosocomial pneumonia, and a list of these conditions is given in Table 12–4.

The difficulty in diagnosing nosocomial pneumonia was highlighted by a prospective study of 24 patients with acute respiratory distress syndrome, all of whom died and had autopsies. Fever, an abnormal leukocyte count, pathogens cultured from sputum, and asymmetric chest radiographic infiltrates were found as often in those with pneumonia as in those without it.[55] Pneumonia was correctly diagnosed

Table 12–4. **Noninfectious Conditions Causing Focal Infiltrate in Hospitalized Patients**

Underlying diseases
  Cancer
    Lymphagitic spread
    Tumor emboli
    Lymphomas, leukemia
  Connective tissue diseases
  Vasculitis syndromes
  Alveolar hemorrhage
    Thrombocytopenia
    Goodpasture syndrome
    Rapidly progressive glomerulonephritis
    Mitral stenosis
  Sarcoidosis
Iatrogenic conditions
  Drug-induced pneumonitis
  Misplaced feeding tube
  Swan-Ganz catheters
    Pulmonary artery rupture
    Pulmonary infarction
Other causes
  Atelectasis
  Thromboembolic disease
  Aspiration of sterile gastric contents

ante mortem in only 64% of the patients. Clinicians should be alert to the possibility of nosocomial pneumonia in at-risk patients, and deterioration in a patient's condition should prompt the physician to consider pneumonia.

Because clinical findings and routine laboratory tests rarely suggest specific bacteria, blood and sputum frequently are sent for culture. Isolation of a pathogen from blood is considered proof that the blood isolate is causing pneumonia, but most patients have negative results for blood cultures. Sputum sent for culture should be screened by microscopy, and a grossly purulent area of sputum should be selected for Gram staining. Microscopic sputum examination serves two purposes. If the specimen contains more than 10 squamous epithelial cells per low-power field, it is not an adequate sample of the lower respiratory tract, and culture of samples yields only multiple species of oral bacteria. Conversely, culture of sputum containing fewer than 10 squamous cells and more than 25 leukocytes per low-power field usually reveals the same bacterial species as those isolated from the lower respiratory tract by transtracheal aspiration.[56, 57] Because more than one potential pathogen commonly is isolated from sputum culture, sputum cultures have low specificity. Five investigations correlated sputum culture bacteriology with results obtained by more definitive tests. In three studies, one of the bacterial species in sputum also occurred in blood, lung biopsy, or pleural fluid culture, suggesting that sputum usually grows the bacteria causing pneumonia.[58–60] Bryan and colleagues reported that bacteria isolated by blood culture were not found in 51% of sputum cultures obtained from the same patients.[45] Similar results were reported by Barrett-Connor for bacteremic pneumococcal pneumonia.[61] Although the latter results are disturbing, it is not clear whether the sputum samples in these two studies were screened before culture; the lack of screening might explain the low sensitivity. Most of the available evidence suggests that culture of an adequate sputum specimen usually grows the bacterial species in the lung.

Examination of a Gram-stained sputum specimen is a simple and rapid way to make an etiologic diagnosis, days before culture results are available. Finding more than 10 gram-positive diplococci per high-power field in areas with many leukocytes is highly specific, although only 55% sensitive, for the presence of *S. pneumoniae* on culture.[62] Similarly, finding large numbers of small gram-negative rods (eg, *H. influenzae*), large gram-positive cocci in clusters (eg, *S. aureus*), or small gram-negative cocci (eg, *B. catarrhalis*) may allow a presumptive diagnosis and appropriate therapy as early as possible.

In addition to routine sputum, blood, and pleural fluid cultures, there are other methods for obtaining culture material. Transtracheal aspiration can be performed with minimal morbidity but has not been widely used and suffers from the same low specificity as sputum culture.[57, 63] Transthoracic needle biopsy, with passage of the needle directly into the area of pneumonia, has been reported to be highly sensitive and specific for diagnosing nosocomial bacterial pneumonia but is also associated with an appreciable risk of pneumothorax or hemoptysis.[64, 65] A protected specimen brush catheter, inserted through the biopsy channel of a bronchoscope, can be used to obtain uncontaminated specimens from the lower respiratory tract with minimal morbidity. The brush is used to obtain quantitative cultures, with a cutoff of $10^3$ to $10^4$ CFU/mL commonly used to discriminate between contaminating and infecting bacteria. The protected specimen brush has been widely used to diagnose pneumonia in intubated, mechanically ventilated patients, and a wide range of sensitivity and specificity ratings have been reported.[66-70]

Winterbauer used protected specimen brush to diagnose 33 episodes of nosocomial pneumonia in 31 patients, most of whom were not intubated and were not receiving antibiotics at the time of bronchoscopy. Protected brush cultures from 29 to 33 episodes grew more than 4000 CFU/mL of at least one pathogenic bacterial species, but none of the 60 control specimens grew more than 4000 CFU/mL bacteria, giving a sensitivity and specificity of 88% and 100%.[71] However, the diagnosis of pneumonia was made clinically, and only 5 patients had positive pleural fluid, blood, or autopsy cultures to substantiate the protected brush results. Many nosocomial pneumonia patients are already receiving antibiotics, and prior antibiotic administration markedly diminishes the sensitivity of the protected brush.[72]

## Therapy

Rapid administration of antibiotics is important, because many nosocomial pathogens cause rapidly progressive, necrotizing pneumonias. Initial empiric antibiotic regimens are usually chosen to cover the major pathogens—*S. aureus*, Enterobacteriaceae, and *P. aeruginosa*. A second- or third-generation cephalosporin and an aminoglycoside are appropriate initial therapy, especially if *Pseudomonas* pneumonia is a concern; animal models and in vitro studies have shown that β-lactam and aminoglycoside combinations are synergistic against *P. aeruginosa*.[73] Attention should be given to the aminoglycoside dose, as reflected by the peak (1 hour after infusion) aminoglycoside plasma level. One analysis of four series of gram-negative pneumonia cases found that significantly more patients with peak gentamicin and tobramycin levels of 7 μg/mL or more (ie, amikacin levels ≥ 28 μg/mL) had a successful outcome, as judged by survival or resolution of the pneumonia.[74]

Other factors to consider in choosing antibiotics are the local antibiotic resistance profiles of nosocomial pathogens and any unique patient characteristics that may be associated with certain infections. For example, vancomycin should be used instead of a cephalosporin if methicillin-resistant *S. aureus* are common; nosocomial pneumonia in a COPD patient should include drugs active against *H. influenzae*; and erythromycin may be added when treating a patient with risk factors for *Legionella* pneumonia in a hospital where the organism is endemic.

Because of the cost and nephrotoxicity of combined β-lactam and aminoglycoside therapy, several trials have been performed to evaluate monotherapy for nosocomial pneumonia.[75-77] The design of these studies has been poor, and it is difficult to make any firm conclusions from them. Most of the antibiotics used so far in monotherapy trials are not effective in vitro against all of the likely pathogens, especially *S. aureus* and *P. aeruginosa*. A new fluroquinolone compound, ciprofloxacin, is active in vitro against virtually all of the common nosocomial pneumonia pathogens and can be given intravenously. One study reported that 91% of ciprofloxacin-treated nosocomial pneumonias were cured, but some ciprofloxacin-treated patients were excluded from final analysis.[78] Additional clinical trials of monotherapy regimens will be required before they can be recommended for widespread use.

## REFERENCES

1. Haley RW, Hooton TM, Culver DH, Stanley RC, Emori TG: Nosocomial infections in U.S. hospitals, 1975–1976. Am J Med 70:947–959, 1981.
2. Hughes JM, Culver DH, White JW, Jarvis WR, Munn VP, Mosser JL, Emori TG: Nosocomial infection surveillance, 1980–1982. MMWR 32(4SS):1SS–15SS, 1983.
3. Haley RW, Schaberg HR, Crossley R, Allmen DV, McGowan E Jr: Extra charges and prolongation of stay attributable to nosocomial infections: A prospective interhospital comparison. Am J Med 70:51–57, 1981.
4. Gross PA, Neu HC, Aswapokee P, Antwerpen CV, Aswapokee N: Death from nosocomial infections: Experience in a university hospital and a community hospital. Am J Med 68:219–223, 1980.
5. Wenzel RP: Hospital-acquired pneumonia: Overview of the current state of the art for prevention and control. J Clin Microbiol Infect Dis 8:56–60, 1989.
6. Leu H, Kaiser DL, Mori M, Woolson RF, Wenzel RP: Hospital-acquired pneumonia. Am J Epidemiol 129:1258–1267, 1989.
7. Toews GB: Nosocomial pneumonia. Clin Chest Med 8:467–479, 1987.
8. Centers for Disease Control: CDC definitions for nosocomial infections, 1988. Am Rev Respir Dis 139:1058–1059, 1989.
9. Pierce AK, Edmonson EB, McGee G, Ketchersid J, Loudon RG, Sanford JP: An analysis of factors predisposing to gram-negative bacillary necrotizing pneumonia. Am Rev Respir Dis 94:309–313, 1966.
10. Pierce AK, Sanford JP, Thomas GD, Leonard JS: Long-term evaluation of decontamination of inhalation-therapy equipment and the occurrence of necrotizing pneumonia. N Engl J Med 282:528–531, 1970.
11. Huxley EJ, Viroslav J, Gray WR: Pharyngeal aspiration in normal adults and patients with suppressed consciousness. Am J Med 64:564–568, 1978.
12. Johanson WG, Pierce AK, Sanford JP: Changing pharyngeal bacterial flora of hospitalized patients. N Engl J Med 281:1137–1140, 1969.
13. Johanson WG, Pierce AK, Sanford JP, Thomas GD: Nosocomial respiratory infections with gram-negative bacilli. Ann Intern Med 77:701–706, 1972.
14. LeFrock JL, Ellis CA, Weinstein L: The relation between aerobic fecal and oropharyngeal microflora in hospitalized patients. Am J Med Sci 277:275–280, 1979.
15. Maki DG: Control of colonization and transmission of pathogenic bacteria in the hospital. Ann Intern Med 89:777–780, 1978.
16. Kaslow RA, Dixon RE, Martin SM, et al: Staphylococcal disease related to hospital nursery bathing practices—A nationwide epidemiologic investigation. Pediatrics 51:414–425, 1973.
17. Valenti WM, Trudell RG, Bentley DW: Factors predisposing to oropharyngeal colonization with gram-negative bacilli in the aged. N Engl J Med 298:1108–1111, 1978.
18. Harakness GA, Bentley DW, Roghmann KJ: Risk factors for nosocomial pneumonia in the elderly. Am J Med 89:457–463, 1990.
19. Britt MR, Schleupner CJ, Matsumiya S: Severity of underlying disease as a predictor of nosocomial infection. JAMA 239:1047–1051, 1978.
20. Celis R, Torres A, Gatell JM, Almela M, Rodriquez-Roisin R, Agusti-Vidal A: Nosocomial pneumonia: A multivariate analysis of risk and prognosis. Chest 93:318–324, 1988.
21. Verghese A, Berk SL: Bacterial pneumonia in the elderly. Medicine (Baltimore) 62:272–282, 1983.
22. Craven DE, Steger KA, Montecalvo MA: Nosocomial pneumonia in the 1990s: Update of epidemiology and risk factors. Semin Respir Infect 5:157–172, 1990.
23. Gary JL, Brown RB, Garb JR, Tuthill RW: Differences in etiology of

pneumonias in nursing home and community patients. JAMA 240:2169–2172, 1978.

24. Crossley KB, Thurn JR: Nursing home-acquired pneumonia. Semin Respir Infect 4:64–72, 1989.

25. Eickhoff TC: Pulmonary infections in surgical patients. Surg Clin North Am 60:175–183, 1980.

26. Garibaldi RA, Britt MR, Coleman ML, Reading JC, Pace NL: Risk factors for postoperative pneumonia. Am J Med 70:677–680, 1981.

27. Gaynes R, Bizek B, Mowry-Hanley J, Kirsh M: Risk factors for nosocomial pneumonia after coronary artery bypass graft operations. Ann Thorac Surg 52:215–218, 1991.

28. Sprunt K, Redman W: Evidence suggesting the importance of bacterial inhibition in maintaining the balance of normal flora. Ann Intern Med 68:579–590, 1968.

29. Tillotson JR, Finland M: Bacterial colonization and clinical superinfection of the respiratory tract complicating antibiotic treatment of pneumonia. J Infect Dis 119:597–624, 1969.

30. Ortqvist A, Hammers-Berggren S, Kalin M: Respiratory tract colonization and incidence of secondary infection during hospital treatment of community-acquired pneumonia. Eur J Clin Microbiol Infect Dis 9:725–731, 1990.

31. Franklin MA, Skoryna SC: Studies on natural gastric flora. Can Med Assoc J 95:1349–1355, 1966.

32. Drasar BS, Shiner M, McLeod GM: Studies on the intestinal flora. Gastroenterology 56:71–79, 1969.

33. Tryba M, Zevounou F, Torok M, Zenz M: Prevention of acute stress bleeding with sucralfate, antacids, or cimetidine. Am J Med 79:55–61, 1985.

34. DuMoulin GC, Paterson DG, Hedley-Whyte J, and Lisbon A: Aspiration of gastric bacteria in antacid-treated patients: A frequent cause of postoperative colonization of the airway. Lancet 1:242–245, 1982.

35. Atherton ST, White DJ: Stomach as the source of bacteria colonizing respiratory tract during artificial ventilation. Lancet 2:968–969, 1978.

36. Driks MR, Craven DE, Celli BR, et al: Nosocomial pneumonia in intubated patients given sucralfate as compared with antacids or histamine type 2 blockers. N Engl J Med 317:1376–1382, 1987.

37. Olivares L, Segovia A, Revuelta R: Tube feeding and lethal aspiration in neurological patients: A review of 720 autopsy cases. Stroke 5:654–657, 1974.

38. Pingleton, SK: Enteral nutrition as a risk factor for nosocomial pneumonia. [Editorial]. Eur J Clin Microbiol Infect Dis 8:51–55, 1989.

39. Pingleton SK, Hinthorn DR, Liu C: Enteral nutrition in patients receiving mechanical ventilation. Am J Med 80:827–831, 1986.

40. Kirby BD, Snyder KM, Meyer RD, Finegold SM: Legionnaires' disease: Report of sixty-five nosocomially acquired cases and review of the literature. Medicine (Baltimore) 59:188–204, 1980.

41. Arnow PM, Anderson RL, Mainous PD, Smith EJ: Pulmonary aspergillosis during hospital renovation. Am Rev Respir Dis 118:49–53, 1978.

42. Blumenfeld HL, Kilbourne ED, Louria DB, Rogers DE: Studies on influenza in the pandemic of 1957–1958. J Clin Invest 38:199–212, 1959.

43. Centers for Disease Control: Nosocomial infection surveillance 1984. MMWR CDC Surveill Summ 35:17SS–29SS, 1986.

44. Bartlett JG, O'Keefe P, Tally FP, Louis TJ, Gorbach SL: Bacteriology of hospital-acquired pneumonia. Arch Intern Med 146:868–871, 1986.

45. Bryan CS, Reynolds KL: Bacteremic nosocomial pneumonia. Am Rev Respir Dis 129:668–671, 1984.

46. Valenti WM, Hall CB, Douglas RG Jr, Menegus MA, Pincus PH: Nosocomial viral infections. Infect Control Hosp Epidemiol 1:33–37, 1979.

47. Simon HB, Southwick FS, Moellering RC Jr, Sherman E: *Hemophilus influenzae* in hospitalized adults: Current perspective. Am J Med 69:219–226, 1980.

48. Doebbeling BN, Ishak MA, Wade BH, et al: Nosocomial *Legionella micdadei* pneumonia: 10 years' experience and a case-control study. J Hosp Infect 13:289–298, 1989.

49. Grayston JT, Diwan VK, Cooney M, Wang S: Community and hospital-acquired pneumonia associated with *Chlamydia* TWAR infection demonstrated serologically. Arch Intern Med 149:169–173, 1989.

50. Choo PW, Gantz NW: *Branhamella catarrhalis* pneumonia with bacteremia. South Med J 82:1317–1318, 1989.

51. Patterson TF, Patterson JE, Masecar BL, Barden GE, Hierholzer WJ Jr, Zervos MJ: A nosocomial outbreak of *Branhamella catarrhalis* confirmed by restriction endonuclease analysis. J Infect Dis 157:996–1001, 1988.

52. Shapiro ED, Berg AT, Austrian R, et al: The protective efficacy of polyvalent pneumococcal polysaccharide vaccine. N Engl J Med 325:1453–1460, 1991.

53. Albert RK, Condie F: Hand-washing patterns in medical intensive-care units. N Engl J Med 304:1465–1466, 1981.

54. Garibaldi RA: Postoperative pneumonia and urinary-tract infection: Epidemiology and prevention. J Hosp Infect 11:265–272, 1988.

55. Andrews CP, Coalson JJ, Smith JD, Johanson WG Jr: Diagnosis of nosocomial bacterial pneumonia in acute, diffuse lung injury. Chest 80:254–258, 1981.

56. Geckler RW, Gremillion DH, McAllister CK, Ellenbogen C: Microscopic and bacteriological comparison of paired sputa and transtracheal aspirates. J Clin Microbiol 6:396–399, 1977.

57. Murray PR, Washington JA II: Microscopic and bacteriologic analysis of expectorated sputum. Mayo Clin Proc 50:339–344, 1975.

58. Guckian JD, Christensen WD: Quantitative culture and gram stain of sputum. Am Rev Respir Dis 118:997–1005, 1978.

59. Thorsteinsson DB, Musher DM, Fagan I: The diagnostic value of sputum culture in acute pneumonia. JAMA 233:894–895, 1975.

60. Tempest B, Morgan R: The value of respiratory tract bacteriology in pneumococcal pneumonia among Navajo Indians. Am Rev Respir Dis 109:577–578, 1974.

61. Barrett-Connor E: The nonvalue of sputum culture in the diagnosis of pneumococcal pneumonia. Am Rev Respir Dis 103:845–848, 1971.

62. Rein MF, Gwaltney JM Jr, O'Brien WM, Jennings RH, Mandell GL: Accuracy of Gram stain in identifying pneumococci in sputum. JAMA 239:2671–2673, 1978.

63. Barlett JG: Diagnostic accuracy of transtracheal aspiration bacteriologic studies. Am Rev Respir Dis 115:777–782, 1977.

64. Zavala DC, Schoell JE: Ultrathin needle aspiration of the lung in infectious and malignant disease. Am Rev Respir Dis 123:125–131, 1980.

65. Palmer DL, Davidson M, Lusk R: Needle aspiration of the lung in complex pneumonias. Chest 78:16–21, 1980.

66. Villers D, Derriennic M, Raffi F, Germaud P, Baron D, Nicolas F, Courtieu AL: Reliability of the bronchoscopic protected catheter brush in intubated and ventilated patients. Chest 88:527–530, 1985.

67. Torres A, De la Bellacasa JP, Xaubet A, Gonzalez J, Rodriguez-Roisin R, Jimenez de Anta MI, Vidal AG: Diagnostic value of quantitative cultures of bronchoalveolar lavage and telescoping plugged catheters in mechanically ventilated patients with bacterial pneumonia. Am Rev Respir Dis 140:306–310, 1989.

68. Fagon J, Chastre J, Domart Y, Trouillet J, Pierre J, Darne C, Gilbert C: Nosocomial pneumonia in patients receiving continuous mechanical ventilation. Am Rev Respir Dis 139:877–884, 1989.

69. Fagon J, Chastre J, Hance AJ, Guiguet M, Trouillet J, Domart Y, Pierre J, Gilbert C: Detection of nosocomial lung infection in ventilated patients. Am Rev Respir Dis 138:110–116, 1988.

70. Chastre J, Francois V, Brun P, et al: Prospective evaluation of the protected specimen brush for the diagnosis of pulmonary infections in ventilated patients. Am Rev Respir Dis 130:924–929, 1984.

71. Winterbauer RH, Hutchinson JF, Reinhardt GN, et al: The use of quantitative cultures and antibody coating of bacteria to diagnose bacterial pneumonia by fiberoptic bronchoscopy. Am Rev Respir Dis 128:98–103, 1983.

72. Johanson WG Jr, Seidenfeld JJ, De Los Santos R, Coalson JJ, Gomez P: Prevention of nosocomial pneumonia using topical and parenteral antimicrobial agents. Am Rev Respir Dis 137:265–272, 1988.

73. Pennington JE: New therapeutic approaches to hospital-acquired pneumonia. Semin Respir Infect 2:67–73, 1987.

74. Moore RD, Smith C, Lietman P: Association of aminoglycoside plasma levels with therapeutic outcome in gram-negative pneumonia. Am J Med 77:657–662, 1984.

75. Cook JL: Gram-negative bacillary pneumonia in the nosocomial setting. Am J Med 88:34S–43S, 1990.

76. Smith CR, Ambinder R, Lipsky JJ, et al: Cefotaxime compared with nafcillin plus tobramycin for serious bacterial infections. Ann Intern Med 101:469–477, 1984.

77. Mangi RJ, Greco T, Ryan J, Thornton G, Andriole VT: Cefoperazone versus combination antibiotic therapy of hospital-acquired pneumonia. Am J Med 84:68–74, 1988.

78. Khan FA, Basir R: Sequential intravenous-oral administration of ciprofloxacin vs ceftazidime in serious bacterial respiratory tract infections. Chest 96:528–537, 1989.

# CHAPTER 13

# Nosocomial Pneumonia in Critically Ill and Mechanically Ventilated Patients

DONALD E. CRAVEN, KATHLEEN A. STEGER, and ROBERT A. DUNCAN

Nosocomial pneumonia affects about 250,000 patients annually in acute care hospitals in the United States.[1] Critically ill patients hospitalized in medical and surgical intensive care units (ICU) are at high risk of nosocomial pneumonia.[2-5] Critical care patients with the adult respiratory distress syndrome (ARDS) or with respiratory failure requiring mechanical ventilation have a 6- to 20-fold increased rate of hospital-acquired pneumonia.[4, 6, 7]

Accurate data on the rates of nosocomial pneumonia are difficult to obtain because of the obstacles in diagnosing pneumonia.[8-10] In most hospitals, the diagnosis of pneumonia is made clinically. During the last decade, bronchoscopy with bronchoalveolar lavage (BAL) and protected specimen brush (PSB) have been advocated to improve the diagnosis of nosocomial pneumonia in mechanically ventilated patients.[8, 9, 11-17a]

In the critically ill patient, aspiration of bacteria colonizing the oropharynx is the primary route of bacterial entry into the lower respiratory tract;[18-21] hematogenous seeding and translocation of bacteria from the gastrointestinal tract occur less frequently.[22] Gastric colonization, reflux, and aspiration have been closely linked to the pathogenesis of pneumonia in critically ill, mechanically ventilated patients.[23-28a]

Early, appropriate antibiotic therapy of nosocomial pneumonia appears to decrease morbidity and mortality.[3, 4] Despite the availability of potent broad-spectrum antibiotics, the crude mortality rates for patients with nosocomial pneumonia remain high, underscoring the importance of prevention.[3-5, 29-31] Strategies for prevention have focused on infec-tion control, risk reduction, and antibiotic prophylaxis with selective decontamination of the digestive tract.[32-38a]

This chapter provides an overview of the epidemiology and pathogenic mechanisms of nosocomial pneumonia and highlights the controversies about the diagnosis and therapy of nosocomial pneumonia in critically ill patients with ARDS and other types of respiratory failure.

## ETIOLOGIC AGENTS

Bacteria most commonly cause nosocomial pneumonia in critically ill, mechanically ventilated patients (Table 13–1). Bacterial nosocomial pneumonia may be conceptually divided into early- and late-onset disease. Early-onset nosocomial pneumonia occurs during the first 3 to 4 days of the hospital stay and is usually caused by *Streptococcus pneumoniae, Haemophilus influenzae,* and sometimes *Moraxella catarrhalis.*[17, 39, 40] Late-onset pneumonia occurs more than 4 days after admission and is more commonly caused by hospital-acquired aerobic gram-negative bacilli or *Staphylococcus aureus,* which are frequently more resistant to antibiotics.

In most patients, bacterial nosocomial pneumonia is caused by multiple organisms.[24, 39, 41-43] Aerobic gram-negative bacilli, including *Escherichia coli, Klebsiella pneumoniae, Enterobacter* and *Serratia* species, *Pseudomonas aeruginosa,* and *Acinetobacter calcoaceticus,* are part of the host's endogenous flora or were acquired during hospitalization.[42a, 44-46] *S. aureus* is isolated in 20% to 30%

Table 13–1. **Pathogens Associated With Early and Late-Onset Nosocomial Pneumonia**

| Pathogen | Frequency (%)* | Sources |
|---|---|---|
| Early-onset bacteria pneumonia | | |
|   *Streptococcus pneumoniae* | 5–10 | Endogenous |
|   *Haemophilus influenzae* | <5 | Endogenous |
| Late-onset bacterial pneumonia | | |
|   Aerobic gram-negative bacilli | ≥60 | |
|     *Pseudomonas aeruginosa* | | Endogenous, other patients, food and water, |
|     *Enterobacter* spp. | |   enteral feeding, hospital personnel, |
|     *Acinetobacter* spp. | |   equipment or devices |
|     *Klebsiella pneumoniae* | | |
|     *Serratia marcescens* | | |
|     *Escherichia coli* | | |
|   Gram-positive cocci | | |
|     *Staphylococcus aureus* | 20–25 | Endogenous, hospital personnel, environment |
| Early- and late-onset pneumonia | | |
|   Anaerobic bacteria | 35 | Endogenous |
|   *Legionella pneumophila* | 0–10 | Water |
|   Viruses | | |
|     Influenza A and B | Variable | Patients or staff |
|     Respiratory syncytial virus | Variable | Patients or staff |
|   Fungi and protozoa | | |
|     *Aspergillus* | <1 | Air, construction |
|     *Pneumocystis carinii* | <1 | Endogenous |

*Frequency refers to the rate of isolation from sputum.
Data from references 42, 42a, 60, and 155.

of cases and is particularly common in injection drug users, in patients with thermal injury, coma, or wound infection, and in those who have previously received antibiotics or prolonged care in the ICU.[39, 47, 48]

Anaerobic bacteria have been isolated from about 35% of all cases of nosocomial pneumonia but are probably less important in intubated patients and in late-onset disease.[42, 49] *Legionella pneumophila* occurs episodically but may be endemic in hospitals with contaminated cooling towers or colonized water supplies.[50–52a]

Epidemic influenza pneumonia is seasonal and always of concern; respiratory syncytial virus is a common problem in pediatric ICUs.[53–55] *Candida albicans* often colonizes the respiratory tract but is an uncommon cause of nosocomial pneumonia, except in immunocompromised patients. *Aspergillus fumigatus* is a rare source of infection, but it should be considered if the patient is neutropenic or otherwise immunocompromised, especially if there is construction nearby.[56] *Pneumocystis carinii* should be included in the differential diagnosis for immunosuppressed patients or patients hospitalized with human immunodeficiency virus (HIV) infection with CD4 helper T-lymphocyte counts less than 200/mm³. However, hospitalized patients with acquired immunodeficiency syndrome (AIDS) are also at increased risk for pneumonia caused by bacteria.[57, 58]

## EPIDEMIOLOGY

In the United States, pneumonia accounts for 13% to 18% of all nosocomial infections, occurs at a rate of 6 to 10 episodes per 1000 hospitalizations, and constitutes the leading cause of death from nosocomial infections.[31, 59–62] Rates of nosocomial pneumonia vary from 0.8% in medical and surgical patients to almost 18% in postoperative patients.[7, 60, 63] Rates of nosocomial pneumonia are 10- to 20-

fold higher in ICU patients and 7- to 21-fold higher in the intubated patient.[2, 4, 6, 7]

Crude mortality rates for nosocomial pneumonia range from 20% to 50%, with an attributable mortality of 33%.[3–5, 29, 30, 41, 43, 62, 64, 65] Mortality rates for ICU patients with hospital-acquired pneumonia are 2- to 10-fold higher than for patients without pneumonia.[3, 5, 29, 43] Rates are increased among patients with secondary bacteremia or infection caused by organisms such as *P. aeruginosa*.[29, 30, 62, 66, 67] Critically ill patients frequently have shock, coma, high APACHE scores, ultimately fatal underlying disease, infection with organisms such as *P. aeruginosa* and *A. calcoaceticus*, bilateral infiltrates on chest x-ray films, ARDS, and respiratory failure; these are all strong predictors of mortality.[3–5] Although nosocomial pneumonia is significantly associated with mortality, it was not identified as an independent risk factor after multivariate analysis.[5]

## PATHOGENESIS

Although bacterial nosocomial pneumonia may result from bacteremia or translocation of bacteria through or between the gastrointestinal mucosal epithelial cells, aspiration of bacteria from the oropharynx is the most common route of infection (Fig. 13–1).[19, 22, 52a] Approximately 45% of healthy people aspirate during sleep, and aspiration is more frequent in patients who are supine and have pathologically altered consciousness, abnormal swallowing, depressed gag reflexes, delayed gastric emptying, or decreased gastrointestinal motility.[18, 19, 23, 27, 28a, 52a]

In the critically ill, mechanically ventilated patient, local trauma and inflammation are caused by the endotracheal tube and leakage of bacteria around the cuff, which results in colonization or local infection of the upper trachea. The lower respiratory tract is then primed for progressive infec-

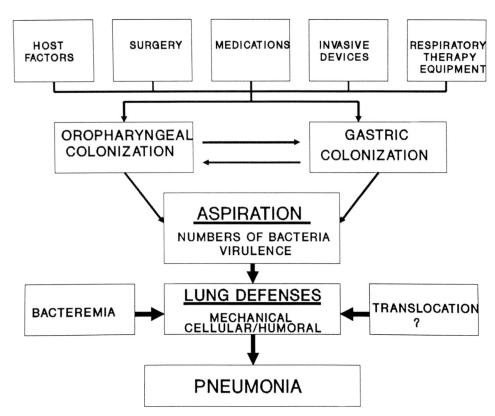

**Figure 13–1.** Factors influencing colonization and infection of the respiratory tract. (From Craven DE, Barber TW, Steger KA, Montecalvo MA: Nosocomial pneumonia in the '90s: Update of epidemiology and risk factors. Semin Respir Infect 5:157–172, 1990.)

tion in the form of tracheobronchitis or pneumonia. In some patients, especially those with ARDS or severe congestive failure, it may be difficult to differentiate among colonization, local infection, purulent tracheobronchitis, and pneumonia.

## Colonization of the Oropharynx

The ability of gram-negative bacilli to adhere to oropharyngeal epithelial cells appears to be pivotal in establishing successful colonization.[68–71] Host factors, body position, types of bacteria colonizing the pharynx, and the use of antibiotics may alter colonization and adherence of gram-negative bacilli.[20, 21, 27, 47, 72] Unlike healthy persons, critically ill patients have high rates of oropharyngeal colonization with aerobic gram-negative bacilli. In one study, gram-negative bacilli colonized 16% of the moderately ill patients and 57% of the critically ill patients, and the rates of pneumonia were increased sixfold in the ICU patients who were colonized.[20, 21]

Oropharyngeal attachment of gram-negative bacilli plays an important role in colonization and is inversely related to the presence of cellular fibronectin.[70, 71] Oral epithelial cells rich in fibronectin bind gram-positive organisms, but those poor in fibronectin preferentially bind gram-negative rods. Bacterial adherence to tracheal cells is associated with high levels of elastase and small amounts of IgA in the sputum.[73]

## Gastric Colonization

In mechanically ventilated patients, the stomach and gastrointestinal tract may contribute to oropharyngeal and tra-

cheal colonization with gram-negative bacilli.[23–28a, 40, 74] The stomach is normally sterile if the pH is low ($<2$) because of the potent bactericidal activity of hydrochloric acid. Studies of *Vibrio cholerae* infection in normal, healthy volunteers demonstrated that the infective dose may be decreased 10,000-fold by prior administration of antacids.[74, 75] Increases in gastric colonization may occur with advanced age, achlorhydria, various gastrointestinal diseases, malnutrition, or the use of antacids and histamine type 2 ($H_2$) blockers.[23–26, 28a, 40, 76] In mechanically ventilated patients, colonization may reach 1 to 100 million gram-negative bacilli per 1 mL of gastric juice if the pH is greater than 4.[24–26, 77] Retrograde colonization of the oropharynx from the stomach may increase the risk of lower respiratory tract infection,[24–26, 28a] constituting the "gastropulmonary route of infection" described by Tryba.[78]

## RISK FACTORS FOR COLONIZATION AND PNEUMONIA

Several risk factors have been associated with increased oropharyngeal bacterial colonization or pneumonia, some of which are amenable to prevention strategies (Fig. 13–2).[20, 21, 65] Host factors, such as advanced age, obesity, poor nutrition, smoking, alcoholism, and intravenous drug use, and the severity of acute and chronic underlying diseases, prior surgery, and entry into the ICU significantly increase the risk of pneumonia but are not effective targets for prevention.

Appropriate targets for prevention include environmental sources of contamination, cross-infection from hospital staff and other patients, medications and mechanical factors

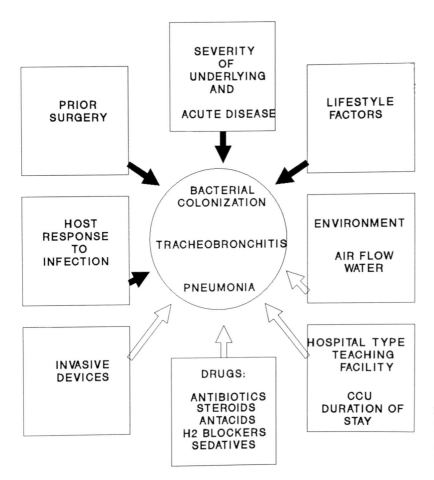

**Figure 13–2.** Factors contributing to bacterial colonization and nosocomial pneumonia. Open arrows indicate areas that should be targeted for prevention. Abbreviations: H₂, histamine type 2; CCU, critical care unit.

that influence gastric colonization and reflux, and the use of invasive devices.[27, 28a, 31] Unrestrained use of antibiotics results in colonization with nosocomial pathogens and increased antibiotic resistance.[47, 72] The use of cytotoxic drugs and steroids may impair the host response to infection in the lung. The selection of stress bleeding prophylaxis prescribed to critical care patients affects colonization and the risk of infection.[24, 26, 40, 76, 79]

Several groups have used multivariate techniques to identify independent risk factors for pneumonia in ventilated and nonventilated patients.[3–5] Variables independently associated with nosocomial pneumonia included age greater than 70 years, depressed consciousness, use of intracranial pressure monitors, chronic lung disease, chest surgery, and duration of mechanical ventilation. More frequent changes of the ventilator circuits (ie, daily versus every 48 hours), reintubation, large-volume tube feedings or documented gastric aspiration, use of H₂-blockers with and without antacids, and fall or winter seasons have been associated with pneumonia. One group recently identified bronchoscopy as an independent risk factor for pneumonia, but further confirmation of these data is needed.[80]

## DIAGNOSIS

### Clinical Diagnosis

Accurate data about etiologic agents, epidemiology, and the treatment of bacterial nosocomial pneumonia are lim-

ited by the lack of a ''gold standard'' for diagnosing infection. The isolation of a pathogen from pleural fluid or blood cultures helps establish the diagnosis of pneumonia, but these findings are relatively uncommon, and culture results are not available to the clinician for 24 to 48 hours.

The clinical diagnosis of nosocomial pneumonia incorporates data on the patient's underlying disease, risk factors for infection, symptoms, and time in the hospital (ie, early-onset or late-onset disease). Information is also garnered from the physical examination and from laboratory data such as blood leukocyte count, blood gases, chest radiographs, sputum Gram stain, and cultures. Pneumonia may be mimicked by atelectasis, pulmonary edema, pulmonary emboli, neoplastic processes, and autoimmune diseases.

Clinical criteria for the diagnosis of pneumonia are used in most hospitals, but this method lacks sensitivity and specificity, particularly in mechanically ventilated patients. Bryant and colleagues followed 60 patients suspected of having pneumonia but found conclusive evidence of pneumonia in only 30%.[10] Similarly, Fagon and coworkers confirmed only 31% of cases of clinically suspected pneumonia in an ICU setting.[8] Joshi and associates were able to eliminate 80% of new infiltrates in ICU patients within 8 hours, using vigorous chest physical therapy alone.[81]

In mechanically ventilated patients, cultures of endotracheal aspirates are commonly used to diagnose pneumonia. Although this technique detected 89% of pneumonias, Torres and colleagues found a specificity of only 14%.[13] Improved diagnostic methods are necessary for optimal management. This is particularly true in patients with ARDS or severe congestive failure, in whom as many as 62% of the pneumonias may be missed by clinical assessment alone.[82, 83]

## Diagnosis by Bronchoscopy With Bronchoalveolar Lavage or Protected Specimen Brush Catheters

PSB and BAL have been advocated for diagnosis in mechanically ventilated patients.[8, 9, 11–16, 17a] The sensitivities of these techniques range from 60% to 95%, with specificities of 80% to 100%.[13, 14] A metanalysis of 18 studies yielded an overall sensitivity of 90% and specificity of 95% for PSB.[84] Sensitivities for BAL ranged from 53% to 100%, with 99% specificity. Further refinement of these methods may be offered by protected BAL.[85]

Despite the seemingly encouraging results of these techniques, false-negative and false-positive rates of 10% to 30% represent a substantial threat to misdiagnosis of patients. Prior antibiotic exposure may have a dramatic effect on quantitative cultures of BAL and PSB.[13, 17a, 85, 86] Interpretation of the many studies of BAL and PSB must remain cautious because of differences in study design, patient populations, definitions of pneumonia, and the effect of prior antibiotic administration. A consensus paper suggested bronchoscopic diagnosis should be used for research studies of ventilator-associated pneumonia,[17a] but in the absence of a gold standard for the diagnosis of pneumonia, application for routine clinical diagnosis is still controversial.

## Nonbronchoscopic Diagnosis

The bronchoscopic diagnosis has correlated well with the clinical pulmonary infection score (CPIS) for the clinical diagnosis of pneumonia.[17] The CPIS incorporates quantitative assessment of the patient's temperature, leukocyte and differential counts, oxygenation, presence of infiltrates or ARDS on chest radiograph, and results of semiquantitative Gram stain and culture of tracheal aspirates. This method is less invasive and may be an alternative to bronchoscopic techniques, but it needs further evaluation. "Blind" BAL or PSB with quantitative bacteriology may be another alternative to bronchoscopic diagnosis, but this technique also needs validation.[17, 87–90]

## CLINICAL MANIFESTATIONS

The history of the patient may provide some nonspecific clues to the diagnosis. Pneumococcal or *Haemophilus* infections are more common early in the hospitalization, especially in patients with advanced age, chronic underlying disease, or head trauma. *S. aureus* usually appears later in the hospital course and should be suspected in insulin-dependent diabetics, injection drug users, or patients with head trauma, coma, or renal failure. Patients with late-onset nosocomial pneumonia who are mechanically ventilated and have chronic underlying diseases, immunosuppression,

alcoholism, or prior antibiotic therapy are at risk for infection with *Klebsiella, P. aeruginosa*, and other gram-negative bacilli.

Most patients with nosocomial pneumonia exhibit fever, malaise, dyspnea, and a productive cough. Critically ill patients are usually tachypneic, tachycardiac, and febrile, and they may be agitated; some may progress to coma, hypotension, or shock. Tracheal deviation may be associated with pneumothorax or empyema, with clinical evidence of consolidation, atelectasis, pleuritis, or pleural effusion.

In patients with fever, leukocytosis, and purulent sputum but without evidence of infiltrates on the chest radiographs, a diagnosis of purulent tracheobronchitis must be entertained. In the intubated patient, it may be difficult to differentiate colonization, tracheobronchitis, and early pneumonia. In most cases, careful observation with aggressive pulmonary toilet is adequate.[81] However, if the patient is critically ill, antimicrobial therapy is often instituted and the clinical response to therapy carefully monitored over the next 48 hours.

The chest radiograph usually shows a localized or diffuse alveolar pattern (Fig. 13–3A). A lung abscess suggests infection with anaerobes, *S. aureus*, or a necrotizing pneumonia due to aerobic gram-negative bacilli. Multiple wedge-shaped infiltrates in the periphery suggest septic emboli, and pneumatoceles are associated with infection due to *S. aureus*. Pleural effusion occurs more commonly with pneumonia caused by pneumococci or *S. aureus* but may occur with gram-negative bacillary pneumonia as well (Fig. 13–3B).[91] Computed tomographic scans may be helpful in the diagnosis of pneumonia or abscess in patients with ARDS or for the management of pneumonia complicated by empyema (Fig. 13–3C). Ultrasound provides similar information and may provide a portable diagnostic and therapeutic tool for patients too unstable to leave the ICU.

In critically ill patients, sputum may be produced spontaneously, induced by nebulized saline, or obtained by transtracheal aspiration or bronchoscopy. Some investigators have used transthoracic thin needle aspiration for diagnosis, but the risk of pneumothorax and a relatively high rate of false-negative results makes this technique less feasible in mechanically ventilated patients.[92]

Examination of sputum often provides ready clues to the diagnosis and may speed the treatment of pneumonia. Adequate Gram-stained sputum samples should reveal multiple inflammatory cells, a paucity of epithelial cells, and a predominant morphology of bacterial types. Highly purulent sputum usually indicates a bacterial source of infection. Gram-positive diplococci suggest pneumococcal pneumonia, and gram-positive cocci in clusters suggest *S. aureus*. Gram-negative coccobacilli (characteristic of *H. influenzae*) and diplococci (eg, *Neisseria* species or *M. catarrhalis*) may be seen early, but gram-negative bacilli (eg, *Klebsiella*, other enteric rods, *Pseudomonas*) may occur early in chronically ill patients or later in nosocomial cases. Because sputum is cultured aerobically, anaerobes should be considered if there are mixed bacterial morphologies revealed by the Gram stain and the culture reveals "normal flora." Pleural fluid, thin needle aspirates, and BAL specimens may be sent for anaerobic culture. If the diagnosis remains unclear, transbronchial or open lung biopsy may be required.

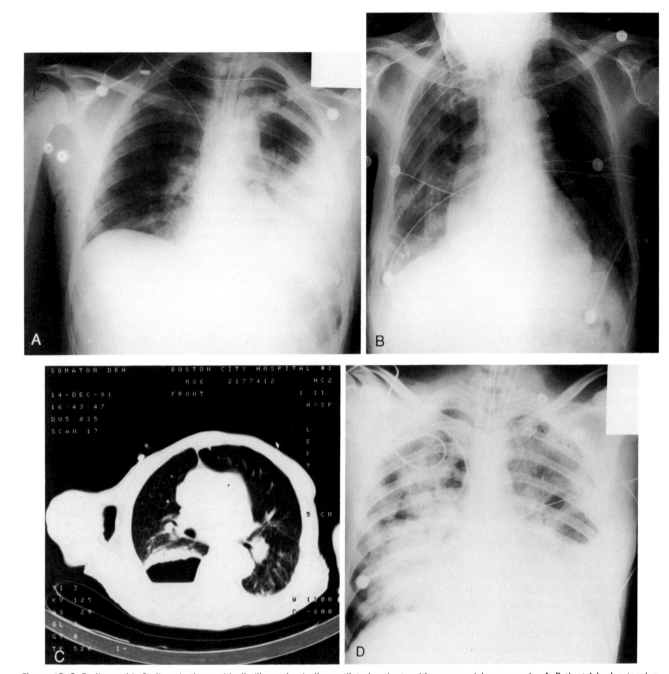

**Figure 13–3.** Radiographic findings in three critically ill, mechanically ventilated patients with nosocomial pneumonia. *A,* Patient 1 had extensive left-sided pneumonia caused by *Pseudomonas aeruginosa,* which responded to therapy with gentamicin and piperacillin. *B,* Patient 2 had right-sided pneumonia caused by anaerobes and *Klebsiella pneumoniae,* which was treated with clindamycin and ceftriaxone after chest tube placement. *C,* Computed tomographic scan of patient 2 on the same day demonstrates the thick peel and undrained pus in the pleural space. After efforts to place a second chest tube, the patient developed acute respiratory distress syndrome and progressive respiratory failure that ended in death. *D,* Patient 3 had diffuse bilateral infiltrates secondary to aspiration pneumonia that progressed to acute respiratory distress syndrome, which was treated with clindamycin, aztreonam, and supportive care. Because of persistent fever, leukocytosis, and sputum cultures with heavy growth of *Acinetobacter calcoaceticus,* therapy was changed to imipenem, which produced a good clinical response.

Some investigators have looked for elastin fibers or antibody-coated bacteria in sputum and for elastolytic activity in pulmonary lavage fluid to aid in the diagnosis of pneumonia, but these methods are not widely available.[93–95]

Legionellosis, *Mycobacterium tuberculosis,* or partially treated bacterial infection should be considered in patients with Gram stains demonstrating polymorphonuclear cells or macrophages but no bacteria. In patients with suspected legionella, sputum should be cultured on charcoal yeast extract or examined by direct immunofluorescent staining. Patients thought to have tuberculosis should have sputum examined by acid-fast stain and cultures planted on Löwenstein-Jensen media.

In intubated patients, serial Gram stains may be useful for monitoring the response to initial antibiotic therapy, and cultures can be used to corroborate the choice of antimicrobial agents. It should be emphasized that microbiologic information reflects only aerobic flora, and antibiotic sensitivity data indicate the minimal inhibitory concentration in serum, not in bronchial secretions. It is prudent to make changes in initial antimicrobial therapy based on the patient's clinical response, rather than altering therapy based purely on the organisms and antibiotic sensitivities in the culture report. If the patient subsequently deteriorates clinically, the antibiotic therapy can be changed to cover a broader spectrum of potential pathogens.

## Adult Respiratory Distress Syndrome

Nosocomial pneumonia occurs in more than 70% of patients with ARDS.[82] ARDS is a form of pulmonary edema that results from increased permeability of the pulmonary capillaries or the alveolar epithelium (Fig. 13–3D).[96, 97] More than 150,000 cases occur annually in the United States, and the mortality rates generally exceed 50%, particularly for patients with infection.[97–99] In a seminal study by Bell and colleagues, the mortality rates were 67% for ARDS patients with infection and 7% for those without infection; the rates were even higher for patients with nosocomial pneumonia.[83]

The incidence of ARDS is high among critically ill patients with shock, ischemia, multiple transfusions, aspiration pneumonia, head and chest trauma, ventilator lung (ie, barotrauma), oxygen toxicity, and bacterial or viral infections.[100–102] Infectious agents can cause ARDS by activating the host inflammatory response.[103–107] Prostaglandins, terminal complement complexes, leukocytes, and platelets have been implicated in the pathogenesis of ARDS. Endotoxin or lipopolysaccharide in the outer membrane of gram-negative bacilli may directly increase capillary permeability or may act indirectly through cytokines or other mediators.[105–108] Isolated bacteremia is associated with a 5% to 15% risk of progressive lung injury, but when combined with shock, thrombocytopenia, or disseminated intravascular coagulation, the risk of ARDS increases to more than 50%.[101, 102] Infection with pneumococci, nonenteric gram-negative bacilli such as *L. pneumophila*, and influenza viruses may also produce ARDS.

Although the specific mechanisms producing ARDS are unknown, the clinical presentation and pathologic changes resulting from various causes are remarkably similar. Histologic examination of lung tissue from patients with ARDS reveals interstitial and intraalveolar edema, diffuse atelectasis, and hemorrhage. The alveolar spaces are filled with denatured plasma proteins that have crossed the interstitial space, giving a hyaline membrane appearance. Inflammatory cells are usually mononuclear, and evidence of fibrosis or secondary infection may also be present.

ARDS produces a diffuse, infiltrative, restrictive lung disease that may be acute or subacute and often results in acute respiratory failure.[97, 98, 100] The chest radiograph shows increased lung markings that are more extensive at the bases and that progress to a reticulonodular pattern in which the nodules become confluent, producing a white-out pattern. Early in the course, arterial blood gases demonstrate hypoxemia and respiratory alkalosis, with pulmonary wedge pressures greater than 18 mm Hg. As the disease progresses, higher fractional concentrations of inspired oxygen ($FIO_2$) are required to maintain an adequate partial pressure of oxygen ($PaO_2$), often requiring positive end-expiratory pressure (PEEP). As the patient's condition declines, alveolar exchange worsens, and respiratory acidosis ensues.

The initial step in the management of acute respiratory failure with ARDS is endotracheal intubation and assisted volume-cycled ventilation.[97] The inspired oxygen should be sufficient to maintain the $PaO_2$ in the range of 60 to 80 mm Hg. PEEP is indicated if ventilation parameters and increases in the $FIO_2$ fail to provide adequate oxygenation. Efforts should be directed at optimizing the patient's hemodynamic status, using a Swan-Ganz catheter to maintain the pulmonary capillary wedge pressure in the range of 10 to 15 mm Hg. Patients should be given stress bleeding prophylaxis and proper nutritional support, and they should have constant monitoring of fluid balances and renal function.

## ANTIBIOTIC TREATMENT

Treatment of nosocomial pneumonia involves supportive care, attention to the underlying disease, and institution of appropriate antimicrobial therapy. Supportive measures include supplemental oxygen, vigorous pulmonary toilet, and appropriate hydration.

Antimicrobial therapy should be directed at the offending pathogen(s). Combination therapy is often prescribed because of the polymicrobial and sometimes cryptic nature of nosocomial pneumonia. The choice of initial antibiotic therapy should be based on the clinical history, severity of underlying disease, time in the hospital, previous culture data, information on indigenous nosocomial pathogens and their antimicrobial sensitivity patterns, and information gained from the Gram stain. Empiric therapy should be broad enough to cover the spectrum of suspected pathogens for the clinical settings outlined in Table 13–2. Although combination antibiotic therapy has been prescribed traditionally, newer data suggest that some patients treated with one drug (eg, ceftazidime, cefoperazone, imipenem) may have similar outcomes to patients treated with combination therapy.[109, 110] Pneumonia due to *P. aeruginosa* should probably be treated with two drugs, and physicians should monitor antimicrobial resistance and superinfection, particularly for pneumonia caused by *Enterobacter* or *Acinetobacter*.[47, 91, 101]

Although aminoglycosides have a wide spectrum of activity against nosocomial gram-negative bacilli, their use may be hampered by a poor toxic-therapeutic ratio, the need for antibiotic peak and trough levels to monitor toxicity, and their low penetration into bronchial secretions.[91, 109] Clinical data suggest that peak levels of 7 µg/mL or higher for gentamicin or tobramycin and 28 µg/mL or higher for amikacin are associated with better outcomes.[111] Alternative therapy with a third-generation cephalosporin such as ceftazidime, ceftriaxone, or imipenem may be preferable if the organisms are sensitive.

In patients who require prolonged therapy and have impaired renal function, aztreonam may be preferable to an aminoglycoside.[91, 109] Quinolones (eg, ciprofloxacin) are particularly useful because of their broad activity against gram-negative bacilli and excellent penetration into respiratory secretions, but additional coverage is needed for pa-

Table 13–2. **Antibiotics for Early- and Late-Onset Ventilator-Associated Pneumonia**

| Setting | Suspected Organism | Antibiotic Therapy* | Comments |
|---|---|---|---|
| Early-onset disease | | | |
| | *Streptococcus pneumoniae* | Penicillin G; ampicillin; clindamycin; erythromycin | Quinolones, third-generation cephalosporins (except ceftriaxone) have less activity and are not recommended. |
| | *Haemophilus influenzae* | Second- or third-generation cephalosporin; TMP-SMX; ampicillin/sulbactam | 15%–30% of strains produce β-lactamase and are resistant to ampicillin |
| | *Moraxella catarrhalis* | Second- or third-generation cephalosporin; TMP-SMX; ampicillin/sulbactam; ciprofloxacin | 50%–70% of strains produce β-lactamase; ampicillin usually ineffective |
| | Anaerobes | Penicillin G; clindamycin | Highly associated with aspiration. Clindamycin has activity against methicillin-sensitive *Staphylococcus aureus*. |
| Late-onset disease | | | |
| Gram-negative bacilli | *Escherichia coli, Klebsiella pneumoniae,* other Enterobacteriaceae | Third-generation cephalosporin ± aminoglycoside; ciprofloxacin; ampicillin/sulbactam; imipenem | Treatment should be based on Gram stain, knowledge of specific flora in hospital, and in vitro antibiotic sensitivity results. Aztreonam may be substituted for aminoglycoside. |
| | *Pseudomonas aeruginosa* | Aminoglycoside + antipseudomonal penicillin; ceftazidime ± aminoglycoside; ciprofloxacin + aminoglycoside or antipseudomonal penicillin; imipenem + aminoglycoside | Two drugs should be used to treat serious infections in critically ill, neutropenic, or intubated patients. Aztreonam may be substituted for aminoglycoside. |
| Gram-positive cocci | *Staphylococcus aureus* | Oxacillin or nafcillin; first-generation cephalosporin; vancomycin | MRSA should be treated with vancomycin. Cefamandole and cefuroxime have good activity. |
| Early- or late-onset disease | *Legionella pneumophila* | Erythromycin | May need > 2 weeks of therapy |

*Second-generation cephalosporin, cefamandole, cefuroxime, cefoxitin; third-generation cephalosporin, ceftriaxone, ceftazidime, cefoperazone, cefotaxime; TMP-SMX, trimethoprim-sulfamethoxazole; aminoglycoside, gentamicin, tobramycin, amikacin; antipseudomonal penicillin, carbenicillin, ticarcillin, mezlocillin, piperacillin, azlocillin; MRSA, methicillin-resistant *Staphylococcus aureus*; PMN, polymorphonuclear leukocytes.

Adapted in part from Sanford JP: Guide to Antimicrobial Therapy 1991. Dallas, TX, Antimicrobial Therapy, 1991.

tients with pneumonia caused by anaerobes or pneumococci,[109] pneumonia due to *P. aeruginosa*, or other resistant nosocomial pathogens.

Studies are in progress using monoclonal antibodies against surface structures of bacteria and cytokines that may increase lung injury. Efforts to bolster lung defenses, such as with granulocyte-stimulating factor, are also under investigation.

## PREVENTION OF NOSOCOMIAL PNEUMONIA

Prevention of nosocomial pneumonia in critically ill patients requires adherence to general principles of infection control and careful attention to the proper use of invasive devices, antibiotics, and equipment (Table 13–3). Aggressive treatment of the patient's acute and underlying disease is critical. The patient with multiple organ system failure, a

Table 13–3. **Summary of Methods to Reduce the Frequency of Nosocomial Pneumonia in Mechanically Ventilated Patients***

**General Principles**
   Treat patient's underlying disease aggressively[31, 45]
   Avoid antacids or H$_2$-blockers for prophylaxis of stress-related bleeding[24, 26, 40, 119–123, 125, 126]
   Keep patient's head elevated at ≥30°[27]
   Use incentive spirometry for postoperative patients
   Assess nutrition and route of feeding[112–114]
   Use caution in prescribing central nervous system depressants.
   Extubate and remove nasogastric tube as clinically indicated[4, 52a, 118]
   Use good chest physiotherapy for patients with chronic obstructive pulmonary diseases
   Control use of antibiotics in the intensive care unit
   Consider use of kinetic therapy[31, 144, 144a]
**Infection Control**
   Maintain surveillance in the intensive care unit[45, 145]
   Education and awareness programs on nosocomial infection[31, 45]
   Use hand-washing and/or barrier precautions[44, 45, 147]
   Change gloves between contact with patients[148–150]
   Assess technique for suctioning patients[142, 143]

**Infection Control** *Continued*
   Evaluate method of condensate disposal
   Use effective methods of disinfection of respiratory devices and equipment
   Consider selective decontamination of the digestive tract with antibiotics for select populations of patients[32–38, 152–153a]
**Respiratory Care Equipment**
   Discriminate between respiratory therapy equipment with nebulizers and humidifiers[129, 130]
   Use circuit changes (tubing and humidifier) >48 h for patients using mechanical ventilators with humidifiers[133, 134]
   Do not use changes for circuits with heat moisture exchangers[5, 132–134]
   Ensure proper removal and attention to methods to reduce tubing condensate and reflux back into the patient's endotracheal tube[132]
   Do not transfer equipment or devices between patients
   Use proper care of in-line medication nebulizers[139]
   Ensure proper disinfection of respiratory tubing, bags, and spirometer[140, 141]

*Revised guidelines for the prevention of nosocomial pneumonia will be published by the Centers of Disease Control and Prevention and the Hospital Infection Control Practices Advisory Committee (Tablon OC, Anderson LJ, Arden NH, et al, in preparation).

Modified from Craven DE, Steger KA, Barber TW: Preventing nosocomial pneumonia: State of the art and perspectives for the 1990's. Am J Med 91(suppl 3B):44S–53S, 1991.

high APACHE II score, and an ultimately or rapidly fatal underlying disease should be targeted for intensive efforts. There are several important areas for intervention. New guidelines for the prevention of nosocomial pneumonia are in preparation by the Centers for Disease Control and Prevention and its Hospital Infection Control Practices Advisory Committee (Tablon OC, Anderson LJ, Arden NH, et al, in preparation).

### Enteral and Parenteral Nutrition

Accurate assessment of the patient's nutritional status and avoidance of unnecessary parenteral nutrition may reduce the risk of nosocomial pneumonia.[112, 113] Early initiation of enteral feeding can help to maintain the integrity of the gastrointestinal epithelium and prevent bacterial translocation,[22] but it may increase the risk of gastric distention, colonization, aspiration, and pneumonia.[113–116] Pingleton and colleagues demonstrated gastric colonization in all of 18 ventilated patients receiving enteral feeding without antacid or $H_2$-blocker therapy, 63% of whom subsequently developed pneumonia.[115] The use of continuous rather than bolus feeding, monitoring and removing residual, and maintaining an upright patient position may decrease this risk of aspiration and pneumonia.[27, 113, 114]

Aspiration and reflux are common in ICU patients. Ibanez and coworkers found that reflux to the oropharynx occurred in approximately 70% of patients receiving tube feedings; 40% had evidence of aspiration.[28] Border and associates emphasized the importance of patient position in the prevention of pneumonia, and Torres and colleagues suggested that aspiration of gastric contents may be reduced by maintaining the patient's head elevation at 30°.[27, 117]

Most patients receiving mechanical ventilation have nasogastric tubes inserted to manage gastric secretions, prevent gastric distention, or provide nutritional support (Fig. 13–4). This tube may increase oropharyngeal colonization or pneumonia by increasing reflux, providing a conduit for bacteria to migrate to the oropharynx, and enhancing stasis and colonization in the oropharynx.[4, 52a, 118] The risks, benefits, and duration of use of nasogastric tubes should receive careful consideration.

### Stress Bleeding Prophylaxis

Although antacids, $H_2$-blockers, and sucralfate have not been approved for stress bleeding prophylaxis by the Food and Drug Administration in the United States, they are frequently prescribed. As shown in Figure 13–5, several studies have found lower rates of pneumonia for patients given a cytoprotective agent (eg, sucralfate) rather than agents that neutralize gastric acids (eg, antacids) or block gastric acid secretion (eg, $H_2$-blockers).[24, 40, 119–126] The rate of gastric colonization with gram-negative bacilli was significantly lower in patients treated with sucralfate than in those given antacid therapy with or without $H_2$-blockers.[24, 40, 121]

In a metanalysis of the efficacy of stress bleeding prophylaxis in ICU patients, respiratory tract infection occurred significantly less frequently ($P<.05$) in patients treated with sucralfate than in patients receiving $H_2$-blockers (nine studies) or antacids (eight studies).[126] These data suggest that sucralfate provides the same protection against stress bleeding in the ICU that $H_2$-blockers and antacids provide, but with less risk of subsequent pneumonia.

### Equipment and Devices

Endotracheal and nasotracheal tubes compromise host defenses against infection by causing increased local trauma, impaired swallowing and ciliary clearance, and

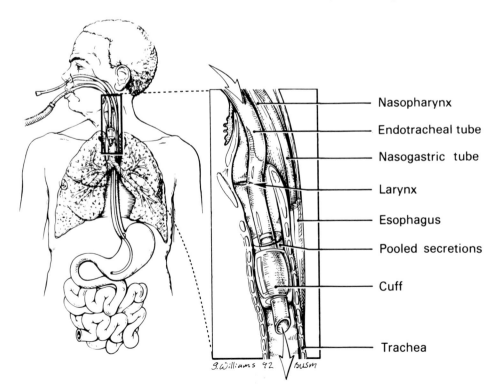

**Figure 13–4.** The diagram depicts the routes of oropharyngeal colonization in the intubated patient with a nasogastric tube. Bacteria may move retrograde from the stomach to the oropharynx, and pooled secretions may leak around the cuff into the trachea. (From Craven DE, Barber TW, Steger KA, Montecalvo MA: Nosocomial pneumonia in the '90s: Update of epidemiology and risk factors. Semin Respir Infect 5:157–172, 1990.)

Nasopharynx

Endotracheal tube

Nasogastric tube

Larynx

Esophagus

Pooled secretions

Cuff

Trachea

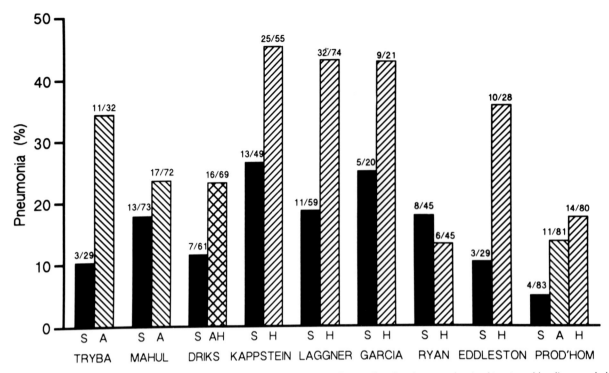

**Figure 13–5.** Summary of reported rates of nosocomial pneumonia in mechanically ventilated patients randomized to stress bleeding prophylaxis with sucralfate *(S)* or antacids *(A)*, antacids with or without H₂-blockers *(AH)*, or H₂-blockers alone *(H)*. (From Craven DE, Steger KA, Duncan RA: Prevention and control of nosocomial pneumonia. *In* Wenzel RP (ed): Prevention and Control of Nosocomial Infections. Baltimore, Williams & Wilkins, 1993:580–599.)

leakage of pooled oral secretions around the endotracheal tube cuff.[64] Because the endotracheal tube is not changed routinely, it may contain large numbers of bacteria covered by biofilm or glycocalyx that may become dislodged and cause focal pneumonia.[127, 128]

Nebulization equipment produces particle aerosols smaller than 4 μm in diameter that, if contaminated, may carry bacteria to the terminal bronchioles and alveoli.[129, 130] Because most ventilators have bubbling or wick humidifiers, no significant aerosol is produced, and bacterial colonization is low because of the high internal temperature.[131] Humidifiers should be filled with sterile water or normal saline.

Ventilator tubing colonization often occurs rapidly after a circuit change and originates primarily from the patient, with the highest concentrations nearest the endotracheal tube.[132] Data suggest that the circuits can be safely changed at intervals of 48 hours or more.[5, 133, 134] We believe that the interval between circuit changes can be prolonged for 5 days or more. This will produce substantial savings in personnel and supplies with little risk to the patient.

Because tubing condensate may contain thousands to millions of gram-negative bacilli per milliliter, reflux into the patient's trachea should be avoided.[132] Turning a patient or raising the bed rail may inoculate the condensate into the lower respiratory tract. Heated tubing reduces formation of condensate, and traps can be used to collect condensate. Inappropriate disposal of contaminated condensate may lead to cross-colonization of personnel and the environment.

Heat-moisture exchangers or hygroscopic humidifiers recycle exhaled moisture and eliminate condensate, but they add dead space to the circuit and may not provide sufficient humidity for critically ill patients.[135–137] The combination of a bacteria-filtering heat-moisture exchanger and an unheated humidifier may be a useful humidification method for selected long-term ventilated patients in the ICU.[138]

Medication nebulizers inserted into the mechanical ventilator circuit may become colonized from contaminated condensate.[139] Resuscitation bags, spirometers, and oxygen analyzers are also potential sources of cross-contamination with nosocomial pathogens.[140, 141] Respiratory therapy devices should not be transferred between patients, and proper disinfection of devices after use is essential for reducing cross-colonization and pneumonia.

Tracheal suction catheters are used on ventilated and nonventilated patients and may carry bacteria directly into the lung, increasing the risk of colonization. Aseptic technique should be followed during suctioning, using gloves and a sterile solution to rinse the catheter. A closed, multiuse suction system may be more convenient than a single-use catheter, and it results in less hypoxia for the patient without increasing the risk of pneumonia.[142] Additional studies are needed to determine whether such devices affect the risks of acquiring or disseminating infection in mechanically ventilated patients.[143]

Investigators have used continuous oscillating beds to prevent pneumonia, decubitus ulcers, and pulmonary emboli in critically ill patients.[144, 144a] Data analyzed in metanalysis suggest that kinetic therapy may reduce pneumonia and atelectasis as well as the length of ICU stay.[144a]

## Infection Control Strategies

Hospitals with effective surveillance and infection control programs have rates of pneumonia 20% lower than hospitals without such programs.[145] Effective surveillance, identification of high-risk patients, staff education, proper isolation techniques, and adherence to infection control practices such as hand washing are cornerstones in the prevention of nosocomial pneumonia.[44, 45]

Gram-negative bacilli and *S. aureus* commonly colonize the hands of health care providers.[45] Hand washing, before and after patient contact, is an effective means of removing transient bacteria, and gloves are particularly useful for medical personnel with open skin lesions or dermatitis. Because of poor compliance with hand-washing protocols among hospital personnel, the use of gloves may be an important strategy to reduce nosocomial infection.[98, 146, 147] However, gloves may become colonized with nosocomial pathogens, and health care workers who follow universal precautions but do not change gloves between patients can increase the risk of cross-colonization and infection.[148–150]

## Selective Decontamination With Antibiotics

Selective decontamination of the digestive tract (SDD) is aimed at preventing oropharyngeal and gastric colonization by aerobic gram-negative bacilli without disturbing the anaerobic flora.[32, 37, 37a, 151, 152] The SDD regimen usually includes systemic antibiotic therapy with cefotaxime, trimethoprim, or a quinolone, and a combination of nonabsorbable local antibiotics, such as an aminoglycoside, polymyxin B, and amphotericin B. The local antibiotics are applied as a paste (Orobase) in the oropharynx, or they may be given orally or through the nasogastric tube.

As shown in Table 13–4, several studies using SDD have demonstrated dramatically reduced rates of nosocomial respiratory tract colonization and infection and a trend toward decreased mortality, but they have had little effect in reducing duration of mechanical ventilation or length of stay in

the ICU.[33–37, 151–153a] One metanalysis suggests that mortality rates randomized to SDD are lower in those receiving a systemic antibiotic in addition to local topical antibiotics alone.[152a] Finally, most studies have few data on antimicrobial resistance and cost effectiveness.[38a]

A large, multicenter, randomized study by Gastinne and colleagues did not show any beneficial effect on overall respiratory infection or mortality rates for patients receiving SDD with no intravenous antibiotic.[154] Interpretation of these data and of Table 13–4 should be cautious, because the 14 cited studies involved diverse patient groups and usually refer to lower respiratory tract infections rather than pneumonia. Gastinne's trial enrolled medical ICU patients, who may constitute the ICU population least likely to benefit from selective decontamination. The disproportionate size of this study obscures the findings of the six other randomized trials, which demonstrated a uniform reduction in respiratory tract infections, but only a modest trend toward reduced mortality. Cockerill and colleagues found decreased rates of gram-negative bacteremia and tracheobronchitis in patients who received SDD plus cefotaxime.[37a] By comparison, Hammond and colleagues, using a double-blind trial, found no benefit of SDD over placebo; both groups were given intravenous cefotaxime.[153a] Currently, it is unclear which patient populations should receive SDD, which regimen is most effective, and what types of antimicrobial selection and whether greater antimicrobial resistance will emerge with long-term use of SDD.[38a]

## CONCLUSION

Significant strides have been made in our understanding of nosocomial pneumonia in critically ill and mechanically ventilated patients. Surveillance data are useful for monitoring changes in etiologic agents and the emergence of new

**Table 13–4. Summary of Trials Using Selective Decontamination of the Digestive Tract to Prevent Nosocomial Lower Respiratory Tract Infection**

| Investigation | Antibiotics* Population | Antibiotics* Local | Antibiotics* Systemic | Respiratory Infections Selective Decontamination (%) | Respiratory Infections Control (%) | Respiratory Infections Odds Ratios (95% CI) | Mortality Selective Decontamination (%) | Mortality Control (%) | Mortality Odds Ratios (95% CI) |
|---|---|---|---|---|---|---|---|---|---|
| **Nonrandomized trials** | | | | | | | | | |
| Stoutenbeek[32] | Trauma | PTA | CTX | 5/63 (8) | 35/59 (59) | 0.06 (0.02–0.18) | 0 (0) | 5 (8) | 0.00 |
| Ledingham[33] | ICU | PTA | CTX | 3/163 (2) | 18/161 (11) | 0.15 (0.05–0.55) | 39 (24) | 39 (24) | 0.98 (0.57–1.69) |
| Brun-Buisson[38] | MICU | PNN | None | 7/36 (20) | 11/50 (22) | 0.86 (0.26–2.78) | 8 (22) | 12 (24) | 0.90 (0.29–2.80) |
| Flaherty[37] | CTICU | PGN | None | 1/51 (2) | 5/56 (9) | 0.20 (0.01–1.91) | NR | NR | NR |
| McClelland[157] | SICU | PTA | CTX | 1/15 (7) | 5/12 (42) | 0.10 (0.01–1.25) | 9 (60) | 7 (58) | 1.07 (0.17–6.60) |
| Total | | | | 17/328 (5) | 74/338 (22) | 0.20 (0.11–0.35) | 56 (17) | 63 (19) | 0.90 (0.59–1.36) |
| **Randomized trials** | | | | | | | | | |
| Unertl[35] | ICU | PGA | None | 1/19 (5) | 9/20 (45) | 0.07 (0.01–0.67) | 5 (26) | 6 (30) | 0.83 (0.17–4.15) |
| Kerver[152] | SICU | PTA | CTX | 6/49 (12) | 40/47 (85) | 0.02 (0.01–0.09) | 14 (29) | 15 (32) | 0.85 (0.33–2.23) |
| Ulrich[36] | ICU | PNA | TMP | 7/48 (15) | 26/52 (50) | 0.17 (0.06–0.49) | 15 (31) | 28 (54) | 0.39 (0.16–0.95) |
| Aerdts[158] | ICU | PNA | CTX | 1/17 (6) | 27/39 (69) | 0.03 (0.00–0.24) | 2 (12) | 6 (15) | 0.73 (0.00–4.84) |
| Godard[159] | ICU | CTA | None | 2/97 (2) | 13/84 (15) | 0.11 (0.03–0.56) | 12 (12) | 15 (18) | 0.65 (0.26–1.59) |
| Pugin[34] | SICU | PNV | None | 4/25 (16) | 21/27 (78) | 0.05 (0.01–0.26) | 7 (28) | 7 (26) | 1.11 (0.28–4.48) |
| Gastinne[154] | MICU | CTA | None | 26/220 (12) | 33/225 (15) | 0.78 (0.43–1.40) | 75 (34) | 67 (30) | 1.22 (0.80–1.85) |
| Hammond[153a] | ICU | CTA | CTX | 25/114 (22) | 28/125 (22) | 0.97 (0.51–1.87) | 21 (18) | 21 (17) | 1.12 (0.53–2.29) |
| Cockerill[37a] | ICU | PGN | CTX | 4/75 (5) | 12/75 (16) | 0.30 (0.08–1.06) | 11 (15) | 16 (21) | 0.63 (0.25–1.59) |
| Total | | | | 76/764 (11) | 209/694 (30) | 0.24 (0.18–0.38) | 162 (24) | 181 (26) | 0.92 (0.69–1.22) |
| Combined total | | | | 93/992 (9) | 283/1032 (27) | 0.24 (0.18–0.38) | 216 (23) | 244 (25) | 0.91 (0.72–1.15) |

*PTA, polymyxin, tobramycin, amphotericin B; CTX, cefotaxime; PGA, polymyxin, gentamicin, amphotericin B; PNN, polimixin, neomycin, nalidixic acid; PNA, polymyxin, norfloxacin, amphotericin B; PGN, polymyxin, gentamicin, nystatin; CTA, colistin, tobramycin, amphotericin B; TMP, trimethoprim; PNV, polymyxin, neomycin, vancomycin; ICU, intensive care unit; MICU, medical intensive care unit; SICU, surgical intensive care unit; CTICU, cardiothoracic intensive care unit; NR, not reported.

Modified from Craven DE, Steger KA, Duncan RA: Prevention and control of nosocomial pneumonia. *In* Wenzel RP (ed): Prevention and Control of Nosocomial Infections. Baltimore, Williams & Wilkins, 1993:580–599.

antibiotic-resistant organisms. The judicious use of antibiotics for treatment and prevention is essential in this regard. In the 1990s, we hope that molecular biologic techniques will help to define the mechanisms of colonization and the interactions between nosocomial pathogens and the mechanical, humoral, and cellular pulmonary defenses.

The diagnosis of nosocomial pneumonia remains a major problem in clinical practice, and research is needed to improve noninvasive diagnostic techniques. Guidelines are needed for the cost-effective use of bronchoscopy with BAL or PSB in mechanically ventilated patients. The need for improved inhalation therapy equipment, safer respiratory care devices, and effective use of nutritional support are subjects for further study.

Studies are needed to define appropriate use, type, and duration of antibiotic therapy in critically ill patients. Improved strategies for the management of ARDS and the use of immunotherapy against nosocomial pathogens or host cytokines may reduce patient morbidity and mortality, but further evaluation of selective decontamination strategies must be undertaken before these measures can be recommended. The need for rigorous infection control practices and strategies to reduce cross-contamination cannot be overemphasized.

## ACKNOWLEDGMENT

The authors thank Maria Tetzaguic and Chris Rolitsky for assistance in the preparation of the manuscript.

## REFERENCES

1. Wenzel RP: Hospital-acquired pneumonia: Overview of the current state of the art for prevention and control. Eur J Clin Microbiol Infect Dis 8:56–60, 1989.
2. Craven DE, Kunches LM, Lichtenberg DA, et al: Nosocomial infection and fatality in medical and surgical intensive care unit patients. Arch Intern Med 148:1161–1168, 1988.
3. Torres A, Aznar R, Gatell JM, et al: Incidence, risk, and prognosis factors of nosocomial pneumonia in mechanically ventilated patients. Am Rev Respir Dis 142:523–528, 1990.
4. Celis R, Torres A, Gatell JM, Almela M, Rodriguez-Roisin R, Augusti-Vidal A. Nosocomial pneumonia: A multivariate analysis of risk and prognosis. Chest 93:318–324, 1988.
5. Craven DE, Kunches LM, Kilinsky V, Lichtenberg DA, Make BJ, McCabe WR: Risk factors for pneumonia and fatality in patients receiving continuous mechanical ventilation. Am Rev Respir Dis 133:792–796, 1986.
6. Cross AS, Roupe B: Role of respiratory assistance devices in endemic nosocomial pneumonia. Am J Med 70:681–685, 1981.
7. Haley RW, Hooton TM, Culver DH, et al: Nosocomial infections in US hospitals, 1975–1976: Estimated frequency by selected characteristics of patients. Am J Med 70:947–959, 1981.
8. Fagon JY, Chastre J, Hance AJ, et al: Detection of nosocomial lung infection in ventilated patients: Use of a protected specimen brush and quantitative culture techniques in 147 patients. Am Rev Respir Dis 138:110–116, 1988.
9. Chastre J, Viau F, Brun P, et al: Prospective evaluation of the protected specimen brush for the diagnosis of pulmonary infections in ventilated patients. Am Rev Respir Dis 130:924–929, 1984.
10. Bryant LR, Mobin-Uddin K, Dillon ML, Griffen WO, Ky L: Misdiagnosis of pneumonia in patients needing mechanical respiration. Arch Surg 106:286–288, 1973.
11. Bartlett JG, Faling LJ, Willey S: Quantitative tracheal bacteriologic and cytologic studies in patients with long-term tracheostomies. Chest 74:635–639, 1978.
12. Chastre J, Fagon JY, Soler P, Bornet M, et al: Diagnosis of nosocomial bacterial pneumonia in intubated patients undergoing ventilation: Comparison of the usefulness of bronchoalveolar lavage and the protected specimen brush. Am J Med 85:499–506, 1988.
13. Torres A, De La Bellacasa JP, Xaubet A, et al: Diagnostic value of quantitative cultures of bronchoalveolar lavage and telescoping plugged catheters in mechanically ventilated patients with bacterial pneumonia. Am Rev Respir Dis 140:306–310, 1989.
14. Chauncey JB, Lynch JP III, Hyzy RC, Toews GB: Invasive techniques in the diagnosis of bacterial pneumonia in the intensive care unit. Semin Respir Infect 5:215–225, 1990.
15. Torres A, De La Bellacasa JP, Rodriguez-Roisin R, Jimenez De Anta MT, Agusti-Vidal A: Diagnostic value of telescoping plugged catheters in mechanically ventilated patients with bacterial pneumonia using the Metras catheter. Am Rev Respir Dis 138:117–120, 1988.
16. Meduri GU: Ventilator-associated pneumonia in patients with respiratory failure: A diagnostic approach. Chest 5:1208–1219, 1990.
17. Pugin J, Auckenthaler R, Mili N, Janssens JP, Lew PD, Suter PM: Diagnosis of ventilator-associated pneumonia by bacteriologic analysis of bronchoscopic and nonbronchoscopic "blind" bronchoalveolar lavage fluid. Am Rev Respir Dis 143:1121–1129, 1991.
17a. Meduri GU, Chastre J: The standardization of bronchoscopic techniques for ventilator-associated pneumonia. Chest 102(suppl 1): 5575–5635, 1992.
18. Amberson JB, Aspiration bronchopneumonia. Int Clin 3:126–134, 1937.
19. Huxley EJ, Viroslav J, Gray WR, et al: Pharyngeal aspiration in normal adults and patients with depressed consciousness. Am J Med 64:564–568, 1978.
20. Johanson WG Jr, Pierce AK, Sanford JP, Thomas GD: Nosocomial respiratory infections with gram-negative bacilli: The significance of colonization of the respiratory tract. Ann Intern Med 77:701–706, 1972.
21. Johanson WG, Pierce AK, Sanford JP: Changing pharyngeal bacterial flora of hospitalized patients: Emergence of gram-negative bacilli. N Engl J Med 281:1137–1140, 1969.
22. Deitch EA, Berg R: Bacterial translocation from the gut: A mechanism of infection. J Burn Care Rehabil 8:475, 1987.
23. Atherton ST, White DJ: Stomach as a source of bacteria colonizing respiratory tract during artificial ventilation. Lancet 2:968–969, 1978.
24. Driks MR, Craven DE, Celli BR, et al: Nosocomial pneumonia in intubated patients given sucralfate as compared with antacids or histamine type 2 blockers; The role of gastric colonization. N Engl J Med 317:1376–1382, 1987.
25. Du Moulin GC, Hedley-Whyte J, Paterson DG, Lisbon A: Aspiration of gastric bacteria in antacid-treated patients: A frequent cause of postoperative colonization of the airway. Lancet 1:242–245, 1982.
26. Daschner F, Kappstein I, Engels I, et al: Stress ulcer prophylaxis and ventilation pneumonia: Prevention by antibacterial cytoprotective agents. Infect Control Hosp Epidemiol 9:59–65, 1988.
27. Torres A, Serra-Batlles J, Ros E, et al: Pulmonary aspiration of gastric contents in patients receiving mechanical ventilation: The effect of body position. Ann Intern Med 116:540–543, 1992.
28. Ibanez J, Penafiel A, Raurich J, et al: Gastroesophageal reflux and aspiration of gastric contents during nasogastric feeding: The effect of posture. [Abstract] Intensive Care Med 14(suppl 2):296, 1988.
28a. Inglis TJJ, Sherratt MJ, Sproat LJ, et al: Gastroduodenal dysfunction and bacterial colonization of the ventilated lung. Lancet 341:911–913, 1993.
29. Stevens RM, Teres D, Skillman JJ, et al: Pneumonia in an intensive care unit: A thirty-month experience. Arch Intern Med 134:106–111, 1974.
30. Graybill JR, Marshall LW, Charache P, et al: Nosocomial pneumonia: A continuing major problem. Am Rev Respir Dis 108:1130–1140, 1973.
31. Craven DE, Steger KA, Barber TW: Preventing nosocomial pneumonia: State of the art and perspectives for the 1990's. Am J Med 91(suppl 3B):44S–53S, 1991.
32. Stoutenbeek CP, van Saene HKF, Miranda DR, et al: The effect of selective decontamination of the digestive tract on colonization and infection rate in multiple trauma patients. Intensive Care Med 10:185–192, 1984.
33. Ledingham IM, Alcock SR, Eastaway AT, et al: Triple regimen of selective decontamination of the digestive tract, sytemic cefotaxime, and microbiological surveillance for prevention of acquired infection in intensive care. Lancet 1:785–790, 1988.

34. Pugin J, Auckenthaler R, Lew DP, Suter PM: Oropharyngeal decontamination decreases incidence of ventilator-associated pneumonia: A randomized, placebo-controlled, double-blind clinical trial. JAMA 265:2704–2710, 1991.

35. Unertl K, Ruckdeschel G, Selbmann HK, et al: Prevention of colonization and respiratory infections in long-term ventilated patients by local antimicrobial prophylaxis. Intensive Care Med 13:106–113, 1987.

36. Ulrich C, Harinck-de Weerd JE, Bakker NC, Jacz K, Doornbos L, de Ridder VA: Selective decontamination of the digestive tract with norfloxacin in the prevention of ICU-acquired infections: A prospective randomized study. Intensive Care Med 15:424–431, 1989.

37. Flaherty J, Nathan C, Kabins A, et al: Nonabsorbable antibiotics versus sucralfate in preventing colonization and infection in a cardiac surgery intensive care unit. J Infect Dis 162:1393–1397, 1990.

37a. Cockerill FR, Muller SM, Anhalt JP, et al: Prevention of infection in critically ill patients by selective decontamination of the digestive tract. Ann Intern Med 117:545–553, 1992.

38. Brun-Buisson C, Legrand P, Rauss A, et al: Intestinal decontamination for control of nosocomial multiresistant gram-negative bacilli: Study of an outbreak in an intensive care unit. Ann Intern Med 110:873–881, 1989.

38a. Craven DE: Use of selective decontamination of the digestive tract: Is the light at the end of the tunnel red or green? Ann Intern Med 117:609–611, 1992.

39. Berk SL, Verghese A: Emerging pathogens in nosocomial pneumonia. Eur J Clin Microbiol Infect Dis 8:11–14, 1989.

40. Prod'hom G, Leutenberger P, Koerfer J, et al: Effect of stress ulcer prophylaxis on nosocomial pneumonia in ventilated patients: A randomized comparative study. *In* Program and Abstracts of the 31st Interscience Conference on Antimicrobial Agents and Chemotherapy, Chicago, October 2, 1991. Washington, DC: American Society for Microbiology, 1991:265.

41. Craig CP, Connelly S: Effect of intensive care unit nosocomial pneumonia on duration of stay and mortality. Am J Infect Control 12:233–238, 1984.

42. Bartlett JG, O'Keefe P, Tally FP, Louie TJ, Gorbach SL: Bacteriology of hospital acquired pneumonia. Arch Intern Med 146:868–871, 1986.

42a. Shaberg DR, Culver DH, Gaynes RP: Major trends in the microbial etiology of nosocomial pneumonia. Am J Med 91(suppl 313):725–755, 1991.

43. Jimenez P, Torres A, Rodriguez-Roisin R, et al: Incidence and etiology of pneumonia acquired during mechanical ventilation. Crit Care Med 17:882–885, 1989.

44. Maki DG: Control of colonization and transmission of pathogenic bacteria in the hospital. Ann Intern Med 89:777–780, 1978.

45. Flaherty JP, Weinstein RA: Infection control and pneumonia prophylaxis strategies in the intensive care unit. Semin Respir Infect 5:191–203, 1990.

46. LaForce FM: Lower respiratory tract infections. *In* Bennett JV, Brachman PS (eds): Hospital Infections, ed 3. Boston, MA: Little, Brown, 1992:611–639.

47. Louria DB, Kaminski T: The effects of four antimicrobial drug regimens on sputum superinfection in hospitalized patients. Am Rev Respir Dis 85:649–665, 1962.

48. Rello J, Quintana E, Ausina V, Puzo C, Net A, Prats G: Risk factors for *Staphylococcus aureus* nosocomial pneumonia in critically ill patients. Am Rev Respir Dis 142:1320–1324, 1990.

49. Fagon JY, Chastre J, Domart Y, et al: Nosocomial pneumonia in patients receiving continuous mechanical ventilation: Prospective analysis of 52 episodes with use of a protected specimen brush and quantitative culture techniques. Am Rev Respir Dis 139:877–884, 1989.

50. Broome CV, Goings SAJ, Thacker SB, et al: The Vermont epidemic of legionnaires' disease. Ann Intern Med 90:570–577, 1979.

51. Kirby BD, Synder KM, Meyer RD, et al: Legionnaires' disease: Report of sixty-five nosocomially acquired cases and review of the literature. Medicine (Baltimore) 59:188–205, 1980.

52. Yu VL, Kroboth FJ, Shonnard J, et al: Legionnaires' disease: New clinical perspective from a prospective pneumonia study. Am J Med 73:357–61, 1982.

52a. Blatt SP, Parkinson MD, Pace E, et al: Nosocomial legionnaires' disease: Aspiration as a primary mode of disease acquisition. Am J Med 95:16–22, 1993.

53. Hoffman PC, Dixon RE: Control of influenza in the hospital. Ann Intern Med 87:725–8, 1977.

54. Valenti WM, Hall CB, Douglas RG, et al: Nosocomial viral infections: Epidemiology and significance. Infect Control Hosp Epidemiol 1:33–37, 1979.

55. Hall CB: Nosocomial viral respiratory infections: Perennial weeds on pediatric wards. Am J Med 70:670–676, 1981.

56. Arnow PM, Anderson RL, Mainous PD, et al: Pulmonary aspergillus during hospital renovation. Am Rev Respir Dis 118:49–53, 1978.

57. Witt DJ, Craven DE, McCabe WR: Bacterial infections in adult patients with the acquired immune deficiency syndrome (AIDS) and AIDS-related complex. Am J Med 82:900–906, 1987.

58. Cohn DL. Bacterial pneumonia in the HIV-infected patient. Infect Dis Clin North Am 5:485–507, 1991.

59. Gross PA, Neu HC, Aswapokee P, Van Antwerpen C, et al: Deaths from nosocomial infection: Experience in a university hospital and a community hospital. Am J Med 68:219–223, 1980.

60. Horan T, Culver D, Jarvis W, et al: Pathogens causing nosocomial infections. CDC: Antimicrob Newsletter 5:65–67, 1988.

61. Wenzel RP, Osterman CA, Hunting KJ, Gwaltney JM Jr: Hospital-acquired infections: I. Surveillance in a university hospital. Am J Epidemiol 103:251–260, 1976.

62. Leu HS, Kaiser DL, Mori M, Woolson RF, Wenzel RP: Hospital-acquired pneumonia: Attributable mortality and morbidity. Am J Epidemiol 129:1258–1267, 1989.

63. Garibaldi RA, Britt MR, Coleman ML, Reading JC, Pace NL: Risk factors for postoperative pneumonia. Am J Med 70:677–680, 1981.

64. Craven DE, Driks MR: Pneumonia in the intubated patient. Semin Respir Infect 2:20–33, 1987.

65. Craven DE, Barber TW, Steger KA, Montecalvo MA: Nosocomial pneumonia in the 90's: Update of epidemiology and risk factors. Semin Respir Infect 5:157–172, 1990.

66. Bryan CS, Reynolds KL: Bacteremic nosocomial pneumonia: Analysis of 172 episodes from a single metropolitan area. Am Rev Respir Dis 129:668–671, 1984.

67. Daschner F, Nadjem H, Langmaack H, Sandritter W: Surveillance, prevention and control of hospital-acquired infections: III. Nosocomial infections as cause of death: Retrospective analysis of 1000 autopsy reports. Infection 6:261–265, 1978.

68. Niederman MS: Gram-negative colonization of the respiratory tract: Pathogenesis and clinical consequences. Semin Respir Infect 5:173–184, 1990.

69. Reynolds HY: Bacterial adherence to respiratory tract mucosa: A dynamic interaction leading to colonization. Semin Respir Infect 2:8–19, 1987.

70. Abraham SN, Beachey EH, Simpson WA: Adherence of *Streptococcus pyogenes*, *Escherichia coli*, and *Pseudomonas aeruginosa* to fibronectin-coated and uncoated epithelial cells. Infect Immun 41:1261–1268, 1983.

71. Woods DE, Straus DC, Johanson WG Jr, et al: Role of fibronectin in the prevention of adherence of *Pseudomonas aeruginosa* to buccal cells. J Infect Dis 143:784–790, 1981.

72. Lepper MH, Kofman S, Blatt N, et al: Effect of antibiotics used singly and in combination on the tracheal flora following tracheostomy in poliomyelitis. Antibiot Chemother 4:829–833, 1954.

73. Niederman MS, Merrill WW, Polomski LM, et al: Influence of sputum IgA and elastase on tracheal cell bacterial adherence. Am Rev Respir Dis 133:255–260, 1986.

74. Giannella RA, Broitman SA, Zamcheck N: Influence of gastric acidity on bacterial and parasitic enteric infections: A perspective. Ann Intern Med 78:271–276, 1973.

75. Hornick RB, Music SI, Wenzel R, et al: The broad street pump revisited; response of volunteers to ingested cholera vibrios. Bull N Y Acad Med 47:1181–1191, 1971.

76. Donowitz LG, Page MC, Mileur BL, Guenthner SH: Alteration of normal gastric flora in critical care patients receiving antacid and cimetidine therapy. Infect Control Hosp Epidemiol 7:23–26, 1986.

77. Reusser P, Zimmerli W, Scheidegger D, et al: Role of gastric colonization in nosocomial infections and endotoxemia: A prospective study in neurosurgical patients on mechanical ventilation. J Infect Dis 160:414, 1989.

78. Tryba M: The gastropulmonary route of infection—Fact or fiction? Am J Med 91(suppl 2A):135S–146S, 1991.

79. Gourdin TG, Smith BF, Craven DE: Prevention of stress bleeding in critical care patients: Current concepts on risk and benefit. Perspect Crit Care 2:44–70, 1989.

80. Joshi N, Hamory BH, Localio AR: A predictive model for nosocomial pneumonia in intensive care units. *In* Program and Abstracts of

the 31st Interscience Conference on Antimicrobial Agents and Chemotherapy, Chicago, October 2, 1991. Washington, DC: American Society for Microbiology, 1991:264.

81. Joshi M, Ciesla N, Caplan E: Diagnosis of pneumonia in critically ill patients. [Abstract] Chest 94:4S, 1988.

82. Andrews CP, Coalson JJ, Smith JD, Johanson WG Jr: Diagnosis of nosocomial bacterial pneumonia in acute, diffuse lung injury. Chest 80:254–258, 1981.

83. Bell RC, Coalson JJ, Smith JD, Johanson WG Jr: Multiple organ system failure and infection in adult respiratory distress syndrome. Ann Intern Med 99:293–298, 1983.

84. Cook DJ, Fitzgerald JM, Guyatt GH, Walter S: Evaluation of the protected brush catheter and bronchoalveolar lavage in the diagnosis of nosocomial pneumonia. Intensive Care Med 6:196–205, 1991.

85. Meduri GU, Beals DH, Maijub AG, Baselski V: Protected bronchoalveolar lavage: A new bronchoscopic technique to retrieve uncontaminated distal airway secretions. Am Rev Respir Dis 143:855–864, 1991.

86. Montravers P, Fagon J, Chastre J, et al: Follow up protected specimen brushes to assess treatment in nosocomial pneumonia. Am Rev Respir Dis 147:38–44, 1993.

87. Piperno D, Gaussorgues P, Bachmann P, Jaboulay JM, Robert D: Diagnostic value of nonbronchoscopic bronchoalveolar lavage during mechanical ventilation. Chest 93:223, 1988.

88. Gaussorgues P, Piperno D, Bachmann P, et al: Comparison of non-bronchoscopic bronchoalveolar lavage to open lung biopsy for the bacteriologic diagnosis of pulmonary infections in mechanically ventilated patients. Intensive Care Med 15:94–98, 1989.

89. Nitenberg G, Casetta M, Antoun S, Leclercq B, Escudier B: Comparison of two methods of bacteriologic sampling of the lower respiratory tract in diagnosing nosocomial pneumonia (NP) in intubated patients. In Program and Abstracts of the 31st Interscience Conference on Antimicrobial Agents and Chemotherapy, Chicago, October 2, 1991. Washington, DC: American Society for Microbiology, 1991:255.

90. Pham LH, Brun-Buisson C, Legrand P, et al: Diagnosis of nosocomial pneumonia in mechanically ventilated patients. Am Rev Respir Dis 143:1055–1061, 1991.

91. Pennington JE: Nosocomial respiratory infection. In Mandell GL, Douglas RG Jr, Bennett JE (eds). Principles and Practice of Infectious Diseases, ed 3. New York, Churchill Livingstone, 1990:2199–2204.

92. Bartlett JG: Invasive diagnostic techniques in pulmonary infections. In Pennington JE (ed). Respiratory Infections: Diagnosis and Management, ed 2. New York, Raven Press, 1989:69–96.

93. Wunderink RG: Detection of nosocomial lung infection in ventilated patients. Am Rev Respir Dis 139:1302–1303, 1989.

94. Wunderink RG, Russell J, Mezger E, Adams J, Popovich JC Jr: The diagnostic utility of antibody-coated bacteria test in intubated patients. Am Rev Respir Dis 131:A81, 1985.

95. Lee CT, Fein A, Lippmann M, Holtzmann H, Kimbel P, Weinbaum G: Elastolytic activity in pulmonary lavage fluid from patient with adult respiratory distress syndrome. N Engl J Med 304:192–196, 1981.

96. Ashbaugh DC, Petty TL: Sepsis complicating the acute respiratory distress syndrome. Surg Gynecol Obstet 135:865–868, 1972.

97. Ingram RH Jr, Fanta CH: Respiratory failure. In Rubenstein E, Federman DD (eds). Medicine. New York, Scientific American, 1991:14.1–14.9.

98. Seidenfeld JJ, Pohl DF, Bell RC, Harris GD, Johanson WG Jr: Incidence, site, and outcome of infections in patients with the adult respiratory distress syndrome. Am Rev Respir Dis 134:12–16, 1986.

99. Montgomery AB, Stager MA, Carrico C, Hudson L: Causes of mortality in patients with the adult respiratory distress syndrome. Am Rev Respir Dis 132:485–489, 1985.

100. Pepe PE, Potkin RT, Reus DH, Hudson LD, Carrico CJ: Clinical predictors of adult respiratory distress syndrome. Am J Surg 144:124–130, 1982.

101. Fein A, Lippmann M, Holtzman H, Eliraz A, Goldberg SK: The risk factors, evidence and prognosis of ARDS following septicemia. Chest 83:40–42, 1983.

102. Fowler AA, Hamman RF, Good JT, et al: Adult respiratory distress syndrome: Risk with common predispositions. Ann Intern Med 98:593–597, 1983.

103. Niederman MS, Craven DE, Fein AM, Schultz DE: Pneumonia in the critically ill hospitalized patient. Chest 97:170–181, 1990.

104. Dubaybo BA, Carlson RW: Postinfectious ARDS: Mechanisms of lung injury repair. Crit Care Med 4:229–243, 1988.

105. Weinberg P, Matthay M, Webster R, Roskos K, Goldstein I, Murray J: Biologically active products of complement and acute lung injury in patients with septic syndrome. Am Rev Respir Dis 130:791–796, 1984.

106. Solomkin J, Cotta L, Satoh P, Hurst J, Nelson R: Complement activation and clearance in acute illness and injury: Evidence for C3 as a cell directed mediator of the adult respiratory distress syndrome in man. Surgery 97:668–678, 1985.

107. Langlois P, Gawryl M: Accentuated formation of the terminal C5b-9 complement complex in patient plasma precedes development of the adult respiratory distress syndrome. Am Rev Respir Dis 138:368–375, 1988.

108. Sherry B, Cerami A: Cachectin/tumor necrosis factor exerts endocrine, paracrine, and autocrine control of inflammatory responses. J Cell Biol 107:1269–1277, 1988.

109. LaForce FM: Systemic antimicrobial therapy of nosocomial pneumonia: Monotherapy versus combination therapy. Eur J Clin Microbiol Infect Dis 8:61–68, 1989.

110. Smith CR, Ambinder R, Lipsky JJ, et al: Cefotaxime compared with nafcillin plus tobramycin for serious bacterial infections: A randomized, double-blind trial. Ann Intern Med 101:469–477, 1984.

111. Moore RD, Smith CR, Lietman PS: Association of aminoglycoside plasma levels with therapeutic outcome in gram-negative pneumonia. Am J Med 77:657–662, 1984.

112. Veterans Affairs Total Parenteral Nutrition Cooperative Study Group. Perioperative total parenteral nutrition in surgical patients. N Engl J Med 325:525–532, 1991.

113. Heymsfield SB, Bethel RA, Ansley JD, Nixon DW, Rudman D: Enteral hyperalimentation: An alternative to central venous hyperalimentation. Ann Intern Med 90:63–71, 1979.

114. Pingleton SK: Enteral nutrition as a risk factor for nosocomial pneumonia. Eur J Clin Microbiol Infect Dis 8:51–55, 1989.

115. Pingleton SK, Hinthorn DR, Liu C: Enteral nutrition in patients receiving mechanical ventilation: Multiple sources of tracheal colonization include the stomach. Am J Med 80:827–832, 1986.

116. Montecalvo MA, Steger KA, Farber HW, et al: Nutritional outcome and pneumonia in critical care patients randomized to gastric versus jejunal tube feedings. Crit Care Med 20:1377–1387, 1992.

117. Border J, Hassett J, LaDuca J, et al: The gut origin septic states in blunt multiple trauma (ISS + 40) in the ICU. Ann Surg 206:427–448, 1987.

118. Cheadle WG, Vitale GC, Mackie CR, Cuschieri A: Prophylactic postoperative nasogastric decompression: A prospective study of its requirement and the influence of cimetidine in 200 patients. Ann Surg 202:361–366, 1985.

119. Tryba M: Risk of acute stress bleeding and nosocomial pneumonia in ventilated intensive care unit patients: Sucralfate versus antacids. Am J Med 83(suppl 3B):117–124, 1987.

120. Mahul PH, Auboyer C, Jospe R, et al: Prevention of nosocomial pneumonia (NP) in mechanically ventilated patients: Respective role of mechanical sub-glottic secretions drainage (SSD) and stress ulcer prophylaxis (antacids vs sucralfate). Intensive Care Med 16(suppl 1):S19, 1990.

121. Kappstein I, Friedrich T, Hellinger P, et al: Incidence of pneumonia in mechanically ventilated patients treated with sucralfate or cimetidine as prophylaxis for stress bleeding: Bacterial colonization of the stomach. Am J Med 91(suppl 2A):125–131, 1991.

122. Laggner AN, Lenz K, Graninger W, et al: Stress ulcer prophylaxis in a general intensive care unit: Sucralfate versus ranitidine. Anaesthesist 37:704–710, 1988.

123. Garcia-Labattut A, Rodriguez-Munoz S, Boebernado-Serrano M, et al: Sucralfate versus cimetidine in the stress bleeding prophylaxis. Intensive Care Med 16(suppl 1):S19, 1990.

124. Ryan P, Dawson J, Teres D, Navab F: Continuous infusion of cimetidine vs sucralfate: Incidence of pneumonia and bleeding compared. Crit Care Med 18(suppl 4):S253, 1990.

125. Eddleston JM, Vohra A, Scott P, et al: A comparison of the frequency of stress ulceration and secondary pneumonia in sucralfate- or ranitidine-treated intensive care unit patients. Crit Care Med 19:1491–1496, 1991.

126. Tryba M: Sucralfate versus antacids or H₂-antagonists for stress ulcer prophylaxis: A meta-analysis on efficacy and pneumonia rate. Crit Care Med 19:942–949, 1991.

127. Sottile FD, Marrie TJ, Prough DS, et al: Nosocomial pulmonary

infection: Possible etiologic significance of bacterial adhesion to endotracheal tubes. Crit Care Med 14:265–270, 1986.

128. Inglis TJJ, Millar MR, Jones JG, Robinson DA: Tracheal tube biofilm as a source of bacterial colonization of the lung. J Clin Microbiol 27:2014–2018, 1989.

129. Reinarz JA, Pierce AK, Mays BB, et al: The potential role of inhalation-therapy equipment in nosocomial pulmonary infection. J Clin Invest 44:831–839, 1965.

130. Pierce AK, Sanford JP, Thomas GD, Leonard JS: Long-term evaluation of decontamination of inhalation-therapy equipment and the occurrence of necrotizing pneumonia. N Engl J Med 282:528–531, 1970.

131. Goularte TA, Craven DE: Bacterial colonization of cascade humidifier reservoirs after 24 and 48 hours of continuous mechanical ventilation. Infect Control Hosp Epidemiol 8:200–204, 1987.

132. Craven DE, Goularte TA, Make BJ: Contaminated condensate in mechanical ventilator circuits: A risk factor for nosocomial pneumonia? Am Rev Respir Dis 129:625–628, 1984.

133. Craven DE, Connolly MG Jr, Lichtenberg DA, Primeau PJ, McCabe WR: Contamination of mechanical ventilators with tubing changes every 24 or 48 hours. N Engl J Med 306:1505–1509, 1982.

134. Dreyfuss D, Djedaini K, Weber P, et al: Prospective study of nosocomial pneumonia and of patient and circuit colonization during mechanical ventilation with circuit changes every 48 hours versus no change. Am Rev Respir Dis 143:738–743, 1991.

135. MacIntyre NR, Anderson HR, Silver RM, et al: Pulmonary function in mechanically ventilated patients using 24-hour use of a hydroscopic condenser humidifier. Chest 84:560–564, 1983.

136. Branson RD, Campbell RS, Davis KJ, et al: Humidification in an intensive care unit. Prospective study of a new protocol utilizing heated humidification and a hygroscopic humidifier. Chest 1993 (in press).

137. Misset B, Escudier B, Rivara D, et al: Heat and moisture exchanger versus heated humidifier during long-term mechanical ventilation: A prospective randomized study. Chest 100:160–163, 1991.

138. Suzukawa M, Usuda Y, Numata K: The effects on sputum characteristics of combining an unheated humidifer with a heat-moisture exchanging filter. Respir Care 34:976–984, 1989.

139. Craven DE, Lichtenberg DA, Goularte TA, Make BJ, McCabe WR: Contaminated medication nebulizers in mechanical ventilator circuits: A source of bacterial aerosols. Am J Med 77:834–838, 1984.

140. Weber DJ, Wilson MB, Rutala WA, Thomann CA: Manual ventilation bags as a source for bacterial colonization of intubated patients. Am Rev Respir Dis 4:892–894, 1990.

141. Craven DE, Steger KA: Nosocomial pneumonia in the intubated patient: New concepts on pathogenesis and prevention. Infect Dis Clin North Am 3:843–866, 1989.

142. Deppe SA, Kelly JW, Thoi LL, et al: Incidence of colonization, nosocomial pneumonia, and mortality in critically ill patients using a Trach Care closed-suction system versus an open-suction system: A prospective, randomized study. Crit Care Med 18:1389–1394, 1990.

143. Mayhall CG: The Trach Care closed tracheal suction system: A new medical device to permit tracheal suctioning without interruption of ventilatory assistance. Infect Control Hosp Epidemiol 9:125–126, 1988.

144. Fink MP, Helsmoortel CM, Stein KL, et al: The efficacy of an oscillating bed in the prevention of lower respiratory tract infection in critically ill victims of blunt trauma: A prospective study. Chest 197:132–137, 1990.

144a. Choi SC, Nelson LD: Kinetic therapy in critically ill patients: Combined results based on meta-analysis. J Clin Care 7:57–62, 1992.

145. Haley RW, Culver DH, White JW, Morgan WM, Emori TG: The nationwide nosocomial infection rate: A new need for vital statistics. Am J Epidemiol 121:159–167, 1985.

146. Leclair JM, Freeman J, Sullivan BF, et al: Prevention of nosocomial respiratory syncytial virus infections through compliance with glove and gown isolation precautions. N Engl J Med 317:329–334, 1987.

147. Klein BS, Perloff WH, Maki DG, et al: Reduction of nosocomial infection during pediatric intensive care by protective isolation. N Engl J Med 320:1714–1721, 1989.

148. Maki DG, McCormick RD, Zilz MA, et al: An MRSA outbreak in a SICU during universal precautions: New epidemiology for nosocomial MRSA. *In* Program and Abstracts of the 30th Interscience Conference on Antimicrobial Agents and Chemotherapy, Atlanta, October 21–24, 1990. Washington, DC: American Society for Microbiology, 1990:165.

149. Doebbeling BN, Pfaller MA, Houston AK, Wenzel RP: Removal of nosocomial pathogens from the contaminated glove: Implications for glove reuse and handwashing. Ann Intern Med 109:394–398, 1988.

150. Patterson JE, Vecchio J, Pantelick EL, et al: Association of contaminated gloves with transmission of *Acinetobacter calcoaceticus* var. *anitratus* in an intensive care unit. Am J Med 91:479–483, 1991.

151. Stoutenbeek CP, van Saene HKF, Miranda DR, et al: Nosocomial gram-negative pneumonia in critically ill patients: A 3-year experience with a novel therapeutic regimen. Intensive Care Med 12:419–423, 1986.

152. Kerver AJH, Rommes JH, Mevissen-Verhage EAE, et al: Prevention of colonization and infection in critically ill patients: A prospective randomized study. Crit Care Med 16:1087–1093, 1988.

152a. Selective Decontamination of the Digestive Tract Trialists' Collaborative Group: Meta-analysis of randomised controlled trials of selective decontamination of the digestive tract. BMJ 307:525–532, 1993.

153. Vandenbroucke-Grauls CMJE, Vandenbroucke JP: Effect of selective decontamination of the digestive tract on respiratory tract infections and mortality in the intensive care unit. Lancet 338:859–862, 1991.

153a. Hammond JM, Potgieter PD, Saunders, GL: A double blind study of selective decontamination in intensive care. Lancet 340:5–9, 1992.

154. Gastinne H, Wolff M, Delatour F, Faurisson F, Chevret S: A controlled trial in intensive care units of selective decontamination of the digestive tract with nonabsorbable antibiotics. N Engl J Med 326:594–599, 1992.

155. Craven DE, Steger KA, Duncan RA: Prevention and control of nosocomial pneumonia. *In* Wenzel RP (ed): Prevention and Control of Nosocomial Infections. Baltimore, Williams & Wilkins, 1993:580–599.

156. Sanford JP: Guide to Antimicrobial Therapy 1991. West Bethesda, MD, Antimicrobial Therapy, 1991.

157. McClelland P, Murray AE, Williams PS, et al: Reducing sepsis in severe combined acute renal and respiratory failure by selective decontamination of the digestive tract. Crit Care Med 18:935–939, 1990.

158. Aerdts SJA, van Dalen R, Clasener HAL, Festen J, Van Lier HJJ, Vollaard EJ: Antibiotic prophylaxis of respiratory tract infection in mechanically ventilated patients: A prospective, blinded, randomized trial of the effect of a novel regimen. Chest 100:783–791, 1991.

159. Godard J, Guillaume C, Reverdy ME, et al: Intestinal decontamination in a polyvalent ICU: A double-blind study. Intensive Care Med 16:307–311, 1990.

160. Craven DE, Steger KA, Duncan RA: Preventing nosocomial pneumonia: Strategies for the critical care unit patient. *In* Maki DG (ed). Prevention of Nosocomial Infection in the ICU—Contemporary Management in Critical Care. New York, Churchill Livingstone (in press).

# CHAPTER 14

# Immunocompromised Patients

## NONTRANSPLANT CHEMOTHERAPY IMMUNOSUPPRESSION
M. Patricia Rivera, Kethy M. Jules-Elysee, and Diane E. Stover

## SOLID ORGAN AND BONE MARROW TRANSPLANTATION
Neil A. Ettinger

## NONTRANSPLANT CHEMOTHERAPY IMMUNOSUPPRESSION
M. Patricia Rivera, Kethy M. Jules-Elysee, and Diane E. Stover

There is an expanding immunosuppressed population in whom respiratory illness is common.[1] This group includes patients with solid tumors or hematologic malignancies who are on chemotherapy, recipients of organ transplants, patients on corticosteroid therapy and cytotoxic therapy for nonmalignant diseases, and patients with congenital or acquired immunodeficiencies. This chapter discusses respiratory bacterial, mycobacterial, fungal, viral, and parasitic infections in patients who are immunosuppressed by chemotherapy.

Patients who are immunosuppressed by chemotherapy are a nonhomogeneous group in terms of their susceptibility to infections. Recognition of the general category of the immunologic defect can help predict a likely organism (Table 14–1).[2, 3] Other considerations important in formulating a differential diagnosis include the duration and severity of the immunologic defect and the time the infection occurs after the initial insult. For example, a patient receiving intensive cytotoxic chemotherapy for acute myelogenous leukemia in whom the neutrophil count has dropped below 500/mm³ for many weeks has a substantial risk of developing a fungal pneumonia rather than a viral pulmonary process.[4]

The radiologic pattern helps to focus the differential diagnosis on a subset of likely agents. A distinction is often made between processes localized to a lobe or segment and those that involve multiple lobes bilaterally, commonly described as "diffuse." In patients with infectious processes, segmental or lobar infiltrates favor the diagnosis of bacterial pathogens, and diffuse infiltrates more often suggest opportunistic infections such as *Pneumocystis carinii* (PCP) or cytomegalovirus (CMV) pneumonia.[5] Although the clinician should be acquainted with the typical radiographic presentations of various pulmonary pathogens, she or he should also be aware that pulmonary disorders in the immunocompromised host (ICH) may present with atypical radiographic features (Table 14–2). For example, in a neutropenic leukemic patient, multiple nodules suggest disseminated aspergillosis rather than metastatic disease, or a febrile dyspneic patient who recently underwent a steroid taper may have pneumocystis despite a normal chest radiograph. The latter patient would need more sensitive physiologic tests, such as measurement of the diffusing capacity or a rest and exercise blood gas determination, which would help to detect an interstitial process. A specific etiologic diagnosis may not always be possible in the ICH with pulmonary disease.[6–8] Because of the many variables involved in evaluating the immunosuppressed, the approach to these patients should be individualized but based on the general principles that are outlined here.

### BACTERIAL PNEUMONIAS

The occurrence of bacterial pneumonia in the ICH depends on many factors, including the underlying immuno-

**Table 14–1. Immune Defects Associated With Pulmonary Infections**

| Immune Defect | Examples of Disease | Organisms Commonly Seen |
|---|---|---|
| B-cell defect (decreased quantity or impaired humoral function) | Some lymphoproliferative disorders (especially acute and chronic lymphatic leukemia), multiple myeloma, some drugs (especially corticosteroids, antimetabolites and alkylating agents) | Common: *Streptococcus pneumoniae, Haemophilus influenzae, Pseudomonas aeruginosa,* other gram-negative bacilli<br>Uncommon: *Pneumocystis carinii, Mycoplasma pneumoniae* |
| T-cell defect (impaired cell-mediated immunity) | Some lymphoproliferative disorders (especially Hodgkin disease), renal insufficiency, some drugs (especially corticosteroids) | Common: *P. carinii, Mycobacterium tuberculosis, Cryptococcus* and the pathogenic fungi, herpesviruses, especially cytomegalovirus<br>Uncommon: *Legionella* species, *Nocardia* species |
| Granulocytes defect (decrease in number or impaired function) | Myeloproliferative disorders (especially acute myelogenous leukemia), most chemotherapeutic agents | Common: *Staphylococcus aureus,* gram-negative bacilli, enteric bacilli, opportunistic fungi (especially *Aspergillus*) |

logic defect, duration of the immunocompromised state, and whether the infection is community acquired or nosocomial. Pneumonias in the immunocompetent are commonly caused by *Streptococcus pneumoniae, Haemophilus influenzae,* and less commonly by *Legionella pneumophila* and *Moraxella catarrhalis,* but most bacterial pneumonias in cancer patients are the result of gram-negative organisms, including *Pseudomonas aeruginosa, Escherichia coli, Klebsiella* species, and some gram-positive organisms, especially *Staphylococcus aureus.*[3, 8] *Serratia marcescens, Enterobacter* species, and *Proteus* species occasionally cause pneumonia in these patients.[9] The major risk factors for the common bacterial pneumonias in the ICH include neutropenia, corticosteroid administration, and inadequate pulmonary drainage from obstructing tumor or decreased cough.[3] Patients with globulin defects, such as those with multiple myeloma, have a high incidence of *S. pneumoniae* and *H. influenzae* pneumonias.

Clinical signs and symptoms of pneumonia in the immunocompromised patient may be atypical or absent, especially in the setting of granulocytopenia. Cough is a common finding, but 30% of patients report no cough. Sputum production is seen in fewer than 60% of patients and in patients with absolute neutrophil counts of less than 100/mm³; purulent sputum has been reported in only 8%. The most sensitive sign of bacterial pneumonia, although nonspecific, is fever, which occurs in almost 100% of patients; rales and signs of consolidation occur inconsistently.[10] The

chest radiograph is abnormal for 93% to 97% of patients, and most radiographs show localized infiltrates.[2, 5]

Tachypnea, diastolic hypotension, and an elevated blood urea nitrogen were factors associated with death from community-acquired pneumonia in hospitalized immunocompetent patients.[11] There are no comparable studies of ICH, but the incidence of bacteremia is higher, as is mortality in patients with an absolute neutrophil count of less than 110/mm³ compared with those with higher counts.[10, 12, 13]

Because bacterial pneumonias in the immunocompromised host may progress rapidly, empiric broad-spectrum antibiotic coverage should be initiated as soon as the diagnosis is suspected. An aminoglycoside with a third-generation cephalosporin or an extended-spectrum penicillin (eg, β-lactam) are favored combinations. Imipenem and an aminoglycoside are also acceptable.[14] In patients with renal insufficiency, aztreonam may be substituted for an aminoglycoside, but the known synergistic killing of many bacteria by an aminoglycoside with a third-generation cephalosporin or β-lactam penicillin has not been demonstrated with aztreonam and a β-lactam.

The duration of antibiotic therapy for treatment of bacterial pneumonias is controversial. A 2-week course of parenteral antibiotics may be sufficient in many patients, especially if there is rapid clinical improvement and leukocyte recovery. If neutropenia is prolonged, longer courses may be required.[14]

Protection against bacterial pneumonia by vaccination has not been demonstrated in the ICH, but prophylactic intravenous immune globulin has significantly decreased the number of episodes of pneumonia and other infections in patients with certain immunodeficiency syndromes, including patients with chronic lymphocytic leukemia who develop progressive hypogammaglobulinemia.[15] Similar results have been seen in patients with multiple myeloma and small cell carcinoma of the lung.[16, 17] The optimal dosing regimens, frequency, and its use in other immunocompromised patients requires further study. Prospective controlled clinical trials are required to evaluate the usefulness of growth factors and immunomodulators in the ICH with bacterial and other types of infectious processes.

**Table 14–2. Radiographic Appearance Associated With Pulmonary Infections in the Immunocompromised Host**

| Segmental or Lobar Infiltrates | Cavitation |
|---|---|
| Bacteria<br>Mycobacteria (especially tuberculosis)<br>Fungi (opportunistic and pathogenic) | Bacteria (gram-negative bacilli, anaerobes, *Nocardia, Actinomyces, Legionella*)<br>Atypical mycobacteria<br>Septic emboli (bacterial or fungal) |
| **Diffuse Infiltrates** | **Pleural Effusion** |
| *Pneumocystis carinii*<br>Viral pneumonia<br>*Mycoplasma pneumoniae*<br>*Legionella* species<br>Sepsis (with bacteria or fungi) | Bacteria<br>Tuberculosis<br>Fungi (occasionally) |
| **Hilar or Mediastinal Adenopathy** | **Nodules** |
| Tuberculosis and atypical mycobacteria<br>Pathogenic fungi<br>Cryptococcosis (occasionally) | *Nocardia* and *Actinomyces*<br>Atypical mycobacteria<br>Opportunistic fungi (especially *Aspergillus*) |

## Aspiration Pneumonia

Aspiration pneumonia is a term used to describe anaerobic bacterial infections of the lung and pulmonary disease resulting from aspiration of gastric juice or solid particles. Predisposing factors to aspiration of oropharyngeal or gastric contents include drug ingestion, alcohol-related coma or seizures, general anesthesia, and acute cerebrovascular accidents. Dysphagia related to surgery and radiation therapy for head and neck tumors or to mucositis due to infection, chemotherapy, or radiation therapy places the cancer patient at risk for aspiration.[18]

The acute complications of aspiration include bronchospasm and chemical pneumonitis, which presents with fever, tachypnea, cough, hypoxemia, and leukocytosis. Pulmonary infections after aspiration usually occur days after the acute event. Anaerobes are the most common isolates for out-of-hospital aspiration, but in hospitalized patients, anaerobes, gram-negative bacilli, and *S. aureus* are common.[19]

The diagnosis of infection shortly after aspiration of gastrointestinal contents can be difficult, because fever, leukocytosis, and pulmonary infiltrates can be caused solely by the chemical injury. Persistent fever, radiographic abnormalities, or any other sign of infection after aspiration warrants the prompt use of empiric antibiotic therapy. Because of the polymicrobial nature of aspiration-related pneumonias and the abnormal oral flora of immunosuppressed patients, initial empiric therapy should include at least two antibiotics directed toward coverage of anaerobes, gram-negative bacilli, and *S. aureus.*

## Uncommon Bacterial Pneumonias

### Moraxella catarrhalis

*M. catarrhalis,* formerly known as *Neisseria* or *Branhamella catarrhalis,* is a large, gram-negative diplococcus. Although once considered a nonpathogen, it has been identified as a cause of pulmonary infections in patients on corticosteroids and in those with chronic pulmonary disease, malignancy, diabetes, alcoholism, or gammaglobulin dyscrasias such as multiple myeloma and hypogammaglobulinemia.[20, 21] Respiratory infections have nondistinctive features and may vary from an acute febrile tracheobronchitis to frank bacterial pneumonia to a rapidly deteriorating course leading to death.[21, 22] Diagnosis usually can be made on the basis of Gram stain and culture of a good-quality sputum sample. In one study, when large gram-negative diplococci were seen on the Gram stain, *M. catarrhalis* was cultured 87% of the time.[23] Because as many as 75% of isolates of *M. catarrhalis* produce penicillin β-lactamase, cephalosporins, erythromycin, tetracycline, and trimethoprim-sulfamethoxazole (TMP-SMX) are the antibiotics of choice.[24]

### Legionella

There have been more than 25 species of *Legionella* isolated, and 18 of these have been implicated in human pneumonias.[25] The organism responsible for most cases of legionnaires disease is *L. pneumophila,* which has 12 serogroups. *Legionella* organisms are small, aerobic, gram-negative bacilli that are facultative intracellular pathogens. Because of the branched-chain fatty acids predominating in their cell wall, they are poorly stained by the Gram

method,[26] but the Dieterle silver stain demonstrates the organism in fixed specimens. In the lung, the initial site of bacterial replication is the alveolar macrophage. Its ability to replicate within monocytes corresponds to its virulence,[27] and clearance from the lung requires an intact humoral and cellular immune system.[28]

The reservoir for *Legionella* is water. The organism can be found in fresh water sources, such as lakes and ponds, and in water heaters, air-conditioning cooling towers, humidifiers, and nebulizers with contaminated tap or distilled water. The organism occasionally is found in the soil.

Risk factors associated with legionnaires disease include male sex, age over 50, renal failure requiring dialysis or transplantation, chronic obstructive pulmonary disease, diabetes mellitus, smoking, cancer, and the use of immunosuppressive drugs, including corticosteroids.[29] Sporadic cases and outbreaks (ie, community acquired, nosocomial) have been reported, but immunocompromised patients more commonly acquire infection from a nosocomial source.

The clinical manifestations of legionnaires disease include systemic and pulmonary symptoms. The systemic manifestations of the disease may be accounted for by extrapulmonary infection or toxin release. Although immunosuppressed patients comprise about a third of the reported cases of *L. pneumophila,*[29, 30] few studies have evaluated legionnaires disease in these patients. Saravolatz[31] reported fever and malaise in all the patients in one study, a productive cough in 66%, and hemoptysis in 38%. Relative bradycardia was seen in half of the cases, and mental status abnormalities, especially confusion and disorientation, occurred in 25%. Gastrointestinal complaints were infrequent. Pulmonary signs included scattered rales, rhonchi and small pleural effusions early in the disease, and signs of consolidation as the disease progressed.

Radiographically, the initial unilobar, patchy alveolar infiltrate progresses to a consolidation involving contiguous and noncontiguous areas of the lung and to bilateral infiltrates in 70% of patients.[26] Cavitation is relatively frequent in the ICH,[32] and an expanding nodule in the absence of respiratory symptoms or fever has also been described.[33]

A specific diagnosis of *Legionella* infection can be made by various laboratory techniques. The "gold standard" is culture of the organism from respiratory tract secretions, blood, tissue, or pleural fluid. Immunofluorescent antigen tests (eg, DFA) can detect *Legionella* from clinical specimens quicker than culturing (within 1 to 3 hours), but these tests are serogroup dependent, require expertise to read the slides, and have a sensitivity between 70% and 80%.[34] With the use of polyvalent reagents, the specificity of the DFA is high, but some false-positive reactions do occur. Other rapid methods of diagnoses include the use of monoclonal antibody reagents, which reduces false-positive results; the use of a DNA probe, which has a sensitivity similar to that of the DFA but is only available for detection of *L. pneumophila*; and the use of the urinary antigen, which has serogroup specificity.[35, 36] Indirect immunofluorescent testing for *Legionella* is less helpful in the ICH, because lack of a fourfold rise in titer or a low titer does not rule out the diagnosis.

The treatment of *Legionella* infection requires antibiotics capable of intracellular killing by entering alveolar macrophages. Erythromycin is the mainstay of therapy for *Legionella.*[29] With its use, the mortality rate for ICHs has decreased from 80% to 24%. Although smaller doses are sometimes effective, the recommended dose is 4 g each day for at least 3 weeks to prevent relapse, which has been described in some patients given shorter courses. Rifampin at a dose of 600 mg twice daily in addition to erythromycin has been advocated for use in the immunosuppressed, the critically ill, and those with cavitary disease. Other agents that have been successful in experimental models of *Legionella* pneumonia include doxycycline, TMP-SMX, and the fluoroquinolones, especially ciprofloxacin.[37] In humans, successes and failures[38] with these regimens have been reported, and their efficacy in the ICH is unproven.

### Chlamydia

For many years, the chlamydiae were considered to be viruses; they now are thought to be a special type of bacteria. *Chlamydia psittaci* is acquired from many species of birds, and *Chlamydia trachomatis* and *Chlamydia pneumoniae* (formerly known as TWAR) are transmitted from human to human. It is not known if immunocompromised humans have a higher risk than normal hosts of developing psittacosis, which is acquired by inhaling aerosolized bird excreta contaminated with *C. psittaci.*

Although *C. trachomatis* is a common cause of sexually transmitted disease in adults, several investigations have documented that it is an etiologic agent of pneumonia in immunocompetent and immunocompromised adults.[39, 40] More studies are needed to determine the frequency, mode of acquisition, and etiologic significance of recovering *C. trachomatis* from immunocompromised patients. The severity of disease caused by the chlamydiae seems to correlate with the degree of immunosuppression. Concurrent infection with CMV or Epstein-Barr virus is frequently found.[41] Respiratory infections caused by *C. pneumoniae* have been associated with epidemics of pneumonia among military recruits and college students.

Infection with chlamydial organisms cannot be differentiated clinically from other infections. Fever, chills, pleuritic chest pain, headache, and productive cough may be seen.[42] It is not uncommon to have an episode of pharyngitis followed by the development of lower respiratory tract symptoms several weeks later. Chest radiographs may show subsegmental, segmental, or patchy infiltrates in one or more lobes, and pleural effusions can be seen.[42]

The diagnosis of *Chlamydia* pneumonia can be confirmed only by culture of the organism, which requires special media or serologic testing. Fluorescein-conjugated monoclonal antibodies to *Chlamydia* species[43] and enzyme-linked immunosorbent assays (ELISA)[44] have been useful for detecting the *Chlamydia* antigen. The demonstration of seroconversion, a fourfold rise in the titer, or the presence of IgM antibody suggests recent infection. In the ICH, these tests have limited usefulness, because diagnostic titers often require 3 to 6 weeks, and their sensitivity is unknown. Tetracycline and erythromycin are the most effective drugs for chlamydial species.[45, 46] Ten to 14 days of treatment with 2 g per day of tetracycline or erythromycin is recommended. Doxycycline (100 mg orally twice daily for 2 weeks) should be effective and may be associated with a higher compliance rate. Immunosuppressed patients have a higher fatality rate than immunocompetent patients; in some series, it has been as high as 50%. The higher fatality rate may reflect delayed diagnosis and treatment or coincident morbid infection.[41, 47]

### Nocardia and Actinomyces

*Nocardia* can occur in patients without any serious underlying illnesses, however, ICH are particularly susceptible to this type of infection. The organisms are found in soil and decaying vegetable matter. They are gram-positive, aerobic, partially acid-fast bacilli appearing as beaded, branching filaments.[48] Human infection has a wide geographic distribution and is presumed to occur by inhalation of aerosolized organisms.[48] *Nocardia asteroides, Nocardia brasiliensis,* and *Nocardia caviae* are clinically relevant. *N. asteroides* accounts for 80% of the pulmonary infections. Nocardiae are considered true bacteria by virtue of their structure and reproductive characteristics and their susceptibility to antibiotics.

Serious underlying conditions exist in 50% to 80% of patients with nocardiosis.[48] These conditions most often include defects in cell-mediated immunity, alterations in serum immunoglobulins, and decreases in circulating granulocytes. In animals, T lymphocytes and neutrophils play important roles in the defense against *Nocardia.*[49, 50] The lung is the primary site of infection; other organs commonly involved include the brain, skin, spleen, kidney, liver, bone, and lymph nodes.[48]

After acquisition of this organism, some patients may be completely without symptoms, and others may have only fever.[51, 52] Malaise, dry or productive cough, hemoptysis, or chest pain may develop. The chest pain can be severe and usually is caused by extension of infection to the pleura or, less often, to the pericardium.

There are no diagnostic chest radiographic findings for *Nocardia* infection. Segmental or lobar infiltrates, single or multiple nodules, miliary abscesses, thick-walled cavitary lesions, and lobar pneumonia with bulging fissures have been observed.[53] In one series, half of the patients had unilateral or bilateral pleural effusions and more than one third had hilar or mediastinal adenopathy.[53] Empyema and sinus tract formation with chest wall perforation has also been reported.[54] Because nodular lesions with or without cavitation and upper lobe infiltrates are frequently seen, *Nocardia* infection can mimic aspergillosis and tuberculosis.[51, 52]

Sputum smears and cultures determine a diagnosis in fewer than 30% of cases.[48] If the organism is suspected, all specimens should be examined by Gram and modified acid-fast smears, and cultures should be maintained for an extended time, because it can take several weeks to recognize and speciate colonies of *Nocardia.* Multiple specimens should be obtained, because *Nocardia* colonies can be obscured by other organisms. Although simple colonization and subclinical infection can occur, isolation of *Nocardia* from the sputum of an ICH should always be considered diagnostically significant.[55]

Complement fixation and precipitation tests for *Nocardia* lack specificity, because they often crossreact with other organisms. An ELISA test, which is sensitive and specific, has been developed but is not available clinically.[56]

If an immunocompromised patient has a sputum culture

positive for *Nocardia* and a normal appearing chest radiograph, the skin and central nervous system should be thoroughly evaluated, because a normal-appearing chest x-ray film does not rule out extrapulmonary infection.[51] Treatment should be strongly considered if immunosuppressed drugs have been or are being used, if there are neurologic signs or mental changes, or if subcutaneous nodules are detected and more common pathogens are not isolated.[57]

Sulfonamides are the mainstay of therapy. Sulfisoxazole should be administered at a dose of 6 to 8 g in divided doses. Other alternatives include sulfadiazine, triple sulfonamides, or TMP-SMX. A serum sulfa level of 12 to 15 mg/dL is desirable, and sulfa levels specific to the agent used must be measured and doses adjusted appropriately.[50] If patients cannot tolerate sulfonamides or the agents fail to produce a response, successful treatment has been accomplished with minocycline alone (600 mg/d) or in combination with cefotaxime (12 g/d).[58, 59] In experimental models of infection with *Nocardia,* the combination of amikacin and imipenem was superior to other drug combinations.[60]

Because relapse after cessation of therapy is common, prolonged treatment for at least 6 to 12 months is indicated, and parenteral therapy should be continued for 4 to 8 weeks.[61] Despite effective treatment for nocardiosis, extrathoracic disease, especially with brain abscesses, has a poor prognosis, with a fatality rate as high as 70%.

*Actinomyces,* which belongs to the order, Actinomycetales, that includes *Nocardia,* is a gram-positive, aerobic, branching, filamentous bacillus that rarely causes disease in the ICH. There are four species: *A. israelii, A. naeslundii, A. viscosus* and *A. odontolyticus. A. israelii* is the cause of most human infections. Because it is part of the normal human flora, pulmonary infections are usually caused by aspiration of this organism from the oropharynx. Infections typically are chronic and suppurative and tend to form external sinuses. The treatment is high-dose penicillin, and in penicillin-allergic patients, tetracycline, erythromycin, and clindamycin have been used successfully.[62] After initial intravenous therapy for 2 to 6 weeks, oral antibiotics should be continued for 6 to 12 months to prevent recurrences.

### Rhodococcus equi

*Rhodococcus equi,* previously known as *Corynebacterium equi,* is an aerobic, gram-positive, variably acid-fast, nonmotile, pleomorphic bacillus classified as a diphtheroid.[63] The organism can be isolated from soil, vegetable matter, and animals. A common cause of pneumonia in horses, *R. equi* also can cause disease in humans, usually in the severely immunocompromised. Van Etta and colleagues[63] reviewed 12 cases of human *R. equi* and found that it generally presents as an asymptomatic or minimally symptomatic illness in a patient with a nodular infiltrate, often with cavitation, seen on a chest radiograph. Unlike other diphtheroids, *R. equi* is not sensitive to penicillin, and in vitro, erythromycin is the most potent antibiotic against the organism. Although the optimal duration of treatment is unknown, prolonged therapy seems to be indicated in most cases, because relapse after 8 weeks of antibiotics has been reported.[64]

### Mycoplasma pneumoniae

Although infections with *Mycoplasma pneumoniae* in normal adults are common and relatively mild, severe pulmonary disease has been described in patients with sickle cell anemia,[65] those with profound antibody deficiencies, and those with malignancy.[66] The initial host immune response is production of IgM antibodies, followed by IgA and IgG. Patients with γ-globulin defects may be at higher risk for mycoplasmal infections, because secretory IgA may prevent attachment of *Mycoplasma* to the respiratory epithelium.[67]

Clinical manifestations of infection include headache, fever, myalgias, malaise, and anorexia, followed by sore throat and a dry, protracted cough, which sometimes yields nonpurulent sputum.[68] Although earache is common, bullous myringitis is seen only occasionally. The radiographic findings are variable. Lower lobe patchy or reticular interstitial infiltrates usually are seen. Hilar adenopathy, lobar consolidation, and pleural effusions have been reported less often. The most specific means of diagnosis is culture of the organism from throat swabs or bronchial specimens. Because few laboratories culture for *Mycoplasma,* the most frequent diagnostic study compares paired sera; in the ICH, there may be no antibody response. Cold agglutinin assays may support the diagnosis, but they lack specificity. Because therapeutic decisions must be made before diagnostic titers are achieved, the diagnosis of *Mycoplasma* pneumonia is rarely established, and the patient usually is treated empirically. The antibiotics with proven efficacy are tetracycline and erythromycin, which are equally effective.[68]

## MYCOBACTERIA

The genus *Mycobacterium* includes the tubercle bacilli (ie, *M. tuberculosis, M. bovis*), the Hansen bacillus (*M. leprae*), and the nontuberculous or atypical mycobacteria. All members of the genus are immotile, non–spore-forming, obligate aerobic bacilli. A distinctive feature of the mycobacteria is the high lipid content of their cell walls, which approaches 50% by weight and is responsible for the difficulty in staining them, their acid fastness, and their relative resistance to antibody and complement.

### Mycobacterium tuberculosis

The prevalence of tuberculosis is higher in patients with cancer, particularly in those with lung cancer, head and neck cancers, and lymphoproliferative disorders.[69–71] In patients with lung, head, or neck cancers, tuberculosis typically develops early in the course of the neoplastic disease, and in those with lymphoproliferative diseases, the infection develops when the underlying malignancy is advanced and requires intensive antineoplastic therapy.[72]

In most immunocompromised patients, tuberculosis develops from reactivation of latent infection.[72] The underlying neoplastic disease may be responsible for activation of existing tuberculosis or for increased susceptibility to exogenous, nosocomial infection. Invasion of dormant tuberculous lesions by carcinoma may lead to active infection.[72]

The severe malnutrition and weight loss associated with advanced cancer increase the susceptibility to active infections acquired from exogenous or endogenous sources.

Immunocompromised patients are at increased risk for rapidly progressive pulmonary tuberculosis. In a series of 201 cancer patients with tuberculosis, 9 developed tuberculous pneumonia, which was uniformly fatal.[72] Thirty-four patients in the same series developed disseminated tuberculosis, which killed 91% of them. Patients at greatest risk for developing severe tuberculosis were those receiving antineoplastic therapy at the time mycobacterial infection was diagnosed. Although miliary dissemination occurs in patients with lung cancer, pulmonary infection is the rule.

The differential diagnosis of pulmonary tuberculosis in immunocompromised patients may be broad, depending on the radiographic presentation. Tuberculosis can produce masses or nodules that can mimic cancer or complicate the staging of neoplastic disease.[72, 73] Opportunistic infections such as histoplasmosis, nocardiosis, and cryptococcosis are diagnostic possibilities when tuberculosis presents with nodular infiltrates or solitary cavitary lesions. Although anergy due to underlying disease may interfere with the purified protein derivative (PPD) tuberculin test, it is positive in 60% to 75% of ICHs.[70, 72, 74] To increase sensitivity, tuberculin skin tests should be performed before immunosuppressive therapy is instituted, and a reaction size of 5 mm of induration should be used to define a positive reaction. Pulmonary tuberculosis can be confirmed in most cases by sputum examination. In miliary tuberculosis, sputum cultures are positive for only two thirds of cases and smears for less than a third.[75] In some patients, bronchoscopy may be necessary, and this technique can be highly productive for smear and culture diagnoses.[76, 77] Specimens of sputum obtained immediately after bronchoscopy are also valuable.

There are no controlled studies of the treatment of tuberculosis in immunocompromised patients. Although the combination of isoniazid and rifampin administered for 9 months has been successful in patients with cancer and those who are on corticosteroid therapy,[78] some authorities recommend that a third drug, ethambutol, pyrazinamide, or streptomycin, be added for the first 2 months of therapy with isoniazid and rifampin continued for an additional 7 to 10 months.[79]

Immunocompromised patients with a history of positive tuberculin reactions who are young, have recently converted to tuberculin reactivity, have radiographic evidence of previous tuberculosis, or have a history of inadequately treated tuberculosis should receive chemoprophylaxis with isoniazid (300 mg/d) for 1 year.[80] If prophylaxis was previously administered, another course is not necessary. All other immunocompromised patients with known tuberculin reactivity should be considered for chemoprophylaxis, if they are expected to survive for a prolonged period. Bacillus Calmette-Guérin (BCG), an attenuated vaccine strain of *M. bovis*, which is used in some parts of the world for prophylaxis against tuberculosis, rarely causes serious complications in the normal host but may cause disseminated disease and death in the immunocompromised host.[81, 82] BCG vaccine is not recommended for tuberculosis prophylaxis in the ICH.

## Nontuberculous Mycobacteria

The nontuberculous mycobacteria are widely distributed in nature and easily isolated from environmental sources such as water, soil, dust, aerosols, and wild and domestic animals and birds.[83] Infection is acquired from these environmental sources rather than by person-to-person spread.

The pathogenesis of adult pulmonary disease is obscure. Skin tests suggest that infection occurs in childhood, but active pulmonary disease is rare early in life.

Pulmonary infection with nontuberculous mycobacteria usually arises in patients with previous tuberculosis, chronic obstructive lung disease, bronchiectasis, and chronic lung disease due to pneumoconiosis. Patients with underlying malignancy, particularly those with lung cancer, head and neck cancers, leukemia, or lymphoma are also at increased risk.[70, 71, 84]

Chronic pulmonary disease resembling tuberculosis represents the most important clinical problem associated with nontuberculous mycobacteria, and *M. avium-intracellulare*, *M. kansasii*, and *M. fortuitum* are the most commonly isolated organisms in patients with cancer.[70, 71, 83, 84]

Cell-mediated immune defects related to an underlying malignant disease or iatrogenically induced with immunosuppressive therapy predispose patients to disseminated infection with nontuberculous mycobacteria.[83, 85] Patients with hairy cell leukemia, which is associated with a defect in cell-mediated immunity, are particularly at risk for developing disseminated nontuberculous mycobacterial infections.[86]

Clinical signs and symptoms are nonspecific and include cough, dyspnea, and weight loss. Fever and hemoptysis are less common. The chest radiograph may show nodules, thin-walled cavities in the upper lobes (ie, posterior and apical segments), infiltrates, and intrathoracic adenopathy. The treatment of these organisms in the ICH is generally the same as in the immunocompetent host.

## FUNGI

A useful way to consider pulmonary fungal infections in the ICH is to separate them on the basis of the patient's underlying immunologic defects. Patients with neutropenia as their major immunologic abnormality more commonly develop infections with *Aspergillus*, Mucorales, and *Candida* species. These organisms are called opportunistic fungi because they usually infect only patients with abnormal host defenses to infection. Patients who have primarily T-cell defects, such as those on corticosteroids or with Hodgkin disease, more often develop infections with *Cryptococcus neoformans*, *Histoplasma capsulatum*, *Coccidioides immitis*, and *Blastomyces dermatitidis*. These organisms are called pathogenic fungi because they also infect immunologically normal persons.

## Opportunistic Fungi

Opportunistic fungal species have emerged as a major cause of complicating infection in the ICH. Infections caused by these fungi have proven difficult to diagnose antemortem and to manage effectively. Early diagnosis and treatment may improve the outcome, although the overall prognosis remains poor.

## Aspergillus

*Aspergillus* was first recognized by Michele in 1729, and it was described as a human pathogen by Sluyter in 1847.[87] The fungus is ubiquitous, commonly found in soil, water, and decaying vegetation. Several species of *Aspergillus* can cause disease in humans. *Aspergillus fumigatus* is the most common, with *Aspergillus flavus* an important second.

Besides prolonged granulocytopenia, other risk factors for *Aspergillus* infection include chronic administration of corticosteroids, especially at high doses, antibiotic therapy, chemotherapy, a prior history of *Aspergillus* pneumonia, prosthetic devices, and tissue damage by a prior infection or trauma.[88, 89]

The in vivo defenses against *Aspergillus* infection are thought to be the macrophage and the neutrophil.[90] Normal macrophages ingest and kill *Aspergillus* spores, and normal neutrophils kill mycelia and halt hyphal growth and dissemination. In animal studies, the administration of corticosteroids impairs macrophage lysosomal function, allowing spores to germinate, and induction of neutropenia with nitrogen mustard permits the growth of mycelia.[90]

The most common form of *Aspergillus* infection in the ICH is a rapidly invasive, necrotizing bronchopneumonia or a hemorrhagic infarction because of its propensity for invading blood vessels (Table 14–3). These infections may present with the classic signs and symptoms of acute pulmonary embolus, with pleuritic chest pain, fever, hemoptysis, a friction rub, or a wedge-shaped infiltrate apparent on the chest roentgenograph. Unfortunately, this classic syndrome occurs in fewer than 30% of patients.[87] Often, the only evidence of infection is prolonged fever with noncharacteristic pulmonary infiltrates that fail to respond to antibacterial therapy. Other commonly observed but nonspecific clinical features include dyspnea, nonproductive cough, rales, and bronchospasm. Massive hemoptysis is a rare complication and tends to occur during the stage of bone marrow recovery and cavity formation.[91] The pulmonary manifestations of aspergillosis are listed in Table 14–3.

The chest radiograph appears abnormal in 75% to 100% of patients with invasive pulmonary aspergillosis.[92] The earliest lesions are single or multiple nodules. As the disease progresses, the chest radiograph may show one of three patterns: cavitation of existing nodules; progression and enlargement of the nodules to produce single or multiple areas of homogeneous consolidation, sometimes in the form of "round" pneumonia; or the rapid development of large, wedge-shaped, pleural-based lesions, mimicking pulmonary infarction. Cavitation may occur, and sometimes a distinctive pattern consisting of "air crescents" partly or completely surrounding a central homogeneous mass (ie, mycetoma) develops.

Computed tomographic (CT) scans of the chest can show the CT "halo sign," which consists of a pulmonary mass or nodule surrounded by a halo of attenuation less than the center of the mass but greater than air in the surrounding uninvolved lung. Although this sign is characteristic of *Aspergillus* and can be seen weeks before the chest radiograph appears abnormal, it occurs in only 20% of these patients.[93]

The diagnosis of invasive aspergillosis usually requires a biopsy of the infected tissue. Because the organism is ubiquitous and a common laboratory contaminant, cultures are not specific for invasive disease. However for a patient who is at high risk epidemiologically for this infection, positive cultures of sputum, bronchoalveolar lavage (BAL), or bronchial washings may be a reliable method of diagnosis.[94–96] The success rate of fiberoptic bronchoscopy in establishing the diagnosis of invasive pulmonary aspergillosis is about 50%.[96] Although transbronchial and bronchial biopsy add little to the yield obtained by bronchial washing, brushing, and lavage, it can establish the diagnosis of tissue invasion as opposed to simple colonization in questionable cases. The isolation of *Aspergillus* from surveillance nasal cultures of immunocompromised patients significantly correlates with concurrent or subsequent invasive aspergillosis, but negative results do not exclude the diagnosis.[97] Serologic tests, which include immunodiffusion, precipitin, counterimmunoelectrophoresis, ELISA, and complement fixation tests may be useful for the diagnosis of noninvasive forms of pulmonary aspergillosis but are not reliable for the ICH. Although detection of *Aspergillus* antigenemia by radioimmunoassay has proved to be highly specific and moderately sensitive in controlled, double-blind trials,[98] a simple, reliable test kit is not commercially available.

Amphotericin B is the drug of choice for the treatment of invasive aspergillosis, with dosages in the range of 0.6 to 1.25 mg/kg/d, depending on the severity of infection. By attaching amphotericin B to a liposomal vehicle, higher drug doses can be given with enhanced efficacy and reduced toxicity. When treating systemic fungal infections in neutropenic patients who fail to respond to or cannot tolerate conventional amphotericin B,[99] liposomal amphotericin B is an alternative. The synergistic possibilities of rifampin or 5-fluorocytosine are poorly documented in vivo. Of the azoles, itraconazole appears to be promising in animal studies.[100] There are also reports of success in treating the ICH, but there is considerable hesitancy to use itraconazole in patients with acute invasive disease, because it has a relatively slow onset of action. Surgical resection should be considered for patients with acute aspergillosis who develop hemoptysis or for leukemic patients who need additional chemotherapy or bone marrow transplants and who

Table 14–3. **Clinical Manifestations of Invasive Pulmonary Aspergillosis**

Acute necrotizing bronchopneumonia
  Localized
  Diffuse
Hemorrhagic pulmonary infarction
  Single wedge-shaped infarct
  Single or multiple nodular infarcts
Lung abscess
Lobar pneumonia
Solitary granuloma
Aspergilloma
Invasive tracheobronchitis
Pleural infection

have residual disease, especially with mycetoma after treatment with amphotericin B.

Because more than 90% of cases of invasive disease involve the lungs,[92] infection is thought to occur from inhalation of airborne spores (ie, conidia). Prophylaxis with amphotericin B nasal spray,[101] and isolation of the susceptible patients in units equipped with high-efficiency particulate air (HEPA) filters have been advocated.[102] However, the efficacy of topical amphotericin B is unknown, and isolation units, because of their expense, are not routinely available. Another source of fungal infection may be the proliferation of endogenous organisms. Patients who recover from invasive aspergillus pneumonia may be at risk of developing asymptomatic colonization. With subsequent episodes of granulocytopenia, clinically apparent pneumonia can recur. It might be prudent to start amphotericin B when chemotherapy is begun or no later than the onset of neutropenia in patients with a history of *Aspergillus* pneumonia.

The clearest correlation with survival of patients with invasive aspergillosis seems to be remission of the underlying hematologic malignancy with recovery of functioning neutrophils.[103]

### Mucorales

Mucormycosis or zygomycosis refers to infections produced by fungi of the order Mucorales, which includes *Mucor, Absidia,* and *Rhizopus.* Rhizopus accounts for about 60% of human infections. In tissue, these organisms appear as broad, frequently irregular, nonseptate hyphae that branch at various angles up to 90°. In nature, the hyphae produce large sporangia that liberate sporangiospores into the air; most human infections probably are acquired by inhalation of sporangiospores. The fungi are ubiquitous and distributed worldwide. They are found in soil, foodstuffs (eg, fruit, breads), and dried, decaying leaves.

Mucorales organisms share several common clinical and histologic features with *Aspergillus* species, including a predilection for infecting the lung and vasculature and for extending along natural surfaces, such as nerves and musculofacial planes. Unlike aspergillosis, mucormycosis is uncommon in immunocompromised cancer patients. Predisposing factors include prolonged neutropenia, impaired cell-mediated immunity caused by underlying disease or chemotherapy, corticosteroid therapy, severe burns, diabetes, and renal failure.

The clinical manifestations of mucormycosis include rhinocerebral, gastrointestinal, cutaneous, pulmonary, and disseminated disease; the latter two are more common in the ICH.[104] Regardless of the anatomic site, the characteristic findings of mucormycosis include invasion of vessel walls with subsequent infarction and production of black, necrotic pus.

The radiographic findings of pulmonary mucormycosis include a patchy, nonhomogeneous infiltrate, consolidation, cavitary lesions, solitary nodules, and rarely, pleural effusions and mycetoma.[105] The propensity for Mucoraceae to invade blood vessels explains why massive hemoptysis may complicate pulmonary mucormycosis, particularly in cases of cavitary disease.[106]

As with *Aspergillus* infections, the antemortem diagnosis of mucormycosis is difficult to confirm. Sputum cultures are rarely positive, even in cases of disseminated disease.[104] However, if one of the Mucoraceae is isolated from sputum of the ICH, it should be considered presumptive evidence of invasive disease. Serologic tests are of little value.

The only reliable antifungal therapy for mucormycosis is amphotericin B. For localized pulmonary mucormycosis, the threat of fatal hemoptysis makes surgical resection combined with amphotericin B the preferred therapy whenever surgery is feasible.[107] Response rates in mucormycosis complicating neoplastic disease are less than 10% and they largely depend on early diagnosis, aggressive surgical debridement, remission in the underlying neoplastic disease, and high cumulative doses of amphotericin B.

### Candida

Candidiasis is caused by yeasts of the genus *Candida.* Although *Candida albicans* is the most frequently isolated species from invasive or disseminated infections, there is increasing incidence of *C. tropicalis* and *C. krusei* among immunosuppressed patients.[108] The closely related yeast, *Torulopsis glabrata,* rarely produces pulmonary infections.[109]

*Candida* species are small, oval, thin-walled cells that reproduce by budding or by producing filamentous growth forms. The organisms possess three morphologically distinct forms in tissue: yeast, pseudohyphae, and hyphae (*C. albicans* only).

*Candida* organisms are part of the normal oropharyngeal and gastrointestinal flora and, in the ICH, can cause a variety of infectious syndromes, including mucocutaneous, intravascular device-associated, and disseminated disease. Other conditions that favor the development of visceral *Candida* infection include extensive burns, extensive surgery, and prolonged antibiotic therapy.[108]

In vitro, the neutrophil ingests and kills *C. albicans,* and neutropenia is an important predisposing factor to disseminated candidiasis.[110] Pneumonia can result from the aspiration of infected secretions or, more commonly, by hematogenous dissemination to the lungs. Documented *Candida* pneumonitis is rare, even in severely neutropenic patients. It is reported in fewer than 3% of autopsied cases from major cancer treatment centers.[111] The rarity of pulmonary candidiasis, even in cases of severe neutropenia, is in part attributable to the alveolar macrophage. Compared with neutrophils, macrophage precursors from bone marrow cultures bind more effectively to yeast-phase organisms, maintain fungicidal activity longer in culture, and are more resistant to damage from ingested yeast.[112] Peterson and colleagues showed that, when alveolar macrophages were mixed in vitro with *Candida* blastospores, the organisms that were engulfed by the macrophages failed to produce germ tubes, and after 4 hours of incubation, 93% of the organisms were killed.[113] The efficient removal of *Candida* by the hepatic reticuloendothelial system is another host defense mechanism against *Candida* pneumonia.

There is nothing distinctive about the clinical manifestations of pulmonary candidiasis, and fever is usually the only evidence of infection. Radiographic findings include patchy, bilateral alveolar infiltrates with an interstitial component and patchy, unilateral or bilateral, lobar or segmental densities.[111, 114] Pleural effusions are rare, as are cavitation, intrathoracic adenopathy, and nodular or mass-like opacities. Because pulmonary candidiasis most often occurs by hematogenous dissemination, extrapulmonary involvement is common.

The diagnosis of pulmonary candidiasis should be considered in ICHs with nonspecific pulmonary infiltrates who have repeated, heavy growth of *Candida* in sputum that is otherwise pathogen free.[108] Because the isolation of *Candida* from secretions is extremely common, conclusive diagnosis requires confirmation by a lung biopsy. Although the utility of bronchoscopy and BAL in the diagnosis of pulmonary candidiasis is unknown, two groups have reported that finding large numbers of *Candida* in BAL specimens correlates with the presence of pulmonary candidiasis.[115, 116] Serologic tests are not useful in the diagnosis of pulmonary candidiasis.[108] When *Candida* is isolated from sputum of neutropenic patients at risk for invasive disease, empiric antifungal therapy should be considered only if there is no other cause for the pulmonary infiltrates, if there is progressive or unresponsive disease despite antibiotics, and if the risk of bronchoscopy or open lung biopsy is too high.

The treatment of choice is amphotericin B. The addition of flucytosine should be considered in a patient with *Candida* pneumonia due to hematogenous spread from an infected tricuspid valve or from thrombophlebitis of a large vein. In vitro, the addition of rifampin to amphotericin B does not improve the treatment of *Candida* infection.[117]

### Cryptococcus neoformans

Cryptococcosis is an uncommon cause of fungal pneumonia in patients with cancer. It is commonly associated with defects in cell-mediated immunity, as in patients with the acquired immunodeficiency syndrome (AIDS), those given chronic corticosteroids,[118] and patients with neoplastic diseases such as chronic lymphocytic leukemia, chronic myelogenous leukemia, and Hodgkin disease.[119] *C. neoformans* may cause asymptomatic colonization of the respiratory tract, especially in patients with underlying pulmonary disease, but in the ICH, recovery of the organism usually indicates invasive disease.[120]

The organism is an encapsulated budding yeast that is ubiquitous in a variety of environmental sites, but the most important natural habitat is dried pigeon excreta, in which the fungi do not have a capsule and are small enough to reach the alveoli if inhaled. After *C. neoformans* enters the lung, it acquires a polysaccharide capsule that is capable of reducing leukocytic phagocytosis, a factor that contributes to the pathogenicity of the organism.

Disseminated cryptococcosis, clinically dominated by the occurrence of meningitis, is the most frequent presentation in the immunocompromised patient.[119] Pulmonary involvement may occur in as many as 50% of patients with disseminated infections and typically presents as a miliary or interstitial process, reflecting the secondary spread of infection to the lung.[120] Isolated pulmonary cryptococcosis occurs less frequently in immunocompromised patients and may present as an acute, subacute, or chronic illness. The clinical manifestations, which are usually minimal or ab-

sent, include fever, cough, scanty sputum, hemoptysis, and pleuritic pain.[119] In some patients, acute fulminating cryptococcosis has been reported to initiate acute respiratory distress syndrome (ARDS).

Radiographically, cryptococcal pneumonia usually presents as a single, well-defined mass, 2 to 10 cm in diameter,[121] and it can mimic primary lung cancer. Solitary or multiple nodules or miliary densities may be seen on the chest roentgenograms. Cavitation is uncommon, occurring in only 10% of patients. Intrathoracic adenopathy and pleural effusions are rare and are usually associated with disseminated or advanced disease. Because disease is usually disseminated, cerebrospinal fluid (CSF), urine, and blood cultures, provide an excellent means of diagnosis. During infection, CSF cultures are positive for 61% of patients, as are urine cultures for 27% of patients and blood cultures for 10% to 40% of patients.[119] In patients with localized pulmonary cryptococcosis, sputum cultures are positive for only 20% of patients. The latex agglutination test for cryptococcal polysaccharide antigen is one of the most useful serologic tests for the ICH and has a sensitivity and specificity for invasive *C. neoformans* of more than 90%. If the cryptococcal antigen is detected in serum, the patient should be evaluated for disseminated disease, including a CSF analysis.[118]

Amphotericin B is the mainstay of therapy in immunocompromised patients with pulmonary cryptococcosis. Recommended treatment regimens include a combination of amphotericin B (0.4 mg/kg/d) and flucytosine (150 mg/kg/d) for 4 weeks or amphotericin B alone (0.4–0.6 mg/kg/d) for 1 to 3 months.[122] For cryptococcal meningitis, the combination of low-dose amphotericin B (0.3 mg/kg/d) and flucytosine (150 mg/kg/d) for 6 weeks has been shown to be more effective than amphotericin B alone, and it has fewer side effects.[123] Intraventricular amphotericin B in addition to systemic amphotericin B and flucytosine may improve the outcome of cryptococcal meningitis in cancer patients.[124] The role of azoles, such as fluconazole, has not been defined for the ICH.

The prognosis for disseminated cryptococcal infection in immunocompromised patients is poor. Of 46 patients with cancer and disseminated cryptococcosis, none survived for more than 2 years.[119]

### Pathogenic Fungi

Although the pathogenic fungi can present in acute and chronic forms, disseminated disease is the rule in the ICH. These fungi have occurred sporadically as pathogens in patients with primary T-cell defects, those receiving corticosteroids or other immunosuppressive therapies, those receiving organ transplantation, and those with AIDS.

### Histoplasma capsulatum

Histoplasmosis, a disease of varied clinical and roentgenographic manifestations caused by *H. capsulatum,* is a common and usually self-limited disease. It is endemic in the river valleys of the central and southeastern United States.[120] Disseminated disease is a rare but well-recognized manifestation occurring primarily in patients with impaired cell-mediated immunity.[125] The most common malignancies associated with histoplasmosis are Hodgkin disease, chronic lymphocytic leukemia, and acute lymphocytic leukemia.[120]

*H. capsulatum* is a dimorphic fungus that exists in mycelial forms in nature and in a yeast phase at the body temperature of mammals. The natural habitat of the organism is soil that has a high nitrogen content, and moderate temperatures favor its growth. The infecting agent is an airborne spore, which may be encountered at times in small numbers almost anywhere in heavily endemic areas. Dusty conditions greatly increase the number of airborne spores, and chicken houses, pigeon roosts, hollow trees, and bat-infested caves are notoriously infectious.[126]

Human infection occurs through inhalation exposure, and the lung is the site of primary infection and reinfection.[126] Although exogenous reinfection occurs frequently in endemic areas, endogenous reactivation of latent disease is rare in histoplasmosis.[127]

In the ICH, histoplasmosis is characterized by a progressive illness with evidence of extrapulmonary spread of infection. Clinical manifestations include fever, weight loss, malaise, hepatosplenomegaly, and cough. In disseminated disease, bone marrow cultures have the highest yield, reported to be positive in 75% of patients, followed by urine (40%–70%) and sputum (60%).[127] More than 50% of the blood cultures obtained by the lysis-centrifugation method may be positive.[128] BAL and transbronchial biopsies have disclosed *H. capsulatum* in 25% to 70% of patients, most of whom have AIDS.[128] A diagnosis of fungemia can be established quickly by visualization of the characteristic organisms on the buffy coat of peripheral blood smears after Wright or Geimsa staining. Although no data are available in non-AIDS patients, as many as 30% of the cases of disseminated histoplasmosis in AIDS patients can be diagnosed by this technique.

Radioimmunoassay of the *H. capsulatum* antigen offers a rapid method for diagnosing disseminated histoplasmosis. The antigen can be detected in the blood in 50% and in the urine in 90% of patients with disseminated histoplasmosis.[127] This test could prove particularly useful in the management of patients with disseminated disease because titers fall with effective therapy.

In the immunosuppressed cancer patient with histoplasmosis, therapy with amphotericin B at a total dose of at least 35 mg/kg is indicated.[125] Clinical improvement is expected within the first 2 weeks of therapy.[125] Relapsing infection, which occurs in 5% to 20% of treated cases,[125, 129] is more frequent in patients receiving less than 30 mg/kg of amphotericin, patients with AIDS,[129] those with underlying immunosuppression, endocarditis, or meningitis,[127, 129] and possibly those with adrenal insufficiency.[129] Although ketoconazole may have some value in the management of immunocompetent patients with histoplasmosis, it is not effective in the ICH.[130] Fluconazole and itraconazole are promising for treating *H. capsulatum,* but studies are still in progress. The major use for these drugs ultimately may be for chronic suppressive therapy in patients at risk of relapse.

### Coccidioides immitis

*C. immitis* is a dimorphic fungus endemic in the southwestern United States, northern Mexico, and portions of Central and South America. Most infections that appear outside the endemic zones are thought to be related to recent travel within an endemic area.[131, 132] The fungus grows in nature and on culture media as a mycelium of septate hyphae that produces numerous arthrospores when it matures. The arthrospores are resistant to drying and are highly virulent.[133] Within tissue, the organism takes the form of endosporulating spherules.[133]

Most infections occur in endemic areas by inhalation of arthrospores, and acquisition of coccidioidomycosis is traditionally associated with outdoor activities in which soil is disturbed, such as excavation and farming.[133]

Cell-mediated immunity is the principal host defense mechanism against *C. immitis;* activated macrophages inhibit spherules and kill endospores.[120] Neutrophils have little activity against spherules or endospores. Because *C. immitis* does not colonize tissues, isolation of the fungus signifies active infection.[120]

Disseminated coccidioidomycosis may occur as a complication of the primary illness or as a result of reactivation of latent disease.[133] Dissemination to skin, bone, lymph nodes, or meninges occurs in 30% to 50% of patients with underlying lymphoreticular malignancies or drug-related impairment of cell-mediated immunity.[120, 131, 133] ICHs tend not to have a localized presentation, and the illness commonly presents as a fever of unknown origin.[131, 132] Cellulitis or disseminated verrucous skin lesions may occur. The chest radiograph may be normal or show diffuse reticulonodular or miliary infiltrates, reflecting hematogenous spread.[131, 134] Rare instances of ARDS have been attributed to acute miliary coccidioidomycosis.

The isolation of *C. immitis* from a clinical specimen is the definitive means of establishing a diagnosis. Sputum smears or cultures are positive in only 20% to 30% of patients with pulmonary coccidioidomycosis.[133] Blood cultures may be positive in patients with hematogenous dissemination and usually are associated with a poor prognosis.[132] Fiberoptic bronchoscopy has a diagnostic yield of about 50% for coccidioidal pneumonia, but the yield is lower for a solitary pulmonary nodule.[135] For solitary nodules, percutaneous needle aspiration or open lung biopsy may be required. CSF samples should be examined in all patients with suspected disseminated coccidioidomycosis. Eosinophils in the CSF suggest *C. immitis* infection.[133]

Serologic tests, including tube precipitin and complement fixation, may be of value in the diagnosis and management of coccidioidomycosis, because titers usually fall with successful treatment.[133] Coccidioidin skin tests are not diagnostically helpful in immunosuppressed patients.[133]

Amphotericin B is recommended for the treatment of all forms of coccidioidomycosis in the ICH. Patients with disseminated disease may require a total dose of 30 to 60 mg/kg of amphotericin B before clinical stabilization is achieved.[120] Coccidioidal meningitis requires treatment with intravenous and intrathecal amphotericin B.[133]

### Blastomyces dermatitidis and Paracoccidioides brasiliensis

Blastomycosis and paracoccidioidomycosis, caused by the dimorphic fungi *B. dermatitidis* and *P. brasiliensis,* respectively, have occurred sporadically among immunocompromised patients with impaired cell-mediated immunity.[136–138]

Blastomycosis occurs most commonly in the Western Hemisphere, mainly in the central and southeastern United States, where endemic areas include states surrounding the Mississippi and Ohio Rivers. Paracoccidioidomycosis is found principally in South and Central America and southern Mexico. Unlike histoplasmosis, these organisms may cause disease decades after a patient has left an endemic area.

In blastomycosis and paracoccidioidomycosis, the primary pulmonary infection is acquired by inhalation of spores[137] and may present as a flu-like illness with constitutional symptoms of fever, malaise, fatigue, and weight loss,[137] or as pneumonia associated with pleuritis, cavitation, and intrathoracic adenopathy. Chronic pulmonary blastomycosis is characterized by a systemic illness of 2 to 6 months' duration[139] and single or multiple mass-like pulmonary infiltrates that can mimic primary carcinoma. Sputum production is more pronounced with infection due to *B. dermatitidis* than with other fungi. Dissemination most commonly occurs to skin (ie, large verrucous ulcers with heaped-up edges), bone, and the male genitourinary tract.[139] Progressive pulmonary paracoccidioidomycosis can mimic tuberculosis, but the diagnosis usually can be made by sputum examination. Dissemination to any organ can occur, and chronic, nonhealing, mucocutaneous lesions in the mouth are typical of extrapulmonary dissemination.

The diagnosis of blastomycosis and paracoccidioidomycosis depends on visualization of the fungi on smear, in tissue, or in culture.[120, 139] Precipitin antibodies can occur early in the course of paracoccidioidomycosis, but they can persist for years after successful therapy of the disease and do not indicate current infection. Complement fixation antibodies occur later in the course of the disease, and titers are directly proportional to the severity of the illness.[120]

Ketoconazole has been successful in the treatment of these infections, but severely immunocompromised patients should be treated with 30 to 40 mg/kg of amphotericin B.[120, 139, 140]

### *Sporothrix schenckii*

Sporotrichosis, caused by the dimorphic fungus *S. schenckii*, is a rare infection in patients with impaired cellular immunity.[120] The organism is a common saprophyte of worldwide distribution, but it has rarely been found in the normal human respiratory tract.[141] Most cases of sporotrichosis are fixed cutaneous infections or lymphangitic cutaneous infections.[142] Dissemination to joints, bone, central nervous system, and genitourinary system most commonly occurs in patients with impaired cell-mediated immunity.[120]

Respiratory disease caused by this fungus may result from primary inhalation of spores or as a result of dissemination from cutaneous disease.[142] The usual clinical presentation is that of progressive pneumonitis with or without intrathoracic adenopathy. Fibrocavitary disease strongly resembling tuberculosis may be seen.[142]

The diagnosis of pulmonary sporotrichosis can readily be made by sputum culture, but bronchoscopic or open lung biopsies may be required.[120] Amphotericin B to a total dose of 2 g remains the drug of choice for pulmonary sporotri-

chosis.[143] The efficacy of amphotericin B is greatly improved with the combination of surgical excision.[142]

## VIRUSES

### Herpesviruses

There are six human herpesviruses. These include herpes simplex (HSV) type I and type II, CMV, varicella-zoster virus, Epstein-Barr virus (EBV), and human herpesvirus type VI. Primary infections with these agents occur early in life and are subclinical or associated with self-limited signs and symptoms. After a primary infection, herpesviruses establish a life-long latent infection within the host. Reactivation of these agents may be asymptomatic, as is the case with CMV or EBV, or it may be associated with clinical symptoms, as seen with varicella-zoster virus and HSV. Infections with these viruses are usually well tolerated by immunocompetent persons. In patients who are immunocompromised, especially by virtue of deficiencies in cellular immunity, severe morbidity and mortality can occur during primary infection or reactivation of herpesviruses. Pulmonary diseases due to each of these viruses have been reported with immunodeficiencies; CMV is the most common, and EBV is the least common. Studies suggest that there may be an association between herpesvirus type VI and idiopathic pneumonitis in some immunocompromised patients.[143a]

Diagnosing CMV pneumonia is difficult because the organism is ubiquitous and the clinical findings are nonspecific. Significant clinical pneumonitis appears to be uncommon in ICHs other than those with organ transplants. There have been several autopsy reports of CMV inclusion disease associated with neoplastic disorders.[144, 145] In these series, Hodgkin disease was a common underlying malignancy, and the administration of corticosteroids was a major predisposing factor.[145, 146] Whether these patients had CMV pneumonia is difficult to ascertain. Clinical information is scant, and simultaneous infections with other organisms, especially *P. carinii*, were often found.[145]

Few data are available on treatment of groups other than transplant recipients. The combined use of ganciclovir and intravenous immune globulin has significantly decreased mortality from CMV pneumonia in the bone marrow transplant population.[147] Whether this is true for other immunocompromised populations is unknown.

HSV is a frequent cause of mucocutaneous disease in the ICH, but lung involvement is uncommon. Pulmonary HSV disease varies from tracheobronchitis to pneumonia. HSV may reach the lung from oropharyngeal aspiration of the organism or through disseminated infection with hematogenous spread in the lung. In one study, mucocutaneous lesions occurred in 85% of patients with pulmonary disease; facial, oral, or esophageal herpetic lesions may be clues to the diagnosis.[148] Cough, dyspnea, and fever are common but nonspecific symptoms. Chest radiographs can show focal lesions, which often denote the aspiration of organisms into the lung, and diffuse infiltrates correlate with dissemination and hematogenous spread to the lung.[148]

The diagnosis of pulmonary HSV infection depends on isolation of the organism from respiratory specimens in the absence of contamination from oral or upper airway lesions. Bronchoscopy may suggest the diagnosis if a necrotizing tracheitis is found.[149] Because patients with HSV pneumonia usually have severe immunosuppression, simultaneous infection with other opportunistic organisms is common, found in 50% of patients with HSV pneumonia reported by Ramsey and colleagues.[148]

Acyclovir is the drug of choice for the treatment of herpetic infections. Acyclovir-resistant isolates have been reported in bone marrow allograft recipients and in AIDS patients, but most of these isolates remain susceptible to foscarnet or vidarabine.

Varicella-zoster virus can be manifested as a primary infection, which is most commonly seen in children as chicken pox, or a reactivation of the virus clinically associated with shingles, usually seen in adults. In the ICH, primary or reactivated varicella can be a devastating illness and is associated with hematogenous visceral dissemination in as many as 20% of patients. Although the histologic and cytologic features of varicella pneumonia are identical to HSV, the diagnosis of varicella pneumonia is usually straightforward, because the signs and symptoms usually occur 3 to 7 days after the onset of the characteristic vesicular cutaneous lesions.

Treatment of varicella pneumonia is recommended for immunocompetent and immunocompromised patients because of the high mortality rate. Acyclovir has efficacy in both groups and is preferred over lymphoblastoid interferon or vidarabine because it has the lowest toxicity.[150] Because untreated primary varicella and shingles may rapidly disseminate and cause death in the ICH, prompt treatment is highly recommended. Reducing the level of immunosuppressive therapy may hasten the resolution of lesions and limit dissemination. Several studies have shown postexposure prophylaxis with varicella-zoster immune globulin is highly effective in decreasing morbidity in the ICH.[151]

### Influenza Viruses

Influenza virus types A, B, and C occur in humans. Their differences are based on the antigenic characteristics of nuclear and matrix protein antigens.[152] These viruses are single-stranded RNA viruses with a lipid envelope containing surface hemagglutinin and neuraminidase glycoproteins. Although the major determinant of immunity is antibody against the hemagglutinin glycoprotein, which undergoes antigenic changes periodically, cell-mediated immunity probably plays a role in halting viral shedding and in recovery.

Influenza, which usually presents as an acute respiratory illness manifested by cough, sore throat, fever, and severe myalgias, has not been thoroughly studied in the ICH population. Some centers have reported a higher incidence of influenza A among children with cancer,[153] and others have reported a more prolonged illness[154] and excess mortality[155] among patients with a variety of neoplasms.

In the normal host, influenza can be diagnosed on clinical grounds. In the immunocompromised patient, the spectrum of diagnoses is wide, and laboratory studies must be done to determine a specific diagnosis. Influenza can be isolated from respiratory secretions, pulmonary tissue, or throat cultures within 1 to 3 days after they are obtained. To detect viruses sooner, immunofluorescent techniques can be used with tissue culture or directly in exfoliated nasopharyngeal cells.[156] Diagnostic methods that depend on elevations in serum antibody titers are not reliable in immunosuppressed patients.

Prevention of influenza A and B involves the use of inactivated influenza vaccines. Although the immune responses in ICHs vary, the Centers for Disease Control recommend that such patients receive vaccination.[157] Antiviral treatment with amantadine or rimantadine has beneficial effects on the symptoms of influenza A infections,[158] but the drugs' effectiveness in treating uncomplicated influenza and influenza pneumonia has not been studied in the immunocompromised population.

### Adenovirus

Adenovirus is a double-stranded DNA virus that is ubiquitous. Infection is acquired by inhalation of aerosolized virus, by viral inoculation in conjunctival sacs, or by fecal-oral contamination. Although uncommon, it has been recognized in the immunocompromised population and seems particularly severe in bone marrow and renal transplant patients.[159] In a study reported by Zahradnik and colleagues, 15 immunosuppressed patients who had adenovirus infection were described.[160] Fever was universal. Fatigue, malaise, chills, or night sweats were observed in 80%; respiratory symptoms, which included cough, tachypnea, or dyspnea with hypoxemia, were observed in 72%; bilateral diffuse infiltrates were revealed on the chest radiographs of 75%; and the mortality rate was 60%.

The diagnosis can be made by isolation of the organism in tissue culture from conjunctiva, oropharynx, sputum, urine, or stool. For measurement of serum antibody titers, complement fixation, neutralization ELISA, or radioimmunoassays are available but have limited use in the ICH.[161]

Specific treatment is not available. The live vaccines that have been developed to control this illness in military recruits are unsuitable for use in the ICH. Administration of intravenous γ-globulin containing high titers of a type specific neutralizing antibody may have therapeutic efficacy, but other than one case report, no other data are available.[162]

### Respiratory Syncytial Virus

Respiratory syncytial virus (RSV) is a single-stranded RNA virus and a member of the Paramyxoviridae family. The virus is ubiquitous and annual outbreaks tend to occur in late fall, winter or spring.

RSV infection in immunocompromised children and adults is more severe than in normal hosts, and viral shedding is prolonged.[163] The clinical symptoms include cough, anorexia, tachypnea, chest pain, and fevers.[164] Rhinorrhea (82%), sinusitis (45%), otalgia (36%), sore throat (27%), and otitis media (18%) may occur. One investigator suggested that otitis media or sinusitis concomitant with interstitial pneumonitis in the ICH should alert the physician to the possibility of RSV infection.[165] The physical examination findings are nonspecific, but rales are detected in most patients,[164] and wheezing can be heard in as many as 36% of these patients.[165] Radiographically, bilateral interstitial infiltrates are most commonly seen, but lobar infiltrates and pleural effusions have been described.[164, 165]

The diagnosis in the ICH usually requires laboratory confirmation. Respiratory secretions, throat swabs, or nasopharyngeal washes can be cultured.[166] Virus can be detected from these specimens using a rapid immunofluorescence technique with a sensitivity and specificity of 95%.[167] ELISA techniques and serologic diagnoses are less sensitive in the immunosuppressed patient.

Ribavirin is the treatment of choice for infants hospitalized with lower respiratory tract disease caused by RSV.[168] Its use in the treatment of the ICH has produced inconsistent results.[165, 169, 170] The use of hyperimmune immunoglobulin to RSV shows some promise for treating this infection in the ICH.[165]

## PARASITES

### *Pneumocystis carinii*

*P. carinii* has been recognized since the 1940s as a cause of severe pneumonia in immunosuppressed patients. It was first described in the epidemics of pneumonia among the severely malnourished infants in wartime Europe.[171] Since then, it has occurred in patients with congenital and acquired immunodeficiencies, those with underlying malignancies, organ transplant recipients, and those with nonmalignant diseases receiving immunosuppressive agents or corticosteroids.

The organism is considered global in its distribution, because cases of human disease have been reported on all continents and in all climates. Numerous mammalian species harbor *P. carinii,* including chimpanzees, cats, dogs, mice, rats, cows, horses, sheep, goats, and monkeys. The natural habitat of the organism and the mode of acquisition are not known, although human data support respiratory transmission as an important route of spread. Extensive study of *P. carinii* has been hampered by the inability to grow the organism in vitro. For many years, the organism was thought to be a protozoan parasite, but there is evidence suggesting that *P. carinii* may be a fungus.[172]

Based entirely on morphology, three forms of the organism have been identified. The cyst, approximately 6 to 7 μm in diameter, is the most commonly identified form in human tissue; it stains with methenamine silver nitrate, Gram, Weigert, or toluidine blue. The sporozoite, which is an intracystic structure, is about 1 to 2 μm in diameter and has poorly defined cell membranes. Trophozoites, 2 to 5 μm in diameter, are the free-floating forms of the organism. Although trophozoites are more abundant in tissue, they are often clumped together in masses, and they are difficult to identify because of their amorphous shapes. These organisms are only visible with special stains, such as the Geimsa or Wright stains. The life cycle of these forms has not been correlated with the expression of disease.

Because the serologic studies of normal children have shown that 66% to 100% of those younger than 4 years of age have antibodies to *Pneumocystis,* asymptomatic infection in the normal host appears common.[173] Active disease with pneumonia is thought to occur only when an infected person becomes immunosuppressed months or years after the primary infection. However, studies using monoclonal antibody binding and other techniques to screen postmortem lungs of immunosuppressed patients who died of causes other than pneumonia have failed to detect *P. carinii.*[174, 175] Unless there is some other site for dormant organisms, primary infection and reinfection with a new strain may be important causes for PCP. Reports of person-to-person spread and cluster outbreaks in hospitals suggest that horizontal transmission may occur.[176]

PCP rarely occurs in a patient whose immune function is normal. There was a report of 5 patients within one hospital who were found to have bronchoscopic evidence of PCP without obvious immune defects.[177] Because tissue confirmation from open lung biopsy was not made for any of the patients who underwent the procedure, it remains questionable whether these patients were infected with *Pneumocystis* or recovery of the organism from BAL represented a contaminant from the bronchoscope or the laboratory.

Although B- and T-cell functions are important for the host defense against *Pneumocystis,* intact cellular immunity seems to provide most protection against active disease.[178] Neutrophils do not appear to play an important role in host defense as assessed in vitro or in human experience. Besides the human immunodeficiency virus (HIV)-infected patient, PCP occurs most commonly in children and adults who have underlying malignancies with cell-mediated defects and those who have undergone organ transplantation or are receiving immunosuppressive drugs, especially cyclosporine or corticosteroids. The natural history of PCP is characterized by progressive involvement of the lungs, culminating in death if untreated.

Nonproductive cough, shortness of breath, and fever are the typical symptoms of PCP. Temperature elevations can be low or high and spiking, but rigors are unusual. The clinical course can be subclinical or chronic in HIV-infected patients or rapidly progressive in cancer and transplant patients. The results of examination of the lungs are often normal, but dry rales can be detected. Wheezing and signs of consolidation have been reported, although these findings are unusual. Routine laboratory and radiographic studies do not provide specific information for the diagnosis of PCP. In HIV- and non–HIV-infected patients, the lactate dehydrogenase level is usually abnormal and is considered a sensitive but nonspecific marker for the disease.[179] Arterial blood gases may show normal oxygenation or hypoxemia, which can be quite severe. Measurement of the diffusing capacity or the alveolar-to-arterial oxygen gradient from rest to exercise have been helpful in evaluating HIV-infected patients for *Pneumocystis* infection.[180] In the non-AIDS patient, a normal diffusing capacity and lack of desaturation with exercise virtually rules out PCP as a diagnostic possibility.[181]

The typical radiographic appearance of PCP is one of diffuse bilateral symmetric interstitial infiltrates, which characteristically progress to fluffy alveolar infiltrates as the disease worsens. Solitary and multiple nodules, a miliary pattern, lobar or asymmetric bilateral infiltrates, upper lobe infiltrates, pneumothoraces, and normal chest radiographs have been reported.[182]

The diagnosis of PCP can be established only by demonstrating the organism in the respiratory secretions or body tissues. Although induced sputum has had a high yield for diagnosing PCP in HIV-infected patients, its usefulness in other immunosuppressed populations has been limited to a few centers.[183] Despite using the collection techniques and laboratory methods recommended by these centers, it has been our experience that induced sputum for the diagnosis of PCP in non–HIV-infected adults has a low sensitivity. The high sensitivity of DNA amplification used to detect *Pneumocystis* on induced sputum raises the possibility that this technique, even applied to saliva, may provide an effective means of diagnosing PCP.[184] Bronchoscopic diagnosis is more sensitive than induced sputum, and it remains the procedure of choice for the diagnosis of PCP in the non–HIV-infected patients.

The introduction of BAL has increased the sensitivity for detecting *P. carinii* to over 80% for ICHs[95] and the use of bilateral lavage has an even higher yield.[185] Transbronchial biopsy is a useful adjunct to BAL, and in skilled hands, the frequency of pneumothorax and bleeding is well below 2.5%. Biopsy occasionally shows *Pneumocystis* organisms that were not seen on lavage and vice versa. The decision about whether transbronchial biopsy should be performed depends on the risk of the biopsy procedure and the range of treatable pathogens that are likely to be found. Open lung biopsy is the reference standard for establishing a diagnosis of PCP. Because of the high bronchoscopic yield, open lung biopsy is rarely necessary. Whenever *Pneumocystis* organisms are recognized in respiratory secretions, lung tissue, or other body fluids, active pneumonia should be presumed, and therapy should be initiated.

There are two conventional drugs for the treatment of PCP: TMP-SMX and parenteral pentamidine. Hughes and coworkers performed a controlled study that showed that a 21-day course of intramuscular pentamidine was as effective for pediatric cancer patients as a 14-day course of intravenous TMP-SMX; however, pentamidine was the more toxic drug.[186] Based on this study, TMP-SMX is the drug of choice for non–HIV-infected patients. Some clinicians are reluctant to use TMP-SMX in neutropenic patients because of the possibility of worsening or prolonging the neutropenia. Intravenous pentamidine is a reasonable therapeutic choice in this setting, although it is not clear if TMP-SMX really affects neutropenia. Since Hughes' original study of children, there have been no controlled studies comparing intravenous or oral TMP-SMX with intravenous pentamidine. If a patient does not respond to initial anti-PCP therapy, there are no controlled studies indicating the best approach. Most clinicians switch from TMP-SMX to intravenous pentamidine and vice versa.

Investigational agents such as trimetrexate and difluoromethylornithine have had some efficacy against pneumocystis, but major toxicity, especially with bone marrow suppression, limits their usefulness in the ICH. Some of the newer quinolones show some promise in the treatment of PCP with less toxicity than conventional agents.

In HIV-infected patients with pneumocystis pneumonia and an arterial PaO$_2$ of less than 70 mm Hg on room air, the addition of corticosteroids to anti-PCP agents has decreased the likelihood of respiratory failure, mechanical ventilation, and death.[187] Controlled, randomized trials adding corticosteroids to conventional agents are not available for the non–HIV-infected population, but it has been our experience that adding or increasing corticosteroids in non-AIDS patients with severe PCP is beneficial.

In the late 1970s, Hughes and coworkers showed that effective prophylaxis against PCP could be achieved by administrating TMP (150 mg/m$^2$/d) and SMX (750 mg/m$^2$/d) orally in two daily doses.[188] The team led by Hughes later showed that TMP (150 mg/m$^2$) and SMX (750 mg/m$^2$) in two divided oral doses on 3 consecutive days provided prophylaxis for PCP in children with cancer that was as effective as 7 days each week.[189] Based on these studies, oral TMP-SMX is considered to have a high degree of efficacy in preventing PCP and should be the regimen of choice for patients who are at risk for developing the disease, including cancer patients with cell-mediated defects, organ transplant patients, and those with solid tumors who are on high doses of corticosteroids.[190, 191] The use of aerosolized pentamidine and oral agents such as dapsone alone or in combination with trimethoprim have been effective and well tolerated in HIV-infected patients. There are no studies of other immunosuppressed patient populations.

## Other Parasites

*Strongyloides stercoralis* is an organism that can cause a spectrum of clinical disease, ranging from asymptomatic autoinfection to symptomatic multiple-organ spread of disease.[192] The latter condition is called the "hyperinfection syndrome" and should be anticipated in patients who have been exposed to *Strongyloides* infection and then develop illness or receive treatment that affects helper T-cell function.[193, 194] People do not have to be in an endemic area to develop the disease, because the carrier state can last for many years.

Infection is initiated by skin penetration of the filariform larvae, which migrate through the venous blood system into the right side of the heart. From the pulmonary vessels, they penetrate intact tissue into the alveoli. To infect the immunocompetent host, the larvae must first transform in the soil or feces to the infective type. In the ICH, the rhabditiform larvae can transform into filariform larvae within the bowel and penetrate its wall, migrating through the circulation into the alveolar spaces to produce pneumonia. The pneumonia produced can be of two types. An eosinophilic pneumonia can occur with cough, wheezing, and diffuse infiltrates seen on the chest radiographs; there is usually peripheral eosinophilia. This pattern of infection is self-limited. The hyperinfection syndrome usually occurs in the immunosuppressed patient and is accompanied by severe and progressive pulmonary disease, usually caused by a large number of filariform larvae and accompanying bacteria from the bowel.

Although the pulmonary signs and symptoms of disseminated strongyloidiasis are nonspecific, the diagnosis should be entertained for an immunosuppressed patient who comes from an endemic area and develops vague abdominal symptoms of pain, diffuse tenderness, or distention and then develops pneumonia. Pulmonary infiltrates may be focal at first, but they usually progress to diffuse bilateral infiltrates. Blood cultures may be positive for one or more bacteria of the gut flora. The diagnosis is made by demonstrating the filariform larvae in sputum or other respiratory tract speci-

## CHEST RADIOGRAPHIC PRESENTATION

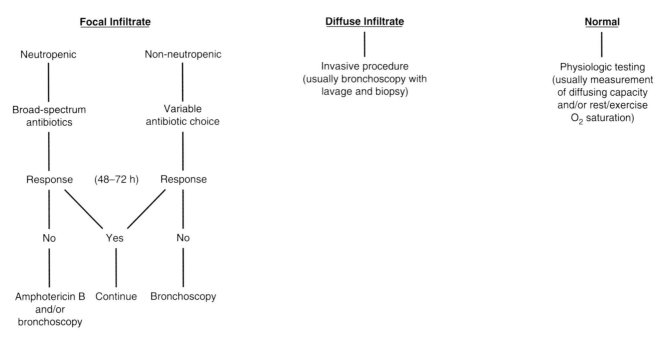

**Figure 14–1.** Management schema for the immunocompromised host suspected of having a pulmonary infection.

mens, especially BAL. The larvae may be found in feces and CSF if meningitis occurs. The value of serologic testing in the immunocompromised patient is unknown.

Standard therapy for gastrointestinal strongyloidiasis is thiabendazole (25 mg/kg orally), administered twice daily for 2 days. For the hyperinfection syndrome with pneumonia or central nervous system involvement the duration should be lengthened to between 10 and 14 days; the optimal treatment time is unknown. If sputum is positive for filariform larvae, it should be monitored after treatment is discontinued to ensure the conversion to a negative status remains. If a patient is receiving corticosteroids while hyperinfection syndrome occurs, it may be wise to taper the drug as soon as possible. If an infection with *Strongyloides* is proven or highly suspected before immunosuppression is started, treatment with thiabendazole (25 mg/kg twice daily for 2 days) should be given.

In our experience, toxoplasmosis is an uncommon cause of pulmonary infiltrates in the ICH. When it does occur, it is usually in the setting of HIV infection or organ transplantation.

## CONCLUSIONS

Although the spectrum of infectious pathogens that occur in the lungs of immunocompromised patients is quite broad, a general strategy for management of these patients is possible. Recognition of the underlying disease with its accompanying immunologic defect, consideration of the presenting radiologic pattern, and the timing of the pulmonary disease in the patient's illness can often narrow the differential diagnosis of infectious pulmonary pathogens. Depending on the clinical setting, this may mean initiating

empiric antibiotic therapy or proceeding to an invasive procedure. A schema illustrating these diagnostic and therapeutic options appear in Figure 14–1.

Developments in analyzing blood and urine specimens for evidence of infectious diseases are likely to decrease the reliance on empiric forms of treatment. Newer therapies, particularly for fungal and viral infections, will broaden the potential therapeutic options available to the clinician and necessitate more specific diagnoses. The development of growth factors and immunomodulators may provide effective methods for augmenting the host defenses against infectious diseases, and advances in effective methods of prophylaxis may prevent many of the infectious diseases that now plague the ICH.

## REFERENCES

1. Rosenow EC, Wilson WR, Cockerill FR: Pulmonary disease in the immunocompromised host. Mayo Clin Proc 60:473, 1985.
2. Singer C, Armstrong D, Rosen PP, et al: Diffuse pulmonary infiltrates in immunocompromised patients: Prospective study of 80 cases. Am J Med 66:110, 1979.
3. Matthay RA, Greene WH: Pulmonary infections in the immunocompromised patient. Med Clin North Am 64:529, 1980.
4. Pizzo PA, Robichaud KJ, Gill FA, et al: Empiric antibiotic and antifungal therapy for cancer patients with prolonged fever and granulocytopenia. Am J Med 72:101, 1982.
5. Tenholder MF, Hooper RG: Pulmonary infiltrates in leukemia. Chest 78:468, 1980.
6. Canham EM, Kennedy TC, Merrick TA: Unexplained pulmonary infiltrates in the immunocompromised patient: An invasive investigation in a consecutive series. Cancer 52:325, 1983.
7. Cockerill FR, Wilson WR, Carpenter HA, et al: Open lung biopsy in immunocompromised patients. Arch Intern Med 145:1398, 1985.
8. Polsky B, Armstrong D: Infectious complications of neoplastic disease. Am J Infect Control 13:199, 1985.
9. Valdivieso M, Gil-Extremera B, Zornoza J, et al: Gram-negative

bacillary pneumonia in the compromised host. Medicine (Baltimore) 56:241, 1977.

10. Sickles EA, Young VM, Greene WH, et al: Pneumonia in acute leukemia. Ann Intern Med 79:528, 1973.

11. Farr BM, Sloman AJ, Fisch MJ: Predicting death in patients hospitalized for community acquired pneumonia. Ann Intern Med 115:428, 1991.

12. Sickles EA, Greene WH, Wiernik PH: Clinical presentation of infection in granulocytopenic patients. Arch Intern Med 135:715, 1975.

13. Singer C, Kaplan MH, Armstrong D: Bacteremia and fungemia complicating neoplastic disease: A study of 364 cases. Am J Med 62:731, 1977.

14. Lynch JP: Managing pulmonary infiltrates in immunocompromised patients. J Respir Dis 9:11, 1988.

15. Chapel HM, Bunch C: Mechanisms of infection in chronic lymphocytic leukemia. Semin Hematol 24:291, 1987.

16. Schedel I: Application of immunoglobulin preparations in multiple myeloma. *In* A Morell, UE Nydeger (eds): Clinical Use of Intravenous Immunoglobulins. New York, Academic Press, 1986:123.

17. Schmidt RE, Hartlapp JH, Niese D, et al: Reduction of infection frequency by intravenous gammaglobulins during intensive induction therapy for small cell carcinoma of the lung. Infection 12:167, 1984.

18. Logemann J: Aspiration in head and neck surgical patients. Ann Otol Rhinol Laryngol 94:373, 1985.

19. Rotstein C, Cummings K, Nicolaou A, et al: Nosocomial infection rates at an oncology center. Infect Control Hosp Epidemiol 9:13, 1988.

20. Slevin NJ, Aitken J, Thornley PE: Clinical and microbiological features of *Branhamella catarrhalis* bronchopulmonary infections. Lancet 1:782, 1984.

21. Diamond LA, Lorber B: *Branhamella catarrhalis* pneumonia and immunoglobulin abnormalities: A new association. Am Rev Respir Dis 129:876, 1984.

22. McNeely DJ, Kitchens CS, Kluge RM: Fatal *Neisseria* (*Branhamella*) *catarrhalis* pneumonia in an immunodeficient host. Am Rev Respir Dis 114:399, 1976.

23. Nicotra B, Rivera M, Luman I, et al: *Branhamella catarrhalis* as a lower respiratory tract pathogen in patients with chronic lung disease. Arch Intern Med 146:890, 1986.

24. Doern CV, Siebers KG, Hallick LM, et al. Antibiotic susceptibility of beta-lactamase-producing strains of *Branhamella* (*Neisseria*) *catarrhalis*. Antimicrob Agents Chemother 17:24, 1980.

25. Fang GD, Yu VL, Vickers RM: Disease due to the Legionellaceae (other than *Legionella pneumophila*): Historical, microbiological, clinical, and epidemiological review. Medicine (Baltimore) 68:116, 1989.

26. Carrington CB: Pathology of legionnaires' disease. Ann Intern Med 90:496, 1979.

27. Jacobs RF, Locksley RM, Wilson CB, et al: Interaction of primate alveolar macrophages and *Legionella pneumophilia*. J Clin Invest 73:1515, 1984.

28. Finegold SM: Legionnaires' disease—Still with us. N Engl J Med 318:571, 1988.

29. Kirby BD, Snyder KM, Meyer RD, et al: Legionnaires' disease: report of sixty-five nosocomially acquired cases and review of the literature. Medicine (Baltimore) 59:188, 1980.

30. Helms CM, Viner JP, Weisenburger DD, et al: Sporadic legionnaires' disease: Clinical observations on 87 nosocomial and community-acquired cases. Am J Med Sci 288:2, 1984.

31. Saravolatz LD, Burch KH, Fisher E, et al: The compromised host and legionnaires' disease. Ann Intern Med 90:533, 1979.

32. Meyer RD, Edelstein PH, Kirby BD, et al: Legionnaires disease. Unusual clinical and laboratory features. Ann Intern Med 93:240, 1980.

33. Ellis AR, Mayers DL, Martone WJ, et al: Rapidly expanding pulmonary nodule caused by Pittsburgh pneumonia agent. JAMA 245:1558, 1981.

34. Winn WC, Cherry WB, Frank RO, et al: Direct immunofluorescent detection of *Legionella pneumophila* in respiratory specimens. J Clin Microbiol 11:59, 1980.

35. Kohorst WR, Schonfeld SA, Macklin JE, et al: Rapid diagnosis of legionnaires' disease by bronchoalveolar lavage. Chest 84:186, 1983.

36. Edelstein PH, Meyer RD: *Legionella* pneumonias. *In* Pennington JE (ed): Respiratory Infections: Diagnosis and Management. New York, Raven Press, 1988:381.

37. Edelstein PH, Calarco K, Yasui VK: Antimicrobial therapy of experimentally induced legionnaire's disease in guinea pigs. Am Rev Respir Dis 130:849, 1984.

38. Kurz RW, Graninger W, Egger TP, et al: Failure of treatment of *Legionella* pneumonia with ciprofloxacin. [Letter] J Antimicrob Chemother 22:389, 1988.

39. Komaroff AL, Aronson MD, Schachter J: *Chlamydia trachomatis* infection in adults with community acquired pneumonia. JAMA 245:1319, 1981.

40. Samra A, Pik A, Guidetti SA, et al: Severe *Chlamydia trachomatis* pneumonia in a patient with immune deficiency. Arch Intern Med 148:1345, 1988.

41. Meyers JD, Hackman RC, Stamm WE: *Chlamydia trachomatis* infection as a cause of pneumonia after human marrow transplantation. Transplantation 36:130, 1983.

42. Marrie TJ, Grayston JT, Wang SP, et al: Pneumonia associated with the TWAR strain of *Chlamydia*. Ann Intern Med 106:507, 1987.

43. Nowinski RC, Tam MR, Goldstein LC, et al: Monoclonal antibodies for diagnosis of infectious diseases in humans. Science 219:637, 1983.

44. Hammerschlag MR, Roblin PM, Cummings C, et al: Comparison of enzyme immunoassay and culture for diagnosis of chlamydial conjunctivitis and respiratory infections in infants. J Clin Microbiol 25:2306, 1987.

45. Beem MO, Saxon E, Tipple MA: Treatment of chlamydial pneumonia of infancy. Pediatrics 63:198, 1979.

46. Centers for Disease Control: *Chlamydia trachomatis* infections: Policy guidelines for prevention and control. Washington, DC, U.S. Department of Health and Human Services, August 1985:1.

47. Shaffner W, Drutz DJ, Duncan GW, et al: The clinical spectrum of endemic psittacosis. Arch Intern Med 119:433, 1967.

48. Palmer DL, Harvey RL, Wheeler JK: Diagnostic and therapeutic considerations in *Nocardia asteroides* infection. Medicine (Baltimore) 53:391, 1974.

49. Beaman BL, Black C: Interaction of *Nocardia asteroides* in BALB/c mice: Modulation of macrophage function, enzyme activity and the induction of immunologically specific T-cell bactericidal activity. Curr Top Microbiol Immunol 122:138, 1985.

50. Filice GA, Niewoehner DE: Contribution of neutrophils and cell-mediated immunity to control of *Nocardia asteroides* in murine lungs. J Infect Dis 156:113, 1987.

51. Frazier AR, Rosenow EC III, Roberts GD: Nocardiosis—A review of 25 cases occurring during 24 months. Mayo Clin Proc 50:657, 1975.

52. Krick JA, Stinson EB, Remington JS: *Nocardia* infection in heart transplant patients. Ann Intern Med 82:18, 1975.

53. Feigin DS: Nocardiosis of the lung: Chest radiographic findings in 21 cases. Radiology 159:9, 1986.

54. Balikian JP, Herman PG, Kopit S: Pulmonary nocardiosis. Radiology 126:569, 1978.

55. Simpson GL, Stinson EB, Egger MJ, et al: Nocardial infections in the immunocompromised host: A detailed study in a defined population. Rev Infect Dis 3:492, 1981.

56. Angeles AM, Sugar AM: Rapid diagnosis of nocardiosis with an enzyme immunoassay. J Infect Dis 155:292, 1987.

57. Young LS, Armstrong D, Blevins A, et al: *Nocardia asteroides* infection complicating neoplastic disease. Am J Med 50:356, 1971.

58. Petersen EA, Nash ML, Mammana RB, et al: Minocycline treatment of pulmonary nocardiosis. JAMA 250:930, 1983.

59. Fried J, Hinthorn D, Ralstin J, et al: Cure of brain abscess caused by *Nocardia asteroides* resistant to multiple antibiotics. South Med J 81:412, 1988.

60. Gombert ME, Aulicino TM, du Bouchet L, et al: Therapy of experimental cerebral nocardiosis with imipenem, amikacin, trimethoprim-sulfamethoxazole, and minocycline. Antimicrob Agents Chemother 30:270, 1986.

61. Jonsson S, Wallace RJ, Hull SI, et al: Recurrent *Nocardia* pneumonia in an adult with chronic granulomatous disease. Am Rev Respir Dis 133:932, 1986.

62. Peabody JW, Seabury JH: Actinomycosis and nocardiosis. A review of basic differences in therapy. Am J Med 28:99, 1960.

63. Van Etta LL, Filice GA, Ferguson RM, et al: *Corynebacterium equi*: A review of 12 cases of human infection. Rev Infect Dis 5:1012, 1983.

64. Williams GD, Flanigan WJ, Campbell GS: Surgical management of localized thoracic infections in immunosuppressed patients. Ann Thorac Surg 12:471, 1971.

65. Schulman ST, Bartlett J, Clyde WA Jr, et al: The unusual severity of mycoplasmal pneumonia in children with sickle-cell disease. N Engl J Med 287:164, 1972.

66. Perez CR, Leigh MW: *Mycoplasma pneumoniae* as the causative agent for pneumonia in the immunocompromised host. Chest 100:860, 1991.

67. Roifman CM, Rao CP, Lederman HM, et al: Increased susceptibility to mycoplasma infection in patients with hypogammaglobulinemia. Am J Med 80:590, 1986.

68. Murray HW, Masur H, Senterfit LB, et al: The protean manifestations of *Mycoplasma pneumoniae* infection in adults. Am J Med 58:229, 1975.

69. Gapalakrishnan P, Miller JE, McLaughlin JS: Pulmonary tuberculosis and coexisting carcinoma. A 10 year experience and review of the literature. Am Surg 41:405, 1975.

70. Feld R, Bodey GP, Groschel D: Mycobacteriosis in patients with malignant disease. Arch Intern Med 136:67, 1976.

71. Ortbals DW, Marr JJ: A comparative study of tuberculosis and other mycobacterial infections and their associations with malignancy. Am Rev Respir Dis 117:39, 1978.

72. Kaplan MH, Armstrong D, Rosen P: Tuberculosis complicating neoplastic disease. Cancer 33:850, 1974.

73. Pitlik SD, Fainstein V, Bodey GP: Tuberculosis mimicking cancer— A reminder. Am J Med 76:822, 1984.

74. Sahn SA, Lahshminarayan S: Tuberculosis after corticosteroid therapy. Br J Dis Chest 70:195, 1976.

75. Munt PW: Miliary tuberculosis in the chemotherapy era: With a clinical review of 69 American adults. Medicine (Baltimore) 51:139, 1971.

76. Willcox PA, Benatar SR, Potgieter PD: Use of the flexible fiberoptic bronchoscope in diagnosis of sputum-negative pulmonary tuberculosis. Thorax 37:598, 1987.

77. Sarkar SK, Sharma TN, Puroket SD, et al: The diagnostic value of routine culture of bronchial washings in tuberculosis. Br J Dis Chest 76:358, 1982.

78. Dutt AK, Moers D, Stead W: Short-course chemotherapy of tuberculosis in patients with associated disease. Chest 78(suppl):514, 1988.

79. Kuritzkes DR, Simon HB: Pneumonia due to *M. tuberculosis* and to atypical mycobacteria. *In* Shelhammer J, Pizzo PA, Parrillo JE, Masur H (eds): Respiratory Diseases in the Immunosuppressed Host. Philadelphia, JB Lippincott, 1991:312.

80. American Thoracic Society: Treatment of tuberculosis and tuberculosis infection in adults and children. Am Rev Respir Dis 134:355, 1986.

81. Aungst CW, Sokal JE, Jager BV: Complications of BCG vaccination in neoplastic disease. Ann Intern Med 82:666, 1975.

82. Hon JK, Hammer RW, Bailey WC, et al: Metastatic melanoma complicated by disseminated BCG. South Med J 75:1263, 1982.

83. Wolinsky E: Nontuberculous mycobacteria and associated diseases. Am Rev Respir Dis 119:107, 1979.

84. Rolston KVI, Jones PG, Fainstein V, et al: Pulmonary disease caused by rapidly growing mycobacteria in patients with cancer. Chest 87:503, 1985.

85. Horsburgh CR Jr, Mason UG III, Farhi DC, et al: DIsseminated infection with *Mycobacterium avium-intracellulare*. A report of 13 cases and a review of the literature. Medicine (Baltimore) 64:36, 1985.

86. Bennet C, Vardiman J, Golomb HM: Disseminated atypical mycobacterial infection in patients with hairy cell leukemia. Am J Med 80:891, 1986.

87. Bodey GP, Vartinarian S: Aspergillosis. Eur J Clin Microbiol Infect Dis 8:413, 1983.

88. Schwartz R, Mackintosh F, Schrier S, et al: Multivariate analysis of factors associated with invasive fungal disease during remission induction therapy for acute myelogenous leukemia. Cancer 53:411, 1984.

89. Gerson SL, Talbot G, Hurwitz S, et al: Prolonged granulocytopenia: The major risk factor for invasive pulmonary aspergillosis in patients with acute leukemia. Ann Intern Med 100:345, 1984.

90. Schaffer A, Douglas H, Braude A: Selective protection against conidia by mononuclear macrophages and resistance to *Aspergillus*. J Clin Invest 69:617, 1982.

91. Albelda SM, Talbot GH, Gerson SL, et al: Pulmonary consolidation and massive hemoptysis in invasive pulmonary aspergillosis. Influence of bone marrow recovery in patients with acute leukemia. Am Rev Respir Dis 131:115, 1985.

92. Pennington JE: Aspergillosis pneumonia in hematologic malignancy. Improvements in diagnosis and therapy. Arch Intern Med 137:769, 1977.

93. Kulhman JE, Fishman EK, Siegelman SS: Invasive pulmonary aspergillosis in acute leukemia: Characteristic findings on CT. The CT halo sign, and the role of CT in early diagnosis. Radiology 157:611, 1985.

94. Yu VL, Muder RR, Poorsattar A: Significance of isolation of *Aspergillus* from the respiratory tract in diagnosis of invasive pulmonary aspergillosis: Results from a three-year prospective study. Am J Med 81:249, 1986.

95. Stover DE, Zaman MB, Hajdu SI, et al: Bronchoalveolar lavage in diagnosing diffuse pulmonary infiltrates in the immunosuppressed host. Ann Intern Med 101:1, 1984.

96. Freeberg G, Stover DE, Levine S, et al: Spectrum of pulmonary aspergillosis in immunocompromised hosts. Chest 98:31S, 1990.

97. Aisner J, Murillo J, Schimpff SC, et al: Invasive aspergillosis in acute leukemia: Correlation with nose cultures and antibiotic use. Ann Intern Med 90:4, 1979.

98. Weiner MH, Talbot GH, Gerson SL, et al: Antigen detection in the diagnosis of invasive aspergillosis. Utility in controlled, blinded trials. Ann Intern Med 99:777, 1983.

99. Lopez-Berenstein G, Bodey GP, Fainstein V, et al: Treatment of systemic fungal infections with liposomal amphotericin B. Arch Intern Med 149:2533, 1989.

100. Longman LP, Martin MV: A comparison of the efficacy of itraconazole, amphotericin B and 5 fluorocytosine in the treatment of *Aspergillus fumigatus* endocarditis in the rabbit. J Antimicrob Chemother 20:719, 1987.

101. Meunier-Carpentier F, Shoeck R, Gerain J, et al: Amphotericin B nasal spray as prophylaxis against aspergillosis in patients with neutropenia. N Engl J Med 311:1056, 1984.

102. Sherertz RJ, Belani A, Kramer BS, et al: Impact of air filtration on nosocomial aspergillosis infections: Unique risk of bone marrow transplant recipients. Am J Med 83:709, 1987.

103. Burch PA, Karp JE, Merz WG, et al: Favorable outcome of invasive aspergillosis in patients with acute leukemia. J Clin Onc 5:1985, 1987.

104. Meyer RD, Rosen P, Armstrong D: Phycomycosis complicating leukemia and lymphoma. Ann Intern Med 77:871, 1972.

105. Bartrum RJ Jr, Watnick M, Herman PG: Roentgenographic findings in pulmonary mucormycosis. Am J Roentgenol Radium Ther Nucl Med 117:810, 1973.

106. Murray HW: Pulmonary mucormycosis with massive fatal hemoptysis. Chest 68:65, 1975.

107. DeSouza R, MacKinnon S, Spagnola SV, et al: Treatment of localized pulmonary phycomycosis. South Med J 72:609, 1979.

108. Bodey P: The emergence of fungi as major hospital pathogens. J Hosp Infect 11:411, 1988.

109. Aisner J, Sickles EA, Schimpff SC, et al: *Torulopsis glabrata* pneumonitis in patients with cancer. Report of three cases. JAMA 230:584, 1974.

110. Lehrer RL, Cline MJ: Leukocyte candidacidal activity and resistance to systemic candidiasis in patients with cancer. Cancer 27:1211, 1971.

111. Dubois PJ, Myerowitz RL, Allen CM: Pathological correlation of pulmonary candidiasis in immunosuppressed patients. Cancer 40:1026, 1977.

112. Baccari MA, Bistoni F, Lohmann-Mathes ML: In vitro natural and cell-mediated cytotoxicity against *Candida albicans*: Macrophage precursors as effector cells. J Immunol 134:2658, 1985.

113. Peterson EM, Calderone RA: Growth inhibition of *Candida albicans* by rabbit alveolar macrophages. Infect Immun 15:1910, 1977.

114. Buff SJ, McLelland R, Gallis HA, et al: *Candida albicans* pneumonia: Radiographic appearance. Am J Roentgenol 138:645, 1982.

115. Kahn FW, Jones JM: Diagnosis of bacterial respiratory infection by bronchoalveolar lavage. J Infect Dis 155:862, 1987.

116. Saito H, Anaissie EJ, Morice RC, et al: Bronchoalveolar lavage in the diagnosis of pulmonary infiltrates in patients with acute leukemia. Chest 94:745, 1988.

117. Graybill JR, Ahrens J: Interaction of rifampin with other antifungal agents in experimental murine candidiasis. Rev Infect Dis 5:20, 1983.

118. Perfect JR: Cryptococcosis. Infect Dis Clin North Am 3:77, 1989.

119. Kaplan MH, Rosen PP, Armstrong D: Cryptococcosis in a cancer hospital. Clinical and pathological correlates in 46 patients. Cancer 39:22, 1977.

120. Drutz DJ: Pneumonia due to endemic fungi. *In* Shelhamer J, Pizzo PA, Parrillo JE, Masur H (eds): Respiratory Disease in the Immunosuppressed Host. Philadelphia, JB Lippincott, 1991:335.

121. Gordonson J, Birbaum W, Jacobson G, et al: Pulmonary cryptococcosis. Radiology 112:557, 1974.

122. Diamond RD, Levitz SM: *Cryptoccocus neoformans* pneumonia. *In* Pennington JE (ed): Respiratory Infections: Diagnosis and Management. New York, Raven Press, 1989:457.

123. Dismukes WE, Cloud G, Gallis HA, et al: Treatment of cryptococcal meningitis with combination amphotericin B and flucytosine for 4 weeks compared with 6 weeks. N Engl J Med 317:334, 1987.

124. Polsky B, Depman MR, Gold JWM, et al: Intraventricular therapy for cryptococcal meningitis via a subcutaneous reservoir. Am J Med 81:24, 1986.

125. Sathapatayovongs B, Batterger BE, Wheat J, et al: Clinical and laboratory features of disseminated histoplasmosis. Medicine (Baltimore) 62:263, 1983.

126. Goodwin RA, Des Prez RA: Histoplasmosis. State of the art. Am Rev Respir Dis 117:929, 1978.

127. Wheat LJ: Histoplasmosis. Infect Dis Clin North Am 3:843, 1989.

128. Prechter GC, Prakash VBS: Bronchoscopy in the diagnosis of pulmonary histoplasmosis. Chest 95:1033, 1989.

129. Paya CV, Hermans PE, Van Scoy RE, et al: Repeatedly relapsing disseminated histoplasmosis. Clinical observations during long-term follow-up. J Infect Dis 156:308, 1987.

130. Dismukes WE, Cloud G, Bowles C, et al: Treatment of blastomycosis and histoplasmosis with ketoconazole. Ann Intern Med 103:861, 1985.

131. Deresinski SC, Stevens DA: Coccidioidomycosis in compromised hosts: Experience at Stanford University Hospital. Medicine (Baltimore) 54:377, 1974.

132. Ampel NM, Ryan KJ, Carry PJ, et al: Fungemia due to coccidioidomycosis immitis: An analysis of 16 episodes in 15 patients and a review of the literature. Medicine (Baltimore) 65:312, 1986.

133. Drutz DJ, Cantanzaro A: Coccidioidomycosis. Part I. Am Rev Respir Dis 117:559, 1978.

134. Ampel NM, Wieden MA, Galgiani JN: Coccidioidomycosis: Clinical update. Rev Infect Dis 11:897, 1989.

135. Wallace JM, Cantanzaro A, Moser KM, et al: Flexible fiberoptic bronchoscopy for diagnosing pulmonary coccidioidomycosis. Am Rev Respir Dis 123:286, 1981.

136. Recht LD, Davies SF, Eckman MR, et al: Blastomycosis in immunosuppressed patients. Am Rev Respir Dis 125:359, 1982.

137. Sarosi GA, Davies SF: Blastomycosis. State of the art. Am Rev Respir Dis 120:911, 1979.

138. Musatti CC, Rezkallah MT, Mendes C, et al: In vivo and in vitro evaluation of cell-mediated immunity in patients with paracoccidioidomycosis. Cell Immunol 24:365, 1976.

139. Bradsher RW: Blastomycosis. Infect Dis Clin North Am 2:877, 1988.

140. Saag MS, Dismukes WE: Treatment of histoplasmosis and blastomycosis. Chest 93:848, 1988.

141. Evers RH, Whereatt RR: Pulmonary sporotrichosis. Chest 66:91, 1974.

142. Winn RE: Sporotrichosis. Infect Dis Clin North Am 2:899, 1988.

143. Pluss JL, Opal SM: Pulmonary sporotrichosis: Review of treatment and outcome. Medicine (Baltimore) 65:143, 1986.

143a. Cone RW, Hackman RC, Huang MW: Human herpesvirus 6 in lung tissue from patients with pneumonitis after bone marrow transplantation. N Engl J Med 329:156, 1993.

144. Duval CP, Casozza AR, Grimley PM: Recovery of cytomegalovirus from adults with neoplastic disease. Ann Intern Med 64:531, 1966.

145. Rosen P, Hajdu S: Cytomegalovirus inclusion disease at autopsy of patients with cancer. An J Clin Pathol 55:756, 1971.

146. Evans DJ, Williams ED: Cytomegalovirus inclusion disease in adults. J Clin Pathol 21:311, 1968.

147. Emanuel D, Cunningham I, Jules-Elysee K, et al: *Cytomegalovirus* pneumonia after bone marrow transplantation successfully treated with the combination of ganciclovir and high-dose intravenous immune globulin. Ann Intern Med 109:777, 1988.

148. Ramsey PG, Fife KH, Hackman RC, et al: Herpes simplex virus pneumonia: Clinical, virologic and pathologic features in 20 patients. Ann Intern Med 97:813, 1982.

149. Sherry MK, Klainer AS, Wolff M, Gerhard H: Herpetic tracheobronchitis. Ann Intern Med 109:229A, 1988.

150. Shepp DH, Dandliker PS, Meyers JD: Treatment of varicella-zoster virus infection in severely immunocompromised patients: A randomized comparison of acyclovir and vidarabine. N Engl J Med 314:208, 1986.

151. Centers for Disease Control: Varicella-zoster immune globulin for the prevention of chickenpox: Recommendations of the Immunization Practices Advisory Committee. Ann Intern Med 100:859, 1984.

152. Murphy B, Webster RG: Influenza viruses. *In* Fields BN (ed): Virology. New York, Raven Press, 1985:1170.

153. Kempe A, Hall CB, MacDonald NE, et al: Influenza in children with cancer. J Pediatr 115:33, 1989.

154. Feldman S, Webster RG, Sugg M. Influenza in children and young adults with cancer. Cancer 39:350, 1977.

155. Smith TF, Burgert EO, Dowdle WR, et al: Isolation of swine influenza virus from autopsy lung tissue of man. N Engl J Med 294:708, 1976.

156. Dowdle W, Kendal AP, Noble GR: Influenza viruses. *In* Lennette EH, Schmidt NJ (eds): Diagnostic Procedures for Viral, Rickettsial and Chlamydial Infections. Washington, DC, American Public Health Association, 1979:585.

157. Centers for Disease Control: Prevention and control of influenza. MMWR 37:361, 1988.

158. Soo W: Clinical effectiveness of rimantadine in prophylaxis and treatment. J Respir Dis 8(suppl 11A):S73, 1987.

159. Rodriguez FH, Liuzza GE, Gohd RH: Disseminated adenovirus serotype 31 infection in an immunocompromised host. Am J Clin Pathol 82:615, 1984.

160. Zahradnik JM, Spencer MJ, Porter DD: Adenovirus infection in the immunocompromised patient. Am J Med 68:725, 1980.

161. Baum SG: Adenovirus. *In* Mandell G, Douglas RG, Bennett JE (eds): Principles and practice of infectious diseases. New York, Churchill Livingstone, 1989:1185.

162. Bagen R, Schwartz RH, Insul RA, et al: Severe diffuse adeno 7A pneumonia in a child with combined immunodeficiency: Possible therapeutic effect of the human serum globulin containing specific neutralizing antibody. Pediatr Infect Dis 3:246, 1984.

163. Hall CB, Powell KR, MacDonald NE, et al: Respiratory syncytial viral infection in children with compromised immune function. N Engl J Med 315:77, 1986.

164. Brugman S, Hutter JJ: Respiratory syncytial virus pneumonia in acute leukemia. Am J Pediatr Hematol Oncol 2:371, 1980.

165. Englund JA, Sullivan CJ, Jordan MC, et al: Respiratory syncytial virus infection in immunocompromised adults. Ann Intern Med 109:203, 1988.

166. Hall CB, Douglas RG: Clinically useful method for the isolation of respiratory syncytial virus. J Infect Dis 131:1–5, 1975.

167. Jacobsen D, Ackerman P, Payne NR: Rapid identification of respiratory syncytial virus infections by direct fluorescent antibody testing: Reliability as a guide to patient cohorting. Am J Infect Control 19(2):73, 1991.

168. Hall CB, McBride JT, Walsh EE, et al: Aerosolized ribavirin treatment of infants with respiratory syncytial viral infections. A randomized double blind study. N Engl J Med 308:1443, 1983.

169. McIntosh K, Kurachek SC, Cairns LM, et al: Treatment of respiratory viral infection in an immunodeficient infant with ribavirin aerosol. Am J Dis Child 138:305, 1984.

170. Gelfand EW, McCurdy D, Rao CP, et al: Ribavirin treatment of viral pneumonitis in severe combined immunodeficiency disease. Lancet 2:732, 1983.

171. Vanek J: Atypical interstitial pneumonia of infants produced by *Pneumocystis carinii*. Cas Lek Cesk 90:1121, 1951.

172. Edman JC, Kovacs JA, Masur H, et al: Ribosomal RNA sequences show *Pneumocystis carinii* to be a member of the fungi. Nature 334:519, 1988.

173. Pifer LL, Hughes WT, Stagno S, Woods D: *Pneumocystis carinii* infection: Evidence for high prevalence in normal and immunosuppressed children. Pediatrics 61:35, 1978.

174. Millard PR, Heryet AR: Observations favouring *Pneumocystis carinii* pneumonia as a primary infection: A monoclonal antibody study on paraffin sections. J Pathol 154:365, 1988.

175. Peters SE, Wakefield AE, Sinclair K, et al: A search for *Pneumocystis carinii* in postmortem lungs by DNA amplification. J Pathol 166:195, 1992.

176. Singer C, Armstrong D, Rosen PP, et al: *Pneumocystis carinii* pneumonia: A cluster of eleven cases. Ann Intern Med 82:772, 1975.

177. Jacobs JL, Libby DM, Winters RA, et al: A cluster of *Pneumocystis carinii* pneumonia in adults without predisposing illness. N Engl J Med 324:246, 1991.

178. Masur H. *Pneumocystis carinii* pneumonia: *In* Shelhamer J, Pizzo PA, Parrillo JC, Masur H (eds): Respiratory Disease in the Immunocompromised Host. Philadelphia, JB Lippincott, 1991:409.

179. Zaman MK, White DA: Serum lactate dehydrogenase levels and *Pneumocystis carinii* pneumonia: Diagnostic and prognostic significance. Am Rev Respir Dis 137:3402, 1988.

180. Stover DE, Greeno RA, Gagliardi AJ: The use of a simple exercise test for the diagnosis of *Pneumocystis carinii* pneumonia in AIDS patients. Am Rev Respir Dis 139:1343, 1989.

181. Jules-Elysee K, Santamauro J, Vander Els R, et al: Use of noninvasive tests in the diagnosis of PCP in non-AIDS patients. Am Rev Respir Dis 145:A543, 1992.

182. Forrest JV: Radiological findings in *Pneumocystis carinii* pneumonia. Radiology 103:539, 1972.

183. Masur H, Gill VJ, Ognibene FP et al: Diagnosis of pneumocystis pneumonia by induced sputum technique in patients with immunologic disorders other than acquired immunodeficiency syndrome. Ann Intern Med 109:755, 1988.

184. Wakefield AE, Guiver L, Miller RF, et al: DNA amplification on induced sputum samples for diagnosis of *Pneumocystis carinii* pneumonia. Lancet 337:1370, 1991.

185. Meduri GU, Stover DE, Greeno RA, et al: Bilateral bronchoalveolar lavage in the diagnosis of opportunistic pulmonary infection. Chest 100:1272, 1991.

186. Hughes WT, Feldman S, Chaudhary SC, et al: Comparison of pentamidine isethionate and trimethoprim-sulfamethoxazole in the treatment of *Pneumocystis carinii* pneumonia. J Pediatr 92:285, 1978.

187. Bozzette SA, Sattler FR, Chiu J, et al: A controlled trial of early adjunctive treatment with corticosteroids for *Pneumocystis carinii* pneumonia in the acquired immunodeficiency syndrome. N Engl J Med 323:1451, 1990.

188. Hughes WT, Kuhn S, Chandhary S, et al: Successful chemoprophylaxis for *Pneumocystis carinii* pneumonia. N Engl J Med 297:1419, 1977.

189. Hughes WT, Rivera GK, Schell MJ, et al: Successful intermittent chemoprophylaxis for *Pneumocystis carinii* pneumonitis. N Engl J Med 316:1627, 1987.

190. Hanson J, Jalal J, Stover DE, et al: *Pneumocystis carinii* pneumonia in patients with primary brain tumors. Arch Neurol 48:406, 1991.

191. Sepkowitz KA, Brown AE, Telzak EE, et al: *Pneumocystis carinii* pneumonia among patients with AIDS at a cancer hospital. JAMA 267:832, 1992.

192. Kaye D: The spectrum of strongyloidiasis. Hosp Pract 23:111, 1988.

193. Igra-Siegman Y, Kapila R, Sen P, et al: Syndrome of hyperinfection with *Strongyloides stercoralis*. Rev Infect Dis 3:397, 1981.

194. Rogers W, Nelson B: Strongyloidiasis and malignant lymphoma. JAMA 195:173, 1966.

# SOLID ORGAN AND BONE MARROW TRANSPLANTATION

## Neil A. Ettinger

The last decade has seen dramatic improvement in the outcome of organ transplantation. The introduction of cyclosporine, refinements in surgical technique, and improvements in organ preservation have contributed to 1-year survival rates, which approach 70% to 80% at experienced transplant centers. In 1990, there were 15% more solid organ transplantations performed in the United States than in 1989 (Table 14–4), and the indications for the various types of procedures broadened.[1]

Despite the favorable survival rates, organ transplant recipients continue to face a variety of complications that limit the success of these procedures. Chief among these complications are infectious and noninfectious pulmonary disorders. In this chapter, the respiratory infections that are common to solid organ and bone marrow transplant recipients are reviewed. The diagnostic approaches to these infections are discussed in Section IV of this book.

### CLINICAL APPROACH

Although pulmonary infections often present in a similar manner and frequency in recipients of different types of organs, the experience of one organ transplant population is not necessarily applicable to that of the next, and the standard therapies for these infections may not apply equally to the different subsets of patients. It is important to understand the unique characteristics of each type of organ transplant recipient, including the nature of the surgical procedure, the impact of prior organ dysfunction, the clinical presentation of various infections, and the reported therapeutic efficacy of different treatment strategies. Efforts to provide a predictable temporal framework for the occurrence of opportunistic infections after organ transplantation (Fig. 14–2) are useful but are not infallible, and the guide-

Table 14–4. **Transplantation Statistics, 1990**

| Type of Transplant | No. of Patients |
| --- | --- |
| Kidney | 9886 |
| Liver | 2682 |
| Heart | 2107 |
| Bone marrow | 2200 |
| Pancreas | 537 |
| Heart-lung | 52 |
| Isolated lung | 202 |

Adapted from the 1993 Annual Report of the US Scientific Registry for Transplant Recipients and the Organ Procurement and Transplantation Network—Transplant Data: 1988–1991. UNOS, Richmond, VA, and the Division of Organ Transplantation, Health Resources and Services Administration, Bethesda, MD; and United Network for Organ Sharing, Transplantation statistics, 1990 (press release).

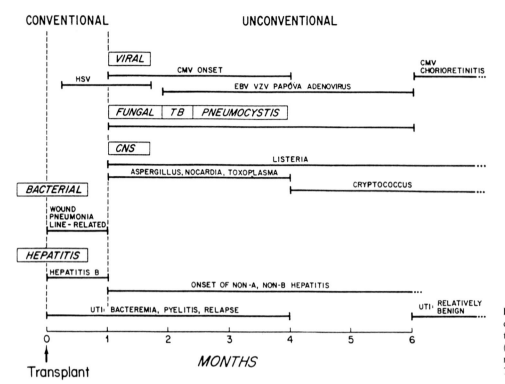

**Figure 14–2.** Framework for the occurrence of opportunistic infections after organ transplantation. (From Rubin RH: Infection in the renal transplant patient. Am J Med 70:405–411, 1981.)

lines should not be relied on in place of making a specific diagnosis.

The clinical presentations of noninfectious pulmonary complications are often identical to those of infectious complications, making a noninvasive approach to diagnosis difficult in many circumstances (Table 14–5). A specific diagnosis should be made for each pulmonary complication. The early diagnosis and treatment of pulmonary infections appear to provide a survival advantage.[2]

## HOST DEFENSE

Factors that influence the organ transplant patient's state of immunosuppression and susceptibility to infectious complications include the type and the amount of immunosuppressive drugs administered and the conditions associated with immunosuppression, such as neutropenia, uremia, hyperglycemia, or malnutrition. Disruption of the mucocutaneous barrier by intravenous catheters and bypassing the upper airway defense mechanisms by endotracheal intubation further enhance the risk of infection in an already susceptible host.[3] Infection with cytomegalovirus (CMV) probably adds immunosuppressive effects to those of immunosuppressive drugs.[4] Coinfection with bacterial or other opportunistic pathogens often complicate CMV disease and reduce the chances for a successful outcome.

The use of high doses of corticosteroids and the development of leukopenia are important risk factors for infection in organ transplant recipients. Corticosteroids inhibit all aspects of polymorphonuclear leukocyte activation and recruitment,[5] inhibit early phases of B-cell activation,[6] selectively inhibit a variety of T-cell functions, and lyse T cells.[7] Corticosteroids prevent alveolar macrophages from eradicating inhaled fungal spores and inhibiting fungal spore germination. Adequate numbers of neutrophils are

required to destroy fungal hyphae that escape alveolar macrophage surveillance.[8]

The specific alterations that occur in host defense mechanisms during organ transplantation depend on the type of

Table 14–5. **Noninfectious Pulmonary Complications of Organ Transplantation**

**Bone Marrow Transplantation**
Intersitial pneumonitis
Mucositis and aspiration
Alveolar hemorrhage
Adult respiratory distress syndrome (ARDS)
Pulmonary edema
Thromboembolism
Mediastinal emphysema
Bronchiolitis obliterans and airway obstruction

**Renal Transplantation**
Pulmonary edema
Thromboembolic disease
Pulmonary calcification
Recurrent renal-pulmonary syndrome

**Liver Transplantation**
Atelectasis
Diaphragmatic dysfunction
Pleural effusions and hemothorax
ARDS
Pulmonary calcification

**Heart Transplantation**
Atelectasis
Pleural effusions
ARDS
Pulmonary edema
Pulmonary hypertension

**Heart-Lung and Lung Transplantation**
Airway dehiscence
Acute rejection
Pulmonary edema
ARDS
Obliterative bronchiolitis

transplant. In bone marrow recipients, the use of high doses of chemotherapeutic agents during the conditioning regimen may result in severe mucositis, predisposing the patient to impaired clearance of secretions, localized mucosal infection, and aspiration.[9] Chemotherapeutic agents and ionizing radiation cause severe neutropenia, lasting approximately 2 to 3 weeks, in all marrow recipients. After neutrophil recovery (ie, engraftment), profound impairment of the cellular and humoral arms of the immune response persists for 4 to 5 months. Complete immunologic recovery may not occur for as long as 1 year, assuming that malignant relapse or graft-versus-host disease (GVHD) does not develop in the interim.[10] Marrow transplantation significantly affects local lung defense mechanisms. The alveolar macrophages of marrow recipients exhibit defective phagocytosis and chemotaxis and an impaired ability to kill bacteria and fungi. These changes persist for 6 to 12 months after transplantation.[11]

In heart-lung and isolated lung transplant recipients, several factors operate in concert to abrogate the ability of the lung allograft to resist infection. First, the lung allograft is usually obtained from donors that have undergone mechanical ventilation for days or weeks, and the lung is often colonized with bacteria before implantation. Second, the lung allograft undergoes periods of ischemia that may last for 4 to 9 hours. Imperfect lung preservation techniques, interstitial edema as a result of reimplantation, and impaired cough and mucociliary clearance due to denervation amplify the risk of pulmonary infection.[12, 13] Superimposed episodes of allograft rejection that require augmentation of immunosuppression further compromise the protective mechanisms of the pulmonary allograft.

In liver and kidney recipients, residual host defects arising as a result of uremia or hepatic failure may exist during the early postoperative period. Uremia is associated with increased susceptibility to infection,[14] as is diabetes mellitus,[15] which is a complicating condition in many patients undergoing renal transplantation. Hepatic insufficiency also impairs cell-mediated immunity and phagocytic function, which may cause persistent endotoxemia in patients with fulminant hepatic failure or severe cirrhosis.[16]

The state of immunosuppression in an organ transplant recipient is the sum of a combination of factors that determine susceptibility to infection. Commonly used methods of assessing the degree of immunosuppression include cutaneous manifestations of delayed hypersensitivity, absolute lymphocyte counts, T-lymphocyte helper-suppressor ratios, in vitro lymphocyte stimulation tests, and flow cytometric analysis of multiple phenotypic markers.[17] However, these methods are quantitatively imprecise, poorly reproducible, and fail to predict reliably whether one patient is more susceptible to infection than another.

## BONE MARROW TRANSPLANTATION

A growing list of hematologic and malignant diseases are successfully treated with bone marrow transplantation. The 2-year, disease-free survival rate exceeds 60% for some forms of leukemia and aplastic anemia,[18] and the results of marrow replacement in nonmalignant disorders such as aplastic anemia or Gaucher disease are promising.[19] Bone

marrow transplantation is a relatively simple procedure, but pulmonary complications occur in 40% to 60% of marrow recipients[18] and are a major obstacle to its success.

## Bacterial Pneumonia

Although bacterial pneumonia is common during the first 2 weeks after marrow transplantation, it is infrequently diagnosed because of the empiric use of broad-spectrum antibiotics,[20, 21] the reliance on radiologic criteria for the diagnosis of pneumonia, and the reluctance to use invasive diagnostic methods during the early pancytopenic period. In a review of the infectious complications in 60 marrow transplant recipients, Winston observed bacterial pneumonia in 12%.[20] However, in two other reviews, a 20% to 50% incidence of bacterial pneumonia was reported.[18, 22]

Gram-negative organisms, particularly *Pseudomonas aeruginosa,* are the predominant causes of pneumonia during the early granulocytopenic period. However, some gram-positive pathogens are identified, and they should be considered when selecting empiric antibiotic coverage.[20, 23] Pneumonia due to *Legionella pneumophila* has been described in nosocomial outbreaks.[24]

Bacterial pneumonia and sinusitis are the most common late infections (>6 months) after marrow transplantation. These infections are associated with chronic GVHD, are caused predominantly by *Streptococcus pneumoniae* and are often accompanied by bacteremia.[25, 26] Impaired opsonic activity for *S. pneumoniae* and a variety of other humoral immune deficits are postulated.[21, 25] Routine prophylaxis with penicillin or trimethoprim-sulfamethoxazole (TMP-SMX) has reduced the incidence of these late infections.[18, 21, 25] Vaccination with pneumococcal vaccine is unlikely to provide significant protection when administered within the first year.[27]

## Cytomegalovirus Pneumonitis

CMV infection occurs in 50% to 70% of allogeneic bone marrow recipients, and approximately one third of infected patients develop CMV pneumonia.[21, 28] CMV pneumonitis occurs in 15% of all marrow recipients, usually 50 to 60 days after transplantation. Patients usually present with pulmonary infiltrates, fever, and hypoxemia. CMV pneumonitis may also be associated with alveolar hemorrhage (Fig. 14–3). Before the availability of ganciclovir or CMV hyperimmune globulin, the devastating consequences of this infection were illustrated by the 85% or greater case fatality rate.[28]

The risk factors associated with the development of CMV pneumonitis after marrow transplantation include CMV seropositivity, advanced age, total body irradiation, and severe GVHD.[29, 30] The infusion of marrow or granulocytes from seropositive donors into seronegative recipients is associated with increased risks of CMV infection and pneumonitis.[31] Recipients of autologous or syngeneic grafts rarely develop CMV pneumonia despite a similar incidence of CMV infection. This observation may be explained by the absence of GVHD in these patients, the lower intensity of immunosuppression, the residual host cellular immunity,

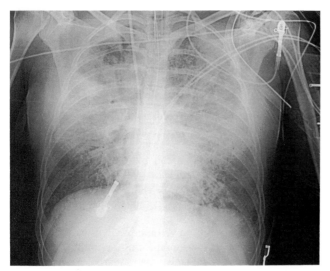

**Figure 14–3.** Chest radiograph of a 26-year-old woman who underwent an allogeneic bone marrow transplant for acute myelogenous leukemia was obtained the day after the patient developed acute dyspnea and hypoxemia, requiring 50% supplemental oxygen to maintain SaO₂ > 90%. Fiberoptic bronchoscopy revealed alveolar hemorrhage. Cytomegalovirus was detected in bronchoalveolar fluid by a shell-vial assay. The patient subsequently died of respiratory failure.

or a combination of these factors.[32, 33] However, the similar incidence of CMV infection and pneumonitis in recipients of T-cell-depleted marrow (ie, low incidence of GVHD) confirms that CMV pneumonitis may occur independently of GVHD.

Marrow transplant recipients experience higher mortality from CMV pneumonia than recipients of solid organ transplants. Early attempts at antiviral therapy with vidarabine, interferon, and high-dose acyclovir were uniformly unsuccessful.[34, 35] Ganciclovir, the first therapeutic agent with good in vitro anti-CMV activity, demonstrated excellent antiviral activity in vivo but little clinical efficacy.[36] In early studies, only 10% to 17% of patients with CMV pneumonitis survived.[36–38] Later series had a 44% to 48% survival rate (Table 14–6), probably reflecting the early diagnosis and treatment of patients with milder disease.[39–41] The potential for ganciclovir toxicity in marrow recipients is appreciable, with a 30% to 60% incidence of reversible neutropenia. An alternative drug, foscarnet, has produced mixed results in this patient population.[42, 43]

The most promising approach to the treatment of CMV pneumonitis in marrow recipients has been the combined use of ganciclovir and high-titer, CMV-specific immune globulin. Two reports describe survival rates of 52% to 70%,[44, 45] but the use of hyperimmune globulin alone is not recommended, because the 67% survival rate observed by Blacklock and coworkers was not substantiated in a subsequent study by Reed.[46, 47] In these studies, different immune globulin preparations were used, the sample sizes were small, and the patients differed in terms of severity of illness at the time of treatment.

The high mortality rate associated with CMV pneumonia in marrow recipients has led to the development of a variety of prophylactic strategies.[28] The use of CMV-seronegative blood products in CMV-seronegative marrow recipients has substantially reduced the incidence of CMV pneumonitis

and is an important initial approach.[48] In one large study, CMV hyperimmune globulin reduced the incidence of CMV infection and viremia but had no impact on symptomatic CMV disease or survival.[49] On the basis of available studies, routine immunoprophylaxis of patients at risk for primary infection cannot be recommended if the ultimate aim is to prevent CMV pneumonitis.[49]

The prophylactic use of antiviral agents has been studied in marrow recipients, and the results are extremely promising. Meyers[50] observed a significant reduction in the incidence and severity of CMV pneumonitis in seropositive patients treated with high-dose intravenous acyclovir.[50] The survival rate was greater for the treated patients, virus excretion occurred later, and the incidence of death due to other infectious causes was reduced. Schmidt and coworkers randomized allogeneic marrow recipients who had CMV detected in bronchoalveolar lavage (BAL) fluid at day 35 to observation alone or to 2 weeks of full-dose ganciclovir followed by maintenance therapy until 120 days after transplantation.[51] The incidence of CMV pneumonitis or death in the prophylaxis group was 25% and 70% among controls. No patient who received the full course of ganciclovir prophylaxis developed CMV pneumonitis. The drug was well tolerated despite a high incidence of reversible neutropenia. These findings suggest that ganciclovir provides effective prophylaxis in asymptomatic marrow recipients shedding CMV in BAL fluid and that further studies of preemptive therapy in viremic patients is indicated.

## Herpes Simplex Pneumonia

Herpes simplex virus (HSV) is excreted by 80% of seropositive marrow recipients, usually between the second and third week after transplantation. Most infections represent viral reactivation, involve the oropharyngeal mucosa, and aggravate the severity of chemotherapy-related mucositis.[21] Positive HSV cultures from the upper or lower respiratory tract in a patient with pulmonary infiltrates does not imply causality and requires histologic confirmation if the need for antiviral therapy is in question.

In a review of 525 patients, Meyers and coworkers found that HSV pneumonitis accounted for 5% of cases of nonbacterial pneumonia.[30] The low incidence compared with CMV may be related to the poor replication of HSV in alveolar macrophages.[52] HSV pneumonitis may be focal or multifocal. Focal involvement usually arises from contiguous spread from the oropharynx, and diffuse pulmonary involvement usually arises from hematogenous dissemination from oropharyngeal or genital sites.[53] Most episodes of HSV pneumonitis begin during the period of profound neutropenia, and almost all patients have identifiable mucocutaneous involvement.

Histologic confirmation of HSV pneumonitis is difficult because of patchy parenchymal involvement. Open or transbronchial lung biopsies are susceptible to sampling error and may be nondiagnostic. Direct immunoflourescent staining of histologic specimens should be routinely performed.

## Respiratory Syncytial Virus Pneumonitis

Respiratory syncytial virus (RSV) pneumonia has been identified in marrow transplant recipients.[54] As in nonim-

Table 14–6. **Ganciclovir and Immunoglobulin for Treating Cytomegalovirus Pneumonia in Bone Marrow Transplant Recipients**

| Investigation | No. of Patients | Regimen | Survival (%) | Rate of Neutropenia (%) |
|---|---|---|---|---|
| Shepp (1985)[36] | 10 | GCV* | 10 | 30 |
| Erice (1987)[39] | 11 | GCV | 45 | 55 |
| Crumpacker (1988)[40] | 21 | GCV | 38 | 23 |
| Ettinger (1989)[41] | 16 | GCV | 44 | 38 |
| Ho (1989)[37] | 13 | GCV | 15 | 30 |
| Reed (1986)[38] | 6 | GCV + Steroids | 17 | 50 |
| Reed (1988)[44] | 25 | GCV + IG | 52 | 67 |
| Emanuel (1988)[45] | 10 | GCV + IG | 70 | 80 |
| Blacklock (1985)[46] | 9 | IG alone | 67 | 0 |
| Reed (1987)[47] | 14 | IG alone | 21 | 0 |

*GCV, ganciclovir; IG, immunoglobulin.
From Ettinger NA, Trulock EP. Pulmonary considerations of organ transplantation. Part 2. Am Rev Respir Dis 144:213–223, 1991.

munosuppressed patients, most RSV infections in the recipients occur during the winter and spring. Patients typically present with fever, cough, and signs of ear or sinus involvement that precede overt clinical or radiographic illness. Wheezing may be prominent, and bilateral interstitial infiltrates are common. The mortality rate approaches 50% and is highest for patients whose infection begins in the early posttransplant period and for whom the diagnosis is delayed.[54]

The seasonal nature of RSV infection combined with the high frequency of upper respiratory tract symptoms and signs should suggest the possibility of RSV pneumonitis. Detection of virus in cell culture is the diagnostic standard, but immunoflourescent staining or direct examination of lung tissue may permit a rapid diagnosis. Treatment with aerosolized ribavirin, often unnecessary in other immunocompromised patients, is recommended in marrow transplant recipients because of the associated high mortality rate.[54]

## Fungal Pneumonia

The liberal use of broad-spectrum antibiotics for treatment and prophylaxis and the use of treatment strategies that prolong the duration of granulocytopenia are the most likely explanations for a resurgence in invasive fungal infections after marrow transplantation.[55, 56] Invasive fungal disease occurs in as many as 40% of marrow recipients, usually during the first 30 to 40 days after transplantation. Pulmonary infections with *Candida*, *Cryptococcus*, *Histoplasma*, and *Coccidioides* have been reported, but *Aspergillus* species are the most common causes of invasive fungal pneumonia and the most life threatening.[8]

*Aspergillus* is often a nosocomial pathogen in marrow recipients. The risk of infection is quantitatively related to the number of *Aspergillus* spores in the air, and the use of high-efficiency particulate air filters effectively decreases the incidence of infection.[57] Marrow transplant recipients are the most susceptible of all transplant patients to invasive pulmonary aspergillosis because of the intensity and the nature of their immunosuppression.[58] The duration of granulocytopenia and the use of high-dose corticosteroids are clearly identified as the most important risk factors.[8, 59] T-cell depletion of harvested marrow results in delayed en-

graftment, prolonged neutropenia, and a higher incidence of invasive aspergillosis.[56]

Although the clinical presentation of invasive pulmonary aspergillosis is often insidious, it is sometimes distinctive in marrow recipients. Most patients have nonspecific symptoms such as fever, dyspnea, and a dry cough.[20] However, pleuritic chest pain and hemoptysis also occur. In a review of 26 marrow recipients with invasive pulmonary aspergillosis, 38% experienced minor hemoptysis (<50 mL), and 15% had major, life-threatening hemoptysis.[60] In the seriously ill patients, the development of massive hemoptysis usually coincided with resolution of granulocytopenia. Wheezing is another important clinical sign of invasive pulmonary aspergillosis. This finding is particularly prominent in patients who have tracheobronchial involvement.[61] Bronchoscopic examination of the airways of these patients typically reveals ulcerative lesions or pseudomembranes covering the bronchial mucosa.

The radiographic features of invasive pulmonary aspergillosis include diffuse infiltrates, focal infiltrates, cavitary nodules, and pleural effusions (Fig. 14–4). Some patients demonstrate peripheral, wedge-shaped infiltrates arising as a result of vessel invasion and pulmonary infarction.[8] Many patients, even those with disseminated disease, do not have positive sputum cultures. Although tissue is usually required to confirm the diagnosis for marrow recipients, detecting *Aspergillus* species in sputum cultures should be considered evidence of invasive disease and warrants institution of therapy.[29, 62, 63]

The mortality rate for marrow recipients with *Aspergillus* pneumonia approaches 100%.[64] The poor outcome may be attributed partially to late diagnosis,[2] although low survival rates are observed in patients who are treated on the basis of clinical suspicion alone.[55] Early detection and treatment may improve outcome, but therapy is often ineffective if started after the clinical illness is obvious.[2, 8, 21] Amphotericin B is the treatment of choice. High doses (1 mg/kg/d) should be used in all granulocytopenic patients, and prophylactic amphotericin should be provided for patients with previous *Aspergillus* disease who require additional courses of chemotherapy.[65] The reported experience with itraconazole includes one treatment success[66] and one treatment failure,[64] but the preliminary results indicate that itraconazole may be effective when used prophylactically in granulocytopenic patients if high serum levels are maintained.[67]

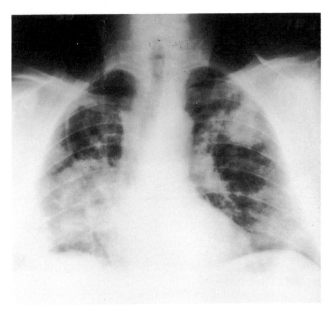

**Figure 14–4.** Chest radiograph of a 46-year-old man 36 days after an allogeneic bone marrow transplantation for ANLL. He initially presented with cough, fever, and nodular infiltrates that were unresponsive to broad-spectrum antibiotics. Bronchoscopic specimens grew *Aspergillus fumigatus*. The infiltrates worsened despite treatment with amphotericin B, and the patient died of respiratory failure 52 days after transplantation.

Granulocyte transfusions have been ineffective and may cause life-threatening respiratory failure if used in conjunction with amphotericin B.[20] Because of the poor response to treatment by marrow recipients, the prevention of infection by reduction of airborne contamination is an important strategy.

### *Pneumocystis* Pneumonia

The incidence of *Pneumocystis carinii* pneumonia (PCP) has dropped sharply since the introduction of routine prophylaxis with TMP-SMX.[29] Most cases of PCP develop in patients who are sulfa allergic or who are noncompliant with the drug regimen. The median time to the onset of PCP is 2 months after transplantation, although cases have developed as early as 2 weeks. In marrow recipients, the onset of PCP is usually fulminant and the progression rapid. The response to treatment is usually good if instituted early.[21]

### KIDNEY TRANSPLANTATION

Patient and renal allograft survival rates have improved over the past decade, and transplantation compares favorably with dialysis as a therapeutic modality for end-stage renal disease.[68, 69] More than 95% of recipients are still alive at 1 year, and the rate of graft survival exceeds 70% for cadaver organs and 90% for organs from living, related donors.[68]

The pulmonary considerations of renal transplantation encompass a variety of infectious and noninfectious disor-

ders. Unlike liver transplantation, in which the surgical procedure itself predisposes the patient to pulmonary complications, the intraoperative pulmonary considerations of renal transplantation are relatively few and are primarily related to anesthesia. There has been a marked decline in the incidence of pulmonary infections in renal transplant recipients during the last 15 years, largely as a result of improved surgical technique and better immunosuppression. At the University of Colorado from 1962 through 1968, 42% of patients undergoing renal transplantation had at least one episode of pneumonia.[70] In more recent surveys, the incidence of pneumonia was 8% to 16%.[71–74]

### Bacterial Pneumonia

Bacterial pneumonia in renal transplant recipients usually develops within the first month after transplantation and is caused by typical nosocomial pathogens. However, outbreaks of pneumonia due to more unusual pathogens, such as *Nocardia asteroides* (Fig. 14–5) or *L. pneumophila*, are well documented.[72, 75] The clinical presentation of bacterial pneumonia may be fulminant,[71] with the sudden onset of fever and pulmonary symptoms over 12 to 24 hours (Fig. 14–6). Malnutrition, a previous pulmonary complication, multiple renal transplants, and the administration of steroids for preventing allograft rejection enhance the risk of developing pneumonia.[76] The response to broad-spectrum antibacterial therapy is generally good if instituted early.[74, 77] However, superinfection with nonbacterial organisms, particularly fungi, is associated with an extremely poor prognosis.[78]

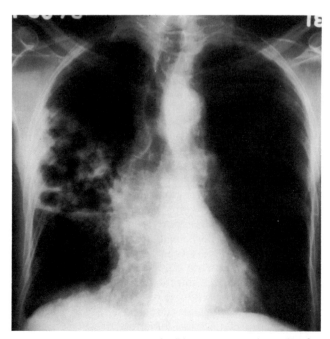

**Figure 14–5.** Chest radiograph of a 54-year-old man 6 months after cadaveric renal transplantation. The patient presented with headache, fever, pleuritic chest pain, and a cavitary infiltrate involving the right lung. Culture of bronchoscopy specimens confirmed the presence of *Nocardia asteroides*. The patient failed to respond to treatment. Postmortem examination revealed disseminated disease involving the brain, spinal cord, heart, kidneys, liver, adrenals, and thyroid.

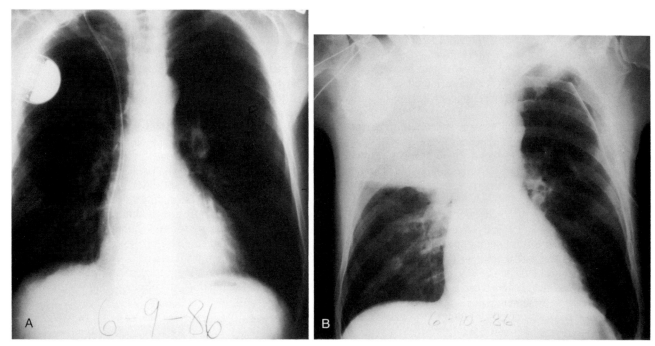

**Figure 14–6.** A 58-year-old man who had received a living-related donor renal transplant 3 months earlier. *A,* Chest radiograph obtained after the acute onset of fever to 40°C, neutropenia, and hypotension. *B,* Chest radiograph obtained 8 hours later, after the rapid development of dense right upper lobe consolidation. The patient died of *Pseudomonas* sepsis the same day. (From Ettinger NA, Trulock EP. Pulmonary considerations of organ transplantation. Part I. Am Rev Respir Dis 143:1386–1405, 1991.)

Gram-positive organisms and *Haemophilus influenzae* are the most common causes of community-acquired pneumonias in renal transplant recipients. These infections in immunosuppressed patients usually respond well to treatment and have a prognosis that is similar to nonimmunosuppressed patients with the same infection.[71]

### Cytomegalovirus Pneumonia

CMV infection is the most common infectious complication after renal transplantation and is a significant cause of morbidity. Although the reported incidence of CMV infection approaches 75%,[79] this figure has declined since the introduction of cyclosporine (CSA)-based immunosuppression.[80] Among infected patients, 20% to 40% develop symptomatic CMV disease within the first 2 months of transplantation. Fever occurs in more than 90%, is frequently high and prolonged, and may be the only clinical sign that appears. Headache, malaise, arthralgias, and diarrhea are common and hematologic abnormalities such as neutropenia or anemia occur most frequently in patients who develop severe CMV disease.[79, 81]

Mild CMV-related symptoms usually precede the onset of CMV pneumonitis by several weeks. Diffuse interstitial and alveolar infiltrates are typical findings, although focal infiltrates, nodules, discoid atelectasis and normal chest radiographs have been described.[79, 81] Coinfection with multiple pathogens, particularly *P. carinii* and *P. aeruginosa,* is common and is associated with high mortality.[81] The failure to seroconvert in the face of a symptomatic infection is reported in 50% of fatal cases of CMV disease in renal transplant recipients.[79]

A variety of prophylactic strategies have been evaluated in renal transplant recipients. Snydman observed a 65% reduction in the incidence of symptomatic CMV disease (including pneumonitis) and other life-threatening opportunistic infections in patients at risk for primary CMV infection who were treated with CMV-specific hyperimmune globulin.[82] This approach has been cost effective for treating patients at risk for primary infection.[83] Polyvalent immune globulin appears to be less effective in this setting.[84–86] Balfour and coworkers demonstrated the ability of high-dose oral acyclovir to reduce the incidence of CMV infection and disease in patients at risk for primary illness. The incidence of CMV pneumonia was markedly reduced, and the drug regimen was well tolerated.[87] The encouraging studies by Balfour and Snydman suggest that some form of prophylaxis is appropriate, particularly in renal transplant patients at risk for primary CMV disease.

Before ganciclovir was available, the mortality rate from CMV pneumonia among renal transplant recipients approached 50% and reached 90% among patients who required mechanical ventilation.[81] However, the data obtained from eight studies in which ganciclovir was used indicate that survival approaches 80% of treated patients, including 40% of patients who require mechanical ventilation.[39, 80, 89–93] Ganciclovir is well tolerated by most renal transplant recipients, with a 20% to 40% incidence of reversible neutropenia that rarely limits the drug's utility.[39, 40, 93] Complete virologic clearing is described in 70% to 90% of patients.

### Fungal Pneumonia

The treatment of allograft rejection is the single most important risk factor for the development of fungal pneumonia after renal transplantation. Many species of fungi cause pneumonia in the renal transplant recipient, including *Aspergillus* sp., *Candida* sp., *Cryptococcus neoformans, Histoplasma capsulatum,* and *Coccidioides immitis.* Survival appears best for patients whose fungal pneumonia is detected and treated early.[71, 94] Fungal infections that are superimposed on another infectious process, particularly CMV infection, have a particularly poor prognosis.[95]

Aspergillosis is the most frequent and the most serious pulmonary mycosis in renal transplant recipients. The peak incidence occurs during the first 4 months after transplantation, but sporadic cases are described throughout the first year.[95] The clinical presentation is usually subacute, with fever, productive cough, and dyspnea evolving over days to weeks.[71] In a review of 25 cases of *Aspergillus* pneumonia in renal transplant recipients, Weiland and coworkers observed focal and diffuse pulmonary involvement. The diagnosis was made antemortem in only 56% of the patients, emphasizing the difficulty in confirming the diagnosis even under optimal circumstances.[95]

The response to treatment with amphotericin B varies among renal transplant patients, although it is much better than in marrow transplant recipients. In Weiland's series, a 16% survival rate was observed, although many patients had multiple pulmonary pathogens that may have significantly affected outcome. Eighty percent of patients in whom *Aspergillus* was the only pathogen responded to combined amphotericin and 5-flucytosine, but none of those with *Aspergillus* infection superimposed on another pulmonary infection survived. The experience with itraconazole in renal transplant recipients has been limited. Of the six cases of invasive pulmonary disease reported in the literature, there have been four clinical cures and two deaths.[64, 66] Surgical resection of localized cavitary disease with or without combined antifungal therapy has been successful in a few patients.[71, 95]

Outbreaks of pneumonia due to *C. immitis* and *H. capsulatum* have been described after renal transplantation. Isolation of either organism from respiratory secretions suggests invasive disease,[72] and dissemination occurs in as many as 75% of patients with either infection.[96, 97] The radiographic features of these pulmonary fungal infections are not predictable. Interstitial, alveolar, and miliary infiltrates have been described,[96–98] but dissemination may occur without any radiographic evidence of pulmonary disease. The response to therapy is also unpredictable. Histoplasmosis is associated with a favorable response to amphotericin B, but pulmonary infection with *C. immitis* is associated with appreciable mortality.[98]

### *Pneumocystis* Pneumonia

Before CSA was available, PCP occurred in fewer than 5% of renal transplant recipients.[71, 72, 74, 76, 78] After the introduction of cyclosporine, a striking increase in the incidence of PCP was reported by several transplant centers.[71, 72, 74, 76, 78, 99–102] Analysis of the potential risk factors identified cyclosporine as the most likely cause of the increased incidence of PCP.

In renal transplant recipients, the onset of infection tends to be acute, with fever and respiratory symptoms developing over several days. The peak incidence occurs 2 to 4 months after transplantation, although later-onset cases have been reported.[99, 100, 102, 103] The mortality rates for various series range from 8% to 80%. Patients with concurrent CMV pneumonitis usually fare the worst.

The use of prophylactic TMP-SMX has markedly reduced the incidence of PCP in centers that had previously reported significant outbreaks.[99–102] The optimal duration of prophylaxis is undetermined, but a 12-month regimen appears appropriate because of the clustering of cases at 2 to 4 months and sporadic episodes occurring during the first year.[101] Indefinite prophylaxis has been suggested because of the favorable effect of TMP-SMX on posttransplant bacterial infections and its relatively low cost.[104] The use of trimethoprim may competitively inhibit creatinine secretion, which may increase serum creatinine without an actual decrease in renal function.[100] In patients in whom the drug is started late after transplantation, this rise in creatinine may be mistaken for allograft rejection. Starting the drug early after transplantation may eliminate this confusion.

### Mycobacterial Pneumonia

The frequency of mycobacterial infections in renal transplant patients ranges from 0.65% to 2.3% of patients,[105, 106] with rates as high as 9.5% for patients reported in areas where tuberculosis is endemic.[107] The onset of infection is usually late, with most patients developing the disease more than a year after transplantation. However, a few cases occurring as early as 2 weeks have been reported.[105, 106, 108, 109]

The clinical presentation of mycobacterial disease is unpredictable in this setting.[108] Although the lung is the most frequently involved organ,[107] there is a high incidence of joint and skin involvement.[105] Respiratory symptoms are often minimal, and a prolonged fever of unknown origin or an abnormal chest radiograph may be the only clue to the infection.[108, 110] Fever, malaise and weight loss are particularly prominent in patients with pulmonary disease.[105] Radiographic manifestations include upper or lower lobe infiltrates or a diffuse miliary pattern.[108] Dissemination is common and often fatal.[106, 109] Although most infections are caused by *Mycobacterium tuberculosis,* infections with nontuberculous mycobacteria are described in 24% to 42% of renal transplant patients with mycobacterial infections.[105, 111]

Mycobacterial disease in renal transplant recipients usually responds to standard antituberculous chemotherapy[110, 112] and short-course therapy with three drugs is usually effective.[110] The possibility of adverse reactions is increased because of the renal excretion of isoniazid, streptomycin, and ethambutol.[108] Drug toxicity may be enhanced during episodes of allograft rejection. Rifampin increases steroid catabolism and reduces the bioavailability of cyclosporine. Either of these effects may precipitate acute allograft rejection.[113] Reduction of immunosuppression during treatment of mycobacterial infection is usually unnecessary unless the infection is life threatening.

### LIVER TRANSPLANTATION

The first orthotopic liver transplantation (OLT) was performed by Starzl in 1963. Subsequent improvements in surgical technique, anesthesia, and immunosuppression have resulted in 1-year survival rates that approach or exceed 70% at major transplant centers.[114–118] These figures compare favorably with the less than 30% 1-year survival rate observed for patients with end-stage liver disease who are treated with medical therapy.[115] OLT is considered an established therapeutic modality for the treatment of end-stage liver disease.[116, 118]

The incidence of infection after OLT approaches or exceeds 70%, a figure that has changed little since the mid-1970s.[119–122] However, the standardization of surgical methods and the introduction of more selective immunosuppression has reduced infection-related mortality. The risk factors for infection after OLT include prolonged operative time, postoperative antibiotic therapy, renal failure, and gastrointestinal or vascular complications.[119, 121]

Bacterial or fungal infections that develop after OLT often arise from the liver or biliary system and are typically caused by aerobic, gram-negative enteric bacteria or *Candida*.[123] Allograft rejection, vascular insult to the liver, or defective biliary drainage facilitates penetration of these microorganisms into the recipient's blood or peritoneum, predisposing the patient to abdominal abscesses and peritonitis. The peak incidence for infection after OLT occurs during the first 2 postoperative months. The use of selective bowel decontamination appears to reduce the morbidity and mortality associated with early infection.[119, 121] After 6 months, infections occur less frequently but may be caused by a wide array of bacterial or opportunistic pathogens.[120, 121]

## Bacterial Pneumonia

Bacterial pneumonia is reported in as many as 25% of OLT recipients and accounts for almost half of all pulmonary infections.[124] The introduction of CSA is associated with a decline in the incidence of bacterial pneumonias (Table 14–7). Most bacterial pneumonias are nosocomial and develop in intubated patients.[124] Atelectasis, aspiration, and prolonged mechanical ventilation are common predisposing factors,[112] and gram-negative enteric organisms are the predominant pathogens. However, gram-positive organisms predominate when selective bowel decontamination is employed.[125] Although the overall incidence of bacterial

pneumonia has decreased, mortality continues to approach 40%.[121]

## Cytomegalovirus Pneumonia

The incidence of CMV infection after OLT approaches 60% in most large series, and symptomatic disease is described in 20% to 70% of infected patients.[120, 122, 126, 127] CMV pneumonia typically occurs during the fourth to sixth postoperative week, although cases occurring as early as the second week are reported. Nonspecific symptoms such as fever, malaise, myalgias, and arthralgias often precede the development of CMV pneumonitis, and CMV hepatitis frequently accompanies pneumonitis.[120, 121] Coinfection with other opportunistic pulmonary pathogens, such as *P. carinii*, is common.[128, 129] The treatment of allograft rejection with anti-lymphocyte antibodies has been associated with a high incidence of disseminated CMV disease in OLT recipients at risk for primary CMV infection. Similar findings have not been observed in patients at risk for reactivation of CMV infection.[127]

Ganciclovir provides effective therapy for CMV pneumonia occurring after OLT. Complete virologic clearing is described in 75% to 100% of patients, and prompt reversal of the clinical, biochemical, and radiographic abnormalities is common. The successful treatment of patients requiring mechanical ventilation has been described.[121, 129–131] The necessity or the effectiveness of combined ganciclovir and CMV-specific immunoglobulin for the treatment of CMV pneumonia has not been established. Passive immunoprophylaxis with CMV-specific immunoglobulin has not been studied in a large, randomized trial, but a retrospective comparison of 42 OLT recipients at risk for primary infection demonstrated dramatic decreases in the incidence of CMV infection and symptomatic disease in those treated with polyvalent immunoglobulin and high-dose acyclovir.[132] Conflicting conclusions were reached by two other studies that addressed this issue.[133, 134]

## Fungal Pneumonia

Before the introduction of CSA, the reported incidence of invasive fungal infections after OLT exceeded 40%.[122] Improvements in surgical technique, decreased total opera-

---

**Table 14–7. Pneumonia After Orthotopic Liver Transplantation**

| Investigation | Total No. of Patients | Patients With Pneumonia | Causative Pathogens† | | | | | | | | |
|---|---|---|---|---|---|---|---|---|---|---|---|
| | | | G(−) | G(+) | AN | CMV | PC | ASP | CAN | HSV | Other |
| Schroeter (1976)[123] | 93 | 40 (43%) | 15 | 2 | 1 | 7 | 11 | 8 | 7 | 4 | 3 (TOXO, *Nocardia*) |
| Dummer (1983)[122] | 24 | 6 (25%) | 2 | 0 | 1 | 1 | 0 | 2 | 0 | 0 | 0 |
| Jensen (1983)[128] | 18 | 6 (33%) | 1 | 1 | 0 | 4 | 1 | 2 | 0 | 1 | 0 |
| Kusne (1988)[121] | 101 | 14 (14%) | 11 | 5 | 0 | 5 | 11 | 3 | 0 | 0 | 0 |
| Thompson (1988)[199] | 46 | 15 (33%) | NR | 2 | NR | 7 | NR | NR | NR | 2 | NR |
| Colonna (1988)*[119] | 35 | 5 (14%) | 4 | 0 | 0 | 1 | 0 | 0 | 0 | 0 | 0 |
| Paya (1989)*[120] | 83 | 14 (17%) | 1 | 3 | 0 | 2 | 5 | 1 | 0 | 0 | 2 (CRYPTO) |

*Used selective bowel decontamination.

†Multiple pathogens often found; NR, not reported; G(−), gram negative; G(+), gram positive; CMV, cytomegalovirus; PC, *Pneumocystis carinii*; ASP, *Aspergillus fumigatus*; CAN, *Candida*; HSV, herpes simplex virus; AN, anaerobe; TOXO, *Toxoplasma gandii*; CRYPTO, *Cryptococcus neoformans*.

From Ettinger NA, Trulock EP: Pulmonary considerations of organ transplantation. Part I. Am Rev Respir Dis 143:1386–1405, 1991.

tive time, selective immunosuppression with cyclosporine, and the use of selective bowel decontamination have contributed to a decline in incidence of invasive fungal infections.[64, 121, 135] Most fungal pneumonias occur within the first month after transplantation and are caused predominantly by *Candida* sp., *Aspergillus* sp., or *C. neoformans* (Fig. 14–7). The recommended treatment is amphotericin B. There is no reported experience with itraconazole or liposomal amphotericin in this patient population. Recovery from invasive pulmonary aspergillosis after OLT has not been reported, and disseminated infection is associated with 70% to 100% mortality.[64, 124]

### *Pneumocystis* Pneumonia

PCP occurs 3 to 5 months after OLT, although episodes occurring within the first few weeks after transplantation have been described. The radiographic presentation is often atypical, with focal instead of diffuse infiltrates.[121] Coinfection with CMV is common and is associated with high mortality rates. Prophylaxis with TMP-SMX has not been studied in a randomized, controlled manner in OLT recipients. However, its effectiveness among other organ transplant recipients recommends its routine use.

### HEART TRANSPLANTATION

During the last decade cardiac transplantation emerged as a standard therapy for end-stage heart disease. Cardio-

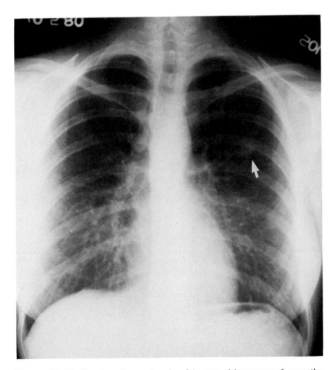

**Figure 14–7.** Chest radiograph of a 21-year-old woman 6 months after orthotopic liver transplantation for chronic active hepatitis. She presented with fever and a focal infiltrate in the left upper lobe. The transthoracic needle aspirate grew *Cryptococcus neoformans,* and the cerebrospinal fluid sample was positive for cryptococcal antigen. She responded to treatment with amphotericin B.

myopathy and coronary artery disease have been the principal indications; less common reasons have included valvular disease and refractory dysrhythmias.[136] From 1987 through 1989, the number of heart transplants reached a plateau at approximately 2500 per year. The 5-year actuarial survival rate after orthotopic heart transplantation exceeds 70%.[137]

The early period after heart transplantation is marked by a variety of noninfectious complications, such as atelectasis, effusions, pulmonary edema, or right ventricular failure.[138, 139] Although most patients experience an uneventful course, the development of these complications may prolong intubation or the intensive care unit stay, increasing the risk of developing infectious complications. During the early era of heart transplantation, infectious complications accounted for more than 50% of patient deaths.[140] The introduction of selective immunosuppression with cyclosporine and the use of endomyocardial biopsy to guide additional immunosuppressive therapy have reduced the incidence and severity of these infections.[141]

### Bacterial Pneumonia

Pneumonia is the leading infectious complication after heart transplantation, occurring in 40% to 60% of patients before the use of cyclosporine[142–144] and in 24% to 40% of patients recently transplanted.[145, 146] The impact of median sternotomy on lung mechanics,[147] the development of acute lung injury after cardiopulmonary bypass,[148] and interstitial pulmonary edema[149] predispose the heart transplant recipient to nosocomial pneumonia. Additional risk factors for pneumonia after heart transplantation include posttransplant reintubation and high doses of corticosteroids.[146]

Most episodes of bacterial pneumonia occur within 2 to 3 weeks after heart transplantation[150] and are usually caused by gram-negative nosocomial pathogens. Multiple pathogens are described in 20% to 35% of pulmonary infections[140, 143, 145] and are responsible for a large proportion of infection related deaths.[142]

*L. pneumophila* has been identified in as many as 2% of heart transplant recipients with bacterial pneumonia.[150] Most episodes are sporadic, but common-source outbreaks are also described.[150] Unlike immunocompetent patients, heart transplant recipients with *Legionella* pneumonia may present with atypical radiographic findings, including nodular infiltrates,[152] effusions, and bronchopleural fistulas.[153, 154] Treatment with erythromycin alone may not be effective, and the addition of rifampin may be required. Clarithromycin, a macrolide antibiotic, appears more effective than erythromycin in preliminary studies and may be useful in patients refractory to standard therapy.[155] Because relapse is common, prolonged therapy for 6 to 12 months may be necessary. Intravenous therapy is preferred during the early stages, because treatment failure is associated with the premature institution of oral therapy.[153, 154]

Nocardial pneumonia occurs sporadically after heart transplantation. Of the first 160 heart transplant recipients at Stanford, 13% developed nocardial pulmonary disease.[156, 157] However, the incidence has fallen to 0% to 6% since the introduction of cyclosporine. The impact of routine prophylaxis with TMP-SMX on the occurrence of this infection is unclear. In the Stanford series, 81% of cases of pulmonary nocardiosis presented as a solitary nodule months to years after transplantation (median, 299; range, 43–982 days). Fever and nonproductive cough were common symptoms, although 40% of all patients were entirely asymptomatic. The lung was the only site of involvement in 80% of patients. Disseminated disease to skin or bone often required surgical debridement. Treatment with sulfamethoxazole was successful in all cases, probably reflecting the aggressive approach to early diagnosis and treatment taken in this series.[156]

The Stanford series also identified an association between nocardial infection and the subsequent development of infection with nontuberculous mycobacteria. Of the 21 heart transplant patients with nocardiosis, 5 subsequently developed infection with nontuberculous mycobacteria (4 had *M. kansasii*, 1 had *M. avium-intracellulare*) at a median of 902 days after the nocardial infection. Intensive analysis of a variety of potential predisposing factors failed to identify an explanation for this.[158]

## Cytomegalovirus Pneumonia

CMV infection has been documented in 67% to 100% of patients after heart transplantation,[150, 159–163] and more than one third of infected patients consistently develop symptomatic CMV disease.[159, 160, 162] The use of CSA-based immunosuppression has decreased the incidence of overall infection and symptomatic disease.[150] Animal studies have verified that the donor heart is capable of transmitting latent CMV infection.[164] Latent virus appears to be harbored by cardiac myocytes,[165] although infection of coronary endothelial cells in association with coronary thrombosis and myocardial infarction can also occur.[166] Direct myocardial injury as a result of CMV infection is rare.[167]

CMV pneumonia occurs in 11% to 16% of heart transplant recipients with CMV infection.[145, 160] Fever is the most common symptom[163] and diffuse pulmonary infiltrates the predominant radiographic finding, although focal infiltrates are described in as many as one third of these patients.[145, 168] Coinfection with bacterial and fungal pathogens is common and is frequently fatal (Fig. 14–8).[160] Viremia has been documented in 62% to 79% of heart transplant recipients and often precedes the development of symptomatic disease and pneumonitis.[122, 159] Before the availability of effective treatment, the mortality rate for patients with CMV pneumonia ranged from 46% to 75%.[145, 160]

Ganciclovir provides effective treatment for CMV pneumonitis in heart transplant recipients, although the number of reported cases is small. Keay and coworkers described response rates of 81% among 16 heart transplant patients with symptomatic CMV disease. Mortality for patients with pulmonary involvement was 14%, which compares favorably with previously published figures.[161] Watson described the successful treatment of CMV pneumonitis in 4 of 4 affected patients.[169]

The prophylactic use of antiviral agents or immunoglobulin has not been studied in large, well-designed trials using heart transplant recipients. Andreone and coworkers observed a lower incidence of symptomatic CMV infections among patients treated with low-dose CSA, azathioprine, and prednisone than the 30% incidence among patients treated with high-dose CSA or conventional immunosuppression. They attributed the low incidence in the first group to the elimination of antilymphocyte preparations from the treatment protocol, the use of lower doses of prednisone, and the use of seronegative blood products and hyperimmune globulin in patients at risk for primary disease.[170]

## Fungal Pneumonia

Pulmonary infection with endemically restricted fungi and invasive fungal species are reported in heart transplant recipients. Although not as lethal as in marrow recipients, mortality, especially with *Aspergillus* pneumonia, remains exceedingly high. Thirty percent of the first 206 heart transplant recipients at Stanford developed invasive fungal disease,[171] with a mortality rate in excess of 50%. The introduction of CSA reduced the incidence of invasive fungal infections[150] to between 0% and 24%, with a mortality rate of 50% to 80%.

Treatment with amphotericin B remains the standard therapy for invasive pulmonary aspergillosis in heart transplant recipients. Liposomal amphotericin has achieved almost tenfold higher plasma levels than free drug with minimal nephrotoxicity and has been used successfully in 3 patients with progressive disease who were not tolerating amphotericin B.[152, 172] Itraconazole has been used successfully in 3 heart transplant recipients.[173, 174] The effectiveness of these agents must be evaluated in larger, controlled studies.

## Protozoal Pneumonia

PCP develops in 3% to 20% of heart transplant recipients, usually within the first 6 months after transplantation.[145] The routine use of prophylactic TMP-SMX and CS-based immunosuppressions have probably reduced these rates substantially.[150] However, no controlled trials addressing this issue have been performed.

PCP may progress rapidly, and the mortality rate has been reported as high as 34% among early heart transplant recipients.[171] Later experience suggests that the outcome is generally good if the diagnosis is made early, treatment is started quickly and if copathogens are not present.[145]

Infection with *Toxoplasma gondii* is of special concern to the heart transplant recipient. After ingestion, *Toxoplasma* organisms disseminate widely to visceral organs such as the heart, where they encyst in a dormant but viable state. The cysts may be transplanted with the allograft,[175] and reactivation may occur under the permissive influence of immunosuppression. The most common clinical manifestations of active *Toxoplasma* infection include fever, chorioretinitis, necrotizing encephalitis, and myocarditis. Pulmonary involvement may be fatal.[176] Prophylaxis with pyrimethamine or TMP-SMX is recommended for patients at risk for primary infection,[177] and the combination of pyrimethamine and sulfadiazine is effective therapy for established disease.[140]

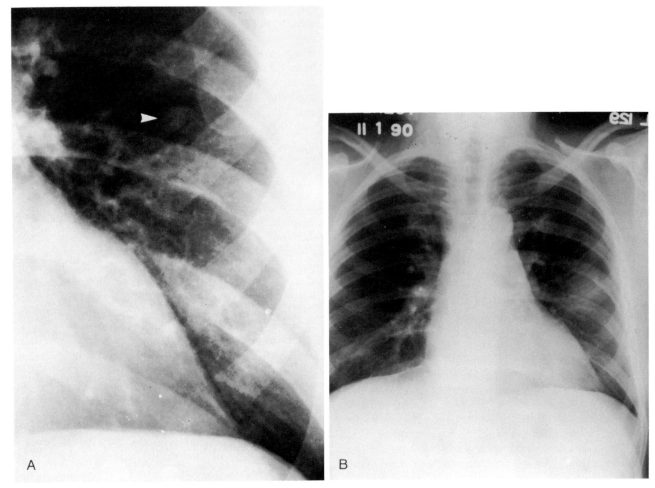

**Figure 14–8.** *A,* Enlargement of a routine chest radiograph of a 49-year-old man 6 weeks after orthotopic heart transplantation. A 1-cm nodule in the left mid-lung field (*arrow*) was missed on review. *B,* A chest radiograph of the same patient 1 week later after the onset of a low-grade fever shows that the nodule has increased dramatically in size. Transbronchial lung biopsy revealed histologic evidence of both cytomegalovirus pneumonitis and invasive *Aspergillus* pneumonia. The patient responded to treatment with ganciclovir and amphotericin B. (From Ettinger NA, Trulock EP: Pulmonary considerations of organ transplantation. Part 3. Am Rev Respir Dis 144:433–451, 1991.)

## HEART-LUNG AND LUNG TRANSPLANTATION

Heart-lung transplantation (HLT) and isolated lung transplantation add another dimension to the pulmonary infectious considerations of organ transplant recipients, because the lung itself becomes an allograft. In addition to the usual spectrum of infectious and noninfectious complications described in recipients of other organs, the clinical and radiographic evaluation is complicated by the possibility of allograft rejection.

After steady growth from 1981 through 1988, HLT activity worldwide plateaued at approximately 200 procedures per year in 1989. The principal indications for HLT include primary pulmonary hypertension, Eisenmenger syndrome, and congenital cardiac defects.[178] However, the annual activity for these indications has decreased, but the annual rates for other pulmonary diseases, such as cystic fibrosis, have increased.

In 1983, isolated lung transplantation became a clinical reality. Unilateral lung transplantation was performed for pulmonary fibrosis,[179] chronic obstructive pulmonary disease (COPD),[180] primary pulmonary hypertension,[181] and selected cases of Eisenmenger syndrome.[182] Bilateral lung transplantation was performed for COPD,[183] antitrypsin-deficiency emphysema,[183] and cystic fibrosis.[184] For many indications, HLT and isolated lung transplantation are now feasible, although the optimal transplant operation for each clinical indication has not been determined. The scarcity of donor heart-lung organ blocks and the more efficient use of donor organs may ultimately favor isolated lung transplantation as the the preferred approach.

Most of the information about the infectious complications of lung transplantation is from HLT recipients, because of the extensive experience with these patients compared with the relatively recent experience with isolated lung transplantation. Although the experience with both types of lung allograft recipients is likely to be similar, this has not been verified.

### Bacterial Pneumonia

Between 1982 and 1989, the overall prevalence of bacterial pneumonia at the University of Pittsburgh was 66%.[185] Bacterial pneumonia was a direct or indirect factor in 42% of all fatalities. The risk of bacterial pneumonia was found to be the highest during the early postoperative period, although the prevalence was rather uniform (35%) throughout posttransplant follow-up periods of 0 to 2 weeks, 2 weeks to 1 year, and longer than 1 year. Since 1988, the early and routine use of ceftazidime and clindamycin has reduced the prevalence of early bacterial pneumonia to only 13%.

Early empiric treatment of bacteria isolated from airway secretions is justified in lung allograft recipients. Although fever and pulmonary infiltrates may have alternative explanations, the susceptibility of the lung allograft to overwhelming infection during the early posttransplant period dictates an aggressive approach. Gram-negative organisms have been the most frequent isolates, although pneumonias due to *Staphylococcus aureus* and *L. pneumophila* also occur (Fig. 14–9).[185–187]

### Cytomegalovirus Pneumonitis

The reported incidence of CMV infection among HLT recipients is 67% to 100%. Of the infected patients, as many as 40% to 50% develop CMV pneumonitis, a much higher rate than for other organ transplant recipients.[185, 188, 189] In the Papworth Hospital experience, the attack rate of CMV pneumonia during primary infection approached

60%, with a case fatality rate of 67%.[189] As a result of considerable CMV-related morbidity and mortality, the Papworth program instituted a policy whereby only D(−) organs are transplanted into R(−) recipients.[189, 190] Although a rigid matching policy is not feasible at most centers because of the shortage of donor organs, seronegative recipients should receive organs from seronegative donors (ie, D−/R− match) whenever possible. Blood product matching is also important. The prevalence of primary CMV infection in seronegative recipients at the University of Pittsburgh declined from 71% to 10% after a blood product matching policy was introduced.[185]

The prevalence of CMV infection in seropositive HLT recipients is 50% to 75%, regardless of the CMV serologic status of the donor.[185, 188, 189] As expected, CMV infection in seropositive recipients is often asymptomatic or mild,[188] and mortality is 6% to 13%.[189]

The clinical presentation of CMV pneumonitis is similar to acute allograft rejection. A definitive diagnosis must be established because of the drastic differences in therapy. Fiberoptic bronchoscopy with transbronchial biopsy has proven useful in this setting.[185, 191] Culture of BAL fluid has a high sensitivity and negative predictive value for the diagnosis of CMV pneumonitis, but a positive culture lacks specificity, and histologic confirmation is required.

Ganciclovir has proved effective in a limited number of

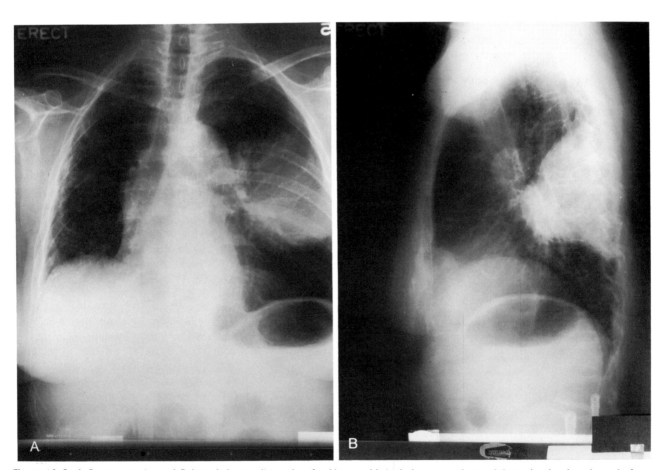

**Figure 14–9.** *A,* Posteroanterior and *B,* lateral chest radiographs of a 61-year-old single-lung transplant recipient who developed cough, fever, and dyspnea 8 months after transplantation. The bronchoalveolar lavage fluid was found to be positive for *Legionella* by DNA probe, and the cultures grew gram-negative coccobacilli, subsequently confirmed to be *Legionella pneumophila.* After failure to respond to the initial treatment with intravenous erythromycin, rifampin was added to the antibiotic regimen, with subsequent resolution of the infection.

HLT recipients with CMV pneumonia.[188, 190, 192] No controlled trials with this agent have been conducted using HLT recipients, and these studies are unlikely because of the widespread availability of the drug and its documented effectiveness in other patient populations. Limited experience with ganciclovir plus hyperimmune globulin has been favorable[188] and appears to be appropriate in refractory or severe cases.

The risk of CMV infection should be minimized by matching CMV seronegative recipients with seronegative donors whenever feasible. No prophylactic regimen has been thoroughly studied in HLT recipients, although CMV hyperimmune globulin is recommended by the Papworth Hospital group based on limited experience.[188] High-dose acyclovir prophylaxis has been adopted by some HLT centers, but a small study of recipients of solid organ transplants did not appear promising.[192a]

### Herpes Simplex Virus Pneumonitis

HLT recipients appear to be at significant risk for HSV pneumonitis if not provided antiviral prophylaxis. Smyth and colleagues observed 6 cases of HSV pneumonitis in 5 HLT recipients.[193] All patients were seropositive for HSV before transplantation, all had intraoral mucosal lesions, and most had been treated for allograft rejection during the previous 10 days. The use of prophylactic acyclovir appears warranted in seropositive HLT recipients, although the optimal duration of prophylaxis has not been determined.[193]

### Pneumocystis carinii Pneumonia

The prevalence of *P. carinii* infection has been low among recipients who have received appropriate prophylaxis.[187, 190] However, the overall risk of infection appears to be high.[185, 186, 194] Before instituting routine prophylaxis, Gryzan and coworkers detected *P. carinii* in the bronchoscopy specimens from 75% of HLT recipients at the University of Pittsburgh. Seventy percent of these infections were asymptomatic and were discovered incidentally. Clinically important episodes of PCP developed less frequently in this series and are rarely described in others.

Despite the use of appropriate prophylaxis, fatal cases of PCP still occur, and PCP must remain in the differential diagnosis of a compatible clinical picture. Asymptomatic infections have responded well to oral treatment with TMP-SMX.[185] TMP-SMX prophylaxis is necessary, although as in other organ transplant populations, the optimal dose or regimen has not been determined. In recipients who are allergic to sulfa drugs, aerosolized pentamidine is the logical alternative because of its documented efficacy in human immunodeficiency virus-infected patients.[195]

### Fungal Pneumonias

Although invasive fungal infections are uncommon after HLT, infections with *Candida* sp., *Aspergillus* sp., and *Cryptococcus* sp. have been documented.[185–187, 190, 196] These fungal infections may be localized or disseminated, and they are frequently life threatening.

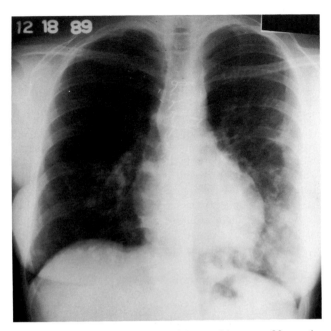

**Figure 14–10.** Chest radiograph of 21-year-old woman 20 months after a heart-lung transplantation for primary pulmonary hypertension. She presented with cough, low-grade fever, and pulmonary infiltrates. Notice the lower lung field involvement and lack of cavitation. Transbronchial biopsy specimens revealed caseating granulomas, and the cultures grew *Mycobacterium avium-intracellulare.* Treatment with isoniazid, rifampin, ethambutol, and streptomycin resulted in resolution of the pulmonary infiltrates and symptoms.

*Candida* frequently colonizes in the donor lung[12, 185] and is often isolated from respiratory tract specimens obtained from the recipient.[187, 196] Although *Candida* may present in the context of disseminated disease or candidemia, intrathoracic presentations also occur and may be dramatic. Infections involving vascular anastomoses may lead to mycotic aneurysm formation and fatal rupture.[185, 196]

Invasive *Candida* infections should be treated with amphotericin B in standard therapeutic doses, although fluconazole may be a suitable alternative. Because of a significant incidence of early *Candida* infection and its attendant morbidity and mortality, a prophylactic regimen of amphotericin (up to 0.3 mg/kg/d for 14 days) was administered to 15 recipients at the University of Pittsburgh to reduce the previously high morbidity and mortality rates associated with early *Candida* infection. This low-dose regimen was effective and produced minimal toxic effects.

Invasive pulmonary aspergillosis has been described in lung transplant recipients.[185, 186, 190] Compared with other organ transplant recipients, lung transplant recipients appear to have a comparatively high frequency of localized airway involvement. Six lung transplant recipients (4 heart-lung and 2 single lung) with ulcerative tracheobronchitis caused by *Aspergillus* species were reported by the Stanford group.[197] All patients were asymptomatic and radiographic changes were uncommon. The bronchoscopic findings included multiple ulcers, tracheobronchial erythema and edema, pseudomembrane formation, and mucus plugging. Only the transplanted lungs were involved in the single lung transplant recipients, and the airway anastomosis was jeopardized in two patients.

The case fatality rate for aspergillosis is high, although

in some cases, *Aspergillus* infection was not the primary cause of death. As in other organ transplant recipients, the diagnosis of invasive aspergillosis can be difficult and is often made postmortem.[185] Amphotericin B is the treatment of choice for invasive fungal infections in lung transplant recipients. However, the initial experience with itraconazole has been encouraging. All 6 patients with ulcerative tracheobronchitis in the Stanford series responded to oral itraconazole,[197] as did an additional HLT recipient reported by Dupont.[66]

## Mycobacterial Pneumonia

Mycobacterial pulmonary infections are rare in lung transplant recipients, although this estimation may reflect underreporting. The only reported case involved infection with a nontuberculous mycobacterium, *Mycobacterium chelonei*.[198] An additional case involving *M. avium-intracellulare* occurred at this institution and was successfully treated (Fig. 14–10).

## REFERENCES

1. United Network for Organ Sharing: Transplantation Statistics, 1990. [Press release] 1991.
2. Aisner J, Schimpff SC, Wiernik PH: Treatment of invasive aspergillosis: Relation of early diagnosis and treatment to response. Ann Intern Med 86:539–543, 1977.
3. Masur H: Infections in critically ill immunosuppressed patients. *In* Parillo JE, Masur H (eds): The Critically Ill Immunosuppressed Patient. Rockville, Aspen Publishers, 1987:215–242.
4. Rubin RH, Cosimi AB, Tolkoff-Rubin NE, et al: Infectious disease syndromes attributable to cytomegalovirus and their significance among renal transplant recipients. Transplantation 24:458–464, 1977.
5. Fauci AS, Dale DC, Balow JE: Glucocorticosteroid therapy: Mechanism of action and clinical considerations. Ann Intern Med 84:304, 1976.
6. Bowen DL, Fauci AS: Positive suppressive effects of glucocorticoids on the early events in the human B cell activation process. Immunology 133:1885, 1984.
7. Zweiman B, Atkins PC, Bedard PM, et al: Corticosteroid effects on circulating lymphocyte subset levels in normal humans. J Clin Immunol 4:151, 1984.
8. Meunier F: Fungal infections in the compromised host. *In* Rubin R, Young L (eds): Clinical Approach to Infection in the Compromised Host. New York, Plenum, 1988:193–220.
9. Champlain RE, Gale RP: The early complications of bone marrow transplantation. Semin Hematol 21:101–108, 1984.
10. Lum LG: The kinetics of immune reconstitution after human marrow transplantation. Blood 69:369–380, 1987.
11. Winston DJ, Territo MC, Ho WG, et al: Alveolar macrophage dysfunction in human bone marrow transplant recipients. Am J Med 73:859–866, 1982.
12. Harjula A, Baldwin JC, Starnes VA, et al: The Stanford experience. J Thorac Cardiovasc Surg 94:874–880, 1987.
13. Dolovich M, Rossman C, Chambers C, et al: Mucociliary function in patients following single lung or lung/heart transplantation. Am Rev Respir Dis 135:A363, 1987.
14. Raska K, Raskova J, Shea SM, et al: T cell subsets and cellular immunity in end stage renal disease. Am J Med 75:734–740, 1983.
15. MacCuish AC, Urbaniak SJ, Campbell CJ, et al: Phytohemagglutinin transformation and a circulating lymphocyte subpopulation in insulin-dependent diabetic patients. Diabetes 23:708–710, 1974.
16. Thomas HC: Immunologic aspects of liver disease. *In* Schiff L, Schiff EC (eds): Diseases of the Liver. Philadelphia, JB Lippincott, 1989:1177–1179.
17. Auchincloss H, Rubin RH: Clinical management of the critically ill renal transplant patient. *In* Parillo JE, Masur H (eds): The Critically Ill Immunosuppressed Patient. Rockville, Aspen Publishers, 1987:347–380.
18. Krowka MJ, Rosenow EC, Hoagland HC: Pulmonary complications of bone marrow transplantation. Chest 87:237–246, 1985.
19. Storb R: Bone marrow transplantation. *In* DeVita VT, Hellman S, Rosenberg SA (eds): Cancer: Principles and Practice of Oncology, ed 3. Philadelphia, JB Lippincott, 1989:2747–2489.
20. Winston DJ, Gale RP, Meyer DV, et al: Infectious complications of human bone marrow transplantation. Medicine (Baltimore) 58:1–31, 1979.
21. Meyers JD, Thomas ED: Infection complicating bone marrow transplantation. *In* Rubin R, Young L (eds): Clinical Approach to Infection in the Compromised host. New York, Plenum, 1988:525–555.
22. Cordonnier C, Bernaudin JF, Bierling P, et al: Pulmonary complications occurring after allogeneic bone marrow transplantation. Cancer 58:1047–1054, 1986.
23. Sullivan KM, Deeg HG, Sanders JE, et al: Late complications after marrow transplantation. Semin Hematol 21:53–63, 1984.
24. Kugler JW, Armitage JW, Helms CM, et al: Nosocomial legionnaires disease: Occurrence in recipients of bone marrow transplants. Am J Med 74:281–288, 1983.
25. Winston DJ, Schiffman G, Wang DC, et al: Pneumococcal infections after human bone marrow transplantation. Ann Intern Med 91:835–841, 1979.
26. Atkinson K, Storb R, Prentice RL, et al: Analysis of late infections in 89 long-term survivors of bone marrow transplantation. Blood 53:720–731, 1979.
27. Winston DJ, Ho WG, Schiffman G, et al: Pneumococcal vaccination of recipients of bone marrow transplants. Arch Intern Med 143:1735–1737, 1983.
28. Meyers JD, Flournoy N, Thomas ED: Risk factors for cytomegalovirus infection after human marrow transplantation. J Infect Dis 153:478–488, 1986.
29. Meyers JD. Infection in bone marrow transplant recipients. Am J Med 81(suppl 1A):27–38, 1986.
30. Meyers JD, Flournoy N, Thomas ED: Nonbacterial pneumonia after allogeneic marrow transplantation: A review of ten years' experience. Rev Infect Dis 4:1119–1132, 1982.
31. Hersman J, Meyers JD, Thomas ED, et al: The effect of granulocyte transfusions on the incidence of cytomegalovirus infection after allogeneic marrow transplantation. Ann Intern Med 96:149–152, 1982.
32. Wingard JR, Sostrin MB, Vriesendorp HM, et al: Interstitial pneumonitis following autologous bone marrow transplantation. Transplantation 46:61–65, 1988.
33. Appelbaum FR, Meyers JD, Fefer A, et al: Nonbacterial nonfungal pneumonia following marrow transplantation in 100 identical twins. Transplantation 33:265–268, 1982.
34. Meyers JD, McGuffin RW, Bryson YJ, et al: Treatment of cytomegalovirus pneumonia after marrow transplant with combined vidarabine and human leukocyte interferon. J Infect Dis 146:80–84, 1982.
35. Wade JC, Hintz M, McGuffin RW, et al: Treatment of cytomegalovirus pneumonia with high-dose acyclovir. Am J Med 73(suppl 1A):249–256, 1982.
36. Shepp DH, Dandliker PS, Miranda P, et al: Activity of 9-[2-hydroxy-1-(hydroxymethyl) ethoxymethyl]-guanine in the treatment of cytomegalovirus pneumonia. Ann Intern Med 103:368–373, 1985.
37. Ho WG, Winston DJ, Champlin RE: Tolerance and efficacy of ganciclovir in the treatment of cytomegalovirus infections in immunosuppressed patients. Transplant Proc 21:3103–3106, 1989.
38. Reed EC, Dandliker PS, Meyers JD: Treatment of cytomegalovirus pneumonia with 9-[2-hydroxy-1-(hydroxymethyl) ethoxymethyl] guanine and high dose corticosteroids. Ann Intern Med 105:214–215, 1986.
39. Erice A, Jordan MC, Chace BA, et al: Ganciclovir treatment of cytomegalovirus disease in transplant recipients and other immunocompromised hosts. JAMA 257:3082–3087, 1987.
40. Crumpacker C, Marlowe S, Zhang JL, et al: Treatment of cytomegalovirus pneumonia. Rev Infect Dis 10:538S–546S, 1988.
41. Ettinger NA, Selby P, Powles R, et al: Cytomegalovirus pneumonia: The use of ganciclovir in marrow transplant recipients. J Antimicrob Chemother 24:53–62, 1989.
42. Apperly JF, Marcus RE, Goldman JM, et al: Foscarnet for cytomegalovirus pneumonitis. Lancet 1:1151, 1985.
43. Ringden O, Lonnqvist B, Paulin T, et al: Pharmacokinetics, safety and preliminary clinical experiences using foscarnet in the treatment

of cytomegalovirus infections in bone marrow and renal transplant recipients. J Antimicrob Chemother 17:373–387, 1986.

44. Reed EC, Bowden RA, Dandliker PS, et al: Treatment of cytomegalovirus pneumonia with ganciclovir and intravenous cytomegalovirus immunoglobulin in patients with bone marrow transplants. Ann Intern Med 109:783–788, 1988.

45. Emanuel D, Cunningham I, Jules-Elysee K, et al: Cytomegalovirus pneumonia after bone marrow transplantation successfully treated with the combination of ganciclovir and high dose intravenous immune globulin. Ann Intern Med 109:777–782, 1988.

46. Blacklock HA, Griffiths P, Stirk P, et al: Specific hyperimmune globulin for cytomegalovirus pneumonitis. Lancet 1:152–153, 1985.

47. Reed EC, Bowden BA, Dandliker PS, et al: Efficacy of cytomegalovirus immunoglobulin in marrow transplant recipients with cytomegalovirus pneumonia. J Infect Dis 156:641–645, 1987.

48. Bowden RA, Sayers M, Flournoy N, et al: Cytomegalovirus immune globulin and seronegative blood products to prevent primary cytomegalovirus infection after marrow transplantation. N Engl J Med 314:1006–1010, 1986.

49. Bowden RA, Fisher LD, Rogers K, et al: Cytomegalovirus (CMV)-specific intravenous immunoglobulin for the prevention of primary CMV infection and disease after marrow transplant. J Infect Dis 164:483–487, 1991.

50. Meyers JD, Reed JC, Shepp DH, et al: Acyclovir for prevention of cytomegalovirus infection and disease after allogeneic marrow transplantation. N Engl J Med 318:70–75, 1988.

51. Schmidt GC, Horak DA, Niland JC, et al: A randomized, controlled trial of prophylactic ganciclovir for cytomegalovirus pulmonary infection in recipients of allogeneic bone marrow transplants. N Engl J Med 324:1005–1011, 1991.

52. Drew WL, Mintz L, Hoo R, et al: Growth of herpes simplex and cytomegalovirus in cultured human alveolar macrophages. Am Rev Respir Dis 119:287–291, 1979.

53. Ramsey PG, Fife KH, Hackman RC, et al: Herpes simplex virus pneumonia. Ann Intern Med 97:813–820, 1982.

54. Englund JA, Sullivan CJ, Jordan C, et al: Respiratory syncytial virus infection in immunocompromised adults. Ann Intern Med 109:203–208, 1988.

55. Peterson PK, McGlave P, Ramsay NKC, et al: A prospective study of infectious diseases following bone marrow transplantation: Emergence of aspergillus and cytomegalovirus as the major causes of mortality. Infect Control 4:81–89, 1983.

56. Pirsch JD, Maki DG: Infectious complications in adults with bone marrow transplantation and T-cell depletion of donor marrow increased susceptibility to fungal infections. Ann Intern Med 104:619–631, 1986.

57. Rhame FS: Lessons from the Roswell Park bone marrow transplant aspergillosis outbreak. [Editorial] Infect Control 6:345–346, 1985.

58. Sherertz RJ, Belani A, Elfenbein GJ, et al: Impact of air filtration on nosocomial *Aspergillus* infections. Am J Med 83:709–718, 1987.

59. Gerson SL, Talbot GH, Hurwitz S, et al: Prolonged granulocytopenia: The major risk factor for invasive pulmonary aspergillosis in patients with acute leukemia. Ann Intern Med 100:345–351, 1984.

60. Albelda SM, Talbot GH, Gerson SL, et al: Pulmonary cavitation and massive hemoptysis in invasive aspergillosis: Influence of bone marrow recovery in patients with acute leukemia. Am Rev Respir Dis 131:115–119, 1985.

61. Pervez NK, Kleinerman J, Kattan M, et al: Pseudomembranous necrotizing bronchial aspergillosis. Am Rev Respir Dis 131:961–963, 1985.

62. Nalesnik MA, Myerowitz RL, Jenkins R, et al: Significance of *Aspergillus* species isolated from respiratory secretions in the diagnosis of invasive pulmonary aspergillosis. J Clin Microbiol 11:370–376, 1980.

63. Treger TR, Visscher DW, Bartlett MS, et al: Diagnosis of pulmonary infection caused by *Aspergillus*: Usefulness of respiratory cultures. J Infect Dis 152:572–576, 1985.

64. Denning DW, Stevens DA: Antifungal and surgical treatment of invasive aspergillosis: Review of 2,121 published cases. Rev Infect Dis 12:1147–1201, 1990.

65. Robertson MJ, Larson RA: Recurrent fungal pneumonias in patients with acute nonlymphocytic leukemia undergoing multiple courses of chemotherapy. Am J Med 84:233–239, 1988.

66. Dupont B: Itraconazole therapy in aspergillosis: Study in 49 patients. J Am Acad Dermatol 23:607–614, 1990.

67. Tricot G, Joosten E, Boogaerts MA, et al: Ketoconazole versus itraconazole for antifungal prophylaxis in patients with severe granulocytopenia: Preliminary results of two non-randomized studies. Rev Infect Dis 9(supp 1):S94–99, 1987.

68. Monaco AP: Clinical kidney transplantation in 1984. Transplantation 17:5–11, 1985.

69. Flye MW: Renal transplantation. *In* Flye W (ed): Principles of Organ Transplantation. Philadelphia, WB Saunders, 1989:264–293.

70. Eickoff TC: Infectious complications in renal transplant recipients. Transplant Proc 5:1233–1238, 1973.

71. Ramsey PG, Rubin RH, Tokoff-Rubin N, et al: The renal transplant patient with fever and pulmonary infiltrates: Etiology, clinical manifestations, and management. Medicine (Baltimore) 59:206–222, 1980.

72. Peterson PK, Ferguson R, Fryd DS, et al: Infectious diseases in hospitalized renal transplant recipients: A prospective study of a complex and evolving problem. Medicine (Baltimore) 61:360–372, 1982.

73. Hesse UJ, Fryd DS, Chatterjee SN, et al: Pulmonary infections: The Minnesota randomized prospective trial of cyclosporine vs azathioprine-antilymphocyte globulin for immunosuppression in renal allograft recipients. Arch Surg 121:1056–1060, 1986.

74. Masur H, Cheigh JS, Stubenbord WT: Infection following renal transplantation: A changing pattern. Rev Infect Dis 4:1208–1219, 1982.

75. Wilczek H, Kallings I, Nystrom B, et al: Nosocomial legionnaires' disease following renal transplantation. Transplantation 43:847–851, 1987.

76. Simmons RL, Uranga VM, LaPlante ES, et al: Pulmonary complications in transplant recipients. Arch Surg 105:260–268, 1972.

77. Peterson PK, Anderson RC: Infection in renal transplant recipients. Am J Med 81:2–10, 1986.

78. Webb WR, Gamsu G, Rohlfing BM, et al: Pulmonary complications of renal transplantation: A survey of patients treated by low-dose immunosuppression. Radiology 126:1–8, 1978.

79. Glenn J: Cytomegalovirus infections following renal transplantation. Rev Infect Dis 3:1151–1178, 1981.

80. Metselaar H, Weimar W: Cytomegalovirus infection and renal transplantation. J Antimicrob Chemother 23:37–47, 1989.

81. Peterson PK, Balfour HH, Marker SC, et al: Cytomegalovirus disease in renal allograft recipients: A prospective study of the clinical features, risk factors and impact on renal transplantation. Medicine (Baltimore) 59:283–300, 1980.

82. Snydman DR, Werner BG, Heinze-Lacey B, et al: Use of cytomegalovirus immune globulin to prevent cytomegalovirus disease in renal transplant recipients. N Engl J Med 317:1049–1054, 1987.

83. Tsevat J, Snydman DR, Pauker SG, et al: Which renal transplant patients should receive cytomegalovirus immune globulin? Transplantation 52:259–265, 1991.

84. Steinmuller DR, Graneto D, Swift C, et al: Use of intravenous immunoglobulin prophylaxis for primary cytomegalovirus infection post living related donor renal transplantation. Transplant Proc 21:2069–2071, 1989.

85. Kasiske BL, Heim-Duthoy KL, Tortorice KL, et al: Polyvalent immune globulin and cytomegalovirus infection after renal transplantation. Arch Intern Med 149:2733–2736, 1989.

86. Khawand N, Light JA, Brems W, et al: Does intravenous immunoglobulin prevent primary cytomegalovirus disease in kidney transplant recipients? Transplant Proc 21:2072–2074, 1989.

87. Balfour HH, Chace BA, Stapleton JT, et al: Randomized, placebo controlled trial of oral acyclovir for the prevention of cytomegalovirus disease in recipients of renal allografts. N Engl J Med 320:1381–1387, 1989.

88. Hecht DW, Snydman DR, Crumpacker CS, et al: Ganciclovir for treatment of renal-transplant associated primary cytomegalovirus pneumonia. J Infect Dis 157:187–190, 1988.

89. Creasy TS, Flower AJE, Veitch PS: Life-threatening cytomegalovirus infection treated with dihydropropoxymethylguanine. [Letter] Lancet 1:675, 1986.

90. Thomson MH, Jeffries DJ: Ganciclovir therapy in iatrogenically immunosuppressed patients with cytomegalovirus disease. J Antimicrob Chemother 23(suppl E):61–70, 1989.

91. Winston DJ, Ho WG, Bartoni K, et al: Ganciclovir therapy for cytomegalovirus infections in recipients of bone marrow transplants and other immunosuppressed patients. Rev Infect Dis 10:S547–553, 1988.

92. Lang PH, Buisson G, Rostoker A, et al: DHPG treatment of kidney

transplant recipients with severe CMV infection. Transplant Proc 21:2084–2086, 1989.

93. Snydman DR: Ganciclovir therapy for cytomegalovirus disease associated with renal transplantation. Rev Infect Dis 10:S554–562, 1988.

94. Bach MC, Adler JL, Breman J, et al: Influence of rejection therapy on fungal and nocardial infections in renal transplant recipients. Lancet 1:180–184, 1973.

95. Weiland D, Ferguson RM, Peterson PK, et al: Aspergillosis in 25 renal transplant patients. Ann Surg 198:622–629, 1983.

96. Wheat LJ, Smith EJ, Sathapatayavongs B, et al: Histoplasmosis in renal allograft recipients. Arch Intern Med 143:703–707, 1983.

97. Yoshino MT, Hillman BJ, Galgiani JN: Coccidioidomycosis in renal dialysis and transplant patients: Radiologic findings in 30 patients. AJR 149:989–992, 1987.

98. Cohen IM, Galgiani JN, Potter D, et al: Coccidioidomycosis in renal replacement therapy. Arch Intern Med 142:489–494, 1982.

99. Hardy AM, Wajszczuk CP, Suffredini AF, et al: *Pneumocystis carinii* pneumonia in renal transplant recipients treated with cyclosporine and steroids. J Infect Dis 149:143–147, 1984.

100. Franson TR, Kauffman M, Adams MB, et al: Cyclosporine therapy and refractory *Pneumocystis carinii* pneumonia. Arch Surg 122:1034–1035, 1987.

101. Santiago-Delpin EA, Mora E, Gonzalez ZA, et al: Factors in an outbreak of *Pneumocystis carinii* in a transplant unit. Transplant Proc 20:462–465, 1988.

102. Talseth T, Holdaas H, Albrechtsen D, et al: Increasing incidence of *Pneumocystis carinii* pneumonia in renal transplant patients. Transplant Proc 20:400–401, 1988.

103. Sterling RP, Bradley BB, Khalil KG, et al: Comparison of biopsy-proven *Pneumocystis carinii* pneumonia in acquired immune deficiency syndrome patients and renal allograft recipients. Ann Thorac Surg 38:494–499, 1984.

104. Fox BC, Sollinger HW, Belzer FO, et al: A prospective, randomized, double-blind study of trimethoprim-sulfamethoxazole for prophylaxis of infection in renal transplantation: Clinical efficacy, absorption of trimethoprim-sulfamethoxasole, effects on the microflora, and the cost-benefit of prophylaxis. Am J Med 89:255–273, 1990.

105. Lloveras J, Peterson PK, Simmons RL, et al: Mycobacterial infections in renal transplant recipients. Arch Intern Med 142:888–892, 1982.

106. Riska H, Gronhagen-Riska C, Ahonen J: Tuberculosis and renal allograft transplantation. Transplant Proc 19:4096–4097, 1987.

107. Malhotra KK, Dash SC, Dhawan IK, et al: Tuberculosis and renal transplantation—Observations from an endemic area of tuberculosis. Postgrad Med J 62:359–362, 1986.

108. Coutts II, Jegarajah S, Stark JE: Tuberculosis in renal transplant recipients. Br J Dis Chest 73:141–148, 1979.

109. Samhan M, Panjwani DD, Dadah SK, et al: Is tuberculosis a contraindication for renal transplantation? Transplant Proc 21:2036–2037, 1989.

110. Dautzenberg B, Grosset J, Fechner J, et al: The management of thirty immunocompromised patients with tuberculosis. Am Rev Respir Dis 129:494–495, 1984.

111. Spence RK, Dafoe DC, Rabin G, et al: Mycobacterial infections in renal allograft recipients. Arch Surg 118:356–359, 1983.

112. Rubin RH: Infection in the renal and liver transplant recipient. *In* Rubin R, Young L (eds): Clinical Approach to Infection in the Compromised Host. New York, Plenum, 1988:657–621.

113. Offerman G, Keller F, Molzahn M: Low cyclosporin A blood levels and acute graft rejection in a renal transplant recipient during rifampin treatment. Am J Nephrol 5:385–387, 1985.

114. Krom RAF, Wiesner RH, Rettke SR, et al: The first 100 liver transplantations at the Mayo Clinic. Mayo Clin Proc 64:84–94, 1989.

115. Maddrey WC, Van Thiel DH: Liver transplantation: An overview. Hepatology 8:948–959, 1988.

116. Wood RP, Rikkers LF, Shaw BW, et al: A review of liver transplantation for gastroenterologists. Am J Gastroenterol 92:593–606, 1987.

117. Iwatsuki S, Starzl T, Gordon RD, et al: Liver transplantation: Selection of patients and results. Transplant Proc 19:2373–2377, 1987.

118. Busuttil RW, Goldstein L, Danovitch GM, et al: Liver transplantation today. Ann Intern Med 104:377–389, 1986.

119. Colonna JD, Winston DJ, Brill JE, et al: Infectious complications in liver transplantation. Arch Surg 123:360–364, 1988.

120. Paya CV, Hermans PE, Washington JA, et al: Incidence, distribution, and outcome of episodes of infection in 100 orthotopic liver transplantations. Mayo Clin Proc 64:555–564, 1989.

121. Kusne S, Dummer JS, Singh N, et al: Infections after liver transplantation: An analysis of 101 consecutive cases. Medicine (Baltimore) 63:132–143, 1988.

122. Dummer JS, Hardy A, Poorsattar A, et al: Early infections in kidney, heart and liver transplant recipients on cyclosporine. Transplantation 36:259–267, 1983.

123. Schroter GPJ, Hoelscher M, Putnam CW, et al: Infections complicating orthotopic liver transplantation: A study emphasizing graft-related septicemia. Arch Surg 111:1337–1347, 1976.

124. Krowka MJ, Cortese DA: Pulmonary aspects of liver disease and liver transplantation. Clin Chest Med 10:593–616, 1989.

125. Wiesner RH, Hermans PE, Rakela J, et al: Selective bowel decontamination to decrease gram negative aerobic bacterial and candida colonization and prevent infection after orthotopic liver transplantation. Transplantation 45:570–574, 1988.

126. Haagsma EB, Klompmaker IJ, Grond J, et al: Herpes virus infections after orthotopic liver transplantation. Transplantation 19:4054–4056, 1987.

127. Singh N, Dummer JS, Kusne S, et al: Infections with cytomegalovirus and other herpes viruses in 121 liver transplant recipients: Transmission by donated organ and the effect of OKT3 antibodies. J Infect Dis 158:124–131, 1988.

128. Jensen WA, Rose RM, Hammer SM, et al: Pulmonary complications of orthotopic liver transplantation. Transplantation 42:484–490, 1986.

129. Harbison MA, DeGirolami PC, Jenkins RL, et al: Ganciclovir therapy of severe cytomegalovirus infections in solid organ transplant recipients. Transplantation 46:82–88, 1988.

130. Paya CV, Hermans PE, Smith TF, et al: Efficacy of ganciclovir in liver and kidney transplant recipients with severe cytomegalovirus infection. Transplantation 46:229–234, 1988.

131. deHemptinne B, Lamy ME, Salizzoni M, et al: Successful treatment of cytomegalovirus disease with 9(1,3-dihydroxy-2-propoxymethyl)-guanine. Transplant Proc 20:652–655, 1988.

132. Stratta RJ, Shaefer MS, Cushing KA, et al: Successful prophylaxis of cytomegalovirus disease after primary CMV exposure in liver transplant recipients. Transplantation 51:90–97, 1991.

133. Saliba F, Gugenheim J, Bismuth SA, et al: Incidence of cytomegalovirus infection and effects of cytomegalovirus immune globulin prophylaxis after orthotopic liver transplantation. Transplant Proc 19:4081–4082, 1987.

134. Rakela J, Wiesner RH, Taswell HF, et al: Incidence of cytomegalovirus infection and its relationship to donor-recipient serologic status in liver transplantation. Transplantation 19:2399–2402, 1987.

135. Kusne S, Dummer JS, Singh N, et al: Fungal infections after liver transplantation. Transplantation 20:650–651, 1988.

136. Kriett JM, Kaye MP: The registry of the International Society for Heart and Lung Transplantation: Eighth official report—1991. J Heart Lung Transplant 10:491–496, 1991.

137. Copeland JG, Mammana RB, Fuller JK, et al: Heart transplantation: Four years' experience with conventional immunosuppression. JAMA 251:1563–1566, 1984.

138. Ettinger NA, Trulock EP: Pulmonary considerations of organ transplantation. Part 3. Am Rev Respir Dis 143:1386–1405, 1991.

139. Ettinger NA, Trulock EP: Pulmonary considerations of organ transplantation. Part 1. Am Rev Respir Dis 144:213–221, 1991.

140. Horn JE, Bartlett JG: Infectious complications following heart transplantation. *In* Baumgartner WA, Reitz BA, Achuff SC (eds): Heart and Heart-Lung Transplantation. Philadelphia, WB Saunders, 1990:220–236.

141. Gentry LO, Zeluff BJ: Diagnosis and treatment of infection in cardiac transplant recipients. Surg Clin North Am 66:459–465, 1986.

142. Stinson EB, Bieber CP, Griepp RB, et al: Infectious complications after cardiac transplantation in man. Ann Intern Med 74:22–36, 1971.

143. Mammana RB, Peterson EA, Fuller JK, et al: Pulmonary infections in cardiac transplant patients: Modes of diagnosis, complications, and effectiveness of therapy. Ann Thorac Surg 36:700–705, 1983.

144. Cooper DKC, Lanza RP, Oliver S, et al: Infectious complications after heart transplantation. Thorax 38:822–828, 1983.

145. Austin JHM, Schulman LL, Mastrobattista JD: Pulmonary infection after cardiac transplantation: Clinical and radiologic correlations. Radiology 172:259–265, 1989.

146. Gorensek MJ, Stewart RW, Keyus TF, et al: A multivariate analysis of risk factors for pneumonia following cardiac transplantation. Transplantation 46:860–865, 1988.

147. Garzon AA, Seltzer B, Karlson KE: Respiratory mechanics following open-heart surgery for acquired valvular disease. Circulation 33–34(suppl 1):57–64, 1966.

148. Rosky LP, Rodman T: Medical aspects of open-heart surgery. N Engl J Med 274:833–840, 1966.

149. Robin ED, Thomas ED: Some relations between pulmonary edema and pulmonary inflammation (pneumonia). Arch Intern Med 93:713–724, 1954.

150. Hofflin JM, Potasman I, Baldwin JC, et al: Infectious complications in heart transplant recipients receiving cyclosporine and corticosteroids. Ann Intern Med 106:209–216, 1987.

151. Redd SC, Schuster DM, Quan J, et al: Legionellosis in cardiac transplant recipients: Results of a nationwide survey. J Infect Dis 158:651–652, 1988.

152. Gentry LO, Zeluff B: Infection in the cardiac transplant patient. *In* Rubin RH, Young LS (eds): Clinical Approach to Infection in the Compromised Host. New York, Plenum, 1988:623–648.

153. Saravolatz LD, Burch KH, Fisher E, et al: The compromised host and legionnaires' disease. Ann Intern Med 90:533–537, 1979.

154. Copeland J, Wieden M, Feinberg W, et al: Legionnaires' disease following cardiac transplantation. Chest 79:669–671, 1981.

155. Hamedani P, Ali J, Hafeez S, et al: The safety and efficacy of clarithromycin in patients with *Legionella* pneumonia. Chest 100:1503–1506, 1991.

156. Simpson GL, Stinson EB, Egger MJ, et al: Norcardial infections in the immunocompromised host: A detailed study in a defined population. Rev Infect Dis 3:492–507, 1981.

157. Krick JA, Stinson EB, Remington JS: *Nocardia* infection in heart transplant patients. Ann Intern Med 82:18–26, 1975.

158. Simpson GL, Remington JS: Association of prior nocardiosis and subsequent occurrence of nontuberculous mycobacteriosis in a defined, immunosuppressed population. J Infect Dis 146:211–219, 1982.

159. Dummer JS, Bahnson HT, Griffith BP, et al: Infections in patients on cyclosporine and prednisone following cardiac transplantation. Transplant Proc 15:2779–2781, 1983.

160. Dummer JS, White LT, Ho M, et al: Morbidity of cytomegalovirus infection in recipients of heart or heart-lung transplants who received cyclosporine. J Infect Dis 152:1182–1191, 1985.

161. Keay S, Petersen E, Icenogle T, et al: Ganciclovir treatment of serious cytomegalovirus infection in heart and heart-lung transplant recipients. Rev Infect Dis 10:S563–S572, 1988.

162. Pollard RB, Arvin AM, Gamberg P, et al: Specific cell-mediated immunity and infections with herpes virus in cardiac transplant recipients. Am J Med 73:679–687, 1982.

163. Preiksaitis JK, Rosno S, Grumet C, et al: Infections due to herpesviruses in cardiac transplant recipients: Role of the donor heart and immunosuppressive therapy. J Infect Dis 147:974–981, 1983.

164. Shanley JD, Billingsley AM, Shelby J, et al: Transfer of murine cytomegalovirus infection by heart transplantation. Transplantation 36:584–586, 1983.

165. Wilson EJ, Medaris DN, Barrett LV, et al: The effects of donor pretreatment on the transmission of murine cytomegalovirus with cardiac transplants and explants. Transplantation 41:781–782, 1986.

166. Min KW, Wickemeyer WJ, Chandran P, et al: Fatal cytomegalovirus infection and coronary arterial thromboses after heart transplantation: A case report. J Heart Transplant 6:100–105, 1987.

167. Pucci A, Grasso M, Arbustini E: Myocardial involvement due to a disseminated cytomegalovirus infection in a heart transplant recipient: A case report. G Ital Cardiol 19:230–233, 1989.

168. Schulman LL: Cytomegalovirus pneumonitis and lobar consolidation. Chest 91:558–561, 1987.

169. Watson FS, O'Connell JB, Amber IJ, et al: Treatment of cytomegalovirus pneumonia in heart transplant recipients with 9(1,3-dihydroxy-2-proproxymethyl)-guanine (DHPG). J Heart Transplant 7:102–105, 1988.

170. Andreone PA, Olivari MT, Elick B, et al: Reduction of infectious complications following heart transplantation with triple-drug immunotherapy. J Heart Transplant 5:13–19, 1986.

171. Jamieson SW, Oyer PE, Reitz BA, et al: Cardiac transplantation at Stanford. J Heart Transplant 1:86–92, 1981.

172. Katz NM, Pierce PF, Anzeck RA, et al: Liposomal amphotericin B for treatment of pulmonary aspergillosis in a heart transplant recipient. J Heart Transplant 9:14–17, 1990.

173. De Laurenzi A: Aspergillosis in a cardiac transplant patient successfully treated with itraconazole. Terasaki PI (ed): Clinical Transplants. UCLA Tissue Typing Laboratory, 1989:321.

174. Faggian G, Bortolotti U, Mazzuco A, et al: Itraconazole therapy for acute invasive pulmonary aspergillosis in heart transplantation. Transplant Proc 21:2506–2507, 1989.

175. Ryning FW, McLeod R, Maddos JC, et al: Probable transmission of *Toxoplasma gondii* by organ transplantation. Ann Intern Med 90:47–49, 1979.

176. Luft BJ, Naot Y, Araujo FG, et al: Primary and reactivated toxoplasma infection in patients with cardiac transplants. Ann Intern Med 99:27–31, 1983.

177. Hakim M, Esmore D, Wallwork J, et al: Toxoplasmosis in cardiac transplantation. Br Med J 292:1108, 1986.

178. Heck CF, Shumway SJ, Kaye MP. The registry of the International Society for Heart Transplant: Sixth official report—1989. J Heart Transplant 8:271–276, 1989.

179. Toronto Lung Transplant Group: Unilateral lung transplantation for pulmonary fibrosis. N Engl J Med 314:1140–1145, 1986.

180. Trulock EP, Egan TM, Kouchoukos NT, et al: Single lung transplantation for severe chronic obstructive pulmonary disease. Chest 96:738–742, 1989.

181. Kaiser LR, Cooper JD, Pasque MK, et al: Single lung transplantation for primary pulmonary hypertension (PPH): A preliminary report. Chest 98:11S, 1990.

182. Theodore J, Lewiston N: Lung transplantation comes of age. [Editorial] N Engl J Med 322:772–774, 1990.

183. Cooper JD, Patterson GA, Grossman R, et al: Double lung transplantation for advanced chronic obstructive lung disease. Am Rev Respir Dis 139:303–307, 1989.

184. Patterson GA: Double lung transplantation. Clin Chest Med 11:227–233, 1990.

185. Dauber JH, Paradis IL, Dummer JS: Infectious complications in pulmonary allograft recipients. Clin Chest Med 11:291–308, 1990.

186. Dummer JS, Montero CG, Griffith BP, et al: Infections in heart-lung transplant recipients. Transplantation 41:725–729, 1986.

187. Brooks RG, Hofflin JM, Jamieson SW, et al: Infectious complications in heart-lung transplant recipients. Am J Med 79:412–422, 1985.

188. Hutter JA, Scott J, Wreghitt T, et al: The importance of cytomegalovirus in heart-lung transplant recipients. Chest 95:627–631, 1989.

189. Smyth RL, Higenbottam TW, Scott JP, et al: Experience of cytomegalovirus infection in heart-lung recipients. Am Rev Respir Dis 141:A410, 1990.

190. Hutter JA, Despins P, Higenbottam T, et al: Heart-lung transplantation: Better use of resources. Am J Med 85:4–11, 1988.

191. Higenbottam T, Stewart S, Penketh A, et al: Transbronchial lung biopsy for the diagnosis of rejection in heart-lung transplant patients. Transplantation 46:532–539, 1988.

192. Burke CM, Theodore J, Baldwin JC, et al: Twenty-eight cases of human heart-lung transplantation. Lancet 1:517–519, 1986.

192a. Bailey TC, Ettinger NA, Storch GA: Failure of high-dose oral acyclovir with or without immunoglobulin to prevent primary cytomegalovirus disease in recipients of solid organ transplants. Am J Med 95:273–278, 1993.

193. Smyth RL, Higenbottam TW, Scott JP, et al: Herpes simplex virus infection in heart-lung transplant recipients. Transplantation 49:735–739, 1990.

194. Gryzan S, Paradis IL, Zeevi A, et al: Unexpectedly high incidence of *Pneumocystis carinii* infection after heart-lung transplantation. Am Rev Respir Dis 137:1268–1274, 1988.

195. Golden JA, Hollander H, Chernoff D, et al: Prevention of *Pneumocystis* pneumonia by inhaled pentamidine. Lancet 1:654–657, 1989.

196. McCarthy PM, Starnes VA, Theodore J, et al: Improved survival after heart-lung transplantation. J Thorac Cardiovasc Surg 99:54–60, 1990.

197. Kramer MR, Denning DW, Marshall SE, et al: Ulcerative tracheobronchitis after lung transplantation. Am Rev Respir Dis 144:552–556, 1991.

198. Trulock EP, Bolman RM, Genton R: Pulmonary disease caused by *Mycobacterium chelonae* in a heart-lung transplant recipient. Am Rev Respir Dis 140:802–805, 1989.

199. Thompson AB, Rickard KH, Shaw BW: Pulmonary complications and disease severity in adult liver transplant recipients. Transplant Proc 20:646S–649S, 1988.

# CHAPTER 15

# Respiratory Infections in Persons Infected With Human Immunodeficiency Virus

JOEL E. GALLANT and RICHARD E. CHAISSON

Human immunodeficiency virus (HIV) infection causes a progressive cellular and humoral immunodeficiency that is associated with the development of many opportunistic infections and malignancies. It is estimated that more than 10 million persons worldwide have HIV infection and that the prevalence will increase to more than 40 million by the year 2000. In the United States by 1993, more than 1 million people were infected with HIV, and 250,000 had developed the acquired immunodeficiency syndrome (AIDS), the advanced stage of the infection. As more HIV-infected persons progress from asymptomatic infection to symptomatic disease, an increasing number of patients will experience HIV-related pulmonary infections.

Infections of the respiratory tract are a prominent feature of HIV infection. Since the first descriptions of AIDS with *Pneumocystis carinii* pneumonia (PCP) in 1981, a variety of opportunistic pulmonary infections have been observed in people with HIV infection. As experience with the full spectrum of HIV-related diseases grows, more respiratory complications of HIV disease are recognized. This chapter reviews the common and unusual infections of the respiratory tract that are associated with HIV infection and the current management strategies for these opportunistic diseases.

## PATHOGENESIS

Infection with HIV produces quantitative and functional defects in cell-mediated immunity that increase the likelihood of disease caused by organisms usually held in check by this arm of the host immune system. Over time, HIV-infected persons experience a decline in the number of circulating $CD4^+$ lymphocytes and become increasingly at risk for opportunistic infections. Functional defects in macrophage function associated with impairment of cytokine production (eg, interferon-$\gamma$, interleukin-2) diminishes the host responses to intracellular pathogens.[1] Other immunologic defects increase the likelihood of disease due to pyogenic bacteria. The spontaneous activation of B lymphocytes leads to a polyclonal gammopathy, which is accompanied by a decreased responsiveness of B lymphocytes to neoantigens and reduced levels of type-specific antibodies.[2] Susceptibility to community-acquired bacteria is enhanced. Neutrophil defects may be seen in HIV infection, including impaired chemotaxis, phagocytosis, and bacterial killing.[3] These changes in immune function contribute to a higher incidence of bacterial pneumonia and invasive bacterial disease in people infected with HIV.

The likelihood that a person with HIV infection will develop opportunistic disease is a function of the host immune defenses, exposure to potential pathogens in the environment, and the relative virulence of the pathogens to which the host is exposed. The $CD4^+$ lymphocyte count is the best surrogate marker of host immune response in the HIV-infected person and is used to stage patients clinically and epidemiologically. In persons with $CD4^+$ lymphocyte counts greater than 500/mm³, opportunistic disease is rare, but common bacterial pulmonary disease, particularly pneumococcal disease, may be seen. As $CD4^+$ cell counts fall lower, infections caused by relatively virulent pathogens such as *Mycobacterium tuberculosis* may appear. When the

CD4$^+$ lymphocyte count falls below 200/mm$^3$, opportunistic infections with organisms that do not cause disease in the normal host, such as *P. carinii,* occur. Evaluating patients with HIV infection and respiratory tract symptoms is significantly aided by knowledge of the host immune status.

## APPROACH TO DIAGNOSIS

An approach to evaluating patients with HIV-related pulmonary disease is shown in Figure 15–1 and is discussed in greater detail in Chapter 41. After confirmation of pulmonary disease by finding abnormalities on a chest radiograph or defects in gas exchange or evidence of pulmonary inflammation with nonspecific tests, examination of respiratory tract secretions for the presence of pathogens is undertaken. Sputum induction is a common procedure with a reasonably high sensitivity for detecting PCP or pyogenic pneumonia. Sputum should be examined for acid-fast bacilli, and mycobacterial cultures should be performed. The negative predictive value of sputum induction for PCP or other respiratory infections is low, and disease cannot be excluded by a negative test result. If a specific diagnosis is not established, bronchoalveolar lavage (BAL) is extremely sensitive and specific for identifying HIV-related pulmonary pathogens. Transbronchial biopsy may increase the yield of bronchoscopy for some diagnoses, although complications of this procedure occur in as many as 10% of patients.

## PROTOZOAN INFECTIONS

### Pneumocystis carinii

Although *P. carinii* was a rare opportunistic pathogen in immunosuppressed patients before the emergence of AIDS, it quickly became one of the most important causes of

morbidity and mortality among patients with HIV infection (see Chap. 36). With the widespread use of antiretrovirals and *Pneumocystis* prophylaxis, the mortality rate for first episodes has dropped to less than 10%, and PCP is no longer a common cause of death among patients with AIDS who receive adequate medical care.[4] Nevertheless, it continues to be one of the most common opportunistic infections in patients with AIDS.

Although *P. carinii* is discussed here under its traditional category as a protozoan infection, newer data suggest that it may be taxonomically closer to a fungus.[5] It is a ubiquitous pathogen, and disease probably occurs as a result of latent infection acquired through the respiratory route early in life.[6]

### Clinical and Laboratory Manifestations

Although *Pneumocystis* infection may occur outside the lungs,[7-10] most infections are pulmonary. The clinical presentation is typically insidious, with initially mild symptoms that progress over weeks or months. The most common symptoms are fever, dyspnea, and a cough, which usually is nonproductive. Other constitutional symptoms, such as fatigue and weight loss, may occur. The physical examination may reveal fever and tachypnea, but findings on chest examination are frequently normal. Radiographic features vary considerably. Most commonly, diffuse, bilateral, interstitial or alveolar infiltrates are seen, but PCP may present with unilateral or focal infiltrates, lobar or segmental consolidation, cavitary or cystic lesions, pleural effusions, or nodular densities.[11, 12] Atypical radiographic features, especially apical infiltrates, are seen more frequently in patients who have received prophylaxis with aerosolized pentamidine.[13, 14] Spontaneous pneumothorax may be associated with concurrent or prior PCP and may be more common in persons who receive aerosol pentamidine prophylaxis.[15, 16] Hilar or mediastinal adenopathy is rare and suggests an

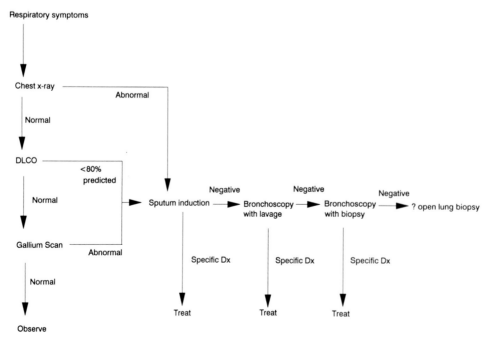

**Figure 15–1.** Algorithm for the evaluation of respiratory symptoms in HIV-infected patients at risk for *Pneumocystis carinii* pneumonia.

alternative or concomitant process. Patients presenting with mild PCP may have normal chest radiographs.[11]

PCP is unusual in HIV-seropositive patients with a CD4+ lymphocyte count greater than 200 to 250/mm³.[6] Laboratory abnormalities are generally nonspecific. The serum lactate dehydrogenase (LDH) level is elevated in most patients with PCP, and the degree of elevation may correlate with severity and outcome.[17] LDH elevations also are seen in other AIDS-related respiratory illnesses. Arterial blood gas determinations may demonstrate hypoxemia, an elevated alveolar-arterial gradient, hypocarbia, or respiratory alkalosis, but normal arterial blood oxygen tension does not exclude PCP. A low oxygen saturation or desaturation with exercise is more common with PCP than with other AIDS-related complications and should prompt consideration of PCP. However, oxygen saturation may be normal.[18] Other tests that are sometimes helpful in supporting the diagnosis of PCP include the diffusing capacity for carbon monoxide and gallium 67 citrate scintigraphy of the lung. Both are highly sensitive for PCP but nonspecific.[19] Because of their high sensitivity and negative predictive value, these tests may be useful in evaluating patients with normal chest radiographs and arterial blood gases to determine the need for further diagnostic procedures.

## Diagnosis

Empiric treatment for *P. carinii* should be avoided. Many other HIV-related conditions can mimic PCP, and toxicity from anti-*Pneumocystis* therapy is common during the 21-day treatment period. The initial diagnostic procedure in patients suspected of having PCP is usually an examination of sputum induced by nebulized hypertonic saline. With proper induction techniques and the use of appropriate stains, the sensitivity of the results of sputum induction can exceed 90%, approaching that of bronchoscopy.[20] Traditional stains used for the diagnosis of PCP are toluidine blue-O and methenamine silver, which stain the cyst wall. Trophozoite stains such as Giemsa (Diff-Quik) are easy to perform, inexpensive, highly accurate, and especially useful for examining sputum specimens (Fig. 15–2). Immunofluorescence stains using direct or indirect monoclonal antibodies are rapid, technically easy to perform, and are sensitive

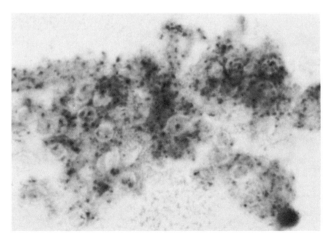

**Figure 15–2.** *Pneumocystis carinii* in a Giemsa-stained induced sputum specimen.

and specific.[20] The use of polymerase chain reaction to detect *P. carinii* in induced sputum samples is highly sensitive[21] and may someday play a role in the routine diagnosis of PCP, especially in patients with sputum samples that are negative by standard staining methods.

The diagnostic yield of sputum examination is not 100%, and varies widely from center to center. When a diagnosis is not established by examination of an induced sputum specimen, fiberoptic bronchoscopy should be performed. BAL alone has a high yield in patients with HIV infection, with sensitivities ranging from 79% to 98%. When combined with transbronchial biopsy, the sensitivity is between 94% and 100%.[22] Bronchial brush biopsies have low diagnostic yield and need not be performed.[11] Repeat bronchoscopy or open lung biopsy should be considered for patients who have had nondiagnostic bronchoscopy and who are clinically deteriorating.[23] However, repeat bronchoscopy usually does not identify other pathogens in patients with bronchoscopically confirmed PCP who appear to be failing therapy.

## Treatment

There are several acceptable treatment options for patients with PCP (Table 15–1). Trimethoprim-sulfamethoxazole (TMP-SMX) given orally or intravenously (15 mg/kg/d of trimethoprim and 75 mg/kg/d of sulfamethoxazole) in three to four divided doses for 2 to 3 weeks is effective in the treatment of *P. carinii* infection and remains the drug of choice for initial therapy in most cases. Adverse reactions are common in AIDS patients and include fever, rash, leukopenia, neutropenia, and hepatic dysfunction. Drug toxicity usually becomes evident after 10 to 12 days of therapy. The traditional alternative to TMP-SMX is parenteral pentamidine (4 mg/kg/d) given intravenously over 1 hour, for 2 to 3 weeks. Pentamidine is associated with a high incidence of adverse reactions, including renal dysfunction, hypoglycemia, hyperglycemia, hypotension, fever, and neutropenia. Intramuscular administration should be avoided, because of the risk of sterile abscesses. In comparative trials, TMP-SMX and pentamidine have had similar degrees of efficacy and toxicity, with 60% to 90% of patients surviving the acute episode of PCP and 25% to 60% experiencing adverse reactions.[24–26] Sattler and colleagues[27] performed a prospective, randomized, noncrossover study and found improved survival (86%) in patients receiving TMP-SMX compared with those receiving pentamidine (61%). Drug doses used in that study were lower than those used in other studies (ie, TMP-SMX, 15 mg/kg/d, adjusted for serum sulfamethoxazole levels, and pentamidine, 3 mg/kg/d), and the frequency and severity of adverse reactions were reduced.

The combination of oral trimethoprim (15–20 mg/kg/d) and dapsone (100 mg/d) for 2 to 3 weeks is an alternative to TMP-SMX and appears to be as effective and better tolerated in patients with mild or moderate PCP.[28, 29] The toxic effects of dapsone include hemolytic anemia in patients with glucose-6-phosphate dehydrogenase (G6PD) deficiency and methemoglobinemia. Dapsone should not be used alone to treat PCP, because it is associated with treatment failures.[30, 31]

A regimen of oral or intravenous clindamycin (1800–2400 mg/d) and oral primaquine (15 mg primaquine base per day) for the treatment of PCP appears promising in early

Table 15–1. **Treatment and Prophylaxis for Common HIV-Related Opportunistic Pulmonary Infections**

| Pulmonary Infection | Preferred Therapy | Alternative Therapy |
|---|---|---|
| ***Protozoan Infections*** | | |
| *Pneumocystis carinii* | | |
| Acute pneumonia | Trimethoprim-sulfamethoxazole (15–20 mg/kg/d of trimethoprim) PO or IV × 21 d in 3–4 doses<br>Trimethoprim, 15–20 mg/kg/d PO or IV + dapsone, 100 mg/d PO | Pentamidine, 3–4 mg/kg/d IV × 21 d<br>Clindamycin, 600 mg IV q 6 h or 300–450 mg PO q 6 h + primaquine (15-mg base PO qd) × 21 d<br>Atovaquone, 750 mg PO tid × 21 d |
| Prophylaxis | Trimethoprim-sulfamethoxazole 1 double-strength PO qd or 3 times/wk or 1 single-strength PO qd | Aerosolized pentamidine, 300 mg q mo<br>Dapsone, 25–100 mg PO qd or 100 mg PO 2 times/wk<br>Pyrimethamine + sulfadoxine (Fansidar), 1–2 per wk<br>Pentamidine (4 mg/kg) IV or IM q 2 wk<br>Atovaquone (investigational—prophylactic dose not established) |
| *Toxoplasma gondii* | | |
| Acute pneumonia | Pyrimethamine, 100–200 mg load then 50–100 mg/d + folinic acid, 10 mg/d + sulfadiazine, 4–8 g/d PO | Pyrimethamine + folinic acid (prior doses) + clindamycin, 600 mg IV q 6 h or 300–450 mg PO q 6 h *or* azithromycin, 1800 mg PO 1st day, then 1200 mg/d PO *or* atovaquone, 750 mg PO tid |
| Maintenance | Not indicated in absence of encephalitis | |
| Prophylaxis (for encephalitis) | Trimethoprim-sulfamethoxazole (see *P. carinii* prophylaxis)<br>Dapsone, 50 mg/d + pyrimethamine, 50 mg/wk | Pyrimethamine, 25 mg PO qd |
| ***Fungal Infections*** | | |
| *Cryptococcus neoformans* | | |
| Acute pneumonia | Accompanying meningitis:<br>Amphotericin B, 0.5–0.8 mg/kg/d IV with or without 5-flucytosine, 100 mg/kg/d in 4 doses | Pneumonia only (no meningitis):<br>Fluconazole, 400 mg/d PO<br>Itraconazole, 200 mg PO bid |
| Maintenance | Fluconazole, 200 mg PO qd | Not indicated in absence of meningitis |
| *Histoplasma capsulatum* | | |
| Acute disease | Amphotericin B, 0.5–1.0 mg/kg/d IV × 4–8 wk, total dose = 1–2.5 g | Itraconazole, 200 mg PO bid (mild disease, normal mental status) |
| Maintenance | Itraconazole 200 mg PO bid<br>Amphotericin B (1.0 mg/kg/wk) | Fluconazole, 200–400 mg/d PO |
| *Coccidioides immitis* | | |
| Acute disease | Amphotericin B, 0.5–1.0 mg/kg/d IV × ≥ 8 wk, total dose = 2–2.5 g | Fluconazole, 400 mg/d PO<br>Itraconazole, 200 mg PO bid |
| Maintenance | Amphotericin B, 1 mg/kg/wk<br>Itraconazole, 200 mg PO bid | Fluconazole, 400–800 mg/d PO |
| ***Mycobacterial Infections*** | | |
| *Mycobacterium tuberculosis* | | |
| Treatment | Isoniazid, 300 mg/d PO + rifampin, 600 mg/d PO + pyrazinamide, 15–30 mg/kg/d PO + ethambutol, 15–25 mg/kg/d PO × 6–9 mo; if isolate sensitive to isoniazid and rifampin, discontinue pyrazinamide + ethambutol after 2 mo | Isoniazid + rifampin + pryazinamide (same doses as for preferred therapy) |
| Prophylaxis | Isoniazid, 300 mg/d PO | Rifampin + pyrazinamide (same doses as for prefered therapy) × 2 mo (investigational) |
| *Mycobacterium kansasii* | | |
| Treatment | Isoniazid + rifampin + ethambutol (same doses as above) | Clarithromycin, 500–1000 mg PO bid + 1 other agent to which organism is susceptible |
| ***Bacterial Diseases*** | | |
| *Streptococcus pneumoniae* | Penicillin | Erythromycin, cephalosporins |
| *Haemophilus influenzae* | Cefuroxime | Trimethoprim-sulfamethoxazole |
| *Rhodococcus equi* | Vancomycin 2 g/d IV ± rifampin, 600 mg PO qd or ciprofloxacin, 750 mg PO bid or imipenem, 0.5 g IV qid × 2–4 wk | Third-generation cephalosporins |

studies.[32–39] Trials in which this regimen has been used for the treatment of mild or moderate PCP have demonstrated favorable responses in more than 90% of patients. When patients with severe PCP requiring mechanical ventilation were treated with clindamycin and primaquine, the failure rate was 20% to 50%, which is similar to the experience with standard regimens. The side effects include rash, diarrhea, leukopenia, and mild methemoglobinemia. Primaquine should be avoided in G6PD-deficient patients.

A new hydroxynaphthoquinone compound, atovaquone, appears to be safe, effective, and well tolerated in the treatment of mild or moderate PCP.[40–42] In a randomized, double-blind study of 322 patients with mild or moderate PCP, 82% of patients assigned to atovaquone responded, and 94% of patients receiving TMP-SMX responded.[43] Treatment-limiting adverse reactions were more frequent with TMP-SMX than with atovaquone (20% versus 7%), so that the overall rate of therapeutic efficacy was similar. Atovaquone is approved for therapy of acute PCP in patients intolerant of TMP-SMX. The recommended dose is 750 mg orally three times daily (see Table 15–1).

Aerosolized pentamidine was initially evaluated for the treatment of PCP.[94] Its use is limited by variability of delivery systems and nonuniform distribution in the lung. Compared with parenteral pentamidine, it is associated with a higher relapse rate and a lower response rate.[45, 46] It may be appropriate for patients who are intolerant of other agents.

Trimetrexate, a new folate antagonist, has been used in patients with refractory PCP or patients who cannot be treated with standard therapies.[47–49] In a multicenter trial comparing trimetrexate with TMP-SMX, significantly more deaths and treatment failures occurred with trimetrexate.[50] The usual dosing regimen is 30 to 45 mg/m$^2$/d, administered as a single dose, combined with leucovorin (30–80 mg/m$^2$/d).[51, 52] The most common adverse effects are neutropenia, thrombocytopenia, and elevations in serum aminotransferase concentrations.

The adjunctive use of corticosteroids with appropriate anti-*Pneumocystis* drugs in patients with moderate or severe PCP is well supported. Three controlled studies of corticosteroids demonstrated reduced short-term mortality rates or respiratory deterioration with the use of corticosteroids.[53–55] Adjunctive steroids are recommended for patients with PCP with an oxygen pressure (Po$_2$) of less than 70 mm Hg or a P(A − a)o$_2$ gradient of more than 35 mm Hg on room air.[56] The recommended regimen, based on the largest of the three studies,[53] is prednisone given as 40 mg twice daily for 5 days, then 20 mg twice daily for 5 days, followed by 20 mg daily for the remaining 11 days of therapy. Preliminary data suggest that corticosteroids may also prevent deterioration and increase the exercise tolerance of patients with mild PCP (ie, baseline oxygen saturation by pulse oximetry ≥90% at rest).[57] There are insufficient data to recommend the institution of corticosteroid therapy for patients who suffer respiratory deterioration after 5 to 10 days of antimicrobial therapy.[56]

The methods of prevention of PCP are discussed in Chapter 50.

### Toxoplasma gondii

Although *T. gondii* is the most common cause of central nervous system mass lesions in patients with AIDS, the lung is the second most common site of disease.[58] The incidence of toxoplasmic pneumonia varies geographically. In France, where there is a high prevalence of *Toxoplasma* infection, 7 (4.1%) of 169 HIV-infected patients who underwent bronchoscopy were found to have pulmonary toxoplasmosis.[59] In a U.S. study, only 1 of 441 patients with AIDS and pneumonia were found to have toxoplasmosis.[60]

Patients with toxoplasmic pneumonitis typically present with dyspnea, nonproductive cough, and fever.[61] Chest radiographs most often demonstrate diffuse interstitial infiltrates. The diagnosis is best made by demonstrating tachyzoites in respiratory specimens by hematoxylin and eosin or Giemsa staining. The demonstration of cysts may suggest the diagnosis, although cysts may persist in tissue after resolution of the infection.[62] As with *Toxoplasma* encephalitis, serologic results are nondiagnostic. IgM antibodies to *T. gondii* are seldom detectable, and although IgG antibody is usually present, diagnostic rises in antibody titers are rare. The absence of IgG antibody makes the diagnosis of toxoplasmosis less likely but does not exclude it.[63–65]

Because no specific studies of therapy of *Toxoplasma* pneumonia have been carried out, patients should be treated with regimens used in *Toxoplasma* encephalitis. The recommendations include the use of pyrimethamine combined with sulfadiazine or clindamycin.

### Other Parasitic Infections

*Cryptosporidium parvum,* a cause of diarrhea and cholecystitis in AIDS patients, has been detected in sputum, bronchial washings, and the lung tissue of AIDS patients.[66–70] Because most had gastrointestinal cryptosporidiosis and concomitant pulmonary infections, it is not clear whether the parasite causes pulmonary disease in AIDS.

*Leishmania donovani,* the agent of visceral leishmaniasis (ie, kala-azar), has caused disseminated disease in HIV-infected persons. Although in most reported cases the clinical presentation is similar to that seen in immunocompetent hosts,[71] some cases of isolated pulmonary disease have been described.[72] A case of *L. donovani* causing pleural effusion in a patient with AIDS has been reported.[73]

The microsporidian *Enterocytozoon bieneusi,* a cause of chronic diarrhea in HIV-infected patients, was detected in the BAL fluid and transbronchial biopsy specimens of a patient with chronic cough, dyspnea, and a pulmonary infiltrate and small pleural effusion.[74] The patient also had chronic diarrhea and intestinal microsporidiosis. No other opportunistic pathogen was found to explain the patient's pulmonary symptoms.

## BACTERIAL INFECTIONS

### Sinusitis

Sinusitis occurs with increased frequency in patients with HIV infection.[75–80] In a retrospective study of 667 patients admitted to the Johns Hopkins Hospital AIDS Ward, 72 (11%) were found to have sinusitis.[80] Most patients (88%) had CD4$^+$ lymphocyte counts less than 200/mm$^3$ at the index episode of sinusitis. Advanced immunosuppression was associated with more extensive and chronic disease. Although 68% of patients had fever, headache, and nasal congestion, many patients had nonspecific symptoms, and the diagnosis was incidental in a third of patients. More than half of the patients had radiographic evidence of sphenoid sinusitis, although no complications were seen. Microbiologic data were limited, because drainage procedures were performed for only 18 patients, all of whom were on antibiotics at the time; however, *Pseudomonas aeruginosa* grew from three of the sinus aspirates. Seventy-nine percent of patients had at least a partial response to antibiotic therapy.

## Bacterial Pneumonia

### Epidemiology

An increased incidence of community-acquired pneumonia among HIV-infected patients was recognized early in the AIDS epidemic. Among 35 patients with AIDS at the New York Veterans Administration Medical Center seen between 1982 and 1983, 4 had community-acquired pneumococcal pneumonia, 2 with bacteremia.[81] At Memorial Sloan-Kettering Cancer Center, 10% of pneumonias in AIDS patients were caused by community-acquired bacteria, with an annual incidence of 17.9 per 1000.[82] Forty-four percent were caused by *Streptococcus pneumoniae* and 44% by *Haemophilus influenzae*. In 59 adult patients with AIDS or AIDS-related complex at Boston City Hospital, 30 patients had 63 episodes of bacterial infection, 52 of which were community acquired.[83] There were 29 episodes of pneumonia, 21 of which were community acquired and eight of which were nosocomial.

The incidence of bacterial pneumonia is higher in certain populations. Witt and colleagues[83] found a higher incidence among intravenous drug users and patients without identified risk factors than among homosexual men. Schlamm and Yancovitz[84] identified 51 cases of *H. influenzae* pneumonia at Beth Israel Hospital in New York. In a retrospective study, they found that 67% were intravenous drug users, 18% were homosexual men, and 15% had both risk factors. The increased incidence of bacterial pneumonia among HIV-infected intravenous drug abusers is not accounted for by drug use alone. Selwyn and colleagues[85] prospectively studied 433 intravenous drug users without AIDS, one third of whom were seropositive for HIV. Over a 12-month period, 9.7% of the seropositive patients developed community-acquired pneumonia, compared with 2% of the seronegative patients. This excess incidence was not attributable to increased use of intravenous drugs. Selwyn and colleagues[86] found that, among HIV-infected intravenous drug users, pyogenic bacterial infections, including pneumonia and sepsis, occurred with an incidence of 8.0 cases per 100 person-years before the diagnosis of AIDS and that bacterial infections were independent predictors of progression to AIDS. Of the 49 cases of bacterial pneumonia, 24 (49%) were caused by *S. pneumoniae,* and 17 (35%) were caused by *H. influenzae*. The median CD4[+] lymphocyte count within the preceding 6 months for patients with bacterial infections was 317/mm[3], compared with 137/mm[3] for patients with AIDS.

### Clinical Manifestations

The clinical presentation of bacterial pneumonia is similar in patients with and without HIV infection.[87, 88] Compared with *P. carinii* pneumonia and other opportunistic infections of the lung, the onset of symptoms is more abrupt, and the patient is more likely to experience a productive cough and pleuritic chest pain.[82, 83, 89, 90] Patients with bacterial pneumonia may have localized findings on chest examinations. A relative leukocytosis and left shift in neutrophil production are common. Radiographic features typically include localized segmental or lobar consolidation, especially in the case of pneumococcal pneumonia.[82, 89, 91–94] Radiographic manifestations of *H. influenzae* pneumonia are variable and may included diffuse bilateral infiltrates, which are characteristic of *P. carinii*.[82] Bacterial pneumonia in patients with HIV infection may be more severe, with a higher incidence of multilobar involvement and a less rapid response to antibiotics.[93]

Bacteremia accompanying pneumonia due to *S. pneumoniae* and *H. influenzae* is much more common in seropositive patients.[82, 83, 91, 95, 96] At Johns Hopkins Hospital, 46% of HIV-infected patients with pneumococcal pneumonia had bacteremia.[96] Empyema, uncommon with pneumococcal pneumonia, has also been reported in HIV-infected patients.[93, 97] HIV-infected patients have a higher rate of recurrent bacterial pneumonia than patients without HIV infection, and relapses or recurrences may occur with the same organism or serotype or with different encapsulated organisms.[88]

### Diagnosis and Treatment

Patients presenting with clinical and radiographic features of pneumonia should have bacterial cultures of blood and sputum performed. Gram stain of the sputum is helpful in making a presumptive diagnosis, particularly if the sputum is purulent. Concomitant pulmonary infection with pyogenic bacteria and *P. carinii* is not uncommon, but the diagnosis of PCP is difficult if the sputum is purulent.

If the diagnostic considerations include *P. carinii* and pyogenic bacteria, treatment with high-dose TMP-SMX should be considered, because it provides excellent coverage against *S. pneumoniae, H. influenzae, Moraxella catarrhalis,* and *P. carinii*. If PCP is less likely, as in a patient with a focal infiltrate or a total CD4[+] count greater than 200/mm[3], the options for empiric treatment include second-generation cephalosporins or ampicillin-clavulanate. If the Gram stain or culture indicate pneumococcal pneumonia, specific therapy with penicillin or erythromycin is preferred. HIV-infected patients with community-acquired pneumonia usually respond rapidly to standard antibiotic therapy.[89, 94] In patients who fail to respond appropriately or who deteriorate after initial improvement, coinfection with another pathogen, especially *P. carinii,* should be considered.[88]

The prevention of bacterial pneumonia in HIV-infected persons is discussed in Chapter 50.

## Other Bacterial Infections

Nosocomial pneumonia in patients with AIDS is usually caused by gram-negative bacilli, including *P. aeruginosa,* or by *Staphylococcus aureus.*[82, 98–102] As with other hospitalized patients, the risk factors include neutropenia, the use of broad-spectrum antibiotics, and the presence of central venous catheters. Nosocomial pneumonia has a higher morbidity and mortality than community-acquired pneumonia.[100]

The incidence of *Pseudomonas* pneumonia may be increasing among HIV-infected patients and does not always appear to be hospital acquired or fulminant. Hollander and Baron[103] described 16 patients with advanced HIV disease (mean CD4$^+$ count, 25/mm$^3$) and *P. aeruginosa* pneumonia, diagnosed by Gram stain and culture of sputum or bronchoscopic washings. In 12 of the 16 patients, the pneumonia was community acquired, and *Pseudomonas* was the sole pathogen in 14 cases. Only 4 patients, 2 of whom had community-acquired pneumonia, presented with fulminant pneumonia and sepsis. The remaining 12, all with community-acquired pneumonia, had a more indolent presentation, with a mean duration of symptoms of 2 weeks. Only 6 of the 16 patients had risk factors for *Pseudomonas* pneumonia (eg, neutropenia, indwelling venous catheters, prior cytotoxic therapy). Fourteen of the patients survived the acute episode, but 12 had relapses, and 6 had multiple relapses.

In a prospective study of patients admitted to Johns Hopkins Hospital with community-acquired pneumonia, Mundy and colleagues[104] reported that gram-negative bacilli were a significantly more common cause of pneumonia in patients with HIV infection than in uninfected patients (9% versus 3%). Yamaguchi and Chaisson conducted a retrospective review of 30 episodes of gram-negative bacteremia in HIV-infected patients at Johns Hopkins Hospital.[105] A pulmonary source was responsible for four of the episodes. *P. aeruginosa* was isolated in 13 of the 30 episodes.

*Salmonella* infections in AIDS patients are often severe, with a high rate of bacteremia.[105, 106] Pneumonia due to *Salmonella typhimurium* has been reported.[107] Other bacterial pathogens reported to cause pneumonia in patients with HIV infection include *Bordetella bronchiseptica,*[108–110] *M. catarrhalis,*[83] group B *Streptococcus,*[82, 83] *Mycoplasma pneumoniae,*[83, 104] and *Streptomyces* species.[111]

Pneumonia due to *Legionella pneumophila* has been described in patients with HIV infection, but is not common.[83, 85, 104, 112, 113] Cavitary pneumonia due to *Legionella micdadei*[114] and *L. pneumophila*[115] has been described.

## Nocardia asteroides

Nocardiosis is unusual in HIV-infected patients, although the actual incidence is unknown, because it is not an indicator disease for AIDS.[116] In most cases, disease occurs in patients with advanced immunodeficiency (ie, CD4$^+$ cell count <200/mm$^3$).[117] Patients typically present with an indolent course and nonspecific constitutional complaints. Pulmonary symptoms, such as cough or dyspnea, may develop. As in patients without HIV infection, the lung is the most common site of disease, although dissemination is common in HIV-infected patients. Roentgenographic changes include nodules, cavities, and diffuse or focal infiltrates.[117–121] A case of pulmonary and disseminated disease due to *Nocardia farcinica* in an HIV-infected patient has been reported.[122]

The diagnosis is suspected if filamentous, beaded, branching, gram-positive, acid-fast rods are seen on Gram stain or modified acid-fast stain of sputum or other respiratory specimens.[118, 123] Because of the slow growth of the organism, cultures should be held for 4 weeks after nocardiosis is suspected. Culturing sputum for mycobacteria and fungi improves the chances of isolating *Nocardia.*

Sulfonamides have been the mainstay of therapy for nocardiosis. Although TMP-SMX is synergistic against *N. asteroides* in vitro, the combination is no more effective than any of the sulfonamides alone.[124] Minocycline is active against *Nocardia* in vitro and has been used successfully in HIV-infected and other patients.[117, 118] Other agents demonstrating in vitro activity against *Nocardia* include cefotaxime, ceftriaxone, imipenem, and amikacin,[125] but clinical experience with these agents is limited.

The optimal duration of therapy for nocardiosis is undetermined for immunocompetent and immunosuppressed patients. Some investigators recommend treatment for 6 to 12 months for patients with pulmonary nocardiosis, regardless of their immune status.[126] Others recommend indefinite therapy for immunosuppressed patients, including those with HIV infection, after an initial course of full-dose therapy.[117, 127]

The use of TMP-SMX for prophylaxis of PCP may help to prevent nocardiosis, although data are limited, and nocardiosis has been described in patients taking TMP-SMX prophylaxis.[117]

## Rhodococcus equi

*R. equi* (formerly *Corynebacterium equi*) was first reported to cause disease in an AIDS patient in 1986.[128] Since then, several cases have been reported.[129–134] The organism is a gram-positive, aerobic, nonmotile, non–spore-forming, pleomorphic bacillus. On Gram stain, its appearance varies from cocci to short rods. Infection typically presents as pneumonia, with unilobar, often upper lobe, pulmonary infiltrates, which progress over several weeks. Multilobar involvement may develop, and cavitation, pleural effusion, empyema, and bacteremia are common. Of 12 HIV-infected patients with *R. equi* infections, 1 had cavitary disease, and 3 had culture-positive pleural effusions.[132, 133] Cavities were distributed throughout the lung fields.

β-Lactam resistance develops frequently. Effective antimicrobial agents include erythromycin, vancomycin, clindamycin, chloramphenicol, and TMP-SMX. Rifampin has been used in combination with other agents and is probably synergistic when given with erythromycin. Prolonged courses of parenteral antibiotics are recommended, and surgical intervention is sometimes necessary for persistent abscesses. Recurrence is not uncommon, even after several weeks of antibiotic therapy.[132, 133]

## MYCOBACTERIAL INFECTIONS

### Mycobacterium tuberculosis

#### Epidemiology

The HIV epidemic has resulted in a rise in the incidence of tuberculosis in developing countries and in the United

States, where the incidence had previously been declining steadily.[135] Epidemiologic data suggest that most cases of tuberculosis in HIV-infected patients are caused by reactivation.[136] Because *M. tuberculosis* is more virulent than many of the other HIV-associated opportunistic pathogens, it often causes disease at an earlier stage of HIV infection and is frequently the initial manifestation. The incidence of tuberculosis is higher in populations with an increased likelihood of prior exposure to *M. tuberculosis,* such as intravenous drug users, blacks, Hispanics, and residents of developing countries.

The natural history of *M. tuberculosis* infection is altered dramatically by HIV infection. In persons with latent *M. tuberculosis* infection who acquire HIV infection, the risk of reactivation is 2% to 8% per year.[137] In HIV-infected persons who acquire new *M. tuberculosis* infection, the risk of progressive primary tuberculosis is extremely high. Daley and coworkers[138] studied an outbreak of tuberculosis in a residential facility for intravenous drug users with AIDS. Within 10 weeks of exposure to an index case, 37% of HIV-infected residents developed culture-proven pulmonary tuberculosis. DNA fingerprinting of isolates with restriction fragment length polymorphisms confirmed that the strains were identical. This acceleration of the natural history of tuberculosis infection underlies institutional outbreaks of tuberculosis among HIV-infected patients.

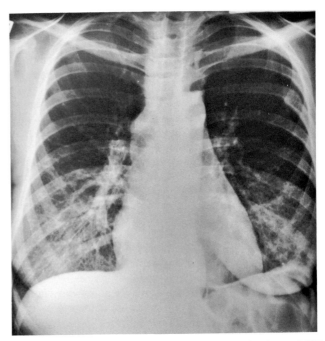

**Figure 15–3.** Pulmonary tuberculosis in a patient with advanced HIV disease, presenting with bilateral interstitial infiltrates in the lower lung fields.

### Clinical Manifestations

The clinical features of tuberculosis in HIV-infected patients depend on the degree of immunosuppression.[136] In patients with mildly or moderately depressed CD4+ counts who present with reactivation tuberculosis preceding the diagnosis of AIDS, the presentation is similar to that seen in other populations.[139, 140] Most have disease confined to the lungs, with upper lobe infiltrates that are sometimes cavitary. Some patients develop tuberculosis at a more advanced stage of HIV infection, often after the development of other opportunistic infections. In these cases, although pulmonary infection is common, the radiographic findings may be atypical or may mimic those of primary tuberculosis (Fig. 15–3). Cavitary disease is unusual, but lower lobe infiltrates or miliary patterns occur frequently. Intrathoracic adenopathy and extrapulmonary dissemination are also common. Some HIV-infected patients with culture-positive pulmonary tuberculosis have normal chest radiographs.[141, 142]

Extrapulmonary tuberculosis is seen in 24% to 48% of HIV-infected patients,[139, 140, 143, 144] although in patients with more advanced stages of immunosuppression, it may occur in more than 70%.[145] As with tuberculosis in other populations, the lymphatic system is the most common site of extrapulmonary involvement.[139, 145–147] HIV-infected patients are more likely to have disseminated, genitourinary, intraabdominal, and mediastinal tuberculosis or concomitant pulmonary disease than patients without HIV infection.[148] Bacteremia occurs in 26% to 42% of HIV-infected patients with tuberculosis.[149, 150] Tuberculous abscesses of the brain parenchyma[151] or spinal cord[152] may occur, appearing as ring-enhancing or hypodense mass lesions. Tuberculous meningitis may be more common in HIV-infected patients,[148, 153] and it has been reported in patients with acellular cerebrospinal fluid.[154]

### Diagnosis and Treatment

Diagnosis of pulmonary tuberculosis is made by examination of sputum for acid-fast bacilli, followed by mycobacterial culture. The diagnostic yield of the sputum smear in less severely immunocompromised patients is comparable to that found in HIV-negative patients,[139, 140, 143, 144] but in more advanced stages of HIV disease, the sensitivity is lower.[155] Sputum culture has a yield of approximately 90%. The sensitivity of smear and culture may be increased by BAL. Because bacteremia occurs in a substantial proportion of patients, blood cultures for acid-fast bacilli should be performed for all patients in whom tuberculosis is suspected. A positive purified protein derivative tuberculin test may support a diagnosis of tuberculosis, but a negative result of the skin test should never be used to exclude tuberculosis, because patients may become anergic with progression of HIV disease and decline in the CD4+ count. Radiographic findings vary considerably, especially in patients with advanced immune suppression.[139, 140] Typical findings of apical, cavitary disease are unusual in these patients.

Patients with acid-fast bacilli found on smears or cultures of respiratory specimens should be treated for presumed tuberculosis until the culture results are obtained. The standard treatment for HIV-infected patients with tuberculosis is effective, and long-term maintenance therapy or prophylaxis is unnecessary.[136, 144] Rates of treatment failure and relapse do not appear to be higher for HIV-infected patients than in patients without HIV infection.[144] Although the 1-year mortality rate for HIV-infected patients with tuberculosis is greater than for HIV-negative patients, it is usually the result of other HIV-related illnesses.[144, 147, 156] Although the optimal regimen has not been determined, based on recommendations by the American Thoracic Society,[157] the

Centers for Disease Control,[158] and the World Health Organization,[159] patients should receive isoniazid (300 mg/d), rifampin (600 mg/d, or 450 mg/d for patients weighing < 50 kg), pyrazinamide (20–30 mg/kg/d), and ethambutol (15–25 mg/kg/d). The four-drug regimen should be continued for 2 months, and therapy with isoniazid and rifampin should be continued for a minimum of 9 months and for at least 6 months after cultures have become negative. Standard 6-month treatment regimens are probably equally effective.[144] Adverse reactions to chemotherapeutic agents, especially rifampin, occur more frequently in HIV-infected patients than in patients without HIV infection.[144, 147]

Prevention is discussed in Chapter 50.

### Multidrug-Resistant Tuberculosis

Several large outbreaks of multidrug-resistant tuberculosis (MDR-TB) have occurred.[160–166] Unlike the smaller outbreaks that occurred in the past, the recent outbreaks involved larger numbers of patients, occurred in institutional settings, and were characterized by rapid propagation and high mortality rates. Virtually all isolates were resistant to isoniazid and rifampin, and most isolates have been resistant to other drugs as well. MDR-TB has been marked by high mortality rates (72%–89%) with rapid progression to death (4–16 weeks). More than 90% of cases have occurred in HIV-infected patients, presumably because they are more likely to develop tuberculosis soon after infection than patients without HIV infection. Several health care workers exposed to patients with MDR-TB developed tuberculin skin test reactivity. At least 8 workers developed active tuberculosis, and 4 of these, all of whom were HIV-seropositive, have died.

There is no satisfactory therapy for MDR-TB. If multidrug resistance is suspected, patients should be treated with a standard four-drug regimen, consisting of isoniazid, rifampin, pyrazinamide, and ethambutol, plus at least two other agents to which local MDR-TB strains are susceptible. The regimen should be modified when susceptibility tests become available.[167] Because of the poor response to treatment of HIV-infected patients with MDR-TB, it is critical that appropriate isolation procedures be used to reduce the risk of nosocomial transmission.[168]

## Other Mycobacteria

*Mycobacterium avium* complex (MAC) is a common cause of morbidity in advanced HIV disease.[169–172] Although it is frequently isolated from sputum or bronchial washings in colonized patients or patients with disseminated infection, it has only rarely been reported to cause lung disease.[173, 174] Endobronchial lesions containing granulomas have been reported.[175] Although it may predict dissemination,[169] the growth of MAC from respiratory specimens without histopathologic evidence of disease is not an indication for treatment.[175] The same is true for many other nontuberculous mycobacterial species, such as *M. gordonae, M. fortuitum, M. chelonei, M. xenopi,* and *M. haemophilum,* which rarely cause isolated pulmonary disease in HIV-infected patients.[174, 176]

*M. kansasii* is a cause of serious pulmonary disease in AIDS patients with advanced immunosuppression. Only disseminated *M. kansasii* infection is an AIDS-defining condition,[151] and it occurs as an index AIDS diagnosis in only 0.44% of cases in highly endemic areas.[177] There are few data on the incidence of pulmonary disease, but it appears to be considerably more common than disseminated infection.[178, 179] In some series, *M. kansasii* was isolated more frequently than *M. tuberculosis* in HIV-infected patients.[179, 180]

Of 19 cases of *M. kansasii* infection reviewed at the Johns Hopkins Hospital, 17 patients had pulmonary disease.[178] The clinical features and response to therapy resembled those of patients with pulmonary tuberculosis. The radiographic features included diffuse interstitial or apical infiltrates, with or without cavities. Thin-walled cavities were common and thought to be an important diagnostic clue in patients with pulmonary disease and advanced HIV infection (Fig. 15–4). No cavities were seen in the 6 patients with pulmonary *M. kansasii* infection in a series at Parkland Hospital.[179] Radiographic findings in that series included nodular, interstitial, or diffuse parenchymal infiltrates, and 1 patient had a pleural effusion. In patients with HIV infection, *M. kansasii* disease is associated with a greater degree of immunosuppression than tuberculosis. In the Johns Hopkins series, all patients with *M. kansasii* disease had CD4+ lymphocyte counts of less than 200 cells/mm³, and the median CD4+ count was 49 cells/mm³.

Extrapulmonary disease due to *M. kansasii* also occurs. In the Hopkins series, 5 patients had extrapulmonary infections, and 3 patients had concomitant pulmonary infections.[178] Other sites from which *M. kansasii* was isolated included bone, urine, stool, lymph nodes, and blood. In the Parkland series, 4 of 9 patients showed evidence of extrapulmonary dissemination, with isolation from blood, lymph nodes, pleural fluid, liver, and cerebrospinal fluid.[179]

A regimen of isoniazid, rifampin, and ethambutol is ef-

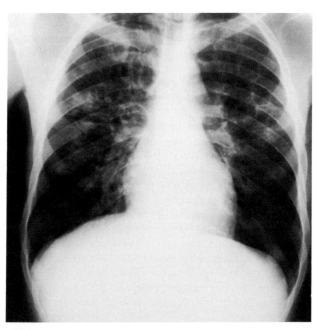

**Figure 15–4.** Bilateral infiltrates and multiple thin-walled cavities in a patient with *Mycobacterium kansasii* infection.

fective in the treatment of pulmonary *M. kansasii* infection.[178–182] Many isolates demonstrate in vitro resistance to isoniazid, but the clinical significance of this resistance pattern is not known.[178] The organisms may be susceptible to sulfonamides and the newer macrolides, and clinical responses have been observed in patients treated with TMP-SMX for presumed or concomitant *P. carinii* pneumonia.[178, 179] Therapy with sulfamethoxazole has been suggested for patients who do not respond to standard regimens.[179]

## FUNGAL INFECTIONS

### Cryptococcus neoformans

Although most patients with disease due to *C. neoformans* present with meningitis, the organism is also the most common cause of fungal pneumonia in AIDS patients. Approximately one quarter to one third of patients with cryptococcal disease present with pulmonary complaints, and in patients without central nervous system infection, as many as two thirds present with cough and dyspnea.[183, 184] Only 18% of patients with documented meningitis have pulmonary symptoms due to *Cryptococcus*.[184] The portal of entry of *C. neoformans* is the lung, and many patients probably develop clinically silent pulmonary infection.

Cryptococcal pneumonia may be an indolent or rapidly progressive disease. Patients usually present with fever and nonspecific constitutional symptoms. At least two thirds have respiratory symptoms, such as productive cough, dyspnea, and pleuritic chest pain.[185–187] Headache may occur, often reflecting concomitant meningeal involvement. The most common radiographic findings are focal or diffuse interstitial infiltrates,[185] but other findings include nodular or miliary infiltrates,[188] alveolar infiltrates,[187] mass lesions,[186] cavitation,[185, 186] pleural effusion,[185–191] and mediastinal adenopathy.[185, 186, 188] An HIV-infected patient from southern California was found to have a cavitary pulmonary nodule due to *C. neoformans gatii*, an unusual variant of *C. neoformans* associated with eucalyptus trees imported into southern California from Australia.[192]

*C. neoformans* is an opportunistic pathogen of relatively low virulence, and cryptococcosis should be considered in patients with advanced immunodeficiency due to HIV.[193] Detection of cryptococcal antigen in the serum is a rapid and highly sensitive screening test for invasive cryptococcal disease,[194] but the result may be negative for pulmonary cryptococcosis. The definitive diagnosis of cryptococcal pneumonia requires culture of *C. neoformans* from respiratory specimens or identification of typical-appearing encapsulated yeast forms in respiratory secretions.

Most data on the treatment of cryptococcosis come from studies of patients with meningitis. The management of cryptococcal meningitis is reviewed elsewhere.[195] Patients should be treated with amphotericin B, with or without 5-flucytosine, for the acute episode. Lifelong maintenance therapy with a triazole agent is indicated, and fluconazole (200 mg/d) is the most widely used and well-studied agent.

### Histoplasma capsulatum

*H. capsulatum* is an important cause of pneumonia and disseminated disease in AIDS patients from endemic areas. The principal endemic regions are the central and south-central United States and Puerto Rico. Disease occurs as a consequence of exogenous exposure, often in the setting of epidemics, and reactivation of latent infection.[196]

The presentation is often chronic or subacute, and progressive constitutional symptoms are more common than pulmonary complaints. Isolated pulmonary disease is uncommon, and most patients present with disseminated disease.[196, 197] Pulmonary infiltrates occur in approximately half of these patients.[196, 197] The most common radiographic findings for patients with pulmonary involvement are diffuse infiltrates, which are usually interstitial but may be reticulonodular or alveolar; localized infiltrates occur less often. Mediastinal adenopathy and calcification, hallmarks of pulmonary histoplasmosis in patients with normal immune function, are rarely seen in HIV-infected patients with disseminated disease. A case of *H. capsulatum* causing pleural effusion has been reported.[198]

A septicemia-like syndrome, with hypotension, coagulopathy, and multiorgan system failure occurs in 10% to 20% of patients.[196] Neurologic manifestations, including encephalopathy, meningitis, and focal brain lesions occur in 5% to 20% of patients.[196, 197, 199] Patients with central nervous system involvement are less responsive to treatment and have a higher mortality rate than other patients with disseminated disease.[196]

Histoplasmosis is diagnosed definitively by culture. The diagnostic evaluation should include fungal cultures of blood and bone marrow and of BAL fluid from those with pulmonary manifestations. Because the growth of *H. capsulatum* may take as long as 6 weeks, a presumptive diagnosis must be made by histopathologic or serologic analysis. Intracellular yeast forms can be demonstrated in the smears of peripheral blood or bone marrow, respiratory specimens, or tissue stained with periodic acid-Schiff or Gomori methenamine silver.[196] Biopsies of the skin lesions, which occur in as many as 18% of patients,[196] may be especially useful in making a rapid diagnosis of disseminated histoplasmosis.[197] Demonstration of *Histoplasma* polysaccharide antigen in serum or urine (available through Histoplasmosis Reference Laboratory, Indianapolis, IN) enables presumptive diagnosis of new infection and relapse.[196, 200–203] Widely available serologic tests for anti-*H. capsulatum* antibodies, such as immunodiffusion and complement fixation, are less sensitive and specific, but they may provide clues to the diagnosis.[196]

Like many opportunistic infections in patients with AIDS, *Histoplasma* infection cannot be eradicated. Effective treatment requires induction therapy and lifelong maintenance.[196] For induction, at least 15 mg/kg of amphotericin B are given over 4 to 6 weeks.[196] Itraconazole also shows promise for the treatment of mild or moderate histoplasmosis.[204] Relapse has been reported in as many as 50% of patients receiving maintenance therapy with ketoconazole and in 10% to 20% of those receiving weekly or biweekly amphotericin B maintenance.[196, 205] Early studies of maintenance therapy with fluconazole (100–400 mg/d)[206] and itraconazole (200 mg twice daily)[207] demonstrated relapse in

7.5% and 0%, respectively, and itraconazole has been approved for therapy of histoplasmosis.

### Aspergillus Species

Despite its importance in other immunocompromised patients, *Aspergillus* is an uncommon cause of pneumonia in AIDS patients. However, invasive aspergillosis and obstructing bronchial aspergillosis have been described as late complications of AIDS. Of 30 patients with invasive pulmonary aspergillosis from a French series,[208] 48% were not neutropenic and had not received steroids. In a series of 13 patients,[209] the potential predisposing factors included drug-induced neutropenia in 6, corticosteroid therapy in 4, and marijuana use in 4. The radiographic findings were variable. In the 10 patients with invasive pulmonary aspergillosis, chest radiographs demonstrated upper lobe cavitation and pleural-based infiltrates or nodules. The diagnosis was confirmed by BAL and transthoracic biopsy of the lesions. Therapy included amphotericin B or itraconazole. Seven patients died, 2 responded to therapy, and 1 survived despite the failure of antifungal therapy. Three patients with obstructing bronchial aspergillosis presented with progressive cough and bilateral infiltrates seen on chest radiography. The diagnosis was made by microscopic examination and culture of expectorated sputum casts. Patients were treated with itraconazole. Two of the 3 patients died, and 1 improved after a large aspergilloma was removed by BAL.

### Coccidioides immitis

*C. immitis* is a soil fungus that is endemic in parts of North, Central, and South America. In the United States, it is found primarily in the deserts of the Southwest. Infection is acquired through inhalation of arthroconidia, and disease is usually a result of reactivation of latent infection.

In patients with AIDS, pulmonary involvement is the most common clinical manifestation, although disseminated or extrapulmonary disease occur more frequently than in patients without HIV infection.[210, 211] Like tuberculosis, coccidioidomycosis may develop in patients with early-stage HIV infection and intact cellular immunity. In these patients, disease is similar to that seen in patients without HIV infection.[211] In patients with CD4$^+$ counts less than 250/mm$^3$, disease is often more severe. Presentation is similar to that of histoplasmosis, with slowly progressive constitutional symptoms, although respiratory symptoms, such as dyspnea, dry or productive cough, and pleuritic chest pain, occur more frequently. Chest radiographs may demonstrate diffuse interstitial or nodular infiltrates, although miliary infiltrates, adenopathy, and nodular and cavitary lesions have also been described. Radiographic findings are often much more extensive than those seen in patients without HIV infection.[210, 211]

In the largest series of HIV-infected patients with coccidioidomycosis,[211] 77 patients were divided into six groups based on clinical characteristics: focal pulmonary disease (20 patients), diffuse pulmonary disease (31), cutaneous disease (4), meningitis (9), lymph node or liver disease (7), and positive serology only (6). Coccidioidal serology by tube precipitin (TP) or complement fixation (CF) was positive in 83% of those with focal pulmonary disease and 69% of those with diffuse pulmonary disease, with mean CF titers of 1:30 and 1:24, respectively. Among patients with diffuse disease, CF was more sensitive than TP. The median CD4$^+$ count for patients with focal pulmonary disease was 143/mm$^3$, and the median CD4$^+$ count was 44/mm$^3$ for those with diffuse pulmonary disease. Patients with diffuse pulmonary disease had the highest mortality rate (70%).

The diagnosis of coccidioidomycosis should be considered in any HIV-infected patient with pulmonary disease who has lived in or traveled to an endemic area. Although serologic determinations may be helpful, false-negative results are not uncommon, and the diagnosis is made definitively by visualization of the coccidioidal spherule on a potassium hydroxide mount of sputum or by culture. As with histoplasmosis, patients should be treated with 1 to 2.5 g of amphotericin B, followed by chronic maintenance therapy with oral triazole agents. Coccidioidomycosis has been reported in patients already taking ketoconazole for other reasons,[211] and the limited data available support the use of the triazoles, itraconazole (200 mg twice daily), or fluconazole (400 mg/d) as maintenance therapy.[212, 213]

### Other Fungi

*Candida* species are infrequent pulmonary pathogens in AIDS patients. When *Candida* is isolated from sputum or bronchial specimens, it usually represents contamination from the oropharynx; the diagnosis of pulmonary candidiasis requires direct visualization and histologic confirmation.[213] Oropharyngeal candidiasis may extend into the larynx and trachea, especially in children.[213] Most cases of true pulmonary candidiasis have been diagnosed at autopsy and reflected disseminated disease.

Blastomycosis, caused by the dimorphic fungus *Blastomyces dermatitidis,* is endemic in the midwestern and south-central United States. Blastomycosis is uncommon in patients with AIDS and is not an AIDS-defining opportunistic infection.[116] In the few cases reported,[214–216] disease has been disseminated or limited to the lungs and pleura. In a series of 15 HIV-infected patients with blastomycosis,[216] 14 patients had CD4$^+$ lymphocyte counts less than 200/mm$^3$. Although the 8 patients with disseminated disease were similar to the 7 patients with pulmonary disease with respect to demographics and CD4$^+$ lymphocyte counts, they had a much higher mortality rate, despite antifungal therapy. All patients with pulmonary blastomycosis presented with fever, weight loss, and cough, and some had pleuritic chest pain and dyspnea. Radiographic abnormalities included focal lobar infiltrates in 3 patients, miliary or diffuse interstitial infiltrates in 3, and bilateral pulmonary nodules in 1. One patient had cavitary disease, and another had a pleural effusion. Therapy should be initiated with amphotericin B. After clinical improvement, chronic suppressive therapy with an oral azole compound is required.[216]

Disseminated infection with the dimorphic fungus, *Penicillium marneffei,* has been reported in HIV-infected patients in Southeast Asia.[217–220] The most common presenting symptoms are fever, anemia, weight loss, and papular skin lesions. Cough is also common, and in the largest series,[220] chest roentgenograms were abnormal for 6 of 21 patients. The radiographic findings included diffuse reticulonodular infiltrates in 3 patients, localized interstitial infiltrates in 2, and localized alveolar infiltrates in 1.

## VIRAL INFECTIONS

### Cytomegalovirus

The importance of cytomegalovirus (CMV) as a pulmonary pathogen in HIV-infected persons is uncertain. Although CMV is an important cause of ocular and gastrointestinal disease, the significance of the isolation of CMV from pulmonary secretions is controversial, because it is often associated with other pathogens and may represent infection without true pneumonitis.[221-224] Patients in whom *P. carinii* and CMV are isolated from respiratory specimens do not have a worse prognosis than patients with PCP alone.[225-228]

When CMV does cause pneumonitis, the clinical features are similar to those seen in PCP: nonproductive cough, progressive dyspnea, hypoxemia, and diffuse interstitial infiltrates. The definitive diagnosis of CMV pneumonitis requires a compatible clinical picture and positive cultures for CMV from lung tissue or BAL, the presence in pulmonary tissue of typical intranuclear inclusion bodies and CMV antigen or nucleic acid, and the absence of other pathogenic organisms, such as *P. carinii*.[222, 224]

For patients thought to have CMV pneumonitis, treatment with ganciclovir should be considered. The standard dose for initial therapy is 5 mg/kg twice daily, although higher doses may be required.[224] Although there are few data regarding therapy of CMV pneumonitis, ganciclovir appears to be less effective against pulmonary infections than for retinitis or gastrointestinal disease, with response rates of 50% to 60%.[224] Unlike other diseases due to CMV, pneumonitis may not require long-term maintenance therapy. In patients with CMV pneumonitis after bone marrow transplantation, the addition of high-dose intravenous immunoglobulin to ganciclovir is more efficacious than ganciclovir therapy alone,[229, 230] but there are no data supporting the use of this combination in patients with AIDS.

### Varicella-Zoster Virus

Varicella pneumonia may complicate primary varicella-zoster virus infection and disseminated secondary infection in patients with HIV infection. Patients may present with mild respiratory symptoms or may develop severe hypoxia and respiratory failure. The clinical findings may be minimal, despite markedly abnormal radiographic findings. These abnormalities include diffuse nodular densities with occasional pleural effusions. Patients should be treated with intravenous acyclovir (30 mg/kg/d).[231]

## REFERENCES

1. Murray HW, Rubin BY, Masur H, Roberts RB: Impaired production of lymphokines and immune (gamma) interferon in the acquired immunodeficiency syndrome. N Engl J Med 310:883–889, 1984.

2. Janoff EN, Douglas JM Jr, Gabriel M, et al: Class-specific antibody response in pneumococcal capsular polysaccharides in men infected with human immunodeficiency virus type I. J Infect Dis 158:983–990, 1988.

3. Ellis M, Gupta S, Galant S, et al: Impaired neutrophil function in patients with AIDS or AIDS-related complex: A comprehensive evaluation. J Infect Dis 158:1268–1276, 1988.

4. Leoung GS, Feigal DW Jr, Montgomery AB, et al: Aerosolized pentamidine for prophylaxis against *Pneumocystis carinii* pneumonia: The San Francisco Community Prophylaxis Trial. N Engl J Med 323:769–775, 1990.

5. Edman JC, Kovacs JA, Masur H, et al: Ribosomal RNA sequence shows *Pneumocystis carinii* to be a member of the fungi. Nature 334:519–522, 1988.

6. Masur H, Lane HC, Kovacs JA, Allegra CJ, Edman JC: *Pneumocystis* pneumonia: From bench to clinic. Ann Intern Med 111:813–826, 1989.

7. Raviglione MC: Extrapulmonary pneumocystosis: The first 50 cases. Rev Infect Dis 12:1127–1138, 1990.

8. Northfelt DW, Clement MJ, Safrin S: Extrapulmonary pneumocystosis: Clinical features of human immunodeficiency virus infection. Medicine (Baltimore) 69:392–398, 1990.

9. Telzak EE, Cote RJ, Gold JWM, Campbell SW, Armstrong D: Extrapulmonary *Pneumocystis carinii* infections. Rev Infect Dis 12:380–386, 1990.

10. Cohen OJ, Stoeckle MY: Extrapulmonary *Pneumocystis carinii* infections in the acquired immunodeficiency syndrome. Arch Intern Med 151:1205–1214, 1991.

11. Levine SJ, White DA: *Pneumocystis carinii*. Clin Chest Med 9:395–423, 1988.

12. Meduri GU, Stein DS: Pulmonary manifestations of acquired immunodeficiency syndrome. Clin Infect Dis 14:98–113, 1992.

13. Conces DJ Jr, Kraft JL, Vix VA, Tarver RD. Apical *Pneumocystis carinii* pneumonia after inhaled pentamidine prophylaxis. AJR 152:1193–1194, 1989.

14. Jules-Elysee KM, Stover DE, Zaman MB, Bernard EM, White DA: Aerosolized pentamidine: Effect on diagnosis and presentation of *Pneumocystis carinii* pneumonia. Ann Intern Med 112:750–757, 1990.

15. Sepkowitz KA, Telzak EE, Gold JWM, et al: Pneumothorax in AIDS. Ann Intern Med 114:455–459, 1991.

16. Leslie J, Gallant JE, Chaisson RE: Pneumothorax in patients with AIDS. Infect Dis Clin Pract 1:308–311, 1992.

17. Zaman MK, White DA: Serum lactate dehydrogenase levels and *Pneumocystis carinii* pneumonia: Diagnostic and prognostic significance. Am Rev Respir Dis 137:796–800, 1988.

18. Smith DE, McLuckie A, Wyatt J, et al: Severe exercise hypoxaemia with normal or near-normal x-rays: A feature of *Pneumocystis carinii* infection. Lancet 2:1049, 1988.

19. Garay SM, Greene J: Prognostic indicators in the initial presentation of *Pneumocystis carinii* pneumonia. Chest 95:769–772, 1989.

20. Kovacs JA, Ng VL, Masur H, et al: Diagnosis of *Pneumocystis carinii* pneumonia: Improved detection in sputum with use of monoclonal antibodies. N Engl J Med 318:589–593, 1988.

21. Lipschik GY, Adrawis VA, Ognibene FP, et al: Improved diagnosis of *Pneumocystis carinii* infections by polymerase chain reaction on induced sputum and blood. Lancet 340:203–206, 1992.

22. Broaddus C, Dake MD, Stulbarg MS, et al: Bronchoalveolar lavage and transbronchial biopsy for the diagnosis of pulmonary infections in the acquired immunodeficiency syndrome. Ann Intern Med 102:747–752, 1985.

23. Fitzgerald W, Bevalaqua FA, Garay SM, Aranda CP: The role of open lung biopsy in patients with acquired immunodeficiency syndrome. Chest 91:659–661, 1987.

24. Wharton JM, Coleman DL, Wofsy CB, et al: Trimethoprim-sulfamethoxazole or pentamidine for *Pneumocystis carinii* pneumonia in the acquired immunodeficiency syndrome. A prospective randomized trial. Ann Intern Med 105:37–44, 1986.

25. Haverkos HW: Assessment of therapy for *Pneumocystis carinii* pneumonia. PCP therapy project group. Am J Med 76:501–508, 1984.

26. Klein NC, Duncanson FP, Lenox TH, et al: Trimethoprim-sulfamethoxazole versus pentamidine for *Pneumocystis carinii* pneumonia in AIDS patients: Results of a large prospective randomized treatment trial. AIDS 6:301–305, 1992.

27. Sattler FR, Cowan R, Nielson DM, Ruskin J: Trimethoprim-sulfa-

methoxazole compared with pentamidine for treatment of *Pneumocystis carinii* pneumonia in the acquired immunodeficiency syndrome: A prospective, noncrossover study. Ann Intern Med 109:280–287, 1988.

28. Medina I, Mills J, Leoung G, et al: Oral therapy for *Pneumocystis carinii* pneumonia in the acquired immunodeficiency syndrome: A controlled trial of trimethoprim-sulfamethoxazole versus trimethoprim-dapsone. N Engl J Med 323:776–782, 1990.

29. Leoung GS, Mills J, Hopewell PC, Hughes W, Wofsy C: Dapsone-trimethoprim for *Pneumocystis carinii* pneumonia in the acquired immunodeficiency syndrome. Ann Intern Med 105:45–48, 1986.

30. Mills J, Leoung G, Medina I, et al: Dapsone treatment of *Pneumocystis carinii* pneumonia in the acquired immunodeficiency syndrome. Antimicrob Agents Chemother 32:1057–1060, 1988.

31. Safrin S, Sattler FR, Lee BL, et al: Dapsone as a single agent is suboptimal therapy for *Pneumocystis carinii* pneumonia. J Acquir Immune Defic Syndr 4:244–249, 1991.

32. Toma E, Fournier S, Poisson M, Morisset R, Phaneuf D, Vega C: Clindamycin with primaquine for *Pneumocystis carinii* pneumonia. Lancet 1:1046–1048, 1989.

33. Queener SF, Bartlett MS, Richardson JD, Durkin MM, Jay MA, Smith JW: Activity of clindamycin with primaquine against *Pneumocystis carinii* in vitro and in vivo. Antimicrob Agents Chemother 32:807–813, 1988.

34. Noskin GA, Murphy RL, Black JR, Phair JP: Salvage therapy with clindamycin/primaquine for *Pneumocystis carinii* pneumonia. Clin Infect Dis 14:183–188, 1992.

35. Vildé JL, Remington JS: Role of clindamycin with or without another agent for treatment of pneumocystosis in patients with AIDS. J Infect Dis 166:694–695, 1992.

36. Black JR, Feinberg J, Murphy RL, Fass RJ, Carcy J, Sattler FR: Clindamycin and primaquine as primary treatment for mild and moderately severe *Pneumocystis carinii* pneumonia in patients with AIDS. Eur J Clin Microbiol Infect Dis 110:204–207, 1991.

37. Black JR, Akil B, Murphy R, et al: Oral clindamycin plus primaquine therapy for *Pneumocystis carinii* pneumonia in AIDS patients. [Abstract ThB42] VII International Conference on AIDS, Florence, 1991.

38. Ruf B, Rohde I, Pohle HD: Efficacy of clindamycin/primaquine versus trimethoprim/sulfamethoxazole in primary treatment of *Pneumocystis carinii* pneumonia. Eur J Clin Microbiol Infect Dis 10:207–210, 1991.

39. Toma E: Clindamycin/primaquine for treatment of *Pneumocystis carinii* pneumonia in AIDS. Eur J Clin Microbiol Infect Dis 10:210–213, 1991.

40. Hughes WT, Kennedy W, Shenep JL, et al: Safety and pharmacokinetics of 566C80, a hydroxynaphthoquinone with anti-*Pneumocystis carinii* activity: A phase I study in human immunodeficiency virus (HIV)-infected men. J Infect Dis 163:843–848, 1991.

41. Falloon J, Kovacs J, Hughes W, et al: A preliminary evaluation of 566C80 for the treatment of *Pneumocystis* pneumonia in patients with the acquired immunodeficiency syndrome. N Engl J Med 325:1534–1538, 1991.

42. Hughes WT: A new drug (566C80) for the treatment of *Pneumocystis carinii* pneumonia. Ann Intern Med 116:953–954, 1992.

43. Hughes W, Leoung G, Kramer F, et al: Comparison of atovaquone (566C80) with trimethoprim-sulfamethoxazole to treat *Pneumocystis carinii* pneumonia in patients with AIDS. N Engl J Med 328:1521–1527, 1993.

44. Montgomery AB, Debs RJ, Luce JM, et al: Aerosolized pentamidine as sole therapy for *Pneumocystis carinii* pneumonia in patients with acquired immunodeficiency syndrome. Lancet 2:480–483, 1987.

45. Soo Hoo GW, Mohsenifar Z, Meyer RD: Inhaled or intravenous pentamidine therapy for *Pneumocystis carinii* pneumonia in AIDS: Randomized trial. Ann Intern Med 113:195–202, 1990.

46. Conte JE Jr, Chernoff D, Feigal DW Jr, Joseph P, McDonald C, Golden JA: Intravenous or inhaled pentamidine for treating *Pneumocystis carinii* pneumonia in AIDS: A randomized trial. Ann Intern Med 113:203–209, 1990.

47. Davey RT, Masur H: Recent advances in the diagnosis, treatment, and prevention of *Pneumocystis carinii* pneumonia. Antimicrob Agents Chemother 34:499–504, 1990.

48. Allegra CJ, Chabner BA, Tuazon CU, et al: Trimetrexate for the treatment of *Pneumocystis carinii* pneumonia in patients with the acquired immunodeficiency syndrome. N Engl J Med 317:978–985, 1987.

49. Feinberg J, McDermott C, Nutter J: Trimetrexate (TMTX) salvage therapy for PCP in AIDS patients with limited therapeutic options. [Abstract B136] VIII International Conference on AIDS, Amsterdam, 1992.

50. Sattler FR, Feinberg J: New developments in the treatment of *Pneumocystis carinii* pneumonia. Chest 101:451–457, 1992.

51. Sattler FR, Allegra CJ, Verdegem TD, et al: Trimetrexate-leucovorin dosage evaluation study for treatment of *Pneumocystis carinii* pneumonia. J Infect Dis 161:91–96, 1990.

52. Amsden GW, Kowalsky SF, Morse GD: Trimetrexate for *Pneumocystis carinii* pneumonia in patients with AIDS. Ann Pharmacother 26:218–226, 1992.

53. Bozzette SA, Sattler FR, Chiu J, et al: A controlled trial of early adjunctive treatment with corticosteroids for *Pneumocystis carinii* pneumonia in the acquired immunodeficiency syndrome. N Engl J Med 323:1451–1457, 1990.

54. Montaner JSG, Lawson LM, Levitt N, Belzberg A, Schecter MT, Ruedy J: Corticosteroids prevent early deterioration in patients with moderately severe *Pneumocystis carinii* pneumonia and the acquired immunodeficiency syndrome (AIDS). Ann Intern Med 113:14–20, 1990.

55. Gagnon S, Boota AM, Fischl MA, Baier H, Kirksey OW, La Voie L: Corticosteroids as adjunctive therapy for severe *Pneumocystis carinii* pneumonia in the acquired immunodeficiency syndrome: Double-blind placebo-controlled trial. N Engl J Med 323:1444–1450, 1990.

56. The National Institutes of Health–University of California Expert Panel for Corticosteroids as Adjunctive Therapy for *Pneumocystis* Pneumonia: Consensus statement on the use of corticosteroids as adjunctive therapy for *Pneumocystis* pneumonia in the acquired immunodeficiency syndrome. N Engl J Med 323:1500–1504, 1990.

57. Quieffin J, Montaner JSG, Guillemi SA, et al: Oral corticosteroids accelerate recovery of mild AIDS-related *Pneumocystis carinii* pneumonia. [Abstract WeB1016] VIII International Conference on AIDS, Amsterdam, 1992.

58. Marche C, Wolff M, Mayorga R, et al: Toxoplasmose pulmonaire au cours du SIDA. [Abstract WBP23] V International Conference on AIDS, Montreal, 1989.

59. Derouin F, Sarfati C, Beauvais B, Garin YJF, Lariviere M: Prevalence of pulmonary toxoplasmosis in HIV-infected patients. [Letter] AIDS 4:1036, 1990.

60. Murray JF, Felton CP, Garay SM, et al: Pulmonary complications of the acquired immunodeficiency syndrome. N Engl J Med 310:1682–1688, 1984.

61. Pomeroy C, Filice GA: Pulmonary toxoplasmosis: A review. Clin Infect Dis 14:863–870, 1992.

62. Weller P: Parasitic pneumonias. *In* Pennington JE (ed): Respiratory Infections. Diagnosis and Management, ed 2. New York, Raven Press, 1988.

63. Catterall JR, Hofflin JM, Remington JS: Pulmonary toxoplasmosis. Am Rev Respir Dis 133:704–705, 1986.

64. Oksenhendler E, Cadranel J, Sarfati C, et al: *Toxoplasma gondii* pneumonia in patients with the acquired immunodeficiency syndrome. Am J Med 88:18N–21N, 1990.

65. Derouin F, Sarfati C, Beauvais B, Iliou M-C, Dehen L, Lariviere M: Laboratory diagnosis of pulmonary toxoplasmosis in patients with acquired immunodeficiency syndrome. J Clin Microbiol 27:1661–1663, 1989.

66. Brady E, Margolis ML, Korzeniowski OM: Pulmonary cryptosporidiosis in acquired immune deficiency syndrome. JAMA 252:89–90, 1984.

67. Hojlyng N, Jensen BN: Respiratory cryptosporidiosis in HIV-positive patients. [Letter] Lancet 1:590–591, 1988.

68. Gross TL, Wheat J, Bartlett M, O'Connor KW: AIDS and multiple system involvement with *Cryptosporidium*. Am J Gastroenterol 81:456–458, 1986.

69. Forgacs P, Tarshis A, Ma P, et al: Intestinal and bronchial cryptosporidiosis in an immunodeficient homosexual man. Ann Intern Med 99:793–794, 1983.

70. Miller RA, Wasserheit JN, Kirihara J, Coyle MB: Detection of *Cryptosporidium* oocysts in sputum during screening for mycobacteria. J Clin Microbiol 20:1992–1993, 1984.

71. Gradon JD, Timpone JG, Schnittman SM: Emergence of unusual opportunistic pathogens in AIDS: A review. Clin Infect Dis 15:134–157, 1992.

72. Ocaña IL, De Luis A, Irreguible D, Vallespi T, Torrebadella M,

Martinez-Vazquez JM: Unusual diagnosis of leishmaniasis in AIDS. [Abstract MBP98] V International Conference on AIDS, Montreal, 1989.

73. Denis M, Chouaid C, Cadranel J, Gonzalez G, Mayaud C: Pleural effusion due to opportunistic infection in AIDS. [Abstract MB2158] VII International Conference on AIDS, Florence, 1991.

74. Weber R, Kuster H, Keller R, Spycher MA, Briner J, Russi E, Lüthy R: Pulmonary *Enterocytozoon bieneusi* microsporidiosis—A new clinical syndrome in patients with AIDS? [Abstract 1088] 32nd Interscience Conference on Antimicrobial Agents and Chemotherapy, Anaheim, CA, 1992.

75. Spech TJ, Rehm J, Longworth DL, Keys TF, McHenry MC: Frequency of sinusitis in AIDS patients. [Abstract 7088] IV International Conference on AIDS, Stockholm, 1988.

76. Sample S, Lanahan GA, Serwonska MH, et al: Allergic diseases and sinusitis in acquired immune deficiency syndrome (AIDS). [Abstract] J Allergy Clin Immunol 83:190, 1989.

77. Hadderingh RJ, Roel J: Recurrent maxillary sinusitis in AIDS patients. [Abstract MBP203] V International Conference on AIDS, Montreal, 1989.

78. Simpson G, Martin M, Cox P, Beck K, Beall G: Bacterial and sinopulmonary infections in HIV infected persons. [Abstract 2044] VI International Conference on AIDS, San Francisco, 1990.

79. Zurlo JJ, Feverstein I, Lebovics R, Lane HC: Sinusitis in HIV-1 infection. [Abstract 1117] 30th Interscience Conference on Antimicrobial Agents and Chemotherapy, Atlanta, 1990.

80. Godofsky EW, Zinreich J, Armstrong M, Leslie JM, Weikel CS: Sinusitis in HIV-infected patients: A clinical and radiographic review. Am J Med 93:163–170, 1992.

81. Simberkoff MS, El Sadr W, Schiffman G, Rahal JJ Jr: *Streptococcus pneumoniae* infections and bacteremia in patients with acquired immune deficiency syndrome with report of a pneumococcal vaccine failure. Am Rev Respir Dis 130:1174–1176, 1984.

82. Polsky B, Gold JWM, Whimbey E, et al: Bacterial pneumonia in patients with the acquired immunodeficiency syndrome. Ann Intern Med 104:38–41, 1986.

83. Witt DJ, Craven DE, McCabe WR: Bacterial infections in adult patients with the acquired immune deficiency syndrome (AIDS) and AIDS-related complex. Am J Med 82:900–906, 1987.

84. Schlamm HT, Yancovitz SR: *Haemophilus influenzae* pneumonia in young adults with AIDS, ARC, or risk of AIDS. Am J Med 86:11–14, 1989.

85. Selwyn PA, Feingold AR, Hartel D, Schoenbaum EE, Alderman MH, Klein RS, Friedland GH: Increased risk of bacterial pneumonia in HIV-infected intravenous drug users without AIDS. AIDS 2:267–272, 1988.

86. Selwyn PA, Alcabes P, Hartel D, et al: Clinical manifestations and predictors of disease progression in drug users with human immunodeficiency virus infection. N Engl J Med 327:1697–1703, 1992.

87. Stover DE, White DA, Romano PA, et al: Diagnosis of pulmonary disease in acquired immune deficiency syndrome (AIDS). Am Rev Respir Dis 130:659, 1984.

88. Janoff EN, Breiman RF, Daley CL, Hopewell PC: Pneumococcal disease during HIV infection. Ann Intern Med 117:314–324, 1992.

89. Gerberding JL, Krieger J, Sande MA: Recurrent bacteremic infection with *S. pneumoniae* in patients with AIDS virus (AV) infection. [Abstract 443] 26th Interscience Conference on Antimicrobial Agents and Chemotherapy, New Orleans, 1986.

90. Kovacs JA, Hiemenz JW, Macher AM, et al: *Pneumocystis carinii* pneumonia: A comparison between patients with the acquired immunodeficiency syndrome and patients with other immunodeficiencies. Ann Intern Med 100:663–671, 1984.

91. Heron CW, Hine AL, Pozniak AL, et al: Radiographic features in patients with pulmonary manifestations of the acquired immune deficiency syndrome. Clin Radiol 36:583, 1985.

92. Stover DE, White DA, Romano PA, Gellene RA, Robeson WA: Spectrum of pulmonary diseases associated with the acquired immune deficiency syndrome. Am J Med 78:429–437, 1985.

93. Murata GH, Ault MJ, Meyer RD: Community-acquired bacterial pneumonias in homosexual men: Presumptive evidence for a defect in host resistance. AIDS Res 1:379–393, 1984–1985.

94. Janoff EN, O'Brien J, Ehret J, Meiklejohn G, Duval G, Dougals JM Jr: Bacteremia, pharyngeal colonization, and immune response to *Streptococcus pneumoniae* in persons with HIV. [Abstract 556] 31st Interscience Conference on Antimicrobial Agents and Chemotherapy, Chicago, 1991.

95. Redd SC, Rutherford GW III, Sande MA, et al: The role of human immunodeficiency virus infection in pneumococcal bacteremia in San Francisco residents. J Infect Dis 162:1012–1017, 1990.

96. Yamaguchi E, Charache P, Chaisson RE: Increasing incidence of pneumococcal infections (PI) associated with HIV infection in an inner-city hospital, 1985–1989. 1990 World Conference on Lung Health, Boston. [Abstract] Am Rev Respir Dis 141:A619, 1990.

97. Rodriguez-Barradas MC, Musher DM, Hamill RJ, Dowell M, Bagwell JT, Sanders CV: Unusual manifestations of pneumococcal infection in human immunodeficiency virus-infected individuals: The past revisited. Clin Infect Dis 14:1920–1929, 1992.

98. Levine SJ, White DA, Fels AO: The incidence and significance of *Staphylococcus aureus* in respiratory cultures from patients infected with the human immunodeficiency virus. Am Rev Respir Dis 141:89–93, 1990.

99. Kielhofner M, Atmar RL, Hamill RJ, Musher DM: Life-threatening *Pseudomonas aeruginosa* infections in patients with human immunodeficiency virus infection. Clin Infect Dis 14:403–411, 1992.

100. Whimbey E, Gold JWM, Polsky B, et al: Bacteremia and fungemia in patients with the acquired immune deficiency syndrome. Ann Intern Med 104:511–514, 1986.

101. Krumholz HM, Sande MA, Lo B: Community-acquired bacteremia in adult patients with acquired immunodeficiency syndrome: Clinical presentation, bacteriology, and outcome. Am J Med 86:776–779, 1989.

102. Rolston KVI, Radentz S, Rodriguez S: Bacterial and fungal infections in patients with the acquired immunodeficiency syndrome. Cancer Detect Prev 14:377–381, 1990.

103. Hollander H, Baron A: Pulmonary *Pseudomonas* infection in late HIV disease—A syndrome of indolent, recurrent disease. [Abstract PoB2891] VIII International Conference on AIDS, Amsterdam, 1992.

104. Mundy L, Auwaerter P, Burton A, Oldach D, Quinn T, Charache P, Bartlett J: Etiology of community acquired pneumonia (CAP): HIV positive vs. HIV negative patients. [Abstract 569] 31st Interscience Conference on Antimicrobial Agents and Chemotherapy, Chicago, 1991.

105. Yamaguchi E, Chaisson RE: Gram-negative bacteremias (GNB) in HIV-infected patients. [Abstract ThB539] VI International Conference on AIDS, San Francisco, 1990.

106. Celum CL, Chaisson RE, Rutherford GW, Barnhart JL, Echenberg DF: Incidence of salmonellosis in patients with AIDS. J Infect Dis 156:998–1002, 1987.

107. Jacobs JL, Gold JWM, Murray HW, et al: *Salmonella* infections in patients with the acquired immunodeficiency syndrome. Ann Intern Med 102:186, 1985.

108. Amador C, Chiner E, Calpe JL, Ortiz de la Table V, Martinez C, Pasquau F: Pneumonia due to *Bordetella bronchiseptica* in a patient with AIDS. [Letter] Rev Infect Dis 13:771–772, 1991.

109. Decker GR, Lavelle JP, Kumar PN, Pierce PF: Pneumonia due to *Bordetella bronchiseptica* in a patient with AIDS. [Letter] Rev Infect Dis 13:1250–1251, 1991.

110. Ng VL, Boggs JM, York MK, Golden JA, Hollander H, Hadley WK: Recovery of *Bordetella bronchiseptica* from patients with AIDS. Clin Infect Dis 15:376–377, 1992.

111. Caron F, Borsa-Lebas F, Boiron P, et al: *Streptomyces* (S) sp. as a cause of nodular pneumonia in an HIV infected patient? [Abstract 1093] 32nd Interscience Conference on Antimicrobial Agents and Chemotherapy, Anaheim, CA, 1992.

112. Murray JF, Felton CP, Gray SM, Gottlieb MS, Hopewell PC, Stover DE, Teirstein AS: Pulmonary complications of the acquired immunodeficiency syndrome. N Engl J Med 310:1682–1688, 1984.

113. Portmore AD, Graman PS: Five cases of *Legionella pneumophila* in patients with advanced HIV disease. [Abstract 374] 32nd Interscience Conference on Antimicrobial Agents and Chemotherapy, Anaheim, CA, 1992.

114. Khardori N, Haron E, Rolston K: *Legionella micdadei* pneumonia in the acquired immune deficiency syndrome. [Letter] Am J Med 83:600–601, 1987.

115. Mirich D, Gray R, Hyland R: *Legionella* lung cavitation. J Can Assoc Radiol 41:100–102, 1990.

116. Centers for Disease Control: Revision of the CDC surveillance case definition for acquired immunodeficiency syndrome. MMWR 36:3S–14S, 1987.

117. Javaly K, Horowitz HW, Wormser GP: Nocardiosis in patients with human immunodeficiency virus infection: Report of 2 cases and review of the literature. Medicine (Baltimore) 71:128–138, 1992.

118. Rodriguez JL, Barrio JL, Pitchenik AE: Pulmonary nocardiosis in the acquired immunodeficiency syndrome: Diagnosis with bronchoalveolar lavage and treatment with non-sulphur containing drugs. Chest 90:912–914, 1986.

119. Holtz HA, Lavery DP, Kapila R: Actinomycetales infection in the acquired immunodeficiency syndrome. Ann Intern Med 102:203, 1985.

120. Cone LA, Polkinghorn GR, Woodard DR, Berk A, Fiala M, Lynch J: *Nocardia asteroides* infections in patients with the acquired immunodeficiency syndrome. [Abstract MBP204] V International Conference on AIDS, Montreal, 1989.

121. Kramer MR, Uttamchandani RB: The radiographic appearance of pulmonary nocardiosis associated with AIDS. Chest 98:382–385, 1990.

122. Parmentier L, Salmon-Ceron D, Boiron P, Paul G, Guez T, Dupont B, Sicard D: Pneumopathy and kidney abscess due to *Nocardia farcinica* in an HIV-infected patient. AIDS 6:891–893, 1992.

123. Mitchell TG: Actinomycetes. *In* Joklik WK, Willet HP, Amos DB, Wilfert CM (eds): Zinsser Microbiology, ed 19. Norwalk, CT, Appleton & Lange, 1988:454–459.

124. Wallace RJ Jr, Septimus EJ, Williams TW Jr, Conklin RH, Satterwhite TK, Bushby MB, Hollowell DC: Use of trimethoprim-sulfamethoxazole for treatment of infections due to *Nocardia*. Rev Infect Dis 4:315–325, 1982.

125. Wallace RJ, Steele LC, Sumter G, Smith JM: Antimicrobial susceptibility patterns of *Nocardia asteroides*. Antimicrob Agents Chemother 32:1775–1779, 1988.

126. Filice GA, Simpson GL: Management of *Nocardia* infections. *In* Remington JS, Swartz M (eds): Current Clinical Topics in Infectious Disease, vol 5. New York, McGraw-Hill, 1988:49–65.

127. Wilson JP, Turner HR, Kirchner KA, Chapman SW: Nocardial infections in renal transplant recipients. Medicine (Baltimore) 68:38–57, 1989.

128. Samies JH, Hathaway BN, Echols RM, Veazey JM Jr, Pilon VA: Lung abscess due to *Corynebacterium equi*—Report of the first case in a patient with acquired immune deficiency syndrome. Am J Med 80:685–688, 1986.

129. MacGregor JH, Samuelson WM, Sane DC, Godwin JD: Opportunistic lung infection caused by *Rhodococcus (Corynebacterium) equi*. Radiology 160:83, 1986.

130. Weingarten JS, Huang DY, Jackman JD Jr: *Rhodococcus equi* pneumonia. An unusual early manifestation of the acquired immunodeficiency syndrome (AIDS). Chest 94:195–196, 1988.

131. Bishopric GA, d'Agay MF, Schlemmer B, Sarfati E, Brocheriou C: Pulmonary pseudotumor due to *Corynebacterium equi* in a patient with the acquired immunodeficiency syndrome. Thorax 43:486–487, 1988.

132. Harvey RL, Sunstrum JC: *Rhodococcus equi* infection in patients with and without human immunodeficiency virus infection. Rev Infect Dis 13:139–145, 1991.

133. Emmons W, Reichwein B, Winslow DL: *Rhodococcus equi* infection in the patient with AIDS: Literature review and report of an unusual case. Rev Infect Dis 13:91–96, 1991.

134. Willsie-Edinger SK, Stanford JF, Salzman GA, Bamberger DM: Spectrum of disease caused by *Rhodococcus equi* in human immunodeficiency virus infection: Report of a case and review of the literature. Can J Infect Dis 1:101–107, 1990.

135. Centers for Disease Control: Update: Tuberculosis elimination—United States. MMWR 39:153–156, 1990.

136. Johnson MP, Chaisson RE: Tuberculosis and HIV disease. *In* Volberding P, Jacobson MA (eds): AIDS Clinical Review 1991. New York, Marcel Dekker, 1991:109–126.

137. Selwyn PA, Hartel D, Lewis VA, et al: A prospective study of the risk of tuberculosis among intravenous drug users with human immunodeficiency virus infection. N Engl J Med 320:545–550, 1989.

138. Daley CL, Small PM, Schecter GF, et al: An outbreak of tuberculosis with accelerated progression among persons infected with the human immunodeficiency virus. An analysis using restriction-fragment-length polymorphisms. N Engl J Med 326:231–235, 1992.

139. Theuer CP, Hopewell PC, Elias D, et al: Human immunodeficiency virus infection in tuberculosis patients. J Infect Dis 162:8–12, 1990.

140. Colebunders RL, Ryder RW, Nzilambi N, et al: HIV infection in patients with tuberculosis in Kinshasha, Zaire. Am Rev Respir Dis 139:1082–1085, 1989.

141. Pitchenik AE, Rubinson HA: The radiographic appearance of tuberculosis in patients with the acquired immune deficiency syndrome (AIDS) and pre-AIDS. Am Rev Respir Dis 131:383–386, 1985.

142. Pedro-Botet J, Gutiérrez J, Miralles R, Coll J, Rubiés-Prat J: Pulmonary tuberculosis in HIV-infected patients with normal chest radiographs. AIDS 6:91–93, 1992.

143. Pitchenick AE, Burr J, Suarez M, et al: Human T-cell lymphotropic virus-III (HTLV-III) seropositivity and related disease among 71 consecutive patients in whom tuberculosis was diagnosed. Am Rev Respir Dis 135:875–879, 1987.

144. Small PM, Schecter GF, Goodman PC, Sande MA, Chaisson RE, Hopewell PC: Treatment of tuberculosis in patients with advanced human immunodeficiency virus infection. N Engl J Med 324:289–294, 1991.

145. Sunderam G, McDonald RJ, Maniatis T, et al: Tuberculosis as a manifestation of the acquired immunodeficiency syndrome (AIDS). JAMA 256:362–366, 1986.

146. Rieder HL, Snider DE Jr, Canthen GM: Extrapulmonary tuberculosis in the United States. Am Rev Respir Dis 141:347–351, 1990.

147. Chaisson RE, Schecter GF, Theuer CP, Rutherford GW, Echenberg DF, Hopewell PC: Tuberculosis in patients with the acquired immunodeficiency syndrome. Clinical features, response to therapy, and survival. Am Rev Respir Dis 136:570–574, 1987.

148. Shafer RW, Kim DS, Weiss JP, Quale JM: Extrapulmonary tuberculosis in patients with human immunodeficiency virus infection. Medicine (Baltimore) 70:384–396, 1991.

149. Kramer F, Modilevsky T, Waliany AR, Leedom JM, Barnes PF: Delayed diagnosis of tuberculosis in patients with human immunodeficiency virus infection. Am J Med 89:451–456, 1990.

150. Shafer RW, Goldberg R, Sierra M, Glatt AE: Frequency of *Mycobacterium tuberculosis* bacteremia in patients with tuberculosis in an area endemic for AIDS. Am Rev Respir Dis 140:1611–1613, 1989.

151. Bishburg E, Sunderam G, Reichman LB, Kapila R: Central nervous system tuberculosis with the acquired immunodeficiency syndrome and its related complex. Ann Intern Med 105:210–213, 1986.

152. Gallant JE, Mueller PS, McArthur JS, Chaisson RE: Intramedullary tuberculoma in a patient with HIV infection. AIDS 6:889–891, 1992.

153. Berenguer J, Moreno S, Laguna F, et al: Tuberculous meningitis in patients infected with the human immunodeficiency virus. N Engl J Med 326:668–672, 1992.

154. Laguna F, Adrados M, Ortega A, Gonzalez-Lahoz JM: Tuberculous meningitis with acellular cerebrospinal fluid in AIDS patients. AIDS 6:1165–1167, 1992.

155. Klein NC, Duncanson FP, Lenox TH III, Pitta A, Cohen SC, Wormser GP: Use of mycobacterial smears in the diagnosis of pulmonary tuberculosis in AIDS/ARC patients. Chest 95:1190–1192, 1989.

156. Soriano E, Mallolas J, Gatell JM, et al: Characteristics of tuberculosis in HIV-infected patients: A case-control study. AIDS 2:429–432, 1988.

157. American Thoracic Society: Mycobacterioses and the acquired immunodeficiency syndrome. Am Rev Respir Dis 136:492–496, 1987.

158. Centers for Disease Control: Tuberculosis and human immunodeficiency virus infection: Recommendations of the Advisory Committee for the Elimination of Tuberculosis (ACET). MMWR 38:236–250, 1989.

159. World Health Organization: Global Programme on AIDS and Tuberculosis Programme—Statement on AIDS and Tuberculosis. Wkly Epidemiol Rec 64:125–131, 1989.

160. Pearson ML, Jereb JA, Frieden TR, et al: Nosocomial transmission of multidrug-resistant *Mycobacterium tuberculosis:* A risk to patients and health care workers. Ann Intern Med 117:191–196, 1992.

161. Fischl MA, Uttamchandani RB, Daikos GL, et al: An outbreak of tuberculosis caused by multiple-drug-resistant tubercle bacilli among patients with HIV infection. Ann Intern Med 117:177–183, 1992.

162. Centers for Disease Control: Nosocomial transmission of multidrug-resistant tuberculosis to health-care workers and HIV-infected patients in an urban hospital—Florida. MMWR 39:718–722, 1990.

163. Centers for Disease Control: Nosocomial transmission of multidrug-resistant tuberculosis among HIV-infected persons—Florida and New York, 1988–1991. MMWR 40:585–591, 1991.

164. Edlin BR, Tokars JI, Grieco MH, et al: Nosocomial transmission of multidrug-resistant tuberculosis among AIDS patients: Epidemiologic studies and restriction fragment length polymorphism analysis. N Engl J Med 326:1514–1521, 1992.

165. Fischl MA, Daikos GL, Uttamchandani RB, et al: Clinical presentation and outcome of patients with HIV infection and tuberculosis caused by multiple-drug-resistant bacilli. Ann Intern Med 117:184–190, 1992.

166. Centers for Disease Control: Transmission of multidrug-resistant tu-

berculosis among immunocompromised persons, correctional system—New York, 1991. MMWR 41:507–509, 1992.

167. Dooley SW, Jarvis WR, Martone WJ, Snider DE: Multidrug-resistant tuberculosis. Ann Intern Med 117:257–258, 1992.

168. Dooley SW, Castro KG, Hutton MD, Mullan RJ, Polder JA, Snider DE: Guidelines for preventing the transmission of tuberculosis in health-care settings, with special focus on HIV-related issues. MMWR 39:1–29, 1990.

169. Jacobson MA, Hopewell PC, Yajko DM, et al: Natural history of disseminated *Mycobacterium avium* complex infection in AIDS. J Infect Dis 164:994–998, 1991.

170. Chaisson RE, Moore RD, Richman DD, Keruly J, Creagh T, Zidovudine Epidemiology Study Group: Incidence and natural history of *Mycobacterium avium* complex infections in patients with advanced human immunodeficiency virus disease treated with zidovudine. Am Rev Respir Dis 146:285–289, 1992.

171. Nightingale SD, Byrd LT, Southern PM, Jockusch JD, Cal SX, Wynne BA: Incidence of *Mycobacterium avium-intracellulare* complex bacteremia in human immunodeficiency virus-positive patients. J Infect Dis 165:1082–1085, 1992.

172. Havlick JA Jr, Horsburgh CR Jr, Metchock B, Williams PP, Fann SA, Thompson SE III: Disseminated *Mycobacterium avium* complex infection: Clinical and epidemiologic trends. J Infect Dis 165:577–580, 1992.

173. Marinelli DL, Albelda SM, Williams TM, Kern JA, Iozzo RV, Miller WT: Nontuberculous mycobacterial infection in AIDS: Clinical, pathologic, and radiographic features. Radiology 160:77–82, 1986.

174. Tenholder MF, Moser RJ III, Tellis CJ: Mycobacteria other than tuberculosis: Pulmonary involvement with acquired immunodeficiency syndrome. Arch Intern Med 148:953–955, 1988.

175. Packer SJ, Cesario T, Williams JH Jr: *Mycobacterium avium* complex infection presenting as endobronchial lesions in immunocompromised patients. Ann Intern Med 109:389–393, 1988.

176. MacDonell KB, Glassroth J: *Mycobacterium avium* complex and other nontuberculous mycobacteria in patients with HIV infection. Semin Respir Infect 4:123–132, 1989.

177. Horsburgh CR Jr, Selik RM: Microbiology of disseminated nontuberculous mycobacterial infection in the acquired immunodeficiency syndrome (AIDS). Am Rev Respir Dis 139:4–7, 1989.

178. Levine B, Chaisson RE: *Mycobacterium kansasii:* A cause of treatable pulmonary disease associated with advanced human immunodeficiency virus (HIV) infection. Ann Intern Med 114:861–868, 1991.

179. Carpenter JL, Parks JM: *Mycobacterium kansasii* infections in patients positive for human immunodeficiency virus. Rev Infect Dis 13:789–796, 1991.

180. Young LS, Inderlied CB, Berlin OG, Gottlieb MS: Mycobacterial infections in AIDS patients, with an emphasis on the *Mycobacterium avium* complex. Rev Infect Dis 8:1024–1033, 1986.

181. Centers for Disease Control: Diagnosis and management of mycobacterial infection and disease in persons with human immunodeficiency virus infection. Ann Intern Med 106:254–256, 1987.

182. Joint Position Paper of the American Thoracic Society and the Centers for Disease Control: Mycobacterioses and the acquired immunodeficiency syndrome. Am Rev Respir Dis 136:492–496, 1982.

183. Chuck SL, Sande M: Infections with *Cryptococcus neoformans* in the acquired immunodeficiency syndrome. N Engl J Med 321:794–799, 1989.

184. Clark RA, Greer D, Atkinson W, et al: Spectrum of *Cryptococcus neoformans* infection in 68 patients infected with human immunodeficiency virus. Rev Infect Dis 12:768–777, 1990.

185. Cameron ML, Bartlett JA, Gallis HA, Waskin HA: Manifestations of pulmonary cryptococcosis in patients with acquired immunodeficiency syndrome. Rev Infect Dis 13:64–67, 1991.

186. Chechani V, Kamholz S: Pulmonary manifestations of disseminated cryptococcosis in patients with AIDS. Chest 98:1060–1066, 1990.

187. Wasser L, Talavera W: Pulmonary cryptococcosis in AIDS. Chest 92:692–695, 1987.

188. Miller WT Jr, Edelman J, Miller WT: Cryptococcal pulmonary infection in patients with AIDS: Radiographic appearance. Radiology 175:725–728, 1990.

189. Newman TG, Soni A, Acaron S, Huang CT: Pleural cryptococcosis in the acquired immunodeficiency syndrome. Chest 91:459–461, 1987.

190. Katz AS, Niessenbaum L, Mass B: Pleural effusion as the initial manifestation of disseminated cryptococcosis in the acquired immunodeficiency syndrome. Chest 96:440–441, 1989.

191. Grum EE, Schwab R, Margolis ML: Case report: Cryptococcal pleural effusion preceding cryptococcal meningitis in AIDS. Am J Med Sci 301:329–330, 1991.

192. Clancy MN, Fleischmann J, Howard DH, Kwon-Chung KJ, Shimizu RY: Isolation of *Cryptococcus neoformans gatii* from a patient with AIDS in southern California. J Infect Dis 161:809, 1990.

193. Masur H, Ogniben F, Yarchoan R, et al: CD4 counts as predictors of opportunistic infections in human immunodeficiency virus (HIV) infection. Ann Intern Med 111:223–231, 1989.

194. Bloomfield N, Gordon M, Elmendorf D Jr: Detection of *Cryptococcus neoformans* antigen in body fluids by latex particle agglutination. Proc Soc Exp Biol Med 114:64–67, 1963.

195. Stansell JD, Sande MA: Cryptococcal infection in AIDS. *In* Sande MA, Volberding PA (eds): The Medical Management of AIDS. Philadelphia, WB Saunders, 1992:297–310.

196. Wheat LJ, Connolly-Stringfield PA, Baker RL, et al: Disseminated histoplasmosis in the acquired immune deficiency syndrome: Clinical findings, diagnosis and treatment, and review of the literature. Medicine (Baltimore) 69:361–374, 1990.

197. Johnson PC, Khardori N, Najjar AF, Butt F, Mansell PWA, Sarosi GA: Progressive disseminated histoplasmosis in patients with acquired immunodeficiency syndrome. Am J Med 85:152–158, 1988.

198. Marshall BC, Cox JK Jr, Carrol KC, Morrison RE: Case report: Histoplasmosis as a cause of pleural effusion in the acquired immunodeficiency syndrome. Am J Med Sci 300:98–101, 1990.

199. Anaissie E, Fainstein V, Samo T, Bodey GP, Sarosi GA: Central nervous system histoplasmosis: An unappreciated complication of the acquired immunodeficiency syndrome. Am J Med 84:215–217, 1988.

200. Wheat LJ, Kohler RB, Tewari RP: Diagnosis of disseminated histoplasmosis by detection of *Histoplasma capsulatum* antigen in serum and urine specimens. N Engl J Med 314:83–88, 1986.

201. Wheat LJ, Connolly-Stringfield P, Blair R, Connolly K, Garringer T, Katz BP: Histoplasmosis relapse in patients with AIDS: Detection using *Histoplasma capsulatum* variety *capsulatum* antigen levels. Ann Intern Med 115:936–941, 1991.

202. Wheat LJ, Connolly-Stringfield P, Kohler RB, Frame PT, Gupta MR: *Histoplasma capsulatum* polysaccharide antigen detection in the diagnosis and management of disseminated histoplasmosis in patients with acquired immunodeficiency syndrome. Am J Med 87:396–400, 1989.

203. Wheat LJ, Connoly-Stringfield P, Blair R, Connolly K, Garringer T, Katz BP: Effect of successful treatment with amphotericin B on *Histoplasma capsulatum* variety *capsulatum* polysaccharide antigen levels in patients with AIDS and histoplasmosis. Am J Med 92:153–160, 1992.

204. Wheat LJ, Hafner RE, Ritchie M, Schneider D: Itraconazole (Itra) is effective treatment for histoplasmosis in AIDS: Prospective multicenter non-comparative trial. [Abstract 1206] 32nd Interscience Congress on Antimicrobial Agents and Chemotherapy, Anaheim, CA, 1992.

205. McKinsey DS, Gupta MR, Riddler SA, Driks MR, Smith DL, Kurtin PJ: Long-term amphotericin B therapy for disseminated histoplasmosis in patients with the acquired immunodeficiency syndrome (AIDS). Ann Intern Med 111:655–659, 1989.

206. Norris S, McKinsey D, Lancaster D, Wheat J: Retrospective evaluation of fluconazole maintenance therapy for disseminated histoplasmosis in AIDS. [Abstract 1207] 32nd Interscience Congress on Antimicrobial Agents and Chemotherapy, Anaheim, CA, 1992.

207. Wheat LJ, Hafner RE, Wulfsohn M, Johnson J, Owens S: Itraconazole (Itra) is effective maintenance treatment for prevention of relapse of histoplasmosis in AIDS: Prospective multicenter non-comparative trial. [Abstract 290] 31st Interscience Congress on Antimicrobial Agents and Chemotherapy, Chicago, 1991.

208. Lortholary O, Meyohas MC, Dupont B, Parrot A: Invasive aspergillosis in patients with AIDS. [Abstract 378] 32nd Interscience Congress on Antimicrobial Agents and Chemotherapy, Anaheim, CA, 1992.

209. Denning DW, Follansbee SE, Scolaro M, Norris S, Edelstein H, Stevens DA: Pulmonary aspergillosis in the acquired immunodeficiency syndrome. N Engl J Med 324:654–662, 1991.

210. Bronnimann DA, Adam RD, Galgiani JN, Habib MP, Petersen EA, Porter B, Bloom JW: Coccidioidomycosis in the acquired immunodeficiency syndrome. Ann Intern Med 106:372–379, 1987.

211. Fish DG, Ampel NM, Galgiani JN, et al: Coccidioidomycosis during human immunodeficiency virus infection: A review of 77 patients. Medicine (Baltimore) 69:384–391, 1990.

212. Tucker RM, Denning DW, Cupont B, Stevens DA: Itraconazole therapy for chronic coccidioidal meningitis. Ann Intern Med 112:108–112, 1990.

213. Diamond RD: The growing problem of mycoses in patients infected with the human immunodeficiency virus. Rev Infect Dis 13:480–486, 1991.

214. Herd AM, Greenfield SB, Thompson GW, Brunham RC: Miliary blastomycosis and HIV infection. Can Med Assoc J 143:1329–1330, 1990.

215. Fraser VJ, Keath EJ, Powderly WG: Two cases of blastomycosis from a common source: Use of DNA restriction analysis to identify strains. J Infect Dis 163:1378–1381, 1991.

216. Pappas PG, Pottage JC, Powderly WG, et al: Blastomycosis in patients with the acquired immunodeficiency syndrome. Ann Intern Med 116:847–853, 1992.

217. Peto TEA, Bull R, Millard PR, et al: Systemic mycosis due to *Penicillium marneffei* in a patient with antibody to human immunodeficiency virus. J Infect 16:285–290, 1988.

218. Piehl MR, Kaplan RL, Haber MH: Disseminated penicilliosis in a patient with acquired immunodeficiency syndrome. Arch Pathol Lab Med 112:1262–1264, 1988.

219. Tsang DNC, Li PCK, Tsui MS, Lau YT, Ma KF, Yeoh EK: *Penicillium marneffei:* Another pathogen to consider in patients infected with human immunodeficiency virus. Rev Infect Dis 13:766–767, 1991.

220. Supparatpinyo K, Chiewchanvit S, Hirunsri P, Uthammachai C, Nelson KE, Sirisanthana T: *Penicillium marneffei* infection in patients infected with human immunodeficiency virus. Clin Infect Dis 14:871–874, 1992.

221. Jacobson MA, Mills J: Serious cytomegalovirus disease in the acquired immunodeficiency syndrome (AIDS). Clinical findings, diagnosis, and treatment. Ann Intern Med 108:585–594, 1988.

222. Jacobson MA, Mills J: Cytomegalovirus infection. Clin Chest Med 8:443–448, 1988.

223. Gallant JE, Moore RD, Richman DD, Keruly J, Chaisson RE, Zidovudine Epidemiology Study Group: Incidence and natural history of cytomegalovirus disease in patients with advanced HIV disease treated with zidovudine. J Infect Dis 166:1223–1227, 1992.

224. Drew WL: Cytomegalovirus infection in patients with AIDS. Clin Infect Dis 14:608–615, 1992.

225. Bower MG, Barton SE, Nelson MR, et al: The significance of the detection of cytomegalovirus in the bronchoalveolar lavage fluid in AIDS patients with pneumonia. AIDS 4:317–320, 1990.

226. Millar AB, Patou G, Miller RF, et al: Cytomegalovirus in the lungs of patients with AIDS: Respiratory pathogen or passenger? Am Rev Respir Dis 141:1474–1477, 1990.

227. Jacobson MA, Mills J, Rush J, et al: Morbidity and mortality of patients with AIDS and first episode *Pneumocystis carinii* pneumonia is unaffected by concomitant pulmonary cytomegalovirus infection. Am Rev Respir Dis 144:6–9, 1991.

228. Bozzette SA, Arcia J, Bartok AE, McGlynn LM, McCutchan JA, Richman DD, Spector SA: Impact of *Pneumocystis carinii* and cytomegalovirus on the course and outcome of atypical pneumonia in advanced human immunodeficiency virus disease. J Infect Dis 165:93–98, 1992.

229. Emanuel D, Cunningham I, Jules-Elysee K, et al: Cytomegalovirus pneumonia after bone-marrow transplantation successfully treated with the combination of ganciclovir and high-dose intravenous immune globulin. Ann Intern Med 109:777–782, 1988.

230. Reed EC, Bowden RA, Dandliker PS, et al: Treatment of cytomegalovirus pneumonia with ganciclovir and intravenous cytomegalovirus immunoglobulin in patients with bone marrow transplants. Ann Intern Med 109:783–788, 1988.

231. Drew WL, Buhles W, Erlich KS: Management of herpes virus infections (CMV, HSV, VZV). *In* Sande MA, Volberding PA (eds): The Medical Management of AIDS. Philadelphia, WB Saunders, 1992:359–382.

# CHAPTER 16

# Mimics of Infectious Pneumonia in Persons Infected With Human Immunodeficiency Virus

JEANNE MARIE WALLACE

Although infections comprise the majority of pulmonary complications in human immunodeficiency virus (HIV)-infected persons, noninfectious processes, which may be clinically indistinguishable, also cause significant morbidity. The recognition of these noninfectious mimics greatly affects the direction of clinical management. Noninfectious pulmonary complications often have a less rapid onset and course than the common HIV-related infections such as *Pneumocystis carinii* or bacterial pneumonia. They may be suspected if sputum collection and bronchoscopy fail to yield evidence of a specific infectious agent. The diagnosis of a noninfectious complication may be difficult, frequently requiring a more invasive procedure, such as open lung biopsy, to obtain a large representative tissue sample.

## MALIGNANT PROCESSES THAT MAY MIMIC PNEUMONIA

### Intrathoracic Kaposi Sarcoma

Kaposi sarcoma (KS) was one of the first clinical manifestations that led to the recognition of acquired immunodeficiency syndrome (AIDS). It occurs most frequently in HIV-infected homosexuals or bisexuals, although persons with other risk factors for AIDS are occasionally affected. Unlike opportunistic infections, KS may occur in HIV-infected persons who have not yet developed severe immunologic dysfunction. In contrast to classic KS, patients with AIDS frequently have significant morbidity because of widespread involvement of the lymph nodes and visceral organs. Intrathoracic involvement has been documented at autopsy in 50% to 75% of patients with AIDS and KS.[1-3]

### Pathologic Features

Intrathoracic KS may involve the lung parenchyma, airways, intrathoracic lymph nodes, and pleura. Within the lung parenchyma, KS may present as nodular masses or a septal angiomatous infiltration.[4] The nodular masses are distributed predominantly in peribronchial and perivascular areas. They contain large numbers of spindle cells. As they enlarge, they obliterate the underlying pulmonary tissue and invade the bronchial or vascular walls. Focal hemorrhage is frequently associated with these lesions. Pulmonary KS may also present as multifocal infiltration of the pulmonary interstitium by the same cellular, vascular, and inflammatory elements. This pattern, which initially may be focal, often affects the distal lung and may extend to the visceral pleura.

Airway involvement by KS is common. Endobronchial KS appears as bright red or violaceous, irregular lesions that are usually flat or only slightly raised. The lesions may occur throughout the tracheobronchial tree or may have a predilection for branching points of the lower airways.[4] Occasionally, extensive endobronchial involvement may compromise the airway.

Invasion by KS is a common cause of mediastinal or

hilar lymph node enlargement in patients with AIDS and KS. Obstruction of the mediastinal lymphatics by KS may retard absorption of pleural fluid and lead to significant pleural effusions.[2]

KS lesions involving the visceral pleura frequently have been demonstrated at autopsy in patients with intrathoracic KS.[3, 4] The appearance was that of hemorrhagic plaques due to thickened pleura, with the characteristic fibroblastic or spindle cell proliferation and vascular slits filled by erythrocytes. Pleural involvement by KS may or may not be accompanied by pleural effusion.[2, 3]

### Clinical Manifestations

**Symptoms and Signs.** Although KS occasionally may originate in the thorax before any cutaneous lesions,[2, 5] most patients have skin or mucous membrane involvement. Pulmonary KS is an important cause of respiratory symptoms and radiographic opacities in patients with AIDS and KS. Several clinical series have described the symptoms associated with pulmonary KS. Moderate to severe dyspnea is the most common symptom. Most patients have extensive parenchymal involvement.[3–6] Nonproductive cough develops in at least half the patients. Wheezing is less common but has occurred in some patients with endobronchial involvement. Patients with pulmonary KS may have fever, although it is often not clear whether these patients have concomitant infections in the lung or elsewhere. One case of persistent fever in a patient with isolated pulmonary involvement with KS resolved after local radiation therapy.[7] Pleuritic chest pain and hemoptysis are sometimes reported by patients with pulmonary KS. Concomitant upper airway involvement has led to hoarseness and occasionally produced stridor.[3, 4]

The physical findings are often unremarkable in patients with pulmonary KS. There may be bilateral diffuse crackles.[3–5] In some patients with endobronchial involvement, wheezing may be heard. Large pleural effusions may be apparent on physical examination.

**Chest Radiographs.** The chest radiographs of patients with pulmonary KS may demonstrate nodular or mixed alveolar-interstitial patterns or both.[3–6] Typically, the alveolar-interstitial infiltrates begin in the perihilar regions and are accompanied by hilar or mediastinal lymphadenopathy.[8] The nodular lesions may be located more peripherally, are irregular and of different sizes, and may coalesce.[8–10] Segmental and lobar consolidations have been reported. These focal findings are usually the result of direct parenchymal involvement with KS rather than collapse or pneumonic infiltration distal to the obstructing airway lesions.[4, 9]

Pleural effusions have been observed on 50% to 89% of the chest x-ray films of patients with intrathoracic KS.[9, 10] They are most often bilateral, although they may be unilateral. Most patients with radiographically apparent pleural effusions have visceral pleural involvement, although some effusions may be caused by mediastinal lymphatic obstruction.[2] Some patients with documented pleural involvement do not have pleural effusions.[2, 3] Occasionally, they are the sole radiographic manifestation of intrathoracic KS.

Intrathoracic KS often involves the mediastinal and hilar lymph nodes. Computed tomographic scans of the chest have been helpful in confirming this finding and, in the proper clinical situation, may provide supportive data for an indirect diagnosis of intrathoracic KS involvement. In some patients with early-stage disease, the chest radiograph may be normal.

**Pulmonary Function Tests.** Patients with pulmonary KS frequently have a low carbon monoxide diffusing capacity.[3, 4] This is a nonspecific finding in patients with AIDS, especially if there is a coexisting pulmonary opportunistic infection. Airway obstruction with a decreased ratio of forced expiratory volume in 1 second to the forced vital capacity ($FEV_1/FVC$) may be demonstrated in patients with pulmonary KS, especially if there is endobronchial involvement. Because these findings do not necessarily correlate with smoking or prior airways disease, it has been suggested that the peribronchial predilection of nodular KS may cause or contribute to the obstruction.[4]

### Diagnostic Tests

The diagnosis of pulmonary KS can be difficult. The results of autopsy series show that as few as 7% to 11% of patients with pulmonary KS were diagnosed during life.[2, 5] Specific radiographic and blood test markers have been lacking. Because visualization of the typical pattern of spindle cell bands intertwined with vascular slits is important for making a histologic diagnosis, adequate-sized tissue specimens are necessary. One of the best diagnostic clues is the presence of skin or mucous membrane lesions. As more experience with pulmonary KS has been gained, the results of a combination of noninvasive tests, such as nuclear scanning techniques and bronchoscopy, and the lack of evidence of other pathologic processes in combination with skin lesions and a consistent clinical presentation have been used as presumptive evidence of pulmonary KS.

**Nuclear Scans.** Gallium 67 scanning has been useful in detecting opportunistic pulmonary infections, especially *P. carinii*. Several studies have shown that KS lesions do not accumulate [67]Ga.[4, 11, 12] Most cases of pulmonary KS with tracer uptake in the lung have had concomitant pathology to which the uptake could be attributed, although some patients with pulmonary KS and no demonstrable pulmonary opportunistic infection have positive [67]Ga scans.[12] The uptake of thallium 201 in KS lesions in various sites, including the lung, has been documented.[13] [201]Tl has been used to evaluate other neoplastic lesions, including lymphomas, thyroid carcinomas, and hepatocellular carcinomas. Although [201]Tl uptake may not be specific for KS, the lack of [67]Ga with the uptake of [201]Tl in a patient with cutaneous KS, dyspnea, cough, and consistent chest radiographic abnormalities should raise the examiner's suspicion of pulmonary involvement.

**Bronchoscopy.** In patients with endobronchial KS, airway involvement may be seen by fiberoptic bronchoscopy as multiple, discrete, slightly raised, violaceous or cherry-red tracheobronchial lesions (Fig. 16–1). Upper airway lesions with a similar appearance, although sometimes more nodular or bulky, are often observed in the mouth and the pharyngeal and laryngeal areas. Endobronchial lesions have been found mostly in the larger airways, and more extensive involvement in the trachea than the bronchial tree has been described.[1, 14] Some series have reported diagnostic bronchial biopsies taken during fiberoptic bronchoscopy,[10]

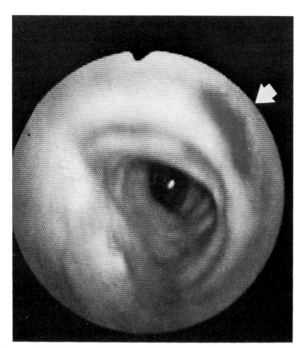

**Figure 16–1.** Bronchoscopic demonstration of endobronchial Kaposi sarcoma. Arrow points to the characteristic plaque-like, cherry-red lesion.

but others have found a very low yield and complications from bleeding.[3, 5, 12, 14] The tendency for the lesions to originate in the peribronchial areas with less involvement of the mucosa may contribute to the difficulty in obtaining diagnostic tissue.[4, 14] A presumptive diagnosis based on the gross appearance of endobronchial KS lesions is accepted by most physicians, especially if the patient has cutaneous lesions. The transbronchial biopsy rarely obtains adequate specimens for the diagnosis of pulmonary KS because of the scattered distribution of the lesions and the need for larger tissue specimens to recognize the diagnostic pattern of the cellular elements. Transbronchial biopsy appears to be a safe procedure in patients with pulmonary KS, and it need not be withheld from patients for whom it would be performed to establish other diagnoses.

**Diagnostic Thoractomy.** Diagnostic thoracotomy is the most definitive means of diagnosing pulmonary KS, although many series have demonstrated that even an open approach frequently fails to provide definitive histopathologic results.[2, 5] Because of the low diagnostic yield and the lack of a significant effect on the management even if the diagnosis is made, diagnostic thoracotomy is usually not performed to document pulmonary KS.

**Thoracentesis and Pleural Biopsy.** In patients with pleural effusions due to KS, thoracentesis and pleural biopsy are useful only for evaluating possible concomitant diseases, such as tuberculosis.[4] KS effusions can be serous or hemorrhagic. The fluid is usually exudative, although transudative effusions have been described.[4, 12] Cytologic specimens and pleural biopsies have been uniformly nondiagnostic in a series of reports,[3–5] probably because of the need for larger intact tissue specimens, localization to the visceral rather than parietal pleura, and the lack of direct pleural involvement in patients in whom the effusions are caused by mediastinal lymphatic obstruction.

## Clinical Course and Treatment

Although most patients with AIDS and KS die of opportunistic infections, pulmonary KS can cause respiratory failure and death. In addition to compromising the pulmonary parenchyma, hemorrhage and upper airway obstruction may contribute to severe respiratory failure. Without treatment, survival may be short, with median survival times of 2.1 to 6 months.[5, 12] Successful palliative measures for pulmonary KS have included conventional chemotherapy and radiation therapy.

Chemotherapy has been the modality most often used to treat pulmonary KS. Combination chemotherapy appears to be more effective than treatment with a single agent. In one study, doxorubicin, bleomycin, and vincristine or bleomycin and vincristine were associated with significant clinical and functional responses in 60% of patients, who had a median survival of 10 months compared with 6 months in nonresponders.[15] Another study reported short-lived but dramatic improvement in 2 patients with respiratory failure due to pulmonary KS that was treated with a combination of doxorubicin, bleomycin, dactinomycin, vincristine, and dacarbazine.[6] Single agents that have been used include vinblastine, vincristine, and etoposide.[16] Biologic response modifiers such as interferon-α have been used in conjunction with chemotherapy.[16, 17]

Radiation therapy has been used for palliation of the respiratory distress due to upper airway KS lesions.[18, 19] There have been a few reports of symptomatic response to whole lung radiation in patients with extensive pulmonary KS.[7, 19]

## Lymphomas

An increased incidence of lymphoid neoplasms is associated with HIV infection. After KS, non-Hodgkin lymphoma, also called AIDS-related lymphoma, is the second most common neoplasm in patients with AIDS. AIDS-related lymphomas have been predominantly high-grade tumors of B-cell origin that are frequently disseminated and involve extranodal sites. Although Hodgkin lymphoma has never been considered an adequate diagnostic criterion for AIDS, it repeatedly has been reported to have an aggressive, atypical course in HIV-infected patients, especially among intravenous drug users.[20–22]

Intrathoracic involvement has not been common in patients with AIDS-related or Hodgkin lymphomas, even if the disease is disseminated. Pulmonary involvement has not been diagnosed frequently during life; it has been reported in no more than 10% of patients,[23] although there have been cases of lymphoma apparently originating in the lung.[23–25] The frequency of pulmonary involvement in AIDS-related lymphoma may be underappreciated, because a number of cases first documented at autopsy were not evident during life.[24]

The symptoms are nonspecific and include cough, dyspnea, chest pain, fever, and weight loss. Generalized lymphadenopathy may or may not occur. The radiographic findings include multiple nodules or infiltration[25] and, in one case of primary pulmonary lymphoma, a solitary nodular lesion.[23] Little has been written on the value of diagnostic procedures for AIDS-related and Hodgkin lymphomas affecting the lung, although the available information suggests that open lung biopsy may be necessary to make a definitive diagnosis.[4, 25] AIDS-related lymphoma can present with unilateral or bilateral pleural effusions, in which case the pleural fluid or biopsy can be diagnostic.[26]

## Primary Pulmonary Malignancies

Primary lung cancer has not occurred with increased frequency among HIV-infected patients. There have been individual reports of small cell[27, 28] and dysplastic carcinoid tumor[29] in patients with AIDS or AIDS-related complex. In these cases, the radiographic presentation was that of a focal infiltrate, cavitating lesion, or anterior mediastinal mass. In one case, small cell carcinoma was found by transbronchial biopsy to coexist with *P. carinii* infection.[27]

## INFILTRATIVE DISORDERS THAT MAY MIMIC PNEUMONIA

### Lymphoid Interstitial Pneumonia

Before the AIDS epidemic, lymphoid interstitial pneumonitis (LIP) was an uncommon disorder that primarily affected middle-aged women and occurred with other immunologically mediated disorders such as Sjögren syndrome. In 1983, LIP, previously a rare pediatric disease, was described in 4 children with AIDS.[30] Since that time, it has been a common pulmonary complication of AIDS in children and a Centers for Disease Control criterion for the diagnosis of AIDS in children younger than 13 years of age. The incidence of LIP among HIV-infected adults has been much lower than among infants and children.

The basis of the association between HIV infection and LIP is unknown. There is evidence to suggest that viral infection, possibly by the Epstein-Barr virus (EBV) or HIV itself, may play a role. In one study, EBV DNA was frequently found in lung biopsy specimens from children with AIDS and LIP and not found in those from children with pulmonary disease other than LIP or adults with AIDS.[31] It was suggested that LIP may have been the result of EBV replication within the lung, leading to infiltration by EBV-infected cells, reactive lymphocytes, and macrophages.

Other reports have suggested that HIV infection of the lung may play a role in the development of LIP.[32, 33] HIV has been isolated in bronchoalveolar lavage fluid from patients with AIDS and LIP in association with IgG antibodies directed specifically at the p24 and gp41 antigens.[32] In another study, a relatively high level of HIV RNA expression was detected by in situ hybridization in lung tissue from a patient with AIDS-related LIP.[33] Retroviruses other than HIV can cause pulmonary disease similar to LIP. HIV has morphologic and genetic similarities to maedi or visna virus, a lenti-retrovirus that causes histologically similar pulmonary disease in sheep. These observations raise the possibility that HIV itself may cause clinically significant lung disease.

Because EBV-infected B cells are more susceptible to in vitro infection by HIV, the pathogenesis of LIP may involve coinfection with EBV and HIV.

### Children Infected With Human Immunodeficiency Virus

**Histopathology.** The pulmonary lymphoid hyperplasia and lymphoid interstitial pneumonia complex (PLH/LIP) is recognized as a distinct pulmonary disorder that occurs in children with HIV infection. This entity appears to be a continuum of invasive lymphoproliferative processes. The PLH component is characterized by multiple pulmonary nodules composed of lymphocytes and plasma cells, with or without germinal centers. The nodular aggregates appear to originate from the bronchus-associated lymphoid tissue and may be of sufficient size to be seen by gross examination.[34, 35] PLH may be associated with mediastinal lymph node hyperplasia and generalized extrathoracic lymphadenopathy. The most important histologic feature of LIP is the diffuse monotonous infiltration of the lung interstitium by lymphocytes and plasma cells. In several pediatric AIDS cases, the pulmonary tissue showed features of PLH and LIP.[36]

**Clinical Manifestations.** The onset of PLH/LIP is usually insidious, with slowly progressive dyspnea. Occasionally, patients have cough or fever or both. The findings of a physical examination of the chest are nonspecific, and adventitial lung sounds are usually absent. There may be peripheral lymphadenopathy, hepatosplenomegaly, or salivary gland enlargement. Digital clubbing frequently occurs.

The most prominent chest radiographic finding of PLH/LIP is diffuse bilateral interstitial or nodular infiltration; occasionally, alveolar filling is seen. There may be widening of the superior mediastinum or hilar enlargement due to lymphadenopathy.

**Diagnostic Tests.** The diagnosis of LIP is important to exclude the need for immediate treatment for infectious pneumonia, particularly *P. carinii* or bacterial pneumonias. Compared with the infectious pneumonias that affect HIV-infected children, the symptoms of LIP are usually mild, and deterioration is slow. In addition to the clinical and radiographic manifestations, certain laboratory findings suggest PHL/LIP. Immunoglobulin levels are usually higher, and although serum lactate dehydrogenase levels may be elevated in PHL/LIP, they tend to be lower than those seen with *P. carinii*. Bronchoscopy with bronchoalveolar lavage has proved to be a useful diagnostic modality for children with AIDS.[37] Although it does not definitively diagnose LIP, not finding a significant infectious agent may suggest that LIP is the primary pathologic process. Most cases of PHL/LIP require open lung biopsies for definitive diagnoses. Because many cases of PLH/LIP have sufficiently characteristic clinical and radiographic features, it has been suggested that invasive procedures are not always needed, particularly if the patient is to be observed rather than receive specific therapy.[34, 35] If there is progressive deterioration and corticosteroid therapy is being considered, the diagnostic confirmation is usually obtained by open lung biopsy.

**Clinical Course and Treatment.** PHL/LIP is a slowly progressive process that may eventually lead to hypoxemia and respiratory failure, although spontaneous resolution has been reported.[35] The course may be accentuated by brief febrile episodes, which may be the result of a superimposed infection, often bacterial. After significant progression has occurred, corticosteroid therapy has been successful in providing symptomatic and radiographic improvement and in reversing hypoxemia.[35, 38] In these cases, high doses of prednisone (2 mg/kg/d) were given initially and subsequently tapered to an alternate day regimen.

### Adults Infected With Human Immunodeficiency Virus

**Histopathology.** The histopathologic findings of LIP in HIV-infected adults consist of diffuse infiltration of the lung interstitium by lymphocytes and plasma cells. There may be perivascular and peribronchial involvement without necrosis or destruction. In more advanced cases, pulmonary fibrosis may develop.

**Clinical Manifestations.** LIP may occur in the earlier stages of HIV infection, before the development of severe immunocompromise, or it may present in patients with AIDS. Initially, symptoms of dyspnea and cough are often mild, but progression to respiratory failure can occur. Examination of the chest may be normal or reveal crackles or rales, especially at the bases. Clubbing, common in children, has not been reported in adults.

LIP may present in adults as part of a diffuse lymphocytic infiltrative syndrome that usually involves the parotid glands but may also include the lymph nodes, liver, kidney, and peripheral nerves.[39–41] In these cases, generalized lymphadenopathy is common. Hepatomegaly, splenomegaly, and parotid gland enlargement may occur. Sicca syndrome has been reported in some patients.

Chest radiographic findings usually include diffuse bilateral reticulonodular or micronodular infiltration that is sometimes more prominent in the lower lobes. Radiographically, LIP may be indistinguishable from *P. carinii* pneumonia. Hilar or mediastinal lymphadenopathy is less common in adults than in children.

**Diagnostic Tests.** Along with the compatible clinical and radiographic findings, some laboratory tests may suggest the presence of LIP in adults. As in children, hypergammaglobulinemia is commonly observed. Lymphocytosis, an unusual finding in HIV-infected patients, has been described in some patients with LIP.[4]

Although open lung biopsy is needed for a definitive diagnosis, demonstration on transbronchial biopsy of the lymphocytic interstitial infiltration without evidence of an infectious agent in a patient with compatible clinical, radiographic, and laboratory findings may be adequate for a presumptive diagnosis of LIP. In such a situation, it may be preferable to defer the open lung biopsy, especially if the patient has mild disease and is to be observed rather than treated.

**Clinical Course and Treatment.** In many HIV-infected adults, LIP remains stable for months or years, and occasionally there may be spontaneous remission.[42] In some patients, there are progression and functional impairment.

In patients with significant respiratory symptoms, corticosteroid treatment with prednisone (60 mg daily) has provided clinical and radiographic improvement.[39–41] In some cases, maintenance therapy was necessary. Improvement with chorambucil therapy has also been reported.[41]

### Lymphocytic Alveolitis

An abnormally high proportion of lymphocytes in bronchoalveolar lavage specimens has been reported in as many as 70% of HIV-infected patients without an infectious diagnosis.[43] Most of these alveolar lymphocytes are CD8 positive and phenotypically identified as cytotoxic cells. Results of further investigation have suggested that cytotoxic cells directed against HIV-infected macrophages may contribute to the development of this lymphocytic alveolitis.[44]

In the series reported by Guillon and colleagues,[43] more than half the patients with lymphocytic alveolitis without pulmonary infections or neoplasms had respiratory symptoms, primarily dyspnea on exertion or cough. Approximately one third had chest radiographic abnormalities described as "diffuse interstitial opacities." Thirty percent to 40% had mild to severe hypoxemia. About one third had decreased carbon monoxide diffusing capacity or an increase of alveolar-arterial difference after exercise. Open lung biopsies from 4 patients demonstrated diffuse lymphocytic infiltration along vascular channels but not involving the alveolar septa.

The relation of lymphocytic alveolitis to PHL or LIP is not understood. It has been suggested that lymphocytic alveolitis might be at one end of a spectrum of invasive lymphoid pulmonary disorders culminating with LIP. Although large numbers of patients with documented lymphocytic alveolitis have not been followed longitudinally, one study suggests that this disorder may resolve with progression of the HIV infection.[44] Whether the symptoms and functional impairment due to lymphocytic alveolitis respond to any form of therapy is unknown.

### Nonspecific Interstitial Pneumonitis

Interstitial pneumonitis that cannot be attributed to any demonstrable cause has been reported in a number of series of HIV-infected patients.[45–47] Because the cause has been unknown, the term nonspecific interstitial pneumonitis (NIP) has been used to describe this diagnostic entity. The relation of NIP to HIV infection and to lymphocytic alveolitis or LIP is unknown. It has been suggested that NIP may be another manifestation of direct HIV infection of the lung, perhaps part of a continuum of HIV-induced pulmonary pathology.

### Histopathology

The histologic findings in lung tissue from HIV-infected patients with NIP have included interstitial mononuclear infiltration, primarily due to lymphocytes and plasma cells; various degrees of diffuse alveolar damage from mild thickening of the alveolar septa, interstitial edema, and focal intraalveolar exudates; and extensive alveolar damage with fibrosis and parenchymal architectural distortion. In one study, vascular changes with medial hypertrophy and intimal thickening were described in a few of the patients.[47]

## Clinical Manifestations

Although many patients considered to have NIP have respiratory symptoms, others have been asymptomatic, and the diagnosis was made by transbronchial biopsy done for research purposes.[46] Symptoms have consisted primarily of cough, dyspnea on exertion, or fever. Radiographic changes may be subtle. The typical chest radiographic abnormality is bilateral, diffuse interstitial or reticulonodular infiltration. In some cases, the chest radiograph was normal.

## Diagnostic Tests

The diagnosis of NIP has been made by transbronchial or open lung biopsy. The characteristic histopathologic findings are required, and other infectious and neoplastic processes that could be responsible for the histologic changes must be excluded by the appropriate microscopic and microbiologic studies.

## Clinical Course and Treatment

NIP usually runs a mild course and resolves or stabilizes without specific therapy. In some cases, there have been exacerbations after initial improvement.

There is no specific treatment recommended for NIP, although the use of corticosteroids has been mentioned.[4]

## OTHER MIMICS OF INFECTIOUS PNEUMONIA

### Complications of Intravenous Drug Use

Most pulmonary complications due to intravenous drug use are infectious and include septic embolic complications, community-acquired pneumonia, and tuberculosis.[48] Less commonly, respiratory symptoms and radiographic findings that may be confused with pneumonia are caused by non-infectious processes such as acute pulmonary edema, pulmonary fibrosis, or atelectasis.[49] Pulmonary talc granulomatosis has been confused with *P. carinii* infection in HIV-infected intravenous drug users,[50] and differentiation can be made by open lung biopsy.

### Iatrogenic Drug-Induced Lung Disease

Drug-induced lung disease has been reported in HIV-infected patients. In many cases, the drug was part of a therapeutic regimen aimed at treating another infectious or neoplastic process that involved the lung. Possible hypersensitivity pneumonitis due to trimethoprim-sulfamethoxazole with fever, rash, hypotension, hypoxemia, and pulmonary infiltration has been reported in patients being treated for *P. carinii* pneumonia.[51] Whether this type of adverse reaction contributes to some cases of *P. carinii* infection that worsen after treatment is begun in unknown.

The cytotoxic drugs used to treat KS or lymphoma may be toxic to the lung. Because bleomycin, a well-known agent of drug-induced pneumonitis, is commonly used to treat both of these neoplasms, secondary pulmonary toxicity may be mistaken for neoplastic invasion of the lung or superinfection.

## REFERENCES

1. Nash G, Fligiel S: Pathologic features of the lung in the acquired immune deficiency syndrome (AIDS): An autopsy study of seventeen homosexual males. Am J Clin Pathol 81:6–12, 1984.
2. Wallace JM, Hannah JB: Pulmonary disease at autopsy in patients with the acquired immunodeficiency syndrome. West J Med 149:167–171, 1988.
3. Meduri GU, Stover DE, Lee M, et al: Pulmonary Kaposi's sarcoma in the acquired immune deficiency syndrome. Am J Med 81:11–18, 1986.
4. White DA, Matthays RA: Noninfectious pulmonary complications of infection with the human immunodeficiency virus. Am Rev Respir Dis 140:1763–1787, 1989.
5. Garay SM, Belenko M, Fazzini E, et al: Pulmonary manifestations of Kaposi's sarcoma. Chest 91:39–44, 1987.
6. Ognibene FP, Steis RG, Macher AM, et al: Kaposi's sarcoma causing pulmonary infiltrates and respiratory failure in the acquired immunodeficiency syndrome. Ann Intern Med 102:471–475, 1985.
7. Bach MC, Bagwell SP, Fanning JP: Primary pulmonary Kaposi's sarcoma in the acquired immunodeficiency syndrome: A cause of persistent pyrexia. Am J Med 85:274–275, 1988.
8. Zibrak JD, Silvestri RC, Costello P, et al: Bronchoscopic and radiologic features of Kaposi's sarcoma involving the respiratory system. Chest 90:476–479, 1986.
9. Sivit CJ, Schwartz AM, Rockoff, SD: Kaposi's sarcoma of the lung in AIDS: Radiologic-pathologic analysis. AJR 148:25–28, 1987.
10. Davis SD, Henschke CI, Chamides BK, et al: Intrathoracic Kaposi sarcoma in AIDS patients: Radiographic-pathologic correlation. Radiology 163:495–500, 1987.
11. Woolfenden JM, Carrasquillo JA, Larson SM, et al: Acquired immunodeficiency syndrome: Ga-67 citrate imaging. Radiology 162:383–387, 1987.
12. Kaplan LD, Hopewell PC, Jaffe H, et al: Kaposi's sarcoma involving the lung in patients with the acquired immunodeficiency syndrome. J Acquir Immune Defic Syndr 1:23–30, 1988.
13. Lee VW, Rosen MP, Baum A, et al: AIDS-related Kaposi sarcoma: Findings on thallium-201 scintigraphy. AJR 151:1233–1235, 1988.
14. Pitchenik AE, Fischl MA, Saldana M: Kaposi's sarcoma of the tracheobronchial tree. Chest 87:122–124, 1985.
15. Gill PS, Akil B, Colletti P, et al: Pulmonary Kaposi's sarcoma: Clinical findings and results of therapy. Am J Med 87:57–61, 1989.
16. Volberding PA: The role of chemotherapy for epidemic Kaposi's sarcoma. Semin Oncol 14:23–26, 1987.
17. Groopman JE, Scadden DT: Interferon therapy for Kaposi sarcoma associated with the acquired immunodeficiency syndrome (AIDS). Ann Intern Med 110:335–337, 1989.
18. Cooper JS, Fried PR, Laubenstein LJ: Initial observations of the effect of radiotherapy on epidemic Kaposi's sarcoma. JAMA 252:934–935, 1984.
19. Nobler MP: Pulmonary irradiation for Kaposi's sarcoma in AIDS. Am J Clin Oncol 8:441–444, 1985.
20. Serrano M, Bellas C, Campo E, et al: Hodgkin's disease in patients with antibodies to human immunodeficiency virus. Cancer 65:2248–2254, 1960.
21. Scheib RG, Siegel RS: Atypical Hodgkin's disease and the acquired immunodeficiency syndrome. Ann Intern Med 102:554, 1985.
22. Knowles DM, Chamulak GA, Subar M, et al: Lymphoid neoplasia associated with the acquired immunodeficiency syndrome (AIDS). Ann Intern Med 108:744–753, 1988.
23. Polish LB, Cohn DL, Ryder JW, et al: Pulmonary non-Hodgkin's lymphoma in AIDS. Chest 96:1321–1326, 1989.
24. Loureiro C, Gill PS, Meyer PR, et al: Autopsy findings in AIDS-related lymphoma. Cancer 62:735–739, 1988.
25. Poelzleitner D, Huebsch P, Mayerhofer S, et al: Primary pulmonary lymphoma in a patient with the acquired immune deficiency syndrome. Thorax 44:438–439, 1989.
26. Sider L, Horton ES: Pleural effusion as a presentation of AIDS-related lymphoma. Invest Radiol 24:150–153, 1989.
27. Moser RJ, Tenholder MF, Ridenour R: Oat-cell carcinoma in transfusion-associated acquired immunodeficiency syndrome. Ann Intern Med 103:478, 1985.
28. Nusbaum NJ: Metastatic small-cell carcinoma of the lung in a patient with AIDS. N Engl J Med 312:1706, 1985.
29. Weitberg AB, Mayer K, Miller ME, et al: Dysplastic carcinoid tumor and AIDS-related complex. N Engl J Med 314:1455, 1986.

30. Oleske J, Minnefor A, Cooper R, et al: Immune deficiency syndrome in children. JAMA 249:2345–2356, 1983.
31. Andiman WA, Eastman R, Martin R, et al: Opportunistic lymphoproliferation associated with Epstein-Barr viral DNA in infants and children with AIDS. Lancet 2:1390–1393, 1985.
32. Resnick L, Pitchenik AE, Fisher E, et al: Detection of HTLV-III/LAV-specific IgG and antigen in bronchoalveolar lavage fluid from two patients with lymphocytic interstitial pneumonitis associated with AIDS-related complex. Am J Med 82:553–556, 1987.
33. Chayt KJ, Harper ME, Marselle LM, et al: Detection of HTLV-III RNA in lungs of patients with AIDS and pulmonary involvement. JAMA 256:2356–2359, 1986.
34. Rubinstein A, Morecki R, Silverman B, et al: Pulmonary disease in children with acquired immune deficiency syndrome and AIDS-related complex. J Pediatr 108:498–503, 1986.
35. Rubinstein A, Morecki R, Goldman H: Pulmonary disease in infants and children. Clin Chest Med 9:507–517, 1988.
36. Joshi VV, Oleske JM: Pulmonary lesions in children with the acquired immunodeficiency syndrome: A reappraisal based on data in additional cases and follow-up study of previously reported cases. Hum Pathol 17:641–642, 1986.
37. Mattey JE, Fitzpatrick SB, Josephs SH, et al: Bronchoalveolar lavage for pneumocystic pneumonia in HIV-infected children. Ann Allergy 64:393–397, 1990.
38. Rubinstein A, Bernstein LJ, Charytan M, et al: Corticosteroid treatment for pulmonary lymphoid hyperplasia in children with the acquired immune deficiency syndrome. Pediatr Pulmonol 4:13–17, 1988.
39. Morris JC, Rosen MJ, Marchevsky A, et al: Lymphocytic interstitial pneumonia in patients at risk for the acquired immune deficiency syndrome. Chest 91:63–67, 1987.
40. Solal-Celigny P, Couderc LJ, Herman P, et al: Lymphoid interstitial pneumonitis in acquired immunodeficiency syndrome-related complex. Am Rev Respir Dis 131:956–960, 1985.
41. Itescu S: Diffuse infiltrative lymphocytosis syndrome in human immunodeficiency virus infection—A Sjogren's-like disease. Rheum Dis Clin North Am 17:99–115, 1991.
42. Grieco MH, Chinoy-Acharya P: Lymphocytic interstitial pneumonia associated with the acquired immune deficiency syndrome. Am Rev Respir Dis 131:952–955, 1985.
43. Guillon JM, Autran B, Denis M, et al: Human immunodeficiency virus-related lymphocytic alveolitis. Chest 94:1264–1270, 1988.
44. Guillon JM, Autran B, Parquin F, et al: Suppressor T lymphocyte alveolitis in HIV-infected patients. Am Rev Respir Dis 139:A618, 1989.
45. Suffredini AF, Ognibene FP, Lack EE, et al: Nonspecific interstitial pneumonitis: A common cause of pulmonary disease in the acquired immunodeficiency syndrome. Ann Intern Med 107:7–13, 1987.
46. Ognibene FP, Masur H, Rogers P, et al: Nonspecific interstitial pneumonitis without evidence of *Pneumocystis carinii* in asymptomatic patients infected with human immunodeficiency virus (HIV). Ann Intern Med 109:874–879, 1988.
47. Ramaswamy G, Jagadha V, Tchertkoff V: Diffuse alveolar damage and interstitial fibrosis in acquired immunodeficiency syndrome patients without concurrent pulmonary infection. Arch Pathol Lab Med 109:408–412, 1985.
48. O'Donnell AE, Pappas LS: Pulmonary complications of intravenous drug abuse. Chest 94:251–253, 1988.
49. Glassroth J, Adams GD, Schnoll S: The impact of substance abuse on the respiratory system. Chest 91:596–599, 1987.
50. Ben-Haim SA, Ben-Ami H, Edoute Y, et al: Talcosis presenting as pulmonary infiltrates in an HIV-positive heroin addict. Chest 94:656–658, 1988.
51. Silvestri RC, Jensen WA, Zibrak JD, et al: Pulmonary infiltrates and hypoxemia in patients with the acquired immunodeficiency syndrome re-exposed to trimethoprim-sulfamethoxazole. Am Rev Respir Dis 136:1003–1004, 1987.

# CHAPTER 17

# Nosocomial Pneumonia in Surgical Patients

MITCHELL P. FINK

## EPIDEMIOLOGY AND PATHOGENESIS

Hospital-acquired lower respiratory tract infections are a common problem in surgical patients, particularly those requiring therapy in an intensive care unit (ICU). Estimates of the incidence of hospital-acquired pneumonia in surgical patients vary widely among studies, presumably because of differences in the diagnositic criteria employed and the populations reviewed. In most epidemiologic studies, the diagnosis of pneumonia has been established using the conventional clinical criteria of fever, leukocytosis, new or progressive infiltrates seen on the chest roentgenogram, and purulent sputum containing a predominant organism on stained smears or cultures. However, these criteria can produce inaccurate conclusions about the incidence of pneumonia, especially among critically ill, mechanically ventilated patients for whom there are often numerous possible causes of pulmonary infiltrates, including cardiogenic pulmonary edema, the adult respiratory distress syndrome, and pulmonary contusion. The microbiologic data obtained from sputum samples aspirated from the colonized tracheas of intubated patients often inaccurately represent the microflora in the more distal airways and pulmonary parenchyma.[1, 2]

The true incidence of nosocomial pneumonia in surgical patients is unknown. In one widely cited study, nosocomial pneumonia was diagnosed in 17.5% of patients undergoing elective abdominal or thoracic procedures,[3] but this study is more than a decade old, and in addition to the possibility of errors caused by the diagnostic problems previously described, these data may not adequately reflect the impact of some of the sweeping changes in surgical practice that have occurred during the past 10 years, such as shorter hospital stays and the use of laparoscopic procedures. Previously

identified risk factors for nosocomial pneumonia, many of which apply to surgical patients, include a history of severe underlying illness, history of smoking, history of chronic obstructive lung disease, prolonged endotracheal intubation, aspiration, recent thoracic or abdominal surgical procedure, long operative procedures, age greater than 70 years, preoperative protein depletion, gastric alkalinization for prophylaxis against stress ulceration, hospitalization during the fall and winter months, requirements for reintubation of the trachea, use of an intracranial pressure monitor, and systemic immunosuppression.[2–10]

## Trauma

Victims of trauma are a subpopulation of surgical patients who are at high risk for the development of lower respiratory tract infections. The incidence of pneumonia in trauma patients has been reported to be as low as 4%,[11] although most studies suggest the incidence is about 20% to 30%.[12–14]

Numerous risk factors for lower respiratory tract infections have been identified in trauma patients, including head injury, a high Injury Severity Score (ie, anatomically based index of the extent of injuries), immobilization in a conventional hospital bed, and a flail chest managed with endotracheal intubation and mechanical ventilation.[6, 14–16, 16a, 16b] In a study of 294 trauma patients requiring endotracheal intubation and admission to an ICU, Rodriguez and colleagues[12] used a multivariate analysis technique (ie, stepwise logistical regression) to identify five mutually independent risk factors for pneumonia: emergency intubation, head injury, hypotension on admission, blunt trauma as the mechanism of injury, and a high Injury Severity

Score. These researchers also showed that the risk of pneumonia is directly related to the duration of intubation, a finding that is consistent with observations made by other investigators.[8]

Although the development of pneumonia has not been definitively associated with excess mortality in trauma patients, the data obtained by Rodriguez and colleagues[12] tend to support this correlation. In their study, the mortality rates for trauma victims were similar for those with and without pneumonia. In the group without pneumonia, most of the deaths occurred early (mean = 3, SEM = 0.5 days), but in the group with pneumonia, most deaths occured later (mean = 22, SEM = 4 days; $P$ = .001). Presumably, most of the early deaths were caused by overwhelming head injuries or uncontrolled hemorrhage, but most of the late deaths were caused by sepsis or multiorgan system failure. The similar rates of mortality observed in the pneumonia and no-pneumonia subgroups may reflect that many of the patients in the latter group died of other causes before having an opportunity to develop pulmonary infection.

The risk of pneumonia in trauma victims is increased by many factors. Some of these factors, such as changes in the microflora of the oropharynx and diminished mucociliary clearance of tracheobrochial secretions, are common to all critically ill patients. Other factors tend to be more specific for trauma victims. For example, trauma leads to marked alterations in immune responsiveness, and the degree of immunosuppression correlates with the risk of infection in these patients.[17-20] A thorough discussion of the pathophysiologic mechanisms responsible for trauma-induced immunosupresion is beyond the scope of this discussion, but soft tissue injury, burns, and even simple hemorrhage have caused derangements in the functioning of mononuclear cells,[21-24] lymphocytes and plasma cells,[25, 26] and polymorphonuclear leukocytes.[27] Blood transfusions, which are commonly necessary in severely injured patients, have been shown to be an independent risk factor for infection after trauma.[27a]

Many blunt trauma victims sustain pulmonary contusions as a result of direct compressive forces acting on the lung. Lung contusion (ie, hemorrhage and edema within the alveoli and interstitium) results from disruption of the integrity of capillaries induced by pressure waves within the pulmonary parenchyma.[28, 29] By increasing the hydrostatic pressure within the pulmonary microvasculature, the degree of edema formation probably can be exacerbated by the injudicious resuscitation of trauma patients with too large a volume of intravenous fluids. Pulmonary contusion decreases bacterial clearance by the lung, an effect that is exacerbated by hypovolemic shock and resuscitation.[30]

In addition to pulmonary contusion, trauma to the chest can lead to other pathologic conditions involving the parenchyma of the lung, including lacerations and pneumatoceles. Lung lacerations result from gross disruption of tissue caused by powerful compressive forces or from the cutting action of bony fragments from fractured ribs or other objects (eg, knives, bullets) penetrating the chest. Pulmonary lacerations usually are accompanied by hemopneumothorax, and creating a direct pathway from the airways to a fluid-filled pleural cavity increases the risk of empyema formation. Posttraumatic pneumatoceles or pseudocysts probably result from the combined effects of compressive and shearing forces on the lung, which lead to bronchial disruption, destruction of pulmonary parenchyma, and formation of a cavity filled with air and fluid.[31-35] Posttraumatic pneumatocele is an uncommon entity that is diagnosed almost exclusively in children and young adults who are victims of major blunt trauma to the chest. Although usually characterized by a benign course, posttraumatic pneumatoceles occasionally become infected and lead to overwhelming, occasionally lethal, sepsis.[31, 35]

Diminished mobility undoubtedly contributes to the increased likelihood of pneumonia in trauma victims by encouraging pulmonary atelectasis and stasis of secretions. This view is supported by data from three studies, which indicate that early operative reduction of fractures, particularly those involving the femur, decreases the incidence of pulmonary complications, including pneumonia, after trauma.[36-38] Two prospective randomized trials have documented a decreased incidence of pulmonary complications, including lower respiratory tract infections, in trauma patients treated on an oscillating hospital bed.[14, 39]

Pain, particularly from rib fracture, is another factor that contributes to the development of pneumonia in trauma victims. Rib fractures are a common injury sustained by victims of blunt chest trauma.[40] Pain from rib fractures leads to splinting, diminished functional residual capacity, and ineffective coughing. When multiple, contiguous ribs are fractured in two or more places, a condition referred to as flail chest results. This term refers to the paradoxic respiratory motion of the involved segment of chest wall that can occur with this kind of injury. Because the involved segment is relatively mobile, it is free to respond to changes in intrapleural pressure, and it moves inward during inspiration and outward during expiration. Formerly, it was thought that flail injuries resulted in impaired ventilation because of a phenomenon called pendelluft (ie, to and fro motion of air from the involved to the uninvolved lung). However, newer data suggest that ipsilateral ventilation is not impaired by flail chest,[41, 42] and the respiratory complications from this injury, including pneumonia, presumably reflect the combined deleterious effects of pain from the rib fractures and the underlying pulmonary contusion, which occurs in most cases.

It increasingly is apparent that most cases of nosocomial pneumonia in mechanically ventilated patients result from microaspiration or macroaspiration of colonized oropharyngeal or upper gastrointestinal secretions.[43, 43a, 43b] Support for this notion derives, in part, from positive results obtained in numerous studies of a concept called selective digestive decontamination (SDD). Although SDD regimens have been evaluated in a variety of patient populations,[44-49] the beneficial effects of this form of therapy have been most evident in trauma victims.[48, 49] SDD is discussed in more detail in Chapter 48. Simply stated, the term refers to a regimen, usually consisting of systemically administered and topically applied antimicrobials, that is designed to eradicate potentially pathogenic microorganisms from the oropharynx and gastrointestinal tract. The term was coined by Stoutenbeek and van Saene,[43] and it refers to species and strains of bacteria and yeast that, although only moderately virulent, are capable of causing invasive infections when one or more normal host antimicrobial defense mechanisms are compromised by breaks in the integrity of the skin, endotracheal intubation, urinary catheterization, or global immunosuppression. According to the classification scheme of Stoutenbeek and van Saene,[43] potentially pathogenic microorganisms include *Staphylococcus aureus*, members of the Enterobacteriaceae, *Pseudomonas aeruginosa*, and *Candida* species.

The data supporting the SDD concept are open to criticism,[50, 51] and this approach to preventing nosocomial pneumonia, although widely used in Europe, has been slow to gain favor in North America. Nevertheless, the weight of evidence suggests that SDD is a valid strategy. The lower respiratory tract infections in trauma and other critically ill surgical patients result from pulmonary contamination by bacteria colonizing the upper digestive tract, and it seems likely that these patients can be helped by applying SDD.

## Burns

Persons with major thermal injuries represent a special type of trauma patient. Respiratory tract infection is the most common complication of thermal injury.[52] Two principal factors contribute to the high risk of pneumonia in this group of patients. First, burns are associated with major derangements in immune responsiveness, lowering host resistance to nosocomial infections of many types, including pneumonia. Second, a substantial percentage of burn victims also sustain inhalation injuries.[53] According to a study by Shirani and coworkers, the incidence of pneumonia among burn victims without inhalation injuries is 8.8%, but in patients with inhalation injuries, the incidence of pneumonia is 38%.[54] The data obtained in this study suggest that inhalation injury and pneumonia independently increase the risk of mortality for victims of burns.

## Intraabdominal Sepsis

Another subpopulation of surgical patients identified as being at high risk for developing pneumonia are persons with intraabdominal sepsis. In a review of 143 patients with intraabdominal abscesses, Richardson and colleagues found that 41 developed pneumonia as a secondary complication.[55] In this study, the mortality rate was 66% in the group of abscess patients with pneumonia, but only 19% of the patients without pneumonia died ($P < .001$). These findings were confirmed in a prospective study of pneumonia complicating intraabdominal sepsis.[56] The study found that 34 of 300 patients had pneumonia at the time of presentation, and among the remaining 266 patients, pneumonia developed postoperatively in 59 (22%). The mortality rate was 58% for patients with intraabdominal sepsis and pneumonia, compared with 20% for patients with only intraabdominal infection.

## MANAGEMENT

### Prevention

As Trunkey pointed out, the best way to treat pneumonia in surgical patients is to prevent it from developing in the first place.[57] Several preventive strategies warrant discussion here, although some are discussed in much greater detail elsewhere in this book.

Endotracheal intubation is a risk factor for pneumonia, and the degree of risk correlates with the duration of intubation.[8] Avoiding prolonged intubation or avoiding intubation altogether assumes paramount importance in the prevention of pneumonia in surgical patients. In the past, most trauma patients with flail chest injuries were intubated and mechanically ventilated, because the goal was to provide internal, pneumatic stabilization of the unstable thoracic wall.[40] This approach was abandoned about 15 years ago as a result of improvements in our understanding of the pathophysiology of this injury and recognition that endotracheal intubation increases the risk of pulmonary infection in these patients.[16] Patients with flail chest injury and pulmonary contusion are managed selectively, avoiding mechanical ventilation except when indicated for other reasons (eg, hypoxemia, head trauma, major operation, shock, upper airway obstruction).[58, 59]

In patients with blunt chest trauma and rib or sternal fractures, pain promotes splinting and atelectasis and is a major factor contributing to the need for intubation. A major advance in the management of these patients has been the development of improved methods for providing durable and satisfactory analgesia, including continuous intercostal nerve blockade using a local anesthetic,[60] intrapleural analgesia using a local anesthetic,[61] and continuous epidural analgesia using local anesthetics or opioids.[62, 63]

Early restoration of patient mobility is an important factor in preventing pulmonary complications after surgery.[64] For most surgical patients, mobilization is best achieved by ensuring that adequate analgesia is provided and that early ambulation is a standard component of the postoperative nursing care. For some patients, such as those with femur fractures or head trauma, ensuring adequate mobilization is more complex. Obtaining early operative stabilization of fractures and limiting continued soft tissue injury improve mobilization. Despite some controversy about the benefit of continuous postural oscillation,[65] most studies suggest that this form of therapy decreases the risk of pneumonia in high-risk patients.[66]

Another controversial issue is the use of gastric alkalinization to prevent stress gastritis and ulceration. Although much has been written about the effect of gastric alkalinization on the incidence of pneumonia,[67] only one study has focused on surgical patients. In a randomized, prospective trial, Simms and associates compared the rates of gastric colonization and pneumonia in 27 critically ill trauma patients treated with antacids, 32 trauma patients treated with continuous intravenous cimetidine, and 30 trauma patients treated with sucralfate.[13] In contrast to data obtained in several other studies,[67] the bacteriologic composition of gastric aspirates was found to be similar among the three groups. Moreover, no differences in the rates of pneumonia were found, and there was no apparent correlation between gastric colonization and the subsequent development of pneumonia.

Another controversial preventive strategy is SDD. One major concern is the expense associated with acquiring and dispensing the antibiotic cocktail used in SDD and performing the requisite microbiologic monitoring.[51] Amphotericin B, the most expensive component of the drug cocktail advocated by Stoutenbeek and coworkers, probably can be purchased in bulk quite inexpensively, and the necessity for performing rigorous, periodic cultures of stool and secretions has not been established. The financial costs of SDD may be lower than previous estimates indicated, and this approach soon may be used more widely in surgical ICUs in North America.

### Diagnosis

The diagnosis of nosocomial pneumonia usually is based on three components: systemic signs of infection, new or worsening infiltrates seen on the chest roentgenogram, and bacteriologic evidence of pulmonary parenchymal infection. Systemic signs of infection, such as fever, tachycardia, and leukocytosis, reflect the release of pyrogenic cytokines, particularly interleukin-1, tumor necrosis factor-α, and interleukin-6. The systemic signs of infection are nonspecific findings and can be caused by any condition that releases cytokines. Hemorrhage, soft tissue trauma, and thermal injury are among the noninfectious conditions that are associated with elevated circulating levels of cytokines.[68–70] In trauma and other surgical patients, fever and leukocytosis should prompt the physician to suspect infection, but in the early posttraumatic or postoperative period (ie, during the first 72 hours), these findings usually are not helpful. Later in the course, fever and leukocytosis are more likely to be caused by infection, but even at this time, other problems associated with an inflammatory response (eg, devitalized tissue, open wounds) can underlie these findings.

The plain (usually portable) chest roentgenogram remains an important component in the evaluation of surgical patients with suspected pneumonia, although it is most helpful when it is normal and rules out pneumonia. When infiltrates are evident, the particular pattern is of limited value for differentiating cardiogenic pulmonary edema, noncardiogenic pulmonary edema, pulmonary contusion, atelectasis (or collapse), and pneumonia. Atelectasis is common in surgical patients. Caplan and colleagues emphasized the value of repeating the chest roentgenogram after vigorous pulmonary physiotherapy to differentiate infiltrates caused by atelectasis from infiltrates due to infection.[71] Recognizing that atelectasis or cardiogenic pulmonary edema often confounds the identification of pneumonic infiltrates, Mock and colleagues devised an objective scoring system evaluating chest roentgenograms in critically ill surgical patients (Table 17–1).[72] In this system, one point is awarded for each of 10 criteria; the radiograph is scored for being

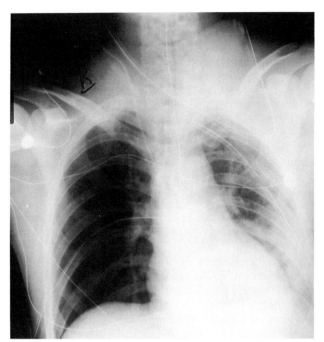

**Figure 17–1.** A portable anteroposterior radiograph of the chest obtained approximately 12 hours after blunt trauma to the thorax shows opacification of the left midlung field.

highly suggestive of pneumonia (8–10 points), moderately suggestive of pneumonia (4–7 points), or minimally suggestive of pneumonia (0–3 points).

Roentgenographic evidence of pulmonary contusion is evident within 1 hour of injury in 70% of cases, and within 6 hours in the remainder (Fig. 17–1).[40] The typical picture is a poorly defined alveolar and interstitial infiltrate that is often most evident near the ipsilateral hilum, perhaps as a result of a concentration of forces in this region.[40] Partial radiographic resolution sometimes is evident within 48 to 72 hours, but complete resolution usually takes several weeks. Pulmonary contusion should be suspected if there is evidence of direct trauma to chest (eg, rib, sternal, clavicular, or scapular fractures; chest wall hematomas or abrasions) and a rapidly developing infiltrate on the plain film of the chest.

Posttraumatic pulmonary cavitary lesions (ie, pneumatoceles) are sometimes evident on the initial plain chest radiographs obtained after blunt chest trauma.[33] More often, cavitation in a region of pulmonary contusion becomes evident in serial films obtained over several days. Moore and associates[31] and our group[35] have emphasized the value of computed tomography for diagnosing this lesion. If adolescent or young adult victims of major blunt chest trauma manifest high fevers and a toxic course over several days, infection of pneumatoceles (which are often multiple) should be strongly suspected, and this diagnosis should be pursued, even if cavitation is not evident on plain films of the chest.

The microbiologic diagnosis of pneumonia, particularly in mechanically ventilated patients, remains a complicated and controversial issue (see Chap. 13). Most authorities agree that Gram-stained smears and cultures of sputum obtained by suctioning through an endotracheal tube lack specificity, although these methods may be sensitive.[1] Data suggest that the diagnostic accuracy can be improved by

**Table 17–1. Criteria for Diagnosing Pneumonia Surgical Patients in the Intensive Care Unit**

Presence of
  New infiltrate
  Acinar shadows
  Air bronchograms
  Segmental infiltrates
  Asymmetric infiltrates
  Infiltrates in nondependent regions of the lung
  Infiltrate with ipsilateral pleural effusion
Absence of
  Volume loss
  Cardiomegaly
  Hilar enlargement

From Mock CN, Burchard KW, Hassan F, Reed M: Surgical intensive care unit pneumonia. Surgery 104:494–499, 1988.

using one or more of several techniques for evaluating distal bronchial secretions that are minimally contaminated by oropharyngeal flora. These techniques include examination of stained smears of fluid obtained by bronchoscopically directed bronchoalveolar lavage (BAL), quantitative cultures of specimens obtained by bronchoscopically directed BAL, quantitative culture of BAL fluid obtained using a blind technique, and quantitative cultures of specimens obtained using a protected specimen brush passed through the suction channel of a bronchoscope.[1] Although there are academic centers that rely extensively on one or more of these methods, these techniques have not been adopted widely by clinicians in North America, presumably because of concerns about financial costs, delays in treatment, and convenience. Controversy persists about which of these methods provides the best compromise in terms of sensitivity, specificity, risk, and cost. No rigorous data support the choice of any one of these methods for making the diagnosis of pneumonia in mechanically ventilated surgical patients.

## Treatment

The mainstay of treatment of nosocomial pneumonia remains the administration of systemic antibiotics. This topic is discussed in greater detail in Chapter 43, and there is little that is different for surgical or medical patients. Infected posttraumatic pseudocysts are a special problem, and we[35] and Moore and colleagues[31] have found that open surgical debridement of infected, devitalized pulmonary tissue is sometimes necessary to effect a cure. For a few patients with necrotizing gram-negative nosocomial pneumonia after blunt trauma, we have used nebulized aminoglycosides as recommended by Klatersky and coworkers,[73] and our experience supports this approach in selected instances. The volume of distribution for aminoglycosides is typically much larger than normal in polytrauma and burn patients, and aminoglycoside clearance rates tend to be supranormal in these patients. The doses of gentamicin or tobramycin that are required to achieve therapeutic circulating levels are often quite large (~3 mg/kg every 8–12 hours), and formal pharmacokinetic monitoring has been valuable in treating these patients.[74] However, once daily dosing of aminoglycosides has been shown to be a safe and effective therapeutic approach, and application of this strategy tends to decrease the need for monitoring of aminoglycoside concentrations in serum, at least in patients with normal renal function.[74a, 74b] We have adopted this approach in our surgical intensive care unit.

I am reluctant to provide firm recommendations for choosing antibiotics to treat pneumonia in postoperative patients or victims of trauma or thermal injury. Truly reliable data regarding the microbiology of the distal airways in these patients are lacking, and there are remarkably few published data comparing the efficacy of different agents or combinations of agents for the treatment of pneumonia in surgical patients.

Despite these concerns, the following suggestions seem to be reasonable. First, in cases of genuine gram-negative pneumonia, as evidenced by positive blood or pleural fluid cultures or the results of cultures obtained from the distal

airways, combination therapy with an aminoglycoside plus an extended spectrum β-lactam agent (eg, third-generation cephalosporin, ceftazidime, monobactam, carbapenem) is a prudent and conservative approach. Second, if there is evidence of staphylococcal infection (eg, positive blood cultures, copious gram-positive cocci on stained smears of sputum), therapy with vancomycin should be initiated. If susequent susceptibility testing indicates that the organism is not methicillin resistant, the antibiotic regimen can be changed to an appropriate antistaphylococcal semisynthetic penicillin or first- or second-generation cephalosporin. Third, in the early period after trauma, when respiratory infections caused by *Haemophilus influenzae, Moraxella (Branhamella) catarrhalis,* and *S. aureus* are common, reasonable empiric therapy consists of a second-generation cephalosporin (eg, cefuroxime), ampicillin-sulbactam, or the combination of vancomycin plus a third-generation cephalosporin; the latter regimen is reserved for the most critically ill.

## REFERENCES

1. Meduri GU: Ventilator-associated pneumonia in patients with respiratory failure; a diagnostic approach. Chest 97:1208–1219, 1990.
2. Fagon J-Y, Chastre J, Domart Y, et al: Nosocomial pneumonia in patients recieving continuous mechanical ventilation: Prospective analysis of 52 episodes with use of a protected specimen brush and quantitative culture techniques. Am Rev Respir Dis 139:877–884, 1989.
3. Garibaldi RA, Britt MR, Coleman ML, Reading JC, Pace NL: Risk factors for post-operative pneumonia. Am J Med 70:677–680, 1981.
4. Haley RW, Hooton TM, Culver DH, et al: Nosocomial infections in U.S. hospitals, 1975–1976: Estimated frequency by selected characteristics of patients. Am J Med 70:947–959, 1981.
5. Windsor JA, Hill GL: Risk factors for postoperative pneumonia: The importance of protein depletion. Ann Surg 208:209–214, 1988.
6. Craven DE, Kunches LM, Kilinsy V, Lichtenberg DA, Make BJ, McCabe WR: Risk factors for pneumonia and fatality in patients receiving continuous mechanical ventilation. Am Rev Respir Dis 133:792–796, 1986.
7. Torres A, Aznar R, Gatell JM, et al: Incidence, risk, and prognosis factors of nosocomial pneumonia in mechanically ventilated patients. Am Rev Respir Dis 142:523–528, 1990.
8. Langer M, Mosconi P, Cigada M, et al: Long-term respiratory support and risk of pneumonia in critically ill patients. Am Rev Respir Dis 140:302–305, 1989.
9. Kingston GW, Phang PT, Leathley MJ: Increased incidence of nosocomial pneumonia in mechanically ventilated patients with subclinical aspiration. Am J Surg 161:589–592, 1991.
10. Celis R, Torres A, Gatell JM, Almela M, Rodriguez-Roisin R, Agusti-Vidal A: Nosocomial pneumonia: A multivariate analysis of risk and prognosis. Chest 93:319–324, 1988.
11. Miller EH, Caplan ES: Nosocomial *Hemophilus* pneumonia in patients with severe trauma. Surg Gynecol Obstet 159:153–156, 1984.
12. Rodriguez JL, Gibbons KJ, Bitzer LG, Dechert RE, Steinberg SM, Flint LM: Pneumonia: Incidence, risk factors, and outcome in injured patients. J Trauma 31:907–914, 1991.
13. Simms HH, DeMaria E, McDonald L, Peterson D, Robinson A, Burchard KW: Role of gastric colonization in the development of pneumonia in critically ill trauma patients: Results of a prospective randomized trial. J Trauma 31:531–537, 1991.
14. Fink MP, Helsmoortel CM, Stein KL, Lee PC, Cohn SM: The efficacy of an oscillating bed in the prevention of lower respiratory tract infection in critically ill victims of blunt trauma: A prospective study. Chest 97:132–137, 1990.
15. Helling TS, Evans LL, Fowler DL, Hays LV, Kennedy FR: Infectious complications in patients with severe head injury. J Trauma 28:1575–1577, 1988.
16. Trinkle JK, Richardson JD, Franz JL, Grover FL, Arom KV, Holms-

trom FMG: Management of flail chest without mechanical ventilation. Ann Thorac Surg 19:355–363, 1975.

16a. Hsien AH-H, Bishop MJ, Kubilis PS, Newell DW, Pierson DJ: Pneumonia following closed head injury. Am Rev Respir Dis 146:290–294, 1992.

16b. Rello J, Ausina V, Castella J, Net A, Prats G: Nosocomial respiratory tract infections in multiple trauma patients: Influence of level of consciousness with implications for therapy. Chest 102:525–529, 1992.

17. Polk HC Jr, George CD, Hershman MJ, Wellhausen SR, Cheadle WG: The capacity of serum to support neutrophil phagocytosis is a vital host defense mechanism in severely injured patients. Ann Surg 207:686–692, 1988.

18. Polk HC Jr, George CD, Wellhausen SR, et al: A systematic study of host defense processes in badly injured patients. Ann Surg 204:282–299, 1986.

19. Keane RM, Birmingham W, Shatney CM, et al: Prediction of sepsis in the multitraumatic patient by assays of lymphocyte responsiveness. Surg Gynecol Obstet 156:163, 1983.

20. O'Mahoney JB, Palder SB, Wood JJ, et al: Depression of cellular immunity after multiple trauma in the absence of sepsis. J Trauma 24:869, 1984.

21. Cheadle WG, Hershman MJ, Wellhausen SR, Polk HC Jr: HLA-DR antigen expression on peripheral blood monocytes correlates with surgical infection. Am J Surg 161:639–645, 1991.

22. Ertel W, Morrison MH, Ayala A, Chaudry IH: Insights into the mechanisms of defective antigen presentation after hemorrhage. Surgery 110:440–447, 1991.

23. Ayala A, Perrin MM, Wagner MA, Chaudry IH: Enhanced susceptibility to sepsis after simple hemorrhage. Arch Surg 125:70–75, 1990.

24. Faist E, Mewes A, Strasser T, et al: Alteration of monocyte function following major injury. Arch Surg 123:287–292, 1988.

25. Grbic JT, Mannick JA, Gough DB, Rodrick ML: The role of prostaglandin $E_2$ in immune suppression following injury. Ann Surg 214:253–263, 1991.

26. Robinson A, Abraham E: Effects of hemorrhage and resuscitation on bacterial antigen-specific pulmonary plasma cell function. Crit Care Med 19:1285–1293, 1991.

27. Maderazo EG, Woronick CL, Hickingbotham N, Jacobs L, Bhagavan HN: A randomized trial of replacement antioxidant vitamin therapy for neutrophil locomotory dysfunction in blunt trauma. J Trauma 31:1142–1150, 1991.

27a. Agarwal N, Murphy JG, Cayten CG, Stahl WM: Blood transfusion increases the risk of infection after trauma. Arch Surg 128:171–177, 1993.

28. Gerblich AA, Kleinerman J: Blunt chest trauma and the lung. Am Rev Respir Dis 115:369–370, 1977.

29. Wilson JV: The pathology of closed injuries of the chest. Br Med J 1:470–474, 1943.

30. Richardson JD, Woods D, Johanson WG Jr, Trinkle JK: Lung bacterial clearance following pulmonary contusion. Surgery 86:730–735, 1979.

31. Moore FA, Moore EE, Haenel JB, Waring BJ, Parsons PE: Posttraumatic pulmonary pseudocyst in the adult: Pathophysiology, recognition, and selective management. J Trauma 29:1380–1385, 1989.

32. Blane CE, White SJ, Wesley JR, et al: Immediate traumatic pulmonary pseudocyst formation in children. Surgery 90:872–875, 1981.

33. Ganske JG, Dennis DL, Vanderveer JB: Traumatic lung cyst: Case report and review of the literature. J Trauma 21:493–496, 1981.

34. Pearl M, Milstein M, Rock GD: Pseudocyst of the lung due to traumatic nonpenetrating lung injury. J Pediatr Surg 8:967–970, 1973.

35. Carroll K, Cheeseman SH, Fink MP, Umali CB, Cohen IT: Secondary infection of post-traumatic pulmonary cavitary lesions in adolescents and young adults: Role of computed tomography and operative debridement and drainage. J Trauma 29:109–112, 1989.

36. Johnson KD, Cadambi A, Seibert GF: Incidence of adult respiratory distress syndrome (ARDS) in patients with multiple musculoskeletal injuries: Effect of early operative stabilization of fractures. J Trauma 25:375–384, 1985.

37. Goris R, Gimbrere J, Van Niewerk J, et al: Early osteosynthesis and prophylactic mechanical ventilation in the multiple trauma patient. J Trauma 22:895–903, 1982.

38. Border JR, Hassett JM, Seibel R, et al: Blunt multiple trauma (ISS 36), femur fracture and the pulmonary failure—septic state. Ann Surg 206:427–448, 1987.

39. Gentilello L, Thompson DA, Tonneson AS, Hernandez D, Kapadia AS, Allen SJ, et al: Effect of a rotating bed on the incidence of

pulmonary complications in critically ill patients. Crit Care Med 16;783–786, 1988.

40. Shackford SR: Blunt chest trauma: The intensivist's perspective. J Intensive Care Med 1:125–136, 1986.

41. Maloney JV, Schmutzer KJ, Raschke E: Paradoxical respiration and "pendelluft." J Thorac Cardiovasc Surg 41:291–298, 1961.

42. Duff JH, Goldstein M, McLean APH, et al: Flail chest. A clinical review and physiological study. J Trauma 8:63–74, 1968.

43. Stoutenbeek CP, van Saene HKF: Infection prevention in intensive care by selective decontamination of the digestive tract. J Crit Care 5:137–156, 1990.

43a. Inglis TJJ, Sherratt MJ, Sproat LJ, Gibson JS, Hawkey PM: Gastroduodenal dysfunction and bacterial colonisation of the ventilated lung. Lancet 341:911–913, 1993.

43b. Heyland D, Mandell LA: Gastric colonization by Gram-negative bacilli and nosocomial pneumonia in the intensive care unit patient: Evidence for causation. Chest 101:187–193, 1992.

44. Aerdts SJA, van Dalen R, Clasener HAL, et al: Antibiotic prophylaxis of respiratory tract infection in mechanically ventilated patients: A prospective, blinded, randomized trial of a novel regimen. Chest 100:783–791, 1991.

45. Blair P, Rowlands BJ, Lowry K, Webb H, Armstrong P, Smilie J: Selective decontamination of the digestive tract: A stratified, randomized, prospective study in a mixed intensive care unit. Surgery 110:303–310, 1991.

46. Kerver AJH, Rommes JH, Mevissen-Verhage EAE, et al: Prevention of colonization and infection in critically ill patients: A prospective randomized study. Intensive Care Med 13:347–351, 1987.

47. Ulrich C, Harinck-de Weerd JE, Bakker NC, et al: Selective decontamination of the digestive tract with norfloxacin in the prevention of ICU-acquired infections: A prospective randomized study. Intensive Care Med 15:424–431, 1989.

48. Ledingham IM, Alcock SR, Eastaway AT, McDonald JC, McKay JC, Ramsay G: Triple regimen of selective decontamination of the digestive tract, systemic cefotaxime and microbiological surveillance for prevention of acquired infection in intensive care. Lancet 1:785–790, 1988.

49. Stoutenbeek CP, van Saene HKF, Miranda DR, Zandstra DF, Langrehr D: The effect of oropharyngeal decontamination using topical nonabsorbable antibiotics on the incidence of nosocomial respiratory tract infections in multiple trauma patients. J Trauma 27:357–364, 1987.

50. Johanson WG: Infection prevention by selective decontamination in intensive care. Intensive Care Med 15:417–419, 1989.

51. Fink MP: Selective digestive decontamination: A gut issue for the nineties. Crit Care Med 20:559–562, 1992.

52. Pruitt BA Jr, Flemma RJ, DiVincenti FC, et al: Pulmonary complications in burn patients. J Thorac Cardiovasc Surg 59:7–20, 1970.

53. Zikria BA, Weston GC, Chodoff M, et al: Smoke and carbon monoxide poisoning in fire victims. J Trauma 12:641–645, 1972.

54. Shirani KZ, Pruitt BA, Mason AD Jr: The influence of inhalation injury and pneumonia on burn mortality. Ann Surg 205:82–87, 1987.

55. Richardson JD, DeCamp MM, Garrison RN, Fry DE: Pulmonary infection complicating intra-abdominal sepsis: Clinical and experimental observations. Ann Surg 195:732–738, 1982.

56. Mustard RA, Bohnen JMA, Rosati C, Schouten BD: Pneumonia complicating abdominal sepsis: An independent risk factor for mortality. Arch Surg 126:170–175, 1991.

57. Trunkey D: Intensive care unit management of blunt chest trauma: A perspective. Intensive Care Med 1:121–122, 1986.

58. Richardson JD, Adams L, Flint LM: Selective management of flail chest and pulmonary contusion. Ann Surg 196:481–486, 1982.

59. Shackford SR, Virgilio RW, Peters RM: Selective use of ventilator therapy in flail chest injury. J Thorac Cardiovasc Surg 81:194–201, 1981.

60. O'Kelly E, Garry B: Continuous pain relief for multiple fracture ribs. Br J Anaesth 53:989, 1981.

61. Rocco A, Reiestad E, Gudman J, et al: Intrapleural administration of local anesthetics for pain relief in patients with multiple rib fractures, preliminary report. Reg Anesth 12:10, 1987.

62. Ullman D, Fortune SB, Greenhouse BB, et al: The treatment of patients with multiple rib fractures using continuous thoracic epidural narcotic infusion. Reg Anesth 14:43, 1989.

63. Rankin APN, Comber REH: Management of five cases of chest injury with a regimen of epidural bupivacaine and morphine. Anaesth Intensive Care 1984; 12:311, 1984.

64. Canavarro K: Early post-operative ambulation. Ann Surg 124:180–181, 1946.
65. Clemmer TP, Green S, Ziegler B, et al: Effectiveness of the kinetic treatment table for preventing and treating pulmonary complications in severely head injured patients. Crit Care Med 18:614–617, 1990.
66. Sahn SA: Continuous lateral rotation therapy and nosocomial pneumonia. Chest 99:1263–1267, 1991.
67. Cook DJ, Laine LA, Guyatt GH, Raffin TA: Nosocomial pneumonia and the role of gastric pH: A meta-analysis. Chest 100:7–13, 1991.
68. Ayala A, Perrin MM, Meldrum DR, et al: Hemorrhage induces an increase in serum TNF which is not associated with increased levels of endotoxin. Cytokine 2:170–174, 1990.
69. Schluter B, Konig B, Bergmann U, Muller FE, Konig W: Interleukin-6—A potential mediator of lethal sepsis after major thermal trauma: Evidence for increased IL-6 production by peripheral blood mononuclear cells. J Trauma 31:1663–1670, 1991.
70. Nijsten MWN, Hack CE, Helle M, ten Duis HJ, Klasen HJ, Aarden LA: Interleukin-6 and its relation to the humoral immune response and clinical parameters in burned patients. 109:761–771, 1991.
71. Joshi M, Ciesla E, Caplan E: Diagnosis of pneumonia in critically ill patients. [Abstract] Chest 94:4S, 1988.
72. Mock CN, Burchard KW, Hassan F, Reed M: Surgical intensive care unit pneumonia. Surgery 104:494–499, 1988.
73. Klatersky J, Carpentier-Meunier F, Kahan-Coppens L, Thys JP: Endotracheally administered antibiotics for gram-negative bronchopneumonia. Chest 75:586–591, 1979.
74. Townsend PL, Fink MP, Stein KL, Murphy SG: Aminoglycoside pharmacokinetics, dosage requirements and nephrotoxicity in trauma patients. Crit Care Med 17:154–157, 1989.
74a. Prins JM, Büller HR, Kuijper EJ, Tange RA, Speelman P: Once versus thrice daily gentamicin in patients with serious infections. Lancet 341:335–339, 1993.
74b. Valcke YJ, Vogelaers DP, Colardyn FA, Pauwels RA: Penetration of netilmicin in the lower respiratory tract after once-daily dosing. Chest 101:1028–1032, 1992.

# Approach to Pneumonia in the Elderly Nursing Home Patient

MICHAEL S. NIEDERMAN

Pneumonia is the second most common infection, after urinary tract infections, among residents of chronic care facilities, but it is the infection with the greatest impact on mortality.[1, 2] The serious and often fatal nature of pneumonia among the elderly has been well known for years and prompted Osler to comment that "pneumonia is the special enemy of old age. In the aged, chances are against recovery. So fatal is it in this group that it has been called the natural enemy of the old man."[3] Pneumonia is a particular problem in the elderly because it is more complicated and more often fatal than in younger persons and because it is frequently characterized by atypical clinical manifestations.

Elderly residents of nursing homes can develop respiratory infections with organisms not seen in many other settings.[4] Clusters of unusual pathogens can be the consequence of two factors. Altered immunity may predispose patients to infection by organisms that are not ordinarily pathogenic in immunocompetent persons, and the closed environment of the nursing home can lead to periodic epidemics with certain pathogens. Among the elderly, unusual pathogens that lead to infection because of altered immune function include nontypable *Haemophilus influenzae, Moraxella catarrhalis,* and group B streptococci. Organisms can cause epidemics in the closed environment of a nursing home because of airborne transmission. Organisms that spread in this manner include influenza, respiratory syncytial virus, *Mycobacterium tuberculosis,* and *Legionella.*[5] It is clear that prevention of pneumonia in the institutionalized elderly requires attention to underlying illness, the use of immune-stimulating vaccines, and the avoidance of airborne transmission of these organisms.

Certain factors common among the institutionalized elderly are responsible for the increased frequency and the altered clinical, bacteriologic, and epidemiologic features of pneumonia in this population. These factors, which lead to malfunction of the normal immune system, include coexisting medical illnesses, certain therapeutic interventions, and to some degree, aging itself.[6]

In this chapter, the epidemiology and risk factors for pneumonia in nursing home patients is discussed with an examination of the common and unusual pathogens for pneumonia. The clinical features of lung infection and approaches to diagnosis, management, and prevention of infections are also discussed.

## EPIDEMIOLOGY

The point prevalence of pneumonia in nursing home residents may be as high as 3.2%.[2, 7] Pneumonia accounts for 13% to 48% of all institutionally acquired infections.[2] This wide range of estimates is a reflection of the diagnostic difficulties associated with pneumonia and the variable rigor with which the diagnosis is pursued in certain clinical settings. In some studies in the nursing home environment, lower respiratory tract infection is diagnosed on clinical grounds, and chest radiographs are not routinely obtained. The incidence of disease also varies with the patient population that resides in a given nursing home. Because the risk for pneumonia is greatest in those with multiple coexisting illnesses, the case mix of different types of chronic illnesses can influence the observed incidence of infection.

Although urinary tract infections are more common in nursing home residents, pneumonia is the most common cause of death from nosocomial infection in this population. Nicolle observed that pneumonia was the only nursing home-acquired infection to be associated with mortality in a study of institutionalized elderly men.[8] In a study of autopsy findings for 234 patients from a chronic care facility, Gross found that pneumonia was the most common cause of death, accounting for 33% of all the deaths.[9] Muder and colleagues reviewed 163 bacteremic infections that arose in a long-term care facility and found that pneumonia was the infection associated with the highest mortality.[10] In that study, bacteremia led to an overall mortality rate of 21.5%, but if pneumonia was the source of infection, the rate rose to 50%. However, because urinary tract infection was more common than pneumonia, it led to more total deaths than respiratory infection, even though the per case mortality was lower. In a study by Marrie and colleagues of patients hospitalized because of nursing home-acquired pneumonia (NHAP), the observed mortality rate was 40%.[11]

The epidemiology of pneumonia in nursing home patients is similar to that of nosocomial pneumonia in the elderly. Among hospitalized patients, pneumonia is the primary cause of death from nosocomial infection,[12] and the incidence of pneumonia is disproportionately high among the elderly after they enter the hospital. In one study, patients older than 60 years of age represented only 23% of all hospitalized patients, but they accounted for 64% of all nosocomial infections.[13] In the National Nosocomial Infection Surveillance data collected between 1986 and 1990, pneumonia was the most common infection to cause death in the elderly, accounting for 48% of the infection-related deaths in this population.[14] Age itself appears to be less important as a risk factor for nosocomial infection than measures of illness severity.[15] Among hospitalized patients, Saviteer documented that the risk of nosocomial infection rose after the eighth hospital day, implying that prolonged exposure to the hospital environment adds to the risk of infection, a conclusion that may have relevance to those living in a chronic care facility.[16]

## RISK FACTORS FOR PNEUMONIA IN NURSING HOME PATIENTS

A review of the altered immune functions associated with aging is beyond the scope of this discussion, but age is not the major factor that predisposes residents of chronic care facilities to pneumonia. Pneumonia results from a convergence of two factors: reduced immune function as a result of impairment in general health, or as a result of certain therapeutic interventions; and increased exposure to large numbers of bacteria as a consequence of serious illness or therapeutic interventions. Other important risk factors for developing pneumonia are the onset of unusual events, such as an episode of confusion or agitation, or the aspiration of a large volume of material into the tracheobronchial tree (Table 18–1).[1, 17]

Impaired immune function can be the result of common diseases such as malignancy, diabetes mellitus, chronic heart or lung disease, renal failure, liver failure, and malnutrition.[18] These illnesses can cause multiple impairments in immune function, and all of these serious illnesses can predispose patients to gram-negative colonization of the oropharynx, a common finding in elderly residents of chronic care facilities.[19] Gram-negative oropharyngeal colonization is considered a risk factor for the development of nosocomial pneumonia, probably because it serves as a

**Table 18–1. Risk Factors for Nursing Home-Acquired Pneumonia**

**Coexisting Medical Illnesses**
Malignancy
Diabetes mellitus
Chronic heart or lung disease
Renal failure
Liver failure
Malnutrition
Serious illness leading to gram-negative oropharyngeal colonization
   Limited ambulation
   Bladder incontinence
   Deteriorating functional status
   Impaired ability to do activities of daily living
Aging (?)
Illnesses leading to aspiration (eg, neurologic, esophageal disorders)

**Therapeutic Interventions**
Endotracheal intubation
Corticosteroid and immunosuppressive therapy
Antibiotic therapy
Sedatives
Tube feedings, nasogastric tube
Neutralization of gastric pH
Common pharmacologic agents (eg, digoxin, calcium channel blockers, aspirin, theophylline)

**Unusual Event**
Confusion
Witnessed aspiration
Agitation
Falling

marker to identify a patient with serious illness and because it represents the presence of potential pathogens in the upper respiratory tract that can easily enter the lung if aspiration occurs.[20]

In the elderly, although oropharyngeal colonization by enteric gram-negative bacteria (EGNB) is common, it may be a transient and variable finding. Irwin and colleagues collected weekly oropharyngeal cultures for 31 weeks from 32 residents of a skilled nursing facility[21] and found gram-negative colonization in 14% of the patients at any given time. However, colonization rates varied on a weekly basis, from as low as 0% to as high as 29%. The most common EGNB in these elderly subjects were *Klebsiella pneumoniae, Escherichia coli,* and *Pseudomonas* species. Valenti and coworkers studied oropharyngeal colonization rates and predisposing factors in 407 elderly subjects.[19] The rates of colonization varied from 19% of those living in independent apartments, to approximately 40% of those living in a health-related facility, and to 60% of those in an acute hospital ward. The severity of illness was not related to the incidence of colonization, and the best predictor of the risk of gram-negative colonization was the patient's ability to function independently. Malignancy, lung disease, and cardiac disease did not promote colonization unless the patient had coexisting functional impairments, such as limited ambulation, deteriorating functional status, inability to do the activities of daily living, or bladder incontinence.

Therapeutic interventions that interfere with immune function include the use of corticosteroids, immunosuppressives, antibiotics, sedatives, and a number of common pharmacologic agents, including digoxin, calcium channel blockers, theophylline, and aspirin.[22] Certain therapeutic interventions serve as risk factors for pneumonia by increasing the size of the potential bacterial inoculum to which patients are exposed. Nasogastric tubes can facilitate gastric content aspiration, sedatives can interfere with airway protection, agents that elevate gastric pH (eg, feedings, antacids, histamine type 2 blockers) can expand the size of the reservoir of gram-negative organisms in the stomach, and antibiotics can promote mucosal overgrowth with bacteria.[6]

Harkness and associates evaluated the risk factors for pneumonia in elderly residents of long-term care facilities and compared these with the risk factors for nosocomial pneumonia in the elderly.[17] They identified 27 cases of pneumonia in a long-term care facility and compared each case with two controls matched for age and place of residence. Individual risk factors were identified, and logistic regression was used to develop a model for predicting the risk of pneumonia. Individual risk factors for pneumonia in residents of a long-term care facility included deteriorating health, malnutrition, recent weight loss, altered level of consciousness, disorientation, aspiration, difficulty with oropharyngeal secretions, presence of a nasogastric tube, need for airway suctioning or inhalation therapy, upper respiratory tract infection, increased confusion, and increased agitation. Active lung disease, previous infection, and previous antibiotic therapy were not found to be risk factors. After a logistic regression model was developed from these findings, the best predictors of pneumonia in the long-term care setting were difficulty with oropharyngeal secretions, deteriorating health, and the occurrence of an unusual event (eg, confusion, agitation, a fall).[17]

Marrie observed that elderly patients with NHAP were more likely to have dementia, chronic obstructive lung disease, and cerebrovascular disease than elderly patients who had community-acquired pneumonia.[23] In another study,[7] pneumonia in patients residing in chronic care facilities was more common in those who had urinary incontinence, decubitus ulcers, or a poor performance status.

The findings in these studies support the theory that the institutionalized elderly develop pneumonia because of the convergence of disease and therapy-associated immune impairments with an increased exposure to bacteria at the time of an unusual event. The elderly patient lives in delicate balance with surrounding bacteria, and pneumonia can occur if an unusual event destabilizes the normal balance between host and organisms.

## CLINICAL FEATURES OF PNEUMONIA

It is difficult to get an exact picture of pneumonia in the institutionalized elderly, because the evaluation and diagnostic criteria for this infection vary widely, depending on the practices in a given nursing home. In some studies, pneumonia is diagnosed by clinical features only, and a radiograph is not obtained. This favors recognition of patients with clear-cut symptoms but may overlook the diagnosis in patients who present with more subtle, nonrespiratory symptoms, which are common in this population. Nonrespiratory presentations of pneumonia include anorexia, weakness, unexplained falling, failure to thrive, and deterioration of a known chronic illness (Table 18–2). A chest radiograph is important, even without obvious pneumonia signs and symptoms, because it leads to the recog-

**Table 18–2. Clinical Features of Nursing Home-Acquired Pneumonia**

**Respiratory Features**
Upper respiratory tract illness
Tachypnea (>20 breaths/min)
Dyspnea
Cough
Sputum production, change in sputum color
Fever, chills, rigors
Pleuritic chest pain

**Nonrespiratory Features**
Anorexia
Failure to thrive
Weakness
Unexplained falling
Deterioration of a known chronic illness
Confusion
Headache
Nausea

nition of pneumonia as the cause of atypical symptoms and because it can provide prognostic information.

Freeman evaluated 17 patients with lung infections developing in a nursing home and found that, although patients with pneumonia and bronchitis had similar features, those with radiographic abnormalities (ie, pneumonia) accounted for all the observed mortalities.[24] In this study, atypical clinical features were common, with fewer than half of all patients having fever, leukocytosis, and dyspnea. However, 70% had a respiratory rate greater than 20 per minute, and 76% had cough.

Marrie evaluated the signs and symptoms of NAHP in 74 elderly patients and compared them with the features of pneumonia in 73 age- and sex-matched controls.[23] Although no statistical differences were seen between the groups, 64% of those with NHAP had fever, 16% had chills, and 62% had cough. Confusion affected 53%, 80% had rales, and 57% had rhonchi. In another study, Marrie compared the features of NHAP in 131 patients with the features of community-acquired pneumonia in 588 persons.[11] Those with NHAP had cough, anorexia, chills, pleuritic chest pain, headache, nausea, sore throat, arthralgias, and rigors less often, but rhonchi detected on physical examination and confusion were more common than in patients with community-acquired pneumonia.

Other studies have documented that atypical clinical features are common in this population. Peterson found that 60% to 70% of those with NHAP had cough, and 75% to 85% had tachypnea, but they had pleuritic chest pain and dyspnea less often.[25] Nonrespiratory presentations of influenza are also common in this population, and symptoms include anorexia, confusion, unexplained fever, and worsening of an underlying chronic illness. In one study of institution-acquired influenza, only two thirds of the patients had cough, fever, or chills.[26]

In many studies, the most common and reliable feature of pneumonia is an elevated respiratory rate.[27, 28] In one study of 15 patients with NHAP, all had a respiratory rate above 25 per minute, although 4 of 15 patients had no localizing respiratory complaints.[27] In another study, an elevated respiratory rate was found to be a sensitive indicator of the presence of pneumonia, commonly preceding the clinical diagnosis.[28] Stable residents of a nursing home had a normal respiratory rate of 16 to 25 per minute, but if pneumonia was present, the respiratory rate exceeded this range, often as early as 48 to 72 hours before clinical recognition of infection.

These observations demonstrate that there must be a high degree of suspicion for pneumonia in the institutionalized elderly and that the diagnosis should be considered, usually by the nonspecific finding of tachypnea with respiratory or nonrespiratory clinical deterioration. In this setting, a chest radiograph should be obtained to establish the diagnosis and to initiate therapy in a timely manner. The atypical features of NHAP can easily lead to a delay in the recognition of infection, and this may account for the observation that atypical presentations of pneumonia in the elderly are associated with enhanced mortality.[29] Among those with NHAP, atypical clinical presentations are common, and this may be related to the finding of high rates of death from this infection. For example, in Marrie's study, the observed mortality rate for NHAP was 40% or more than twice the mortality rate for patients with traditional community-acquired pneumonia, and these findings paralleled the increased frequency of atypical presentations of pneumonia in those with NHAP.[11] In an autopsy study, pneumonia was correctly diagnosed 73% of the time, and in those who had the diagnosis established, fever was present in 95% and leukocytosis was present in 90%.[9] However, in the patients who had this diagnosis missed, and were first diagnosed at autopsy, all had been afebrile, and none had sputum production.

Subtle clinical symptoms can also occur in patients who develop pneumonia from unusual and nonbacterial pathogens. Viral upper respiratory illnesses can cluster in the nursing home environment, and pneumonia may follow an episode of febrile pharyngitis. In one outbreak, 17% to 30% of the patients with parainfluenza virus infection developed pneumonia.[30] Similarly, pneumonia and mortality may complicate infection with respiratory syncytial virus more commonly in the institutionalized elderly than in younger populations.[30] In the setting of an epidemic viral illness in a nursing home, it may be difficult to recognize the onset of pneumonia and to differentiate it from an uncomplicated viral upper respiratory tract infection.

Infection by pathogens such as *M. catarrhalis,* group B streptococci, and enterococci can present without classic pneumonic symptoms and may occur in the nursing home setting. Aspiration pneumonia, common in elderly patients because of illnesses that interfere with swallowing or impair the level of consciousness, can be an indolent and subacute illness, especially if complicated by an anaerobic lung abscess. The atypical presentations are probably a reflection of the abnormal immune function of patients who are infected with these organisms, rather than an indication that the host normally responds to these organisms in an indolent fashion. However, certain organisms can elicit an exuberent host response, even in the institutionalized elderly. For example, group B streptococcal disease can present as a fulminant illness with high fever, leukocytosis, tachypnea, and hypoxemia.[31]

Especially in the nursing home setting, tuberculosis should not be overlooked in patients who have a variety of respiratory or nonrespiratory complaints. Tuberculosis can present without fever, night sweats, or weight loss and may even appear radiographically as a lower lobe process, par-

ticularly in the debilitated patient with progressive primary disease.[32] When elderly tuberculosis patients were compared with younger patients with this illness, fever, night sweats, weight loss, hemoptysis, sputum production, and hepatomegaly occurred less often, but abnormal mentation was more common.[33] Extrapulmonary complications, including meningitis, miliary tuberculosis, and renal tuberculosis, are frequent occurrences in the elderly.

## ETIOLOGIC PATHOGENS

Because of the frequency of gram-negative colonization of the airway in the elderly and the diagnostic difficulties posed by the atypical presentations of NHAP, it is clear that data about the responsible pathogens for pneumonia in the institutionalized elderly are imperfect. Depending on how pneumonia is defined, how extensive the diagnostic workup, and how chronically ill the population being studied, the responsible pathogens vary widely. Many studies have used expectorated sputum to define etiologic pathogens, but these samples can be contaminated by oral flora, which can consist normally of EGNB. The recovery of gram-negative organisms from the sputum of a patient with pneumonia may represent colonization and not the identity of the pathogen causing parenchymal lung infection. A sputum may also fail to reveal the etiologic pathogen because of an inadequate sample, (ie, representing saliva, but not deep respiratory secretions), overgrowth of the pathogen by a colonizing organism, suppression of pathogen growth by prior antibiotics, or inability to identify the pathogen without special testing, such as is needed for *Legionella, Mycoplasma,* and certain viruses. In one study, 7 of 11 patients with NHAP who received prior antibiotics had no identifiable cause, but only 5 of 30 with NHAP and no prior antibiotics had no identifiable cause.[34]

The most common pathogens for NHAP, keeping in mind the methodologic limitations of such data, are pneumococci, *H. influenzae, Staphylococcus aureus* (including methicillin-resistant organisms), EGNB, aspirated oral anaerobes and gram-negative organisms, and viruses. Gram-negative colonization is common in the institutionalized elderly, but NHAP due to EGNB is not as common as in the elderly with nosocomial pneumonia. Factors predisposing to pneumonia with EGNB include severe underlying medical illness and the recent use of broad-spectrum antibiotics.

Garb and colleagues reported one of the earliest studies of the bacteriology of NHAP, using expectorated sputum to define etiologic pathogens.[35] Among 35 patients, some of whom had multiple pathogens simultaneously, *K. pneumoniae* was cultured from 40%, other EGNB from 44%, and *H. influenzae* from 6%. In addition, 50% of the patients also had gram-positive cocci such as pneumococci and *S. aureus.* Marrie used extensive culture and serologic methods to define the cause of NHAP in two studies. In the first, 74 patients were evaluated, and no cause could be defined in 64%.[23] Aspiration was the most common cause found, but others identified included pneumococci, *S. aureus,* and viruses; infections caused by EGNB, *Legionella,* and *Mycoplasma* were uncommon. In another study of 131 patients with NHAP, no organism was found in 59% of patients,

Table 18–3. **Etiologic Pathogens for Nursing Home-Acquired Pneumonia**

No pathogen identified*
Pneumococcus
Aspiration
  Anaerobes
  Enteric gram-negative bacilli
Viruses
  Influenza A and B
  Respiratory syncytial virus
*Staphylococcus aureus*
*Haemophilus influenzae* (including nontypable strains)
Others (<5% of cases)
  *Moraxella catarrhalis*
  *Legionella* species
Chlamydia pneumoniae
Mycobacterium tuberculosis
Enterococcus
Group B streptococci
Unusual gram-negative organisms

*Pathogens are listed in descending order of frequency.

and aspiration was the most common cause of infection.[11] Other commonly identified pathogens included pneumococci, influenza viruses A and B, *S. aureus,* and EGNB.[11] Fang and colleagues used similar methodology in studying 46 cases of NHAP, and an unknown pathogen was present in 26% of patients. Identified pathogens included pneumococci (19.6%), aerobic gram-negative bacilli (10.9%), aspiration (10.9%), *H. influenzae* (8.7%), *Legionella* spp. (6.5%), *Chlamydia pneumoniae* (6.5%), *S. aureus* (6.5%), and *Streptococcus* spp. (4.3%).[34] Other investigators[2, 7, 36] have made similar observations, but *H. influenzae* was seen in as many as 21.7% of all patients, and *S. aureus* was found in as many as 27% of all patients with NHAP. Peterson observed that *M. catarrhalis* and EGNB, including *E. coli, Pseudomonas aeruginosa, K. pneumoniae,* and *Proteus* spp., are often isolated from sputum samples of patients with NHAP, even though pneumococcus was the most commonly identified pathogen from these patients.[25]

Although blood cultures are not positive in most patients with pneumonia, bacteremic isolates are an accurate reflection of the pathogens causing pneumonia. Muder found 18 cases of bacteremic pneumonia among 163 patients with bacteremia in a chronic care facility. In these patients, *Streptococcus pneumoniae* was recovered from 39%, *S. aureus* from 33%, gram-negative organisms and mixed agents from 22%, and *H. influenzae* from 6%.[10]

The most commonly identified causes of NHAP (in descending order of occurrence) are pneumococci, aspirated EGNB, viruses, *S. aureus, H. influenzae,* and other pathogens (Table 18–3). Some of the unusual pathogens of pneumonia that can affect the debilitated elderly who live in chronic care facilities are nontypable *H. influenzae, M. catarrhalis,* enterococci, and group B streptococci.[31] Despite these general patterns, nursing homes can have vastly different spectrums of infection, particularly if there is an epidemic with an airborne organism such as those responsible for tuberculosis, *Legionella* infection, or viral infection.

Epidemic viral infection is common in the closed environment of a nursing home. Morales studied 159 residents of a chronic care facility for 6 months and found rises in

titers to respiratory syncytial virus in 12 patients, influenza A in 14 patients, and influenza B in 18 patients.[37] In other studies, respiratory syncytial virus occurred in 29% of nursing home patients and led to pneumonia in 5% of these.[38] Influenza A occurred in 35% of nursing home patients, causing pneumonia in 24% of these patients.[39] Falsey estimated that 27% of all respiratory infections in nursing home patients are caused by respiratory syncytial virus and that pneumonia complicates 10% to 55% of these cases.[30] Viral infection may be complicated by secondary bacterial pneumonia, a common pattern with influenza and respiratory syncytial viruses.

The other major pathogen spread by the airborne route in a chronic care facility is *M. tuberculosis.* In the Arkansas experience, active tuberculosis was far more common in nursing home residents than in the general population, and among the elderly, the tuberculosis case rate rose fourfold among nursing home residents.[32] Transmission of tuberculosis can occur if there is an active case in the nursing home, and such an event occurred in 32% of Arkansas nursing homes observed for an 8-year period.[32]

## DIAGNOSIS AND THERAPY

### Diagnostic Approach

If a nursing home resident is suspected of having a respiratory tract infection, a diagnostic evaluation should be initiated to answer several questions (Table 18–4). Are the symptoms due to respiratory tract infection, and is that infection pneumonia or bronchitis? What is the most likely etiologic agent? What complications of pneumonia have occurred, and is the patient ill enough to be transferred to a hospital?

The first question is best addressed by obtaining a chest

Table 18–4. **Diagnostic Approach to Nursing Home-Acquired Pneumonia**

**Are the symptoms due to pneumonia?**
Careful physical examination for abnormal lung findings
Obtain a chest radiograph

**What is the likely etiologic agent?**
Obtain expectorated sputum or endotracheal tube suction sample
  Gram stain for predominant pathogen
  Culture to define antibiotic susceptibility patterns
Blood cultures
Sample any pleural fluid for culture
Look for radiographic clues to specific infections
Consider invasive testing if
  Immunosuppressed
  Not responding to therapy
  Pneumonia diagnosis uncertain
  Unusual organism suspected
Consider serologic testing if
  Not responding to therapy
  Epidemic present (define epidemiology)
Consider tuberculin skin testing if active case in the home

**What complications are present, and how ill is the patient?**
Carefully measure respiratory rate and other vital signs
Sample any pleural fluid
Consider lumbar puncture if meningitis possible
Obtain serum electrolytes and blood urea nitrogen
Assess oxygenation (oximetry or blood gas)

radiograph, which can differentiate pneumonia from bronchitis and may have prognostic significance if abnormal. The radiograph is a useful supplement to the physical examination. In one study of patients with organic brain syndrome, the radiograph was abnormal for 76% of those with a new respiratory symptom and for 62% of those with abnormal ausculatory signs in the lungs.[40] An abnormal radiograph does not always mean pneumonia, and processes such as atelectasis, pulmonary embolus with infarction, and congestive heart failure should be considered in the differential diagnosis. Although specific radiographic patterns cannot reliably predict the cause of pneumonia, certain patterns may be helpful in focusing on specific pathogens.[41] Tuberculosis can present in a variety of ways, but it should be considered if a cavitary infiltrate in the upper lobe posterior segment is seen. Aspiration pneumonia is a likely possibility if the patient has appropriate risk factors and a cavitary infiltrate in the superior segment of the lower lobe. The radiograph can also show pneumonic complications such as a pleural effusion, which should be evaluated to eliminate the possibility of an empyema. In some instances, the radiographic pattern can give clues to all of the major diagnostic questions considered in Table 18–4.

The most accurate way to identify an etiologic pathogen is to use a combination of epidemiologic clues and evaluation of respiratory secretions with a Gram stain and culture. The Gram stain can point to a predominant pathogen, which may not dominate in the culture, because the sputum sample can be overgrown by colonizing organisms. Expectorated sputum should be examined. The sample is considered an adequate representation of lower respiratory tract secretions if it has more than 25 neutrophils and fewer than 10 squamous epithelial cells per low-powered field. If the patient is intubated, a direct sputum suction sample can be obtained. If the patient is not intubated and is unable to expectorate, therapy is usually initiated on empiric grounds, because the benefit of invasive sampling (ie, bronchoscopy, transtracheal aspiration) is usually outweighed by the risks. If infection with an unusual organism requiring special therapy is suspected, invasive sampling of respiratory secretions may be considered. Invasive testing may be required if the patient is immunosuppressed by recent chemotherapy, certain underlying illnesses, or certain medications. Invasive testing can be useful if the patient is not responding to empiric therapy or if the diagnosis of pneumonia is uncertain.

Serologic testing for viruses and atypical pathogens should probably not be done for all patients as part of a routine evaluation. These tests should be reserved for the patient not responding to initial therapy or to evaluate the source of a cluster of cases in the nursing home. Similarly, unless there is an active case of tuberculosis in the nursing home, tuberculin skin testing is probably not needed in the evaluation of a new case of pneumonia, although an organized tuberculosis screening program should be part of routine care in all chronic care facilities.

Other tests should be done to evaluate the severity of illness of the patient with pneumonia, and admission to the hospital should be considered for any patient who is dehydrated, hypoxemic, potentially septic, in severe electrolyte imbalance, acutely confused, decompensated from an underlying chronic illness, or with distant infectious complications (eg, meningitis, empyema, endocarditis). Each patient should have a careful recording of respiratory rate and other vital signs (>30 breaths/min is a poor prognostic sign), blood cultures, a complete blood count, measurement of serum electrolytes and blood urea nitrogen, and assessment of oxygenation by oximetry or blood gas measurement.[42]

## Therapeutic Considerations

The severity of illness should be determined to define the adjunctive therapy, including hospitalization. However, for the institutionalized elderly, a decision to hospitalize must be made on the basis of ethical and social considerations as well as on medical grounds. Each patient should be evaluated individually, taking into account all appropriate factors to define the ultimate approach to therapy and the appropriateness of a decision about hospitalization.

Supportive care of the elderly patient with NHAP may necessitate hydration, oxygen, mucolytic and mucokinetic agents (ie, hydration and bronchodilators), and chest physiotherapy. Specific therapy involves the use of antibiotics directed at the likely etiologic pathogen. Because of the limitations of the diagnostic methods for pneumonia, the therapy for NHAP often is empiric, based on knowledge of local epidemiology and specific patient risks.

The antibiotic therapy for NHAP should be directed at *S. pneumoniae*, aspiration involving anaerobes and EGNB, *S. aureus*, and *H. influenzae*. For patients with chronic obstructive lung disease, *M. catarrhalis* may need to be considered. If the patient is to be kept in the nursing home, therapy can be achieved with oral or parenteral agents. Oral therapy can be accomplished with a second-generation cephalosporin (eg, cefuroxime), trimethoprim-sulfamethoxazole, or amoxicillin clavulanate. If *Legionella* infection is an important concern, a macrolide such as erythromycin, clarithromycin, or azithromycin can be added. Another combination of agents that covers most responsible pathogens is ciprofloxacin with penicillin or clindamycin.

If the patient is hospitalized and parenteral therapy is used, treatment can be achieved with a second-generation cephalosporin, imipenem, or ampicillin-sulbactam as monotherapy.[43] Combination therapy can be accomplished with an aminoglycoside plus either clindamycin or a first-generation cephalosporin such as cefazolin. Alternatively, ciprofloxacin can be used with clindamycin. In any of these regimens, ciprofloxacin should not be used alone, because it does not always provide reliable coverage of pneumococci or anaerobes, but it is a useful agent for many of the other likely pathogens, and it penetrates the respiratory secretions exceedingly well.

If the patient has received antibiotics or corticosteroids and is at risk for *P. aeruginosa,* antipseudomonal therapy is needed. If bacteremia is suspected, combination therapy with two antipseudomonal agents is necessary. In the absence of bacteremia, monotherapy may be adequate, but during therapy, cultures should be followed to recognize the emergence of an antibiotic-resistant strain. Antipseudomonal agents that are effective as monotherapy for nonbacteremic infection include the third-generation cephalosporins ceftazidime and cefoperazone and imipenem, aztreonam, and ciprofloxacin.[44, 45] These agents can be combined if bacteremia is suspected, but only the combination of an aminoglycoside and an antipseudomonal β-lactam can achieve synergy against *P. aeruginosa*. In this setting, the antipseudomonal penicillins (eg, piperacillin, azlocillin, mezlocillin) can be used with an aminoglycoside, but not as monotherapy. If two β-lactam antibiotics are combined, there may be antagonism and one agent may promote resistance to the other. The combination of ciprofloxacin and a β-lactam does not achieve synergy but does avoid the concern of a double β-lactam combination regimen.

When parenteral therapy is used, additional agents may be required in specific settings. If *Legionella* infection is a serious concern, a macrolide should be added, and if methicillin-resistant *S. aureus* is suspected, vancomycin may be needed. With all parenteral agents, doses should be adjusted for changes in renal and liver function, interactions with other medications should be considered, and serum levels of some agents, especially aminoglycosides, should be monitored. With the advent of once-daily aminoglycoside dosing, it may be possible to use these agents effectively without monitoring serum levels.[45a]

## PREVENTION

Influenza vaccine should be given yearly to all residents of chronic care facilities, and it is known to be effective in this setting.[46] Similarly, pneumococcal vaccine should be given to all nursing home residents and possibly repeated every 6 years.[47] If a patient is diagnosed as having pneumonia and has not received pneumococcal vaccine, the vaccine should be given after the patient recovers.[48] The effectiveness of these vaccines is discussed elsewhere in this book. If an epidemic of influenza A does occur in a nursing home, all nonimmunized patients should receive amantidine prophylaxis and immediate immunization. Amantidine should be used at a dosage of 100 mg per day (a reduced dosage to avoid central nervous system side effects) for the 2 weeks that it takes for the immunization to become effective.[49]

If an epidemic of respiratory infection caused by an airborne organism does occur, specific measures can be taken to prevent spread to other residents of a nursing home facility. First, the airborne nature of the infection should be recognized, and all infected patients should be isolated from uninfected residents. During an epidemic, it may be necessary to avoid putting many patients in a small room, as occurs with certain social activities. The staff should use particulate respirator masks when contacting infected patients, and the building ventilation should be evaluated.[5] Air from isolation rooms should be vented outside and not recirculated, and air in other rooms should have two room changes of outside air per hour. This level of ventilation reduces the likelihood of airborne infection transmission. The use of high-efficiency particulate air filters is an alternative for removing droplet nuclei from the air of an isolation room if exhaust to the outside is impossible.[5] Upper room air ultraviolet light is another way to achieve air disinfection. If *Legionella* infection is suspected, the water in the institution should be evaluated, and decontamination of this site may be necessary.

Attention to the specific host and environmental factors in the nursing home setting can ultimately be the key to avoiding preventable respiratory tract infections.

## REFERENCES

1. Bentley DW, Mylotte JM: Epidemiology of respiratory infections in the elderly. *In* Niederman MS (ed): Respiratory Infections in the Elderly. New York, Raven Press, 1991:1–23.
2. Crossley KB, Thurn JR: Nursing home-acquired pneumonia. Semin Respir Infect 4:64–72, 1989.
3. Berk SL: Bacterial pneumonia in the elderly: The observations of Sir William Osler in retrospect. J Am Geriatr Soc 32:683–685, 1984.
4. Verghese A, Berk SL: Bacterial pneumonia in the elderly. Medicine (Baltimore) 62:271–282, 1983.
5. Nardell E, Abrams A: Airborne infection in nursing homes: Administrative and environmental interventions. *In* Niederman MS (ed): Respiratory Infections in the Elderly. New York, Raven Press, 1991:325–348.
6. Niederman MS: Nosocomial pneumonia in the elderly. *In* Niederman MS (ed): Respiratory Infections in the Elderly. New York, Raven Press, 1991:207–237.
7. Alvarez S, Shell CG, Woolley TW, Berk SL, Smith JK: Nosocomial infections in long-term facilities. J Gerontol 43:M9–17, 1988.
8. Nicolle LE, McIntyre M, Zacharias H, MacDonell JA: Twelve month surveillance of infection in institutionalized elderly men. J Am Geriatr Soc 32:513–519, 1984.
9. Gross JS, Neufeld RR, Libow LS, Gerber I, Rodstein M: Autopsy study of the elderly institutionalized patient: Review of 234 autopsies. Arch Intern Med 148:173–176, 1988.
10. Muder RR, Brennen C, Wagener MM, Goetz AM: Bacteremia in a long-term care facility: A five-year prospective study of 163 consecutive episodes. Clin Infect Dis 14:647–654, 1992.
11. Marrie TJ, Durant H, Yates L: Community-acquired pneumonia requiring hospitalization: 5-year prospective study. Rev Infect Dis 11:586–599, 1989.
12. Gross PA, Van Antwerpen C: Nosocomial infections and hospital deaths: A case-control study. Am J Med 75:658–662, 1983.
13. Smith PW: Nosocomial infections in the elderly. Infect Dis Clin North Am 3:763–777, 1989.
14. Emori TG, Banerjee SN, Culver DH, et al: Nosocomial infections in elderly patients in the United States, 1986–1990. Am J Med 91 (suppl 3B):289S–293S, 1991.
15. Craven DE, Kunches LM, Lichtenberg DA, Kollisch NR, Barry A, Heeren TC, McCabe WR: Nosocomial infection and fatality in medical and surgical intensive care unit patients. Arch Intern Med 148:1161–1168, 1988.
16. Saviteer SM, Samsa GP, Rutala WA: Nosocomial infections in the elderly: Increased risk per hospital day. Am J Med 84:661–666, 1988.
17. Harkness GA, Bentley DW, Roghmann KJ: Risk factors for nosocomial pneumonia in the elderly. Am J Med 89:457–463, 1990.
18. Skerrett SJ, Niederman MS, Fein AM: Respiratory infections and acute lung injury in systemic illness. Clin Chest Med 10:469–502, 1989.
19. Valenti WM, Trudell RG, Bentley DW: Factors predisposing to oropharyngeal colonization with gram-negative bacilli in the aged. N Engl J Med 298:1108–1111, 1978.
20. Niederman MS: Gram-negative colonization of the respiratory tract: Pathogenesis and clinical consequences. Semin Respir Infect 5:173–184, 1990.
21. Irwin RS, Whitaker S, Pratter MR, Millard CE, Tarpey JT, Corwin RW: The transiency of oropharyngeal colonization of gram-negative bacilli in residents of a skilled nursing facility. Chest 81:31–35, 1982.
22. Esposito AL: Pulmonary host defenses in the elderly. *In* Niederman MS (ed): Respiratory Infections in the Elderly. New York, Raven Press, 1991:25–44.
23. Marrie TJ, Durant H, Kwan C: Nursing home-acquired pneumonia: A case-control study. J Am Geriatr Soc 34:697–702, 1986.
24. Freeman E, Sutton RNP, Cevikbas A: Respiratory infections on long-stay wards. J Infect 4:237–242, 1982.
25. Peterson PK, Stein D, Guay DRP, et al: Prospective study of lower respiratory tract infections in an extended-care nursing home program: Potential role of oral ciprofloxacin. Am J Med 85:164–171, 1988.

26. Mathur U, Bentley DW, Hall CB, Roth FK, Douglas RG: Influenza A/Brazil/78 (H1N1) infection in the elderly. Am Rev Respir Dis 123:633–635, 1981.

27. Berman P, Hogan DB, Fox RA: The atypical presentation of infection in old age. Age Ageing 16:201–207, 1987.

28. McFadden JP, Price RC, Eastwood HD, Briggs RS: Raised respiratory rate in elderly patients: A valuable physical sign. Br Med J 1:626–627, 1982.

29. Starczewski AR, Allen SC, Vargas E, Lye M: Clinical prognostic indices of fatality in elderly patients admitted to hospital with acute pneumonia. Age Ageing 17:181–186, 1988.

30. Falsey AR, Betts RF: The common cold. In Niederman MS (ed): Respiratory Infections in the Elderly. New York, Raven Press, 1991:73–98.

31. Williams EA, Verghese A: Newer or emerging pulmonary pathogens in the elderly. In Niederman MS (ed): Respiratory Infections in the Elderly. New York, Raven Press, 1991:157–188.

32. Dutt AK, Stead WW: Tuberculosis in the elderly. In Niederman MS (ed): Respiratory Infections in the Elderly. New York, Raven Press, 1991:189–206.

33. Alvarez S, Shell C, Berk SL: Pulmonary tuberculosis in elderly men. Am J Med 82:602–606, 1987.

34. Fang GD, Fine M, Orloff J, Arisumi D, et al: New and emerging etiologies for community-acquired pneumonia with implications for therapy: A prospective multicenter study of 359 cases. Medicine (Baltimore) 69:307–316, 1990.

35. Garb JL, Brown RB, Garb JR, Tuthill RW: Differences in etiology of pneumonias in nursing home and community patients. JAMA 240:2169–2172, 1978.

36. Magnussen MH, Robb SS: Nosocomial infections in a long-term care facility. Am J Infect Control 8:12–17, 1980.

37. Morales F, Calder MA, Inglis JM, Murdoch PS, Williamson J: A study of respiratory infections in the elderly to assess the role of respiratory syncytial virus. J Infect 7:236–247, 1983.

38. Osterweil D, Norman D: An outbreak of an influenza-like illness in a nursing home. J Am Geriatr Soc 38:659–662, 1990.

39. Kashiwagi S, Ikematsu H, Hayashi J, Nomura H, Kajiyama W, Kaji M: An outbreak of influenza A (H3N2) in a hospital for the elderly with emphasis on pulmonary complications. Jpn J Med 27:177–182, 1988.

40. Heckerling PS: The need for chest roentgenograms in adults with acute respiratory illness. Arch Intern Med 146:1321–1324, 1986.

41. MacFarlane JT, Miller AC, Smith WHR, Morris AH, Rose DH: Comparative radiographic features of community acquired legionnaires' disease, pneumococcal pneumonia, mycoplasma pneumonia, and psittacosis. Thorax 39:28–33, 1984.

42. Fine MJ, Smith DN, Singer DE: Hospitalization decision in patients with community-acquired pneumonia: A prospective cohort study. Am J Med 89:713–721, 1990.

43. Nolan PE, Bass JB: New drugs for treating lung infections. Chest 94:1076–1079, 1988.

44. Mangi RJ, Greco T, Ryan J, Thornton G, Andriole VT: Cefoperazone versus combination antibiotic therapy of hospital-acquired pneumonia. Am J Med 84:68–74, 1988.

45. Hilf M, Yu VL, Sharp J, Zuravleff JJ, Korvick JA, Muder RR: Antibiotic therapy for *Pseudomonas aeruginosa* bacteremia: Outcome correlations in a prospective study of 200 patients. Am J Med 87:540–546, 1989.

45a. Miyagawa CI: Aminoglycosides in the intensive care unit: An old drug in a dynamic environment. New Horizons 1:172–180, 1993.

46. Patriarca PA, Weber JA, Parker RA, Hall WN, Kendal AP, Bregman DJ, Schonberger LB: Efficacy of influenza vaccine in nursing homes: Reduction in illness and complications during an influenza A(H3N2) epidemic. JAMA 253:1136–1139, 1985.

47. LaForce FM: Respiratory infections in the elderly: Prevention of community-acquired and nosocomial pneumonia. In Niederman MS (ed): Respiratory Infections in the Elderly. New York, Raven Press, 1991:349–363.

48. Fedson DS, Harward MP, Reid RA, Kaiser DL: Hospital-based pneumococcal immunization: Epidemiologic rationale from the Shenandoah study. JAMA 264:1117–1122, 1990.

49. Cate TR: Influenza in the elderly. In Niederman MS (ed): Respiratory Infections in the Elderly. New York, Raven Press, 1991:99–120.

# CHAPTER 19

# Respiratory Tract Infections Among the Economically Disadvantaged

EDWARD A. NARDELL

The poorest of the poor in most societies suffer disproportionately from afflictions of those organs that interface with their often hostile environments. In shelters for the homeless in the United States, skin disorders, foot ailments, frostbite of the extremities in cold climates, trauma, and acute and chronic respiratory infections are among the most common medical problems, often superimposed on mental illness or the complications of substance abuse.[1] In developing countries, respiratory infections account for about a third of all childhood deaths and for substantial morbidity and mortality among adults, especially among the elderly.

Although the causative infectious agents, clinical presentations, pathogenesis, diagnosis, and treatment of respiratory infections among economically and medically disadvantaged persons should be similar to those of their more affluent counterparts, this chapter focuses on some of the important differences rarely discussed in traditional reviews of respiratory infections. Pertussis and measles, for example, should be preventable childhood infections, but the lack of parental understanding and limited access to health care are important barriers to vaccination of disadvantaged children in the United States and in many resource-poor countries. Physicians caring for poor children must be familiar with the clinical presentations of these and other vaccine-preventable infections.

In addition to the usual spectrum of respiratory infections, immigrants and refugees coming to developed countries from different climates may bring with them infections such as melioidosis and infestations such as paragonimiasis that are unfamiliar to physicians practicing in developed countries. Rich and poor immigrants are susceptible to tu-

berculosis, but the probabilities of new infection, especially in congregate living situations, and of reactivation of old foci are much greater among the disadvantaged, and the likelihood of successful prevention and treatment, uncomplicated by noncompliance and drug resistance, is much less.

More than many acute respiratory infections, tuberculosis (TB) depends on socioeconomic factors. The most potent cofactor for TB, coinfection with the human immunodeficiency virus (HIV), disproportionately afflicts the poor of the world, dramatically increasing morbidity and mortality from tuberculosis and other respiratory infections.

## HOST AND ENVIRONMENTAL FACTORS

From street crime to exposure to the elements, the environment is dangerous for the economically disadvantaged. The poor often leave the most hazardous jobs only to return to dwellings in the most polluted parts of cities. To the extent that atmospheric pollutants encountered at work and at home can impair lung defenses, they represent important, potentially reversible causes of excess respiratory infections among the disadvantaged. A list of atmospheric pollutants with the greatest potential to alter host defenses (Table 19–1) ranges from the by-products of unvented kerosene heaters, wood stoves, and gas ovens—often used by the poor—to high concentrations of allergens in infested inner-city apartments.[2]

The epidemiologic evidence linking respiratory infections to atmospheric pollutants is strongest in children. Ex-

Table 19–1. **Atmospheric Pollutants With the Greatest Potential to Alter Host Defense**

| Pollutant | Sources | Effects |
|---|---|---|
| Acidic aerosols | Power plants | Impaired pulmonary function (asthmatics) |
| | Kerosene heaters | Altered mucociliary clearance |
| | | Altered alveolar macrophage function (?) |
| Particles | Tobacco smoke | Depend on particle size and active chemical species |
| | Diesel engines | |
| | Coal or wood stoves | |
| | Fireplaces | |
| Nitrogen dioxide | Automobile exhaust | |
| | Gas stoves | Increased airway reactivity |
| | Kerosene heaters | Impaired pulmonary function (asthmatics) |
| | | Acute respiratory illness in children (?) |
| | | Altered alveolar macrophage function (?) |
| Ozone | Atmospheric photochemical reactions | Impaired pulmonary function |
| | | Airway inflammation |
| | | Increased epithelial permeability |
| Sulfur dioxide | Power plants | Increased airway reactivity |
| | Steel smelting plants | Impaired pulmonary function |
| | Kerosene heaters | Upper airway irritation |
| Sensitizing antigens | Dust mites | Asthma |
| | Cockroach debris | |
| | Mouse urine | |

From Frampton WW, Samet JM, Utell MJ: Environmental factors and atmospheric pollutants. Semin Respir Infect 6:186, 1991.

tensive evidence shows a dose-related correlation between exposure to high levels of environmental tobacco smoke (ie, secondhand smoke) and increased lower respiratory tract infections (LRTI) in children, especially infants.[3] Because of the strong correlation between the prevalence of smoking and socioeconomic status in the United States,[4] the adverse effects of environmental tobacco smoke on respiratory infections is probably greatest among poor children. Nitrogen dioxide ($NO_2$) released from unvented heating and cooking fires has been associated with respiratory infections, primarily in developing countries. The unusual finding of equal prevalence of chronic bronchitis among men and women in Nepal has been attributed to hours spent near wood-burning stoves.[5]

Although experimental evidence linking pollutants to respiratory infections in animals is difficult to extrapolate, human studies of lung function and in vitro studies of lavaged human alveolar macrophages have provided insights. Utell and coworkers found airway hyperresponsiveness in volunteers with uncomplicated influenza who were exposed to nitrate aerosols but not in normal persons or asymptomatic asthma patients.[6] Frampton and colleagues found that lavaged pulmonary alveolar macrophages of patients exposed to $NO_2$ were less able to inactivate influenza virus in vitro.[7] The adverse effects of pollutant exposure on mucociliary defenses have also been demonstrated.[8] Whether host defenses are impaired by atmospheric pollutants or nutritional deficits, the predisposition to pneumonia may be similar. The interactions of host defenses, various pathogens, nutrition, and HIV infection are discussed in the pathogenesis section of this book.

The effects of nutritional deficits on infection in the residents of developed countries are most often considered in the context of critical care. However, many of the underlying concepts are derived from observations of infections among economically disadvantaged populations around the world.[9] Bor and Epstein[9] attribute the first detailed description of the synergy between nutrition and infection to Scrimshaw.[10] Tomkins and Watson described a "malnutrition-infection cycle" in which decreased dietary intake depresses immunity and the integrity of epithelial surfaces, promotes microbial colonization and invasion, and increases the severity and duration of infections.[11] Anorexia, malabsorption, and diarrhea, sometimes worsened by antibiotic treatment, may further reduce nutritional intake, and infection increases the requirements for calories, proteins, and micronutrients. Rapid and complete recovery requires treatment of the infection and nutritional support well in excess of baseline needs. The correlation of poor nutrition with increased mortality and morbidity of respiratory infections in developing countries is well documented and is independent of age and other risk factors.[11]

The beneficial effects of nutritional supplementation have been shown.[12] Vitamin A supplementation appears to be particularly beneficial in preventing respiratory infections and diarrheal illnesses. Vitamin A may work by means of its effects on epithelial integrity and repair, although other mechanisms have been postulated.[13–15] Vitamin D deficiency has been associated epidemiologically and in vitro with impaired host responses to tuberculosis.[16, 17] Before the chemotherapy era, the beneficial effects attributed to sunlight exposure among sanitoria patients may have been mediated by vitamin D metabolism. Deficiencies in micronutrients have been associated with decreased immunity, predisposing patients to various infections.

Obesity is a paradoxic form of malnutrition common among the poor of many developed countries, and it is often associated with non–insulin-dependent diabetes mellitus. Although more frequent respiratory infections have not been firmly associated with obesity or diabetes (except for diabetes and active TB), it is thought that infections may be more complicated. Alcoholism has long been associated with TB, probably because of increased exposure, but also because of malnutrition. Alcoholism impairs host defenses by predisposing the person to aspiration pneumonia. The impoverished around the world have little access to dental care. Tooth loss contributes to malnutrition, and periodontal disease leads to virulent oropharyngeal flora, which, when aspirated, predispose to pneumonia. Stress may be the most common but the hardest to define factor predisposing the disadvantaged of the world to infections. In a review of the role of stress in the pathogenesis of infectious diseases, Peterson and colleagues found evidence that stress impairs immunity, but the impairments were not severe, and the studies required confirmation.[18]

Crowded living conditions among the poor predispose to the transmission of respiratory infections spread by direct contact, by respiratory droplets, and by droplet nuclei. The more people living close together, the greater is the chance that one of them will develop a respiratory infection, and the greater is the potential for spread to others. In the United States, shelters for the homeless protect people from exposure to the elements, but they also increase exposure to a variety of respiratory infections, particularly TB.[19] Person-to-person transmission of pneumococcal pneumonia in a shelter has been reported, and transmission of influenza and other respiratory viruses can be assumed.[20] Jails, prisons, nursing homes, and acute and chronic health care facilities are among the other group settings where transmission of TB and other respiratory infections is likely.[21]

Although transmission of HIV is not facilitated by crowding, HIV coinfection greatly accelerates the transmission of TB in shelters, prisons, residential drug treatment units, and other health care settings.[22] The effects of HIV infection on TB transmission are several and syergistic: greatly facilitated reactivation of latent TB infection, increased susceptibility to new infection (unproven), and rapid progression from new infection to active, communicable disease—often occurring over weeks or months rather than years. Recommendations have been published to help reduce the risk of tuberculosis transmission in shelters, prisons, nursing homes, and health care facilities caring for HIV-infected persons.[23] Crowding itself is perhaps the most obvious risk factor favoring transmission, but it is rarely mentioned in the recommendations, perhaps because crowding is not readily alleviated and is almost never under the control of health care providers.

## RESPIRATORY INFECTIONS AMONG DISADVANTAGED CHILDREN

### Preventing and Treating Respiratory Infections

Acute respiratory infections remain an important cause of childhood morbidity and mortality, especially among the disadvantaged. Although massive international efforts have increased immunization rates in many developing countries, the last decade has witnessed falling vaccination rates among disadvantaged preschool children in the United States, in some cases to rates below those in developing countries. Data from Texas indicate that only 12% of the 2-year-old children in Houston were fully immunized, but the World Health Organization (WHO) data indicate that more than 50% of children in developing countries had received a primary series of diphtheria, pertussis, tetanus (DPT) immunizations by their first birthday.[24, 25] The results of these concomitant changes have been a profound reduction in the

infant mortality rate in large cities in Brazil and Costa Rica while epidemics of vaccine-preventable infections have occurred in poor, urban areas of the United States.

In developing countries, further reductions in morbidity and mortality from the acute respiratory infections of childhood depend on increased vaccination coverage and on access to basic medical care. In the United States, successful vaccination coverage in the past has led to complacency about the threat of what have become largely unknown infections. Parental reeducation about the importance of immunization is necessary for segments of the population. However, access to immunization for families without health insurance is increasingly threatened by the deterioration of publicly funded municipal and state public health programs. At the same time, access to basic medical care for many families is becoming increasingly unaffordable in the United States under the current health care delivery system.

Connelly and Starke reviewed the clinical aspects of the six vaccine-preventable respiratory infections seen in the United States: pertussis, diphtheria, measles, influenza, and pneumonias caused by *Haemophilus influenzae* and *Streptococcus pneumoniae*.[24] In the United States immunization against influenza and *S. pneumoniae* has been reserved for children at high risk because of other medical problems, including HIV infection. A routine immunization schedule is reproduced in Table 19–2. In addition to pneumococcal and influenza vaccines, Connelly and Starke recommend that HIV-infected children receive all routine immunizations except for oral polio vaccine.[24]

Of the vaccine-preventable infections having a resurgence in the United States and in other developed countries, pertussis and measles merit additional comments. Before vaccination against pertussis infection became common in the early 1950s, whooping cough was an important cause of childhood morbidity and mortality. By the early 1980s, the annual attack rate had been reduced from 100 cases to less than 1 case per 100,000 persons.[26] However, public concern about the rare neurologic reactions after vaccinations has contributed to a decline in immunization rates in the United Kingdom, Japan, Sweden, and the United States, with outbreaks of infection following in each country.[27, 28] Although immunization with the standard vaccine is still strongly favored by risk-benefit analyses, an acellular vaccine has had fewer local reactions and may replace conventional DPT vaccine.[29, 30]

The resurgence in measles is more complicated because it is so highly contagious, because it is occurring at an older average age than it had in the prevaccine era but has a higher mortality rate among very young children, and because it is occurring in vaccinated and unvaccinated children.[31] The vaccine has a low failure rate of 5% to 10%, but these failures and a sizable unvaccinated population are apparently sufficient to sustain outbreaks of this highly infectious disease under conditions in which exposure is likely.[32] Revaccination between the ages of 4 and 12 is recommended to regain better control among high school and college age groups.[33, 34] To further reduce transmission, consideration should be given to air disinfection with upper room ultraviolet germicidal irradiation (UVGI) in waiting rooms of pediatric clinics, emergency rooms, and other defined areas where cases have been reported.[35] Measles is

Table 19–2. **Routine Immunization Schedule for Children**

| Schedule | DPT | Polio | MMR | Hib Conjugate* | | | Td |
| | | | | HbOC | | PRP-OMP | |
| --- | --- | --- | --- | --- | --- | --- | --- |
| 2 mo | ✓ | ✓ | | ✓ | or | ✓ | |
| 4 mo | ✓ | ✓ | | ✓ | or | ✓ | |
| 6 mo | ✓ | | | ✓ | | | |
| 12–15 mo | | | ✓ | ✓ (15 mo) | or | ✓ (12 mo) | |
| 15–18 mo | ✓ | ✓ | | | | | |
| 4–6 y | ✓ | ✓ | | | | | |
| Later in childhood | | | ✓† | | | | ✓‡ |

Abbreviations: DPT, diphtheria-pertussis-tetanus; MMR, measles-mumps-rubella; Hib, *Haemophilus influenzae* B; HbOC, *Haemophilus* B diphtheria protein conjugate, Hib TITER (Lederle-Praxis); PRP-OMP, *Haemophilus* B meningococcal protein conjugate, Pedvax HIB (Merck Sharp and Dohme); Td, tetanus-diphtheria.
*Either HbOC or PRP-OMP can be used at the schedule indicated. HbOC requires four doses, PRP-OMP requires three doses.
†The second MMR should be given sometime between ages 4 and 12 years.
‡The Td booster should be given between ages 14 and 16 years.
From Connelly KK, Starke JR: Vaccine-preventable respiratory infections in childhood. Semin Respir Infect 6:205, 1991.

the one airborne infection for which the efficacy of UVGI can be supported by good field trial data.[36]

Although children in developed and developing countries are subject to similar numbers of respiratory infections each year caused by the same spectrum of microorganisms, disadvantaged children are more likely to have severe infections involving the lower respiratory tract, especially pneumonia due to *H. influenzae* or *S. pneumoniae*. As a complement to efforts toward universal basic immunization, including bacillus Calmette-Guérin vaccine in some areas, the WHO launched its international acute respiratory infection case management program in 1983.[37] The program is part of the WHO's larger primary health care strategy, and it is based on the premise that the timely availability of oxygen and antibiotics can reduce mortality from acute respiratory infections, even in the absence of socioeconomic advances. The case management approach depends heavily on educational programs for mothers and grass-roots health care workers and on improvements in primary and referral health services. According to Douglas, the

WHO's most important contribution has been the development of simplified guidelines for the diagnosis and treatment of respiratory infections (Tables 19–3 and 19–4).[37] They are designed to allow mothers and health care workers to make treatment decisions based on simple observations, without using a stethoscope or laboratory tests. Despite imperfections in the guidelines, ongoing logistic problems in training, and maldistribution of antibiotics and oxygen in remote areas, there is already evidence that the program is saving children, and there is reason to believe that it can be further refined and more broadly applied.[38]

## Long-term Consequences of Lower Respiratory Tract Infections

The substantial mortality and morbidity of acute respiratory infections in children around the world may not reflect their full long-term consequences. In developing countries, untreated bacterial LRTI still result in chronic bronchiec-

Table 19–3. **Pneumonia Management at the Small Hospital for the Child 2 Months to 5 Years of Age With Cough or Difficult Breathing**

| Clinical Signs | Classification* | Summary of Treatment |
| --- | --- | --- |
| Central cyanosis or not able to drink | Very severe pneumonia | Admit; give oxygen; give an antibiotic: chloramphenicol; treat fever, if present; treat wheezing, if present; give supportive care; reassess twice daily† |
| Chest indrawing; no central cyanosis; able to drink | Severe pneumonia; if child is wheezing, assess further before classifying | Admit; give an antibiotic: benzylpenicillin; treat fever, if present; treat wheezing, if present; give supportive care; reassess daily |
| No chest indrawing; fast breathing‡ | Pneumonia | Advise mother to give home care; give an antibiotic (at home): cotrimoxazole, amoxycillin, ampicillin or procaine penicillin; treat fever, if present; advise the mother to return in 2 days for reassessment or earlier if the child's condition becomes worse |
| No chest indrawing and no fast breathing | No pneumonia: cough or cold | If coughing more than 30 days, assess for causes of chronic cough; assess and treat for ear problem or sore throat, if present; assess and treat other problems; advise mother to give home care; treat fever, if present; treat wheezing, if present |

*These classifications include some children with bronchiolitis and asthma.
†If oxygen supply is ample, also give oxygen to a child with (1) restlessness (if oxygen improves the condition), (2) severe chest indrawing, or (3) breathing rate of ≥ 70 breaths per minute.
‡Fast breathing is (1) ≥ 50 breaths per minute in a child aged 2 months to 12 months, or ≥ 40 breaths per minute in a child aged 12 months to 5 years.
Modified from Douglas RM: Acute respiratory infections in children in the developing world. Semin Respir Infect 6:220, 1991.

Table 19–4. **Management of Cough or Difficult Breathing at the Small Hospital for the Infant Younger Than 2 Months of Age**

| Clinical Signs | Classification† | Summary of Treatment |
|---|---|---|
| Stopped feeding well, or abnormally sleepy or difficult to wake; stridor in calm child; wheezing; fever (≥38°C) or low body temperature (<35.5°C); fast breathing*; severe chest indrawing; central cyanosis; grunting; apnoeic episodes or distended and tense abdomen | Severe pneumonia or very severe disease | Admit; give oxygen if central cyanosis is present or infant is not able to drink; give antibiotics: benzylpenicillin and gentamicin; careful fluid management; maintain a good thermal environment; specific management of wheezing or stridor |
| No fast breathing; no sign of pneumonia or very severe disease | No pneumonia: cough or cold | Advise mother to give the following home care: Keep young infant warm; breastfeed frequently; clear nose if it interferes with feeding. Return quickly if breathing becomes difficult, breathing becomes fast, feeding becomes a problem, or the young infant becomes sicker |

*Fast breathing is ≥ 60 breaths per minute in the young infant (<2 months of age); repeat the count.
†If oxygen supply is ample, also give oxygen to a young infant with restlessness (if oxygen improves the condition), severe chest indrawing, or grunting.
Modified from Douglas RM: Acute respiratory infections in children in the developing world. Semin Respir Infect 6:221, 1991.

tasis, but in developed countries, viral infections have been implicated in the subsequent development of asthma and chronic airway obstruction. Brown and Weiss reviewed the evidence linking asthma with LRTI in childhood.[39] They conclude that respiratory infections do not actually cause asthma but that infections may promote predisposed persons to greater levels of airway reactivity. Although atopy is not causally associated with respiratory infections, data suggest that respiratory illness is likely to be more severe among persons (among young males in particular) with allergic disease.

The complex associations among respiratory infection, asthma, and allergy are further complicated in the United States by racial and socioeconomic differences in asthma prevalence, increasing asthma morbidity (especially among poor black children), inadequate access to health care, exposure to environmental tobacco smoke and household allergens, and the effects of urban air pollution.[40–42] Although complex, these associations are undoubtedly worth elucidating, because in the United States, asthma is the most common chronic respiratory disease of childhood and the most common cause of pediatric hospitalizations.[43] For children who survive acute respiratory infections in developing countries, similar long-term consequences can be assumed, but data are unavailable.

## PULMONARY INFECTIONS AMONG IMMIGRANTS AND REFUGEES

The United States and other developed countries have long attracted immigrants and refugees from economically disadvantaged and politically oppressed regions of the world, and they have brought with them a burden of increased respiratory infections. In the early 1980s, refugees from Southeast Asia contributed heavily to the TB case rate in the United States, but as they became integrated into this society, their case rate rapidly decreased. In Massachusetts in 1990, foreign-born persons accounted for 46.5% of 438 TB cases; of these, 21% were from Haiti, 10% from Cambodia, 9% from Viet Nam, 8% from Cape Verde, 8% from China, and fewer than 2% from each of 36 other countries of origin.[44]

Legal immigrants and refugees to the United States are

screened for active TB before departure but not for latent TB infection, which may reactivate at a later time. By definition, illegal arrivals are not screened. Entrance screening procedures are directed at diseases that pose potential public health risks: active TB, HIV infection, and a few other infections. Agencies sponsoring immigrants are asked to be sure new arrivals have medical evaluations, with a special focus on TB, hepatitis, infestations, and a few other conditions, but compliance is not enforced.

Although TB and most other common respiratory infections are likely to be recognized and treated in this country, certain infections acquired abroad may not be within the clinical experience of primary care physicians in the United States. Iralu and Maguire reviewed the clinical features of unusual respiratory infections seen among immigrants and refugees.[45] Table 19–5 organizes the infections into three useful categories: those that resemble TB, those associated with eosinophilia, and latent infections that can reactivate after immigration. Readers are referred to this review and to other sources of information on tropical infections.[46]

Although TB is often missed, growing awareness of the recent resurgence of the disease in the United States may also lead to overdiagnosis. Several unusual diseases are easily confused with TB. Any physician seeing patients

Table 19–5. **Special Considerations in the Diagnosis of Pulmonary Infections in Immigrants**

| Infections That May Resemble Tuberculosis | Parasitic Infections With Peripheral Blood Eosinophilia | Latent Infections That Can Become Active After Immigration |
|---|---|---|
| Melioidosis | Ascariasis | Tuberculosis |
| Paracoccidioidomycosis | Hookworm infection | Melioidosis |
| Histoplasmosis | Strongyloidiasis | Paracoccidioidomycosis |
| Coccidioidomycosis | Tropical pulmonary eosinophilia | Histoplasmosis |
| Paragonimiasis | Visceral larva migrans | Coccidioidomycosis |
| | Trichinosis | Strongyloidiasis |
| | Schistosomiasis | Amebiasis |
| | Echinococcosis | |
| | Paragonimiasis | |

From Iralu JV, Maguire JH: Pulmonary infections in immigrants and refugees. Semin Respir Infect 6:125, 1991.

from Southeast Asia and other tropical regions may have seen but not recognized melioidosis—a disease with highly variable clinical features that may resemble chronic TB with fever, weight loss, hemoptysis, and cavitary upper lobe disease seen on the chest radiograph. The causative agent is the gram-negative bacillus, *Pseudomonas pseudomalei,* which grows readily on routine laboratory media but is often discounted as a contaminant. Like TB, melioidosis may remain subclinical for years and reactivate in response to immunosuppressive illnesses or therapy. Serologic results can suggest latent or active infection. Serologic studies have found elevated titers in as many as 29% of Southeast Asian immigrants.[47,48] Treatment of active disease is at least a 2-month course of conventional antibiotics, such as ceftazidime or trimethoprim-sulfamethoxazole, guided by susceptibility tests.

Paragonimiasis is another infection found among immigrants from Southeast Asia and similar tropical areas that can be confused with TB because of the clinical features of cough, hemoptysis, pleuritic pain, and chest radiographic findings, which include pleural effusions, pleural thickening, lung infiltrates, calcifications, nodular densities, and midlung cavities. The causative agent is a lung fluke, most often ingested in the larval stage in raw or undercooked crabs. Eosinophilia is characteristic and is not a feature of TB, but the diagnosis is based on the examination of stool for the characteristic eggs. Serologic tests are also useful. Treatment is a 2-day course of praziquantel, even for asymptomatic cases. Any of the fungal infections listed in Table 19–5 may resemble TB and may present in immigrants from endemic areas. Diagnosis usually requires biopsy or bronchial lavage, although serologic tests can be helpful.

## RESPIRATORY INFECTIONS AMONG THE HOMELESS

Homeless men and women in the United States are heterogeneous in age, race, and ethnicity. Some are alcoholic, some use illicit drugs, some are mentally ill, and others are simply homeless. They have little in common, except for the uncertainties of day-to-day survival on the streets, the disapproval of passers-by, the ritual of waiting in food and bed lines, the chaos of crowded shelters, and for many, the solitary gratification of cigarettes. Smoking is pervasive among the homeless, and the respiratory complications of smoking—lung cancer, emphysema, and respiratory infections—account for about 40% of their medical complaints, according to a review by O'Connell, and lead to about 20% of all deaths in this population.[49] The effects of smoking on host defenses are compounded by various forms of substance abuse, by increased exposure to respiratory pathogens inherent in congregate living, and increasingly by the devestating consequences of HIV infection.

Table 19–6 lists the causes of respiratory-related deaths among the homeless of Boston from 1986 to 1988. Not represented in this mortality survey are the countless exacerbations of bronchitis and other respiratory infections, which add greatly to the misery of day-to-day life but do not directly lead to death. TB accounted for 6 of the 36

**Table 19–6. Respiratory Deaths Among the Homeless of Boston, 1986–1988**

| Cause | No. of Deaths* |
|---|---|
| Infectious causes | |
| Pulmonary tuberculosis | 6 |
| Pneumonia | 16 |
| *Pneumocystis carinii* | 5 |
| *Streptococcus pneumoniae* | 4 |
| Aspiration | 1 |
| Unknown organism | 4 |
| Total | 22 |
| Noninfectious causes | |
| Cancer | 6 |
| End-stage chronic obstructive pulmonary disease | 5 |
| Pulmonary embolus | 2 |
| Obstructive sleep apnea | 1 |
| Total | 14 |

*There were 36 (20%) deaths due to respiratory causes among a total of 184 deaths during this period.
Modified from O'Connell JJ: Nontuberculous respiratory infections among the homeless. Semin Respir Infect 6:249, 1991.

deaths in this series, a disturbing figure in an age when most cases should be cured.

### Nontuberculous Respiratory Infections

In contrast to TB, relatively little has been written about bacterial and viral respiratory infections among the homeless. It is likely that only a minority of homeless persons suffering from severe upper respiratory infections or from acute or chronic bronchitis seek medical care. However, data on nontuberculous respiratory infections has been reported for 6800 Boston area homeless men, women, and children receiving care through the Boston Health Care for the Homeless Program (BHCHP).[49] Of 14,762 physician and nurse practitioner encounters in 1990, respiratory illness was the primary or secondary diagnosis for 10.5%, and of those, 54% were respiratory infections (Table 19–7).

Influenza is a predominantly airborne infection and presumably spreads through crowded shelters as it does through nursing homes and other congregate living situations, but this has been poorly documented. Coordinated efforts at mass vaccination against influenza have been car-

**Table 19–7. Respiratory Diagnoses of the Boston Health Care for the Homeless Program in 1990**

| | |
|---|---|
| Total medical encounters | 14,762 |
| Primary secondary respiratory diagnoses | 1,555 (10.5%) |
| Acute infections | |
| Bronchiolitis | 30 |
| Bronchitis | 226 |
| Pneumonia | 108 |
| Upper respiratory tract infection | 483 |
| Total | 847/1,555 (54%) |
| Chronic conditions | |
| Asthma | 332 |
| Chronic obstructive pulmonary disease | 240 |
| Other | 136 |
| Total | 708/1,555 (46%) |

From O'Connell JJ: Nontuberculous respiratory infections among the homeless. Semin Respir Infect 6:250, 1991.

ried out annually by the BHCHP, achieving a 32% coverage rate among the estimated 1600 homeless to whom it was offered in 11 Boston shelters in 1988. Transmission of type 1 capsular pneumococcal pneumonia within a large Boston shelter was reported in 1978.[20] Nose and throat cultures on regular residents of the shelter found an unusually high (10%) carriage rate, a precondition to the aspiration of pneumococci, which are droplet-born rather than airborne organisms. The BHCHP attempts to administer polyvalent pneumococcal vaccine to all shelter residents, but coverage is far from complete. Unfortunately, the efficacy of immunization against influenza and pneumococcus infections among the homeless are unknown and are difficult to assess. Outbreaks of infection due to invasive type b *H. influenzae* have also been associated with shelters, and increased pharyngeal carriage has been found.

## Tuberculosis Transmission and Pathogenesis Among the Homeless

Shelters for the homeless have long been associated with tuberculosis. A large shelter in Boston has taught us much about TB pathogenesis and transmission among the homeless, with implications for housing the homeless, for TB control, and for shelter-worker safety.

In 1971, 41 of Boston's 299 cases were users of one large shelter. In 1973, a full-time public health nurse was hired to work at the shelter, and on-site x-ray screening was instituted in an effort to achieve control. In 1980, a newly renovated, larger shelter temporarily relieved overcrowding, and for the first 3.5 years, only 2 to 4 TB cases per year were diagnosed. Late in 1983, however, the first of an ongoing outbreak of epidemiologically and bacteriologically linked TB cases was diagnosed at the shelter.[19] Similar outbreaks were soon reported from New York and other large cities. The index case in the Boston outbreak was subsequently identified as an alcoholic man with a 10-year history of previously treated isoniazid- and streptomycin-resistant TB. He had resided at the shelter for a period of 11 months before the first of the secondary cases was diagnosed. Over the next several years, the TB rate among the homeless of Boston soared (Fig. 19–1), with roughly half

of the cases caused by organisms resistant to isoniazid and streptomycin.

For several years thereafter, subcultures of all isoniazid- and streptomycin-resistant isolates in the state were sent to the Centers for Disease Control in Atlanta for phage typing, and all doubly-resistant isolates associated with the shelter were found to be the same phage type. Based on the preepidemic prevalence of the drug-resistance pattern and phage-type markers in Massachusetts, it was estimated that the probability of the spontaneous occurrence of both markers in a single case, independent of another case, was approximately 1 in 500. The probability of two such cases occurring in the same shelter, unrelated to one another, would be about 1 in 250,000 ($\frac{1}{500} \times \frac{1}{500}$). Finding almost 50 cases associated with one shelter, linked by two independent bacteriologic markers, constituted definitive proof of transmission within the shelter, originating with a single index case.

Closer scrutiny of the linked cases led to insights into the pathogenesis and transmission of TB among the homeless in shelters. Many of the epidemiologically linked shelter cases presented with upper lobe cavitary disease, a pattern usually associated with disease reactivation, long believed to be the predominant pathogenic mechanism for cavitary TB in low-prevalence countries. However, the epidemic pattern and the bacteriologic markers strongly favored recent transmission rather than coincidental, spontaneous reactivations of old TB foci. Progressive primary infection can present with lung cavitation, but that mechanism would have required all of the patients to have been previously uninfected; however, the prevalence of tuberculin reactivity among homeless men had been as high as 50%.[50] Exogenous reinfection of previously infected persons is the one mechanism that resolved the contradictory data, a mechanism that had been proven in only a handful of case reports in this country, but has been postulated as an important, ongoing cause of cavitary TB in high-prevalence countries.

According to Smith, repeated exposure is necessary, because previously infected persons are usually resistant to disease from reinfection.[51] Foci of reinfecting organisms are usually destroyed by rapidly recalled cell mediated immunity. Reinfection is thought to require implantation of organisms in the vulnerable upper lung zones, where sterilization is incomplete. Because inhaled organisms follow the

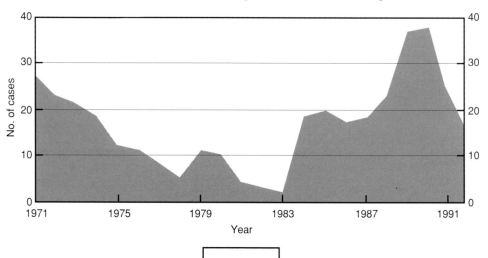

**Figure 19–1.** Incidence of tuberculosis among the homeless in Massachusetts, 1971–1992. (From the Massachusetts Department of Public Health, Division of Tuberculosis Control.)

MDPH TB SURVEILLANCE PROGRAM

CASES

distribution of ventilation, predominantly to the lower lobes, clinical disease after reinfection is usually a low-probability event. If reinfection does occur, liquefaction necrosis and cavitation appear accelerated because of preexisting hypersensitivity to tuberculoproteins. Although medical histories of the homeless are often unavailable or unreliable, 7 of an initial 25 linked patients had convincing evidence of previous TB infection or disease, proving exogenous reinfection. Exogenous reinfection probably led to accelerated epidemic transmission within the shelter through rapid lung cavitation, a pathologic event associated with greater infectivity. Nonspecific impairments in systemic and local lung defenses and recurrent exposure in the shelter were probably risk factors favoring exogenous reinfection.

HIV-infected persons are increasingly being forced into homelessness, as reflected in an increasing proportion of shelter-related tuberculosis cases with HIV infection. As with exogenous reinfection among immunocompetent hosts, an accelerated pattern of epidemic transmission has been observed in shelters, drug treatment facilities, and hospitals.[22, 52, 53] Immunodeficiency predisposes the patient to TB reactivation, leading to increased transmission, especially to other immunodeficient hosts, and more active disease. Exogenous reinfection with drug-resistant organisms has also been demonstrated in a hospital outbreak.[53] This pattern of accelerated transmission has profound implications for the use of congregate housing for HIV-infected persons, for the safety of shelter and health care workers, and for the feasibility of conventional contact tracing and preventive strategies for tuberculosis. Small group living arrangements are preferable to large shelters, because they should be less conducive to widespread transmission. Secondary cases may develop before contacts are tested and treated preventively. Because HIV-infected persons may be anergic to skin tests, preventive therapy may need to be based on estimates of group risk rather than on evidence of individual infection. UVGI air disinfection may be necessary to help reduce transmission among residents and staff in shelters. Environmental interventions have been the subject of several recent articles.[23, 35, 54]

## OBSTACLES TO TUBERCULOSIS TREATMENT AND CONTROL

### Resource-Rich and Resource-Poor Countries

Disadvantaged persons around the world are more likely to become infected and reinfected with TB, and to reactivate latent infection. They are also less likely to be successfully treated than more advantaged groups. In many developing countries, adequate medical care is not available, especially outside the large cities. Among the homeless in the United States, where treatment is generally available, noncompliance often accounts for treatment failures. Where TB treatment is incomplete or erratic, the failure is often as much that of the treatment strategy, itself dependent on available resources, as it is of patients' adherence to treatment. Poor adherence to conventional treatments has motivated a series of clinical trials of shorter and shorter treatment regimens, culminating in regimens of 6 months'

duration for smear-positive disease caused by drug-susceptible organisms. Even in developing countries, high rates of success under field conditions have been achieved if resources permit directly observed treatment.[55]

In some of the world's poorest countries, good tuberculosis control has been shown to be among the most cost-effective public health interventions.[56] Farmer and colleagues reported data from a community-based research project in rural Haiti that challenges the conventional view that health beliefs are the important determinants of compliance with therapy, especially in cultures with strong traditions of folk medicine.[57] Two similar groups of patients were studied. One group received free medicine only, and the other group received free medicine, financial aid, incentives to attend a monthly clinic, and aggressive home follow-up visits by trained village health workers. Although there were no differences in health beliefs between the two groups, those receiving financial aid and other services had fewer missed appointments, a higher sputum conversion rate, greater weight gain, higher cure rates, and a quicker return to work than the group with free medication but fewer support services (Table 19–8). The investigations conclude that in developing countries, "higher cure rates can be achieved if the primacy of economic causes of TB is acknowledged and addressed." Travel to distant clinics in rural areas to obtain medication often means losing valuable income for the family. After the symptoms of TB respond to treatment, the economic price for continued therapy, even "free" therapy, may be too great for disadvantaged persons to sustain. Among the homeless in developed countries, TB treatment often competes with personal safety, shelter, care for acute ailments, the demands of substance abuse, and obstacles such as incarceration and mental illness.

In a provocative article, Brudney compared the success of a well-conceived and executed TB control program in impoverished, war-torn Nicaragua with the near-total failure of current TB control efforts in one of the world's richest cities, New York.[58] Nicaragua's TB program focused on active cases, had available on-site microscopy for

**Table 19–8. Characteristics of Tuberculosis in Sector 1 and Sector 2 Patients**

| Characteristic | Sector 1* | Sector 2 |
|---|---|---|
| Mortality from TB during 18 mo after diagnosis | 0 (0%) | 3 (10%) |
| Sputum positivity for acid-fast bacilli 6 mo after diagnosis | 0 (0%) | 4 (13.3%) |
| Persistent pulmonary symptoms after 1 y of treatment | 2 (6.7%) | 13 (43.3%) |
| Average weight (lb) gained/patient/y | 10.4 | 1.7 |
| Return to work after 1 y of treatment | 28 (93.3%) | 14 (46.7%) |
| Average no. of clinic visits/patient/y | 11.4 | 5.8 |
| Average no. of home visits/patient/y | 37.9 | 1.4 |
| Seropositivity to HIV | 1 (3.3%) | 2 (6.7%) |
| No. of patients who denied possible role of sorcery in illness | 5 (16.7%) | 4 (13.3%) |
| Cure rate | 30 (100%) | 17 (56.7%) |

Abbreviations: HIV, human immunodeficiency virus; TB, tuberculosis.
*The patients in sector 1 had financial aid; those in sector 2 had none.
From Farmer P, Robin S, Ramilus SL, Kim JV: Tuberculosis, poverty and "compliance" lessons from rural Haiti. Semi Respir Infect 6:256, 1991.

Table 19–9. **Changing Characteristics of Tuberculosis Patients Treated Under Court Order in Massachusetts**

| Characteristic | 1968 to 1978 (10 y) | 1985 to 1989 (5 y) | January 1990 to May 1991 (5 mo) |
|---|---|---|---|
| Admission (total) | 21 | 26 | 26 |
| Age 20–39 y (%) | 38 | 54 | 68 |
| Female (%) | 10 | 18 | 16 |
| Boston cases (%) | 28 | 58 | 64 |
| Homeless (%) | 10 | 50 | 60 |
| Substance abusers (%) | 41 | 77 | 80 |

From Etkind S, Boutotte J, Ford J, et al: Treating hard-to-treat tuberculosis patients in Massachusetts. Semin Respir Infect 6:280, 1991.

rapid diagnosis, and employed a combination of directly observed therapy and close supervision of therapy through outreach workers, achieving cure rates as high as 75% using cohort analysis. New York City dramatically reduced its TB control program in the 1970s. Well before the HIV-associated increases in the mid-1980s, the TB case rate in New York was no longer decreasing, as it was in most American cities. In 1980, there were approximately 1500 new cases in New York City, but by 1986, there were 2500, and by 1990, there were 3500–a case rate of almost 50 per 100,000 persons.[59] The increases since the mid-1980s have reflected the profound effect of HIV infection on TB and the gross inadequacy of control efforts. In nearby Massachusetts, which has smaller populations at high risk for TB and HIV infections, there were only 438 cases in 1990, a case rate of 7.45 per 100,000.[44]

In Brudney and Dopkin's 1988 study of TB cases admitted to Harlem Hospital, 89% of 178 patients discharged on antituberculous therapy failed to complete therapy, with most never making it to their first follow-up appointment.[59] Within 12 months of discharge, 48 of the 178 were readmitted with active TB, but most were again lost to follow-up. Although short-course regimens are probably prescribed most often, the resources for directly observed therapy have not been available for New York City's hard-to-treat patients, who are often young, black or Hispanic, male, homeless, drug using, HIV infected, disadvantaged, or mentally ill.

The consequences of incomplete and erratic TB treatment are not fully reflected in New York City's TB case rate. In addition to an explosion of cases, current conditions in New York have fostered the development and transmission of organisms resistant to all or most effective drugs.

Table 9–10. **Advantages of Long-Term Hospitalization for Hard-to-Treat Tuberculosis Patients**

Achieves cures not otherwise possible because of patient noncompliance
Definitively interrupts transmission in institutions
Cost effective in terms of cases prevented
Allows concurrent medical, behavioral, psychiatric, social, and economic issues to be addressed more effectively than in the outpatient setting
Fewer treatment interruptions due to concurrent alcohol or drug use; lower risk of treatment complications
Permits effective use of compulsory treatment under court order for uncooperative patients considered public health threats

From Etkind S, Boutotte J, Ford J, et al: Treating the hard-to-treat tuberculosis patients in Massachusetts. Semin Respir Infect 6:278, 1991.

Inadvertent genetic engineering of this kind was predicted in an editorial accompanying a report on the introduction of a modern multidrug regimen in Peru in the absence of the resources to ensure compliance.[60] A similar scenario occurred in the Philippines.[61] Conditions in New York City may be worse than in some developing countries because of the accelerating effect of HIV infection on transmission and disease progression, especially in shelters, jails, prisons, hospitals, and other institutional settings.

In central Africa, the prospects for TB control have dimmed, not because of drug resistance or because of non-compliance, but because the vast number of cases is rapidly outstripping the capacity of otherwise highly effective programs, with no additional resources expected.[62] Ironically, in the late twentieth century, the prospects for tuberculosis control in some of the richest and poorest places on Earth are equally bad, largely because of the HIV pandemic, but also because of the lack of adequate resources to ensure complete TB treatment under the conditions extant in each area.

## Hard-to-Treat Tuberculosis in Developed Countries

In Massachusetts, TB is under good control by world standards, but among subpopulations such as the disadvantaged, homeless persons, recent arrivals from high incidence countries, and HIV-infected drug users, case rates remain unacceptably high. Although they represent a minority of cases, persons who fail even directly observed therapy are making use of a large and growing proportion of TB control resources. In Massachusetts, Etkind and co-workers reported the increasing use of long-term hospitalization to ensure completion of therapy for selected hard-to-treat patients who are potential sources of ongoing transmission, often of drug-resistant disease.[44] Long-term hospitalization has been used in Massachusetts for treating TB patients who also suffer from chronic alcoholism, mental illness, or homelessness, patients whom public health nurses, outreach workers, and shelter staff have concluded could not be successfully treated as outpatients, even with directly observed therapy. These traditionally difficult patients have been joined by even harder-to-treat patients, chronic users of injectable drugs or cocaine, who are involved in antisocial or criminal activities, often HIV infected, and homeless (Table 19–9). The advantages of long-term hospitalization for hard-to-treat tuberculosis patients are summarized in Table 19–10.

## REFERENCES

1. Nardell EA: Respiratory infections among the economically and medically disadvantaged. Semin Respir Infect 6:183, 1991.
2. Frampton MW, Samet JM, Utell MJ: Environmental factors and atmospheric pollutants. Semin Respir Infect 6:185, 1991.
3. Wu-Williams AH, Samet JM: Environmental tobacco smoke: Exposure response relationships in epidemiologic studies. Risk Anal 10:39, 1990.
4. U.S. Department of Health and Human Services: Reducing the Health Consequences of Smoking: 25 Years of Progress. A Report of the Surgeon General. Washington, DC, U.S. Government Printing Office, 1989.

5. Prandey MR: Domestic smoke pollution and chronic bronchitis in a rural community of the hill region of Nepal. Thorax 39:337, 1984.
6. Utell MJ, Aquillina AT, Hall WJ, et al: Development of airway reactivity to nitrates in subjects with influenza. Am Rev Respir Dis 121:233, 1980.
7. Frampton MW, Finkelstein JN, Roberts NJ Jr, et al: Nitrogen dioxide exposure in vivo and human alveolar macrophage inactivation in influenza virus in vitro. Environ Res 48:179, 1989.
8. Foster WM, Costa DL, Langenback EG: Ozone exposure alters tracheobroncheal mucociliary function in humans. J Appl Physiol 63:996, 1987.
9. Bor DH, Epstein PR: Pathogenesis of respiratory infection in the disadvantaged. Semin Respir Infect 6:194, 1991.
10. Scrimshaw NS, Taylor CE, Gordon JE: Interactions of nutrition and infection. Geneva, World Health Organization, 1968.
11. Tupasi TE, Mangubat NV, Sunico MES, et al: Malnutrition and acute respiratory infections in Filipino children. Am Rev Respir Dis 12:1047, 1990.
12. Kielmann AA, Taylor CE, Parker RI: The Narangwal nutrition study: A summary review. Am J Clin Nutr 31:2040, 1978.
13. Sommer A, Katz H, Tarwotjo I: Increased risk of respiratory disease and diarrhea in children with preexisting mild vitamin A deficiency. Am J Clin Nutr 40:1090, 1984.
14. Keutsch GT: Vitamin A supplements—Too good not to be true. N Engl J Med 323:985, 1990.
15. Hussey GD, Klein M: A randomized, controlled trial of vitamin A in children with severe measles. N Engl J Med 323:160, 1990.
16. Davis PDO: A possible link between vitamin D deficiency and impaired host defence to *Mycobacterium tuberculosis.* Tubercle 66:301, 1985.
17. Rook GAS: The role of vitamin D in tuberculosis. Am Rev Respir Dis 138:768. 1988.
18. Peterson PK, Chao CC, Molitor T, et al: Stress and the pathogenesis of infectious disease. Rev Infect Dis 13:710, 1991.
19. Nardell EA, McInnis B, Thomas B, et al: Exogenous reinfection with tuberculosis in a shelter for the homeless. N Engl J Med 315:1570, 1986.
20. DeMaria A, Browne K, Berk SL, et al: An outbreak of type 1 pneumococcal pneumonia in a men's shelter. JAMA 244:1446, 1980.
21. Nardell EA: Tuberculosis in homeless, residential care facilities, prisons, nursing homes, and other closed communities. Semin Respir Infect 4:206, 1989.
22. Daley CL, Small PM, Schecter GF, et al: An outbreak of tuberculosis with accelerated progression among persons infected with the immunodeficiency virus. N Engl J Med 326:231, 1992.
23. Centers for Disease Control: Guidelines for preventing the transmission of tuberculosis in health care settings, with special focus on HIV-related issues. MMWR 39(RR-17):1, 1990.
24. Connelly KK, Starke JR: Vaccine-preventable respiratory infections in childhood. Semin Respir Infect 6:204, 1991.
25. Bart KJ, Lin KF: Vaccine-preventable diseases and immunization in the developing world. Pediatr Clin North Am 37:735, 1990.
26. Cherry JD: The epidemiology of pertussis and pertussis immunization in the United Kingdom and the United States: A comparative study. Curr Probl Pediatr 14:1, 1984.
27. Centers for Disease Control: Pertussis surveillance—United States, 1984 and 1985. MMWR 36:168, 1987.
28. Centers for Disease Control: Pertussis surveillance—United States, 1986–1988. MMWR 39:57, 1990.
29. Blumberg DA, Mink CM, Cherry JD, et al: Comparison of an acellular pertussis component diphtheria-tetanus-pertussis (DPT) vaccine with a whole cell pertussis component DPT vaccine in 17- to 24-month-old children, with measurement of 69-kilodalton outer membrane protein antibody. J Pediatr 117:46, 1990.
30. Morgan CM, Blumberg DA, Cherry JD: Comparison of acellular and whole-cell pertussis-component DPT vaccines: A multicenter double-blind study in 4- to 6-year-old children. Am J Dis Child 144:41, 1990.
31. Centers for Disease Control: Measles—United States, 1990. MMWR 40:369, 1991.
32. Krober MS, Stracener CE, Bass JW: Decreased measles antibody response after measles-mumps-rubella vaccine in infants with colds. JAMA 265:2095, 1991.
33. American Academy of Pediatrics, Committee on Infectious Diseases: Measles: Reassessment of the current immunization policy. Pediatrics 84:1110, 1989.
34. Centers for Disease Control: Measles prevention: Recommendations of the Immunization Practices Advisory Committee (ACIP). MMWR 38:1, 1989.
35. Riley RL, Nardell EA: Clearing the air—The theory and application of ultraviolet air disinfection. Am Rev Respir Dis 139:1286, 1989.
36. Wells WF, Wells MW, Wilder TS: The environmental control of epidemiologic study of radiant disinfection of air in day schools. Am J Hyg 35:97, 1942.
37. Douglas RM: Acute respiratory infections in children in the developing world. Semin Respir Infect 6:217, 1991.
38. World Health Organization: ARI Programme for Control of Acute Respiratory Infections—Fourth Programme Report 1988–1989. Geneva, World Health Organization, 1990.
39. Brown RW, Weiss ST: The influence of lower respiratory illness on childhood asthma: Defining risk and susceptibility. Semin Respir Infect 6:225, 1991.
40. Gergen PJ, Weiss KB: Changing patterns of asthma hospitalization among children: 1979 to 1987. JAMA 264:1688, 1990.
41. Sly RM: Mortality from asthma in children, 1979–1984. Ann Allergy 60:433, 1988.
42. Sly RM: Mortality from asthma, 1979–1984. J Clin Allergy Immunol 82:705, 1988.
43. Wissow LS, Gittelsohn AM, Szklo M, et al: Poverty, race and hospitalization for childhood asthma. Am J Public Health 78:777, 1988.
44. Etkind S, Boutotte J, Ford J, et al: Treating hard-to-treat tuberculosis patients in Massachusetts. Semin Respir Infect 6:273, 1991.
45. Iralu JV, Maguire JH: Pulmonary infections in immigrants and refugees. Semin Respir Infect 6:235, 1991.
46. Wilson ME: A World Guide to Infections—Diseases, Distribution, and Diagnosis. New York, Oxford University Press, 1991.
47. Koponen MA, Zlock D, Palmer DL, et al: Melioidosis, forgotten but not gone. Arch Intern Med 151:605, 1991.
48. Ashdown LR, Guard RW: The prevalence of human melioidosis in Northern Queensland. Am J Trop Med Hyg 33:474, 1984.
49. O'Connell JJ: Nontuberculous respiratory infections among the homeless. Semin Respir Infect 6:247, 1991.
50. McAdam J, Brickner PW, Glickman R, et al: Tuberculosis in the SRO/homeless population. *In* Brickner PW, Scharer LK, Conanan B, et al (eds): Health Care of Homeless People. New York, Springer, 1985:155.
51. Smith DW, Wiengeshaus EH: What animal models can teach us about the pathogenesis of tuberculosis in humans. Rev Infect Dis 11(suppl 2):385, 1989.
52. DePerri G, Danzi ML, DeChecchi G, et al: Nosocomial epidemic of active tuberculosis among HIV-infected patients. Lancet 2:1502, 1989.
53. Centers for Disease Control: Nosocomial transmission of multidrug-resistant tuberculosis to health care workers and HIV-infected patients in an urban hospital—Florida. MMWR 39:718, 1990.
54. Nardell EA. Dodging droplet nuclei—Reducing the probability of nosocomial tuberculosis transmission in the AIDS era. Am Rev Respir Dis 142:501, 1990.
55. Committee on Treatment of the International Union Against Tuberculosis and Lung Disease: Antituberculosis regimens of chemotherapy. Bull Int Union Tuberc Lung Dis 63:60, 1988.
56. Murray CJL, Styblo K, Rouillon A: Tuberculosis in developing countries: Burden, intervention and cost. Bull Int Union Tuberc Lung Dis 65:6, 1990.
57. Farmer P, Robin S, Ramilus SL, Kim JY: Tuberculosis, poverty and ''compliance'': Lessons from rural Haiti. Semin Respir Infect 6:254, 1991.
58. Brudney K, Dobkin J: A tale of two cities: Tuberculosis control in Nicaragua and New York City. Semin Respir Infect 6:261, 1991.
59. Brudney K, Dobkin J: Resurgent tuberculosis in New York City. Am Rev Respir Dis 144:745, 1991.
60. Iseman MD: Tailoring a time-bomb: Inadvertent genetic engineering. Am Rev Respir Dis 132:735, 1985.
61. Manalo F, Tan F, Sbarbaro JA, Iseman MD: Community-based short-course treatment of pulmonary tuberculosis in a developing nation. Am Rev Respir Dis 142:1301, 1990.
62. Sandford JL, Grange JM, Pozniak A: Is Africa lost? Lancet 338:557, 1991.

# CHAPTER 20

# Cystic Fibrosis and Respiratory Infections

ROBERT B. FICK, JR., RICHARD C. AHRENS, and WENDY COLIN

Cystic fibrosis (CF) is a multisystem, autosomal recessive disease characterized by a defect in sodium and chloride transport in various epithelial and exocrine glands. *Pseudomonas aeruginosa* infections of the lungs, occurring in 90% of adolescent and adult CF patients, prominently influence the clinical course. The outlook for patients diagnosed today is greatly improved, but CF remains the most common fatal disease among Caucasians. The disease incidence in the North American white population is 1 in 1900 to 3700 live births. The incidence among nonwhites is much less: 1 in 17,000 U.S. blacks and an estimated 1 in 90,000 Asian live births.[1]

In the summer of 1989, the gene for CF was identified and sequenced.[2] A single defect in this gene, located on chromosome 7, has been called ΔF508 and is present in 70% of CF patients. Many additional mutations, each accounting for a small percentage of CF patients, have been reported. The gene appears to code for a 150 to 180 kd membrane protein, the CF transmembrane regulator (CFTR). CFTR is predicted to possess 12 membrane-spanning domains, two nucleotide binding folds, and a potential regulatory domain.[3] Based on close amino acid homology and modeling studies, it is proposed that CFTR belongs to a family of traffic ATPases and transport proteins, which include those associated with multidrug resistance. Other evidence indicates that CFTR functions as a cyclic AMP-regulated chloride channel. Rich and coworkers[4] successfully demonstrated that defective cAMP-mediated stimulus-response coupling of chloride permeability in a CF respiratory cell line was corrected in most cells when these cells were transfected with a vaccinia virus CFTR cDNA plasmid. Although the precise function of CFTR is argued and other mutations in this CF protein remain undiscovered, these reports provide insight into the pathogenesis of CF

disease and offer hope for dramatic new therapies in the next 5 years.

Abnormal fluid and electrolyte transport occurs across CF epithelial tissues, accompanied by widespread dysfunction involving salivary, sweat, bronchiolar, pancreatic, and biliary glands. All fields of medicine may be affected by this disease, and it is possible for the astute physician to find adult patients with CF while evaluating chronic sinusitis, asthma, pancreatic insufficiency, sprue-like symptoms, azoospermia, or cirrhosis and portal hypertension. Although CF is a systemic disorder, it is the pulmonary disease—recurrent pulmonary bacterial infections superimposed on chronic infection of the airways caused most prominently by *Staphylococcus aureus, Haemophilus influenzae,* and *P. aeruginosa* and resultant inflammation leading to destructive disease of the airways (bronchiectasis)[5]—that causes most of the morbidity. Ninety percent of CF patients die of respiratory failure.

## CYSTIC FIBROSIS AIRWAYS

Patients with CF present an abnormal respiratory epithelium to potential bacterial pathogens. In healthy, normal persons, the epithelium actively transports $Cl^-$ from the submucosal to the mucosal surface, driving fluid secretion. By this means, transepithelial electrolyte transport controls the quantity and composition of the respiratory tract fluid and is important in effecting normal mucociliary clearance. CF epithelia provide insufficient water to surface liquids to prevent inspissation of periciliary fluids and airway mucus. Several alterations in the mucociliary apparatus of CF patients have been described (Table 20–1). Many of the de-

Table 20–1. *Pseudomonas* **Infection and the Cystic Fibrosis Mucociliary Apparatus**

| Characteristics | Action | Investigation |
|---|---|---|
| Cl⁻ conductance | Secondarily inhibited by *Pseudomonas aeruginosa* (PA) | Stutts (1986)[6] |
| Mucus | Exocrine gland ducts obstructed | Matthews (1963)[7] |
| | Decreased water content | |
| | Mucus glycoprotein: changed composition and increased amounts | Boat (1976)[8] |
| | PA proteinases induce hypersensitivity and lower-molecular-weight | Klinger (1984)[9] |
| | mucins | Rose (1987)[10] |
| Clearance kinetics | Direct visualization of Teflon discs | Wood (1976)[11] |
| | 10.5 mm/min, normal | |
| | 3.2 mm/min, CF | |
| | PA phenazine pigments inhibit ciliary beat frequency | Wilson (1987)[12] |
| Microtubules | No primary ciliary structural abnormalities | Reid (1977)[13] |
| | PA proteinases secondarily disrupt dynein | Hingley (1986)[14] |

Adapted from Fick RB. Pathogenesis of the *Pseudomonas* lung lesion in cystic fibrosis. Chest 96:158–164, 1989.

fects reported are secondarily acquired, and of these, many are caused by the exoproducts of *Pseudomonas*.

The details of *Pseudomonas* affinity for CF respiratory epithelial cells have not been described, although it is known that potential receptors include amino sugars in the mucous layer and plasma membrane constituents exposed when airway proteases release surface fibronectin.[14a] Relevant to CF patients are the studies demonstrating that the gelatinous exopolysaccharide produced by CF mucoid variants of *Pseudomonas* appears to be the adhesin binding *Pseudomonas* to tracheal cells.[15] Although it appears that all *P. aeruginosa* strains contain the gene for "mucoidy," the phenotype is unstable and rapidly lost in culture. Several experimental conditions favor selection of the mucoid phenotype in CF airways. Media containing carbenicillin have been used to prolong the mucoid state in vitro, and others have suggested that the particular $Fe^{2+}:Fe^{3+}$ ratio thought to be present in the CF airway fosters the expression of the mucoid phenotype. Studies by Krieg and co-workers[16] indicated that culture conditions thought to represent the CF airway physiologic state (ie, limited aeration, nitrogen, and phosphate) favored the growth of mucoid strains. The *Pseudomonas* exopolysaccharide receptor in the respiratory tract involves a carbohydrate-containing moiety such as *N*-acetylneuraminic acid or *N*-acetylglucosamine.[15] Both of these amino sugars are normal constituents in respiratory mucus. *N*-acetylglucosamine may be incorporated in glycolipids, such as gangliosides. Data strongly suggest that it is epithelial cellular glycolipids to which *Pseudomonas* cells adhere.[17]

## PERMISSIVE DEFECTS IN PULMONARY HOST DEFENSES

Systemic host defenses in CF patients have been demonstrated repeatedly to be intact.[18] However, in the CF airways, bacterial and phagocytic cell proteases overwhelm the antiprotease screen, permitting proteolytic activity to act on local host defenses. Alterations in local humoral and cellular immune responses (reviewed later) allow the persistence of *S. aureus, H. influenzae,* and *P. aeruginosa* in the airway and, as a result, foster continued destruction of the CF airways and the development of respiratory failure characteristic of this disease.

IgG-opsonizing antibodies with *Pseudomonas* lipopolysaccharide (LPS) specificity and pulmonary macrophages (PM) armed with Fc receptors (FcR) are required for optimal clearance of *Pseudomonas* from the distal human airway. *Pseudomonas* LPS-reactive IgG antibodies have been isolated from the respiratory secretions of CF patients suffering from chronic *Pseudomonas* infections and studied in vitro.[19] These immunoglobulins do not support the uptake of *Pseudomonas* by normal, healthy macrophages. Detailed immunochemical analyses indicate that IgG is largely fragmented in the CF airway fluids.[20] Phagocytic clearance becomes ineffectual. Similar observations have been made for secretory IgA derived from CF sputum.

The contribution complement components make to phagocytic cell clearance of *Pseudomonas* from distal airways in humans remains unsettled. Many complement proteins are difficult to identify in these secretions, but it is known that *Pseudomonas* elastase is capable of hydrolyzing C3 and C5.[21] The C3b molecule is an effective opsonin. A report has linked deficiency of the C3b receptor (called CF1 on neutrophils)[22] to recurrent *Pseudomonas* infections of the airways. The hydrolysis of C3 peptides may be important in the pathogenesis of the chronic *Pseudomonas* lung lesion.

An IgG antibody response to *P. aeruginosa*, which is largely restricted to a subclass (IgG2) in the CF airway,[23] binds poorly to human PM and cannot effectively contribute to phagocytic clearance. This appears to be the case in CF lung fluids. It has been postulated that the IgG2-bacterial antigen complexes are poorly cleared, which may contribute to immune complex-mediated destruction of the CF airways. Immune complexes have been detected in CF lung fluids and pulmonary tissues by many investigators, and high levels of circulating immune complexes correlate with a poor prognosis[24] and increased severity of lung function abnormalities. The immunoglobulin component subclass has been characterized, and this information suggests that IgG2 occurs in significant quantities in circulating CF immune complexes.[25]

Several well-defined chemoattractants move sheets of neutrophils and maturing monocytic phagocytes into the airways.[26] These cells augment the proteolytic and oxidative damage to the CF lung. Bronchoalveolar lavage (BAL) of CF airways reveals greatly increased numbers of cells and an abnormal cell differential count. The BAL fluids obtained from healthy volunteers generally yield 86% to 90% PMs, up to 12% lymphocytes, and less than 3% neutrophils. The predominant cell found in CF lavage fluids is the neutrophil (30%–90%), depending on the clinical state of the patient, with a greatly decreased percentage of PMs, few lymphocytes, and poor cell viability. Many studies have examined circulating neutrophils in CF patients, but few investigators have scrutinized phagocytes in CF airways. Nevertheless, no consistent primary defects in cellular immunity have been described.

## CLINICAL COURSE OF CYSTIC FIBROSIS LUNG DISEASE

CF lung disease is marked by extensive variability. The age of onset of pulmonary symptoms varies, and not all patients evidence the same rate of decline, despite similar aggressive management provided in a CF center. Based on the histologic appearance of neonates dying of meconium ileus in the first few weeks of life, the lungs of newborns with CF appear to be normal or nearly normal.[27, 28] Although abnormalities in the size of mucous glands have been described, work with age-matched controls has not uncovered consistent abnormalities. Careful light and electron microscopic studies[29] have failed to identify a single lesion specific for CF. However, within a few weeks to months of life, pulmonary abnormalities and symptoms may develop. This earliest lung histopathologic lesion has been described as a terminal bronchiolitis (Fig. 20–1), evidenced by metaplasia of the bronchiolar epithelium and mucopurulent plugging of these small airways. The role infection plays in the earliest CF lung lesion is an area of active investigation.[30]

### Pulmonary Mechanics and Evolution of Lung Disease

The first respiratory symptom of CF is usually cough that begins with a viral respiratory infection but fails to clear. About 40% of patients with CF initially seek medical atten-

tion because of respiratory symptoms. Twenty percent present signs or symptoms of malabsorption. The remainder present because of meconium ileus, siblings with cystic fibrosis, or symptoms arising from other organ systems.

The initial respiratory symptoms are accompanied by and may be preceded by decreased forced expiratory flow rates, air trapping, and increased airway resistance.[31, 32] The first radiologic change in the chest tends to be hyperinflation. This may be accompanied by segmental or lobar atelectasis, which usually occurs in the upper lobes.[33, 34] When this combination of atelectasis and hyperinflation is seen in infancy, it is associated with a poor prognosis.[35] As time passes, bronchiectasis becomes established in virtually all CF patients. Airway damage progresses to saccular bronchiectasis and to peripheral abscesses and large cystic bronchiectatic lesions. This progression can be readily identified on the chest radiograph. Spirometry shows initial declines in the forced expiratory flow (FEF 25%–75%) followed by declines in forced expiratory volume ($FEV_1$) and forced vital capacity (FVC). Lung volume measurement shows progressive air trapping. As the disease progresses, arterial hypoxemia and hypercapnea ensue.

There is a high degree of interpatient variability in the rate of decline in respiratory function.[36] Some patients have minimal signs of lung disease even into adulthood, but other patients die of respiratory failure in the first year of life. There is some evidence that pulmonary function deteriorates more rapidly in females than in males, especially after puberty.[37] After hypercapnea and cor pulmonale associated with hypoxemia develop, the prognosis for prolonged survival is poor.[38]

### Terminal Pulmonary Disease

By the time patients with CF enter adulthood, only 2% lack evidence of pulmonary disease by history, chest radiographic examination, or pulmonary function tests. As the airway disease becomes established, patchy areas of parenchymal involvement (ie, bronchopneumonia) become more

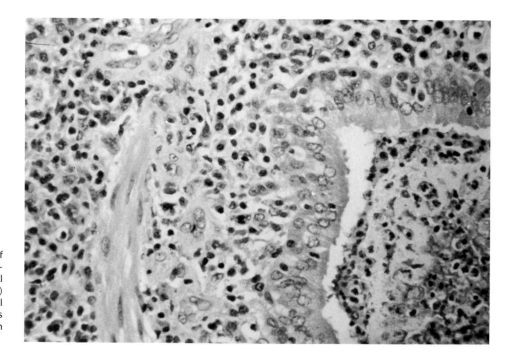

**Figure 20–1.** Earliest lung lesion of cystic fibrosis. Shown is a light microscopic photograph (original magnification × 1000; H&E stain) of lung tissue displaying terminal bronchiolitis. Small airway debris and peribronchiolar inflammation are present.

apparent. Respiratory infections in CF follow a smoldering course, punctuated by acute exacerbations in part caused by viral agents. These exacerbations are superimposed on a baseline of chronic productive cough and bacterial infection most commonly caused by mucoid *P. aeruginosa*. Omnipresent infection and airway inflammation eventually destroy the supporting structures of the airway walls, resulting in bronchiectasis (Fig. 20–2).[39] Despite frequent antibiotic interventions, progressive bronchiectasis and increasingly frequent acute exacerbations are followed by a gradual loss of pulmonary reserve, cor pulmonale, and respiratory failure. Morphometric work performed on lungs from patients with CF obtained at autopsy indicate that the airways disease and pulmonary remodeling are irregularly distributed and that the upper lobe segments are disproportionately involved.[40] In 98% of patients beyond the neonatal period, death occurs from respiratory complications, usually progressive respiratory and right-sided heart failure.

## Noninfectious Respiratory Complications

Chronic inflammatory disease of the upper airways results in an extremely high frequency of sinusitis and nasal polyposis (Table 20–2). Lower respiratory tract complications in CF adults are common. Five percent to 10% of adults with CF have clinically evident pneumothoraces; 25% of these are multiple, and 60% subside spontaneously, not requiring tube drainage. Hypertrophic pulmonary osteoarthropathy (ie, ossifying periostitis) occurs as a complication in older children with severe CF lung disease and causes long bone pain and occasionally causes joint effusions. Although wheezing is reported in as many as 63% of patients,[35] a confirmed propensity to asthma with hyperactive airways disease and a demonstrated response to bron-

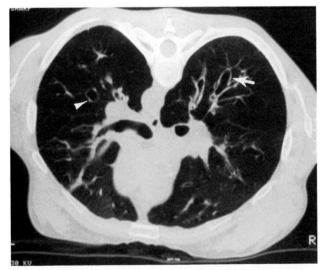

**Figure 20–2.** The computed tomographic (CT) signs of bronchiectasis include a distended linear airway in the periphery with thickened bronchial mucosa *(white arrow)*, peribronchial thickening *(white arrowhead)*, and numerous areas of cystic dilation. Cine CT allows a more thorough evaluation of the lung (3-mm sections) in less time and with less discomfort to the patient than conventional CT. (Reprinted with permission from Fick RB: Cystic fibrosis and bronchiectasis. *In* Stein JH, Kohler PO, Hutton JJ, et al (eds): Internal Medicine, ed 3. Boston, Little, Brown, and Company, copyright 1990:715.)

**Table 20–2. Noninfectious Respiratory Complications of Cystic Fibrosis**

| Manifestations | Frequency (%) |
|---|---|
| Upper tract | |
| Chronic sinusitis | 100 |
| Nasal polyposis | 29–61 |
| Lower tract | |
| Bronchiectasis | 80 |
| Hemoptysis | |
| Streaking | 51–76 |
| Massive | 10–23 |
| Atelectasis | 16–40 |
| Intermittent wheezing | 36 |
| Pneumothorax | 10 |
| Cor pulmonale and respiratory failure | 90 |

chodilators occurs in a smaller percentage of CF patients. In reports of short-term bronchodilator therapy and small numbers of subjects studied with methacholine challenges, 20% to 60% of CF adolescents and adults were found to have asthma.[41] Hemoptysis usually amounts to blood streaking of sputum but may be massive (>300 mL/episode). There is disagreement about the prognosis portended by hemoptysis, but there is no disagreement that pulmonary disease appears in most patients with CF, frequently dominates the clinical picture, is progressive, and determines the fate of most patients.

## AIRWAY PATHOGENS IN CYSTIC FIBROSIS

Viral infections (Table 20–3) may play an important role in the development of the early lung pathology. It may be that in the CF airway staphylococcal bronchitis and bronchopneumonia appear as complications of antecedent viral infections, just as in the non-CF airway bacterial infections frequently follow influenza pneumonia. The widely accepted theory is that the respiratory microbiologic flora in CF patients undergoes a characteristic evolution from *S. aureus* infection, accompanied commonly by infections due to nontypable *H. influenzae* and *Streptococcus pneumoniae*. As these pathogens are treated, *P. aeruginosa* infection follows. However, this sequence (ie, virus followed by bacteria) has not been convincingly demonstrated in CF, and preliminary studies indicate that nonmucoid *P. aeruginosa* may be the first pathogen demonstrated in neonatal airway secretions.[42]

The precise sequence of pathogens contributing to the early progression of the CF lung lesion remains in doubt, primarily because obtaining airway secretions representative of the distal CF airway is problematic. In CF patients unable to spontaneously produce sputum specimens, a throat swab may have acceptable specificity for *P. aeruginosa; Pseudomonas* is recovered from 86% of CF throat cultures, and the same pathogen is present in specimens obtained bronchoscopically.[43] The sensitivity of throat swabs is poor. When *P. aeruginosa* is obtained from bronchoscopic aspirates of the distal airway, the organism is grown only 50% of the time. The spontaneously produced sputum specimens in patients with bronchiectasis largely reflect the predominant pathogens in the distal human airway. This accuracy is increased through the use of quanti-

Table 20–3. **Nonbacterial Pathogens in the Cystic Fibrosis Airway**

| Group | Specific Agents | Comment |
|---|---|---|
| Viruses | Respiratory syncytial virus, influenza A and B, adenovirus, rhinovirus, parainfluenza | Debatable initiators of the bronchiolar lesion; greater likelihood that viral agents contribute to undefined percentage of respiratory exacerbations |
| Fungi | *Candida albicans* | Frequently isolated, but tissue invasion or dissemination rarely occurs |
| | *Aspergillus fumigatus* | Serologic responses may contribute to clinical picture of asthma and central bronchiectasis |
| Mycobacteria | *Mycobacterium tuberculosis, M. chelonei, M. fortuitum* | Uncommonly may cause picture of fever and night sweats associated with worsening of respiratory symptoms |

tative cultures,[43] because oropharyngeal contaminants are generally present in densities of less than $10^3$ colony-forming units per gram of sputum.

## Staphylococcal Species

The classic pathogen in CF is *S. aureus*. This organism was responsible for most of the CF lung morbidity and mortality until the introduction of penicillin, which contributed to a significant increase in CF survival and to the emergence of resistant pathogens, including *P. aeruginosa* and, more recently, methicillin-resistant *S. aureus* (MRSA). Staphylococcal species, including *S. aureus* and *S. epidermidis*, remain the most frequent gram-positive organisms cultured from sputa and throat swabs of CF patients (Table 20–4), with incidences of 29% to 37%, although a figure as high as 72% has been reported.[44] No particular phage type predominates. The prevalence of *S. aureus* infection decreases with age, but it is more persistent than the transient finding of *S. epidermidis* in cultures of CF respiratory secretions.

## Haemophilus influenzae

*H. influenzae* is commonly isolated with other pathogens from sputum during an acute exacerbation of CF lung disease, although chronic carriage seems to be considerably lower, 1.4% to 11.8%.[44] The ability to culture this pathogen in the presence of a heavy growth of *P. aeruginosa* is problematic, and selective inhibition of *Pseudomonas* is necessary. *H. influenzae* strains are usually not encapsulated and therefore not serotypable, although biotyping is possible. The potentially more virulent biotype I (also found in non-CF patients with meningitis and septicemia) is much more common than biotype II.[45] However, the same researchers obtained sequential isolates over 2 years from CF patients and observed rapid changes in these biotypes from month to month in a given patient, with up to four types present at one time.

## Pseudomonas aeruginosa

*Pseudomonas* is the dominant pathogen recovered from sputum culture and lung tissue obtained at thoracotomy or postmortem. Seventy percent to 90% of CF patients are chronically infected with *Pseudomonas*. Chronic indolent *Pseudomonas* infections contrast with the acute and rapidly

progressive pulmonary infections typical of immunosuppressed patients. The weight of evidence supports the concept that *P. aeruginosa* in the CF airways is not acquired from environmental sources and is not easily spread from patient to patient. Exactly when in the natural history of the progression of this destructive pulmonary infection *P. aeruginosa* is acquired is still unknown. It is thought that the CF patient is infected with *S. aureus* during the early years of life and that the nonmucoid variant of *P. aeruginosa* follows. Older studies found that the mucoid phenotype appeared infrequently during the first year of life, with only 2 of 8455 CF infants affected in one series.[46] Later information suggests that mucoid *P. aeruginosa* may be found in CF airway secretions earlier than previously thought. Two case reports describe lethal respiratory failure in pre-term CF infants complicated by *P. aeruginosa* lung infections,[47] and preliminary reports of bronchoscopically obtained specimens from CF neonates indicate that *P. aeruginosa* is an important pathogen at that very early age.[42] Despite raised serum levels of antibodies against *P. aeruginosa*, this mucoid transformation is associated with progressive disease and a poor prognosis.[48]

Table 20–4. **Bacteria in the Pathogenesis of the Cystic Fibrosis Lung Lesion**

| Agent | Comment |
|---|---|
| *Staphylococcus aureus* | Gram positive with the highest incidence and prevalence in younger patients; low incidence of MRSA |
| *Haemophilus influenzae* | Nonencapsulated, biotype I most frequently associated with respiratory exacerbations |
| *Pseudomonas aeruginosa* | Unclear at what age acquired and propensity for mucoid phenotype in CF, but once sputum infected, PA persists, responds poorly to antibiotics |
| *Burkholderia cepacia* (formerly *Pseudomonas cepacia*) | A low-incidence pathogen with resistance to multiple antibiotics but may be associated with fulminant decline |
| *Pseudomonas gladioli* *Xanthomonas aeruginosa* (formerly *P. maltophilia*) *Pseudomonas fluorescens/ putida* and *P. stutzeri* | Isolation not convincingly associated with respiratory exacerbations |
| *Escherichia coli* | Isolated in up to 16% of CF sputum samples; 12% present with unusual mucoid phenotype |

Abbreviations: CF, cystic fibrosis; MRSA, methicillin-resistant *S. aureus*; PA, *Pseudomonas aeruginosa*.

## ANTIBIOTIC THERAPIES

Because it is chronic bacterial growth in the airways that causes the progressive bronchiectasis universally seen in patients with CF, it is desirable to eliminate this infection. Although it is possible with intensive courses of intravenous antibiotic therapy to transiently eliminate pathogens from the sputum of some patients, infection is rapidly reestablished after the antibiotic therapy is completed. The approach adopted by the clinicians is to use antibiotic therapy at selected points in the clinical course. This is intended to reduce the bacterial load of the airways and to slow, although not completely prevent, the progression of CF-related bronchiectasis.[49, 50] It is widely held that improved antibiotic therapy and improved nutrition are primarily responsible for the progressive improvement in the prognosis of cystic fibrosis over the past five decades.[51] If comprehensive care is provided at a CF center, the clinical outcome is significantly better than if patients are managed in other clinical settings.[52]

Strategies for antibiotic therapy for patients with CF can be divided into three general categories: identification and aggressive treatment at periods of accelerated decline in respiratory function ("acute exacerbations"), which are a characteristic part of the waxing and waning course of CF-related lung disease; continuous or regularly scheduled antibiotic administration to prevent acute exacerbations and slow the overall decline in respiratory function; and vigorous treatment to eradicate a newly acquired bacterial pathogen (usually *S. aureus* or *P. aeruginosa*) regardless of other clinical findings.

### Treatment of Acute Exacerbations of Lung Disease With Oral Antibiotics

Exacerbations of CF lung disease evolve over days, weeks, or months. Truly acute pneumonic episodes (ie, evolving over hours) are rare. Exacerbations may be accompanied by increased cough and sputum production, dyspnea, fatigue, crackles or wheezes on pulmonary physical examination, decline in spirometric values (ie, FVC, $FEV_1$, and $FEF_{25\%-75\%}$), and increased lung volumes. Fever and leukocytosis may or may not be present.

When an exacerbation of CF-related lung disease is identified, it has been common practice to initiate a trial of several weeks of oral antibiotic therapy. This widespread practice has not been extensively evaluated in clinical trials. The choice of antibiotic regimen depends on the specific organism cultured, the antibiotic sensitivity of cultured organism, and concentrations of antibiotics that are achievable in bronchial secretions.[53]

*S. aureus* is commonly present in the airway during the initial episodes of bronchopulmonary infection.[54–56] The orally administered penicillinase-resistant penicillins, including dicloxacillin, cloxacillin, and oxacillin, are commonly used to treat *S. aureus* airway infections. First-generation cephalosporins, (including cephalexin and cephradine) and the fluoroquinolone ciprofloxacin have activity against *S. aureus* in vitro and in vivo. In a study by Harrison and colleagues,[57] cephalexin was associated with better

patient compliance and more frequent elimination of *S. aureus* from the sputum than dicloxacillin, although the cephalexin-treated group had a higher incidence of secondary fungal infections. Oral clindamycin therapy may have theoretic advantages (eg, better tissue penetration), and its use is associated with clinical improvement.[58]

*Haemophilus* species (eg, *H. influenzae, H. parainfluenzae*) are frequent and early pathogens in the airway of the CF patient.[54, 59, 60] Amoxicillin-clavulanic acid, trimethoprim-sulfamethoxazole, and broad-spectrum cephalosporins (eg, cefixime, cefuroxime axetil) have good in vitro activity against *Haemophilus* spp. and have been commonly prescribed for CF patients colonized with these organisms.

The development of an orally active antipseudomonal fluoroquinolone, ciprofloxacin, has been a major advance in the treatment of acute exacerbations while allowing the patient to remain at home. Unlike most orally administered antibiotic agents, this drug selectively concentrates in pulmonary secretions.[61] Several studies have documented that 78% to 100% of patients with *Pseudomonas* infections of the lower respiratory tract improve on oral ciprofloxacin doses of 1.0 to 1.50 g/d in treatment periods ranging from 10 days to 8 weeks.[62] Compared with conventional therapy (ie, aminoglycoside plus an antipseudomonal β-lactam), ciprofloxacin has demonstrated comparable clinical efficacy,[63–65] although Jensen and colleagues[66] observed that the most seriously affected patients showed significantly greater improvement after receiving conventional therapy than after receiving treatment with a quinolone. A parenteral dosage form of ciprofloxacin has been approved by the U.S. Food and Drug Administration (FDA). This formulation offers no additional benefit, because the oral dosage formulation is 70% to 85% bioavailable.[67, 68] Strandvik[69] observed better clinical efficacy and tolerance with the oral formulation than with the intravenous formulation.

Ciprofloxacin has not been FDA approved for use in children, because it has been shown to interfere with cartilage formation in young dogs, but it has been widely used in children with CF without important apparent adverse effects.[70, 71] Two of the newer fluoroquinolones, ofloxacin and fleroxacin, have shown good in vitro activity against *P. aeruginosa*. Although they may achieve higher serum concentrations than ciprofloxacin, they are also associated with higher minimal inhibitory concentrations. Ciprofloxacin was eightfold more active against *P. aeruginosa* and twofold more active against *S. aureus* than the other quinolones.[72] Enoxacin, perfloxacin, and ofloxacin have better penetration into the sputum than ciprofloxacin.[73] Ofloxacin has shown comparable effectiveness compared with ciprofloxacin in improving pulmonary function.[74] No other clinical studies of these quinolones are available.

The absorption of the fluoroquinolones is markedly reduced by the concomitant administration of products containing iron, aluminum, magnesium, zinc, or calcium.[75] Theophylline elimination is inhibited by concurrent use of ciprofloxacin, enoxacin, or perfloxacin. This can result in increased serum theophylline concentrations and associated theophylline toxicity. Reports on the effect of ofloxacin on theophylline metabolism are conflicting.[76, 77] Theophylline doses should be reduced by 50% at the initiation of quinolone antibiotic therapy to avoid potential theophylline toxicity.

## Treatment of Exacerbations of Lung Disease With Intravenous Antibiotic Therapy

Hospitalization for intravenous antibiotic treatment is required if the oral antibiotics fail to achieve the desired goals of reduction of symptoms and return of pulmonary functions to baseline levels or if the exacerbation is too severe (criteria not clearly defined) to treat with oral drugs. The reasoning behind this decision includes the ability to achieve antibiotic concentrations in serum and respiratory secretions that are at least one order of magnitude greater than can be achieved by oral administration of the same agents (quinolones excepted) and the ability to administer multiple antibiotics at frequent intervals to achieve synergistic suppression of bacterial growth.

In randomized studies, patients who harbor *P. aeruginosa* are more likely to improve if treated with intravenous antibiotics directed specifically at the organism than if they are treated empirically.[78, 79] However, this has not been a consistent finding.[80] Gold and colleagues[81] found no difference between intravenous treatment and placebo when the exacerbation was objectively judged to be mild to moderate (criteria include ESR $\leq$ 50 mm/h and fewer than three of the following other abnormalities: leukocyte count $\leq$ 15,000/dL; pulse $\leq$ 100 bpm; respirations $\leq$ 30/min, and temperature $\leq$ 38.5°C). This study suggests that patients who present with recent, mild increases in respiratory symptoms may not always require hospitalization for antibiotic therapy. The increase in symptoms may be caused by viral or mycoplasmal infections. More severely involved patients may fail to survive without aggressive in-hospital antibiotic therapy.[78]

Numerous studies have compared the efficacy of various intravenous antibiotic regimens. Single-drug therapy (eg, tobramycin or ceftazidime) has been compared with multi-drug therapy (eg, one or two β-lactam antibiotics plus an aminoglycoside). Different combination regimens have been compared. Virtually all of these studies document efficacy primarily by evaluating symptoms and pulmonary functions measured at the beginning and completion of 1 to 2 weeks of intravenous therapy during hospitalization. Few of these studies show important clinical differences in outcome among the therapeutic regimens. Although it is possible to conclude that one regimen is as good as another, it seems likely that these results reflect the insensitivity of the methods used in these studies.

Winnie and associates[82] compared the efficacy of administering intravenous tobramycin on an every 6- or 8-hour basis. Doses were adjusted based on sampling of plasma concentrations to achieve peak concentrations of 8 to 10 µg/mL (level drawn at 1 hour after the end of the infusion). No difference was seen between these regimens in improvement in symptoms or pulmonary function during the hospitalization, but those on the 8-hour regimen subsequently required another hospitalization for intravenous antibiotics significantly sooner (mean, 17.8 weeks) than those patients treated with 6-hour doses of tobramycin (mean, 32.1 weeks). To determine which antibiotic regimen is optimal for treatment during hospitalization, it may be necessary to examine clinical outcomes other than changes in pulmonary function and symptoms during the hospitalization. Those that have been proposed include rate of long-term decline

in lung function, duration of time until the next hospitalization, and changes in the quantitative bacterial load in the sputum during hospitalization.

Although individual studies rarely provide sufficient guidance for the clinician who is selecting antibiotics for the patient with CF, Michael[83] was able to draw some useful conclusions by carefully summarizing entrance criteria, treatment regimens, and outcomes, including efficacy, toxicity, and development of antibiotic resistance, for all studies published between 1980 and February 1987. Little has been published since that time that would alter Michael's conclusions. A combination of an aminoglycoside and an antipseudomonal β-lactam should be used rather than a single antibiotic. This is based on minimizing the probability of selecting resistant organisms and in vitro evidence of antibiotic synergism.[84] No clear-cut differences in efficacy can be identified between antipseudomonal β-lactam antibiotics. No clear-cut differences between currently available aminoglycosides can be identified, and there is convincing evidence that the aminoglycoside dose should be optimized. Peak serum concentrations of 8 to 12 µg/mL (for tobramycin or gentamicin) should be achieved. The dosing interval should be shortened to the greatest degree possible while maintaining an appropriate trough concentration (1–2 µg/mL for tobramycin and gentamicin). A β-lactam antibiotic with a high level of activity against *S. aureus* should be included if this organism is also recovered from the sputum.

When intravenous antibiotics are required frequently, as is the case in advanced CF lung disease, intravenous access may become a problem. Implantable intravenous catheters are being used with increasing frequency to circumvent this problem.[85, 86] Some investigators have examined the use of an inhaled aminoglycoside in addition to intravenous antibiotic administration during hospitalization.[87] These studies demonstrate that inhaled tobramycin or amikacin do not provide additional efficacy. This approach is not advocated as a part of routine inpatient therapy.

## Chronic Antibiotic Administration to Prevent Progression of Lung Disease

For many years, it has been routine to administer chronic oral antibiotics to slow the progression of bronchiectasis. Antibiotics that are effective against *S. aureus* and *Haemophilus* species such as dicloxacillin, trimethoprim-sulfa, and cephalexin are often used, but there are few studies evaluating this practice. In a double-blind, placebo-controlled, crossover study, patients who were colonized with *S. aureus* had improved clinical courses while on a first-generation cephalosporin[59] compared with the placebo. However, this and other studies suggest that daily, chronic oral antibiotic administration hastens the acquisition of *Pseudomonas* spp. in the airway and promotes resistant organisms.

Clinicians at the National Cystic Fibrosis Center in Copenhagen, Denmark, have employed scheduled, in-hospital, intravenous antibiotic administration for 2 weeks every 3 months for all patients who harbor *Pseudomonas,* with improved 5- and 10-year survival rates. Although clinical experience at this center provides some support for this approach in delaying the progression of bronchiectasis, this practice has not become widespread.

Chronic administration of inhaled antibiotics is used with increasing frequency, although this practice is actually quite old. The use of inhaled sulfonamides to treat bronchiectasis was first recorded in 1941 and 1943.[88] In 1946, di'Saint'Agnese and Andersen described the administration of inhaled penicillin for the treatment of staphylococcal infection in patients with cystic fibrosis.[89] After this, use of inhaled antibiotics for treating cystic fibrosis apparently fell out of favor, and little appeared in the literature until Hodson and colleagues[90] published the first controlled trial addressing this issue in 1981. The specific purpose for treating patients in this trial was to ''benefit CF patients by halting the decline in lung function and reducing the frequency of hospital admission.'' In this blinded, crossover trial, treatment with aerosolized carbenicillin and gentamicin twice each day for 6 months was associated with better pulmonary function and fewer hospitalizations than the placebo treatment.

Confirmation that inhaled antibiotics are capable of reducing the frequency of hospitalization and improving other measures of clinical course, including pulmonary functions and weight gain, come from four additional placebo-controlled trials[91–94] and several uncontrolled case series.[95–98] Only one study which used 80 mg of tobramycin nebulized three times each day, failed to demonstrate efficacy in this setting.[99]

No study has found any evidence of ototoxicity or nephrotoxicity during periods of inhaled antibiotic administration that range from 3 months to 2.5 years. However, acquisition of *Pseudomonas* organisms with antibiotic resistance remains a concern. Acquisition of resistance does not appear to correlate with duration of therapy, but the choice of antibiotics may play a role. Smith and associates[97] reported this occurrence in 73% of the patients treated with inhaled tobramycin for 3 months. MacLusky and colleagues[100] reported antibiotic resistance in 33% of the patients treated chronically with inhaled tobramycin for a mean of 32 months. Hodson[90] found no resistance during 6 months of treatment with carbenicillin and gentamicin. With the exception of Wall and coworkers,[95] who described 1 of 8 patients developing resistance to ticarcillin while being treated with ticarcillin and tobramycin, all of the studies demonstrating acquisition of drug resistance used inhalation of a single aminoglycoside (ie, gentamicin or tobramycin).

Most evidence indicates that chronic use of inhaled antibiotics is effective in the advanced pulmonary disease of cystic fibrosis. However, certain issues should be resolved, including what drug or combination of drugs is optimal and what kind of nebulizer system should be used.[94, 100–102]

## Treatment to Eradicate Newly Acquired *Staphylococcus aureus* or *Pseudomonas aeruginosa*

Littlewood and coworkers[103] in a small, uncontrolled study, used inhaled antibiotics to eliminate colonization with *P. aeruginosa*. Inhalation of colimycin (500 U twice daily), given to patients who had only recently acquired *P.*

*aeruginosa* in their sputum, reduced the subsequent positive culture from 42% to 6%. A later controlled study found that initiation of inhaled colistin in combination with oral ciprofloxacin after the first recovery of *Pseudomonas* from CF sputum reduced the transition to chronic *P. aeruginosa* carriage to 14%, compared with 58% transition in an untreated group.[104] This therapeutic strategy requires further investigation before it can be advocated as part of routine therapy.

For several years, 2 weeks of dicloxacillin plus fusidic acid has been prescribed at the Danish Cystic Fibrosis Center after *S. aureus* is cultured from the sputum. This has reduced the chronic carriage rate of this organism to less than 10%.[105]

## Appearance of Antibiotics in Bronchial Secretions

One factor that hinders treatment of CF-related airway infection is the limited access that many antibiotics have to airway secretions. This is one of the reasons that relatively high doses of antibiotics are necessary to treat CF-related airway disease. Penicillins are weak organic anions that exhibit poor diffusibility across the lipid membrane layers and penetrate poorly into the bronchial secretions. Aminoglycosides, as polar polycations, also penetrate poorly into bronchial secretions. Of the available aminoglycosides, tobramycin appears to have the greatest penetration into bronchial secretions. For β-lactam and aminoglycoside antibiotics, concentration of the antibiotic in the airways is only 20% to 30% of the concentration that can be obtained in the serum.[106] Fluoroquinolones are an exception to this rule, with sputum concentrations greater than those found in plasma.

## Pharmacokinetics in Cystic Fibrosis

Many studies have documented the altered pharmacokinetics for several antibiotics used in the treatment of CF pulmonary exacerbations. The antimicrobial agents that have been best studied include the β-lactams and aminoglycosides. Juske and colleagues[107] were the first to demonstrate the increased renal clearance of dicloxacillin in CF patients. Subsequent studies have shown that CF patients exhibit reduced plasma concentrations[108] and areas-under-the-curve[109] of β-lactam and aminoglycoside antibiotics because of increased clearance. Increases in glomerular filtration rate and tubular secretion have been implicated. The increased distribution of aminoglycosides has also been observed in CF patients,[110] although this finding has not been consistent in all studies.[111] Tailoring patient dosing by monitoring serum concentrations of aminoglycosides is mandatory in the CF population to overcome the effects of increased clearance and volume of distribution.

Several studies have suggested improved efficacy for antibiotics administered in higher doses or as the result of increased dosing frequency. A slower decline in respiratory function after 6-hour tobramycin administration was discussed previously.[82] Li and colleagues had similar findings.[112] The pharmacokinetic studies demonstrated that β-lactam antibiotics such as azlocillin[113] and ticarcillin[114] should also be administered at higher doses than commonly used in other diseases.[115]

## IMMUNOTHERAPY AND CLINICAL INVESTIGATION OF NOVEL THERAPIES

In an effort to modulate the immune-mediated inflammatory process, a 4-year trial of alternate-day prednisone (2 mg/kg to a maximum of 60 mg/d) was undertaken in CF children with mild or moderate pulmonary disease.[116] Patients in the prednisone-treated group showed better growth and pulmonary function and reduced morbidity than the placebo-treated group. In a multicenter trial to further evaluate this approach, patients were randomized to alternate-day prednisone at a dose of 2 mg/kg (high dose) or 1 mg/kg (low dose) or to placebo. A high incidence of complications, including an increased frequency of cataracts, growth retardation, and glucose abnormalities, was revealed in the high-dose prednisone group after 3 years of study participation, and the high-dose study treatment was discontinued.[117] Results concerning efficacy are not yet available. Short-term corticosteroid therapy (prednisone, 20 to 30 mg/d for 3 weeks) does not significantly improve pulmonary function in adult patients and may expose the patients to increased risk for the development of pneumothorax.

### Mucolytics

High concentrations of DNA, derived from inflammatory cell degradation, are found in the secretions of CF patients, and this chromosomal material contributes to the viscous, tenacious nature of CF sputa. Recombinant human deoxyribonuclease (DNase) applied in vitro cleaves the DNA in sputum of CF patients to reduce this viscosity. Hubbard and coworkers[118] studied the clinical efficacy of aerosolized DNase given at a dose of 10 mg twice daily for 7 days. The DNase subjectively improved ease of breathing and significantly improved FVC. $FEV_1$ and FVC returned toward the baseline values, and there was no significant difference between the treatment groups at 1 week after the completion of the study. Additional studies have determined that the long-term treatment of the CF patient with DNase (2.5 mg nebulized daily for 6 months), significantly decreased airway infections.[118a] Various mucolytic treatment modalities have been studied in an attempt to enhance mucus clearance. In most cases, mucolytics and expectorants have been ineffective in clearing mucus.[119]

### Amiloride

Based on in vitro and in vivo studies,[120, 121] there is hope that the sodium channel blocker, amiloride, can reverse the dehydration of airway secretions that is characteristic of patients with cystic fibrosis. App and associates[122] studied the effects of single doses of inhaled amiloride in 23 patients and found that mucociliary clearance improved immediately. This effect was maintained in 9 patients who inhaled amiloride twice daily for 3 weeks. Sputum visco-elasticity decreased, and sputum sodium content increased in the CF patients who received single inhaled doses of amiloride. Knowles and coworkers[123] administered similar doses of amiloride to 18 patients for 25 weeks and concluded that amiloride slowed the decline in FVC in the adult patients with CF. Although these preliminary studies are encouraging, significant questions concerning efficacy and potential side effects remain.[124] The Cystic Fibrosis Foundation is conducting a large multicenter trial to further examine these issues. Whether twice-daily administration of amiloride, with each dose having effects that last less than 1 hour,[125, 126] can sufficiently alter sputum characteristics to affect the long-term course of CF patients must be determined.

### Protease Inhibitors

Excess neutrophil and bacterial elastases lead to a protease-antiprotease imbalance in the CF airway and significantly contribute to host defense abnormalities and pathogenesis of the CF lung lesion. Efforts to correct this imbalance with exogenously administered antiproteases are actively being explored. Secretory leukocyte protease inhibitor (SLPI) is the main antiprotease of the upper bronchial tree, and $\alpha_1$-protease inhibitor is the most important antiprotease of the terminal respiratory tract. Recombinant SLPI has an advantage over $\alpha_1$-protease inhibitor as a potential therapy, because it is a low-molecular-weight antiprotease and binds more elastase per unit weight.[127] Preliminary studies have demonstrated safety and decreased BAL elastase levels after aerosolized SLPI.[128] Other agents in clinical trials include $\alpha_1$-proteinase inhibitor[129] and a low-molecular-weight inhibitor of the trifluoromethylketone class (ICI Americas, Inc.). Ongoing clinical trials will probably establish the effectiveness of aerosolized SLPI or other antiproteases in slowing the progression of CF lung disease.

### Immunotherapy

Because of the central role infectious agents play in the pathogenesis of CF lung disease, there are two forms of immunotherapy to consider: active therapy (vaccination) and passive immunization. Parenteral administration of polyvalent *Pseudomonas* vaccines to children before acquisition of *Pseudomonas* and to adults with CF who are colonized with *Pseudomonas* fails to delay the onset of *Pseudomonas* infection in children and does not clear the adult CF airways of this bacterium.[130] Similarly, local respiratory immunization by intranasal administration of a *Pseudomonas* antigen preparation to a small number of adult patients with CF who were troubled by chronic *Pseudomonas* infections did not result in clinical improvement or eradication of this pathogen.[131] Although many different *Pseudomonas* vaccines are in preparation, it seems unlikely that any will be widely used in the treatment of patients with CF in the near future.

Passive immunotherapy has been used to successfully treat pneumococcal and meningococcal diseases. Several investigators have described fragmented immunoglobulins in CF airway fluids, providing a rationale for evaluating passive immunotherapy of *Pseudomonas* airway infections in patients with CF. A commercial preparation of polyclonal immunoglobulins, modified for safe intravenous use with high titers to *Pseudomonas* lipopolysaccharides, is well tolerated by humans, has been shown to be effective against experimental *P. aeruginosa* pneumonia, and is therapeutic in a burned mouse model.[106] However, *Pseudomonas* in CF airways converts to a smooth, nontypable O lipopolysaccharide, making inappropriate some of the commercial preparations of *Pseudomonas* antibodies used for passive immunotherapy.

Additional thought must be given to the proper protocol for administration of passive immunotherapy in the CF population. Ideally, young patients who are newly identified carriers of *P. aeruginosa* should be enrolled while the bacterial burden is low and alterations in the architecture of the airways are minimal. Alternatively, patients with CF may receive monthly intravenous *Pseudomonas* immunotherapy in combination with oral anti-*Pseudomonas* antibiotics beginning immediately after a vigorous course of intravenous antibiotic treatment. Additional in vitro studies of this potentially beneficial therapy must be completed before the risk-benefit analysis for patients with CF can be accomplished. It remains an experimental therapy that should not yet be applied to patients with CF but may hold promise for use in the future.

## ACKNOWLEDGMENTS

The authors wish to acknowledge the support of a Veterans Administration research grant and express appreciation for the secretarial assistance of Tanya Teets, Jackie Hand, Margaret Weatherford, and Donna Reihman.

## REFERENCES

1. Steinberg AG, Brown DC: On the incidence of cystic fibrosis of the pancreas. Am J Hum Genet 12:416, 1960.
2. Rommens JM, Iannuzzi MC, Kerem B, et al: Identification of the cystic fibrosis gene: Chromosome walking and jumping. Science 245:1059, 1989.
3. Riordan JR, Rommens JM, Kerem B, et al: Identification of the cystic fibrosis gene: Cloning and characterization of complementary DNA. Science 245:1066–1073, 1989.
4. Rich DP, Anderson MP, Gregory RJ, et al: Expression of cystic fibrosis transmembrane conductance regulator corrects defective chloride channel regulation in cystic fibrosis airway epithelial cells. Nature 347:358–363, 1990.
5. Hata JS, Fick RB: *Pseudomonas aeruginosa* and the airways disease of cystic fibrosis. Clin Chest Med 9:679–691, 1988.
6. Stutts MJ, Schwab JH, Chen MG, Knowles MR, Boucher RC: Effects of *Pseudomonas aeruginosa* on bronchial epithelial ion transport. Am Rev Respir Dis 134:17–21, 1986.
7. Matthews LW, Specter S, Lemm J, Potter JL: Studies on pulmonary secretions. I. The overall chemical composition of pulmonary secretions from patients with cystic fibrosis, bronchiectasis, and laryngectomy. Am Rev Respir Dis 88:199–203, 1963.
8. Boat TF, Chen PW, Iyer RN, Carlson DM, Polony I: Human respiratory tract secretions: Mucous glycoproteins of non-purulent tracheobronchial secretions and sputum of patients with bronchitis and cystic fibrosis. Arch Biochem Biophys 177:95–104, 1976.
9. Klinger JD, Tandler D, Liedtke CM, Boat TF: Proteinases of *Pseudomonas aeruginosa* evoke mucin released by trachial epithelium. J Clin Invest 74:1669–1678, 1984.
10. Rose MC, Brown CS, Jacoby JZ, Lynn WS, Kaufman B: Biochemi-

cal properties of tracheobronchial mucins from cystic fibrosis and non-cystic fibrosis individuals. Pediatr Res 22:545–551, 1987.
11. Wood RE, Boat TF, Doershuk CF: Cystic fibrosis: State of the art. Am Rev Respir Dis 113:833–878, 1976.
12. Wilson R, Pitt T, Taylor G, Watson D, McDermott J, Sykes D, et al: Piocyanin and 1-hydroxyphenazine produced by *Pseudomonas aeruginosa* inhibit the beating of human respiratory cilia in vitro. J Clin Invest 79:221–229, 1987.
13. Reid L: Gap Conference San Diego, CA, report: Chronic bronchitis and cystic fibrosis. Two chronic obstructive lung diseases of adults. Cystic Fibrosis Foundation, Atlanta, February 1–2, 1977:6–7.
14. Hingley ST, Hostie AT, Kueppers F, Higgins ML: Disruption of respiratory cilia by proteinases including those of *Pseudomonas aeruginosa*. Infect Immun 54:379–385, 1986.
14a. Woods DE, Straus DC, Johanson WG Jr, Bass JA: Role of salivary protease activity in adherence of Gram-negative bacilli to mammalian buccal epithelial cells in vivo. J Clin Invest 68:1435, 1981.
15. Hata JS, Fick RB: Airway adherence of *Pseudomonas aeruginosa:* Mucoexopolysaccharide binding to human and bovine airway proteins. J Lab Clin Med 117:410–422, 1991.
16. Krieg DP, Bass JA, Mattingly SJ: Aeration selects for mucoid phenotype of *Pseudomonas aeruginosa*. J Clin Microbiol 24:986–990, 1986.
17. Krivan HC, Ginsberg G, Roberts DD: Communication: *P. aeruginosa* and *P. cepacia* isolated from cystic fibrosis patients binds specifically to gangliotetraosylaceramide (asialo GM₁) and gangliotrisylceramide (asialo GM₂). Arch Biochem Biophys 260:493, 1988.
18. McCubbin M, Fick RB: Pathogenesis of the *Pseudomonas* lung disease in cystic fibrosis. *In* Fick RB (ed): Pathogenesis of *Pseudomonas aeruginosa* Infections. Boca Raton, FL, CRC Press, 1992:189–212.
19. Fick RB, Naegel GP, Squier SU, Wood RE, Gee JBL, Reynolds HY: Proteins of the cystic fibrosis respiratory tract: fragmented immunoglobulin-G opsonic antibody causing defective opsonophagocytosis. J Clin Invest 14:236–248, 1984.
20. Fick RB, Baltimore RS, Squier SU, Reynolds HY: IgG proteolytic activity of *Pseudomonas aeruginosa* in cystic fibrosis. J Infect Dis 151:589–598, 1985.
21. Fick RB, Robbins RA, Squier SU, et al: Complement activation in cystic fibrosis respiratory fluids: in vivo and in vitro generation of C5a and chemotactic activity. Pediatr Res 20:1258–1268, 1986.
22. Tosi MF, Zakem H, Berger M: Neutrophil elastase cleaves C3bi on opsonized *Pseudomonas* as well as CR1 on neutrophils to create a functionally important optimum receptor mismatch. J Clin Invest 86:300, 1990.
23. Fick RB, Olchowski J, Squier SW, Merrill WW, Reynolds HY: IgG subclasses in cystic fibrosis: IgG2 response to *Pseudomonas* lipopolysaccharide. Am Rev Respir Dis 133:418–422, 1986.
24. Moss RB, Hsu Y-P, Lewiston NJ: Association of systemic immune complexes, complement activation, and antibodies to *P. aeruginosa* lipopolysaccharide and exotoxin A with mortality in cystic fibrosis. Am Rev Respir Dis 133:648–652, 1986.
25. Hornick DB, Fick RB: The IgG subclass composition of immune complexes and the pathogenesis of cystic fibrosis lung disease. J Clin Invest 86:1285, 1990.
26. Smits WL, Sonoda F, Fick RB: Attraction of host cells: *Pseudomonas*-stimulated neutrophil chemotaxins, *In* Pathogenesis of *Pseudomonas aeruginosa* Infections. Boca Raton, FL, CRC Press, 1992:95–112.
27. Sturgess J, Imrie J: Quantitative evaluation of the development of tracheal submucosal glands in infants with cystic fibrosis and control infants. Am J Pathol 106:303, 1982.
28. Claireaux AE: Fibrocystic disease of the pancreas in the newborn. Arch Dis Child 31:22, 1956.
29. Simel DL, Mastin JP, Pratt PC, et al: Scanning electron microscopic study of the airways in normal children and in patients with cystic fibrosis and other lung diseases. J Submicrosc Cytol Pathol 21:521–534, 1989.
30. Balough K, Fick RB, Weinberger M, McCubbin M, Ahrens R: Inflammation in the early cystic fibrosis lung lesion: Lack of correlation with infection. Am Rev Respir Dis 14S:A689, 1992.
31. Godfrey S, Bar-Yishay E, Arad I, Landau LI, Taussig LM: Flow-volume curves in infants with lung disease. Pediatrics 72:517–522, 1983.
32. Godfrey S, Mearns M, Howlett G: Serial lung function studies in

cystic fibrosis in the first 5 years of life. Arch Dis Child 53:83–85, 1978.

33. di'Saint'Agnese PA: Bronchial obstruction with lobar atelectasis and emphysema in cystic fibrosis of the pancreas. Pediatrics 12:178–190, 1953.

34. Hodson CJ, France NE: Pulmonary changes in cystic fibrosis of the pancreas. A radio-pathological study. Clin Radiol 13:54–61, 1962.

35. Lloyd-Still JR, Khaw KT, Shwachman H: Severe respiratory disease in infants with cystic fibrosis. Pediatrics 30:389–396, 1974.

36. Corey ML: Longitudinal studies in cystic fibrosis. In Sturgess J (ed): Perspectives in Cystic Fibrosis. Proceedings of the 8th International Congress on Cystic Fibrosis. Toronto, Canadian Cystic Fibrosis Foundation, 1980:246–255.

37. Corey M, Levison H, Crozier D: Five to seven year course of pulmonary function in cystic fibrosis. Am Rev Respir Dis 114:1085–1092, 1976.

38. Wagener SJ, Taussig LM, Burrows B, Hernried L, Boat T: Comparison of lung function and survival patterns between cystic fibrosis and emphysema or chronic bronchitis patients. In Sturgess J (ed): Perspectives in Cystic Fibrosis. Proceedings of the 8th International Congress on Cystic Fibrosis Foundation, Toronto, Cystic Fibrosis Foundation, 1980:236–295.

39. Bedrossian CM, Greenberg SD, Singer DB, et al: The lung in cystic fibrosis. A quantitative study including prevalence of pathologic findings among different age groups. Hum Pathol 7:195, 1976.

40. Tomashefski JF, Bruce M, Goldberg HI, Dearborn DG: Regional distribution of macroscopic lung disease in cystic fibrosis. Am Rev Respir Dis 133:535–540, 1986.

41. Eggleston PA, Rosenstein DJ, Stackhouse CM, Mellitis ED, Baumgardner RA: A controlled trial of long-term bronchodilator therapy in cystic fibrosis. Chest 99:1088–1092, 1991.

42. Ramsey BW, Wentz KR, Smith AL, et al: Predictive value of oropharyngeal cultures for identifying lower airway bacteria in cystic fibrosis. Am Rev Respir Dis 144:331–337, 1991.

43. Smith AL, Ramsey B, Redding G, Haas J: Endobronchial infection in cystic fibrosis. Acta Paediatr Scand Suppl 363:31–36, 1989.

44. Bauernfeind A, Bretele RM, Harms K, Horol G, Jungrith R: Qualitative and quantitative microbiological analysis of sputa of 102 patients with cystic fibrosis. J Infect 15:270–277, 1987.

45. Watson KC, Kerr EJC, Baillie M: Temporal changes in biotypes of *Haemophilus influenzae* isolated from patients with cystic fibrosis. J Med Microbiol 26:129–132, 1988.

46. Huang NN, Doggett RG: *Pseudomonas aeruginosa:* Clinical Manifestations of Infection and Current Therapy. Academic Press, New York, 1979.

47. Sharples PM, Colditz PB, Wilkinson AR: Lethal respiratory failure in preterm infants due to cystic fibrosis. The first care reports. Acta Paediatr Scand 78:641–643, 1989.

48. Fick RB: *Pseudomonas* in cystic fibrosis: Sylph or sycophant? Clin Chest Med 2:91–102, 1981.

49. Rabin HR, Harley FL, Bryan LE, Elfring GL: Evaluation of a high dose tobramycin and ticarcillin treatment protocol in cystic fibrosis based on improved susceptibility criteria and antibiotic pharmacokinetics. In Sturgess J (ed): Perspectives in Cystic Fibrosis. Proceedings of the 8th International Congress on Cystic Fibrosis. Toronto, Canada, Canadian Cystic Fibrosis Foundation, 1980:370–395.

50. Regelmann WE, Elliott GR, Warwick WJ, Clawson CC: Reduction of sputum *Pseudomonas aeruginosa* density by antibiotics improves lung function in cystic fibrosis more than do bronchodilators and chest physiotherapy alone. Am Rev Respir Dis 141:914–921, 1990.

51. Mouton JW, Kerrebijn KF: Antibacterial therapy in cystic fibrosis. Med Clin North Am 74:837–850, 1990.

52. Nielsen OH, Thomsen BL, Green A, Andersen PK, Hauge M, Schiotz PO: Cystic fibrosis in Denmark 1945 to 1985. Acta Paediatr Scand 77:836–841, 1988.

53. Kelly HW, Lovato C: Antibiotic use in cystic fibrosis. Drug Intell Clin Pharm 18:772–783, 1984.

54. Mearns MB, Hunt GH, Rushworth R: Bacterial flora of respiratory tract in patients with cystic fibrosis, 1950–1971. Arch Dis Child 47:902–907, 1972.

55. Iacocca VG, Sibinga MS, Barbero GJ: Respiratory tract bacteriology in cystic fibrosis. Am J Dis Child 106:315–324, 1963.

56. Huang NN, Van Loon EL, Sheng KT: The flora of the respiratory tract of patients with cystic fibrosis of the pancreas. J Pediatr 59:512–521, 1961.

57. Harrison CJ, Marks MI, Welch DF, Sharma BB, Baker D, Dice J: Collaborative CF antibiotic study group. Pediatr Pharmacol 5:7–16, 1985.

58. Shapera RM, Warwick WJ, Matsen JM: Clindamycin therapy of staphylococcal pulmonary infections in patients with cystic fibrosis. J Pediatr 99:647–650, 1981.

59. Loening-Baucke VA, Mischler E, Myers MG: A placebo-controlled trial of cephalexin therapy in the ambulatory management of patients with cystic fibrosis. J Pediatr 95:630–637, 1979.

60. Hoiby M, Killian M: *Haemophilus* from the lower respiratory tract of patients with cystic fibrosis. Scand J Respir Dis 57:103–107, 1976.

61. Goldfarb J, Stern RC, Reed MD, Yamashita TS, Myers CM, Blumer JL: Ciprofloxacin monotherapy for acute pulmonary exacerbations of cystic fibrosis. Am J Med 2:174–179, 1987.

62. LeBel M: Fluoroquinolones in the treatment of cystic fibrosis: A critical appraisal. Eur J Clin Microbiol Infect Dis 10:316–324, 1991.

63. Bosso JA, Black PG, Matsen JM: Ciprofloxacin versus tobramycin plus azlocillin in pulmonary exacerbations in adult patients with cystic fibrosis. Am J Med 82:180–184, 1987.

64. Rubio TT: Ciprofloxacin: Comparative data in cystic fibrosis. Am J Med 882:185–188, 1987.

65. Hodson MR, Roberts CM, Butland RJA, Smith MJ, Batten JC: Oral ciprofloxacin compared with conventional intravenous treatment for *Pseudomonas aeruginosa* infection in adults with cystic fibrosis. Lancet 1:235–237, 1987.

66. Jensen T, Pederson SS, Hoiby N, Kock C: Efficacy of oral fluoroquinolones versus conventional intravenous antipseudomonal chemotherapy in treatment of cystic fibrosis. Eur J Clin Microbiol Infect Dis 6:618–622, 1987.

67. Davis RL, Koup JR, Williams-Warren J, Weber A, Heggen L, Stempel D, et al: Pharmacokinetics of ciprofloxacin in cystic fibrosis. Antimicrob Agents Chemother 31:915–918, 1987.

68. Bergan T, Thorsteinsson SB, Solberg R, Bjornskau L, Kolstad IM, Johnson S: Pharmacokinetics of ciprofloxacin: Intravenous and increasing oral doses. Am J Med 82:97–102, 1987.

69. Strandvik B, Hjelte L, Lindblad A, Ljungberg B, Malmborg AS, Nilsson-Ehle I: Comparison of efficacy and tolerance of intravenously and orally administered ciprofloxacin in cystic fibrosis patients with acute exacerbations of lung infection. Scand J Infect Dis (suppl) 60:84–88, 1989.

70. Chysky V, Kapila K, Hullman R, Arcieri G, Schacht P, Echols R: Safety of ciprofloxacin in children: Worldwide clinical experience based on compassionate use. Emphasis on joint evaluation. Infection 19:289–296, 1991.

71. Schaad UB, Stoupis C, Wedgwod J, Tschaeppeler H, Vock P: Clinical, radiologic, and magnetic resonance monitoring for skeletal toxicity in pediatric patients with cystic fibrosis receiving a three-month course of ciprofloxacin. Pediatr Infect Dis J 10:723–729, 1991.

72. Akaniro JC, Vidaurre CE, Stutuman HR, Marks MI: Comparative in vitro activity of a new quinolone, fleroxacin, against respiratory pathogens from patients with cystic fibrosis. Antimicrob Agents Chemother 34:1880–1884, 1990.

73. Davies BL, Maesen FPV, Geraedts WH, Baur C: Penetration of ofloxacin from blood to sputum. Drugs 34:26–32, 1987.

74. Jensen T, Pedersen SS, Nielsen CH, Hoiby N, Koch C: The efficacy and safety of ciprofloxacin and ofloxacin in chronic *Pseudomonas aeruginosa* in infection in cystic fibrosis. J Antimicrob Chemother 20:585–594, 1987.

75. Janknegt R: Drug interactions with quinolones. J Antimicrob Chemother 26:7–29, 1990.

76. Wijnands WJA, Vree TB, Baars AM, van Herwaarden CLA: Steady-state kinetics of the quinolone derivatives ofloxacin, enoxacin, ciprofloxacin and pefloxacin during maintenance treatment with theophylline. Drugs 34:159–169, 1987.

77. Gregoire SL, Grasela TJ, Freer JP, Tack KJ, Schentag JJ: Inhibition of theophylline clearance by coadministered ofloxacin without alteration of theophylline effects. Antimicrob Agents Chemother 31:375–378, 1987.

78. Wientzen R, Prestidge CB, Kramer RI, McCracken GH, Nelson JD: Acute pulmonary exacerbations in cystic fibrosis. A double-blind trial of tobramycin and placebo therapy. Am J Dis Child 134:1134–1138, 1980.

79. Hyatt AC, Chipps BD, Kumor KM, Mellits D, Lietman PS, Rosenstein BJ: A double-blind controlled trial of anti-*Pseudomonas* chemotherapy of acute respiratory exacerbations in patients with cystic fibrosis. J Pediatr 99:307–311, 1981.

80. Beaudry PH, Marks MI, McDougall D, Desmond K, Rangel R: Is anti-*Pseudomonas* therapy warranted in acute respiratory exacerbations in children with cystic fibrosis? J Pediatr 97:144–147, 1980.

81. Gold R, Carpenter S, Heurter H, Corey M, Levison H: Randomized trial of ceftazidime versus placebo in the management of acute respiratory exacerbations in patients with cystic fibrosis. J Pediatr 111:907–913, 1987.

82. Winnie GB, Cooper JA, Witson J, Cowan RG, Mayer D, Lepow M: Comparison of 6 and 8 hourly tobramycin dosing intervals in the treatment of pulmonary exacerbations in patients with cystic fibrosis. Pediatr Infect Dis J 10:381–386, 1991.

83. Michael BC: Antibacterial therapy in cystic fibrosis: A review of the literature published between 1980 and February 1987. Chest 94:S1295–S1405, 1988.

84. Bertrou A, Marty N, Henry S, Agueda L, Chabanon G: In vitro bactericidal activity of tobramycin and amikacin alone or in combination against *Pseudomonas aeruginosa* isolated from patients with cystic fibrosis. Pathol Biol (Paris) 38:366–375, 1990.

85. Morris JB, Occhionero ME, Gauderer MW, Stern RC, Doershuk CF: Totally implantable vascular access devices in cystic fibrosis: A four-year experience with fifty-eight patients. J Pediatr 117:82–85, 1990.

86. Ball AB, Duncan FR, Foster FJ, Davidson TI, Watkins RM, Hodson ME: Long-term venous access using a totally implantable drug delivery system in patients with cystic fibrosis and bronchiectasis. Respir Med 83:429–431, 1989.

87. Schaad UB: Pulmonary infection and treatment in cystic fibrosis: Aerosol therapy: Discussion. Chest 94:S161–162, 1988.

88. Stacey JW: Inhalation of nebulized solutions of sulfonamides in the treatment of bronchiectasis. Dis Chest 9:302–306, 1943.

89. di'Saint'Agnese PEA, Andersen DH: Celiac syndrome IV. Chemotherapy in infection of the respiratory tract associated with cystic fibrosis of the pancreas: Observations with penicillin and drugs of the sulfonamide group, with special reference to penicillin aerosol. Am J Dis Child 72:17–61, 1946.

90. Hodson ME, Pendeth ARL, Batten JC: Aerosol carbenicillin and gentamicin treatment of *Pseudomonas aeruginosa* infection in patient with cystic fibrosis. Lancet 2:1137–1139, 1981.

91. Kun P, Landau LI, Phelan PD: Nebulized gentamicin in children and adolescents with cystic fibrosis. Aust Paediatr J 20:43–45, 1984.

92. Jensen T, Pedersen SS, Garne S, Heilmann C, Hoiby N, Koch C: Colistin inhalation therapy in cystic fibrosis patients with chronic *Pseudomonas aeruginosa* lung infection. J Antimicrob Chemother 199:831–838, 1987.

93. Stead RJ, Hodson ME, Batten JC: Inhaled ceftazidime compared with gentamicin and carbenicillin in older patients with cystic fibrosis infected with *Pseudomonas aeruginosa*. Br J Dis Chest 81:272–279, 1987.

94. MacLusky IB, Gold R, Corey M, Levison H: Long-term effects of inhaled tobramycin in patients with cystic fibrosis colonized with *Pseudomonas aeruginosa*. Pediatr Pulmonol 7:42–48, 1989.

95. Wall MA, Terry AB, Eisenberg J, McNamara M: Inhaled antibiotics in cystic fibrosis. [Letter] Lancet 1:1325, 1983.

96. Steinkamp G, Burkhard T, Gappa M, et al: Long-term tobramycin aerosol therapy in cystic fibrosis. Pediatr Pulmonol 6:91–98, 1989.

97. Smith AL, Ramsey BW, Hedges DL, et al: Safety of aerosol tobramycin administration of 3 months to patients with cystic fibrosis. Pediatr Pulmonol 7:265–271, 1989.

98. Jenkins ST, Kelly WC, Mason WG, et al: Aerosolized amikacin administration to cystic fibrosis patients chronically infected with *Pseudomonas aeruginosa*. Cystic Fibrosis Club Abstracts 16:147, 1985.

99. Nathanson I, Cropp GJA, Li P, et al: Efficacy of aerosolized gentamicin in cystic fibrosis. Cystic Fibrosis Club Abstracts 26:145, 1985.

100. MacLusky I, Levison H, Gold R, McLaughlin FJ: Inhaled antibiotics in cystic fibrosis: Is there a therapeutic effect? J Pediatr 108:861–865, 1986.

101. Newman SP, Pellow PGD, Clarke SW: Choice of nebulisers and compressors for delivery of carbenicillin aerosol. Eur J Respir Dis 69:160–168, 1986.

102. Newman SP, Woodman G, Clarke SW: Deposition of carbenicillin aerosols in cystic fibrosis: Effects of nebuliser system and breathing pattern. Thorax 43:318–322, 1988.

103. Littlewood JM, Miller MG, Choneim AT, Ramsden CH: Nebulised colomycin for early *Pseudomonas* colonisation in cystic fibrosis. Lancet 1:865, 1985.

104. Valerius NH, Koch C, Hoiby N: Prevention of chronic *Pseudomonas aeruginosa* colonisation in cystic fibrosis by early treatment. Lancet 338:725–726, 1991.

105. Hoiby N, Friis B, Jensen K, Koch C, Moller NE, Stovring S, Szaff M: Antimicrobial chemotherapy in cystic fibrosis patients. Acta Paediatr Scand (suppl) Vol:301:75–100, 1982.

106. Fick RB, Stillwell PC: Controversies in the management of pulmonary disease due to cystic fibrosis. Chest 95:1319–1327, 1989.

107. Juske WJ, Mosovich LL, Gerbracht LM, Mattar ME, Yaffee SL: Enhanced renal excretion of dicloxacillin in patients with cystic fibrosis. Pediatrics 56:1038–1044, 1975.

108. Hedman A, Adan-Abdi Y, Alvan G, Strandvik B, Arvidsson A: Influence of the glomerular filtration rate on renal clearance of ceftazidime in cystic fibrosis. Clin Pharmacokinet 15:57–65, 1988.

109. Yaffe SJ, Gerbracht LM, Mosovich LL, Mattar ME, Danish M, Jusko WJ: Pharmacokinetics of methicillin in patients with cystic fibrosis. J Infect Dis 135:828–831, 1977.

110. Kearns GL, Hilman BC, Wilson JT: Dosing implication of altered gentamicin disposition in patients with cystic fibrosis. J Pediatr 100:312–319, 1982.

111. Finkelstein E, Hall K: Aminoglycoside clearance in patients with cystic fibrosis. [Letter] J Pediatr 94:163–164, 1979.

112. Li SC, Bowes G, Ioannides-Demos LL, et al: Dosage adjustment and clinical outcomes of long-term use of high-dose tobramycin in adult cystic fibrosis patients. J Antimicrob Chemother 28:561–568, 1991.

113. Rosselli P, Marianelli L, Valenza T, Bartolozzi G: Azlocillin in the treatment of pulmonary infections in patients with cystic fibrosis: Plasma concentrations and therapeutic indications. Pediatr Med Chir 11:389–391, 1989.

114. De Groot R, Hack BD, Weber A, Chaffin D, Ramsey B, Smith AL: Pharmacokinetics of ticarcillin in patients with cystic fibrosis: A controlled prospective study. Clin Pharmacol Ther 47:73–78, 1990.

115. Strandvik B: Antibiotic therapy of pulmonary infections in cystic fibrosis: Dosage schedules and duration of treatment. Chest 94:146S–149S, 1988.

116. Auerback HS, Williams M, Kirkpatrick JA, Colten HR: Alternate-day prednisone reduces morbidity and improves pulmonary function in cystic fibrosis. Lancet 2:686–688, 1985.

117. Rosenstein BJ, Eigen H: Risks of alternate-date prednisone in patients with cystic fibrosis. Pediatrics 87:245–246, 1991.

118. Hubbard RC, McElvaney NG, Birrer P, et al: A preliminary study of aerosolized recombinant human deoxyribonuclease I in the treatment of cystic fibrosis. N Engl J Med 326:812–815, 1992.

118a. Fuchs H, Borowitz D, Christiansen D, et al: Aeorsolized recombinant human DNase reduces pulmonary exacerbations and improves pulmonary function in patients with cystic fibrosis. Abstract presented at 36th Annual Intermountain Thoracic Society Meeting, 1993.

119. Dietzsch JH, Gottschalk B, Heyne K, Leupoid W, Wunderlich P: Cystic fibrosis: Comparison of two mucolytic drugs for inhalation treatment (acetylcysteine and arginine hydrochloride). Pediatrics 55:96–100, 1975.

120. Knowles M, Murray G, Shallal J, et al: Bioelectric properties and ion flow across excised human bronchi. J Appl Physiol 56:868–877, 1984.

121. Knowles M, Gatzy J, Boucher R: Increased bioelectric potential difference across respiratory epithelia in cystic fibrosis. N Engl J Med 305:1489–1495, 1981.

122. App EM, King N, Helfesrieder R, Kohler D, Matthys H: Acute and long-term amiloride inhalation in cystic fibrosis lung disease. Am Rev Respir Dis 141:605–612, 1990.

123. Knowles MR, Church NL, Waltner WE, et al: A pilot study of aerosolized amiloride for the treatment of lung disease in cystic fibrosis. N Engl J Med 332:1189–1194, 1990.

124. Henkin J: Aerosolized amiloride for the treatment of lung disease in cystic fibrosis. [Letter] N Engl J Med 323:997, 1990.

125. Waltner WE, Church NL, Gatzy JT, Boucher RC, Knowles MR: Toxicity and pharmacokinetics of acute amiloride aerosol in normal and cystic fibrosis subjects. [Abstract] Cystic Fibrosis Club Abstr 27:121, 1986.

126. Waltner WE, Church NL, Gatzy JT, Boucher RC, Knowles MR: Deposition, pharmacokinetics, and toxicity of amiloride aerosol in normal and cystic fibrosis (CF) subjects. [Abstract] Am Rev Respir Dis 135(suppl):A288, 1987.

127. Vogelmeier C, Hubbard RC, Fels GA, Schnebli H, et al: Anti-neutrophil elastase defense of the normal human respiratory epithelial surface provided by secretory leukoprotease inhibitor. J Clin Invest 87:482–488, 1991.

128. Vogelmeier C, Buhl R, Hoyt RF, Wilson E, Fells GA, et al: Aerosolization of recombinant secretory leukoprotease inhibitor as a strategy to augment the anti-neutrophil elastase protective screen of the pulmonary epithelial surface. Am Rev Respir Dis 141:847, 1990.

129. McElvaney NG, Hubbard RC, Birrer P, et al: Aerosol α-1-antitrypsin treatment for cystic fibrosis. Lancet 337–393, 1991.

130. Pennington JE, Reynolds HY, Wood RE, et al: Use of a *Pseudomonas aeruginosa* vaccine in patients with acute leukemia and cystic fibrosis. Am J Med 58:629–636, 1975.

131. Wood RE, Pennington JE, Reynolds HY: Intranasal administration of a *Pseudomonas* lipopolysaccharide vaccine in cystic fibrosis patients. Pediatr Infect Dis 2:367–369, 1983.

# CHAPTER 21

# Pneumonia and Empyema

JOHN E. HEFFNER

Radiographically apparent pleural effusions develop in 20% to 60% of patients with bacterial pneumonia.[1, 2] More than 90% of these parapneumonic effusions remain sterile or minimally infected (ie, uncomplicated) and resolve with effective antibiotic therapy of the underlying pulmonary infection. The remaining patients develop a complicated parapneumonic effusion that progresses to intrapleural loculation and abscess formation unless adequately drained.[2] Complicated parapneumonic effusions that have already undergone suppuration and contain viscous pleural fluid with the physical features of frank pus are called empyemas.

The incidence of empyema has decreased during the last several decades because of improved medical management of pneumonia and the advent of increasingly effective antibiotics. However, empyema remains a major source of morbidity and mortality, with death rates as high as 27% to 70% for patients with advanced age,[3–8] chronic debilitation from coexistent disease,[6, 9] malnutrition, or socioeconomic factors that delay antibiotic therapy for pulmonary infections. Prompt recognition of empyema and urgent initiation of vigorous and complete drainage of infected pleural fluid remain the most effective measures in improving patient outcome.[10]

## EMPYEMA FORMATION

Empyema results most commonly from direct extension of bacteria from a region of acute bacterial pneumonia, from a lung abscess, or from septic pulmonary embolization to the pleural space. Less frequent causes include malignant or congenital abnormalities that predispose the pleura to chronic infections, mediastinal suppuration, subphrenic collections of pus, blunt and penetrating chest trauma, esophageal rupture, infections of the neck and thoracic spine, and postthoracotomy bronchopleural fistulas.

After infection, the pathophysiologic events within the pleural space evolve to produce three major stages in the formation of a frank empyema.[11] An understanding of the clinical features of each stage assists in developing patient treatment plans. The initial exudative stage occurs during the first several days of bacterial contamination of the pleural space and is characterized by thin, free-flowing, protein-rich pleural fluid that contains a low concentration of polymorphonuclear leukocytes. The inflamed pleural surfaces remain pliable, and the adjacent lung retains the capacity to reexpand to the chest wall after drainage of the pleural fluid. Patients with parapneumonic effusions in the exudative stage have the greatest opportunity to fully recover after pleural fluid drainage through a closed intercostal chest tube.

The fibrinopurulent stage develops several days later and is characterized by intense pleural inflammation and pleural fluid that becomes turbid and progressively more viscous. Fibrin deposits coat the pleural surfaces, establishing the foundations of a pleural peel that can eventually encase the lung and prevent pulmonary reexpansion (ie, trapped lung). Fibrin strands crisscross the pleural space, creating intrapleural adhesions, fluid loculations, and a scaffold for ingrowing fibroblasts. The progression of multiple intrapleural loculations complicates effective drainage of the pleural space.

The organizing stage of empyema formation is characterized by an influx of fibroblasts that reenforces the pleural peel and further restricts pulmonary reexpansion. Multiple loculations exist in local regions of the pleural space or throughout the hemithorax. Pleural fluid becomes highly viscous and purulent, containing mixed cellular debris that prevents adequate drainage through a closed thoracostomy tube. Depending on the virulence of the pathogen and the severity of the pneumonia, progression to an organized empyema occurs 7 to 14 days after the onset of pneumonia. Occasionally, patients with rupture of a parenchymal lung abscess into the pleural space may rapidly develop intrapleural collections of frank pus (Fig. 21–1).

## MICROBIOLOGY

Most empyemas occur after pneumonias caused by *Streptococcus pneumoniae, Staphylococcus aureus,* or anaerobic bacteria.[12] *S. pneumoniae* was the most common cause of empyema in the preantibiotic era, accounting for 60% of all intrapleural infections.[13] The incidence of pneumococcal empyemas has diminished to 10% because the typically abrupt onset and systemic toxicity of pneumococ-

cal pneumonia cause patients to present early in the course of infection and receive antibiotic therapy. Pneumococcal empyema in the postantibiotic era usually represents neglected disease and delayed medical intervention.

Estimates of the incidence of pleural infection in patients with pneumonia caused by *S. aureus* range from 10% to 25%.[13] As many as 48% of patients with staphylococcal pneumonia have associated pleural effusions, and one half of the effusions are empyemas.[14]

Anaerobic pleuropulmonary infections are the most common cause of empyema in some centers,[15] with anaerobes causing between 17% and 71% of all empyemas.[6, 13, 15] The frequency of detection of anaerobic bacteria in empyemas

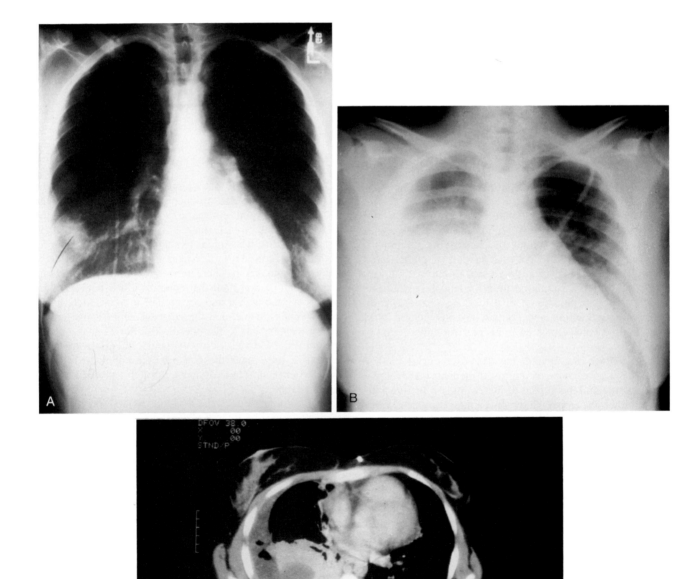

**Figure 21–1.** Rapid, 48-hour progression to frank empyema. *A,* The admission chest radiograph demonstrates a right lower lobe infiltrate due to *Staphylococcus aureus* pneumonia. *B,* Two days later, a repeat radiograph (panel) showed a large right pleural effusion. *C,* Thoracentesis demonstrated frank pus. A computed tomographic scan revealed a right lower lobe lung abscess that ruptured into the pleural space. (From Heffner JE: A successful approach to empyema. Contemp Intern Med 3:94–104, 1991.)

correlates with the expertise of an institution's microbiology laboratory in culturing and identifying anaerobic species.[13] Institutions caring for indigent or alcoholic patients observe a higher incidence of anaerobic empyemas. Pleural fluid isolates from patients with anaerobic empyema are often polymicrobial and harbor *Bacteroides melaninogenicus,* anaerobic streptococci (eg, peptostreptococci), and *Fusobacterium nucleatum.* Anaerobic pathogens coexist with aerobic bacteria, such as *S. aureus* and *S. pneumoniae,* in patients with empyema.[16]

Aerobic gram-negative bacteria, such as *Haemophilus influenzae, Klebsiella pneumoniae,* and *Pseudomonas aeruginosa,* and unusual pathogens, such as *Rhodococcus equi, Nocardia asteroides,* and *Actinomyces* species, are important causes of empyema in certain clinical settings. Almost every bacterium that can produce pneumonia has been identified as an etiologic pathogen for thoracic empyema. In many instances, pleural pathogens are never identified, because 57% of patients who present with empyema after having received a partial course of antibiotics have sterile pleural fluid cultures.[9]

## CLINICAL MANIFESTATIONS

The clinical manifestations of empyema usually merge with the signs and symptoms of the underlying pneumonia. Pleuritic chest pain is a nonspecific marker but heightens clinical suspicion of pleural infection. The physical examination may demonstrate diminished or absent breath sounds and decreased fremitus over the region of the effusion, unlike the tubular nature of breath sounds with preserved or increased fremitus over a consolidated pneumonia. Occasionally, patients treated with corticosteroids may have suppression of the signs and symptoms of infection and present with a ''silent'' empyema.[17]

Patients with anaerobic empyema frequently have a history of aspiration, an underlying comorbid condition, or poor dental hygiene as a source of bacteria-laden oral debris.[18] Anaerobic empyemas may follow an indolent course, and the patients may present with weight loss, anemia, and chronic productive cough, simulating cancer or pulmonary tuberculosis.[18] This nonspecific presentation typically delays medical evaluation and the prompt initiation of therapy with antibiotics and pleural fluid drainage until intrapleural loculation occurs. This delayed presentation is the major cause of prolonged morbidity in patients with anaerobic empyema.[16, 19] Extensive pulmonary necrosis causes lung abscesses and bronchopulmonary fistulas in 30% to 40% of patients with anaerobic pleuropulmonary infections.[13]

## DIAGNOSIS

Any patient with a bacterial pneumonia, regardless of the nature or severity of symptoms, should be considered at risk for empyema. The empyema may already exist when the patient seeks medical attention for the underlying pneumonia, or it may develop during the course of antibiotic therapy. A careful radiographic evaluation for a parapneumonic effusion and diagnostic thoracentesis if pleural fluid is detected are the initial diagnostic measures. The clinical evaluation emphasizes the importance of thoracentesis and pleural fluid analysis, because no clinical features or imaging technique differentiate with adequate reliability pleural effusions that resolve with antibiotic therapy from those that require pleural drainage.[20, 21]

The posteroanterior and lateral chest radiographs are sensitive but nonspecific screening tests for pleural fluid in patients with pneumonia. Unobscured diaphragmatic margins visible on both projections exclude clinically important parapneumonic effusions if nondependent pleural loculations do not exist elsewhere in the chest. Patients with clear diaphragms can undergo antibiotic therapy for the underlying pneumonia and careful observation for delayed onset of parapneumonic effusions. Patients with clear diaphragms but radiographic evidence of nondependent loculations should undergo thoracic ultrasound evaluation or computed tomography (CT) and image-guided thoracentesis if fluid is detected (Fig. 21–2).

Indistinct diaphragmatic contours may represent free or loculated pleural fluid, pleural thickening, or an area of consolidated pneumonia adjacent to the diaphragm. These radiographic appearances require right- and left-lateral decubitus chest radiographs. The decubitus view with the affected side positioned up layers free fluid against the mediastinum, allowing a better evaluation of the radiographic features of the pneumonia. The decubitus view with the affected side down can detect layering of free fluid against the lateral chest wall (Fig. 21–3). Light and coworkers[2] have shown that patients with pneumonia and less than 10 mm of pleural fluid layering do not require thoracentesis

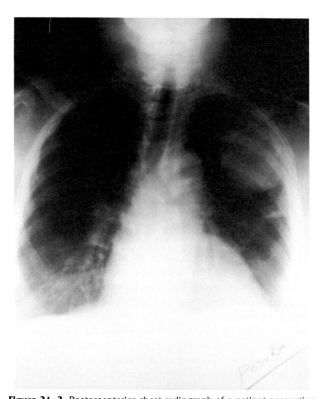

**Figure 21–2.** Posteroanterior chest radiograph of a patient presenting with a 3-week history of low-grade fever and cough. The pleural-based density in the left upper lung zone suggested a pleural-based mass or a loculated pleural effusion. Ultrasound-directed thoracentesis revealed frank pus that grew anaerobic pathogens in culture.

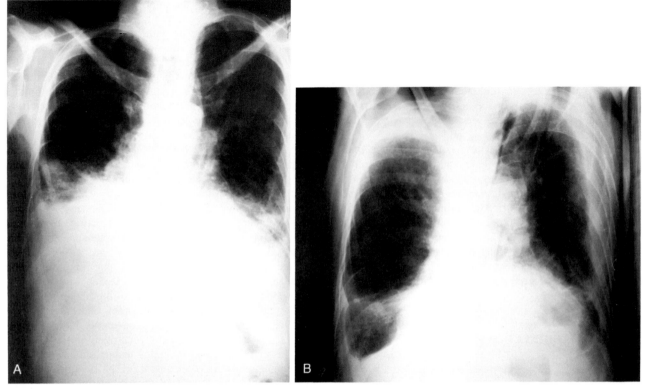

**Figure 21–3.** *A*, The admission chest radiograph of an elderly patient with pneumococcal pneumonia shows bibasilar infiltrates with indistinct diaphragmatic margins. *B*, A left lateral decubitus view better defines the right lower lobe infiltrate and demonstrates a sufficient volume of free-flowing fluid on the left to warrant thoracentesis.

because they respond to antibiotic therapy. Thoracentesis is indicated and considered safe in patients with more than 10 mm layering to exclude a complicated parapneumonic effusion.

If no layering occurs but the admission chest radiograph suggests pleural loculation adjacent to the diaphragm, the patient should undergo evaluation with thoracic ultrasound,[22, 23] which can detect as little as 5 mL of pleural fluid, or have CT scans. If fluid is found, an image-guided thoracentesis should be performed. Specialized imaging techniques are particularly important in patients with extensive pulmonary consolidation that may obscure pleural fluid. Loculated pleural effusions may simulate other processes, such as pleural-based masses, and be demonstrable only by ultrasound or CT in as many as 30% of patients.[20, 23, 24]

CT has evolved as the primary technique for imaging pleural disease in many institutions. In patients with parapneumonic effusions, CT scans can define loculations adjacent to or extending into the mediastinum and guide therapeutic interventions.[20, 25–27] CT scans can also differentiate parenchymal lung abscesses from empyema with bronchopleural fistulas in patients with large cavities containing air-fluid levels.[20, 25, 28] The use of intravenous contrast with CT can characterize underlying pulmonary pathology, such as coexistence of a lung abscess with empyema, the extent of necrosis within a pneumonia, and the presence of pulmonary infarctions. The radiographic thickness of contrast-enhanced pleural membranes and the presence of edema in extrapleural tissues can assist in the differential diagnosis

of empyema from a transudative or malignant pleural effusion.[21, 29]

The clinical role for magnetic resonance (MR) imaging in the evaluation of parapneumonic effusions is not yet established. Initial reports indicate that MR signals correlate with the composition of pleural fluid, with exudative effusions appearing as higher-intensity images than transudative effusions.[30] MR scans may be helpful for detecting pleural loculations and underlying lung pathology in patients with contraindications to intravenous contrast that limit the value of CT.

## PLEURAL FLUID ANALYSIS AND DECISION FOR DRAINAGE

Diagnostic thoracentesis provides fundamentally important information for guiding the management of patients with parapneumonic effusions. Gross inspection and laboratory analysis of the pleural fluid may establish the presence of an empyema, identify the etiologic pathogen of the pneumonia if sputum and blood cultures are unrevealing, and define by chemical criteria the probability that a non-purulent effusion will follow a complicated course and require chest tube drainage. Although the risk of pneumothorax varies from 5% to 19%, depending on the skills of the operator, most instances of pneumothorax are inconsequential, and the incidence of pleural space contamination is extraordinarily low.[31, 32]

Between 30 and 50 mL of fluid should be aspirated for

inspection of gross characteristics, such as color, purulence, viscosity, and odor. Nonpurulent fluid is analyzed for glucose, protein, lactate dehydrogenase (LDH), amylase, pH, and total and differential leukocyte count. Except for amylase, which can detect a ruptured esophagus as the cause of empyema,[33] these laboratory studies do not add additional diagnostic information that affects therapy when frank pus is aspirated. All pleural samples should be submitted for aerobic and anaerobic culture and Gram stain (ie, spun specimens if initial unspun Gram stains are negative). Special studies, such as cytologic analysis, mycobacterial culture and stains, and fungal culture and smears, should be performed if clinically indicated.

Frank pus confirms the presence of an empyema and establishes an absolute indication for urgent drainage of the pleural space. Gram stain detection of pleural fluid bacteria similarly indicates the need for pleural fluid drainage. Although malodorous pus identifies anaerobic pleuropulmonary infection, 50% to 60% of anaerobic empyemas are not foul smelling.[18] The total leukocyte count offers little diagnostic utility because of the low specificity for empyema,[34] but the predominance of polymorphonuclear cells in parapneumonic effusions may assist in decreasing the likelihood of some noninfectious causes of exudative pleural effusions that often have a mononuclear cell predominance, such as malignant pleural effusions.

The most difficult decision in managing parapneumonic effusions is determining whether Gram-negative, nonpurulent pleural fluid should be drained by a chest tube. CT or ultrasound evidence of pleural loculations favors pleural drainage, because only 30% of patients with loculated effusions respond to conservative therapy with antibiotics alone, compared with 90% of patients with free-flowing effusions.[20] Patients with loculated effusions are more likely to require decortication or to die of sepsis. The presence of loculations by themselves, however, is not an absolute indication for chest tube drainage.[20]

Clinical experience indicates that chemical analysis of pleural fluid can assist in the differentiation of uncomplicated parapneumonic effusions that respond to antibiotic therapy alone from complicated parapneumonic effusions that require pleural drainage.[2, 10, 35] The chemical criteria are

based on observations that pleural fluid pH and glucose decrease and LDH increases proportionally with the severity of pleural inflammation. These changes result from the metabolism of glucose to carbon dioxide and lactate by activated leukocytes and bacteria and the subsequent lysis of phagocytic cells.[36–39] Uncontrolled, observational studies have suggested the utility of these assays if combined with other features of the patient's clinical presentation, in identifying the necessity for chest tube drainage of nonpurulent parapneumonic effusions.[2, 10, 35, 37, 40, 41]

The threshold values of pleural fluid pH and glucose that indicate a need for chest tube placement vary among investigative groups (Table 21–1).[2, 10, 35, 37, 40, 41] The criteria used by Light and coworkers[2] can be applied to patients with nonpurulent parapneumonic effusions with or without intrapleural loculations. These investigators recommend that a pleural fluid glucose level below 40 mg/dL or a pleural fluid pH below 7.00 is an absolute indication for chest tube drainage. If the pleural fluid glucose is above 40 mg/dL and the pH above 7.20, tube thoracostomy is not indicated, even in patients with pleural loculations. Patients with pH values above 7.20 should be monitored for enlarging pleural effusions or inadequate systemic response to antibiotics.

Patients with pleural fluid glucose levels above 40 mg/dL combined with a pleural fluid pH between 7.00 and 7.20 or a pleural fluid LDH greater than 1000 IU/L are at intermediate risk for progression to empyema. Light and coworkers[2] recommend individualization of therapy. If the effusion is large, the patient poorly able to tolerate progression to empyema, and the pH closer to 7.00, chest drainage should be initiated. If the effusion is small and the pH closer to 7.20 in a more vigorous patient, careful observation is indicated, with intervention if the patient fails to improve. Repeat thoracentesis within 12 to 24 hours in uncertain instances may assist the decision, with placement of chest tubes if the pH decreases or the LDH increases.[2]

The pleural fluid chemical criteria established by Sahn's group apply to patients with free-flowing pleural effusions (see Table 21–1).[42] Pleural fluid pH is considered the most important determinant for drainage, because a fall in pH precedes the decrease in the pleural fluid glucose level.[39]

There are exceptions to the chemical criteria for pleural

**Table 21–1. Guidelines for Chest Tube Insertion in Patients With Nonpurulent, Gram-Negative Parapneumonic Effusions**

| Pleural Fluid Result | Management |
| --- | --- |
| *Light Recommendations** | |
| pH <7.00 *or* glucose <40 mg/dL | Placement of chest tube for drainage in most patients |
| pH 7.00–7.20 *or* LDH† >1000 IU/L | Consider chest tube for drainage if the pleural effusion is loculated or large |
| pH >7.20 *and* glucose >40 mg/dL *and* LDH <1000 IU/L | Chest tube not indicated, even for loculation; reevaluate with repeat thoracentesis if patient does not respond clinically or if effusion increases |
| *Sahn Recommendations‡* | |
| pH <7.10, usually with glucose <40 mg/dL, LDH >1000 IU/L | Placement of chest tube for drainage |
| pH 7.10–7.29, glucose 40–60 mg/dL, LDH 500–1000 IU/L | Repeat thoracentesis in 6–8 hours; if pH decreases and clinical status worsens, placement of chest tube indicated |
| pH ≥7.30, pleural fluid to serum glucose ratio >0.5, LDH <1000 IU/L | No indication for chest tube drainage; continue close observation |

*Recommendendations apply regardless of the presence of pleural loculations. Pleural fluid pH should be ≥0.30 lower than arterial pH to confirm pleural fluid acidosis. Data from Light RW: Management of parapneumonic effusions. Chest. 100:892–893, 1991.

†LDH, lactate dehydrogenase.

‡Recommendations apply to free-flowing effusions. Pleural fluid pH should be ≥0.15 lower than arterial pH to confirm pleural fluid acidosis. Data from Strange C, Sahn S. Management of parapneumonic pleural effusions and empyema. Infect Dis Clin North Am 5:539–559, 1991.

fluid drainage. The pleural fluid pH should be at least 0.15 to 0.30 unit below arterial pH to serve as an indicator of chest tube drainage, because pleural fluid pH mirrors systemic acidosis (see Table 21–1).[35, 42] Empyema caused by *Proteus mirabilis* may have pleural fluid with a high pH, because this pathogen has a urease enzyme that splits urea to produce ammonia, resulting in higher pH.[43, 44] Nonempyemal causes of low pleural pH must be excluded, such as tuberculous pleural effusion, pleural malignancy, and rheumatoid pleurisy.[33] Some investigators have suggested that complicated parapneumonic effusions due to *S. pneumoniae,* are more likely to respond than other pyogenic pathogens to antibiotic therapy without pleural drainage.[41]

Some reports have challenged the clinical utility of pleural fluid chemical analysis in determining the need for chest tube drainage.[45, 46] Berger and Morganroth[45] retrospectively reviewed the course of 62 patients with complicated parapneumonic effusions as defined by nonpurulent fluid with any one of three features: pH less than 7.20, positive Gram stain, or a positive culture. Of the 26 patients with complicated effusions, 16 were initially treated with antibiotics alone, and 10 received chest tube drainage at the discretion of the attending physician. Although the duration of hospitalization, fever, and leukocytosis tended to be longer in the 16 patients treated with antibiotics alone, no statistically significant differences existed in clinical outcome between the two groups.

Nine of the 16 patients with complications who were treated with antibiotics alone had pleural fluid pH determinations. Five of these patients had pH values between 7.00 and 7.20 and recovered without pleural drainage. Four patients had a pleural fluid pH less than 7.00; of these, 1 patient subsequently required drainage and 3 patients recovered with antibiotics (ie, 2 patients with pneumococcal pneumonia and 1 patient with negative culture results). The investigators concluded that some patients with complicated parapneumonic effusions may be treated with antibiotics alone and that reliance on pleural fluid characteristics (ie, Gram stain, culture, and pH) may result in unnecessary chest tube placements.[45]

Poe and coworkers[46] retrospectively reported the course of 91 patients with parapneumonic effusions (some of whom had frank empyemas) who received early chest tube placement or antibiotic therapy at the discretion of the attending physician. They analyzed the predictive value, sensitivity, and specificity for determining need of chest tube drainage of the following pleural fluid findings: positive Gram stain, pH less than 7.00, glucose concentration less than 40 mg/dL, and LDH level greater than 1000 IU/L. They found that each of the four criteria had a high specificity, ranging from 82% to 96%, but a low sensitivity, ranging from 18% for a positive Gram stain to 53% for a pleural fluid LDH level greater than 1000 IU/L. They conclude that pleural fluid Gram stain, pH, glucose, and LDH have limited usefulness in predicting the need for eventual chest tube drainage.

Data from these two reports are difficult to analyze because of the retrospective study design, which has inherent weaknesses for validating clinical practice recommendations. Designed to test the predictive accuracy of the pleural fluid drainage guidelines of Light and coworkers, the two studies used different definitions of complicated pleural effusions. Incomplete data collection hampered the conclu-

sions; only a minority of patients had complete sets of pH, glucose, and LDH values. The study by Poe and coworkers[41] included an unknown number of children, a high proportion of patients partially treated with antibiotics, and patients with frank empyema who should undergo pleural drainage regardless of pleural fluid chemical results. Attending physicians in both studies made decisions for chest tube placement based on incompletely described clinical parameters that introduced hidden selection bias into group comparisons.

No prospective, controlled studies exist to validate the predictive accuracy of pleural fluid pH, glucose, and LDH in selecting patients for chest tube drainage. On the basis of available observational data,[2, 10, 35, 37, 40, 41] pleural fluid chemical analysis appears clinically useful in identifying patients with nonpurulent parapneumonic effusions at increased risk for progression to intrapleural loculation unless adequately drained. Considering that chest tubes are well tolerated during the initial phases of empyema formation and that delayed drainage increases morbidity and the duration of hospitalization,[10, 18, 20, 47] pleural fluid analysis tends to encourage early chest tube placement. Management decisions based on pleural fluid chemical findings should be tempered by the patient's complete bacteriologic, radiographic, and clinical presentation and subsequently modified as needed by careful patient follow-up and monitoring.[42, 48]

## TREATMENT

### Antibiotic Therapy

General principles guide the selection and delivery of antibiotics for the primary pneumonia, incorporating the patient's clinical presentation, epidemiologic setting, and microbiologic data collected from lower airway secretions, pleural fluid, and blood. A parapneumonic effusion does not require extension of the antibiotic spectrum or selection of combination regimens that would not be indicated for the underlying pneumonia. Although correct antibiotic selection improves patient outcome, initiating prompt pleural fluid drainage in patients with complicated parapneumonic effusions equals drug therapy in importance.

Most antibiotics, including newer agents such as the quinolones, penetrate the pleural space well and achieve concentrations in pleural fluid within 75% of serum levels.[49, 50] No need exists for direct intrapleural instillation of antibiotics in complicated parapneumonic effusions or for the use of higher drug doses than those required for the underlying pneumonia. Aminoglycosides may represent special considerations in drug selection for patients with frank empyema. Although they effectively penetrate exudative pleural effusions, measurable levels of gentamicin may be undetectable in empyema pus.[51] The possibility exists that conditions within a thoracic empyema are unfavorable for aminoglycoside bioactivity because of drug inactivation by pleural pus or poor penetration across severely inflamed and fibrin-coated empyema membranes.[51]

The duration of antibiotic therapy is dictated by the underlying pneumonia and the adequacy of pleural drainage in patients with complicated pleural effusions. After the pleural space infection is controlled, antibiotics are no longer needed if the pneumonia has responded to the 10 to 14 days of therapy. Patients with uncomplicated parapneumonic effusions require no alteration of the duration of antibiotic therapy directed at the underlying pneumonia.

Anaerobic pleuropulmonary disease has classically relied on penicillin for achieving effective therapy.[52] Data from patients with anaerobic lung abscesses, empyema, or necrotizing pneumonia suggest that clindamycin may be a more effective agent because of the 15% to 20% incidence of *B. melaninogenicus* resistance to penicillin.[52–55] Metronidazole is recommended for use in patients with anaerobic pulmonary infection only in combination with penicillin[56] because of the resistance to metronidazole frequently shown by microaerophilic streptococci and *Peptostreptococcus;* as many as 43% of patients with anaerobic pulmonary infections treated with metronidazole alone fail to respond to therapy.[52–57]

## Pleural Fluid Drainage

Many methods can provide adequate drainage of the infected pleural space (Table 21–2). Each method has an appropriate role in the management of complicated parapneumonic effusions.[58] The proper drainage procedure depends on the pathophysiologic stage of the empyema, the nature of the infecting pathogen, the existence of comorbid disease, the patient's ability to tolerate an aggressive operative procedure, and the patient's ability to tolerate potential delays from inadequate conservative measures before definitive drainage is established. Local experience and expertise with interventional techniques greatly influence the adopted therapeutic approach.

In patients with established empyemas, selected drainage techniques should fulfill the following treatment goals: eradication of the empyema, reexpansion of the lung, restoration of the chest wall and diaphragmatic mobility, return of respiratory function to normal, elimination of the

Table 21–2. **Methods for Achieving Drainage of a Complicated Parapneumonic Effusion and Closure of Empyema Cavities**

**Effusion Drainage**
Nonsurgical methods
  Thoracentesis
  Closed intercostal chest (thoracostomy) tube
  Image-guided percutaneous chest catheter
  Intrapleural instillation of fibrinolytic agents
Surgical methods
  Formal decortication
  Partial decortication
  Thoracoscopy
  Open drainage with rib resection
  Open window thoracostomy
**Closure of Empyema Cavities***
Surgical methods
  Transposition of muscle or omental flaps
  Clagett procedure: two-stage drainage with open window thoracostomy
    followed by instillation of antibiotic solution and thoracostomy
    closure
  Thoracoplasty

*Closure is performed after control of pleural sepsis.

potential for chronic pleural space infection, and reduction to a minimum of the duration of hospital stay.[59]

### Thoracentesis

Approximately 25% of patients presenting with primary pneumonia and culture-positive parapneumonic effusions respond to complete thoracentesis drainage of the pleural fluid and systemic antibiotics.[54] The fluid must be compatible with the exudative phase of empyema formation: nonpurulent, nonviscous, free flowing, and completely drained from the pleural space. Reports about thoracentesis do not describe the microbiologic, chemical, or cellular features of the pleural fluid used to better characterize the clinical features or severity of illness of the successfully drained patient population.

If complete thoracentesis is attempted as the primary drainage procedure in patients with infected pleural fluid, the following clinical features should not exist: viscous pleural fluid, frank empyematous pus, intrapleural loculations, virulent or loculation-forming pathogens such as anaerobic species or *S. aureus,* incomplete thoracentesis drainage, or severe toxicity. Most authorities recommend chest tube drainage in all patients during the early exudative phase of empyema formation because of the acceptable morbidity of intercostal thoracostomy and the low (36%) success rate of thoracentesis in some patient series.[60, 61]

### Chest Tube Drainage

Blind placement of a large bore (28–30 Fr) intercostal chest tube is the primary method of pleural space drainage for complicated parapneumonic effusions. Proper patient selection is important, because only 26% to 60% of closed thoracostomy tube placements successfully drain the pleural space and avoid subsequent decortication.[12, 61–68] Patients should be in the acute exudative or early fibrinopurulent stage of empyema formation, in which pleural fluid retains sufficient fluidity to flow through an intercostal tube but resists drainage by simple thoracentesis. The effusion should be posteriorly dependent and free flowing or minimally loculated, as demonstrated by fluid layering, with clear pleural margins on left and right lateral decubitus chest radiographs. Improved success rates during the early phases of empyema formation underscore the urgency of prompt diagnosis and drainage of complicated parapneumonic effusions.

The factors underlying failure of chest tube drainage include tube clogging by viscous fluid, multiple pleural loculations, improper tube position, and tube kinking.[69] Detection of thick empyema pus at thoracentesis obviates the benefit from chest tube placement and supports a surgical drainage procedure as initial therapy, as is described later in this chapter. Specialized imaging techniques assist in excluding the possibility of multiple loculations before the chest tube is placed. At the time of thoracentesis, radiocontrast instilled into the pleural space (ie, empyemagram) can define the distribution of pleural fluid and identify the extent of loculations.[60, 70] Thoracic CT can see the distribution of pleural fluid and identify anterior, paramediastinal, or apical loculations that respond poorly to chest tubes (Fig. 21–4).[25, 71, 72] Thoracic ultrasound can demonstrate fibrin

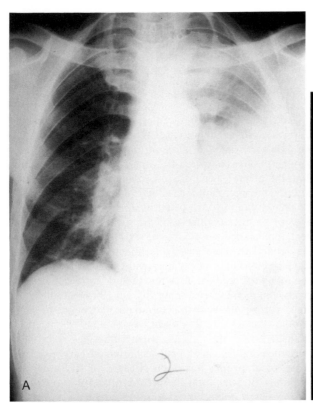
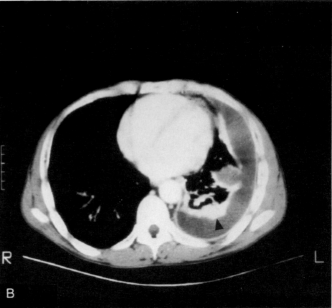

**Figure 21–4.** *A*, Admission chest radiograph and *B*, computed tomographic (CT) scan of a patient with pneumonia and parapneumonic effusion. Infusion of intravenous contrast allowed CT visualization of a thick pleural peel *(arrowhead)*. The patient underwent early decortication and experienced full lung expansion immediately after surgery. (From Heffner JE: A successful approach to empyema. Contemp Intern Med 3:94–104, 1991.)

webs within fluid collections, indicating the presence of a loculated pleural space.[20]

After chest tube insertion, serial radiographs should confirm the adequacy of tube position, because placement into the major fissure or away from remaining loculations markedly decreases success. If the plain radiograph shows resolution of pleural fluid with clear pleural margins and the patient clinically improves, no additional imaging is necessary. If fluid persists or a pulmonary consolidation obscures the pleural margins, follow-up imaging with CT or ultrasound can detect undrained fluid collections and tube misplacement (Fig. 21–5).[23, 73]

The major complications of intercostal chest tube include malpositioning with chest wall hematoma, pulmonary laceration, pulmonary infarction, and trauma to the liver, spleen, or stomach.[74] The overall mortality rate is as high as 5%, emphasizing the importance of preinsertion thoracic imaging in the absence of clear-cut evidence of free pleural fluid.[62, 75]

Successfully placed chest tubes that adequately drain the pleural space can be removed when drainage decreases to less than 50 to 100 mL each day. A chest tube draining more than this volume for longer than 14 days can be converted to an empyema tube if the patient is not a candidate for an open surgical drainage procedure. If the chest tube is cut several centimeters from the insertion site, it becomes an "empyema tube" and can be retracted during the following months as the lung expands to the chest wall and obliterates the empyema cavity.[54]

### Fibrinolytic Therapy

Intrapleural instillation of fibrinolytic agents may benefit patients with complicated parapneumonic effusions who fail chest tube therapy because viscous pleural fluid or loculations prevent adequate drainage.[76–83] The fibrinolytic enzymes can promote drainage and lung reexpansion by debriding the pleural surface, thinning pleural fluid, and lysing intrapleural adhesions. First reported in 1950 with the use of partially purified streptococcal concentrates by Sherry and coworkers,[84] the efficacy of intrapleural streptokinase has been supported by multiple observational reports since 1977.[76–83]

Intrapleural streptokinase appears most effective in the exudative or early fibrinopurulent stages of a complicated parapneumonic effusion, before extensive pleural space organization and frank empyema develop.[76] The technique involves daily instillation of 250,000 U of streptokinase with 100 mL of saline into the chest tube, which is clamped for 4 hours. Treatment continues until the drainage from the chest tube has decreased to 100 mL or radiographic clearing of pleural fluid occurs. Although antibodies can limit the success of streptokinase, no major complications or laboratory evidence of systemic fibrinolysis have been reported.[83, 85] Urokinase has been suggested as an alternative therapy because of its low antigenicity, but the high cost of urokinase limits its widespread application.[81]

Contraindications to intrapleural instillation of streptokinase include suspected allergies, bronchopleural fistula, fibrothorax, and a large empyema with obvious trapped lung.

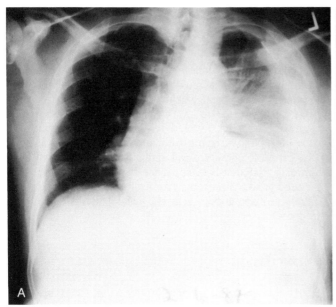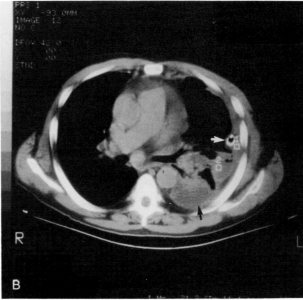

**Figure 21–5.** *A,* The chest radiograph shows the placement of a left-sided chest tube for thoracic empyema. *B,* The computed tomographic scan demonstrated a large posterior loculation *(black arrow)* distant from the region drained by the chest tube *(white arrow)*. The patient underwent decortication and was discharged 8 days after surgery.

Multiple intrapleural loculations may be less likely to respond to therapy. Some reports suggest the utility of percutaneous instillation of streptokinase through a thoracentesis needle into pleural loculations that do not communicate with a chest tube.[79] Although designed to promote pleural fluid drainage and circumvent decortication, prolonged trials of partially effective fibrinolytic therapy should be avoided to prevent delays in proceeding to surgical drainage.

### Image-Guided Percutaneous Catheter Drainage

Many institutions have reported the efficacy of image-guided 10- to 14-gauge catheters placed percutaneously by a trocar or Seldinger technique for draining parapneumonic effusions.[25, 73, 86–91] Direct guidance by fluoroscopic, CT, or ultrasound imaging allows accurate catheter placement into loculated pleural effusions in apical, anterior, and paramediastinal locations that are difficult to access by standard large-bore chest tubes.[89]

Most centers reserve percutaneous catheters as an initial thoracic drainage technique for patients in the exudative or early fibrinopurulent stages of empyema formation who have relatively thin pleural fluid.[86, 87] Primary drainage by percutaneous catheters may be prolonged for 1 week or longer in many patients, with treatment failures resulting from clotted tubes, thick fluid, and pleural peels that prevent lung reexpansion.[73, 86–88] If placed for initial therapy, image-guided catheters should not delay surgical intervention in good operative candidates if adequate drainage does not rapidly occur. Image-guided catheters are best used as an adjunctive measure to cannulate loculated empyemas in patients who fail chest tube drainage and present excessive risks for surgical therapy.[25]

### Surgical Drainage Techniques

Patients with late fibrinopurulent or organized empyemas associated with thick intrapleural pus and multiple locula-

tions have a low probability of prompt adequate drainage by closed thoracostomy tube. These patients require more aggressive surgical procedures to break up loculations, initiate adequate drainage, and promote lung reexpansion.[61, 70] Early recognition and surgical management of patients unlikely to respond to catheter drainage or those who have failed several days of a chest tube trial improves outcome by avoiding extensive pleural fibrosis, lengthy duration of illness, and prolonged hospitalization.[6, 9, 71, 92, 93] Furthermore, the complexity of the eventual operative procedure is compounded by the preceding duration of unsuccessful nonsurgical management efforts.[92]

Many surgical procedures are available for treatment of thoracic empyema. Selection of an operative approach depends on anatomic considerations, such as the extent and location of the empyema, degree of loculation, presence of bronchopleural fistulae, and the capacity of the lung to reexpand against the chest wall. The ability of the patient to tolerate extensive surgery and local experience and expertise further influence selection of the operative procedure. The underlying principle centers on establishing early effective drainage to avoid a persistent empyema cavity and prolonged morbidity.[61, 92, 94]

Initial thoracic drainage by decortication accelerates recovery in patients with organized empyemas characterized by thick and gelatinous pus or multiple loculations.[59, 93, 95–98] This procedure requires a good operative candidate because it entails a thoracotomy incision under general anesthesia to remove intrapleural pus and the thick pleural peel that restricts lung reexpansion. The procedure is termed an empyemectomy when the entire empyema sac is removed en toto.

Patient selection for primary decortication is assisted by thoracentesis examination of the pleural fluid and CT or ultrasound thoracic imaging to determine the extent of pleural organization (see Fig. 21–4).[99] Unfortunately, the CT-determined thickness of the parietal pleura does not correlate with the subsequent need for decortication.[100] Patients who fail several days of initial chest tube drainage with or without instillation of streptokinase benefit from early decortication to control pleural sepsis and avoid persistent or recurrent empyemas.[92, 101] Empyemas of long duration or uncertain onset can also undergo successful decortication.[101, 102] Patients do not require decortication for management of pulmonary restriction alone; thick pleural peels adequately treated by chest tube drainage and antibiotics resolve in most patients without surgical resection.[100, 103]

Partial decortication is a well-tolerated variation of the formal procedure and can be applied initially or after unsuccessful chest tube drainage in patients with localized loculations.[104] Performed through a 4-inch (10-cm) limited thoracotomy incision, pleural space debridement and partial decortication with placement of two to three chest tubes in dependent regions can promote lung reexpansion. The incision can be extended for patients who appear on intraoperative inspection to require formal decortication because of extensive pleural peels. Although investigators have successfully used a thoracoscope to break down loculations, promote chest tube drainage, and avoid decortication,[105] recovery appears prolonged compared with surgical drainage.[47]

The mortality rate after decortication approaches 11% for patients of advanced age and with severe debilitation.[9, 106] However, patients too old or sick to undergo decortication experience a mortality rate as high as 58% if resigned to nonsurgical therapy for loculated and inadequately draining empyemas.[6] In such clinical situations, open drainage with rib resection presents a less aggressive surgical alternative to decortication. The procedure requires resection of segments from one to three ribs overlying the dependent region of the empyema, allowing regional intrapleural debridement. Chest tubes are inserted into the empyema cavity under direct visualization to promote maximal drainage, and the incision is closed. After adequate pleurodesis occurs to prevent pneumothorax, the chest tubes are cut, and the distal ends are inserted into collecting bags to promote patient mobility. Over weeks or months, the chest tubes are progressively retracted as the empyema cavity is obliterated by ingrowing granulation tissue.

Open drainage can also be performed as an open window thoracostomy that avoids chest tube placement in patients with empyema and provides control of pleural infection in patients with bronchopleural fistulas.[107–110] The procedure was originally reported by Robinson in 1915[111, 112] and subsequently ascribed to Eloesser, who performed a similar operation for tuberculous empyema.[113, 114] Two to three 5-cm rib segments overlying the empyema cavity are resected, and a skin flap from the U-shaped skin incision is sutured to the parietal pleura to prevent closure of the drainage channel.[107, 114] Open drainage continues until granulation tissue grows into the empyema cavity.

Persistent empyema cavities or bronchopleural fistulas in patients with open window thoracostomies can be managed with a second procedure that obliterates the space by the transposition of muscle or omental flaps.[115–120] Clagett and Geraci[121] described another two-stage procedure for patients with empyemas and trapped lungs[107] or postpneumonectomy space infections. In this operation, the pleural infection is first controlled with an open window thoracostomy.

Weeks or months later, an antibiotic solution is instilled into the cavity, which is then closed at the chest wall.

Thoracoplasty is useful for selected patients with chronic empyemas and trapped lungs or bronchopleural fistulas.[122] The goal of thoracoplasty is to collapse the chest wall over the mediastinum by multiple rib resections. Originally described in the management of tuberculosis, thoracoplasty has been adapted to the management of nontuberculous empyema. Patients should have adequate nutritional and cardiorespiratory status with intrapleural sepsis controlled by chest tube drainage and antibiotics for several weeks or months.[123] Extensive experience with the procedure is required to avoid postoperative scoliosis, chronic pain, progressive respiratory insufficiency, and a mutilating cosmetic appearance.[122]

## CONCLUSION

Despite the availability of effective antimicrobial agents, thoracic empyema remains a challenging clinical problem with a persistent capacity for producing morbidity and mortality. Although the specific approaches for the evaluation and treatment of parapneumonic effusions may vary between institutions, the fundamental principles of early detection of infected pleural fluid and urgent initiation of adequate pleural drainage achieve consensus.

## REFERENCES

1. Taryle DA, Potts DE, Sahn SA: The incidence and clinical correlates of parapneumonic effusions in pneumococcal pneumonia. Chest 74:170–173, 1978.
2. Light WL, Girard WM, Jenkinson SG, et al: Parapneumonic effusions. Am J Med 69:507–512, 1980.
3. Finland M, Barnes MW: Changing etiology of acute bacterial empyema: Occurrence and mortality at Boston City Hospital during 12 selected years from 1935–1972. J Infect Dis 137:274–291, 1978.
4. De la Rocha AG: Empyema thoracis. Surg Gynecol Obstet 155:839–845, 1982.
5. Grant DR, Finley RJ: Empyema: Analysis of treatment techniques. Can J Surg 28:449–451, 1985.
6. Smith JA, Mullerworth MH, Westlake GW, et al: Empyema thoracis: 14-year experience in a teaching center. Ann Thorac Surg 51:39–42, 1991.
7. Varkey B, Rose HD, Kutty CP, et al: Empyema thoracis during a ten-year period. Arch Intern Med 141:1771–1776, 1981.
8. Jess P: Mortality in thoracic empyema. Scand J Thorac Cardiovasc Surg 18:85–90, 1981.
9. Forty J, Yeatman M, Wells FC: Empyema thoracis: A review of a 4 1/2 year experience of cases requiring surgical treatment. Respir Med 84:147–153, 1990.
10. Potts DE, Levin DC, Sahn SA: Pleural fluid pH in parapneumonic effusions. Chest 70:328–331, 1976.
11. Andrews NC, Parker EF, Shaw RR, et al: Management of nontuberculous empyema. Am Rev Respir Dis 85:935–936, 1962.
12. Wehr CJ, Adkins R Jr: Empyema thoracis: A ten-year experience. South Med J 79:171–176, 1986.
13. Bartlett JG: Bacterial infections of the pleural space. Semin Respir Infect 3:308–321, 1988.
14. Kaye MG, Fox MJ, Bartlett JG, et al: The clinical spectrum of *Staphylococcus aureus* pulmonary infection. Chest 97:788–792, 1990.
15. Bartlett J, Thadepalli H, Gorbach S, et al: Bacteriology of empyema. Lancet 1:338–340, 1974.
16. Bartlett JG, Gorbach SL, Thadepalli H, et al: Bacteriology of empyema. Lancet 1:338–340, 1974.

17. Sahn S: ''Silent'' empyema in patients receiving corticosteroids. Am Rev Respir Dis 107:873–876, 1973.
18. Bartlett JG, Finegold SM: Anaerobic infections of the lung and pleural space. Am Rev Respir Dis 110:56–77, 1974.
19. Bartlett JG: Treatment of anaerobic pleuropulmonary infections. Ann Intern Med 83:376–377, 1975.
20. Himelman RB, Callen PW: The prognostic value of loculations in parapneumonic pleural effusions. Chest 90:852–856, 1986.
21. Waite RJ, Carbonneau RJ, Balikian JP, et al: Parietal pleural changes in empyema: Appearances at CT. Radiology 175:145–150, 1990.
22. Rasmussen OS, Boris P: Ultrasound guided puncture of pleural fluid collections and superficial thoracic masses. Eur J Radiol 9:91–92, 1989.
23. O'Moore PV, Mueller PR, Simeone JF, et al: Sonographic guidance in diagnostic and therapeutic interventions in the pleural space. AJR 149:1–5, 1987.
24. Mirvis SE, Tobin KD, Kostrubiak I, et al: Thoracic CT in detecting occult disease in critically ill patients. AJR 148:685–689, 1987.
25. vanSonnenberg E, Nakamoto SK, Mueller PR, et al: CT- and ultrasound-guided catheter drainage of empyemas after chest-tube failure. Radiology 151:349–353, 1984.
26. Leung AN, Müller NL, Miller RR: CT in differential diagnosis of diffuse pleural disease. AJR 154:487–492, 1990.
27. Carrol CL, Brooke J, Federle MP, et al: CT evaluation of mediastinal infections. J Comput Assist Tomogr 11:449–454, 1987.
28. Stark DD, Federle MP, Goodman AE, et al: Differentiating lung abscess and empyema: Radiography and computed tomography. AJR 141:163–167, 1983.
29. Takasugi JE, Godwin DJ, Teefey SA: The extrapleural fat in empyema: CT appearance. Br J Radiol 64:580–583, 1991.
30. Davis SD, Henschke CI, Yankelevitz DF, et al: MR imaging of pleural effusions. J Comput Assist Tomogr 14:192–198, 1990.
31. Collins TR, Sahn SA: Thoracentesis: Clinical value, complications, technical problems, and patient experience. Chest 91:817–822, 1987.
32. Grogan DR, Irwin RS, Channick R, et al: Complications associated with thoracentesis: A prospective, randomized study comparing three different methods. Arch Intern Med 150:873–877, 1990.
33. Sahn SA: State of the art. The pleura. Am Rev Respir Dis 138:184–234, 1988.
34. Stogner SW, Campbell GD, Paulson ZD, et al: Diagnostic value of the white blood cell count in pleural effusions. Chest 100(suppl) 2:39S, 1985.
35. Light RW, MacGregor MI, Ball WC, et al: Diagnostic significance of pleural fluid pH and $Pco_2$. Chest 64:591–596, 1973.
36. Taryle DA, Good JT Jr, Sahn SA: Metabolic activity of pleural fluid: Possible role in production of pleural fluid acidosis. J Lab Clin Med 93:1041–1046, 1979.
37. Good JT Jr, Taryle DA, Maulitz RM, et al: The diagnostic value of pleural fluid pH. Chest 78:55–59, 1980.
38. Sahn SA, Reller B, Taryle DA, et al: The contribution of leukocytes and bacteria to the low pH of empyema fluid. Am Rev Respir Dis 128:811–815, 1983.
39. Sahn SA, Taryle DA, Good JT: Time course and pathogenesis of pleural fluid acidosis and low pleural fluid glucose. Am Rev Respir Dis 120:355–361, 1979.
40. Potts DE, Taryle DA, Sahn SA: The glucose-pH relationship in parapneumonic effusions. Arch Intern Med 138:1378–1380, 1978.
41. Light RW: Management of parapneumonic effusions. Chest 100:892–893, 1991.
42. Strange C, Sahn S: Management of parapneumonic pleural effusions and empyema. Infect Dis Clin North Am 5:539–559, 1991.
43. Isenstein D, Honig E: *Proteus vulgaris* empyema and increased pleural fluid pH. Chest 97:511, 1990.
44. Pine JR, Hollman JL: Elevated pleural fluid pH in *Proteus mirabilis* empyema. Chest 84:109–111, 1983.
45. Berger H, Morganroth ML: Immediate drainage is not required for all patients with complicated parapneumonic effusions. Chest 97:731–735, 1990.
46. Poe RH, Marin MG, Israel RH, et al: Utility of pleural fluid analysis in predicting tube thoracostomy decortication in parapneumonic effusions. Chest 100:963–967, 1991.
47. Wells FC: Empyema thoracis: What is the role of surgery? Respir Med 84:97–99, 1990.
48. Light RW: Pleural Disease, ed 2. Philadelphia, Lea & Febiger, 1990:139.
49. Taryle DA, Good JT, Morgan JT, et al: Antibiotic concentrations in human parapneumonic effusions. J Antimicrob Chemother 7:171–177, 1981.
50. Morgenroth A, Pfeuffer PH, Seelmann R, et al: Pleural penetration of ciprofloxacin in patients with empyema thoracis. Chest 100:406–409, 1991.
51. Thys JP, Vanderhoeft P, Herchuelz A, et al: Penetration of aminoglycosides in uninfected pleural exudates and in pleural empyemas. Chest 93:530–532, 1988.
52. Bartlett JG: Anaerobic bacterial infections of the lung. Chest 91:901–909, 1987.
53. Gudiol F, Manresa F, Pallares R, et al: Clindamycin vs penicillin for anaerobic lung infections. Arch Intern Med 150:2525–2529, 1990.
54. Mandal AK, Thadepalli H: Treatment of spontaneous bacterial empyema thoracis. J Thorac Cardiovasc Surg 94:414–418, 1987.
55. Levison ME, Mangura CT, Lorber B, et al: Clindamycin compared with penicillin for the treatment of anaerobic lung abscess. Ann Intern Med 98:466–471, 1983.
56. Eykyn SJ: The therapeutic use of metronidazole in anaerobic infection: Six years' experience in a London hospital. Surgery 93:209–214, 1983.
57. Tally FP, Sutter VL, Finegold SM: Treatment of anaerobic infections with metronidazole. Antimicrob Agents Chemother 7:672–675, 1983.
58. Miller JI: Empyema thoracis. Ann Thorac Surg 50:343–344, 1990.
59. Mayo P, Saha SP, McElvein RB: Acute empyema in children treated by open thoracotomy and decortication. Ann Thorac Surg 34:401–407, 1982.
60. Orringer MB: Thoracic empyema—Back to basics. Chest 93:901–902, 1988.
61. Lemmer JH, Botham MJ, Orringer MB: Modern management of adult thoracic empyema. J Thorac Cardiovasc Surg 90:849–855, 1985.
62. Sherman MM, Subramanian V, Berger RL: Management of thoracic empyema. Am J Surg 133:474–479, 1977.
63. Light RW: Parapneumonic effusions and empyema. Clin Chest Med 6:55–62, 1985.
64. Cohn LH, Blaisdell EW: Surgical treatment of nontuberculous empyema. Arch Surg 100:376–381, 1970.
65. Varkey B, Rose HD, Kutty CP, et al: Empyema thoracis during a ten-year period. Analysis of 72 cases and comparison to a previous study (1952–1967). Arch Intern Med 141:1771–1776, 1981.
66. Benfield GFA: Recent trends in empyema thoracis. Chest 75:358–366, 1981.
67. Sullivan KM, O'Toole RD, Fisher RH, et al: Anaerobic empyema thoracis. Arch Intern Med 131:521–527, 1973.
68. Geha AS: Pleural empyema. Changing etiologic, bacteriologic, and therapeutic aspects. J Thorac Cardiovasc Surg 61:626–635, 1971.
69. Stark DD, Federle MP, Goodman PC: CT and radiographic assessment of tube thoracostomy. AJR 141:253–258, 1983.
70. Nakaoka K, Nakahara K, Iioka S, et al: Postoperative preservation of pulmonary function in patients with chronic empyema thoracis: A one-stage operation. Ann Thorac Surg 47:848–852, 1989.
71. vanSonnenberg E, Ferrucci JT Jr, Mueller PR, et al: Percutaneous drainage of abscesses and fluid collections: Techniques, results, and applications. Radiology 141:1–10, 1982.
72. Cohen AM: Magnetic resonance imaging of the thorax. Radiol Clin North Am 22:829–846, 1984.
73. Stavas J, vanSonnenberg E, Casola G, et al: Percutaneous drainage of infected and noninfected thoracic fluid collections. J Thorac Imaging 2:80–87, 1987.
74. Milliken JS, Moore EE, Steiner E, et al: Complications of tube thoracostomy for acute trauma. Am J Surg 140:738–741, 1980.
75. Benfield GF: Recent trends in empyema thoracis. Br J Dis Chest 75:358–366, 1981.
76. Mitchell ME, Alberts WM, Chandler KW, et al: Intrapleural streptokinase in management of parapneumonic effusions: Report of series and review of literature. J Fla Med Assoc 76:1019–1022, 1989.
77. Lysy Y, Gavish A, Werczberger A, et al: Intrapleural instillation of streptokinase in the treatment of organizing empyema. Isr J Med Sci 25:284–287, 1989.
78. Aye RW, Froese DP, Hill LD: Use of purified streptokinase in empyema and hemothorax. Am J Surg 161:560–562, 1991.
79. Ogirala RG, Williams HM: Streptokinase in a loculated pleural effusion. Effectiveness determined by site of instillation. Chest 94:884–886, 1988.
80. Bergh NP, Ekroth R, Larsson S, et al: Intrapleural streptokinase in

the treatment of haemothorax and empyema. Scand J Thorac Cardio-vasc Surg 11:265–268, 1977.

81. Moulton JS, Moore PT, Mencini RA: Treatment of loculated pleural effusions with transcatheter intracavitary urokinase. AJR 153:941–945, 1989.

82. Willsie-Ediger SK, Salzman G, Reisz G, et al: Use of intrapleural streptokinase in the treatment of thoracic empyema. Am J Med Sci 300:296–300, 1990.

83. Fraedrich G, Hoffman D, Effenhauser P, et al: Instillation of fibrinolytic enzymes in the treatment of pleural empyema. J Thorac Cardiovasc Surg 30:36–38, 1982.

84. Sherry S, Tillett WS, Read CT: The use of streptokinase-streptodornase in the treatment of haemothorax. J Thorac Cardiovasc Surg 20:393–419, 1950.

85. Berglin W-O E, Ekroth R, Teger-Nilsson AC, et al: Intrapleural instillation of streptokinase effects on systemic fibrinolysis. Thorac Cardiovasc Surg 29:124–126, 1981.

86. Hunnam GR, Flower CD: Radiologically-guided percutaneous catheter drainage of empyemas. Clin Radiol 39:121–126, 1988.

87. Silverman SG, Mueller PR, Saini S, et al: Thoracic empyema: Management with image-guided catheter drainage. Radiology 169:5–9, 1988.

88. Merriam MA, Cronan JJ, Dorfman GS, et al: Radiographically guided percutaneous catheter drainage of pleural fluid collections. AJR 151:1113–1116, 1988.

89. Kerr A, Vasudevan VP, Powell S, et al: Percutaneous catheter drainage for acute empyema. Improved cure rate using CAT scan, fluoroscopy, and pigtail drainage catheters. N Y State J Med 91:4–7, 1991.

90. Crouch JD, Keagy BA, Delany DJ: ''Pigtail'' catheter drainage in thoracic surgery. Am Rev Respir Dis 136:174–175, 1987.

91. Westcott JL: Percutaneous catheter drainage of pleural effusion and empyema. AJR 144:1189–1193, 1985.

92. Ashbaugh DG: Empyema thoracis. Chest 99:1162–1165, 1991.

93. Muskett A, Burton NA, Karwande SV, et al: Management of refractory empyema with early decortication. Am J Surg 156:529–532, 1988.

94. Ali I, Unruh H: Management of empyema thoracis. Ann Thorac Surg 50:355–359, 1990.

95. Fishman NH, Ellertson DG: Early pleural decortication for thoracic empyema in immunosuppressed patients. J Thorac Cardiovasc Surg 74:537–541, 1981.

96. Spagnuolo PJ, Payne VD: Clostridial pleuropulmonary infection. Chest 78:622–625, 1980.

97. Mayo P: Early thoracotomy and decortication for nontuberculous empyema in adults with and without underlying disease: A twenty-five year review. Am J Surg 51:230–236, 1985.

98. Frimodt-Møller PC, Vejlsted H: Early surgical intervention in non-specific pleural empyema. J Thorac Cardiovasc Surg 33:41–43, 1985.

99. Muskett AD, Burton NA, Gay WA: Improved diagnostic accuracy in surgical pleural disease with computed tomography and ultrasound. Chest 89(suppl):483, 1986.

100. Neff CC, vanSonnenberg E, Lawson DW, et al: CT follow-up of empyemas: Pleural peels resolve after percutaneous catheter drainage. Radiology 176:195–197, 1990.

101. Morin JE, Munro DD, MacLean LD: Early thoracotomy for empyema. J Thorac Cardiovasc Surg 64:530–536, 1972.

102. Hoover EL, Hsu HK, Ross MJ, et al: Reappraisal of empyema thoracis. Surgical intervention when the duration of illness is unknown. Chest 90:511–515, 1986.

103. Hoff SJ, Neblett WW III, Heller RM, et al: Postpneumonic empyema in childhood: Selecting appropriate therapy. J Pediatr Surg 24:659–664, 1989.

104. Van Way III C, Narrod J, Hopeman A: The role of early limited thoracotomy in the treatment of empyema. J Thorac Cardiovasc Surg 96:436–439, 1988.

105. Ridley PD, Braimbridge MV: Thoracoscopic debridement and pleural irrigation in the management of empyema thoracis. Ann Thorac Surg 51:461–464, 1991.

106. Snow N, Lucas A, Gray LA Jr: Thoracic empyema. J Ky Med Assoc 80:653–659, 1982.

107. Bayer AJ, Wilson JAS, Chiu RCJ, et al: Clagett open-window thoracostomy in patients with empyema who had and had not undergone pneumonectomy. Can J Surg 30:329–331, 1987.

108. Adebo OA, Osinowo O: Management of empyema and broncho-pleural fistula. Trop Doct 17:26–29, 1987.

109. Weissberg D: Empyema and bronchopleural fistula. Chest 82:447–437, 1982.

110. Iverson LI, Young JN, Ecker RR, et al: Closure of bronchopleural fistulas by an omental pedicle flap. Am J Surg 152:40–42, 1986.

111. Robinson S: The treatment of chronic non-tuberculous empyema. Collect Pap Mayo Clin 7:618–644, 1915.

112. Robinson S: The treatment of chronic non-tuberculous empyema. Surg Gynecol Obstet 22:557–571, 1916.

113. Eloesser L: An operation for tuberculous empyema. Surg Gynecol Obstet 60:1096–1097, 1935.

114. Hurvitz RJ, Tucker BL: The Eloesser flap: Past and present. J Thorac Cardiovasc Surg 92:958–961, 1986.

115. Pairolero PC, Arnold PG, Trastek VF, et al: Postpneumonectomy empyema: The role of intrathoracic muscle transposition. J Thorac Cardiovasc Surg 99:958–968, 1990.

116. Stafford EG, Clagett OT: Postpneumonectomy empyema: Neomycin instillation and definitive closure. J Thorac Cardiovasc Surg 63:771–775, 1972.

117. Arnold PG, Pairolero PC: Intrathoracic muscle flaps. An account of their use in the management of 100 consecutive patients. Ann Surg 211:656–662, 1990.

118. Pairolero PC, Trastek VF: Surgical management of chronic empyema: The role of thoracoplasty. Ann Thorac Surg 50:689–690, 1990.

119. Cicero R, Del Vecchyo C, Porter JK, et al: Open window thoracostomy and plastic surgery with muscle flaps in the treatment of chronic empyema. Chest 89:374–377, 1986.

120. Shirakusa T, Ueda H, Takata S, et al: Use of pedicled omental flap in treatment of empyema. Ann Thorac Surg 50:420–424, 1990.

121. Clagett OT, Geraci JE: A procedure for the management of postpneumonectomy empyema. J Thorac Cardiovasc Surg 45:141–145, 1963.

122. Horrigan TP, Snow JN: Thoracoplasty. A current application to the infected pleural space. Ann Thorac Surg 50:695–699, 1990.

123. Gregoire R, Deslauriers, Beaulieu M, et al: Thoracoplasty: Its forgotten role in the management of nontuberculous postpneumonectomy empyema. Can J Surg 30:343–345, 1987.

# CHAPTER 22

# Nonresolving, Slowly Resolving, and Recurrent Pneumonia

STEVEN H. FEINSILVER, ALAN M. FEIN,
and MICHAEL S. NIEDERMAN

The clinician is often faced with a patient who has clinical signs consistent with infection and a radiologic infiltrate that suggests pneumonia but does not respond to treatment in the expected way. Much of the problem is related to our inability to diagnose pneumonia definitively; usually, a specific causative organism is not identified, and our treatment remains empiric, based on clinical clues and the epidemiologic setting. It is difficult to be certain about the etiologic agent, and it is often difficult to be certain that the problem is pneumonia. The clinician is often frustrated by a pneumonia that is slow to resolve, that appears not to be resolving, or that recurs.

A slowly resolving pneumonia is one that responds to optimal therapy but in a period considered excessively long. This includes slow resolution of clinical signs and symptoms or slow clearing of the chest radiograph. This definition requires some agreement about the expected rate of resolution for pneumonia, but data for rates of resolution of pneumonia are available only for some of the more common causes.

Nonresolving pneumonia is defined as focal, radiographic infiltrates that begin with clear clinical signs of acute pulmonary infection (eg, fever, sputum production, malaise, dyspnea) and do not resolve radiographically in the expected time.[1] A knowledge of the natural history of pneumonia is required, because nonresolution and slow resolution are overlapping problems. These are addressed together for most of this chapter, although the distinction is sometimes useful in formulating a differential diagnosis and approach to the problem.

Recurrent pneumonia can be defined as distinct episodes of pneumonia with fever, infiltrates, and leukocytosis, occurring in the same patient at least twice within 1 year. The definition requires complete resolution for at least 1 month between bouts to differentiate recurrent from relapsing or nonresolving pneumonia. By limiting the definition to pneumonias recurring within 1 year, it is more likely that recurrences will be related pathophysiologically.

## PATTERNS OF SLOWLY RESOLVING AND NONRESOLVING PNEUMONIAS

At the Winthrop-University Hospital in Mineola, New York, approximately 15% of all pulmonary consultations and 10% of fiberoptic bronchoscopies are done to evaluate focal radiographic infiltrates that have failed to resolve or are resolving atypically. These investigations represent a substantial expenditure of resources, compounded by lengthy hospitalizations, other diagnostic studies, and prolonged antibiotic therapy. Pneumococcal pneumonia, the most common cause of community-acquired pneumonia, accounts for 400,000 to 500,000 cases each year.

This problem is not new. In Osler and McCrae's *Modern Medicine* (1913), Norris writes, "The duration of lobar pneumonia ranges from one day to three weeks. . . . In contradistinction to brief or abortive pneumonia we have delayed resolution, migratory and recurrent pneumonias. . . . Delayed resolution was reported in 105 among 2548 cases."[2] This observation was based on clinical signs, because radiographs were infrequently available. Norris observed delayed resolution "chiefly in old and debilitated subjects." He appropriately cautioned that delayed resolution may be simulated by diseases other than lobar pneumonia, which at that time was primarily tuberculosis. The main issues in the approach to slowly resolving or nonresolving pneumonia were well formulated in 1913. How fast should pneumonias resolve, and when should other diagnoses be considered?

Several decades later, Amberson[3] wrote, "If the patient survives pneumonia, due to pneumococcus, it should be expected to resolve in the usual way. If it does not, pneumococcus as such is not primarily implicated." Amberson divided the possible causes for nonresolution into four categories: complicated pneumococcal infection (eg, abscess, empyema), other infections (eg, anaerobes, tuberculosis, fungi), poor bronchial clearance (eg, bronchiectasis, foreign body), and inherent disease of the pulmonary parenchyma. His differential diagnosis remains essentially valid. Failure of an infiltrate to resolve may be caused by failure of host defenses, an unusual or virulent pathogen, or a noninfectious problem.

What is normal resolution? Establishing a specific cause for pneumonia is difficult. Bacteremia is uncommon in pneumococcal pneumonia and *Haemophilus* pneumonia, and it is extremely rare in atypical pneumonia.[4-6] Sputum is often unobtainable because of ineffective expectoration or uninterpretable because of upper airway contamination. History, a chest radiograph, and epidemiology may be the only way to establish a working diagnosis. Definitive data on the rate of resolution of pneumonia are not available, but our current estimates are given in Table 22–1. What is known about the natural history of some of the more common pneumonias follows.

## Pneumococcal Pneumonia

*Streptococcus pneumoniae* still accounts for between 40% and 60% of cases of community-acquired pneumonia.[7-10] The resolution for pneumonia in general is often measured against our knowledge of the natural history of pneumococcal pneumonia.

Several studies have demonstrated that microaspiration is probably the most important cause of community-acquired and institutionally acquired pneumonia.[11, 12] Structural neu-

rologic disease, metabolic encephalopathy, and the use of sedative and hypnotic medications increase the risk of aspiration. Acute pneumonia frequently starts in the most dependent pulmonary segments, where aspiration is most likely to occur.

Failure of the host defenses to control the replicating organism in the lung leads to spread to the bloodstream or thoracic duct, eventually reaching other sites, including the pleura, meninges, or valvular endothelium. With these complications, recovery is often prolonged, and mortality is increased, particularly in the elderly.[8, 13, 14] The cellular and molecular biologic factors responsible for normal resolution are being investigated. Neutrophils are found in the early lesion. Macrophages appear and later take up and degrade potential leukocyte mediators and enzymes and degrade fibrin. In animal models of pneumococcal pneumonia, the persistence of organisms in the lung appears to interfere with transformation of type II cells and inhibition of fibroblast proliferation, delaying resolution and promoting fibrosis.[15]

Although clinical and radiologic improvements are often expected shortly after the initiation of antibiotic therapy, they usually do not occur. Abnormal physical signs and fever were reported even after 2 weeks in the preantibiotic era.[16-18] Delayed radiographic resolution of *S. pneumoniae* infection is now most frequently seen in the elderly, whose radiographs often remain abnormal although the patient no longer has signs of systemic illness.[19-21] In MacFarlane's series, bacteremic pneumococcal pneumonia was more common in older patients, most of whose radiographs worsened after the initiation of therapy.[20] Although only 50% of all chest roentgenograms in this study were normal at 9 weeks, younger, nonbacteremic patients usually had normal chest roentgenograms by 5 weeks. Residual atelectasis and pleural-based abnormalities were present at 2 months in approximately one third of patients in the older group but occurred in fewer than 10% of younger patients.

The resolution of bacteremic pneumococcal pneumonia was compared in patients older or younger than 50 years of age by Jay and associates.[22] Chronic obstructive pulmonary disease (COPD) was more common in those older than 50, but alcoholism was common in those younger than 50 years of age. However, 40% of the younger patients without host defense impairment had abnormal chest roentgenograms at 2 weeks. Consolidation was seen at 1 month in approximately one third of the patients. Persistent fever, leukocytosis beyond 1 week, COPD, and alcoholism were significantly associated with delayed radiographic resolution (Fig. 22–1). Age com-

Table 22–1. **Resolution of Common Pneumonias**

| Infecting Organism | Initial Radiographic Worsening | Time to Resolution (months) | Residual Radiographic Abnormalities |
|---|---|---|---|
| *Streptococcus pneumoniae* | | | |
|   Bacteremic | Majority | 3–5 | 25%–35% |
|   Nonbacteremic | Occasional | 1–3 | Rare |
| Group B streptococci | Common | 1–3 | Common |
| *Staphylococcus aureus* | Majority | 3–5 | Common |
| *Haemophilus influenzae* | Occasional | 1–5 | Occasional |
| *Legionella* | Majority | 3–5 | 25% |
| *Chlamydia* TWAR | Rare | 1–3 | Occasional |
| *Moraxella catarrhalis* | Rare | 1–3 | Uncommon |
| Enteric gram-negative organisms | Occaisonal | 3–5 | 10%–20% |
| Viruses | Variable | Variable | Occasional fibrosis, bronchiolitis obliterans organizing pneumonia (?) |

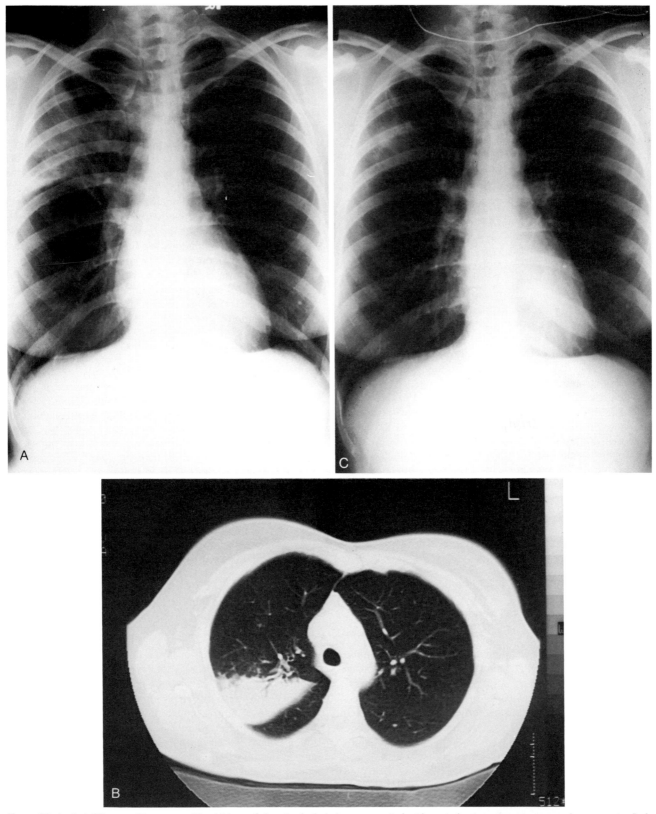

**Figure 22–1.** *A,* A 39-year-old woman with a history of chronic alcohol abuse presented with acute bacteremic pneumococcal pneumonia. *B,* A computed tomographic scan performed 3 weeks after discharge demonstrated a persistent right upper lobe infiltrate. The infiltrate persisted for 12 weeks despite clinical improvement. *C,* The diagnosis was slowly resolving bacteremic pneumococcal pneumonia.

pounded host defense impairments. At 14 weeks, 60% of those older than 50 with alcoholism and COPD had abnormal chest roentgenograms, compared with 10% of those younger than 50 years of age. Bronchogenic carcinoma was not found as the cause of delayed resolution in any patient.

In our series, abnormal resolution of community-acquired pneumonia (ie, delayed >1 month) was highly associated with increased age (>55 years), unilateral infiltrates, and smoking.[23]

*S. pneumoniae* is probably responsible for most slowly resolving pneumonias. Initially, the chest roentgenogram may worsen despite appropriate antibiotic chemotherapy. Age, smoking, and comorbid illness, especially alcoholism and COPD, often delay resolution of the chest radiograph beyond 4 weeks. Most patients will have normal chest radiographs within 12 weeks.

## *Legionella* Pneumonia

*Legionella pneumophila* has a spectrum of presentation, ranging from atypical pneumonia to severe sepsis and multiorgan failure. The latter syndrome is more common in elderly and immunocompromised patients in hospitals and in the community. *Legionella* infection is more common in smokers and those with underlying pulmonary, cardiac, renal, or neoplastic disease.[20, 24–26] Multiorgan involvement and electrolyte disturbance are characteristic of severe *Legionella* infection. Patchy infiltrates may progress to confluence, often bilaterally. There appear to be no radiologic features that reliably differentiate *Legionella* from other causes of pneumonia.[25, 27] Radiologic deterioration occurred in two thirds of patients with *Legionella* infections and persisted for as long as 2 weeks in one series.[25] Macfarlane reported that only 50% of chest roentgenograms were normal at 10 weeks.[20] Radiographic resolution rarely occurs after 2 weeks of illness, but it can take as long as 1 year. Fibrosis may result, and generalized weakness and fatigue can persist for months.[20, 27]

## *Haemophilus influenzae* Pneumonia

*H. influenzae* is a special threat to the elderly and immunosuppressed.[4, 6, 28] COPD patients and alcoholics are particularly prone to *H. influenzae* infection. Encapsulated strains are more likely to produce severe sepsis and death, and unencapsulated strains cause febrile tracheobronchitis. In one surveillance study, 71% of *H. influenzae* pneumonias occurred in patients who were severely immunocompromised. Most who developed a severe course were 50 years of age or older.[8] Nontypable organisms (ie, unencapsulated) are associated with a more chronic course and lower initial mortality rate.[29]

Because *H. influenzae* pneumonia is more common in the elderly and immunosuppressed, resolution and hospitalization are often prolonged for 2 to 3 weeks. Approximately one half do not return to their previous level of functioning after 6 weeks.[8, 29]

## Enteric Gram-Negative Rod Pneumonia

Pneumonia caused by enteric gram-negative organisms is common in the elderly in community, nursing home, and hospital settings.[30–33] Oropharyngeal colonization with gram-negative organisms increases with decreasing physiologic function and increasing age. Comorbid illnesses, especially COPD, bronchiectasis, malignancy, and diabetes, increase the risk of colonization with these organisms.[12] In these infections, gram-negative organisms are frequently mixed with other organisms.[31, 34]

No radiologic picture of pneumonia caused by enteric gram-negative organisms is characteristic, although upper lobe consolidation with ''bulging fissures'' was reported initially as a classic finding in *Klebsiella* pneumonia. Of community-acquired pneumonias caused by enteric organisms, *Klebsiella* pneumonia has probably been best described and may account for up to 10% of pneumonias in some debilitated populations (eg, nursing homes). Abscess formation is common (15%–50%) and develops within 2 weeks. Resolution is likely to be prolonged because of the virulence of the organism and impaired state of most afflicted patients. Necrosis occurs frequently, and residual fibrosis commonly develops.

## *Staphylococcus aureus* Pneumonia

The incidence of *S. aureus* pneumonia may be increasing. In the community, infection with this organism often follows influenza or other viral upper respiratory infections.[35] It is a common pathogen causing community-acquired pneumonia requiring intensive care.[36] Kaye and co-workers reported that 87% of cases of staphylococcal pneumonia occurred in patients older than 50 years of age and that 81% of cases were nosocomial.[37] Bilateral lower lobe involvement with pleural effusion was the most common radiographic pattern. Cavitary infiltrates may lead to confusion with gram-negative rod pneumonia, and the pattern of resolution with residual fibrosis and scarring is similar for both.

## Viral Pneumonia

Viruses cause infection in the lung, and they may facilitate the acquisition or delay the resolution of bacterial pneumonia, especially in very young and very old patients. Respiratory syncytial virus (RSV) infection has been identified as a cause of severe pneumonia in elderly patients with COPD.[38, 39] Prolonged fever (5–10 days) is common, although death is unusual unless bacterial superinfection occurs. Viral infection may be atypical in the elderly, causing cough, headache, and pneumonia more frequently than chills, fever, and myalgias.[35] Superinfection with pneumococcus, *S. aureus,* and *H. influenzae* often complicates influenza, obscuring assessment of the cause and delaying resolution.

Viral pneumonia can result in bronchitis, bronchiolitis, bronchiectasis, and pulmonary fibrosis. Bronchiolitis obliterans organizing pneumonia (BOOP) may be the result of abnormal healing of viral pulmonary infection, which is discussed later in this chapter.

## Other Organisms Causing Pneumonias

Mycoplasmal pneumonia is the classic atypical pneumonia and a common cause of community-acquired pneumonia. Interstitial infiltrates progress to confluent involvement of multiple lobes in most patients. Resolution is usually rapid compared with other common lower respiratory infections. Complete resolution usually occurs by 8 weeks, and residual fibrosis is an unusual finding.

Chlamydial infection with the TWAR strain is also a common cause of community-acquired pneumonia, especially in young adults. Involvement of a single lobe is usual, but pleural effusion and atelectasis occur sporadically.[40] Data on the resolution of TWAR pneumonia may be estimated from studies on psittacosis, another chlamydial infection. Although psittacosis is generally associated with contact with infected birds, as many as one third of patients have no history of contact. Resolution of psittacosis can be faster than for *Legionella* infection, with 50% of chest roentgenograms appearing normal by 4 weeks.[20] However, in another study, 45% of patients took longer than 6 weeks to clear infections, and approximately 20% took longer than 9 weeks.[41]

*Branhamella (Moraxella) catarrhalis* leads to an atypical pneumonia syndrome in the elderly, in smokers, and in those with COPD, cancer, or malnutrition.[42] Infection generally affects those in the seventh and eighth decades of life. Dyspnea, cough, and chest pain are common, but severe sepsis and respiratory failure are uncommon. Interstitial and alveolar infiltrates usually develop. Typical lobar consolidation and pleural effusion also occur. Most patients have associated obstructive lung disease, atelectasis, or tumor, making resolution of the pneumonia difficult to assess. The mortality rate is high during the first 3 months after the onset of infection. Resolution is slow, and evaluation is compounded by underlying pulmonary pathology.

Group B streptococci produce severe infection in very elderly and debilitated patients, particularly those with diabetes, heart failure, or neurologic disease. Bacteremia is common, and the mortality rate exceeds 50%.[43] The disease of survivors may be expected to resolve in a fashion similar to that of *S. aureus* infection.

## NONRESOLUTION

### Unusual Infectious Causes

If an infiltrate fails to resolve, the process may be caused by an infectious organism that is not diagnosed or treated by the usual methods. We include in this group the higher-order bacteria and fungi (Table 22–2). It would be unreasonable to search for these organisms in all patients with pneumonia. The workup must be guided by knowledge of the presentation and natural history of these infections.

### Tuberculosis

The incidence of tuberculosis in the United States is increasing.[44] Because a frequent presentation of tuberculosis is that of a pneumonia with a poor response to antibiotics, attention should be paid to this possibility, particularly in the elderly and in persons infected with the human immunodeficiency virus.

The typical radiographic presentation is a cavitary infiltrate in the apical or posterior segments of one or both upper lobes. Khan and colleagues[45] found that 34% of all patients with newly diagnosed tuberculosis presented with atypical radiographs in a series that predated the recognition of the acquired immunodeficiency syndrome (AIDS). Unusual localized interstitial and miliary infiltrates are especially common in tuberculosis complicating AIDS. Skin testing and sputum examination remain the principal clinical tools for diagnosing tuberculosis, but the results of tuberculin testing may be negative in 10% to 20% of patients with active disease, especially in the elderly.[46]

### Atypical Mycobacteria

The presentation of atypical mycobacterial infection may be indistinguishable from *Mycobacterium tuberculosis*. However, atypical mycobacteria rarely cause disease in a host with normal lungs and normal host defenses. Except among patients with AIDS, disease from the atypical mycobacteria is predominantly seen in middle-aged or elderly patients with preexisting chronic lung disease, and dissemination is extremely rare. Because elderly patients with chronic lung disease may be colonized with atypical organisms, the diagnosis of infection generally requires culturing the organism from sputum at least three times for a patient with a compatible chest radiograph. Treatment is difficult and may require multiple drugs and surgery.

### Nocardia and Actinomyces

*Nocardia* and *Actinomyces*, which are higher-order bacteria, behave clinically in ways more typical of the fungi. Their diagnosis can be made by sputum culture, but the clinician must be aware of some specific culture requirements to facilitate the diagnosis.

*Nocardia* is a gram-positive and variably acid-fast orga-

**Table 22–2. Unusual Infectious Causes of Nonresolving or Slowly Resolving Pneumonia**

| Organism | Clinical Clues |
| --- | --- |
| *Mycobacterium tuberculosis* | Tuberculin skin test, acid-fast smear and culture of sputum |
| Atypical mycobacteria | Rare with normal lungs and normal host defenses |
| *Nocardia* | Branching filamentous pseudohyphae; culture aerobically for 4 weeks |
| *Actinomyces* | "Sulfur granules" in sputum; may invade chest wall and drain |
| Endemic fungi (eg, *Histoplasma*) | Serologic testing may be useful; skin test for histoplasmosis |
| Nonendemic fungi (eg, *Aspergillus*) | Can culture but may be colonization; invasive disease in severely immunocompromised patients |

nism with branching filamentous pseudohyphae. It is grown aerobically, but culture may take as long as 4 weeks; the microbiology laboratory should be informed if this organism is suspected. Chest radiographs most typically show a localized alveolar infiltrate that is nonsegmental and may cavitate.[47] The clinical presentation is a chronic illness with cough, purulent sputum, and low-grade fever. The most common nonpulmonary infection is brain abscess. *Nocardia* may be seen in immunocompromised persons, and the organism frequently infects those with pulmonary alveolar proteinosis.

Clinical actinomycosis is most commonly caused by *Actinomyces israelli,* which is found in the normal oropharynx. Like *Nocardia, Actimomyces* is a gram-positive organism, but it is less likely to be acid fast. ''Sulfur granules'' in sputum may suggest the diagnosis. The organism spreads through the lung without regard to the usual anatomy of lobes or fissures, and it may spread to or through the chest wall. Culture requires strict anaerobic conditions and enriched media. Other clinical and radiographic features are similar to those of *Nocardia.*

### Fungi

The common fungal diseases occur in specific endemic areas but share many clinical characteristics. *Histoplasma capsulatum* is found along the Mississippi River valley and other river valleys throughout the world; *Coccidioides immitis* is confined to California and the U.S. Southwest; and *Blastomyces dermatitidis* is endemic to the U.S. Southeast. In endemic areas, most inhabitants have immunologic evidence of previous infection but remain asymptomatic.

Each of these fungi may cause an acute, nonspecific illness with fever, chills, and cough (eg, San Joaquin Valley fever). Because serologic confirmation is required for a specific diagnosis, many cases are initially confused with community-acquired bacterial pneumonia. The greatest diagnostic difficulties are caused by the development of chronic pulmonary infiltrates. These usually affect the upper lobe and are cavitary, and they are easily confused with tuberculosis. Coccidiodomycosis classically produces a thin-walled cavity near the pleural surface. The radiographic appearance of blastomycosis frequently mimics that of pneumonia.[48, 49] These fungi cannot be reliably separated radiographically. The diagnosis can be made by potassium hydroxide smear and culture of sputum in many cases. Serologic testing may be useful. In coccidiodomycosis, IgM antibodies become positive in the first few weeks of an infection and disappear in about 1 month. Complement-fixing IgG appears late in primary disease or several months later. High or rising antibody titers carry a poor prognosis. Skin testing for histoplasmosis reflects past or current infection and is positive in more than 90% of the population in highly endemic areas.

*Aspergillus* may cause several distinct forms of pulmonary disease that may result in a nonresolving pneumonia. Chronic necrotizing aspergillosis, a semiinvasive form of infection,[50] shares some features of invasive aspergillosis and mycetoma formation and is most commonly seen in elderly patients with underlying chronic lung disease. The disease appears most commonly as a necrotizing upper lobe infiltrate that slowly progresses. Diagnosis is based on culture of the fungus bronchoscopically or by percutaneous needle aspiration in a patient with a compatible radiograph and clinical course. Serologic tests are supportive but not diagnostic; *Aspergillus* precipitins are positive in almost all cases.

Invasive pulmonary aspergillosis is usually seen in severely neutropenic patients undergoing chemotherapy for leukemia. However, some reports have stressed that nonresolving or progressive pneumonia caused by *Aspergillus* may develop in the community setting in elderly COPD patients receiving corticosteroids. In one series, patients were treated for an average of 18 days with multiple broad-spectrum antibiotics for presumed bacterial pneumonia.[51] *Aspergillus* was recognized only postmortem in most cases.

## Noninfectious Causes

Almost every diagnostic entity in pulmonary medicine has at some time been confused with a slowly resolving or nonresolving pneumonia. We consider here some of the more common differential diagnostic possibilities for persistent radiographic abnormalities that may begin with fever, cough, or sputum production (Table 22–3).

### Neoplasm

Bronchogenic carcinoma presenting with a totally or partially occluding mass and postobstructive pneumonia is the most important possibility in this category (Fig. 22–2). However, bronchogenic carcinoma is a distinctly uncommon finding in all series of nonresolving pneumonia. Patients in a high-risk group for carcinoma with nonresolving or slowly resolving pneumonia should have fiberoptic bron-

Table 22–3. **Noninfectious Diagnoses Confused With Nonresolving Pneumonia**

| Diagnosis | Clinical Clues |
| --- | --- |
| Neoplasm | |
|   Bronchogenic carcinoma | Risk factors (eg, smoking, age) |
|   Bronchoalveolar cell carcinoma | Bronchorrhea; lavage cytology produces high yield |
|   Lymphoma | Associated mediastinal or hilar adenopathy; fever, weight loss |
| Immunologic and idiopathic disorders | |
|   Wegener granulomatosis | Sinus, upper airway, or renal disease; antineutrophil cytoplasmic antibodies |
|   Bronchocentric granulomatosis | Wheezing |
|   Bronchiolitis obliterans organizing pneumonia | May follow viral illness |
| Thromboembolism | Slowly shrinking infiltrate |
| Inhalational conditions (eg, foreign body, lipid) | History |
| Drug-induced lung disease | History |

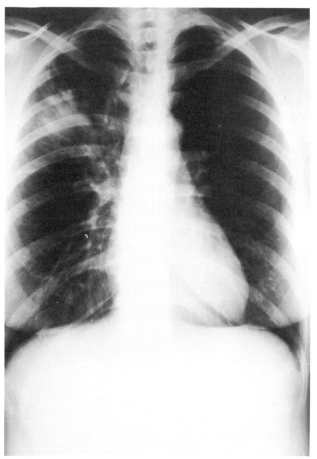

**Figure 22–2.** A 75-year-old woman presented with a nonresolving pulmonary infiltrate. Her illness had begun 2 months previously with cough, purulent sputum, and a low-grade fever. The failure of the chest roentgenogram to show any improvement prompted bronchoscopy, which revealed squamous cell carcinoma occluding the right upper lobe bronchus. The diagnosis was bronchogenic carcinoma.

choscopy performed. Unless there are compelling clinical reasons, the procedure is best delayed for at least a few weeks while antibiotic therapy is given. Benign lesions such as adenomas and papillomas may also present this way, and a few tumors, especially breast, renal cell, and gastrointestinal carcinomas, may metastasize endobronchially.

Bronchoalveolar cell carcinoma in about one third of cases presents with lobar consolidation, frequently with air bronchograms.[52] Most patients present with cough, which may be copious (ie, bronchorrhea). Because the tumor grows as a thin layer inside the alveoli, endobronchial masses are not seen at bronchoscopy, but lavage for cytology is a sensitive test.

The lymphomas are commonly associated with disease in the chest, but parenchymal lung disease is seen in fewer than 12% of cases of Hodgkin disease and 4% of non-Hodgkin lymphomas at time of the initial diagnoses.[53] Associated mediastinal or hilar adenopathy is an important clue; in one series, all patients with Hodgkin disease and parenchymal involvement also had adenopathy in the chest.[54] Lung disease is seen in five patterns: direct extension from involved nodes, poorly defined small nodules extending from the hila, cavitating masses, segmental and lobar infiltrates, and interstitial disease. Segmental or lobar infiltrates in lymphoma can easily be mistaken for pneumonia, especially because most patients have fever. Bronchoscopic biopsies are rarely adequate for the diagnosis of lymphoma, and open lung biopsy usually is required.

### Immunologic and Idiopathic Disorders

Wegener granulomatosis is most often thought of as presenting with multiple nodules that may cavitate, but a review of the experience of the National Institutes of Health shows slightly more patients present with infiltrates than with nodules.[55] Almost one half of the episodes of Wegener granulomatosis in this series were associated with cough, fever occurred in about one half of patients during the course of their illness, and most had leukocytosis. This disease could easily be confused with acute pneumonia, and our own experience suggests this may be common.[56] A helpful radiographic clue is the tendency of some lesions to spontaneously regress while others worsen. Sinus, upper airway, or renal disease should point to this diagnosis.[57] Serologic testing for antineutrophil cytoplasmic antibodies appears to be a sensitive and specific tool for this disorder.[58]

Bronchocentric granulomatosis denotes an intense inflammatory reaction surrounding proximal bronchi or bronchioles with granuloma formation. The pathologic findings are similar, if not identical, to allergic bronchopulmonary aspergillosis in which the inflammation represents a reaction to *Aspergillus*.[59] Wheezing is a common finding in both illnesses. Nodules are most commonly seen on chest radiographs, but alveolar infiltrates and consolidation are also commonly seen, particularly in upper lung fields.[60]

Patients with idiopathic BOOP commonly present with several weeks of cough, dyspnea, and fatigue.[61] Persistent symptoms and infiltrates may suggest a slowly resolving viral pneumonia. Although BOOP may represent a nonspecific pattern of dysfunctional resolution of lung injury, it is likely that in some cases it is the sequela of a viral or mycoplasma infection.[62] Radiographs generally show alveolar filling and nodular infiltrates in two thirds of patients, but diffuse interstitial opacities are also seen in one third. In one series, 10 of 14 patients showed consolidation on computed tomographic scans of the chest.[63] Recurrent infiltrates are common. Because there are no specific laboratory tests, a definitive diagnosis requires an open lung biopsy. The prognosis with steroid treatment is thought to be considerably better than in the other interstitial diseases,[64] and an empiric trial of corticosteroids may be warranted.

### Thromboembolism

Segmental infiltrates can be caused by pulmonary embolism with infarction, although a clear chest roentgenogram is more common. Infiltrates are commonly peripheral, abutting the pleural surface, and are more likely in the elderly and those with heart failure. The classic "Hampton's hump," a truncated cone pointing at the hilum, is rarely seen. The resulting infiltrate may resolve gradually over several weeks and has been described as shrinking slowly, like a melting ice cube, rather than breaking up like a typical pneumonia.[65]

## Inhalational Conditions

Aspiration of a foreign body may cause postobstructive atelectasis and consolidation (Fig. 22–3). Aspiration of exogenous lipid (eg, mineral oil, oily nose drops) can cause chronic or recurrent lipid pneumonia. The pulmonary reaction to lipid depends on the aspirated material, with mineral oil and animal fats leading to inflammation and fibrosis. Cough is more common than systemic complaints.[66] Atelectasis and mixed interstitial and alveolar infiltrates, usually in the lower lobes, are seen. Fat droplets in macrophages can be recovered by bronchial lavage.

## Drug-Induced Pulmonary Disease

The mechanisms and pattern of drug-induced pulmonary disease are enormously varied. Alveolar consolidation is easily confused with pneumonia. One example of a drug that may cause a picture of alveolar consolidation is amiodarone; pulmonary toxicity from this drug is becoming increasingly common as it is more widely used. Because the drug is frequently used for life-threatening arrhythmias, the clinician may be willing to accept substantial toxicity. In these patients, differentiating pulmonary toxicity from congestive heart failure is difficult. Two radiologic patterns

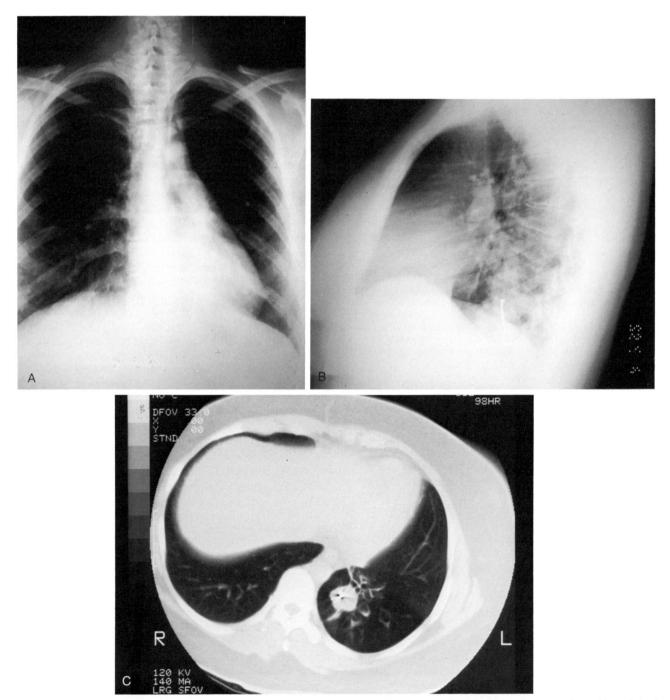

**Figure 22–3.** *A,* A 25-year-old woman presented with a history of chronic cough and sputum production. *B,* The posteroanterior and lateral chest roentgenograms revealed a left lateral lobe infiltrate and an aspirated nail. *C,* The computed tomographic scan performed 3 weeks later demonstrated a dense area of consolidation and bronchiectasis adjacent to a foreign body. The diagnosis was foreign body aspiration.

are seen: diffuse interstitial disease and localized alveolar filling. These may occur simultaneously.[67] Fever and leukocytosis occur, suggesting an acute infectious pneumonia. Although a reduced diffusion capacity is a sensitive indicator of amiodarone lung toxicity, it lacks specificity, and the diagnosis is often one of exclusion. Bronchoscopy may reveal foamy alveolar macrophages.

## Approach to Managing Nonresolution

Before embarking on a workup for a slowly resolving or nonresolving pneumonia, two questions should be addressed. Is the rate of resolution really abnormal? This determination assumes that a definitive diagnosis has been made, which is often not the case, and that the natural history of the pneumonia is well understood. Radiographic resolution of many common pneumonias is actually a slower process than is generally appreciated, and resolution generally lags behind clinical improvement. The second question is whether deficient host defenses are to blame. They may range from obvious problems such as cystic fibrosis to more subtle conditions such as diabetes or alcoholism. Slow resolution is more likely to be caused by a defect in host defenses than by a noninfectious disorder or bronchial obstruction.

Nonresolving pneumonia is a relatively common indication for fiberoptic bronchoscopy. We reviewed our experience with 35 consecutive patients bronchoscoped because of failure of pneumonia to improve after what was considered adequate antibiotic therapy.[23] All had radiographic infiltrates, cough, and either fever, leukocytosis, or sputum production. Fourteen ultimately had a specific diagnosis made that accounted for the prolonged course (Table 22–4). Bronchoscopy was diagnostic for 12 (86%) of these patients. The remaining 21 had no specific diagnosis other

Table 22–4. **Final Diagnoses in 35 Patients With Nonresolving Pneumonia**

| Diagnosis | No. of Patients |
| --- | --- |
| *Pneumocystis carinii* pneumonia | 3 |
| Tuberculosis | 2 |
| Bronchoalveolar carcinoma | 2 |
| Adenocarcinoma | 2 |
| Cytomegalovirus | 1 |
| Actinomycosis | 1 |
| Eosinophilic pneumonia | 1 |
| Wegener granulomatosis | 1 |
| Bronchiolitis obliterans organizing pneumonia | 1 |
| Slowly resolving pneumonia (ie, no other diagnosis) | 21 |

From Feinsilver SH, Fein AM, Niederman MS, Schultz E, Faegenburg DH: Utility of fiberoptic bronchoscopy in non-resolving pneumonia. Chest 98:1322–1326, 1990.

than infectious pneumonia. We concluded that fiberoptic bronchoscopy was useful in establishing a cause for failure of apparent pneumonia to resolve. The yield for a specific diagnosis was highest in patients who were young nonsmokers and who had multilobar radiographic abnormalities and symptoms present for at least 4 to 6 weeks. Older patients with a history of smoking, COPD, or immune defect and lobar or segmental infiltrates could be observed without bronchoscopy, because the diagnostic yield for this substantial subset of patients was minimal. Our recommended approach to the problem of slowly resolving or nonresolving pneumonia is summarized in Figure 22–4.

## RECURRENT PNEUMONIA

Many systemic and thoracic diseases associated with nonresolving or slowly resolving pneumonia may also cause recurrent lower respiratory tract infection. Often the

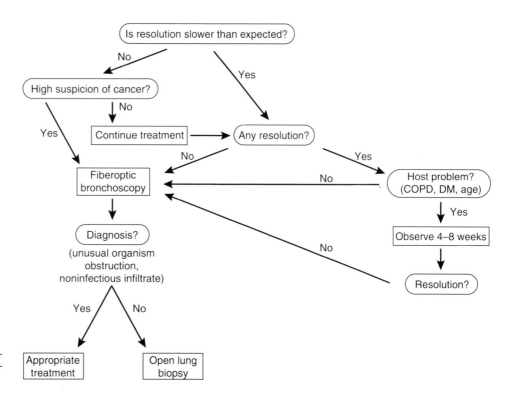

**Figure 22–4.** The approach to nonresolving or slowly resolving pneumonia.

Table 22–5. **Causes of Recurrent Pneumonia**

| Location | Pathophysiology | Examples |
|---|---|---|
| Single lobe | Obstruction | Foreign body, cancer, lymph node |
| | Parenchymal disease | Bronchiectasis, sequestration, bronchogenic cyst |
| Multiple lobes | Aspiration | Central nervous system disease, neuromuscular disease, esophageal pathology |
| | Immunodeficiency | Antibody deficiency, complement deficiency |
| | Mucociliary dysfunction | Cystic fibrosis, primary ciliary dyskinesia |
| | Congenital | Tracheobronchomegaly |
| | Inflammatory | Asthma, allergic bronchopulmonary aspergillosis |
| | Systemic illness | Diabetes |

distinction between nonresolving and recurrent pneumonia depends more on the acuity of the clinical observation than on the pathophysiology. In this section, some of the processes that are more likely to cause recurrent pneumonia are discussed.

## Causes and Patterns of Disease

The problem of recurrent pneumonia is not sufficiently addressed by modern studies. Much of the older literature dealt with recurrent community-acquired infectious pneumonia, rather than the inflammatory and immunologic processes that have assumed greater significance in recent years.

In 1969, Winterbauer and colleagues described 158 adults with infectious causes of recurrent pneumonia, defined as fever, infiltrates, and leukocytosis with at least 1 month between bouts.[68] One quarter of the patients had three or more episodes. More than one half were older than 50 years of age; younger patients were more likely to have systemic than local thoracic host defense impairment associated with recurrent pneumonia. Alcoholism, congestive heart failure, and diabetes were the most common systemic host defense impairments. Bronchiectasis and COPD were the most common local defense impairments.

Recurrent pneumonia also affects children. In one report, multiple episodes of pneumonia (primarily pneumococcal) were approximately twice as common in children younger than 15 years of age as in adults, with the outcome related to the number of comorbid illnesses.[69] In another study of 18 children with recurrent pneumonia (average age, 5.7 years), 44% had inherited immune or metabolic disorders.[70] Only 4 of 18 had structural diseases of the lung.

The presentation of recurrent pneumonia depends on the nature of the underlying predisposition. Finland[71] could find no difference in the clinical presentation between initial and recurrent infections. The incidence of bacteremia in recurrent infections was reduced. In an animal model of recurrent pneumococcal infection, the durations of illness and bacteremia were decreased, but the neutrophil response was increased in the episode of reinfection.[72]

The bacteriology of recurrent pneumonia depends on the underlying cause. Recurrent aspiration pneumonia may be caused by anaerobic organisms in the community setting or mixed anaerobic and gram-negative flora in the hospital setting. One report described the risk of recurrent *Pseudomonas* infection in the intensive care unit in COPD patients who required prolonged mechanical ventilation.[73] Recurrent infection by encapsulated organisms may occur in the setting of asplenia, alcoholism, or multiple myeloma. Patients with AIDS are at increased risk for recurrent *Pneumocystis carinii* and bacterial pneumonia (encapsulated organisms).[74–77] Oseasohn and Winterbauer reported pneumococcus to be the most common cause of recurrent pneumonia, but there have been no studies to confirm these observations.[68, 69]

A useful clinical distinction can be made between pneumonias that recur in a single area of the lung and those that involve multiple areas. An outline of some of the more common causes of recurrent pneumonia is given in Table 22–5.

Recurrence in the same lobe often implies local thoracic pathology. Intraluminal obstruction as typified by foreign body aspiration is a common problem in children younger than 3 years of age and usually involves aspiration of vegetable material, such as peanuts, corn, and carrots.[78, 79] The aspiration may be unrecognized because weeks may elapse before the first episode of pneumonia occurs. Because of bronchial anatomy, adults more frequently aspirate on the right side than children. A case report described a 14-year-old boy with recurrent episodes of lobar pneumonia and hemoptysis, which on biopsy proved to be caused by the aspiration of a plastic component of a pen that had occurred approximately 2 years before the first episode.[80] Other causes of intraluminal obstruction include bronchial adenomas[81] and endobronchial lipomas. Any long-standing process obstructing a bronchus may result in secondary bronchiectasis and recurrent infection. Although endobronchial obstruction caused by carcinoma may produce a similar process, patients generally have nonresolving rather than recurrent infection, which is perhaps a reflection of the limited life expectancy.

Mediastinal or hilar adenopathy secondary to tuberculosis or fungal infections may cause extraluminal bronchial narrowing leading to recurrent pneumonia. This right middle lobe syndrome results in recurrent lobar consolidation due to impaired drainage of the right middle lobe by surrounding lymph nodes.[82, 83] Localized bronchiectasis may cause recurrent pneumonia. The chronically inflamed area cannot be effectively cleared, leading to repeated episodes of bacterial infection. Previous episodes of pertussis, tuberculosis, adenovirus infection, or measles have been associated with secondary bronchiectasis.[84]

Bronchopulmonary sequestrations and bronchial cysts are malformations of lung parenchyma that lack drainage to major bronchi. In the most common form, intralobar sequestrations receive their vascular supply from the aorta. Most are found in the posterior segments of the left lower lobe. Recurrent pneumonia is a common feature of these malformations, sometimes with frequent hemoptysis and chest pain.

Multilobar recurrent pneumonia suggests a broader differential diagnosis. Systemic immune dysfunction is more likely than a localized problem.[65, 85] Aspiration is the most common cause of recurrent bilateral pneumonia. Gastroesophageal reflux has been associated with recurrent wheezing and asthma in adults and children[86] and may be a cause of recurrent pneumonia as well.

Structural abnormalities of the tracheobronchial tree rarely cause recurrent pneumonia. One report identified an 86-year-old man with recurrent pneumonia secondary to tracheobronchomegaly, also known as Mounier-Kuhn disease.[87] This syndrome is characterized by dilatation of the trachea and major bronchi. It is thought to be caused by a congenital defect of tracheobronchial elastic tissue. Frequent episodes of pneumonia and bronchiectasis occur.

Mucociliary dysfunction leading to recurrent pneumonia is seen in cystic fibrosis and in the immotile cilia syndromes, now called primary ciliary dyskinesias.[88] Cystic fibrosis should be considered in an adult patient with recurrent pneumonia, although the disease occurs in childhood. Cystic fibrosis and the primary ciliary dyskinesias share many features, including recurrent infections, sinusitis, and infertility. Kartagener syndrome is an example of primary ciliary dyskinesia associated with dextrocardia.

Mucoid impaction in asthma can cause a recurrent lobar infiltrate, leading to confusion with pneumonia or malignancy (Fig. 22–5). In pediatric patients with recurrent pneumonia, almost one half had a family history of asthma or atopy, and one third had wheezing.[89]

Allergic bronchopulmonary aspergillosis often presents with pulmonary infiltrates and fever that may be confused with infectious pneumonia. The characteristic features of this hypersensitivity reaction to the *Aspergillus* fungus include almost exclusive affliction of patients with asthma, involvement of central bronchi, peripheral eosinophilia, and dramatically elevated levels of IgE. Infiltrates may involve any lobe and are similar to those seen with mucoid impaction. These infiltrates slowly resolve and are likely to recur.

Immunodeficiency syndromes are a rare cause of recurrent pneumonia in the pediatric age group.[66, 67] Most frequently seen is the variable hypogammaglobulinemia subclass deficiency of IgG and IgA. Many rare causes of

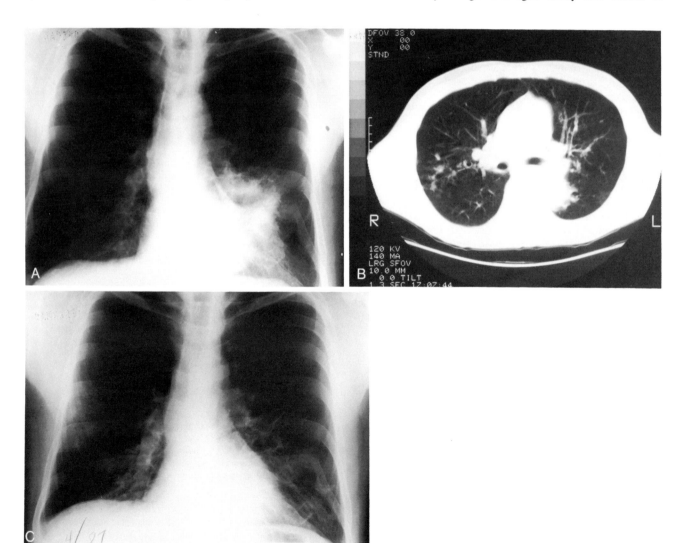

**Figure 22–5.** *A*, A 39-year-old man with long-standing asthma and bronchiectasis presented with fever, weight loss, and a chest roentgenogram with a left lower lobe infiltrate, which persisted for more than 1 month. *B*, The chest computed tomographic scan shows a dense consolidation of the left lower lobe and bilateral bronchiectasis. *C*, The consolidation resolved after treatment with high-dose corticosteroids. The diagnosis was mucoid impaction.

immunodeficiency have been associated with recurrent lower respiratory tract infection.[90, 91] Rare causes of recurrent pneumonia include chronic granulomatous disease and hyper-IgE levels.

The differential diagnosis of recurrent pneumonia must include AIDS. Although *Pneumocystis* is the most common recurrent pneumonia in AIDS, infections with common encapsulated organisms such as pneumococcus and *H. influenzae* may also recur.[72] Patients with iatrogenic immunodeficiency may develop recurrent pneumonia. Patients with acute nonlymphocytic leukemia may develop recurrent fungal pneumonia (predominantly *Aspergillus*) during episodes of granulocytopenia.[92]

Many noninfectious illnesses may cause slowly resolving or recurrent pneumonia. Two syndromes mentioned earlier deserve special consideration: BOOP and chronic eosinophilic pneumonia.[84, 93] BOOP results in infiltrates that may wax and wane for weeks or months. Chronic eosinophilic pneumonia is a syndrome of migratory peripheral pulmonary infiltrates and eosinophilia, affecting predominantly middle-aged women.[94] The process usually is chronic or subacute, although an acute, rapidly progressive course associated with adult respiratory distress syndrome has been described.[95] Bronchospasm associated with chronic eosinophilic pneumonia often follows the development of pulmonary infiltrates. Wegener granulomatosis and other pulmonary vasculitides are also associated with recurrent pulmonary infiltrates, which may masquerade as infectious pneumonia.

### Evaluation of Recurrent Pneumonia

To evaluate recurrent pneumonia, demographic, clinical, and radiologic features must be considered. If the infection is recurrent in a single lobe, intraluminal or extraluminal bronchial obstruction must be suspected. Foreign body aspiration remains the most common ''remediable'' cause of pneumonia. Computed tomography and bronchoscopy are most useful in the preliminary evaluation of localized obstruction to bronchial drainage and diffuse abnormalities such as bronchiectasis and tracheobronchomegaly. Perfusion lung scanning may be a good screening test for localized structural disease in children with recurrent pneumonia.[96] Normal or diffusely nonhomogeneous patterns are associated with an excellent prognosis. Lobar or multisegmental perfusion defects suggest disorders such as bronchiectasis, bronchomalacia, agenesis, and sequestration. If pneumonia recurs in the lower lobes, especially in the posterior segments, bronchopulmonary sequestration should be considered. Evaluation should include an aortogram to look for a feeding vessel from the abdominal or thoracic aorta. This study is diagnostic and provides information required for surgical resection.

If the recurrent pneumonia involves multiple lobes, aspiration must be considered first. An esophagogram or endoscopy should provide information about functional or anatomic obstruction to the esophagus. Patients who present with recurrent diffuse pulmonary infiltrates and wheezing should be evaluated for allergic bronchopulmonary aspergillosis, chronic eosinophilic pneumonia, and asthma. In the pediatric age group, immunoglobulin deficiency, although

rare, must be evaluated. Immunoglobulins, using age-appropriate standards, should be measured. A sweat chloride determination can provide information about the likelihood of cystic fibrosis, although genetic testing will be available soon. If the patient has sinus disease, a nasal brush biopsy or scraping can be done to assess ultrastructural abnormalities of primary ciliary dyskinesia. AIDS should be considered for all patients with recurrent pneumonias, even if the standard risk factors are not elicited in the history.

## REFERENCES

1. Fein AM, Feinsilver SH, Niederman MS, Fiel S, Pai PB: When the pneumonia doesn't get better. Clin Chest Med 8:529–541, 1987.
2. Norris GW: Lobar pneumonia. *In* Olser W, McCrae T (eds): Modern Medicine. Philadelphia, Lea & Febiger, 1913:241.
3. Amberson JB: Significance of unresolved organizing or protracted pneumonia. J Mich State Med Soc 42:599–603, 1943.
4. Crowe H, Levitz R: Invasive *Haemophilus influenzae* in adults. Arch Intern Med 147:241–244, 1987.
5. Esposito A: Community acquired bacteremic pneumococcal pneumonia: Effect of age on manifestations and outcome. Arch Intern Med 144:945–948, 1984.
6. Musher D, Kubitschek K, Crennan J, Baughn R: Pneumonia and acute febrile tracheobronchitis due to *Haemophilus influenzae*. Ann Intern Med 99:444–450, 1983.
7. Niederman MS, Fein AM: Pneumonia in the elderly. Geriatr Clin North Am 2:241–268, 1986.
8. Venkatesan P, Gladman J, MacFarlane J, Barer D, Berman P, Kinnear W, Finch R: A hospital study of community acquired pneumonia in the elderly. Thorax 45:254–258, 1990.
9. Verghese A, Berk S: Bacterial pneumonia in the elderly. Medicine (Baltimore) 62:271–285, 1983.
10. Woodhead M, MacFarlane J, Rodgers F, Laverick A, Pilkington R, Macrae A: Aetiology and outcome of severe community-acquired pneumonia. J Infect 10:204–210, 1985.
11. Harkness G, Bentley D, Roughman K: Risk factors for nosocomial pneumonia. Am J Med 89:457–463, 1990.
12. Skerett S, Niederman MS, Fein AM: Respiratory infections and acute lung injury in systemic illness. Clin Chest Med 10:469–502, 1989.
13. Marrie T, Haldane V, Faulkner R, Durant H, Kwan C: Community acquired pneumonia requiring hospitalization: Is it different in the elderly? J Am Geriatr Soc 33:671–680, 1985.
14. Starczewski A: Clinical prognostic indices of fatality in elderly patients admitted to the hospital with acute pneumonia. Age Ageing 17:181–186, 1988.
15. Rhodes GC, Lykke AWJ, Tapsall JW, et al: Abnormal alveolar epithelial repair associated with failure of resolution in experimental streptococcal pneumonia. J Pathol 159:245–253, 1989.
16. Chatard J: Analytic study of lobar pneumonia. Johns Hopkins Hospital from May 15th, 1889 to May 15th, 1905. Johns Hopkins Hosp Rev 15:55–60, 1910.
17. McRae T: Delayed resolution in lobar pneumonia. Johns Hopkins Hosp Rev 15:277–280, 1910.
18. Musser J: Lobar pneumonia. *In* Osler W (ed): Modern Medicine, vol 2. Philadelphia, Lea & Febiger, 1914:537–545.
19. Graham W, Bradley D: Efficacy of chest physiotherapy and intermittent positive pressure breathing in the resolution of pneumonia. N Engl J Med 293:624–627, 1978.
20. MacFarlane J, Miller A, Smith W, et al: Comparative radiographic features of community acquired legionnaires' disease, pneumococcal pneumonia, mycoplasma pneumonia, and psittacosis. Thorax 39:28–33, 1984.
21. Van Metre T: Pneumococcal pneumonia treated with antibiotics. N Engl J Med 25:1048–1052, 1954.
22. Jay S, Johanson W, Pierce A: The radiographic resolution of *Streptococcus pneumoniae* pneumonia. N Engl J Med 293:798–801, 1975.
23. Feinsilver SH, Fein AM, Niederman MS, Schultz E, Faegenburg DH: Utility of fiberoptic bronchoscopy in non-resolving pneumonia. Chest 98:1322–1326, 1990.
24. Finegold S, Johnson C: Legionnaires' disease: Still with us. N Engl J Med 318:517–536, 1988.

25. Kirby B, Snyder K, Meyer R, Finegold S: Legionnaires' disease: Report of 65 nosocomially acquired cases and review of the literature. Medicine (Baltimore) 59:188–205, 1980.
26. Lattimer G, Rhodes L, Salent J, et al: The Philadelphia epidemic of legionnaires' disease: Clinical, pulmonary and serologic findings two years later. Ann Intern Med 90:522–526, 1979.
27. Helms C, Viner J, Sturm R, Renner E, Johanson W: Comparative features of pneumococcal, mycoplasmal, and legionnaires' disease pneumonia. Ann Intern Med 90:543–547, 1979.
28. Levin D, Schwarz M, Matthay R, LaForce F: Bacteremic *Hemophilus influenzae* pneumonia in adults. Am J Med 62:219–222, 1977.
29. Takala A, Eskola J, van Alphen J: Spectrum of invasive *Hemophilus influenzae* type b disease in adults. Arch Intern Med 150:2573–2576, 1990.
30. Ebright J: Bacterial pneumonia in the elderly. J Am Geriatr Soc 28:220, 1980.
31. Fein AM, Feinsilver SH, Niederman MS: Atypical manifestations of pneumonia in the elderly. Clin Chest Med 12:319–337, 1991.
32. Garb J, Brown R, Tuthill R: Differences in etiology of pneumonias in nursing home and community patients. JAMA 240:2169–2175, 1978.
33. Johanson W, Pierce A, Sanford J: Changing pharyngeal bacterial flora of hospitalized patients. Emergence of gram-negative bacilli. N Engl J Med 281:1138–1140, 1969.
34. Bentley D: Bacterial pneumonia in the elderly: The observations of Sir William Osler in retrospect. Gerontology 30:297–307, 1984.
35. Rubin F, Cate T: Influenza pneumonia. Semin Respir Infect 2:122–129, 1987.
36. Woodhead M, MacFarlane J, Rodgers F, Laverick A, Pilkington R, Macrae A: Aetiology and outcome of severe community-acquired pneumonia. J Infect 10:204–210, 1985.
37. Kaye MG, Fox MJ, Bartlett JG, et al: The clinical spectrum of *Staphylococcus aureus* pulmonary infection. Chest 97:788–792, 1990.
38. Freeman E, Sutton N, Cevikbas A: Respiratory infections on long-stay wards. J Infect 4:237–242, 1982.
39. Morales F, Calder M, Inglis J, et al: A study of respiratory infections in the elderly to assess the role of respiratory syncytial virus. J Infect 7:236–247, 1983.
40. Marrie TJ, Grayston JT, Wang SP, Kuo CC: Pneumonia associated with the TWAR strain of *Chlamydia*. Ann Intern Med 106:507–511, 1987.
41. Stengstrom R, Jansson E, Wager O: Ornithoses pneumonia with special reference to roentgenological lung findings. Acta Med Scand 171:349–356, 1962.
42. Wright P, Wallace R Jr, Shepperd J: A descriptive study of 42 cases of *Branhamella catarrhalis* pneumonia. Am J Med 88:2–8, 1990.
43. Verghese AC, Berk SL, Boelen LJ, Smith JK: Group B streptococcal pneumonia in the elderly. Arch Intern Med 142:1642, 1982.
44. Centers for Disease Control: Update: Tuberculosis elimination: United States. MMWR 39:153–156, 1990.
45. Kahn MA, Kovnat DN, Bachus B, et al: Clinical and roentgenographic spectrum of tuberculosis in the adult. Am J Med 62:31–38, 1977.
46. Kent DC, Schwartz R: Active pulmonary tuberculosis with negative tuberculin skin reactions. Am Rev Respir Dis 95:411–418, 1967.
47. Grossman CB, Bragg DG, Armstrong D: Roentgen manifestations of pulmonary nocardiosis. Radiology 96:325, 1970.
48. Brown LR, Swensen SJ, Van Scoy RE, Prakash UB, Coles DT, Colby TV: Roentgenologic features of pulmonary blastomycosis. Mayo Clin Proc 66:29–38, 1991.
49. Winer-Muram HT, Beals DH, Cole FH Jr: Blastomycosis of the lung: CT features. Radiology 182:829–832, 1992.
50. Binder RE, Faling LJ, Pugatch RD, et al: Chronic necrotizing pulmonary aspergillosis: A discrete clinical entity. Medicine (Baltimore) 61:109–124, 1982.
51. Rodrigues J, Niederman MS, Fein AM, Pai PB: Non-resolving pneumonia in steroid-treated patients with obstructive lung disease. Am J Med 93:29–34, 1992.
52. Ludington LG, Verska JJ, Howard T et al: Bronchiolar carcinoma (alveolar cell), another great imitator; a review of 41 cases. Chest 61:622–628, 1972.
53. Blank N, Castellino RA: The intrathoracic manifestations of the malignant lymphomas and the leukemias. Semin Roentgenol 15:227–245, 1980.
54. Filly R, Blank N, Castellino RA: Radiographic distribution of intrathoracic disease in previously untreated Hodgkin's disease and non-Hodgkin's lymphoma. Radiology 120:277–281, 1976.
55. Hoffman GS, Kerr GS, Leavitt RY, et al: Wegener's granulomatosis: An analysis of 158 patients. Ann Intern Med 116:488–498, 1992.
56. Sklarek H, Narain S, Feinsilver S, Niederman M, Fein A: Wegener's granulomatosis mimics acute bacterial pneumonia. Chest 92:111S, 1987.
57. Israel HL, Patchefsky AS, Saldana MJ: Wegener's granulomatosis, lymphomatoid granulomatosis, and benign lymphocytic angiitis and granulomatosis of the lung. Ann Intern Med 87:691–699, 1977.
58. Nolle B, Specks U, Ludemann J, Rohrbach MS, DeRemee RA, Gross WL: Anticytoplasmic autoantibodies: Their immunodiagnostic value in Wegener's granulomatosis. Ann Intern Med 111:28–40, 1989.
59. Churg A: Pulmonary angiitis and granulomatosis revisited. Hum Pathol 14:868–883, 1983.
60. Koss MN, Robinson RG, Hochholzer L: Bronchocentric granulomatosis. Hum Pathol 12:632–638, 1981.
61. Epler GR, Colby TV, McLoud TC, et al: Bronchiolitis obliterans organizing pneumonia. N Engl J Med 312:152–158, 1985.
62. Nikki P, Meretoja O, Valtonen V, et al: Severe bronchiolitis probably caused by varicella-zoster virus. Crit Care Med 10:344–346, 1982.
63. Muller NL, Staples CA, Miller RR: Bronchiolitis obliterans organizing pneumonia: CT features in 14 patients. AJR 154:983–987, 1990.
64. McLoud TC, Epler GR, Colby TV, Gaensler EA, Carrington CB: Bronchiolitis obliterans. Radiology 159:1–8, 1986.
65. Woesner ME, Sanders I, White GW: The melting sign in resolving transient pulmonary infarction. Am J Roentgenol 111:782, 1971.
66. Wright BA, Jeffery PH: Lipoid pneumonia. Semin Respir Infect 5:314–321, 1990.
67. Kennedy JI, Myers JL, Plumb VJ, et al: Amiodarone pulmonary toxicity: Clinical, radiologic and pathologic correlations. Arch Intern Med 147:50–55, 1987.
68. Winterbauer RH, Bedon GA, Ball WC Jr: Recurrent pneumonia. Ann Intern Med 70:689–700, 1969.
69. Oseasohn R, Skipper BE, Tempest B: Pneumonia in a Navajo community. Am Rev Respir Dis 117:1003–1009, 1978.
70. Adam KAR: Persistent or recurrent pneumonia in Saudi children seen at King Khalid University Hospital, Riyadh: Clinical profile and some predisposing factors. Ann Trop Paediatr 11:129–135, 1991.
71. Finland M, Winkler AW: Recurrences in pneumococcus pneumonia. Am J Med Sci 188:309–321, 1934.
72. Coggeshall LT, Robertson OH: A study of repeated attacks of experimental pneumococcus lobar pneumonia in dogs. J Exp Med 61:213–233, 1935.
73. Silver DR, Cohen IL, Weinberg PE: Recurrent *Pseudomonas aeruginosa* in an intensive care unit. Chest 101:194–198, 1992.
74. Castro R, Klein J, Padmalingam R, Eppes SC: Recurrent/persistent pneumonia in a 3 1/2 year old girl due to acquired immune deficiency syndrome. Del Med J 61:455–458, 1989.
75. Shanley DJ, Luyckx BA, Haggerty MF, et al: Spontaneous pneumothorax in AIDS patients with recurrent pneumocystis carinii pneumonia despite aerosolized pentamidine prophylaxis. Chest 99:502–504, 1991.
76. Tamura SS, Shimomura S, Takahashi S, et al: Recurrent *Pneumocystis carinii* pneumonia with long interval showing disparate radiographic findings. Jpn J Med 30:346–350, 1991.
77. Wachter RM, Luce JM, Hopewell PC: Critical care of patients with AIDS. JAMA 267:541–548, 1992.
78. Cohen SR, Lewis GB, Herber WI, et al: Foreign bodies in the airway: A 5 year retrospective study with special reference to management. Ann Otol Rhinol Laryngol 89:437–442, 1980.
79. Moazam JF, Talbert JL, Rodgers EM: Foreign bodies in the pediatric tracheobronchial tree. Clin Pediatr 22:148–151, 1983.
80. Case Records of the Massachusetts General Hospital: Weekly clinicopathological exercise 48—1983: A 14-year-old boy with recurrent hemoptysis and a right lower lobe infiltrate. N Engl J Med 309:1374–1381, 1983.
81. Bradham RR: Bronchial adenoma: A cause of recurrent and persistent pneumonia. J S C Med Assoc 77:107–111, 1981.
82. Abrutyn E: Recurrent pneumonia. *In* Levinson ME (ed): The Pneumonias: Clinical Approaches to Infectious Diseases of the Lower Respiratory Tract. Littleton, MA, John Wright PSH, 1984:153–166.
83. Livingston GL, Holinger LD, Luck SR: Right middle lobe syndrome in children. Int J Pediatr Otorhinolaryngol 13:11–23, 1987.
84. Lewiston NJ: Bronchiectasis in children. Pediatr Clin North Am 31:865–878, 1984.
85. Kirtland SH, Winterbauer RH: Slowly resolving, chronic and recurrent pneumonia. Clin Chest Med 12:303–318, 1991.

86. Chen PH, Chang MH, Hsu SC: Gastroesophageal reflux in children with recurrent bronchopulmonary infection. J Pediatr Gastroenterol Nutr 13:16–22, 1991.

87. Geppert EF: Recurrent pneumonia. Chest 98:739–744, 1990.

88. Rooklin AR, McGeady SJ, Mikaelian DO, et al: The immotile cilia syndrome: A cause of recurrent pulmonary diseases in children. Pediatrics 66:526–531, 1980.

89. Eigen H, Laughlin JJ, Homrighausen J: Recurrent pneumonia in children and its relationship to bronchial hyperreactivity. Pediatrics 70:698–704, 1982.

90. Alper CA, Colten HR, Rosen ES, et al: Homozygous deficiency of C3 in a patient with repeated infections. Lancet 2:1179–1181, 1972.

91. Cazzola G, Valletta EA, Ciaffoni S, et al: Neutrophil function and human immunity in children with recurrent infections of the lower respiratory tract and chronic bronchial suppuration. Ann Allergy 63:213–218, 1989.

92. Robertson MJ, Larson RA: Recurrent fungal pneumonias in patients with acute nonlymphocytic leukemia undergoing multiple courses of intensive chemotherapy. Am J Med 84:233–239, 1988.

93. Gross TJ, Chavis AD, Lynch JP: Noninfectious pulmonary diseases masquerading as community acquired pneumonia. Clin Chest Med 12:365–393, 1991.

94. Carrington CB, Addington WW, Goff AM, et al: Chronic eosinophilic pneumonia. N Engl J Med 280:787–798, 1969.

95. Allen JN, Pacht ER, Gadek JE, et al: Acute eosinophilic pneumonia: A hypersensitivity phenomenon? Am Rev Respir Dis 139:242–245, 1989.

96. Hardoff R, Rivlin J, Front A: The contribution of perfusion scintigraphy in the evaluation of children suffering from recurrent localized pneumonia. Eur J Nucl Med 17:152–155, 1990.

# CHAPTER 23

# Lung Abscess and Other Subacute Pulmonary Infections

EUGENE F. GEPPERT

A subacute lung infection is a febrile illness of at least 2 weeks' duration that produces changes on the chest roentgenogram. This definition excludes a large number of acute pneumonias that evolve rapidly and cause the patient to seek help within a few days of onset. The subacute lung infections have a more gradual onset, and the patient may delay coming to a physician or receive one or more courses of empiric antimicrobial drugs without benefit before a diagnosis is made.

A lung abscess is a type of subacute pulmonary infection for which the chest roentgenogram shows a cavity within the lung parenchyma.

In the discussion that follows, the subacute lung infections are divided into groups according to their roentgenographic patterns. The infections with noncavitary lung infiltrates show a focal or diffuse patchy ground glass pattern. Diffuse lung lesions are those with a diffuse infiltration in all lobes without areas of normal lung. A roentgenographic cavity is a gas-filled space within a zone of pulmonary consolidation, mass, or nodule.[1]

This chapter describes the clinical approach to subacute pulmonary infections and lung abscess, including the noninfectious conditions that can mimic them.

## SUBACUTE PULMONARY DISEASES WITH NONCAVITARY FOCAL INFILTRATES

### Differential Diagnosis

#### Infectious Causes

The typical patient with a subacute pulmonary infection has a fever of more than 2 weeks' duration, respiratory symptoms, and unifocal or multifocal ground glass infiltrates on the chest roentgenogram. The list of infections with this presentation is given in Table 23–1.

All of these diseases are noncavitary during their early stages. After some weeks, they may undergo necrosis and appear as infiltrates with multiple, small lucencies or cavities on the chest roentgenogram. These patients typically have an intermittently febrile course, although fever is not constant, and it is not rare for the patient to be afebrile at the time of presentation to a physician. Also common are cough, chest pain, dyspnea, weight loss, malaise, and night sweats. The physical findings vary, but in patients without bronchial obstruction, there are focal bronchial breath sounds over the diseased lung segment. Patients with an obstructed bronchus have no breath sounds over the obstructed lobe.

The typical roentgenographic finding is a focal ground glass infiltrate, often with indistinct borders. The location of the infiltrate on the chest x-ray film can be helpful in formulating the differential diagnosis. The infiltrates of fibrocaseous tuberculosis are usually found in the apical and posterior regions of the upper lobes or in the superior seg-

Table 23–1. **Subacute Pulmonary Infections With Focal Infiltrates**

| |
|---|
| Fungal pneumonia |
| Actinomycosis |
| Nocardiosis |
| Tuberculosis |
| Mycobacterial infection other than tuberculosis |
| Infected bronchopulmonary sequestration |
| Bacterial pneumonia with obstructed bronchus |
| Anaerobic pneumonia (some cases) |
| Bronchiectasis |

ments of the lobar lobes, and they may be unilateral or bilateral. The infiltrates of anaerobic pneumonia are the result of aspiration of oropharyngeal contents and are usually located in the most dependent regions of the lungs: segments of the lower lobes and sometimes in the upper lobes. Bronchopulmonary sequestration may occur in any segment, but classically it is found in the posterior basilar segment of the left lower lobe. Obstructive pneumonia, mycobacterial disease other than tuberculosis, actinomycosis, nocardiosis, and fungal pneumonia can be found anywhere in the bronchopulmonary tree. The clinical features of all these diseases are described elsewhere in this book. The case described in Figure 23–1 provides an example of a patient with a subacute infection with a noncavitating, focal ground glass infiltrate revealed on the chest roentgenogram.

Infectious causes of noncavitary infiltrates usually present with signs and symptoms that are less severe than those of acute bacterial pneumonia. The patient may or may not have fever or an elevated leukocyte count. There is often a predisposing disease process. Some patients are completely asymptomatic, and their lung lesions are found when a chest roentgenogram is obtained for some other purpose.

### Noninfectious Diseases

Several conditions that are not respiratory infections can mimic subacute lung diseases. They are listed in Table 23–2.

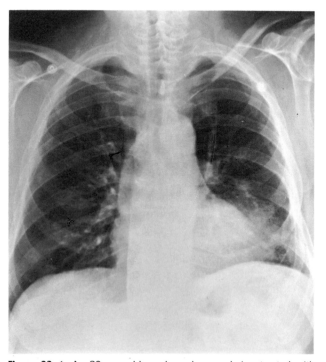

**Figure 23–1.** An 80-year-old smoker who was being treated with prednisone and azathioprine for idiopathic thrombocytopenic purpura presented to the hospital with a 9-week illness characterized by cough, without dyspnea, chest pain, or chills. Empiric therapy for community-acquired pneumonia with an aminoglycoside and a β-lactam antibiotic led to improvement, and he was discharged on oral therapy. Three weeks later, he returned with fever and right knee pain. Fluid from the knee contained *Nocardia brasiliensis*. Therapy was initiated with trimethoprim-sulfamethoxazole for 6 months.

**Table 23–2. Conditions That Mimic Subacute Infections With Focal Infiltrates**

| |
|---|
| Bronchiolitis obliterans organizing pneumonia |
| Chronic eosinophilic pneumonia |
| Allergic bronchopulmonary aspergillosis |
| Exogenous lipoid pneumonia |
| Radiation pneumonitis |

Bronchiolitis obliterans organizing pneumonia (BOOP) can present as a subacute infection with persistent fever and respiratory symptoms. BOOP has several patterns on the chest x-ray film. One of them is a focal ground glass infiltrate.[2] Although BOOP is occasionally caused by a microbial agent such as *Legionella pneumophila* or *Nocardia asteroides,* most cases are idiopathic, even when they have a febrile course. Diagnosis usually requires an open lung biopsy or transbronchial biopsy.

Chronic eosinophilic pneumonia is often a febrile disease with focal pulmonary infiltrates that persist for weeks or months before a diagnosis is made, and it is usually mistaken at first for a subacute infection.[3] In the review by Jederlinic, Sicilian, and Gaensler of 19 cases of chronic eosinophilic pneumonia, many of the patients presented with nonproductive cough, dyspnea, accompanying fever, and weight loss that often exceeded 10 kg. In some cases, the diagnosis is strongly suggested by the roentgen pattern, in which the patchy ground glass infiltrates are located in the periphery of the lung on the chest x-ray film or computed tomographic (CT) scan. Diagnosis often requires transbronchial or open lung biopsy.

Fever and focal pulmonary infiltrates often are found in patients with allergic bronchopulmonary aspergillosis,[4] a disease that is usually characterized by asthma, blood eosinophilia, infiltrates on the chest roentgenogram, high serum levels of IgE, and a positive immediate hypersensitivity scratch test to *Aspergillus fumigatus* antigen.

Subacute fever and patchy, ground glass infiltrates on the chest roentgenogram are seen for patients with exogenous lipoid pneumonia, an illness usually caused by aspiration of mineral oil. The history of mineral oil ingestion as a cause of their aspiration may not become evident until after they have undergone invasive biopsy procedures.[5]

The diagnosis of radiation pneumonitis as a cause for prolonged fevers and infiltrates can be made for irradiated patients in whom a true subacute infection is carefully ruled out by diagnostic studies. Overall, fewer than 20% of irradiated patients develop radiation pneumonitis. The fever of radiation pneumonitis may at times be high and spiking.[6] The illness often begins between 6 and 12 weeks after completion of radiation therapy, but some cases appear as soon as 2 weeks afterward. Systemic symptoms of drenching sweats and weight loss may also be seen. The most frequent symptom is cough, which varies from mild to very severe. Dyspnea is also a common symptom of radiation pneumonitis. Although the history of recent chest irradiation is helpful in identifying radiation pneumonitis as the cause of the patient's symptoms, a complicating subacute pneumonia should be ruled out in all cases by cultures of blood, sputum, and in some cases, cultures of samples obtained at bronchoscopy. The bronchial mucosa at bronchoscopy in patients with radiation pneumonitis may appear normal, but if major bronchi have received appreciable radiation, the mucosa shows atrophy with scattered telangiectatic blood vessels on the mucosal surface.

## Diagnostic Approach

### History

Patients should be questioned about possible exposure to persons with active tuberculosis. A careful geographic history should be taken to determine whether the patient has been exposed to regional fungi such as coccidioidomycosis (Southwest United States), blastomycosis (North Central North America), or histoplasmosis (river valleys). Homeless alcoholic patients are at risk for tuberculosis, anaerobic pneumonia (due to alcoholic stupor accompanied by aspiration), and the rarer subacute infection pulmonary sporotrichosis.[7] Patients who suffer from epileptic seizures, patients who have had recent dental surgery, and patients with known esophageal disease are especially at risk for anaerobic pneumonia. Dental disease is a risk factor for actinomycosis, because the causative organism normally lives on the surface of teeth.[8] Old chest roentgenograms can help in diagnosing a bronchopulmonary sequestration if the telltale unresolving segmental infiltrate can be shown to have existed for years.

### Physical Examination

Physical examination findings for patients with subacute pulmonary infections are similar to those for acute pneumonias. Crackles and bronchial breath sounds may be heard over the consolidated lobe unless bronchial obstruction exists, in which case breath sounds are decreased. Patients with severe periodontal disease should be examined by a dentist, but gross findings include red, inflamed gums and recession of the gums with exposure of the base of the teeth. Patients who have severe periodontal disease are most at risk of developing anaerobic pneumonia or actinomycosis, but edentulous patients are least likely to develop anaerobic pneumonia. Putrid breath odor is practically diagnostic of anaerobic lung infection.[9]

### Expectorated Sputum Analysis

Sputum should be collected and sent for acid-fast smear and culture for tuberculosis and nocardiosis, periodic acid-Schiff stain for fungi, Gram stain for bacterial infection and actinomycosis, and cytologic analysis (ie, cytologists sometimes diagnose fungal disease). Sputum should be cultured for mycobacteria, *Nocardia,* and fungi but not for anaerobes, because the specimens are always contaminated by anaerobes in the mouth. If mineral oil aspiration is suspected, a sputum wet prep should be obtained to search for lipid-laden alveolar macrophages.[10] Sputum is expected to show eosinophils in allergic bronchopulmonary aspergillosis. The sputum of patients with anaerobic pneumonia is putrid in about 60% of cases, and the Gram stain shows a high density of gram-positive and gram-negative organisms with myriad neutrophils and degenerating cells.

### Fiberoptic Bronchoscopy

If the cause of a subacute pulmonary infection is not evident after the history, physical examination, and sputum analysis, it is best to proceed promptly with bronchoscopy and transbronchial biopsy. Fiberoptic bronchoscopy is capable of finding bronchial obstruction, mycobacterial disease,[11–14] fungal organisms, and some cases of actinomycosis[15] and nocardiosis.[16, 17] The yield from fiberoptic bronchoscopy varies for different pathogens. In pulmonary histoplasmosis, the yield was about 50% in one study after solitary pulmonary nodules were excluded from consideration.[18] Pulmonary blastomycosis and pulmonary aspergillosis often are diagnosed by bronchoscopy, but this technique fails for some cases. *Cryptococcus neoformans* lung infection is often diagnosed by cultures from fiberoptic bronchoscopy, and the detection of cryptococcal antigen in bronchoalveolar lavage fluid may enhance the usefulness of bronchoscopy in detecting this infection.[19]

### Computed Tomography

In this group of diseases, CT scans may show areas of necrosis within the infiltrate that were not visible on plain chest roentgenograms. CT may better define the pleural or chest wall involvement with actinomycosis[20] or nocardiosis. CT is also helpful in diagnosing bronchopulmonary sequestration,[21] and CT often reveals the exact site of obstruction in an obstructed bronchus.

### Special Studies

When coccidioidomycosis is suspected, it may be reasonable to order an immunodiffusion test for the fungus if fewer than 2 months have passed since the patient was infected or a complement fixation titer if 2 months have passed since the patient was infected. In many cases, it is appropriate to do a serologic test for human immunodeficiency virus (HIV). An intermediate-strength purified protein derivative tuberculin skin test should be done on all these patients, together with control tests such as *Candida albicans* and *Trichophyton* skin tests.

### Aspiration and Surgery

Transthoracic needle aspiration is often worthwhile in making a microbiologic diagnosis and obviating thoracotomy.

After all other efforts have failed to produce a diagnosis, thoracotomy and biopsy are indicated. This is especially true if the patient's condition is deteriorating.

## SUBACUTE PULMONARY INFECTIONS WITH DIFFUSE LUNG LESIONS

### Differential Diagnosis

The number of infections in which the patient presents with at least 2 weeks of fever and a diffuse lung lesion seen on a chest roentgenogram is small. The most striking example in this category is miliary tuberculosis, which typically has a gradual febrile onset. Another frequent pneumonia in this category is that caused by *Pneumocystis carinii*. Rarely, fungal diseases such as histoplasmosis and coccidioidomycosis can present with a fever and diffuse lung lesion on the chest x-ray film, but their course is usually faster, and they reach a crisis within 2 weeks. Several conditions that are not infectious can mimic a subacute pulmonary infection, because they are characterized by subacute fever, respiratory symptoms, and a diffuse lung lesion on chest roentgenogram. These conditions and the infectious diseases in this category, are listed in Table 23–3.

If the physician is faced with a febrile patient with a subacute course and a diffuse lung lesion seen on the chest radiograph, a description of the roentgenographic pattern can be helpful. With miliary tuberculosis, the shadows are typically small, circular, water-density shadows smaller than 3 mm in diameter. Discovering a patient like this requires quick action, because miliary tuberculosis is a life-threatening emergency that is frequently complicated by tuberculous meningitis; delayed treatment is associated with increased mortality.[22] In most cases, the preferred manner of diagnosis is fiberoptic bronchoscopy with transbronchial biopsy.

The noninfectious diseases in this category often require biopsies. Although most cases of BOOP have a roentgenographic pattern that is diffuse and patchy (with areas of normal lung between), some cases are diffuse and spare no segment. These cases usually require open lung biopsy for diagnosis. BOOP is considered here because it is often associated with fever, at least during a part of its clinical course. Pulmonary sarcoidosis can present as a subacute infection, and approximately 20% of patients with this disease have fevers. Sarcoidosis often requires fiberoptic bronchoscopy with transbronchial biopsy for diagnosis. The subacute variety of hypersensitivity pneumonitis is a febrile disease that is usually mistaken for recurrent community-acquired pneumonia. It is caused by the inhalation of organic dust and the patient's immunologic response to that dust. If a history of exposure to a typical organic dust (eg, hay, home humidifier, bird droppings) can be obtained, biopsy need not be done. In many cases, a biopsy is obtained before the history is obtained or appreciated, and the biopsy result shows granulomatous inflammation of the alveolar walls without a particular predilection for areas rich in lymphatics, as is seen in sarcoidosis.

Alveolar proteinosis is an idiopathic disease in which the alveolar spaces are infiltrated with phospholipids. Many of the patients present with a subacute febrile illness although they do not have a superinfecting organism. Although alveolar proteinosis has been associated with many organisms

(eg, *Nocardia, Aspergillus, Cryptococcus, Mucor, Histoplasma, Mycobacterium, Pneumocystis,* cytomegalovirus), some patient series have emphasized the absence of superinfecting microbes in lavage fluid.[23, 24] The diagnosis of alveolar proteinosis usually requires lung biopsy. The chest x-ray film may show infiltrates that are diffuse, diffuse patchy, or focal. Superinfection should be ruled out by cultures obtained by fiberoptic bronchoscopy or open lung biopsy.

### Diagnostic Approach

#### History

In miliary tuberculosis, there is typically no history of previous tuberculosis or exposure. In disseminated fungal disease, the dissemination most often follows a previous infection, and the history of recent illness can be useful in suggesting that dissemination is a complication. The history in BOOP is usually that of an abrupt, flu-like illness followed by subacute fever and respiratory symptoms. In hypersensitivity pneumonitis, the physician must ask about possible exposure to organic antigens, especially taking into account household humidifiers, birds, and any other possible source of organic dust. The history may reveal important risk factors, such as possible infection with HIV, an important predisposing condition for *P. carinii* pneumonia, fungal pneumonia, tuberculosis, and infection with *Mycobacterium avium-intracellulare*. Risk factors for developing active tuberculosis include silicosis, diabetes, immunosuppression, past gastrectomy or other bowel surgery with subsequent weight loss, infection with HIV, and drug therapy with immunosuppressive agents.

#### Physical Examination

The physical examination is not helpful in this class of diseases, but any skin or mucosal lesions should be biopsied to detect fungal disease.

#### Sputum Analysis

Sputum should be sent for acid-fast stain, silver stain, and fungal stains.

#### Bronchoscopy

Bronchoscopy should be done in most patients as a first step. Miliary tuberculosis can be diagnosed by biopsy in a high percentage of cases. Fewer data are available for disseminated fungal disease. Bronchoscopy is good for diagnosing sarcoidosis, and transbronchial biopsies can suggest the diagnosis of hypersensitivity pneumonitis if the history has not yet suggested this diagnosis. Bronchoscopy has succeeded in diagnosing alveolar proteinosis, but open lung biopsy is often needed.

#### High-Resolution Computed Tomography

High-resolution CT (HRCT) scans of the lung can show patterns of abnormality that are sometimes not visible on

Table 23–3. **Subacute Respiratory Illnesses With Diffuse Infiltrates**

| |
|---|
| Infections |
|     Miliary tuberculosis |
|     Miliary or disseminated fungal disease |
|     *Pneumocystis carinii* pneumonia |
| Noninfectious causes |
|     Bronchiolitis obliterans organizing pneumonia |
|     Sarcoidosis |
|     Hypersensitivity pneumonitis |
|     Alveolar proteinosis |

plain chest roentgenograms. HRCT is especially good in suggesting sarcoidosis because of the concentration of micronodules distributed along the bronchovascular bundles.[25] Alveolar proteinosis and BOOP show a ground glass pattern on CT scans, and hypersensitivity pneumonitis may show a fine nodular or reticulonodular pattern during its acute or subacute phases.[26]

### Special Studies

If disseminated fungal disease is suspected, serologic testing can be helpful. For histoplasmosis, the best test is radioassay of blood and urine for *Histoplasma capsulatum* antigen.[27] For disseminated coccidioidomycosis, blood should be sent for determination of complement-fixing antibody. If sarcoidosis is suspected, blood should be sent for angiotensin-converting enzyme assay, because this value sometimes is elevated in this disease. Although elevated values on the angiotensin-converting enzyme assay are not diagnostic, they can influence the probability that a patient has sarcoidosis if a biopsy is not possible.

### Open Lung Biopsy

If a fiberoptic bronchoscopy and transbronchial biopsy does not yield an immediate diagnosis, open lung biopsy should be done promptly to make a definitive diagnosis. If miliary tuberculosis is strongly suspected, a bone marrow biopsy or liver biopsy can substitute for an open lung biopsy. The therapies for the various diseases are so different that a correct diagnosis is imperative.

## CAVITIES

### Differential Diagnosis

The differential diagnosis of cavitary lung disease can be subdivided into cavitary infectious diseases and cavitary diseases that are not infections. Tables 23–4 and 23–5 list the main elements of the differential diagnosis.

### Diagnostic Approach

#### History

Historic data can be useful in determining the cause of a lung cavity by shedding light on the patient's risk factors for different illnesses. For example, most patients with an-

Table 23–4. **Infectious Causes of Cavities**

| | |
|---|---|
| Tuberculosis | *Klebsiella* |
| Histoplasmosis | *Pseudomonas* |
| Blastomycosis | Melioidosis |
| Coccidioidomycosis | *Streptococcus pneumoniae* |
| Mucormycosis | Anaerobes |
| Sporotrichosis | *Pneumocystis carinii* |
| Cryptococcosis | Actinomycosis |
| Aspergillosis | Nocardiosis |
| *Staphylococcus aureus* | Infected pulmonary infarct |
| *Legionella* | Infected bulla |

Table 23–5. **Noninfectious Causes of Cavities**

| |
|---|
| Bland pulmonary infarct |
| Lung cancer |
| Metastatic cancer |
| Hodgkin disease |
| Wegener granulomatosis |
| Sarcoidosis (rare) |

aerobic lung abscess have some known predisposition for aspirating oropharyngeal contents. Some of the more common causes of aspiration are listed in Table 23–6. A history of an underlying debilitating disease is also common in many patients with cavitary lung disease, including chronic illnesses such as diabetes mellitus, immunosuppression for an organ transplant or during cancer chemotherapy, chronic obstructive pulmonary disease, and steroid therapy.[28-30] Patients with a lung cavity should be questioned about exposure to persons known to have active tuberculosis and about travel to regions of the world where coccidioidomycosis, blastomycosis, and histoplasmosis are endemic. Melioidosis is a rare cause of cavitary disease that is usually seen in patients who have spent time in the endemic region (ie, in Indochina and in latitudes between 20° N and 20° S), and patients who have been in the region have developed lung abscess after returning to North America.[31] Melioidosis has a variable time course after endemic exposure, with an acute pneumonia or a presentation that occurs years later as ''recrudescent melioidosis,''[31] and almost any past history of travel to Southeast Asia may be relevant.

### Physical Examination

For the lung infections that cause cavities, there are few helpful physical findings outside the chest. Skin lesions should be sought that can be biopsied to help diagnose disseminated infections such as blastomycosis, cryptococcosis, or *Pseudomonas* infection. Swelling and redness along the chest wall, or even frank fistula formation, may be seen in cases of advanced actinomycosis or nocardiosis. Signs of gum disease greatly increase the chances of anaerobic lung infection after aspiration of oropharyngeal contents.

### Sputum Analysis

Because sputum is important for diagnosis, it should be obtained by expectoration or by using a catheter to obtain a nasotracheal sample. Sputum should be induced if none is readily obtainable. The putrid sputum odor of an anaerobic lung abscess is so offensive that it is unlikely to be over-

Table 23–6. **Causes of Aspiration**

| |
|---|
| Alcoholic stupor |
| Seizure disorder |
| Dental or oropharyngeal surgery |
| Gastric or esophageal surgery |
| Esophageal diseases (eg, diverticulum) |
| Neurologic disease with bulbar dysfunction |
| General anesthesia |
| Drug abuse with stupor |

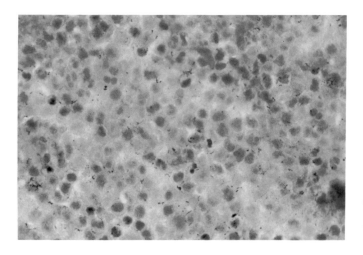

**Figure 23–2.** Gram stain of pleural fluid from an empyema complicating anaerobic lung abscess. The inflammatory cells are neutrophils, some in a state of degeneration. There is a dense population of organisms; most are gram positive with an occasional gram-negative bacillary form. The pleural fluid was brown and feculent.

looked. In anaerobic lung abscess, a Gram stain shows many neutrophils mixed with a dense population of gram-positive and gram-negative bacteria, including rods, cocci, and elongated forms. This is the classic polymicrobial Gram stain result for an anaerobic lung abscess (Fig. 23–2). For a lung abscess caused by aerobic bacteria, the Gram stain shows neutrophils mixed with one type of organism (ie, monomicrobial stain). A silver stain can be done if fungal disease, *Nocardia*, or *P. carinii* is suspected. Fungal diseases can sometimes be diagnosed by special stains of sputum (eg, periodic acid-Schiff stain), and some fungal organisms can be picked up on a Papanicolaou stain submitted for cytologic analysis.

All sputum should be sent for examination for acid-fast bacilli. Sputum should be cultured for mycobacteria, fungi, aerobic organisms, and *Legionella.* Sputum is not an appropriate specimen to send for culture for *Actinomyces* infection, because it is contaminated by oral flora that may normally contain this species. If *Actinomyces* is suspected, a sample of material not contaminated by oral secretions must be sent to the laboratory, such as a transthoracic needle aspirate, a telescoping plugged catheter from bronchoscopy,[32] or an open lung biopsy specimen. These same techniques are good for making a diagnosis of *Nocardia* species, but ordinary sputum occasionally may be adequate to make a diagnosis if the clinical setting supports the diagnosis.[33, 34] In some immunocompromised patients, a sputum culture positive for *Nocardia* may represent colonization.[33] Sputum for Gram stain helps in diagnosing abscesses caused by *Staphylococcus aureus.*[35] Sputum should also be cultured for *Legionella,* and direct fluorescent antibody testing should be performed, because this organism sometimes causes lung abscess.[36, 37] If unusual infections are suspected (eg, melioidosis), it is best to advise the microbiology laboratory of the suspected diagnosis, because special testing may be necessary.

Sputum is useful in diagnosing many of the noninfectious conditions that cause lung cavity. Many cases of bronchogenic carcinoma can be diagnosed from sputum cytology. Expectorated sputum often fails to yield a diagnostic cytologic result if the disease is metastatic cancer or Hodgkin disease; for these, transthoracic needle aspiration or lung biopsy is preferable.

### Radiographic Analysis

Roentgenographic cavities are the end result of a pathologic process that causes tissue necrosis. Before full-blown cavitation, these lesions are focal infiltrates that start to change in such a way that small black spaces appear in the infiltrates (Figs. 23–3 and 23–4). The roentgenographic and clinical aspects of lung cavitation are graphically illustrated in the patient with anaerobic lung abscess described in Figure 23–5. This patient had a complicated lung abscess that probably began many weeks earlier with aspiration of oropharyngeal contents during the extraction of two teeth. A lung abscess starts as a focal anaerobic pneumonia. Treatment can be effective at this stage, but if therapy is terminated too soon, the infection can produce necrosis of lung tissue and form a cavity. Despite adequate medical therapy, the lung abscess can become complicated by rupture into the pleural space with severe empyema. Surgical therapy is necessary in this situation to ensure proper healing of the empyema and to promote normal expansion of the involved lung. This type of severe subacute lung infection can only be cured by a combination of antimicrobials and surgical drainage.

Roentgenographic cavities that are questionable on pos-

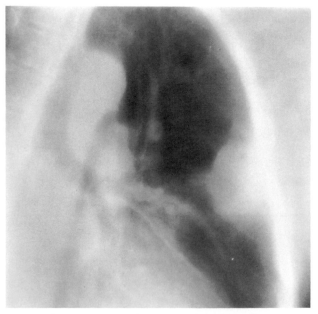

**Figure 23–3.** Early evidence of necrosis within a focal infiltrate is seen in this tomogram of the left upper lobe of a patient infected with *Actinomyces israelii.* The small black spot represents air within a necrotic portion of the abscess.

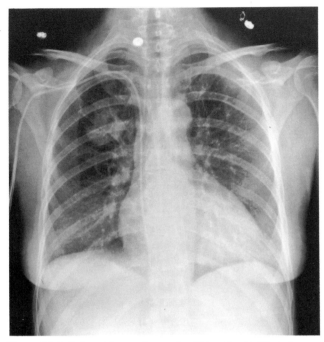

**Figure 23–4.** Early evidence of necrosis within a focal infiltrate is seen in this plain posteroanterior chest x-ray film of a patient infected with *Nocardia asteroides*. The patient was the recipient of a renal transplant; a central venous catheter had been placed for administration of medications. The diagnosis was made by transthoracic needle aspiration (see Fig. 23–12).

teroanterior and lateral views can be confirmed with a thoracic CT scan. Figure 23–6 shows an example of a lung cavity in the posterior basilar segment of the left lower lobe that was caused by *S. aureus*. In this case, it is evident on the CT scan that the lesion is located in the lung parenchyma; in some cases, CT scans are needed to differentiate a lung abscess from an empyema on the plain chest roentgenogram. CT helps differentiate these two lesions in most cases. Table 23–7, based on the work of Stark and associates,[38] summarizes the differences between a lung abscess and empyema on an infusion CT study of the thorax with lung and mediastinal window settings. Stark and associates point out that an additional benefit of CT scanning is that the extension of an actinomycotic abscess into the chest wall can be visualized. Other than this sign, CT scans offer little to suggest the microbial cause of an abscess.

A cavity located in the posterior basilar segment of the left lower lobe should raise the question of whether the lesion is a secondarily infected congenital bronchopulmonary sequestration. CT scanning can help to support the diagnosis of bronchopulmonary sequestration, and magnetic resonance scanning has been proposed as a substitute for aortography to search for an aberrant systemic feeding artery to the sequestered segment.[21, 39]

### Bronchoscopy

If sputum analysis fails to yield a diagnosis of the cause of a lung cavity after three separate sputum samples have been sent for acid-fast stain, fungal stain, Gram stain, silver stain, and cytologic analysis, bronchoscopy should be done in many cases. Sosenko and Glassroth[40] suggested that patients with lung cavities should undergo fiberoptic bronchoscopy if they have certain clinical findings that make the diagnosis of bronchogenic carcinoma more likely. These criteria for bronchoscopy are listed in Table 23–8. In addition to these clinical criteria, the investigators point out the differences in the roentgenographic appearance of lung abscess and cavitary bronchogenic carcinoma. An extensive inflammation surrounding the cavity is more common in lung abscess (Fig. 23–7); in bronchogenic carcinoma, there is distinctly less ground glass infiltrate surrounding the cavity (Fig. 23–8). If a diagnosis of anaerobic lung abscess is supported by the clinical and laboratory findings, bronchoscopy need not be done as long as the patient shows signs of responding to treatment within the first week. Bronchoscopy can be dangerous when it is performed on a patient with a giant anaerobic lung abscess (> 4 cm in diameter), because the passage of a brush or biopsy forceps into the abscess cavity can result in massive endobronchial spillage of pus with disastrous results.[41] When it is considered necessary to perform bronchoscopy on a patient with a giant anaerobic lung abscess, it is best to delay until the patient is no longer toxic and the abscess has decreased somewhat in size or drained spontaneously.

Most patients with anaerobic lung abscess expectorate large volumes of sputum, usually more than 60 mL per day. If a patient is thought to have possible anaerobic lung abscess but is not coughing up any sputum, bronchial obstruction is probable, and the patient should undergo fiberoptic bronchoscopy.

Cavitary disease caused by aerobic bacteria can be diagnosed by bronchoscopy if a telescoping plugged catheter (ie, microbiology brush) is passed into the area of the cavity and the brush sample then yields a pure culture of one organism, such as *Klebsiella pneumoniae*. In some hospitals, quantitative culture of bronchoalveolar lavage fluid is available as a service, and a yield of greater than $10^3$ colony-forming units per milliliter of fluid is considered diagnostic of infection rather than colonization.[42] For cavities

Table 23–7. **Lung Abscess and Empyema Characteristics on Computed Tomographic Scans**

| Feature | Lung Abscess | Empyema |
| --- | --- | --- |
| Wall | Thick | Thin |
|   Luminal margin | Irregular | Smooth |
|   Exterior wall | Irregular | Smooth |
| Chest wall angles | Acute | Obtuse |
| Shape | Round | Lenticular |
| Compression of uninvolved lung | Absent | Present |
| Separate pleural layers seen | Absent | Present |

Table 23–8. **Criteria for Bronchoscopy in Patients With Lung Cavities***

| |
| --- |
| Low-grade fever (<100°F) |
| Leukocyte count < 11,000/mm³ |
| Minimal systemic complaints |
| No factors that predispose to aspiration |

*Patients with three or more of these criteria should undergo bronchoscopy. A patient with fewer than three of the criteria who has a minimal infiltrate surrounding the cavity should also have bronchoscopy.

Modified from Sosenko A, Glassroth J: Fiberoptic bronchoscopy in the evaluation of lung abscesses. Chest 87:489–494, 1985.

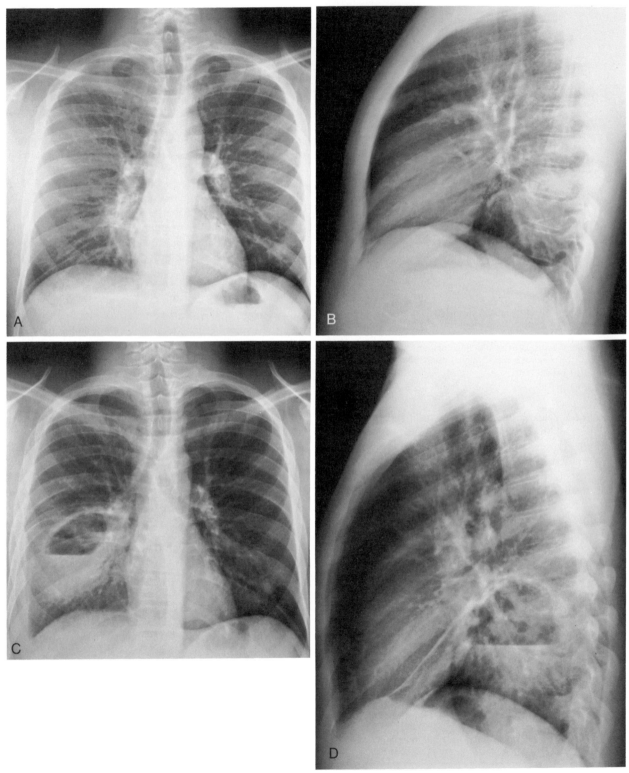

**Figure 23–5.** *A* and *B*, Posteroanterior (PA) and lateral chest roentgenograms of a patient with anaerobic pneumonia secondary to aspiration of oropharyngeal contents during extraction of teeth. The abnormality is a focal water-density infiltrate seen on the PA view next to the right heart border. On the lateral view, the infiltrate overlies vertebral body T-8 and is located in the superior segment of the right lower lobe. *C* and *D*, PA and lateral chest roentgenograms taken 5.5 weeks after those in *A* and *B*. A cavity 6 cm in diameter is seen in the superior segment of the right lower lobe, where there had formerly been a focal ground glass infiltrate. The cavity contains an air-fluid level; the actual cavity is surrounded by an infiltrate. A pleural effusion is on the right side.

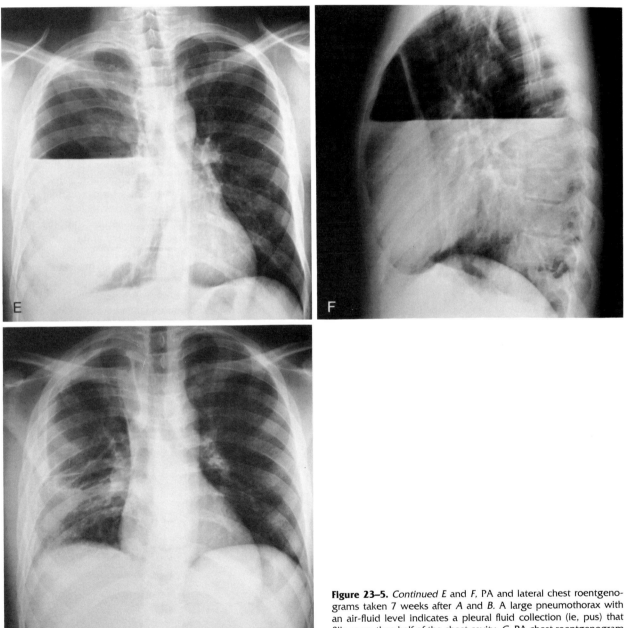

**Figure 23–5.** *Continued E* and *F,* PA and lateral chest roentgenograms taken 7 weeks after *A* and *B.* A large pneumothorax with an air-fluid level indicates a pleural fluid collection (ie, pus) that fills more than half of the chest cavity. *G,* PA chest roentgenogram taken 9 weeks after *A* and *B* and 1 week after right-sided thoracotomy for surgical drainage of anaerobic empyema. The lung is fully expanded, and a band of pleural thickening represents the growth of fibrous tissue into the obliterated right pleural space.

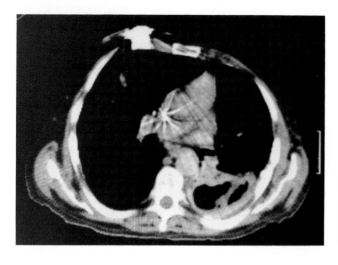

**Figure 23–6.** Thoracic computed tomographic scan of a patient with lymphoma who had a lung abscess in the basilar segment of the left lower lobe caused by *Staphylococcus aureus.* The abscess has a thick wall, and the cavity is traversed by a septum. It has irregular luminal and exterior margins, it forms an acute angle with the chest wall, and it does not compress the surrounding lung.

occurring with diffuse lung lesions in patients infected with HIV, *P. carinii* is a possible cause, and this infection can be diagnosed in most cases by bronchoscopy.[43, 44]

Bronchoscopy in patients with cavitary disease due to fungus is most useful when it produces diagnostic stains of bronchoalveolar lavage, brush, or biopsy material. Testing for cryptococcal antigen in bronchoscopy specimens is often valuable.[19]

If actinomycosis or nocardiosis is suspected, it is important for the bronchoscopist to instruct the microbiology laboratory staff to incubate the cultures for a long enough period. Many microbiology laboratories discard simple bacterial culture specimens after 3 days, and *N. asteroides,* for example, often requires 2 weeks for colonies to appear on ordinary culture media. Fortunately, *Nocardia* grows on fungal media (eg, Sabouraud) and tuberculosis media (eg, Löwenstein-Jensen), and this means that the organism is often found on specimens submitted for ''TB and fungus.'' *Actinomyces* species require special handling that cannot be done routinely for all specimens. If a bronchial brush is passed into a lung segment infected with *Actinomyces,* it is best to transfer the brush into anaerobic holding medium until it can be processed in anaerobic culture in the microbiology laboratory.

If tuberculosis or fungal disease is suspected from the clinical situation and the result of sputum analysis is negative, fiberoptic bronchoscopy has been useful.[44, 45] Stains and cultures of bronchoalveolar lavage fluid yield most of the diagnoses, although some transbronchial biopsies have provided the sole diagnostic finding.

Cavitary lung diseases that are not infections can be diagnosed by fiberoptic bronchoscopy. Approximately 80% of lung cancer cases can be diagnosed by this means.[40] The rare examples of cavitary sarcoidosis[46] can be diagnosed by

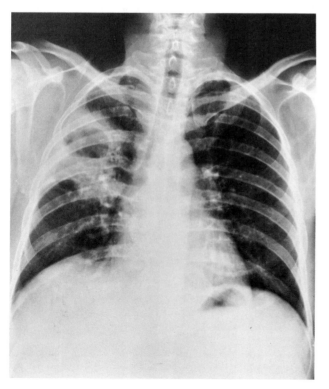

**Figure 23–7.** Posteroanterior chest roentgenogram of a patient with chronic lymphocytic leukemia who has a lung abscess in the right upper lobe caused by *Staphylococcus aureus.* Notice the cavity which contains an air-fluid level. There is a substantial ground glass infiltrate surrounding the wall of the cavity.

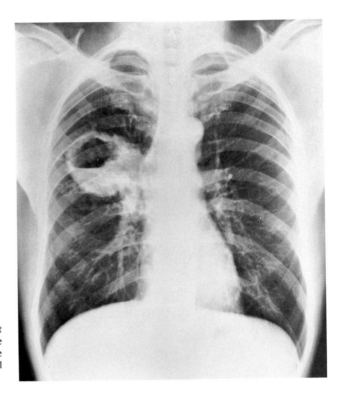

**Figure 23–8.** Posteroanterior chest roentgenogram of a patient without clinical signs of infection. The patient had been a heavy cigarette smoker. The diagnosis was cavitating squamous cell carcinoma of the lung. Notice the cavity that contains an air-fluid level and the minimal ground glass infiltrate surrounding the wall of the cavity.

transbronchial biopsy (Fig. 23–9). Cavitary diseases that usually cannot be diagnosed by bronchoscopy include most cases of cavitary metastatic cancer and Hodgkin disease, bland pulmonary infarct (Fig. 23–10),[47] and Wegener granulomatosis (Fig. 23–11).

### Needle Aspiration

Transthoracic needle aspiration provides a useful alternative to fiberoptic bronchoscopy, and needle aspiration frequently leads to a diagnosis in cases in which bronchos-

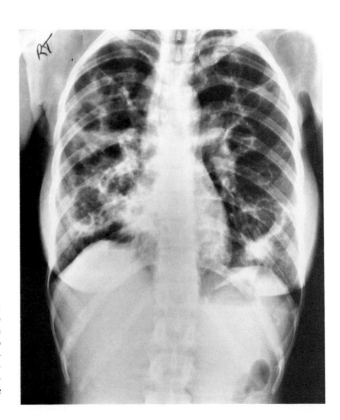

**Figure 23–9.** Posteroanterior chest roentgenogram of a patient with cavitary sarcoidosis. The patient was a 30-year-old black woman who presented with productive cough and dyspnea on exertion and with night sweats, chills, and a 5-kg weight loss. She was afebrile, with no crackles or wheezes in her chest. The blood level of angiotensin-converting enzyme was strikingly elevated. A transbronchial biopsy revealed noncaseating granulomas. The chest film revealed bilateral multiple cavities without air-fluid levels and a ground glass infiltrate surrounding some of the cavities.

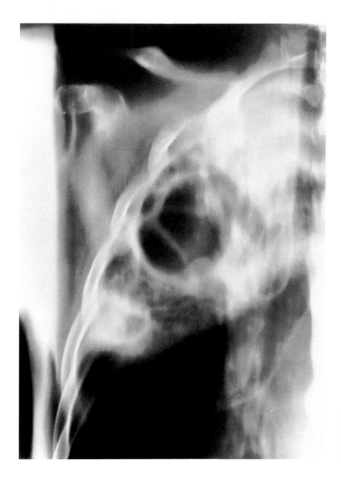

**Figure 23–10.** Chest tomogram of the right upper lobe of a patient with a bland pulmonary infarction and secondary infection. The large cavity contains no air-fluid level and is surrounded by extensive ground glass infiltrate. This case was fatal and proved at autopsy.

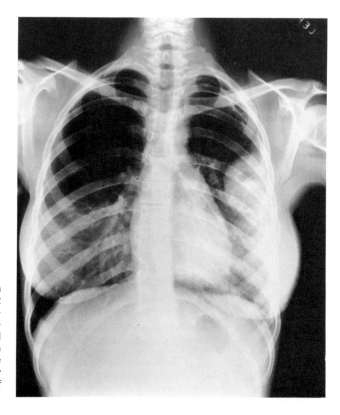

**Figure 23–11.** Posteroanterior chest roentgenogram of a patient with Wegener granulomatosis. The patient was a 16-year-old girl who first presented with arthralgias, fatigue, and weight loss. Later she developed a nonproductive cough, fever, dyspnea, and intermittent hemoptysis. She was febrile and tachycardic and had nasal congestion and diffuse crackles on lung examination. Initially, her chest x-ray film showed a focal ground glass infiltrate that over 1 year changed into the focal cavitary lesion seen here. Notice the central, thick-walled cavity and air-fluid level. Anticytoplasmic antibodies were present at titer of 1:32. The open lung biopsy was diagnostic.

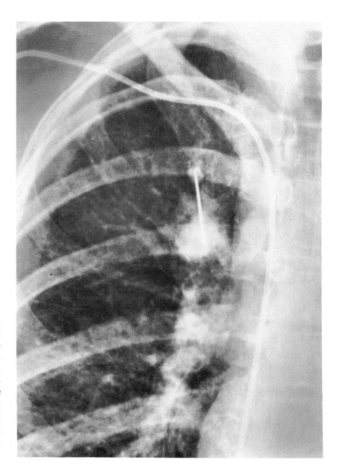

**Figure 23–12.** Roentgenogram of the right upper lobe taken at fluoroscopy for transthoracic needle biopsy. The patient was a 38-year-old woman, a non-smoker who suffered from chronic renal failure secondary to chronic glomerulonephritis. She had received a cadaveric renal transplant and was being treated with the immunosuppressives prednisone, azathioprine, and cyclosporine when she presented with fever and chest pain of 10 days' duration. The physical examination revealed a fever of 38.9°C and clear lungs. The posteroanterior chest film showed a right subclavian catheter and a new abscess nodule containing a small amount of central cavitation (see Fig. 23–3). Shown here is a film documenting the transthoracic needle in the lesion. Gram stain suggested *Nocardia*, and culture confirmed *N. asteroides*.

copy has failed. Transthoracic needle aspiration can successfully diagnose a wide variety of organisms causing subacute pulmonary infection (Fig. 23–12).[48] Unlike the samples obtained at bronchoscopy, samples obtained by transthoracic needle biopsy are not mixed with much local anesthetic, and local anesthetics are known to inhibit growth in culture of some organisms, such as *Mycobacterium tuberculosis*.

### Cultures and Serology

In addition to sending sputum, bronchoscopic specimens, and needle aspirations for culture, blood cultures should be performed for patients with cavitary disease, and if pleural fluid is present, a thoracentesis should be done and sent for culture, cytologic analysis, and staining for microbes.

A limited number of serologic studies may be helpful in the differential diagnosis of cavitary lung disease. Serologic tests for the fungal diseases include the radioassay for *H. capsulatum* and the complement fixation test for *Coccidioides immitis*. If the initial steps in the diagnostic workup have not yielded a diagnosis, a consideration of more unusual causes of lung cavities makes it worthwhile to submit serum for other serologic studies. In a patient with Wegener granulomatosis, the serum contains anticytoplasmic antibodies that are quite sensitive and specific for the disease.[49] The angiotensin-converting enzyme assay of serum can provide good support for the diagnosis of cavitary sarcoidosis.[46]

### Thoracotomy

The previous list of studies determines the cause of most cases of lung cavities, but a small percentage of cases do not yield a diagnosis. In these patients, thoracotomy with lobectomy or segmentectomy must be considered, but this should be the procedure of last resort.

### CONCLUSION

Subacute lung infections can be classified according to the roentgenographic abnormality that is seen on the chest x-ray film when the patient comes to the physician. The simplest clinical problems to solve are those in which the patient has a known risk factor and classic complaints, physical findings, and chest roentgenogram. Cavitary tuberculosis, for example, may require no more than a carefully taken history, physical examination, chest x-ray film, and sputum stain and culture for diagnosis. More challenging diagnoses require more extensive investigations, and individual cases may benefit from CT scanning, bronchoscopy, transthoracic needle aspiration, and in the most difficult cases, thoracotomy and open biopsy or lobectomy.

### REFERENCES

1. Fleischner Society: Glossary of terms for thoracic radiology: Recommendation of the nomenclature committee of the Fleischner Society. AJR 55:363–374, 1984.

2. Cordier JF, Loire R, Brune J: Idiopathic bronchiolitis organizing pneumonia. Definition of characteristic clinical profiles in a series of 16 patients. Chest 96:999–1004, 1989.

3. Jederlinic PJ, Leonard S, Gaensler EA: Chronic eosinophilic pneumonia. A report of 19 cases and a review of the literature. Medicine (Baltimore) 67:154–162, 1988.

4. Hinson KFW, Moon AJ, Plummer NS: Bronchopulmonary aspergillosis. A review and report of eight cases. Thorax 7:317–333, 1952.

5. Kennedy JD, Costello P, Balikian JP, Herman PG: Exogenous lipoid pneumonia. AJR 136:1145–1149, 1981.

6. Fennessy JJ: Irradiation damage to the lung. J Thorac Imaging 2:68–79, 1987.

7. Pluss JL, Opal SM: Pulmonary sporotrichosis: Review of treatment and outcome. Medicine (Baltimore) 65:143–153, 1986.

8. Williams RC: Periodontal disease. N Engl J Med 322:373–382, 1990.

9. Bartlett JG: Anaerobic bacterial infections of the lung. Chest 91:901–909, 1987.

10. Epstein RL: Constituents of sputum. A simple method. Ann Intern Med 77:259–265, 1972.

11. Jett JR, Cortese DA, Dines DE: The value of bronchoscopy in the diagnosis of mycobacterial disease. A five year experience. Chest 80:575–578, 1981.

12. Stenson W, Aranda C, Bevelaqua FA: Transbronchial biopsy culture in pulmonary tuberculosis. Chest 83:883–884, 1983.

13. De Gracia J, Curull V, Vidal R, et al: Diagnostic value of bronchoalveolar lavage in suspected pulmonary tuberculosis. Chest 93:329–332, 1988.

14. Wallace JM, Deutsch AL, Harrell JH, Moser KE: Bronchoscopy and transbronchial biopsy in evaluation of patients with suspected active tuberculosis. Am J Med 70:1189–1194, 1981.

15. Ariel I, Breuer R, Kamal NS, et al: Endobronchial actinomycosis simulating bronchogenic carcinoma. Diagnosis by bronchial biopsy. Chest 99:493–495, 1991.

16. Rodriguez JL, Barrio JL, Pitchenik AE: Pulmonary nocardiosis in the acquired immunodeficiency syndrome. Diagnosis with bronchoalveolar lavage and treatment with non-sulphur-containing drugs. Chest 90:912–914, 1986.

17. Henkle JQ, Nair V: Endobronchial pulmonary nocardiosis. JAMA 256:1331–1332, 1986.

18. Prechter G, Prakash U: Bronchoscopy in the diagnosis of pulmonary histoplasmosis. Chest 95:1033–1036, 1989.

19. Baughman R, Rhodes J, Dohn M, Henderson H, Frame P: Detection of cryptococcal antigen in bronchoalveolar lavage fluid: A prospective study of diagnostic utility. Am Rev Respir Dis 145:1226–1229, 1992.

20. Kwong J, Müller N, Godwin J, Aberle D, Grymaloski M: Thoracic actinomycosis: CT findings in eight patients. Radiology 183:189–192, 1992.

21. Chan KC, Hyland RH, Gray RR, et al: Diagnostic imaging of intralobar bronchopulmonary sequestration. Chest 93:189–192, 1988.

22. Maartens G, Wilcox P, Benatar S: Miliary tuberculosis: Rapid diagnosis, hematologic abnormalities, and outcome in 109 treated adults. Am J Med 89:291–296, 1990.

23. Kariman K, Kylstra J, Spock A: Pulmonary alveolar proteinosis: Prospective clinical experience in 23 patients for 15 years. Lung 162:223–231, 1984.

24. Claypool W, Rogers R, Matuschak G: Update on the clinical diagnosis, management, and pathogenesis of pulmonary alveolar proteinosis (phospholipidosis). Chest 85:550–558, 1984.

25. Grenier P, Valeyre D, Cluzel P, Brauner MW, Lenoir S, Chastang C: Chronic diffuse interstitial lung disease: Diagnostic value of chest radiography and high-resolution CT. Radiology 179:123–132, 1991.

26. Müller N, Miller R: Computed tomography of chronic diffuse infiltrative lung disease. Am Rev Respir Dis 142:1206–1215; 1440–1448, 1990.

27. Wheat LJ, Kohler RB, Tewari RP: Diagnosis of disseminated histoplasmosis by detection of *Histoplasma capsulatum* antigen in serum and urine specimens. N Engl J Med 314:83–86, 1986.

28. Estrera AS, Platt MR, Mills LJ, et al: Primary lung abscess. J Thorac Cardiovasc Surg 79:275–282, 1980.

29. Pohlson EC, McNamara JJ, Char C, et al: Lung abscess: A changing pattern of disease. Am J Surg 150:97–101, 1985.

30. Neild JE, Eykyn SJ, Phillips I: Lung abscess and empyema. Q J Med 57:875–882, 1985.

31. Carruthers MM: Recrudescent melioidosis mimicking lung abscess. Am Rev Respir Dis 124:756–758, 1981.

32. Bordelon JY, Legrand P, Gewin WC, et al: The telescoping plugged catheter in suspected anaerobic infections. A controlled series. Am Rev Respir Dis 128:465–468, 1983.

33. Filice GA: Nocardiosis. *In* Sarosi GA, Davies SF (eds): Fungal Diseases of the Lung. Orlando, Grune & Stratton, 1986:238.

34. Wilson JP, Turner HR, Kirchner KA, et al: *Nocardia* infections in renal transplant recipients. Medicine (Baltimore) 68:38–57, 1989.

35. Kaye MG, Fox MJ, Bartlett JG, et al: The clinical spectrum of *Staphylococcus aureus* infection. Chest 97:788–792, 1990.

36. Venkatachalam KK, Saravolatz LD, Cristopher K: Legionnaires' disease. A cause of lung abscess. JAMA 241:597–598, 1979.

37. Lewin S, Brettman LR, Goldstein EJC, et al: Legionnaires' disease. A cause of severe abscess-forming pneumonia. Am J Med 67:339–341, 1979.

38. Stark DD, Federle MP, Goodman PC, et al: Differentiating lung abscess and empyema: Radiography and computed tomography. AJR 141:163–167, 1983.

39. Oliphant L, McFadden RG, Carr TJ, et al: Magnetic resonance imaging to diagnose intralobar pulmonary sequestration. Chest 91:500–502, 1987.

40. Sosenko A, Glassroth J: Fiberoptic bronchoscopy in the evaluation of lung abscesses. Chest 87:489–494, 1985.

41. Hammer DL, Aranda CP, Galati V, Adams FV: Massive intrabronchial aspiration of contents of pulmonary abscess after fiberoptic bronchoscopy. Chest 74:306–307, 1978.

42. Henriquez AH, Mendoza J, Gonzalez PC: Quantitative culture of bronchoalveolar lavage from patients with anaerobic lung abscess. J Infect Dis 164:414–417, 1991.

43. Klein JS, Warnock M, Webb WR, et al: Cavitating and noncavitating granulomas in AIDS patients with *Pneumocystis carinii* pneumonitis. AJR 152:753–754, 1989.

44. Chechani V, Zaman MK, Finch PJP: Chronic cavitary *Pneumocystis carinii* pneumonia in a patient with AIDS. Chest 95:1347–1348, 1989.

45. Baughman RP, Kohn MN, Loudon RG, et al: Bronchoscopy with bronchoalveolar lavage in tuberculosis and fungal infections. Chest 99:92–97, 1991.

46. Biem J, Hoffstein V: Aggressive cavitary pulmonary sarcoidosis. Am Rev Respir Dis 143:428–430, 1991.

47. Libby LS, King TE, LaForce M, et al: Pulmonary cavitation following pulmonary infarction. Medicine (Baltimore) 64:342–348, 1985.

48. Conces DJ, Schwenk GR, Doering PR, et al: Thoracic needle biopsy. Improved results utilizing a team approach. Chest 91:813–816, 1987.

49. Nölle B, Specks U, Lüdemann J, et al: Anticytoplasmic autoantibodies: Their immunodiagnostic value in Wegener granulomatosis. Ann Intern Med 111:28–40, 1989.

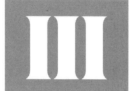
# Pathogens Causing Pneumonia

# CHAPTER 24

# Pneumococcal Pneumonia

SCOTT F. DAVIES

Pneumococcal pneumonia is the most common bacterial pneumonia in humans, accounting for one third to one half of cases. Lobar consolidation is strongly associated with this infection but actually occurs in a minority of cases.[1] The etiologic agent is *Streptococcus pneumoniae,* an encapsulated α-hemolytic *Streptococcus* that is characteristically ovoid or lancet shaped and is arranged in pairs and in chains. Like other streptococci, it is gram positive. More than 80 types of pneumococci have been identified and sequentially numbered, based on variation in the carbohydrate capsule. Serotype-specific IgG antibodies are protective against infection and cause capsular swelling in vitro (ie, Quellung reaction), permitting identification of the clinical isolates. Serotypes differ in virulence, and most infections are caused by a relatively few, low-numbered serotypes.[2]

## HISTORY

Evidence of lobar pneumonia has been observed in Egyptian mummies from 1200 BC. The clinical features of the illness were described well by Hippocrates in the fourth century BC. In the early nineteenth century, Corvisart popularized percussion to localize consolidation or effusion. His student Laennec invented the stethoscope and combined percussion and auscultation to differentiate consolidation from pleural effusion. Laennec introduced most of the terms used in physical diagnosis of chest abnormalities, including rales, crepitations, rhonchi, bronchophony, and egophony.[3]

The concept of a specific infectious cause for a given disease arrived with the germ theory in the late 1800s. Pasteur isolated the pneumococcus in 1880, and it was more fully identified by Frankel in 1884.[3] Frankel named the organism *Diplococcus pneumoniae* and recognized that it was the usual cause of lobar pneumonia. In the interim, Friedlander had identified *Klebsiella pneumoniae,* a gram-negative rod, after growing it from an infected human lung, proving that there were multiple causes of lobar pneumonia. Most microbiologic techniques, including Gram stains, sputum cultures, and blood cultures, originated in the late nineteenth and early twentieth centuries.[3] Chest roentgenograms became available about 1900 and improved diagnostic capabilities.

Study of the bacterial capsule led to serotyping of pneumococci and was soon followed by the development of type-specific antisera for treatment. Serotherapy, introduced in 1912 by Dubos, increased in popularity during the next few decades.[3] The mortality rate of bacteremic pneumococcal pneumonia decreased with serotherapy from 80% to about 50%.[4] The use of oxygen as supportive therapy began in 1918.[3] The introduction of truly effective chemotherapy—penicillin—in the mid-1940s further reduced the mortality of bacteremic pneumococcal pneumonia to about 15%.[5] Penicillin made serotherapy obsolete, and serotyping is of interest only for epidemiologic research.

## EPIDEMIOLOGY

Pneumococci colonize the upper respiratory tract of as many as 20% of healthy adults and a higher percentage of children. Carriage rates are highest in the winter. Transmission of nasopharyngeal bacteria occurs from person to person by droplet nuclei and is facilitated by crowded housing, but it is difficult to "catch" pneumonia directly from airborne bacteria because of the highly effective lung defenses against aerosolized particles. Usually, a person is colonized first and acquires pneumonia after microaspiration of pharyngeal material, which presents a larger inoculum of bacteria to a smaller segment of the lung. A colonized adult carries the organism for a few weeks to 1 year, with an average duration of colonization of about 6 weeks. Few colonized persons develop pneumonia, most of them in the first week of colonization.[6] Long-term carriers may be protected by local and systemic immune responses, including the production of IgG.[7]

Pneumococcal pneumonia is common in infants and children (estimated 6.4 cases/year/1000 persons), uncommon in healthy young adults (estimated 0.2 case/year/1000 persons), and common again in the elderly (estimated 2.8 cases/year/1000 persons > 70 years of age).[7]

Most patients with pneumococcal pneumonia have some predisposing factors. The likelihood of pneumonia increases if a large bolus of pharyngeal material is aspirated (eg, anesthesia, alcohol intoxication, coma, seizure, other loss of airway protection) or if the local lung defenses are impaired (eg, excess mucus, excess of other secretions, impaired cilia from smoking, recent viral infection). Congestive heart failure is a major factor predisposing the patient to bacterial pneumonia if there is chronic edema fluid in the lung. Potent loop diuretics generally can dry the alveolar spaces and reduce this risk.

A reduced IgG response predisposes the patient to pneumococcal pneumonia. This occurs in patients with hypogammaglobulinemia, multiple myeloma, chronic lymphocytic leukemia, and other conditions.

Absence of the spleen or functional hyposplenism (eg, sickle cell anemia) increases the chance that a pneumococcal infection will become fulminant. The spleen enhances antibody production and helps clear bacteria from the blood.

In the acquired immunodeficiency syndrome (AIDS), the annual incidence of bacteremic pneumococcal pneumonia is 10 per 1000 persons, with total pneumococcal pneumonia cases at least double that rate.[8] Colonization rates are not increased. The increased incidence of pneumonia may reflect poor local antibody responses to colonization or other local and systemic immune defects.[8]

## PATHOGENESIS

Colonization of the nose and throat can lead to microaspiration. The presence of specific IgG antibody to the colonizing serotype prevents infection, whether the antibody developed in response to colonization, in response to a previous infection, or in response to vaccination. Even without specific antibody, pulmonary clearance mechanisms usually prevent infection unless there is a large inoculum or there are impaired mechanical defenses.

Under the right conditions in the absence of specific anticapsular antibody, the pneumococci proliferate in the lung. All humans have antibodies to cell wall antigens.[9] These antibodies attach to the cell wall and bind complement. The C-reactive protein, an acute phase reactant, binds to phosphocholine (ie, component of the "C carbohydrate" of the pneumococcal cell wall). This complex can activate the classic complement pathway.[10] The alternate pathway is activated directly by the cell wall and particularly by capsular antigens. All these immune responses release C5a, a potent chemoattractant for neutrophils, which flood the lung. Other cytokines, including interleukin-1 (IL-1) and

tumor necrosis factor (TNF), are released, causing fever and other manifestations of sepsis and recruiting more neutrophils. Pneumolysin, the only toxin produced by pneumococci, is released when bacteria lyse. This toxin has chemoactive and proinflammatory properties.[11]

Despite these immune responses, the neutrophils cannot efficiently phagocytose the bacteria because the antibody and the opsonic fragments of complement (ie, C3b) are sitting on the cell wall, blocked by the carbohydrate capsule from interacting with the appropriate receptors on the phagocytes. The outcome is determined by the balance between the bacterial killing accomplished by this inefficient inflammatory response and the growth rate of the organism. As the bacteria multiply, protein-rich edema fluid and erythrocytes leak into alveolar spaces. Edema is followed by an influx of neutrophils that fill the alveoli. The process spreads centrifugally through the lung, with the leading edge of red hepatization (ie, hemorrhagic edema) surrounding the more established gray hepatization (ie, intense neutrophilic exudate). The process often stops at the pleura or at fissures, resulting in lobar consolidation. Alternatively, the pleura can become inflamed, leading to parapneumonic effusions or empyema.

As pneumococcal pneumonia evolves, bacteria invade the lymphatics. If the draining lymph nodes cannot remove enough bacteria, the organisms spread to the bloodstream. The resultant bacteremia can lead to meningitis, septic arthritis, endocarditis, and other distant manifestations. The spleen has an important role in clearing bacteria that reach the bloodstream. In asplenic patients, the density of the organisms may reach $10^6/1$ mL of peripheral blood. The high-grade bacteremia is often accompanied by septic manifestations, including purpura fulminans, disseminated intravascular coagulation, acute lung injury, and septic shock.[12, 13] Many of these features are caused by immune mediators, including IL-1, TNF, activated components of complement, and platelet activating factor, which are designed for host defense but are capable of local and systemic injury.[10]

In self-limited cases, the neutrophils limit further proliferation of bacteria, because they overcome the inefficient uptake caused by the capsule or because specific anticapsular IgG antibodies develop that coat the exterior of the bacteria, allowing the neutrophils to efficiently ingest them when their Fc receptors attach to fully exposed Fc fragments of the anticapsular antibody. Despite the enormous number of neutrophils that fill the lung during lobar pneumonia, necrosis of the lung is unusual, and scarring of the lung seldom occurs. The proteolytic enzymes of the neutrophils may be neutralized by serum components that leak into the lung. The inflammatory debris is removed by alveolar macrophages, and normal lung architecture is restored. The macrophages do not signal for an influx of fibroblasts as they do in some other lung conditions by release of platelet-derived growth factor and other cellular modulators.

## CLINICAL MANIFESTATIONS

Most patients with pneumococcal pneumonia have abnormal vital signs, including fever, tachycardia, and tachypnea. Hypotension is unusual and is a marker of severe infection. Abrupt onset (within hours) is characteristic, with a shaking chill followed by fever, cough producing purulent or rusty sputum, pleuritic chest pain, and dyspnea. In most cases, this symptom complex evolves over 1 to several days. In the elderly, the clinical findings may be subtle, with a change in mental status the only clue.[14] Cough, sputum production, and fever may be absent.

During an outbreak of influenza A, a biphasic illness is sometimes seen with a viral prodrome (ie, fever, myalgias, headache, nonproductive cough), rapidly turning worse with higher fever, chest pain, productive cough, and dyspnea, usually after an interval of 3 to 7 days.

Classic physical findings of lobar pneumonia include dullness to percussion and increased transmission of all sounds through the fluid-filled lung, which is not as efficient at filtering high-frequency sounds as is the air-filled lung. The breath sounds generated by turbulent flow in central airways are loud and harsh over the affected lobe (ie, bronchial breath sounds). Voice sounds are transmitted better to the hand (ie, increased tactile fremitus) and to the stethoscope (ie, egophony, whispered pectoriloquy). Rales are common because of secretions in the distal airways. Percussion reveals a dull note because the fluid-filled lung is less resonant than the air-filled lung. If there is a pleural effusion or if the lobar bronchus is totally obstructed by pus or other secretions, a decrease in breath sounds and a decrease in tactile and vocal fremitus accompanies the dullness.

An elevated leukocyte count with a shift toward immature forms is common. Other patients have a low leukocyte count, usually with a similar shift toward immature forms. Hypoxemia is common, largely because of shunting through the consolidated lobe. An acute respiratory alkalosis usually occurs. A modest elevation of serum bilirubin may occur. Serum glutamic-oxaloacetic transaminase and alkaline phosphatase are usually only one to two times normal. Some patients have increased blood urea nitrogen levels. Disseminated intravascular coagulation can develop in fulminant cases.

Lobar consolidation is the characteristic finding on the chest roentgenogram (Fig. 24–1). It is more common in bacteremic cases than in nonbacteremic cases. However, more than half of all patients have only a small infiltrate involving less than one segment.[1] Many patients have multifocal infiltrates or patchy infiltrates rather than dense consolidation. If there is underlying emphysema, there is seldom a uniform consolidation, because the abnormal air spaces do not fill with exudate in a uniform manner. The result is a less homogeneous infiltrate (Fig. 24–2). It takes a beautiful lung to produce a ''beautiful'' lobar pneumonia with uniform density and branching air bronchograms. Cavitation of lung parenchyma is unusual. The proposed explanations for lung necrosis have included the high virulence of some serotypes, a large inoculum of organisms, and mixed infection with pneumococci and anaerobic bacteria.[15]

The complications of pneumococcal pneumonia include empyema, meningitis, endocarditis, and septic arthritis. All but empyema have become rare since penicillin has been available. Diffuse infiltrates with the development of the adult respiratory distress syndrome (ARDS) can evolve rapidly in floridly septic patients, or they can develop over

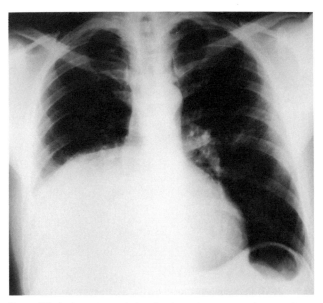

**Figure 24–1.** A posteroanterior chest roentgenogram shows a dense consolidation of the right lower and right middle lobes. The consolidation stops at the lobar boundary. The patient is a 44-year-old man predisposed by alcohol abuse who presented with acute fever, shaking, chills, productive cough, and right-sided pleuritic chest pain. The blood cultures were positive.

several days in less ill patients with less initial hypotension (Fig. 24–3).

Five percent of all patients with pneumococcal pneumonia and 15% of bacteremic patients die of their disease. Estimates of mortality for bacteremic cases vary from 10% to more than 30% and depend greatly on the patient population. A 15% mortality rate is widely accepted as a reasonable estimate, but it may be optimistic. The risk factors for

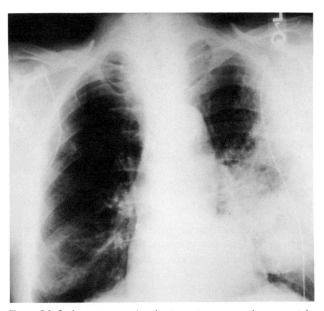

**Figure 24–2.** A posteroanterior chest roentgenogram shows a patchy infiltrate in the left lower lobe. The patient is a 73-year-old man with chronic obstructive lung disease who presented with acute fever, shaking, chills, productive cough, and left-sided pleuritic chest pain. The blood cultures were positive.

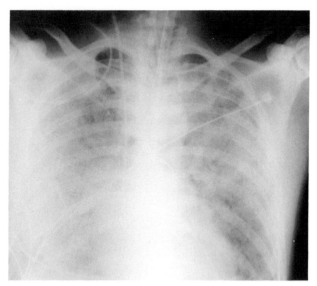

**Figure 24–3.** A posteroanterior chest roentgenogram shows bilateral diffuse infiltrates characteristic of acute lung injury in the same patient as shown in Figure 24–1. He was bacteremic but was never hypotensive. Despite prompt antibiotic therapy, he developed diffuse infiltrates over a 3-day period. He required ventilatory support for 14 days and recovered fully.

death include old age, a very high or very low leukocyte count, tachypnea, hypotension, diffuse infiltrates, severe hypoxemia, and confusion.[16] Patients who develop ARDS have a mortality rate greater than 50%. Approximately half of these deaths occur in the first 4 days, and there is evidence that this incidence of early deaths from overwhelming infection has not been altered much by antibiotic therapy.[5]

Pneumococcal pneumonia in AIDS patients has several different features. Bacteremia occurs in more than 50% of these patients, compared with a rate of 20% for non-AIDS patients. The mortality rate for bacteremic patients is low (6% in one large series), probably significantly lower than for immunocompetent patients. The mortality rate may be lower because bacteremia occurs in milder cases of pneumonia, or it may be lower because of a blunting of the expected immune response that in normal hosts contributes to systemic manifestations of sepsis. Patients with AIDS can have relapses of infection or recurrent infections with different serotypes. In one series, 13% of patients had a second episode of pneumococcal disease within 6 months.[8]

## DIAGNOSIS

The diagnosis of pneumonia is usually imprecise, largely because all coughed respiratory secretions are expelled through the mouth, which is a virtual cesspool. Infected respiratory secretions and infected lung tissue have approximately $10^5$ organisms per 1 mL of secretions or per 1 g of tissue. Oral secretions have $10^8$ or more organisms per 1 mL, and all coughed specimens are contaminated by oral flora. Only positive cultures from the blood or from other normally sterile body fluids can give a certain diagnosis. Blood cultures are positive for 20% of cases of pneumococ-

cal pneumonia. Positive cultures of pleural fluid are uncommon ($\le$ 1%).

Sputum must be screened to make sure it is of good quality. One common guideline is that it must show more than 25 neutrophils and less than 10 epithelial cells per low-powered field.[17] Good-quality sputum is examined directly after Gram staining and is cultured.

A Gram stain shows gram-positive diplococci for 15% to 30% of cases. Although the sensitivity is poor, the specificity is fairly good. One study showed a positive predictive value of 78%.[16] False-positive results occur for colonized patients and patients with acute and chronic bronchitis. Gram-positive organisms from the mouth can also appear on the slide, even if the sample meets the criteria for "good quality."

Sputum cultures are positive in 25% to 50% of all cases. About 10% of control patients and a higher percentage of patients with chronic bronchitis grow pneumococcus from upper or lower respiratory secretions.

Counterimmunoelectrophoresis (CIE) of sputum is controversial. In most hands, the sensitivity is higher than that of sputum culture.[16] There is disagreement about whether there are more false-positive results from colonization and from chronic bronchitis than there are with sputum cultures.

Prior treatment with antibiotics decreases the yield of all tests by 50% or more, and about half of all patients who are hospitalized with pneumonia have already received an antibiotic before admission.[16] The mortality rate of patients with pneumococcal pneumonia who have received antibiotics before admission may be less than that of patients who have not.[16]

Transtracheal aspiration can reliably diagnose pneumococcal pneumonia. A negative result for a culture before any antibiotic treatment is strong evidence against pneumococcal pneumonia. Most of the information about transtracheal aspirates comes from research studies. The test is seldom performed today and is unlikely to be done before any antibiotic is given.

A negative culture result for a protected catheter brush sample obtained during fiberoptic bronchoscopy virtually excludes pneumococcal pneumonia if the specimen is obtained before administration of antibiotics,[18] but a negative test result is likely after antibiotics have been started. In practice, diagnostic bronchoscopy is seldom done before antibiotic treatment. It is usually done late to diagnose unusual infections, including those of *Legionella,* mycobacteria, and fungi, rather than early to diagnose pneumococcal infection.

Transthoracic aspiration has a fairly good yield before antibiotic treatment has begun, and it has almost perfect specificity. Transthoracic aspiration has a high risk of pneumothorax and is seldom done, especially before any antibiotic is given. There is a need for more sensitive and more specific tests for pneumococcal pneumonia.

## TREATMENT

Penicillin is the treatment of choice for sensitive isolates. Hospitalized patients can be given 1 to 2 million units intravenously every 4 hours. Procaine penicillin, administered intramuscularly in a dosage of 1.2 million units twice daily, is also appropriate treatment. Patients who do not require hospitalization can be treated with oral penicillin or with oral amoxicillin. About 50% of patients have a marked decrease in temperature within 36 hours, and a very high percentage have a similar response within 72 hours. Therapy should continue until the patient has been afebrile for 48 hours. The total course usually is 5 to 7 days. Patients with AIDS should be treated for 10 to 14 days.[8]

Because the diagnosis of pneumonia is imprecise and often delayed, most patients with pneumococcal pneumonia are initially treated with a broad-spectrum cell wall antibiotic that covers *S. pneumoniae, Haemophilus influenzae, Moraxella catarrhalis,* and *K. pneumoniae* and that has some activity against *Staphylococcus aureus.* A variety of broad-spectrum agents cover this range of organisms. Second- and third-generation cephalosporins are used most often, sometimes in combination with other agents. If the blood cultures are positive for *S. pneumoniae,* the patient should be switched to penicillin. If blood cultures are negative and sputum cultures grow *S. pneumoniae,* another likely pathogen, or "oral flora," it is reasonable if the patient is clinically improving to complete the treatment course with the initial antibiotic. If the patient is still not improving, additional diagnostic tests or additional empiric therapy, guided by the clinical situation, will be necessary.

The minimal inhibitory concentration (MIC) for strains of pneumococcus has gradually increased since the introduction of penicillin, from less than 0.02 μg/1 mL of penicillin to the current range of 0.05 to 1.0 μg/mL. In the United States, 10% of the strains have MICs between 0.1 and 1.0 μg/mL. These strains have intermediate resistance but can still be treated with penicillin. Only 1% of strains have MICs greater than 2.0 μg/mL. These strains are highly resistant to penicillin and usually are resistant to other antibiotics. Reports of the spread of resistant strains in South Africa, Spain, and Hungary[19-21] have caused concern that similar problems are ahead in the United States. It is prudent to screen all isolates for penicillin resistance, using an oxacillin disk.

Therapy should include ventilatory support and hemodynamic support for appropriate critically ill patients. Large pleural effusions should be tapped, and those that are very inflammatory or grossly infected should be drained by chest tube, thoracoscopy, or thoracotomy. The diagnostic tests to rule out meningitis (including spinal tap) should be done for headache or stiff neck, because higher doses of penicillin are used for meningitis and the duration of therapy is longer.

## PREVENTION

The vaccine contains antigens from 23 serotypes. Healthy adults develop protective antibodies against at least 75% of the serotypes. In immunocompetent adults with indications for the vaccine, the protective efficacy is 61% (47%–72% for a 95% confidence interval).[22]

Patients with serious underlying diseases, postsplenectomy patients, and immunosuppressed patients including those with AIDS have less uniform and less predictable antibody responses.[23] The number of responses and the magnitude of the responses are greatly reduced, but there is little to lose from vaccinating all high-risk patients as early as possible in the course of the illness that places them at risk. Prophylactic oral penicillin is used for high-risk postsplenectomy patients and may also be appropriate in some particularly high-risk patients with AIDS.[8]

## REFERENCES

1. Ort S, Ryan JL, Barden G, D'Esopo N: Pneumococcal pneumonia in hospitalized patients: Clinical and radiographical presentations. JAMA 249:214–218, 1983.
2. Gray BM, Dillon HC Jr: Clinical and epidemiologic studies of pneumococcal infection in children. Pediatr Infect Dis 5:201–207, 1986.
3. Duffin J: Pneumonia. *In* Kipple KF (ed): The Cambridge World History of Human Disease. Cambridge, Cambridge University Press, 1993:938–941.
4. Tilghman RC Jr, Dowdle WR, Marine RC, Finland M: Clinical significance of bacteremia in pneumococcal pneumonia. Arch Intern Med 59:602–619, 1937.
5. Austrian R, Gold J: Pneumococcal bacteremia with special reference to bacteremic pneumococcal pneumonia. Ann Intern Med 60:759–776, 1964.
6. Gray BM, Dillon HC Jr: Natural history of pneumococcal infections. Pediatr Infect Dis J 8:S23–S25, 1989.
7. Musher DM: Infections caused by *Streptococcus pneumoniae:* Clinical spectrum, pathogenesis, immunity, and treatment. Clin Infect Dis 14:801–809, 1992.
8. Janoff EN, Breiman RF, Daley CL, Hopewell PC: Pneumococcal disease during HIV infection. Ann Intern Med 117:314–324, 1992.
9. Musher DM, Watson DA, Baughn RE: Does naturally acquired IgG antibody to cell wall polysaccharide protect human subjects against pneumococcal infection? J Infect Dis 161:736–740, 1990.
10. Johnston RB Jr: Pathogenesis of pneumococcal pneumonia. Rev Infect Dis 13:S509–S517, 1991.
11. Berry AM, Yother J, Briles DE, et al: Reduced virulence of a defined pneumolysin-negative mutant of *Streptococcus pneumoniae.* Infect Immun 57:2037–2042, 1989.
12. Bisno AL, Freeman JC: The syndrome of asplenia, pneumococcal sepsis and disseminated intravascular coagulation. Ann Intern Med 72:389–393, 1970.
13. Torres J, Bisno AL: Hyposplenism and pneumococcemia: Visualization of *Diplococcus pneumoniae* in the peripheral blood smear. Am J Med 55:851–855, 1973.
14. Verghese A, Berk SL: Bacterial pneumonia in the elderly. Medicine (Baltimore) 362:271–285, 1983.
15. Leatherman JW, Iber C, Davies SF: Cavitation in bacteremic pneumococcal pneumonia: Causal role of mixed infection with anaerobic bacteria. Am Rev Respir Dis 129:317–321, 1984.
16. British Thoracic Society Research Committee and the Public Health Laboratory Service: Community acquired pneumonia in adults in British hospitals in 1982–1983. A survey of aetiology, mortality, prognostic factors and outcome. Q J Med 62:195–220, 1987.
17. Murray PR, Washington JA II: Microscopic and bacteriologic analysis of expectorated sputum. Mayo Clin Proc 50:339–344, 1975.
18. Windely NW, Bass JB, Boyd BW, et al: Use of a bronchoscopic protected catheter brush for the diagnosis of pulmonary infections. Chest 81:556–562, 1982.
19. Klugman KP: Pneumococcal resistance to antibiotics. Clin Microbiol Rev 3:171–196, 1990.
20. Ward J: Antibiotic-resistant *Streptococcus pneumoniae.* Clinical and epidemiological aspects. Rev Infect Dis 3:254–266, 1981.
21. Marton A, Gulyas M, Munoz R, Tomasz A: Extremely high incidence of antibiotic resistance in clinical isolates of *Streptococcus pneumoniae* in Hungary. J Infect Dis 163:542–548, 1991.
22. Shapiro ED, Berg AT, Austrian R, et al: The protective efficacy of polyvalent pneumococcal polysaccharide vaccine. N Engl J Med 325:1453–1460, 1991.
23. Simlerkoff MS, Cross AP, Al-Ibralian M, et al: Efficacy of pneumococcal vaccine in high risk patients. Results of a VA cooperative study. N Engl J Med 325:1318–1327, 1986.

# Haemophilus influenzae as a Cause of Acute Tracheobronchitis or Pneumonia

DANIEL M. MUSHER

*Haemophilus influenzae* is second only to *Streptococcus pneumoniae* as a cause of acute bacterial infection of the lungs and lower airways in adults. Unencapsulated, nontypable organisms are responsible for most of these infections, and they also cause otitis media and acute sinusitis. The more highly virulent, encapsulated *H. influenzae* type b (HITB), the organism that, before widespread vaccination, was the most common cause of bacterial meningitis in infants and toddlers, occasionally causes pneumonia in adults.

## HISTORIC CONTEXT

*H. influenzae* organisms were first seen in lung tissue obtained at autopsy during an influenza virus pandemic, and it was isolated by growth on a medium containing blood. The organism derived its name from the growth requirement for blood and because it was thought to be the etiologic agent of epidemic influenza. Although by the 1950s British physicians considered nontypable *H. influenzae* (NTHI) to play a major role in the pathogenesis of chronic bronchitis, the importance of this organism was largely overlooked in the United States. In 1967, Turk and May[1] summarized data from papers published mainly in Great Britain in the 1950s and 1960s, showing that the average rate of isolation of *H. influenzae* from purulent sputum of patients with chronic bronchitis was 65%, compared with 15% from mucoid specimens. The studies in-

volving antibiotic therapy for chronic bronchitis showed that after the *Haemophilus* was eliminated, the purulent quality of the sputum disappeared, sometimes accompanied by an improvement in breathing. Symptoms recurred at the end of therapy, coincident with the reappearance of the *Haemophilus* infection. The investigators used these data to support the theory that NTHI plays a causative role in chronic bronchitis and in acute exacerbations. However, they failed to recognize the importance of NTHI in adult infection, stating, "It is certain that capsulated type b strains can cause pneumonia but there is no clear evidence that noncapsulated strains ever do so."[1]

In the United States, three errors contributed to the failure to recognize the role of *H. influenzae* in pulmonary disease: sputum was not always cultured on chocolate agar; blood cultures were not read as positive unless the broth turned turbid; and isolates were assumed to be type b or were typed incorrectly by the agglutination technique. As a result, *H. influenzae* was regarded as a relatively uncommon cause of pneumonia in the United States, and HITB was thought to be responsible.

In the early 1970s, the routine use of chocolate agar for culturing sputum became accepted, and laboratories began to subculture blood culture onto chocolate agar routinely after 48 hours of incubation, whether they were cloudy or not. In 1981, Wallace and colleagues[2] showed that incorrect serotyping was responsible for systematic errors in which unencapsulated isolates were said to be encapsulated. As a result of this work, it became apparent that most cases of pneumonia, meningitis, and bacteremia in adults are caused by nontypable rather than type b *H. influenzae*. We[3] were able to demonstrate that *H. influenzae* is a common cause of pneumonia or acute purulent tracheobronchitis in adults and that nontypable strains are responsible for most cases. Of the typable strains, HITB is by far most commonly implicated in pulmonary disease, although other serotypes may cause disease, as described by Slater and coworkers.[4] For a review of NTHI, the reader is referred to the work of Murphy and Apicella.[5]

## MICROBIOLOGY

*H. influenzae* organisms appear on Gram stain as tiny, gram-negative coccobacilli. For growth, these organisms require nicotinamide adenine dinucleotide (ie, V factor), which diffuses out of erythrocytes, and hemin (ie, X factor), which is only released after erythrocytes are lysed. Isolation of *H. influenzae* on an agar medium requires the erythrocytes to be broken up, as occurs when the blood is heated to make chocolate agar or when hemolytic bacteria form colonies that are surrounded by a zone of lysed erythrocytes; in the latter instance, *H. influenzae* grows as tiny colonies around the hemolytic organism in a satellite pattern. *Haemophilus parainfluenzae*, which is occasionally implicated as a cause of a bronchopulmonary infection in adults, does not require X factor and can grow on blood agar and on chocolate agar. Recent observations suggest that many isolates identified as *H. parainfluenzae* should be properly designated as *H. paraphrophilus*.

*H. influenzae* can be separated into encapsulated or typable strains, based on the antigenic nature of the capsular polysaccharide, and unencapsulated or nontypable strains. There are seven serotypes of *H. influenzae*, types a through f and e'. The serotypes were originally identified by an agglutination reaction using antisera raised in rabbits, but with this method, crossreactions with somatic antigens may cause nontypable strains to be designated as typable, the systematic error that occurred in the United States until the late 1970s. Counterimmunoelectrophoresis eliminates this problem because, under the influence of an electric current, somatic (protein) antigens migrate away from the antibody, but capsular (polysaccharide) antigens migrate toward the antibody, forming a line of precipitation. A molecular epidemiologic study[6] of more than 2000 encapsulated isolates of HITB from around the world showed a high degree of genetic conservation, with nine clonal types causing most disease resulting from this serotype. Serotypes a and d are related to HITB, but serotypes c, e, e', and f are not closely related to any other *H. influenzae*. The NTHI are much more genetically and phenotypically diverse.[5]

## EPIDEMIOLOGY

*H. influenzae* colonizes healthy children and adults; the rate of colonization is far greater for NTHI than for HITB, approaching 50% in children, 30% in normal adults, and 50% to 60% in persons who have chronic obstructive pulmonary disease (COPD). These results have been derived from studies that used a variety of methodologies, and no direct comparison among these populations can be made. HITB is found in only 1% to 2% of healthy children and only rarely in adults. The organisms spread among persons by direct contact, transmission of secretions, or by aerosol routes, without a known contribution from environmental sources or animal reservoirs. Families and day care centers are important sources for dissemination of these organisms.[7] Crossinfection of adults within a hospital has also been documented.[8]

Longitudinal studies of children[7, 9] have shown that some children maintain a resident strain of NTHI and others acquire new strains as they are exposed to them. Acute otitis media due to *Haemophilus* (usually NTHI) is associated with the acquisition of a new strain.[9] In their studies of acute exacerbations of chronic bronchitis in adults, Groeneveld and coworkers[10] showed that some are caused by a new strain and others by an older, prevailing strain of *H. influenzae*. After persons have been colonized by *H. influenzae*, they tend to retain the same organisms for weeks to months. Adults who have chronic lung disease keep the same isolate even after treatment with antibiotics to which the organisms are susceptible. A slight degree of antigenic drift has been observed,[11] with changes in outer membrane proteins but not in DNA fingerprinting by restriction enzyme analysis.

## PATHOGENESIS

*H. influenzae* adheres to epithelial cells by means of pili (fimbriae)[12–14] and by other, non–pili-related mechanisms that involve synthesis perhaps of adherence proteins.[15] In vitro studies of tracheal culture[16] show that mucus production increases and epithelial damage occurs as a result of the interaction with NTHI. It is not certain which bacterial component is responsible for this damage, but lipooligosaccharide is probably involved. The more invasive HITB has been shown to penetrate epithelial layers and capillary endothelium by migrating between cells.[17] These observations help to explain why colonization of the upper airways may be followed immediately by bacteremia. Some prior damage may facilitate the process of bacterial adherence to tracheal epithelium.[16] We previously demonstrated that infection of human subjects with attenuated influenza virus increased attachment of NTHI to their epithelial cells.[18]

Pneumonia is thought to occur when colonization of the upper airways is followed by microaspiration or inhalation of nasopharyngeal secretions. The early notion[1] that the lower airways of persons who have chronic lung disease are always colonized with *H. influenzae* may be true for patients who chronically produce purulent sputum,[19] but it is not true of those who do not.[20, 21] Transtracheal aspiration in patients who have stable COPD without purulent sputum reveals few organisms below the trachea, and *Haemophilus* is identified in only a small proportion of such cases.[20] Similarly, longitudinal studies of COPD patients using repeated Gram stain analysis and semiquantitative culture show few or no *Haemophilus* organisms during periods of clinical stability.[21]

Most bacterial pneumonias occur in people who have underlying conditions that alter their ability to clear aspirated microorganisms from the lungs or compromise their

Table 25–1. **Underlying Diseases in Patients With Pneumonia or Febrile Purulent Tracheobronchitis**

| Underlying Diseases | Pneumonia (n = 30) | Febrile Purulent Tracheobronchitis (n = 14) |
|---|---|---|
| Chronic obstructive pulmonary disease | 24 | 11 |
| Severe alcoholism | 8 | 4 |
| Malignancy | 6* | 0 |
| Nosocomial infection | 4† | 0 |
| Diabetes mellitus | 2 | 0 |
| Miscellaneous | 7‡ | 3§ |

*Cancer of lung (3 patients), lung and larynx (1), larynx (1), and esophagus (1).
†Postoperative condition (3 patients), paraplegia (1).
‡Multiple myeloma (1 patient), systemic lupus erythematosus (1), pancytopenia (1), common variable immunodeficiency (1), hepatitis (1), multiple drug addiction (1), and multiple rib fractures (1).
§Meningioma with seizures (1 patient), Felty syndrome (1), and peritoneal dialysis (1).

immunity. Pneumonia caused by *H. influenzae* has received much less clinical attention than that caused by *S. pneumoniae*. In 30 patients who had *H. influenzae* pneumonia, we[3] identified a total of 51 underlying conditions, with at least one found in every person (Table 25–1). Twenty-four patients, some of whom were taking glucocorticosteroids, had a diagnosis of COPD; 16 of these had at least one other major underlying disease. Of the 6 who did not have COPD, 4 patients with NTHI pneumonia had hepatitis, common variable immunodeficiency, pancytopenia, or malnutrition due to alcoholism, and the 2 patients with HITB pneumonia included a multiple-drug abuser and an alcoholic. Arteriosclerotic heart disease was present in several patients but without congestive heart failure, and it was not included as an underlying condition. Four patients had nosocomial infections, of whom 3 had just undergone surgery. The findings in 14 persons who had acute febrile tracheobronchitis were similar; every patient had at least one serious underlying illness. Several other investigators have demonstrated a variety of underlying diseases in patients who have infection caused by *H. influenzae*.[22–25] There has been an enormous increase in *H. influenzae* infection among patients infected with human immunodeficiency virus.[24]

## DIAGNOSIS

### Symptoms and Signs

The average duration of acute symptoms before hospitalization of patients with NTHI pneumonia was 5.1 days, in contrast to the more acute onset of symptoms in patients with pneumonia due to typable *H. influenzae* (mean, 1.5 days). Most patients had a prodromal syndrome of upper or lower respiratory infection for 2 to 4 days, followed by a more acute deterioration that led them to seek medical attention. Almost all patients had cough and sputum production, that was new or increased over their baseline values. The mean temperature (highest recorded value) of all patients with *H. influenzae* pneumonia was 38.5°C. Three patients had temperatures of 37.8°C or less. All had overwhelming infections, 2 died (1 had bacteremia), and 1 sur-

vived (also with bacteremia). The mean leukocyte count was 13,400/mm,[3] although a substantial proportion of patients had counts of less than 11,500/mm.[3]

The clinical findings in 14 patients who had acute, febrile, purulent tracheobronchitis with *H. influenzae* (nontypable in every case) as the sole pathogenic bacterium cultured from sputum were similar to those in pneumonia patients except for the absence of a distinct pulmonary infiltrate. The presenting symptoms and signs of the illness in patients with acute, febrile, purulent tracheobronchitis were indistinguishable from those of patients with pneumonia. The mean duration of symptoms before hospitalization was 5.9 days. The mean temperature was 38.5°C, and the mean leukocyte count was 13,320/mm[3]. These findings suggest that NTHI principally damages bronchi and bronchioles, with secondary involvement of the alveoli. Alternatively, the frequent occurrence of underlying lung disease may have obscured detection of small infiltrates.

### Radiographic Manifestations

In our study,[3] all 30 patients with pneumonia had lower lobe infiltrates. Seven patients had consolidated infiltrates: 3 in the right lower lobe and 4 in the left lower lobe. In 23 patients, the infiltrates were subsegmental; 12 involved the right lower lobe, 7 the left lower lobe, and 4 both lower lobes (Fig. 25–1). Two of the 26 patients with NTHI pneumonia had complicated parapneumonic effusions[18] requiring thoracostomy or thoractomy. One patient with HITB pneumonia had an uncomplicated parapneumonic effusion that resolved after antibiotic therapy alone. By definition,

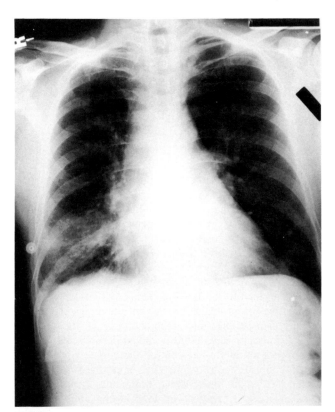

**Figure 25–1.** Radiograph of a patient who had pneumonia in the right lower lobe caused by nontypable *Haemophilus influenzae*.

none of the patients with acute febrile purulent tracheobronchitis had recognizable pulmonary infiltrates.

### Diagnostic Microbiology

*H. influenzae* infection stimulates a vigorous inflammatory response. Most patients who have *Haemophilus* infections of the lower airways already have chronic inflammation of the lungs, and obtaining a valid sputum specimen is usually not a problem. Gram stain and culture of the sputum are central to making the correct diagnosis. *Haemophilus* organisms are present in such profuse numbers that the Gram-stained sputum is characteristic,[3, 26] as is a comparison of the sputum culture on blood and on chocolate agar.[27] Quantitative studies generally reveal $5 \times 10^7$ or more colony-forming units per milliliter of homogenized sputum, a finding that is consistent with Gram stain and culture results. Some strains require increased levels of $CO_2$ for growth; unless a $CO_2$ incubator or candle jar is routinely used for primary isolation, some NTHI isolates will be missed. The rate of coinfection is sufficiently high that the presence of *S. pneumoniae* must be sought by careful inspection of the blood agar plate, even if *H. influenzae* is the obviously predominant colony. With escalating antibiotic resistance of pneumococci, the search for pneumococci is likely to become increasingly important. Blood cultures are positive for about 10% to 15% of patients with pneumonia due to NTHI and in a higher percentage if HITB is responsible. Patients with acute, purulent, febrile tracheobronchitis do not have *Haemophilus* bacteremia.

### ANTIBIOTIC THERAPY

In 1983, when we reported the results of treating bronchopulmonary *Haemophilus* infections,[3] almost all nontypable isolates were susceptible to penicillin (mean minimal inhibitory concentration, 0.5 µg/mL; range, 0.15–1.2 µg/mL), and only about 20% of the type b isolates were penicillin-resistant. There has been a steady increase in the incidence of resistance among *Haemophilus* strains. In 1986, 16% of NTHI and 32% of HITB produced β-lactamase.[28] In 1993, about 20% of NTHI and almost 50% of HITB isolated from infected adults are β-lactamase producers. Treatment with a penicillin, such as ampicillin or amoxicillin, combined with a substance that covalently binds β-lactamase, such as clavulanic acid or sulbactam, is effective. Some second-generation cephalosporins, such as cefaclor, are effective against β-lactamase–producing *H. influenzae*, as are all widely used third-generation cephalosporins. The failure of an isolate to grow in laboratory media can lead to the false appearance of susceptibility to ampicillin; the problem has become more widespread in recent years because microdilutions in wells are routinely used to measure susceptibility. Laboratories must rely on appropriate antibiotic-free controls to avoid this problem.[29]

It is more difficult to generalize about the susceptibility of the rare ampicillin-resistant strains that do not produce β-lactamase and are resistant to β-lactam antibiotics because of decreased transport of antibiotic across the cell membrane. Mendelman and colleagues[29] pointed out a number of problems with the susceptibility testing of typable *H. influenzae* on standard test media. Ampicillin-resistant isolates that are not β-lactamase producers are likely to be reported erroneously as susceptible. It seems reasonable to use ampicillin-sulbactam or a third-generation cephalosporin to treat pneumonia thought to be caused by *H. influenzae*. We change to ampicillin if the organism is not a β-lactamase producer. Treatment is associated with a rapid decline in bacteria, polymorphonuclear leukocytes (PMN), and sputum purulence and with a resolution of symptoms. If this response is not observed, complications (eg, empyema) or infections caused by other organisms are more likely to be responsible than a poorly responsive, β-lactamase–negative, ampicillin-resistant strain. We have seen several patients who were being treated for upper lobe pneumonia that was thought to be caused by *H. influenzae* but was actually caused by *Mycobacterium tuberculosis*.

NTHI has remained uniformly susceptible to trimethoprim-sulfamethoxazole (TMP-SMX) and chloramphenicol and nearly so to tetracycline.[28] These drugs may be reasonable choices to treat acute, febrile, purulent tracheobronchitis, but it is difficult to be enthusiastic about the use of TMP-SMX or tetracycline for pneumonia because of the increasing incidence of *S. pneumoniae* infections resistant to these drugs. These two organisms coexist sufficiently frequently in the sputum of patients with pneumonia to avoid an antibiotic that is not effective against the pneumococcus. Erythromycin is not effective against *H. influenzae*. The notion that this (or any other agent) can be selected ''empirically'' for pneumonia without examining a Gram-stained sputum is erroneous, and physicians daily see the consequences of such poor medical practice. Newer macrolides such as clarithromycin or azithromycin are effective against *Haemophilus* but their usefulness may be limited, because penicillin-resistant pneumococci are likely to be resistant to them as well.

### IMMUNITY

Infants at the time of a first infection caused by NTHI (usually otitis media) lack antibody to the outer membrane proteins and lipooligosaccharides of these organisms, and they have low levels or no bactericidal and opsonizing antibodies. Antibodies to these bacterial components are demonstrable soon after infection by a particular strain, and reinfection is usually caused by a new strain to which antibody is not present.[30, 31] Healthy, young adults tend to have antibodies to many of these bacterial constituents in their serum, although sera exhibit various degrees of bacterial and opsonizing capacities against different isolates of NTHI.[32] Older men with COPD have high levels of bacterial antibody and modest levels of opsonizing activity in their sera at the time *H. influenzae* pneumonia is diagnosed.[3] Opsonizing antibody increases during infection and has been correlated with the appearance of antibody to particular outer membrane proteins.[33]

Antibody that appears after infection is thought to protect toddlers from subsequent infection by that same strain of NTHI, explaining the observation that recurrent infections are often caused by different strains.[5, 30, 31, 34] Murphy and Bartos[35] have shown a representative antibody to the P2 outer membrane protein of NTHI to be bactericidal. An infant rat model has been used successfully to document the emergence and the biologic activity of these antibodies.[36] Because older men with COPD have such high levels of antibody to NTHI, it is thought that anatomic damage to airways is responsible for their susceptibility to pneumonia, although, even higher levels of opsonizing antibody are present after infection. We have shown that sIgA in the respiratory secretions may exert a blocking effect on the interaction between NTHI and IgG,[37] perhaps preventing eradication of NTHI from the bronchial tree during infection.

In the case of HITB, bactericidal antibody is lacking in the serum of infants and toddlers but is present in the serum of about one half of healthy young adults.[38] The principal mode of protection is thought to be by antibody to capsular polysaccharide antigen (PRP), although several studies have shown a role for antibody to lipooligosaccharides and outer membrane proteins.[39] Bactericidal and opsonizing antibodies are thought to be involved, and the literature is difficult to interpret because the demonstration of bactericidal antibody may depend on the methods used. Certainly the effectiveness of a vaccine that contains PRP conjugated to an unrelated protein supports the importance of anti-PRP antibody in immunity. However, vaccines that link PRP to ribosomal or outer membrane proteins of HITB may be even more effective, suggesting a contributing role for other immune determinants.

Infection by HITB is not frequent enough in the adult population to warrant a general recommendation for vaccination. Special consideration should be given to splenectomized persons, those with complement deficiencies, and persons who have deficiencies in humoral immunity but may be able to mount some response.

## SPECIAL PROBLEMS

Because *H. influenzae* can be isolated as a colonizing organism in a substantial proportion of persons who have COPD, how can the physician determine whether it is responsible for a specific illness? How can the physician tell if an exacerbation of COPD is induced by infection, specifically bacterial infection? British investigators related the isolation of *H. influenzae* to increased purulence of sputum. Chodosh[21] used semiquantitative techniques to show that the number of PMNs and the number of bacteria (eg, *Haemophilus, Neisseria,* pneumococci) correlate with the degree of purulence and symptoms of exacerbated chronic bronchitis. The organisms present in the greatest absolute numbers were the *Haemophilus*-like organisms. This correlates with my clinical observations on sputum specimens in pneumonia or acute, purulent tracheobronchitis due to *Haemophilus* or pneumococcus. These findings help to explain the emphasis on microscopic examination of a Gram-stained sputum specimen.

For many years, the medical literature contained conflicting results for the role of antibiotics in prophylaxis and treatment of acute exacerbations of chronic bronchitis. In most studies, the continuous use of prophylactic antibiotics did not appear to be of benefit, although in many instances, the investigators were certain that some patients did much

better while receiving antibiotics. Some authorities suggest that all exacerbations of COPD should be treated with antibiotics; others claim that this should only be done if increased production of purulent secretions is observed and the Gram-stained sputum demonstrates bacteria. Patient identification and selection is the key. If an inflammatory component is included as a major selection feature, it is not surprising that bacterial infection plays an important role in most cases or that the patient improves with antibiotics. The greater the evidence for infection (eg, fever, elevated peripheral leukocyte count), the greater is the likelihood of a beneficial effect. In contrast, if emphasis is placed on increased shortness of breath, if purulent secretions are not a criterion for selection, and if fever leads to exclusion, it is understandable that antibiotics are not beneficial.

## ACKNOWLEDGMENTS

I am deeply indebted to Inez Campbell for secretarial assistance. This work was supported by Merit Review Funding from the Department of Veterans Affairs.

## REFERENCES

1. Turk D, May R: *Haemophilus influenzae:* Its Clinical Importance. London, English Universities Press, 1967.
2. Wallace RJ Jr, Musher DM, Septimus EJ, et al: *Haemophilus influenzae* infections in adults: Characterization of strains by serotypes, biotypes and β-lactamase production. J Infect Dis 144:101–106, 1981.
3. Musher DM, Kubitschek KR, Crennan J, Baughn RE: Pneumonia and acute febrile tracheobronchitis due to *Haemophilus influenzae.* Ann Intern Med 99:444–450, 1983.
4. Slater LN, Guarnaccia J, Makintubee S, Istre GR: Bacteremic disease due to *Haemophilus influenzae* capsular type f in adults: Report of five cases and review. Rev Infect Dis 12:628–635, 1990.
5. Murphy TF, Apicella MA: Nontypable *Haemophilus influenzae.* A review of clinical aspects, surface antigens, and the human immune response to infection. Rev Infect Dis 9:1–15, 1989.
6. Musser JM, Kroll JS, Granoff DM, et al: Global genetic structure and molecular epidemiology of encapsulated *Haemophilus influenzae.* Rev Infect Dis 12:75–111, 1990.
7. Trottier S, Stenberg K, Svanborg-Eden C: Turnover of nontypable *Haemophilus influenzae* in the nasopharynges of healthy children. J Clin Microbiol 27:2175–2179, 1989.
8. Gough J, Kraak WAG, Anderson EC, Nichols WW, Slack MPE, McGhie D: Cross-infection by non-encapsulated *Haemophilus influenzae.* Lancet 336:159–160, 1990.
9. Loos BG, Bernstein JM, Dryja DM, Murphy TF, Dickinson DP: Determination of the epidemiology and transmission of nontypeable *Haemophilus influenzae* in children with otitis media by comparison of total genomic DNA restriction fingerprints. Infect Immun 57:2751–2757, 1989.
10. Groeneveld K, von Alphen L, Eijk PP, Visschers G, Jansen HM, Zanen HC: Endogenous and exogenous reinfections by *Haemophilus influenzae* in patients with chronic obstructive pulmonary disease: The effect of antibiotic treatment on persistence. J Infect Dis 161:512–517, 1990.
11. Groeneveld K, van Alphen L, Voorter C, Eijk PP, Jansen HM, Zanen HC: Antigenic drift of *Haemophilus influenzae* in patients with chronic obstructive pulmonary disease. Infect Immun 57:3038–3044, 1989.
12. Bakaletz LO, Tallan BM, Hoepf T, DeMaria TF, Birck HG, Lim DJ: Frequency of fimbriation of nontypable *Haemophilus influenzae* and its ability to adhere to chinchilla and human respiratory epithelium. Infect Immun 56:331–335, 1988.
13. Loeb MR, Connor E, Penney D: A comparison of the adherence of fimbriated and nonfimbriated *Haemophilus influenzae* type b to human adenoids in organ culture. Infect Immun 56:484–489, 1988.

14. Farley MM, Stephens DS, Kaplan SL, Mason EO Jr: Pilus- and non–pilus-mediated interactions of *Haemophilus influenzae* type b with human erythrocytes and human nasopharyngeal mucosa. J Infect Dis 161:274–280, 1990.

15. St. Geme JW III, Falkow S: *Haemophilus influenzae* adheres to and enters cultured human epithelial cells. Infect Immun 58:4036–4044, 1990.

16. Read RC, Wilson R, Rutman A, et al: Interaction of nontypable *Haemophilus influenzae* with human respiratory mucosa in vitro. J Infect Dis 163:549–558, 1991.

17. Rubin LG, Moxon ER: Pathogenesis of bloodstream invasion with *Haemophilus influenzae* type b. Infect Immun 41:280–284, 1983.

18. Fainstein V, Musher DM: Bacterial adherence to pharyngeal cells in smokers, nonsmokers, and chronic bronchitics. Infect Immun 26:178–182, 1979.

19. Haas H, Morris JF, Samson S, Kilbourn JP, Kim PJ: Bacterial flora of the respiratory tract in chronic bronchitis: Comparison of transtracheal, fiberbronchoscopic, and oropharyngeal sampling methods. Am Rev Respir Dis 116:41–47, 1977.

20. Irwin RS, Erickson AD, Pratter MR, et al: Prediction of tracheobronchial colonization in current cigarette smokers with chronic obstructive bronchitis. J Infect Dis 145:234–241, 1982.

21. Chodosh S, Eichel B, Ellis C, Medici TC: Comparison of trimethoprim-sulfamethoxazole with ampicillin in acute infectious exacerbations of chronic bronchitis: A double-blind crossover study. Rev Infect Dis 4:517–527, 1982.

22. Crowe HM, Levitz RE: Invasive *Haemophilus influenzae* disease in adults. Arch Intern Med 147:241–244, 1987.

23. Fainstein V, Berkey P, Elting L, Bodey GP: *Haemophilus* species bacteremia in patients with cancer: A 13-year experience. Arch Intern Med 149:1341–1345, 1989.

24. Schlamm HT, Yancovitz SR: *Haemophilus influenzae* pneumonia in young adults with AIDS, ARC, or risk of AIDS. Am J Med 86:11–14, 1989.

25. Takala AK, Eskola J, van Alphen L: Spectrum of invasive *Haemophilus influenzae* type b disease in adults. Arch Intern Med 150:2573–2576, 1990.

26. Fine MJ, Orloff JJ, Rihs JD, et al: Evaluation of housestaff physicians' preparation and interpretation of sputum gram stains for community-acquired pneumonia. J Gen Intern Med 6:189–198, 1991.

27. Musher DM: *Haemophilus influenzae* infections. Hosp Pract 18(8):158–173, 1983.

28. Doern GV, Jorgensen JH, Thornsberry C, et al: National collaborative study of the prevalence of antimicrobial resistance among clinical isolates of *Haemophilus influenzae*. Antimicrob Agents Chemother 32:180–185, 1988.

29. Mendelman PM, Wiley EA, Stull TL, Clausen C, Chaffin DO, Onay O: Problems with current recommendations for susceptibility testing of *Haemophilus influenzae*. Antimicrob Agents Chemother 34:1480–1484, 1990.

30. Faden H, Bernstein J, Brodsky L, et al: Otitis media in children. I. The systemic immune response to nontypable *Hemophilus influenzae*. J Infect Dis 160:999–1004, 1989.

31. Faden H, Brodsky L, Bernstein J, et al: Otitis media in children: Local immune response to nontypable *Haemophilus influenzae*. Infect Immun 57:3555–3559, 1989.

32. Musher DM, Hague-Park M, Baughn RE, Wallace RJ Jr: Opsonizing and bactericidal effects of normal human serum on nontypable *Haemophilus influenzae*. Infect Immun 39:297–304, 1983.

33. Hansen MV, Musher DM, Baughn RE: Outer membrane proteins of nontypable *Haemophilus influenzae* and reactivity of paired sera from infected patients with their homologous isolates. Infect Immun 47:843–846, 1985.

34. Murphy TF, Bernstein JM, Dryja DM, Campagnari AA, Apicella MA: Outer membrane protein and lipooligosaccharide analysis of paired nasopharyngeal and middle ear isolates in otitis media due to nontypable *Haemophilus influenzae*: Pathogenetic and epidemiological observations. J Infect Dis 156:723–731, 1987.

35. Murphy T, Bartos LC: Human bactericidal antibody response to outer membrane protein P2 of nontypeable *Haemophilus influenzae*. Infect Immun 56:2673–2679, 1988.

36. McGehee JL, Radolf JD, Toews GB, Hansen EJ: Effect of primary immunization on pulmonary clearance of nontypable *Haemophilus influenzae*. Am J Respir Cell Mol Biol 1:201–210, 1989.

37. Musher DM, Goree A, Baughn RE, Birdsall HH: IgA from bronchopulmonary secretions blocks bactericidal and opsonizing effects of antibody to nontypable *Haemophilus influenzae*. Infect Immun 45:36–40, 1984.

38. Musher D, Goree A, Murphy T, et al: Immunity to *Haemophilus influenzae* type b in young adults: Correlation of bactericidal and opsonizing activity of serum with antibody to ribose ribitol phosphate and lipooligosaccharide, before and after vaccination. J Infect Dis 154:935–943, 1986.

39. Kimura A, Gulig PA, McCracken GH Jr, Loftus TA, Hansen EJ: A minor high-molecular-weight outer membrane protein of *Haemophilus influenzae* type b is a protective antigen. Infect Immun 47:253–259, 1985.

# CHAPTER 26

# *Legionella*

ROBERT R. MUDER and VICTOR L. YU

Legionnaires disease was first recognized at the 1976 American Legion Convention in Philadelphia, during which 221 American Legionnaires contracted pneumonia and 34 persons died. Investigators from the Centers for Disease Control subsequently identified the causative agent as an aerobic, gram-negative bacterium and named it *Legionella pneumophila.*

## MICROBIOLOGY

The legionellae are a group of gram-negative bacilli that are widely distributed in aquatic habitats. They can be readily isolated from fresh water and soil[1, 2] and from artificial aquatic environments, including water distribution systems[3] and heat rejection devices such as cooling towers and evaporative condensers.[4] Many strains of *Legionella* can multiply at temperatures of 40° to 60°,[5] and they are often found in high concentrations in naturally and artificially warmed water. Legionellae exist symbiotically with other environmental microorganisms.[6, 7] *L. pneumophila* is an intracellular parasite of amebas and other aquatic protozoa.[8]

Legionellae are fastidious and do not grow on most microbiologic media. They have an absolute requirement for L-cysteine, and growth is enhanced by availability of ferric ions. Although several supplemented media support growth, buffered charcoal yeast extract agar[9, 10] is most commonly used for clinical and environmental isolation.

## PATHOPHYSIOLOGY

Pneumonia is the presenting clinical syndrome in more than 95% of cases of legionnaires disease. Pathogenic microorganisms can enter the lung by aspiration preceded by oropharyngeal colonization of the organism, direct inhala-

tion, or hematogenous dissemination from another focus of infection. Colonization of the oropharynx has not yet been demonstrated for *Legionella,* suggesting that subclinical aspiration of contaminated water or direct inhalation are more likely modes of entry for this organism.

After organisms have entered the upper respiratory tract, clearance is effected by the cilia on respiratory epithelial cells, and the *Legionella* organisms are probably cleared by the mucociliary process.[11, 12] This theory is supported by the consistent epidemiologic association of increased risk of legionnaires disease in cigarette smokers, patients with chronic pulmonary diseases, and alcoholics—persons with diseases in which mucociliary clearance is impaired.

Alveolar macrophages phagocytose the *Legionella* organisms, although the process is more avid in the presence of specific opsonizing antibody.[13] The organism escapes the microbicidal mechanisms of the lysosomes and multiplies until the cell ruptures.[14] Presumably, the liberated bacteria are phagocytosed by newly recruited cells, and the cycle of ingestion, multiplication, and liberation with cell lysis begins anew. Initially, there is an influx of neutrophils, followed by transformation of the blood monocytes into macrophages.[15] Phagocytosis of *Legionella* is mediated by complement receptors on the monocytes. *Legionella* fixes complement component C3b to its surface through the alternative pathway; C3 acts as a ligand on the bacterial surface and becomes available for binding to the monocyte receptor.[16] A major outer membrane protein appears to be the prominent acceptor molecule for C3.[17]

Susceptibility to *Legionella* infection among different animal species correlates with the macrophage response to *L. pneumophila.*[18, 19] Mutants of *L. pneumophila* that fail to grow intracellularly are also less virulent in animals.[20–22] Interferon-γ–activated human monocytes down-regulate transferrin receptors and inhibit intracellular multiplication of *L. pneumophila* by limiting the availability of iron, an essential growth factor for this organism.[23]

Neutropenic patients do not have an undue susceptibility for *Legionella* infection. Although *L. pneumophila* is susceptible to oxygen-dependent microbicidal systems in vitro,[24] *L. pneumophila* resists killing by polymorphonuclear leukocytes. *L. pneumophila* is ingested efficiently by neutrophils in vitro only in the presence of specific antibody and complement. Unlike monocytes, however, intracellular replication of the organism fails to occur within polymorphonuclear leukocytes.[14, 15] Neutrophils are probably important in limiting *L. pneumophila* growth, because elimination of polymorphonuclear leukocytes by administration of antileukocyte serum has increased the number of *Legionella* bacteria recovered in the lungs of aerosol-infected animals.[25, 26] Leukocytes from nonimmune donors can be activated by interferon-γ and tumor necrosis factor to kill *Legionella* in vitro, and these cytokines can be activated by this bacterium as a response to infection.[27, 28]

Humoral immunity probably plays only a secondary role in host defense; for example, antibody does not promote killing of *L. pneumophila* by complement, promotes only modest killing of *L. pneumophila* by phagocytes (eg, polymorphonuclear leukocytes, monocytes, or alveolar macrophages),[29] and does not inhibit intracellular multiplication in monocytes or alveolar macrophages.[13] However, in patients with legionnaires disease, type-specific anti-*Legionella* antibody, usually IgM initially followed by IgG, is measurable within the first several weeks of infection. Moreover, immunized animals develop a specific antibody response with subsequent resistance to *Legionella* challenge.[30, 31]

Cell-mediated immunity is considered the primary host defense against *Legionella*, as is the case for other intracellular pathogens. Lymphocyte proliferation and cutaneous delayed hypersensitivity to *L. pneumophila* antigens appear within the first 2 weeks of infection.[30, 32–34] Legionnaires disease is more common and more severe for patients with depressed cell-mediated immunity, including transplant recipients and patients receiving corticosteroids. *Legionella* pneumonia has been found frequently in patients with hairy cell leukemia,[35–37] a malignancy associated with monocyte deficiency and dysfunction.

In infected patients and animals, mononuclear cells respond to *L. pneumophila* antigens with proliferation and with the generation of monocyte-activating cytokines, including interferon-γ[38, 39] and interleukin-1.[40] Tumor necrosis factor and lipopolysaccharide potentiate the interferon-γ resistance in alveolar macrophages.[41] Although the activated monocytes and alveolar macrophages inhibit the intracellular multiplication of *L. pneumophila*, killing is not enhanced.[13] Natural killer-like cells triggered by interleukin-2 have been shown to kill mononuclear cells infected by *L. pneumophila*.[27]

*L. pneumophila* strains differ in virulence. Agar-passaged strains that lose their virulence are more serum sensitive, more readily phagocytosed and killed intracellularly, and less likely to kill guinea pigs.[20, 32, 42] *L. pneumophila* serogroup 1 is known to cause most of the cases of legionnaires disease in the United States. Although multiple strains of *L. pneumophila* serogroup 1 may colonize water distribution systems, only a few strains are likely to cause disease in patients exposed to the water.[43, 44] Monoclonal antibody subtyping of strains of *L. pneumophila* serogroup 1 has shown that a surface epitope that is recognized by a mono-

clonal antibody (ie, Mab-2) may be associated with virulence. Virulent strains fail to bind complement components to the cell surface and are resistant to the bactericidal activity of normal human serum, but avirulent strains are serum sensitive and bind C3b to the cell surface.[45] Virulent strains are cytotoxic for guinea pig alveolar macrophages, but avirulent strains exhibit little toxicity. A toxic factor associated with the bacterial cell of *L. pneumophila* inhibits protein systhesis of Chinese hamster ovary cells, U937 cells, and human monocytes.[46]

A 38-kd extracellular metalloprotease exhibits cytotoxic activity[47, 48] and produces pulmonary lesions in guinea pigs.[11, 49] Vaccination with this protease induces cell-mediated and protective immunity.[50, 51] The 58- to 60-kd immunodominant antigen of *L. pneumophila* is a heat shock protein and a major humoral and cellular antigen.[52, 53]

## EPIDEMIOLOGY

### Incidence and Descriptive Epidemiology

Numerous investigations during the past 15 years have demonstrated that *Legionella* species are a significant cause of community-acquired and nosocomial pneumonia. The proportion of community-acquired pneumonias caused by *Legionella* has ranged from 1% to 16% in studies conducted in the United States, Europe, Israel, and Australia.[54–70] Although there are likely to be geographic differences in the relative incidence of *Legionella* infection, the studies differed in clinical setting, population, and intensity of diagnostic evaluation for *Legionella* infection, making direct comparisons difficult. However, in 9 of these studies,[55–57, 59, 65, 67–70] *Legionella* was among the three most frequently identified causes of pneumonia.

In addition to being an important cause of sporadic community-acquired pneumonia, *Legionella* infection occurs in apparent point-source epidemics, with several to several dozen persons infected within days or weeks.[71–73] In several outbreaks, investigators implicated a specific environmental source of *Legionella*.[72, 74, 75] In others, no apparent source of the organism could be found despite detailed investigation.[76, 77]

The risk factors for community-acquired *Legionella* pneumonia include advanced age, cigarette smoking, chronic pulmonary disease, immunosuppression, and chronic illness, including diabetes, liver disease, and renal disease.[71, 78] Patients with acquired immunodeficiency syndrome are surprisingly not at high risk for *Legionella* infection,[79] despite the well-documented association between *Legionella* infection and defects in cell-mediated immunity. *Legionella* infection has been increasingly reported in highly immunocompromised children.[80, 81]

*Legionella* is a common cause of nosocomial pneumonia.[82] Although early reports stressed the occurrence of epidemic disease,[83–85] endemic nosocomial infection is much more common. If the organism is actively sought by the application of specialized diagnostic tests to all cases of nosocomial pneumonia, the proportion of nosocomial pneumonia attributed to *Legionella* ranges from 0% to 46% (Table 26–1).[57, 68, 86–91] Colonization of the hospital water system with *Legionella* appears to be the major predictor of

Table 26–1. **Proportion of Nosocomial Pneumonias Due to *Legionella* Species in Prospective Clinical Studies**

| Investigation | No. of Patients Studied | No. With *Legionella* Infection | Percentage of Nosocomial Pneumonias |
|---|---|---|---|
| Muder[57] | 23 (hospital A) | 4 | 14 |
| | 32 (hospital B) | 15 | 47 |
| Bates[68] | 50 | 3 | 6 |
| Johnson[86] | 27 | 8 | 30 |
| Rudin[87] | 37 | 6 | 16 |
| Yu[88] | 32 | 3 | 9 |
| Brennen[89] | 185 | 26 | 14 |
| Marrie[90] | 813 | 52 | 6 |
| Louie[91] | 135 | 4 | 3 |

nosocomial infection.[86, 88, 92] Patients who are highly immunocompromised, such as organ transplant recipients, appear to be at particularly high risk.[83–96] Recent surgery,[97] endotracheal intubation[57] and use of respiratory therapy equipment[98] have been cited as additional risk factors.

The incidence of nonpneumonic legionellosis (ie, Pontiac fever) is unknown. Most recognized cases have occurred in point-source epidemics related to devices generating contaminated aerosols.[99–101] Because the symptoms are nonspecific and self-limited, the recognition of sporadic cases is difficult.

## Mode of Transmission

Most epidemiologic investigations have identified contaminated water distribution systems as the reservoir of *L. pneumophila*. Reports implicating cooling towers gradually diminished after recognizing that *Legionella* could be ubiquitous within water distribution systems.[3] Muder concluded that the studies linking legionnaires disease to cooling towers all suffered from detection bias and that the conclusions from these studies require reevaluation.[102]

The mode of transmission of *L. pneumophila* from water to man is uncertain, although evidence exists for aerosolization, aspiration, or direct instillation into the lung during respiratory tract manipulation. The strongest evidence for airborne spread is derived from the original Pontiac fever outbreak building in which the central air conditioning system may have been contaminated by aerosols from an evaporative condenser. *L. pneumophila* was isolated from the lungs of sentinel guinea pigs exposed to the air at the facility.[100] An epidemiologic link between showering and acquisition of disease has never been shown in prospective studies, and we are skeptical that this is a major mode of transmission.

Humidifiers have generated aerosols containing *L. pneumophila* and caused subclinical infection in guinea pigs exposed to the aerosols.[103] Inhalation of aerosolized tap water from nebulizers has been linked to hospital-acquired legionnaires disease.[98]

Health care personnel frequently use tap water to rinse respiratory apparatus and tubing for use in mechanical ventilation machines. If the tap water is contaminated with *L. pneumophila,* the organism can be directly instilled into the lung.[104, 105] In two studies, patients with legionnaires disease underwent endotracheal tube placement significantly more often or had significantly longer duration of intubation than patients with other pneumonias.[57, 106]

Aspiration of contaminated water or contaminated oropharyngeal secretions has been suggested as a mode of transmission.[107] This was supported by two prospective studies. *Legionella* infection was found to be the most common cause of nosocomial pneumonia in a population of oncologic head and neck surgery patients.[86] These patients have a propensity for aspiration as a result of their oral surgery and extensive history of cigarette smoking. Blatt concluded that aspiration was the mode of transmission in an endemic situation of nosocomial legionellosis based on a prospective case-control study.[108] Nasogastric tube placement has been implicated as a risk factor in intubated patients; microaspiration of contaminated water was the presumed mode of entry.[108, 109] During the original 1976 outbreak, consumption of water at the implicated hotel was significantly associated with acquisition of disease—an association that has been generally overlooked.[71]

Aerosolization from excavated soil was suggested as a possibility in the outbreaks at Wadsworth Veterans Association Medical Center and St. Elizabeth Hospital, Washington, DC, in the era before knowledge that the organism could be in water distributions systems; contaminated water distribution systems were probably the actual culprit.

## Pneumonia Caused by Nonpneumophila *Legionella* Species

There are 34 named species of *Legionella*,[110, 111] of which 18 have been implicated in human disease.[112] More than 90% of human infections are caused by a single species, *L. pneumophila*. Most of the remaining infections (excluding Pontiac fever) reported in the literature have been caused by *L. micdadei, L. bozemanii, L. dumoffii,* or *L. longbeachae*.[112, 113] Approximately 10% of *Legionella* pneumonias are caused by species other than *L. pneumophila*. Of these, *L. micdadei* (i.e., Pittsburgh pneumoina agent) has caused most of reported cases.[112] Most *L. micdadei* pneumonias have been nosocomial infections occurring in highly immunocompromised patients such as transplant recipients.[87, 114, 115] In one study of 26 consecutive cases,[116] only half of the patients were immunosuppressed; the remainder had a variety of chronic illnesses, including pulmonary, cardiac, and renal diseases. Recognized community-acquired cases are rare, although infection in healthy, ambulatory patients has been documented.[117]

Infections with *L. bozemanii, L. dumoffii,* and *L. longbeachae* follow *L. micdadei* in reported frequency. Most *L. bozemanii* and *L. dumoffii* infections have also been nosocomially acquired by highly immunocompromised patients.[112, 118, 119] *L. longbeachae* may be associated with community-acquired pneumonia.[113, 120] Other *Legionella* species are the subject of limited number of case reports, and extensive epidemiologic data is lacking. Cases of simultaneous infection with more than one *Legionella* species are well documented.[121, 122] As with *L. pneumophila,* nosocomial infection with *L. micdadei, L. bozemanii,* and *L. dumoffii* has been linked to colonization of hospital water systems.[118, 119, 123, 124] In one outbreak of *L. dumoffii* pneumonia, distilled water used in respiratory therapy devices was the apparent source of the organism.[119]

## DISEASE

### Clinical Features

The initial reports of the clinical manifestations of *Legionella* infection presented a picture of severe, progressive pulmonary infection with prominent extrapulmonary complications.[94, 125, 126] In the clinical description of the 1976 Philadelphia outbreak,[126] renal insufficiency (15% of patients), altered sensorium (21%), and gastrointestinal symptoms, particularly diarrhea (41%), were reported. The overall mortality rate was 21%. Because *L. pneumophila* was previously unknown as a pathogen, most patients received therapy with ineffective antibiotics. Studies directly comparing legionnaires disease with pneumonia from other causes have demonstrated that *Legionella* infection is not readily differentiated from other bacterial infections on the basis of clinical presentation.[127–130]

The clinical manifestations of *L. pneumophila* infection are presented in Table 26–2. Based on common source outbreaks, the incubation period after exposure is 2 to 10 days.[71] The patient may experience a brief prodrome of malaise, fever, chills, and a nonproductive cough.[125, 126] Myalgias are often striking.

The symptoms usually progress until the patient presents for medical care. The median period from onset to presentation is 4 days.[126] Ninety percent of patients are febrile at presentation, and half have fever of 103°F or more. Chest pain occurs in one third, and dyspnea affects as many as 60% of patients. Although cough is initially minimally productive, half of the patients produce purulent sputum after several days of illness. Diarrhea is often prominent, occurring in about one third of patients. Nausea and abdominal pain are also common. Respiratory failure requiring ventilatory support is ultimately required for 15% to 50%, illustrating the unusual degree of severity in many patients.[65, 67, 126, 128]

Many extrapulmonary manifestations have been described, including acute renal failure,[131] headache and mental status changes,[132] and jaundice.[133] There are isolated case reports of a diverse spectrum of complications, including rhabdomyolysis,[134] peripheral neuropathies,[132] myocarditis,[135] pericarditis,[136] glomerulonephritis,[137] and thrombotic

thrombocytopenic purpura.[138] The pathologic basis of most of these manifestations is not certain. However, bacteremia occurs in as many as 40% of patients with *Legionella* infection,[139] and organisms have been demonstrated in many different organs, including myocardium, brain, kidney, intestine, spleen, bone marrow, and lymph nodes.[140–143] Extrapulmonary legionellosis diagnosed antemortem is uncommon; wound infection,[144, 145] endocarditis,[146] cellulitis,[147] hemodialysis shunt infection,[148] peritonitis,[141, 149] and colitis[150] have been documented.

Immunocompromised patients may present with atypical symptoms. Fever without respiratory symptoms may occur despite the presence of radiographic infiltrates.[95, 151] The acute onset of dyspnea, hemoptysis, and pleuritic chest pain mimicking pulmonary embolism has also been described.[114, 152, 153]

Laboratory findings are nonspecific. Most patients demonstrate a leukocytosis in excess of 10,000 cells/mm$^3$ with a left shift.[126, 128] We have found thrombocytopenia that resolves with antibiotic therapy to be common. Hyponatremia has been prominent in numerous studies.[94, 126, 127] Although elevated hepatic transaminases, elevated serum creatinine, and metabolic abnormalities have been described, comparative studies with pneumonias resulting from other causes indicate that there are no laboratory findings sufficiently distinctive to suggest a diagnosis of *Legionella* infection.[127]

### Radiographic Manifestations

Most patients presenting with *L. pneumophila* infection have radiographically demonstrable infiltrates; all have abnormal findings by the third day of illness.[154–156] The initial involvement is unilateral in most cases; the lower lobes are more commonly affected initially, although any lung field may be involved. The initial infiltrate is alveolar and may appear segmental, lobar, patchy, or diffuse (Fig. 26–1).[154, 155, 157] The densities may appear as poorly marginated, rounded opacities (Fig. 26–2)[154]; if pleural based, they may resemble pulmonary infarction. During the first several days, the infiltrates tend to progress in the original area of involvement to produce widespread consolidation and involve additional lobes in 25% to 50% of cases.[125, 155, 156, 158] This progression may occur after the institution of appropriate antibiotic therapy and does not necessarily indicate therapeutic failure. Modest pleural effusions are relatively

Table 26–2. **Clinical Manifestations of Legionnaires Disease**

| Clinical Manifestations | Percentage of Cases (%) | | | | |
| --- | --- | --- | --- | --- | --- |
| | *Tsai*[126] (n = 123) | *Kirby*[94] (n = 65) | *Helms*[125] (n = 87) | *Woodhead*[129] (n = 79) | *Fang*[65] (n = 24) |
| Nosocomial acquisition | 0 | 100 | 23 | 0 | 0 |
| Fever | 97 | 99 | 90 | 90 | 67 |
| Chills | 74 | 77 | 51 | | 42 |
| Cough | 86 | 92 | 71 | 94 | 79 |
| Sputum | 50 | 49 | 46 | 53 | 75 |
| Chest pain | 23 | 33 | 26 | 46 | 14 |
| Dyspnea | 59 | 36 | 37 | 45 | 50 |
| Diarrhea | 41 | 47 | 24 | 28 | 21 |
| Mental status change | 21 | 38 | 35 | 45 | 22 |

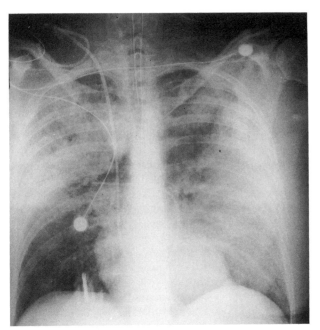

**Figure 26–1.** Fatal community-acquired legionnaires' disease. A 50-year-old woman with a history of cigarette smoking presented to a community hospital with cough, fever, and pulmonary infiltrates. Therapy with cefazolin and erythromycin was begun shortly after admission. She developed hypotension and respiratory failure requiring ventilatory support; she died of multisystem failure 4 days after presentation. The culture of antemortem sputum and lung tissue obtained at autopsy yielded *Legionella pneumophila.*

common and usually require no specific therapy. Loculated effusion and empyema occur occasionally.[159, 160] Hilar adenopathy and pneumatocele formation are rare,[126, 156] as is cavitation in the immunocompetent host.[156, 158] The extent of radiographic findings does not correlate with clinical outcome.[155, 157]

In the immunocompromised patient, an initial radiographic finding of circumscribed, peripheral densities is common (see Fig. 26–2).[161] The pulmonary lesions in immunosuppressed patients have a tendency to cavitate.[162–166] Cavitation may progress even after the institution of therapy and a clinical response.[165–167] Complications such as bronchopleural fistula or massive hemoptysis are unusual.

Radiographic clearing of infiltrates in *L. pneumophila* infection tends to be slow. Clearance rates of 60% at 12 weeks[158] and 29% after more than 100 days[157] have been described. Cavities in immunocompromised patients tend to gradually enlarge over a period of weeks, with a thinning of surrounding infiltration.[152] Most ultimately resolve, and specific intervention is rarely required.

Many infections with other *Legionella* species occur in immunocompromised patients; radiographic findings resemble those described for *L. pneumophila* infection in this patient population.[161, 168]

### Nonpneumonic Legionellosis

Nonpneumonic legionellosis (ie, Pontiac fever) is a self-limited, flu-like illness that results from exposure to aerosols contaminated with *Legionella.*[99, 100] It is characterized by an incubation period averaging 36 hours (range, 6–60

hours) and an exceptionally high attack rate among exposed persons (range, 45%–100%).[99, 100, 169] Symptoms include fever, chills, headache, myalgia, cough, and chest pain. Chest radiographs are normal. Affected patients recover without specific therapy after 2 to 5 days. The disease is characterized by a rise in serum antibody titer to the responsible *Legionella* species; *Legionella* has not been isolated from respiratory secretions. The occurrence of pneumonic and nonpneumonic disease among persons exposed to the same source is unusual. It is by no means clear that nonpneumonic legionellosis is caused by infection; a toxic or immunologic effect of the bacteria has been postulated.[170]

Aerosol-generating devices associated with nonpneumonic legionellosis include air conditioning equipment,[99] whirlpool baths,[170, 171] industrial equipment[101, 172] and decorative fountains.[173] Although most reported outbreaks have been associated with *L. pneumophila, L. feeleii,*[172] *L. micdadei,*[174] and *L. anisa*[173] have also been implicated.

### DIAGNOSIS

Specialized laboratory tests are the key means of diagnosing this infection, because the clinical presentation is nonspecific. The varying incidence of *Legionella* infection in different geographic areas may be a result of the availability of these specialized tests.

The single most important test for legionnaires disease is culture of the organism on selective media. To achieve a high yield (>80%) from sputum, the use of multiple selec-

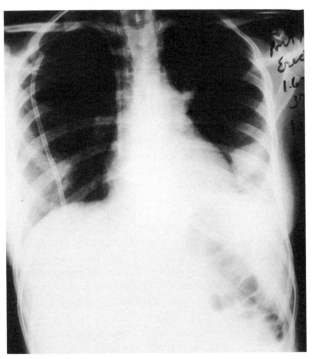

**Figure 26–2.** A 19-year-old woman treated with combination chemotherapy for acute myelomonocytic leukemia developed fever to 40°C while receiving ceftazidime and amphotericin B. A chest radiograph showed a nodular, pleural-based left lower infiltrate. DFA stain of the bronchoalveolar lavage fluid was positive for *Legionella micdadei.* Defervescence and resolution of the infiltrate occurred after the addition of erythromycin and rifampin.

tive media with antibiotics and dyes is required.[175] Pretreatment of the sputum specimens with an acid wash reduces competing flora and can improve the sensitivity by 10% to 20%.

Transtracheal aspirate specimens that bypass the contaminating oropharyngeal flora can have a sensitivity as high as 90%. Specimens obtained by bronchoscopy are useful but do not necessarily provide a higher yield than a good sputum specimen. If sputum is not available, bronchoalveolar lavage can be used. Bronchial washing in which the volume of fluid instilled is lower than that of lavage is not as sensitive. Transbronchial biopsy can yield the organism in tissue by direct fluorescent antibody stains and has been successful when sputum and bronchial washings were unrevealing.[176, 177] Percutaneous needle aspiration of lung abscess has yielded the organism in culture in a patient with negative sputum and bronchoscopy cultures.[178]

The organism can be isolated from blood by biphasic, buffered charcoal, yeast extract agar bottles, a radiometric system (BACTEC, Becton Dickinson, Cockeysville, MD),[139] or isolation lysis centrifugation system (Isolator, Dupont, Wilmington, DE). In one study, 38% of patients with legionnaires disease cases had positive blood cultures when subcultures from BACTEC bottles were plated onto buffered charcoal yeast extract agar.[139]

The sensitivity of the direct fluorescent antibody test has ranged from 25% to 80%. It is highly specific, and the monoclonal antibody (Genetic Systems, Seattle, WA) test has eliminated the rare occurrence of crossreactivity with other gram-negative bacilli.

The commercially available test for *Legionella* antigen in urine (Binax, South Portland, ME) can detect *L. pneumophila* serogroup 1 only, but because this species causes 80% to 90% of clinically apparent *L. pneumophila* infections, the test remains quite useful. Its advantages are its high sensitivity (>90%), its specificity (99%), the relatively low cost, and the persistence of test positivity for weeks despite antibiotic therapy.[179] This test result was positive when applied to pleural fluid of a patient subsequently found to have culture-confirmed legionnaires disease.[180]

Antibody tests have become less important with the advent of cultures and special stains. Maximal sensitivity requires both IgG and IgM tests. Because fourfold seroconversion is the definitive criteria, a repeat serology is required 4 to 6 weeks after convalescence. The sensitivity obtained in the original 1976 legionnaires disease outbreak was 91%,[181] but the sensitivity in later studies has been as low as 43%.[69] Effective antibiotics and suboptimal timing of specimen collection are possible reasons for the decreasing sensitivity.

The commercially available DNA probe (GenProbe, San Diego, CA) is expensive and relatively insensitive, and its applicability has not been validated in rigorous clinical trials.

## THERAPY

Antibiotics active in vitro in broth or agar studies may have little effect in embryonated egg or animal studies. This discrepancy between in vitro and in vivo studies has been attributed to the intracellular location of *Legionella* in phagocytes. Ideally, the most effective drug should be active in vitro, concentrate intracellularly in phagocytic cells, and penetrate into respiratory secretions.

Erythromycin is the drug of choice based on retrospective evaluation of *Legionella* outbreaks.[71, 182] The side effects of erythromycin include phlebitis and fluid management problems, because erythromycin is administered with a large volume of fluid. Nausea and vomiting are common with oral and intravenous preparations. Ototoxicity occurs with the higher 4-g daily dose, although it is reversible with discontinuation of the drug.[184]

Tetracyclines are probably as effective as erythromycin, although experience is limited.[71, 183] Doxycycline and minocycline have been described as effective in anecdotal reports.[185] Because of their high lipid solubility and twice-daily dosing regimen, these agents may be preferred over tetracycline.

Rifampin has high in vitro[186, 187] and in vivo potency, penetrates intracellularly, and achieves high concentrations in the lung. Infected guinea pigs treated with rifampin show the most rapid disappearance of *Legionella* from the lungs.[188] However, rifampin should not be used as sole therapy because of the theoretical possibility of emergence of resistance. Elevations in bilirubin are common, but they resolve with discontinuation of the drug.

Trimethoprim-sulfamethoxazole has been successfully used in patients with legionnaires disease and Pittsburgh pneumonia (ie, *L. micdadei* infection) that failed to respond to erythromycin.[189] This antimicrobial agent is active in vitro and in vivo.[188]

Quinolone agents show excellent activity in vitro[186] and in animals.[190] Patients with legionnaires disease unresponsive to erythromycin have also been successfully treated with ciprofloxacin.[191] One case of endocarditis was successfully treated with intravenous ciprofloxacin and oral rifampin.[146] Ciprofloxacin may be the preferred treatment for patients receiving with cyclosporine because of the interaction of other antibiotics with cyclosporine.[192] Anecdotal cases of the successful use of pefloxacin, ofloxacin, and fleroxacin have been reported.

Azithromycin and clarithromycin are two macrolides that have superior in vivo potency against *L. pneumophila* infection compared with erythromycin. They have excellent pharmacokinetics, allowing once-daily (azithromycin) or twice-daily (clarithromycin) dosing. Clinical experience is limited.

Although anecdotal experience suggests that imipenem may be effective therapy,[193] this antibiotic has been less effective in animal studies.[194]

Antibiotics should be given intravenously for the first 5 to 7 days. We recommend combination therapy, with the addition of rifampin in toxic patients with confirmed legionnaires disease. After the patient has shown objective clinical improvement (eg, defervescence), oral therapy can be substituted. The duration of therapy is 10 to 14 days for the immunocompetent host and 3 weeks for the immunosuppressed host presenting with advanced pneumonia. Prolonged therapy of 4 weeks may be required for lung abscess.

## PREVENTION AND CONTROL

The response to the identification of an environmental source linked to multiple cases of disease is conceptually straightforward. Transmission can be prevented by eliminating the organism, eliminating the conditions under which transmission occurs, or preventing exposure of susceptible persons to the source. In practice, most experience has been with microbiologic decontamination. The water distribution system to which the patients have been exposed should be cultured immediately. Dye-containing selective media with glycine (Gibco, Madison, WI; Remel, Lenexa, KS) are the optimal media. Water should be taken from the bottom of the hot water tanks, and swab samples should be obtained from the faucets and showerheads to which the patients were exposed. Areas with sediment give the highest yield. If the water distribution system cultures prove to be positive, subtyping the environmental and patient isolates by molecular techniques can strengthen the epidemiologic link. Eradication measures can be considered if large numbers of patients are at risk.

In a survey of Pennsylvania hospitals, lower hot water temperature (< 60°C [140°F]), vertical configuration of the hot water tank (presumably leading to temperature strata and accumulation of sediment on the bottom), elevated calcium and magnesium concentrations of the water, and older tanks were significantly associated with *Legionella* contamination.[195]

### Superheat and Flush Method

If eradication of contamination in the water distribution system must be implemented immediately, the superheat and flush method warrants primary consideration.[196] Numerous variations of this method exist, but the basic method requires that hot water tank temperatures be elevated to greater than 70°C (158°F), followed by flushing of all faucets and showerheads to kill the *L. pneumophila* organisms colonizing these sites.

This measure sterilizes the water distribution system, but recolonization gradually occurs. We have minimized recolonization by maintaining hot water tank temperatures at 60°C (140°F); with this additional measure, the heat and flush method is required only once every 2 to 3 years, making this method a cost effective one. The costs are low except those for personnel; if overtime is required, the costs can quickly escalate. We use volunteers for the flushing process.

The main disadvantage is that numerous personnel are involved to monitor distal site and tank water temperatures and flushing times. The potential for scalding exists, although no incidents have occurred in four Pittsburgh hospitals using this method for the past 10 years. The Joint Commission on Accreditation of Health Care Organizations has rescinded its earlier maximum water temperature of 110°F and allows each hospital to establish its own maximum temperature.

### Hyperchlorination

A chlorinator can be inserted without disruption to the rest of the hospital or staff, and chlorine provides a residual concentration throughout the entire water distribution system. This disinfection modality is relatively expensive.

After 5 to 6 years of chlorination, corrosion followed by destruction of the water distribution system can be problematic. A silicate coating for hot water pipes can reduce corrosion.[197] The University of Iowa spent more than $300,000 on maintenance and repairs associated with chlorination.[198] The formation of carcinogenic compounds from chlorine byproducts is now recognized as a public health hazard.

### Instantaneous Steam Heating Systems

Steam heating systems operate by flash-heating water to a temperature greater than 88°C and then blending the hot water with cold water to achieve the desired temperature. In many situations, these systems are less expensive to install than conventional hot water tank systems, but maintenance is more complex. Although these systems appear effective when they are installed as the original heating system in a new building,[195] they are not effective in older systems, because established niches of *Legionella* easily reseed the system.

### Ultraviolet Light

Ultraviolet light kills *Legionella* by disrupting cellular DNA. These systems have proven to be effective if disinfection can be localized (eg, transplant or intensive care unit). Because ultraviolet sterilization provides no residual protection, areas distal to the sterilizer must be disinfected after installation.[199–201] The most common method is to use the heat and flush technique to disinfect the major portion of the system and then to introduce chemical disinfection (eg, metallic ion, chlorine) as an adjunct.[92] Prefiltration is necessary to prevent the accumulation of scale onto the ultraviolet lamps, which renders them useless.

### Metallic Ionization

A commercial system (Liquitech, Burr Ridge, IL) uses copper-silver electrodes that generate ions when an electrical current is applied. The positively charged ions form electrostatic bonds with negatively hypercharged sites on bacterial cell walls, causing cell lysis and death. The system is less expensive than chlorine and provides residual protection throughout the system. Theoretically, microorganisms are killed rather than suppressed, which should minimize the possibility of recolonization. Our preliminary results and those of others suggest that this modality will likely be a major advance in disinfection.[202, 203]

Elimination of *Legionella* from cooling towers and evaporative condensers has been achieved with difficulty by cleaning followed by the addition of biocides. Commonly used biocides, including chlorine, phenolics, and quaternary ammonium compounds, are inconsistently effective under field conditions.[4] The optimal approach is uncertain. Prophylactic treatment of highly immunocompromised patients with erythromycin has been used in a few instances.[204] Trimethoprim-sulfamethoxazole used for *Pneumocystis* prophylaxis in immunosuppressed patients is probably effective against *Legionella* infection.

Although no vaccine is available, laboratory evidence suggests that vaccine development is feasible. The sublethal challenge of animals with virulent or attenuated *L. pneumophila* induces protection from a subsequent challenge; this is associated with evidence of humoral and cell-mediated immunity.[30, 51] Immunization of guinea pigs with a major secretory protein[50] or *L. pneumophila* cell membranes[205] also affords protection.

## Controversies

Because *Legionella* species are ubiquitous in the environment and a limited number of environmental sources are associated with clinical infection, it is not surprising that there is controversy regarding the appropriate approach to environmental *Legionella*.

Microbiologic surveillance of cooling towers and evaporative condensers for *Legionella* is unlikely to offer public health benefits. Many such devices are colonized without evidence of disease transmission. Engineering groups and some public health agencies have recommended that emphasis be given to scrupulous adherence to good engineering maintenance practices to minimize biofouling of these devices.[206] However, such practices are designed to promote efficient operation and heat exchange; their efficacy in eliminating *Legionella* and preventing disease has not been proven, and it is likely that heat exchange devices account for a relatively small proportion of total *Legionella* infections.[102] Nevertheless, several health departments have published explicit policies for cooling tower decontamination aimed at prevention of legionellosis. The public health impact of such policies is questionable.

Some public health authorities do not recommend routine surveillance of potable water for *Legionella*, arguing that the organism is ubiquitous and its presence is of uncertain significance in causing disease.[207] However, measures aimed at reducing *Legionella* colonization of potable water are effective in reducing the risk of *Legionella* infection.[123, 196, 198]

In the case of hospital water supplies, however, there is good evidence to indicate that microbiologic surveillance for *Legionella* is indicated. Hospital patients have many risk factors predisposing them to pneumonia in general and legionellosis in particular. Nosocomial legionellosis has a mortality rate as high as 40%. In prospective studies, *Legionella* colonization of a hospital water system is predictive of the occurrence of nosocomial infection.[57, 86, 88, 92] Because *Legionella* infection is clinically indistinguishable from other pneumonias, cases are unlikely to be recognized unless specialized diagnostic tests are used.

The presence of *Legionella* in a hospital water supply mandates that diagnostic tests for *Legionella* be made available.[208] These tests should include culture on selective media and urinary antigen. A prospective investigation of all nosocomial pneumonias would provide direct evidence of the existence of nosocomial legionellosis. An alternative strategy is to apply these diagnostic tests to patients with nosocomial pneumonia and the highest risk for legionellosis,[90, 209] including those with immunosuppression, those with chronic pulmonary disease, or those requiring surgery with general anesthesia.

The necessity for surveillance of other potential sources of *Legionella*, such as residential or municipal water supplies, is less clear. The magnitude of risk posed by many of these environmental sources is unknown, and extensive surveillance is unlikely to provide useful information without a link to disease. However, careful investigation of the potential exposures in cases of sporadic, community-acquired legionellosis reveals the source of the organism in as many as 40% of cases.[210] Such studies are an important step in defining the risk posed by environmental sources of the organism.

## REFERENCES

1. Fliermans CB, Cherry LH, Orrison SJ, et al: Ecological distribution of *Legionella pneumophila*. Appl Environ Mirobiol 41:9–16, 1981.
2. Joly JR, Boissiot M, Duchaine J, et al: Ecological distribution of Legionellaceae in the Quebec City area. Can J Microbiol 30:63–67, 1984.
3. Stout JE, Yu VL, Vickers RM, et al: Ubiquitousness of *Legionella pneumophila* in the water supply of a hospital with endemic legionnaires' disease. N Engl J Med 306:466–468, 1982.
4. Muraca PW, Stout JE, Yu VL: Environmental aspects of legionnaires' disease. J Am Water Works Assoc 80:78–86, 1988.
5. Tison DL, Baross JA, Seidler RJ: *Legionella* in aquatic habitats in the Mount Saint Helens blast zone. Curr Microbiol 9:345–348, 1983.
6. Stout JE, Yu VL, Best M: Ecology of *Legionella pneumophila* within water distribution systems. Appl Environ Microbiol 49:221–228, 1985.
7. Wadowsky RM, Yee RB: Effect of non-Legionellaceae bacteria on the multiplication of *Legionella pneumophila* in potable water. Appl Environ Microbiol 49:1206–1210, 1985.
8. Rowbotham TJ: Preliminary report on the pathogenicity of *Legionella pneumophila* for freshwater and soil amoebae. J Clin Microbiol 33:1179–1183, 1980.
9. Feeley JC, Gibson RJ, Gorman GW, et al: Charcoal-yeast extract agar: Primary isolation medium for *Legionella pneumophila*. J Clin Microbiol 10:437–441, 1979.
10. Pasculle AW, Feeley JC, Gibson RJ, et al: Pittsburgh pneumonia agent: Direct isolation from human lung tissue. J Infect Dis 241:727–732, 1980.
11. Baskerville A, Fitzgeorge RB, Broster M, et al: Histopathology of experimental legionnaires' disease in guinea pigs, rhesus monkeys and marmosets. J Pathol 139:349–362, 1983.
12. Davis GS, Winn WC, Gump DW, Craighead JE: Legionnaires' pneumonia after aerosol exposure in guinea pigs and rats. Am Rev Respir Dis 126:1050–1057, 1982.
13. Nash TW, Libby D, Horwitz MA: Interaction between the Legionnaires' disease bacterium *(L. pneumophila)* and human alveolar macrophages: Influence of antibody, lymphokines, and hydrocortisone. J Clin Invest 74:771–782, 1984.
14. Horwitz MA: The legionnaires' disease bacterium *(Legionella pneumophila)* inhibits phagosome-lysosome fusion in human monocytes. J Exp Med 158:2108–2126, 1983.
15. Davis GS, Winn W, Gump DW, Beaty H: The kinetics of early inflammatory events during experimental pneumonia due to *Legionella pneumophila* in guinea pigs. J Infect Dis 148:823–835, 1983.
16. Payne NR, Horwitz MA: Phagocytosis of *Legionella pneumophila* is mediated by human monocyte complement receptors. J Exp Med 166:1377–1389, 1987.
17. Bellinger-Kawahara C, Horwitz MA: Complement component C3 fixes selectively to the major outer membrane protein (MOMP) of *Legionella pneumophila* and mediates phagocytosis of lipsome-MOMP complexes by human monocytes. J Exp Med 172:1201–1210, 1990.
18. Yammamoto Y, Klein TW, Newton CA, et al: Differential growth of *Legionella pneumophila* in guinea pig versus mouse macrophage cultures. Infect Immun 55:1369–1374, 1987.
19. Yoshida SI, Mizuguchi Y: Multiplication of *Legionella pneumophila* Philadelphia-1 in cultured peritoneal macrophages and its correlation to susceptibility of animals. Can J Microbiol 32:438–442, 1986.

20. Horwitz MA: Characterization of avirulent mutant *Legionella pneumophila* that survive but do not multiply within human monocytes. J Exp Med 166:1310–1328, 1987.

21. Cianciotto NP, Eisenstein BI, Mody CH, Toews GB, Engleberg NC: A *Legionella pneumophila* gene encoding a species-specific surface protein potentiates initiation of intracellular infection. Infect Immun 57:1255–1262, 1989.

22. Cianciotto NP, Eisenstein BI, Mody CH, Engleberg NC: A mutation in the mip gene results in an attenuation of *Legionella pneumophila* virulence. J Infect Dis 162:121–126, 1990.

23. Byrd TF, Horwitz MA: Interferon gamma-activated human monocytes downregulate transferrin receptors and inhibit the intracellular multiplication of *Legionella pneumophila* by limiting the availability of iron. J Clin Invest 83:1457–1465, 1989.

24. Lochner JE, Friedman RL, Bigley RH, et al: Effect of oxygen-dependent antimicrobial systems on *Legionella pneumophila*. Infect Immun 39:487–489, 1983.

25. Davis GS, Winn W, Christman JW: Role of recruited nonimmuno-specific defenses in Legionnaires' disease. Chest 95:232S–233S, 1989.

26. Fitzgeorge RB, Featherstone ASR, Baskerville A: Effects of poly-morphonuclear leukocyte depletion on the pathogenesis of experimental legionnaires' disease. Br J Exp Pathol 69:105–112, 1988.

27. Blanchard DK, Stewart WE, Klein TW, et al: Cytolytic activity of human peripheral blood leukocytes against *Legionella pneumophila*-infected monocytes: Characterization of the effector. J Immunol 139:551–556, 1987.

28. Blanchard DI, Friedman H, Klein TW, Djen JY: Induction of inter-feron-gamma and tumor necrosis factor by *Legionella pneumophila*: Augmentation of human neutrophil bactericidal activity. J Leuk Biol 45:538–545, 1989.

29. Horwitz MA, Silverstein SC: Interaction of the legionnaires' disease bacterium *(Legionella pneumophila)* with human phagocytes. II. Antibody promotes binding of *L. pneumophila*. J Exp Med 153:398–406, 1981.

30. Breiman RF, Horwitz MA: Guinea pigs sublethally infected with aerosolized *Legionella pneumophila* develop humoral and cell-mediated immune responses. J Exp Med 164:799–811, 1987.

31. Rolstad B, Berdal B: Immune defenses against *Legionella pneumophila* in rats. Infect Immun 32:805–812, 1981.

32. Friedman H, Widen R, Klein T, et al: *L. pneumophila*-induced blastogenesis of murine lymphoid cells in vitro. Infect Immun 43:314–319, 1984.

33. Friedman H, Widen R, Lee I, et al: Cellular immunity to *L. pneumophila* in guinea pigs assessed by direct and indirect migration inhibition; reaction in vitro. Infect Immun 41:1132–1137, 1983.

34. Plouffe JF, Baird IM: Cord blood lymphocyte transformation to *L. pneumophila*. J Clin Lab Immunol 9:119–120, 1982.

35. Cordonnier C, Farcet JP, Desforges L: Legionnaires' disease and hairy-cell leukemia. Arch Intern Med 144:2373–2375, 1984.

36. Fang GD, Stout JE, Yu VL, Goetz A, Rihs JD, Vickers RM: Community-acquired pneumonia caused by *Legionella dumoffii* in a patient with hairy cell leukemia. Infection 18:383–385, 1990.

37. Lang R, Miller I, Manon J, Kazak R, Boldur I: *Legionella longbeachae* in a splenectomized hairy-cell leukemia patient. Infection 18:31–32, 1990.

38. Bhardwaj N, Nash T, Horwitz MA: Interferon-gamma–activated human monocytes inhibit the intracellular multiplication of *Legionella pneumophila*. J Immunol 137:2662–2669, 1986.

39. Blanchard DK, Klein TW, Friedman H, et al: Kinetics and characterization of interferon production by murine spleen cells stimulated with *Legionella pneumophila* antigens. Infect Immun 49:719–723, 1985.

40. Klein TW, Newton CA, Blanchard D, et al: Induction of interleukin 1 by *Legionella pneumophila* antigens in mouse and human mononuclear leukocyte cultures. Zbl Bakt Hyg A 265:462–471, 1987.

41. Skerrett SJ, Maratin TR: Tumor necrosis factor and lipopolysaccharide potentiate interferon-gamma–induced resistance of alveolar macrophages to *Legionella pneumophila*. [Abstract I-9] 1992 International Symposium on *Legionella*. American Society for Microbiology, Orlando, FL.

42. Klein WT, Friedman H, Widen R: Relative potency of virulent versus avirulent *Legionella pneumophila* for indication of cell-mediated immunity. Infect Immun 44:753–755, 1984.

43. Plouffe JF, Para MF, Maher WE, et al: Subtypes of *Legionella pneumophila* serogroup 1 associated with different attack rates. Lancet 2:649–650, 1983.

44. Stout JE, Joly J, Para M, et al: Comparison of molecular methods for subtyping patients and epidemiologically linked environmental isolates of *L. pneumophila*. J Infect Dis 157:486–494, 1988.

45. Caparon M, Johnson W: Macrophage toxicity and complement sensitivity of virulent and avirulent strains of *Legionella pneumophila*. Rev Infect Dis 10:S377–384, 1988.

46. McCusker KT, Braaten BA, Cho MW, Low DA: *Legionella pneumophila* inhibits protein synthesis in Chinese hamster ovary cells. Infect Immun 59:240–246, 1991.

47. Keen MG, Hoffman PS: Characterization of a *Legionella pneumophila* extracellular protease exhibiting hemolytic and cytotoxic activities. Infect Immun 57:732–738, 1989.

48. Quinn FD, Tompkins LS: Analysis of a cloned sequence of *Legionella pneumophila* encoding a 38 kd metalloprotease possessing haemolytic and cytotoxic activities. Mol Microbiol 3:797–805, 1989.

49. Conlan JW, Williams A, Ashworth L: In vivo production of a tissue-destructive protease by *Legionella pneumophila* in the lungs of experimentally infected guinea pigs. J Gen Microbiol 134:143–149, 1988.

50. Blander S, Horwitz MA: Vaccination with the major secretory protein of *L. pneumophila* induces cell-mediated immunity in a guinea pig model of legionnaire's disease. J Exp Med 100:691–705, 1989.

51. Blander SJ, Breiman R, Horwitz MA: A live avirulent mutant *L. pneumophila* vaccine induces protective immunity against lethal aerosol challenge. J Clin Invest 83:810–815, 1989.

52. Sampson JS, O'Connor SP, Holloway BP, et al: Nucleotide sequence of htpB, the *Legionella pneumophila* gene encoding the 58-kilodalton (kDa) common antigen, formerly designated the 60-kDa common antigen. Infect Immun 58:3154–3157, 1990.

53. Hoffman PS, Houston L, Butler CA: *Legionella pneumophila* htpab heat shock operon: Nucleotide sequence and expression of the 60-kilodalton antigen in *L. pneumophila*-infected HeLa cells. Infect Immun 58:3380–3387, 1990.

54. White RJ, Blainey AD, Harrison KJ, Clarke SKR: Causes of pneumonia presenting to a district general hospital. Thorax 36:566–570, 1981.

55. MacFarlane JT, Finch RG, Ward MJ, Macrae AD: Hospital study of adult community-acquired pneumonia. Lancet 2:255–258, 1982.

56. Klimek JJ, Ajemian E, Fonteccio S, Gracewski J, Klemas B, Jimenez L: Community-acquired bacterial pneumonia requiring admission to hospital. Am J Infect Control 11:79–82, 1983.

57. Muder RR, Yu VL, McClure J, et al: Nosocomial legionnaires' disease uncovered in a prospective pneumonia study: Implications for underdiagnosis. JAMA 249:3184–3188, 1983.

58. Marrie TJ, Grayston JT, Wang S, et al: Pneumonia associated with TWAR strain of *Chlamydia*. Ann Intern Med 106:507–511, 1987.

59. Aubertin J, Dabis F, Fleurette J, et al: Prevalence of legionellosis among adults: A study of community-acquired pneumonia in France. Infection 15:328–331, 1987.

60. Community-acquired pneumonia in adults in British hospitals in 1982-1983: A survey of aetiology, mortality, prognostic factors and outcome. Q J Med 62:192–220, 1987.

61. Holmberg H. Aetiology of community-acquired pneumonia in hospital patients. Scand J Infect Dis 19:491–501, 1987.

62. Levy M, Dromer F, Brion N, Leturdu F, Carbon C: Community-acquired pneumonia—Importance of initial noninvasive bacteriologic and radiographic investigation. Chest 92:43–48, 1988.

63. Woodhead MA, MacFarlane JT, McCracken JS, Rose DH, Finch RG: Prospective study of the aetiology and outcome of pneumonia in the community. Lancet 1:671–674, 1987.

64. Lim R, Shaw DR, Stanley DP, Lumb R, McLennan G: A prospective hospital study of the aetiology of community-acquired pneumonia. Med J Aust 151:87–91, 1989.

65. Fang GD, Fine M, Orloff J, et al: New and emerging etiologies for community-acquired pneumonia with implications for therapy: A prospective multicenter study of 359 cases. Medicine (Baltimore) 69:307–316, 1990.

66. Maayan S, Morali G, Engelhard D, et al: Legionellosis at Hadassah University Hospital: A 1-year survey. Isr J Med Sci 27:145–149, 1991.

67. Falco V, Fernandez de Sevilla T, Alegre J, Ferrer A, Vasquez J: *L. pneumophila*—A cause of severe community acquired pneumonias. Chest 100:1007–1011, 1991.

68. Bates JH, Campbell GD, Barron AL, et al: Microbiology of acute pneumonia in hospitalized patients. Chest 101:1005–1012, 1992.

69. Ruf B, Schurmann D, Horbach I, Fehrenbach F, Pohle HD: The

incidence of legionella pneumonia: A 1-year prospective study in a large community hospital. Lung 167:11–22, 1989.

70. Friss-Moller A, Rechnitzer C, Blak F, et al: Prevalence of legionnaires' disease in pneumonia patients admitted to a Danish department of infectious disease. Scand J Infect Dis 18:321–328, 1986.

71. Fraser DW, Tsai T, Orenstein W, et al: Legionnaires' disease: Description of an epidemic of pneumonia. N Engl J Med 297:1183–1197, 1977.

72. Cordes L, Fraser D, Skally P, et al: Legionnaires' disease outbreak at an Atlanta, Georgia, country club: Evidence for spread from an evaporative condenser. Am J Epidemiol 11:425–431, 1980.

73. Schlech WF III, Gorman GW, Payne MC, Broome CV: Legionnaires' disease in the Caribbean: An outbreak associated with a resort hotel. Arch Intern Med 145:2076–2079, 1985.

74. Mahoney FJ, Hoge CW, Farley T, et al: Community-wide outbreak of legionnaires disease associated with a grocery store mist machine. J Infect Dis 165:736–739, 1992.

75. Addiss DG, Davis JP, LaVenture M, Wang PJ, Hutchinson MA, McKinney RM: Community-acquired legionnaires' disease associated with a cooling tower: Evidence for longer-distance transport of *Legionella pneumophila.* Am J Epidemiol 130:355–368, 1989.

76. Monforte R, Cayla J, Sala MR, et al: Community outbreak of legionnaires' disease in Barcelona. Lancet 1:1011, 1989.

77. Redd SC, Yeng F, Lin C, et al: A rural outbreak of legionnaires' disease linked to visiting a retail store. Am J Public Health 80:431–434, 1990.

78. England AC, Fraser DW: Sporadic and epidemic nosocomial legionellosis in the United States. Am J Med 70:707–711, 1981.

79. Bangsborg JM, Jensen BN, Friis-Moller A, Bruun B: Legionellosis in patients with HIV infection. Infection 18:342–346, 1990.

80. Carlson NC, Kuskie MR, Dobyns EL, Wheeler MC, Roe MH, Abzug MJ: Legionellosis in children: An expanding spectrum. Pediatr Infect Dis J 9:133–137, 1990.

81. Brady M: Nosocomial legionnaires' disease in a children's hospital. J Pediatr 115:46–50, 1989.

82. Korvick J, Yu VL, Fang GD: The role of *Legionella* sp. in nosocomial pneumonia. Semin Respir Infect 2:34–47, 1987.

83. Haley CE, Cohen ML, Halter J, Myer RD: Nosocomial legionnaires' disease: A continuing common-source epidemic at Wadsworth Medical Center. Ann Intern Med 90:583–586, 1979.

84. Dondero TJ Jr, Rendtorff RC, Mallison GF, et al: An outbreak of legionnaires' disease associated with a contaminated air-conditioning cooling tower. N Engl J Med 302:365–370, 1980.

85. Thacker SB, Bennet JV, Tsai T, et al: An outbreak in 1965 of severe respiratory illness caused by legionnaires' disease bacterium. J Infect Dis 138:512–519, 1978.

86. Johnson JT, Yu VL, Best M, et al: Nosocomial legionellosis uncovered in surgical patients with head and neck cancer: Implications for epidemiologic reservoir and mode of transmission. Lancet 2:298–300, 1985.

87. Rudin J, Wing E: Prospective study of pneumonia: Unexpected incidence of legionellosis. South Med J 79:417–419, 1986.

88. Yu VL, Beam TR, Lumish R, et al: Routine culturing for *Legionella* in the hospital environment may be a good idea: 3-hospital prospective study. Am J Med Sci 294:97–103, 1987.

89. Brennen C, Vickers RM, Yu VL, et al: Discovery of occult *Legionella* pneumonia in a long-term care facility. Br Med J 297:306–307, 1987.

90. Marrie TJ, MacDonald S, Clarke S, Haldan D: Nosocomial legionnaires' disease: Lessons from a four-year prospective study. Am J Infect Control 19:79–85, 1991.

91. Louie M, Dyck B, Parker S, Sekla L, Nicolle LE: Nosocomial pneumonia in a Canadian tertiary care center: A prospective surveillance study. Infect Control Hosp Epidemiol 12:356–363, 1991.

92. Struelens MJ, Maes N, Deplano A, et al: Genotypic and phenotypic methods for the investigation of a nosocomial *Legionella pneumophila* outbreak and efficacy of control measures. J Infect Dis 166:22–30, 1992.

93. Bock B, Edelstein P, Snyder K, et al: Legionnaires' disease in renal transplant recipients. Lancet 1:410–413, 1978.

94. Kirby BD, Snyder K, Meyer R, Finegold SM: Legionnaires' disease: Report of 65 nosocomially acquired cases and a review of the literature. Medicine (Baltimore) 59:188–205, 1980.

95. Fuller J, Levinson MM, Kline JR, et al: Legionnaires' disease after heart transplantation. Ann Thorac Surg 39:308–311, 1985.

96. LeSaux NM, Sekla L, McLeod J, et al: Epidemic of nosocomial

legionnaires' disease in renal transplant recipients: A case-control and environmental study. Can Med Assoc J 140:1047–1053, 1989.

97. Korvick J, Yu VL: Legionnaires' disease: An emerging surgical problem. Ann Thorac Surg 43:341–347, 1986.

98. Arnow P, Chou T, Weil D, et al: Nosocomial legionnaires' disease caused by aerosolized tap water from respiratory devices. J Infect Dis 146:460–467, 1982.

99. Glick TH, Gregg MB, Berman B, et al: Pontiac fever: An epidemic of unknown etiology in a health department. Clinical and epidemiologic aspects. Am J Epidemiol 107:149–160, 1978.

100. Kaufmann A, McDade J, Patton C, et al: Pontiac fever: Isolation of the etiologic agent *(Legionella pneumophila)* and demonstration of its mode of transmission. Am J Epidemiol 114:337–347, 1981.

101. Fraser DW, Deubner DC, Hill DL, et al: Nonpneumonic short-incubation period legionellosis (Pontiac fever) in men who cleaned a steam turbine condenser. Science 205:691–692, 1979.

102. Muder RR, Yu VL, Woo A: Mode of transmission of *L. pneumophila:* A critical review. Arch Intern Med 146:1607–1612, 1986.

103. Woo AJ, Goetz A, Yu VL: Transmission of *Legionella* by respiratory equipment and aerosol-generating devices: A review. Chest 102:1586–1590, 1992.

104. Bouvet A, Defenoyl O, Desplaces N: Maladie des legionnaires' due au serogroup de *Legionella pneumophila*—contamination d'un domicile par canule de tracheostomie. Presse Med 15:35, 1986.

105. Woo AH, Yu VL, Goetz A: Potential in-hospital mode of transmission for *Legionella pneumophila:* Demonstration experiments for dissemination by showers, humidifiers, and rinsing of ventilation bag apparatus. Am J Med 80:567–573, 1986.

106. Markowitz L, Tompkins L, Wilkinson H, et al: Transmission of nosocomial legionnaires' disease in heart transplant patients. [Abstract 170] Program and Abstracts of the 24th Interscience Conference on Antimicrobial Agents and Chemotherapy, American Society for Microbiology, Washington, DC, 1984.

107. Yu VL, Stout J, Zuravleff JJ: Aspiration of contaminated water may be a mode of transmission for *Legionella pneumophila.* [Abstract 297] Program and Abstracts of the 21st Interscience Conference on Antimicrobial Agents and Chemotherapy, American Society for Microbiology, Washington, DC, 1981.

108. Blatt SP, Parkinson MD, Pace E, et al: Nosocomial legionnaires' disease: Aspiration as a primary mode of disease acquisition. Am J Med 95:16–22, 1993.

109. Marrie TJ, Haldane D, Macdonald S, et al: Control of endemic nosocomial legionnaires' disease by using sterile potable water for high risk patients. Epidemiol Infect 107:591–605, 1991.

110. Brenner DJ. Classification of the Legionellae. Semin Respir Infect 4:190–205, 1987.

111. Benson RF, Thacker WL, Lanser JA, Sangster N, Mayberry WR, Brenner DJ: *Legionella adelaidensis,* a new species isolated from cooling tower water. J Clin Microbiol 29:1004–1006, 1991.

112. Fang GD, Yu VL, Vickers RM: Disease due to the Legionellaceae (other than *Legionella pneumophila*): Historical, microbiological, clinical and epidemiological review. Medicine (Baltimore) 68:116–139, 1989.

113. Cameron S, Roder D, Walker C, Feldheim J: Epidemiological characteristics of Legionella infection in South Australia: Implications for disease control. Aust N Z J Med 21:65–70, 1991.

114. Myerowitz RL, Pasculle AW, Dowling JN, et al: Opportunistic lung infection due to "Pittsburgh pneumonia agent." N Engl J Med 391:953–958, 1979.

115. Rogers BH, Donowitz GR, Walker GK, et al: A clinicopathological study of five cases caused by an unidentified acid-fast bacterium. N Engl J Med 301:959–961, 1979.

116. Muder RR, Yu VL, Zuravleff JJ: Pneumonia due to the Pittsburgh pneumonia agent: New clinical perspective with a review of the literature. Medicine (Baltimore) 62:120–128, 1983.

117. Fumarola D, Miragliotta C, Logroscino G, et al: Simultaneous infection with *Legionella pneumophila* and *Legionella micdadei* in an immunologically intact host. A case report. Boll Ist Sieroter Milan 63:165–166, 1984.

118. Parry MF, Stampleman L, Hutchinson J, et al: Waterborne *Legionella bozemanii* and nosocomial pneumonia in immunosuppressed patients. Ann Intern Med 103:205–210, 1985.

119. Joly JR, Diery P, Gauvreau L, et al: Legionnaires' disease caused by *Legionella dumoffii* in distilled water. Can Med Assoc J 135:1274–1277, 1986.

120. McKinney RM, Porschen RK, Edelstein PH, et al: *Legionella long-*

*beachae* species nova, another etiologic agent of human pneumonia. Ann Intern Med 94:739–743, 1981.

121. Muder RR, Yu VL, Vickers R, et al: Simultaneous infection with *Legionella pneumophila* and Pittsburgh pneumonia agent—Clinical features and epidemiological implications. Am J Med 74:609–614, 1983.

122. Tang PW, Toma S, MacMillan LG: *Legionella oakridgensis:* Laboratory diagnosis of a human infection. J Clin Microbiol 21:462–463, 1985.

123. Best M, Yu VL, Stout J, Goetz A, Muder RR, Taylor F: Legionellaceae in the hospital water supply—Epidemiological link with disease and evaluation of a method of control of nosocomial legionnaires' disease and Pittsburgh pneumonia. Lancet 2:307–310, 1983.

124. Doebbeling BN, Ishak M, Wade B, et al: Nosocomial *Legionella micdadei* pneumonia: 10 years experience and a case control study. J Hosp Infect 13:289–298, 1989.

125. Helms CM, Viner JP, Dennis D, et al: Sporadic legionnaires' disease: Clinical observations on 87 nosocomial and community-acquired cases. Am J Med Sci 288:2–12, 1984.

126. Tsai TF, Finn DR, Pilikaytis B, et al: Clinical features of the epidemic in Philadelphia. Ann Intern Med 90:509–517, 1979.

127. Yu VL, Kroboth FJ, Shonnard J, Brown A, McDearman S, Magnussen MH: Legionnaires' disease: New clinical perspective from a prospective pneumonia study. Am J Med 73:357–361, 1982.

128. Woodhead MA, MacFarlane JT: Legionnaires' disease: A review of 79 community acquired cases in Nottingham. Thorax 41:635–640, 1986.

129. Roig J, Aguilar X, Ruiz J, et al: Comparative study of Legionella pneumophila and other nosocomial-acquired pneumonias. Chest 99:344–350, 1991.

130. Granados A, Podzamczer D, Guidol F, Manresa F: Pneumonia due to *L. pneumophila* and pneumococcal pneumonia: Similarities and differences on presentation. Eur Respir J 2:130–134, 1989.

131. Fenves AZ: Legionnaires' disease associated with acute renal failure: A report of two cases and review of the literature. Clin Nephrol 23:96–100, 1985.

132. Johnson JT, Raff M, Van Arsdall J: Neurologic manifestations of legionnaires' disease. Medicine (Baltimore) 63:303–310, 1984.

133. Van Arsdall JA, Wunderlich HF, Melo JC, et al: The protean manifestations of legionnaires' disease. J Infect 7:51–62, 1983.

134. Posner MR, Caudill A, Brass R, Ellis E: Legionnaires' disease associated with rhabdomyolysis and myoglobinuria. Arch Intern Med 140:848–850, 1980.

135. Gross D, Willens H, Zeldis ST: Myocarditis in legionnaires' disease. Chest 79:232–234, 1981.

136. Mayock R, Skale B, Kohler RB: *Legionella pneumophila* pericarditis proved by culture of pericardial fluid. Am J Med 75:534, 1983.

137. Saleh F, Rodichok LD, Satya-Murti S, Tillotson JR: Legionnaires' disease: Report of a case with unusual manifestations. Arch Intern Med 140:1514–1516, 1980.

138. Riggs SA, Wray NP, Waddell CC, Rossen RD, Ferene G: Thrombotic thrombocytopenic purpura complicating legionnaires' disease. Arch Intern Med 142:2275–2280, 1982.

139. Rihs JD, Yu VL, Zuravleff JJ, et al: Isolation of *Legionella pneumophila* from blood using the BACTEC: A prospective study yielding positive results. J Clin Microbiol 22:422–424, 1985.

140. White H, Felton W, Sun CN: Extrapulmonary histopathologic manifestations of legionnaires' disease. Arch Pathol Lab Med 104:287–289, 1980.

141. Dournon E, Bure A, Kenney J, Pourriat J, Valeyre P: *Legionella pneumophila* peritonitis. [Letter] Lancet 1:1363, 1982.

142. Weisenburger D, Helms C, Viner J, Renner E: Demonstration of the legionnaires' disease bacillus in hilar lymph nodes. [Letter] Arch Pathol Lab Med 103:153, 1979.

143. Monforte R, Maro F, Estruch R, Campo E: Multiple organ involvement by *L. pneumophila* in a fatal case of legionnaires disease. J Infect Dis 159:809, 1989.

144. Brabender W, Hinthorn DR, Asher M, et al: *Legionella pneumophila* wound infection. JAMA 250:3091–3095, 1983.

145. Lowry PW, Blankenship RJ, Gridley W, et al: A cluster of *Legionella* sternal wound infections due to postoperative topical exposure to contaminated tap water. N Engl J Med 324:109–112, 1991.

146. Tompkins LS, Roessler BJ, Redd SC, et al: *Legionella* prosthetic-valve endocarditis. N Engl J Med 318:530–535, 1988.

147. Waldor MK, Wilson B, Swartz M: *Legionella pneumophila* cellulitis. Clin Infect Dis 16:51–53, 1992.

148. Kalweit W, Winn WC, Racco T, Girod J: Hemodialysis fistula infections caused by *Legionella pneumophila.* Ann Intern Med 96:173–175, 1982.

149. Nomura S, Hatta K, Iwata T, Aihara M: *Legionella pneumophila* isolated in pure culture from the ascites of a patient with systemic lupus erythematosus. Am J Med 86:833–834, 1989.

150. Schmidt T, Pfeiffer A, Ehret W, Keiditsch E, Ruckdeschel G, Kaess H: Legionella infection of the colon presenting as acute attack of ulcerative colitis. Gastroenterology 97:751–755, 1989.

151. Copeland J, Weiden BS, Feinberg W, et al: Legionnaires' disease following cardiac transplantation. Chest 79:669–671, 1981.

152. Moore EH, Webb WR, Gamsu G, Golden JA: Legionnaires' disease in the renal transplant patient: Clinical presentation and radiographic progression. Radiology 153:589–593, 1984.

153. Kugler JW, Armitage JO, Helms CM, et al: Nosocomial legionnaires' disease: Occurrence in recipients of bone marrow transplants. Am J Med 74:218, 1983.

154. Dietrich P, Johnson R, Fairbank J, Walke J: The chest radiograph in legionnaires' disease. Radiology 127:577–582, 1978.

155. Kroboth FJ, Yu VL, Reddy S, Yu AC: Clinicoradiographic correlations with the extent of legionnaires' disease. AJR 141:263–268, 1983.

156. Kirby B, Peck H, Meyer R: Radiographic features of legionnaires' disease. Chest 76:562–565, 1979.

157. Fairbank JT, Mamourian AC, Dietrich PA, et al: The chest radiograph in legionnaires' disease. Further observations. Radiology 147:33–34, 1983.

158. MacFarlane JT, Miller AC, Roderick-Smith WH, et al: Comparative radiographic features of community-acquired legionnaires' disease, pneumococcal pneumonia, *Mycoplasma pneumoniae,* psitacossis. Thorax 39:28–33, 1984.

159. Freedman AP, Coodley E, Johnston RF, et al: Loculated pleural effusion caused by *Legionella pneumophila.* Thorax 37:79–80, 1982.

160. Randolph KA, Beckman JF: Legionnaires' disease presenting with empyema. Chest 75:404–406, 1979.

161. Muder RR, Yu VL, Parry M: Radiology of legionella pneumonia. Semin Respir Infect 2:242–254, 1987.

162. Saravolatz LD, Burch KH, Fisher E, Madhavan T, et al: The compromised host and legionnaires' disease. Ann Intern Med 90:533–537, 1979.

163. Gump DW, Frank RO, Winn WC, Foster RS, Broome CV, Cherry WB: Legionnaires' disease in patients with associated serious disease. Ann Intern Med 90:538–542, 1979.

164. Gombert M, Josephson A, Goldstein EJC, et al: Cavitary *Legionella* pneumonitis; nosocomial infection in renal transplant recipients. Am J Surg 147:402–405, 1984.

165. Edelstein PH, Meyer RD, Finegold SM: Long-term follow-up of two patients with pulmonary cavitation caused by *Legionella pneumophila.* Am Rev Respir Dis 124:90–93, 1981.

166. Ebright JR, Tarakji E, Brown WJ, Sunstrum J: Multiple bilateral lung cavities caused by *Legionella pneumophila:* A case report and review of the literature. Infect Dis Clin Pract 2:195–199, 1993.

167. Magnussen CR, Israel RH: Legionnaires' lung abscess. Am J Med Sci 279:117–120, 1980.

168. Muder RR, Reddy S, Yu VL, Kroboth FJ: Pneumonia caused by Pittsburgh pneumonia agent radiologic manifestations. Radiology 150:633–637, 1984.

169. Spitalny KC, Vogt RL, Orciari LA, et al: Pontiac Fever associated with a whirlpool spa. Am J Epidemiol 120:809–817, 1984.

170. Armstrong C, Miller GB: A 1949 outbreak of Pontiac fever-like illness in steam condensor cleaners. Arch Environ Health 40:26–29, 1985.

171. Mangione EJ, Remus RS, Tait KA, McGee HB: An outbreak of Pontiac fever related to whirlpool use, Michigan 1982. JAMA 253:535–539, 1985.

172. Herwaldt LA, Gorman GW, McGrath J, et al: A new *Legionella* species, *Legionella feeleii* species nova, causes Pontiac fever in an automobile plant. Ann Intern Med 100:333–338, 1984.

173. Fenstersheib M, Miller M, Diggins C, et al: Outbreak of Pontiac fever due to *Legionella anisa.* Lancet 336:35–37, 1990.

174. Goldberg DJ, Collier PW, Fallon RJ, et al: Lochgoilhead fever: Outbreak of non-pneumonic Legionellosis due to *Legionella micdadei.* Lancet 1:316–318, 1989.

175. Vickers RM, Stout JE, Yu VL, Rihs JD: Culture methodology for the isolation of *Legionella pneumophila* and other Legionellaceae from clinical and environmental specimens. Semin Respir Infect 2:274–279, 1987.

176. Chiodini P, Williams A, Barker J, et al: Bronchial lavage and transbronchial lung biopsy in the diagnosis of legionnaires' disease. Thorax 40:154–155, 1985.

177. Thomas P, Lang AP, Fong IW: Diagnosis of legionnaires' disease from transbronchial biopsy using the fiberoptic bronchoscope. Can Med Assoc J 122:794–796, 1980.

178. Dobranowski J, Stringer D: Diagnosis of *Legionella* lung abscess by percutaneous needle aspiration. Can Assoc Radiol J 40:43–44, 1989.

179. Kohler RB: *Legionella* antigenuria: Testing and interpretation. Clin Microbiol Newsletter 12:185–188, 1990.

180. Oliverio MJ, Fisher MA, Vickers RM, Yu VL, Menon A: Diagnosis of Legionnaires disease by radioimmunoassay of *Legionella* in pleural fluid. J Clin Microbiol 29:2893–2894, 1991.

181. Wilkinson H, Cruce D, Broome C: Validation of *Legionella pneumophila* indirect immunofluorescence assay with epidemic sera. J Clin Microbiol 13:139–146, 1981.

182. Keys TF: Therapeutic considerations in the treatment of *Legionella* infection. Semin Respir Infect 2:770–273, 1987.

183. Miller AC. Erythromycin in legionnaires' disease: A reappraisal. J Antimicrob Chemother 7:217–222, 1981.

184. Swanson DJ, Sung RJ, Fine MJ, Orloff J, Chu SY, Yu VL: Erythromycin ototoxicity: Prospective assessment with serum concentrations and audiograms in a study of patients with pneumonia. Am J Med 92:61–68, 1992.

185. Nash P, Sideman I, Pidcoe V, Kleger B: Minocycline in legionnaires' disease. [Letter] Lancet 1:45, 1978.

186. Liebers DM, Baltch AL, Smith RP, Hammer MC, Conroy JV: Susceptibility of *Legionella pneumophila* to eight antimicrobial agents including 4 macrolides under different assay conditions. J Antimicrob Chemother 23:37–41, 1989.

187. Moffie BG, Mourton RP: Sensitivity and resistance of *L. pneumophila* to some antibiotics and combination of antibiotics. J Antimicrob Chemother 22:457–462, 1988.

188. Edelstein PH, Calarco K, Yasui VK: Antimicrobial therapy of experimentally induced legionnaires' disease in guinea pigs. Am Rev Respir Dis 130:849–856, 1984.

189. Rudin J, Evans TL, Wing E: Failure of erythromycin in treatment of *Legionella micdadei* pneumonia. Am J Med 76:318–320, 1984.

190. Saito A, Koga H, Shigeno H, Watanabe K, et al: The antimicrobial activity of ciprofloxacin against *Legionella* species and the treatment of experimental *Legionella* pneumonia in guinea pigs. Br Soc Antimicrob Chemother 18:251–260, 1986.

191. Unertl KE, Lenhart FL, Forst H, et al: Brief report: Ciprofloxacin in the treatment of legionellosis in critically ill patients including those cases unresponsive to erythromycin. Am J Med 87(suppl 5A):128S–131S, 1989.

192. Hooper T, Gould F, Swinburn CR, et al: Ciprofloxacin: A preferred treatment for legionella infection in patients receiving cyclosporin A. J Antimicrob Chemother 6:952–953, 1988.

193. Farrell ID, Baher J, Chiodini PL, Hutchinson JGP: The activity of imipenem on *Legionella pneumophila*, with a note on the treatment of two cases. J Antimicrob Chemother 16:61–65, 1985.

194. Fitzgeorge RB: The effect of antibiotics on the growth of *L. pneumophila* in guinea pigs. Alveolar phagocytes infected in vivo by an aerosol. J Infect Dis 10:189–193, 1985.

195. Vickers RM, Yu VL, Hanna S, et al: Determinants of *Legionella pneumophila* contamination of water distribution systems: 15-hospital prospective study. Infect Control 8:357–363, 1987.

196. Muraca PW, Yu VL, Goetz A: Disinfection of water distribution systems for *Legionella:* A review of application procedures and methodologies. Infect Control Hosp Epidemiol 11:79–88, 1990.

197. Snyder MB, Siwicki M, Wireman J, et al: Reduction in *Legionella pneumophila* through heat flushing followed by continuous supplemental chlorination of hospital hot water. J Infect Dis 162:127–132, 1990.

198. Grosserode M, Helms C, Pfaller M, Moyer N, Hall N, Wenzel R: Continuous hyperchlorination for control of nosocomial legionnaires' disease: A ten-year follow-up of efficacy, environmental effects, and cost. [Abstract 23] 1992 International Symposium on *Legionella,* American Society for Microbiology, Orlando, FL, 1992.

199. Makin T, Hart CA: The efficacy of ultraviolet radiation for eradicating *L. pneumophila* from a shower. [Abstract 14] 1992 International Symposium on *Legionella,* American Society for Microbiology, Orlando, FL, 1992.

200. Liu Z, Stout JE, Tedesco L, Boldin M, Hwang CC, Yu VL: Demonstration of the efficacy of ultraviolet light irradiation of potable water for prevention of *Legionella* colonization of hospital water fixtures. [Abstract L8] Meeting of the American Society for Microbiology, New Orleans, LA, 1992.

201. Matulonis U, Rosenfeld CS, Shadduck RK: Prevention of Legionella infections in a bone marrow transplant unit: Multifaceted approach to water system contamination. Infect Control Hosp Epidemiol 14:571–575, 1993.

202. Baker RL, Stevens J, Fish L, Criggar D: Nosocomial legionnaires' disease controlled by UV light and low level silver/copper ions. [Abstract 72] Third International Conference on Nosocomial Infection, Atlanta, GA, 1990.

203. Thomson RB, File TM, Plouffe J, Stephens C, Ricks R: Use of Tarn-Pure to eradicate *L. pneumophila* from a hospital hot water system. [Abstract L18] Meeting of the American Society for Microbiology, Anaheim, CA, 1990.

204. Veerstraeten P, Stolear JC, Schoutens-Serruys E, et al: Erythromycin prophylaxis for legionnaires' disease in immunosuppressed patients in a contaminated hospital environment. Transplantation 41:52–54, 1986.

205. Blander SJ, Horwitz MA: Vaccination with *L. pneumophila* membrane induces cell-mediated and protective immunity in a guinea pig model of legionnaires' disease. J Clin Invest 87:1054–1059, 1991.

206. Mallison GF: Legionellosis: Environmental aspects. Ann N Y Acad Sci 353:67–70, 1980.

207. Redd SC, Cohen ML: Legionella in water: What should be done? JAMA 257:1221–1222, 1987.

208. Yu VL: Nosocomial legionellosis: Current epidemiologic issues. *In* Swartz M, Remington J (eds): Current Clinical Topics in Infectious Diseases. New York, McGraw-Hill, 1986:239–253.

209. Goetz A, Yu VL: Screening for nosocomial legionellosis by culture of the water supply and targeting of high-risk patients for specialized laboratory testing. Am J Infect Control 19:63–66, 1991.

210. Stout JE, Yu VL, Muraca P, Joly J, Troup N, Tompkins LS: Potable water as the cause of sporadic cases of community-acquired legionnaires' disease. N Engl J Med 326:151–154, 1992.

# CHAPTER 27

# Atypical Pneumonia

STEPHEN B. GREENBERG and ROBERT L. ATMAR

In the past 100 years, there has been a tremendous increase in our understanding of the causes and pathogenesis of pneumonia. Advances in bacteriologic methods, recognition of the utility of serotherapy for the treatment of pneumococcal pneumonia, and the discovery and use of sulfonamides in the treatment of bacterial infections led to the recognition of nonbacterial pneumonia as a discrete clinical entity.[1–3] These pneumonias, which came to be called atypical pneumonias, were characterized by distinctive clinical features and by their failure to respond to sulfonamide therapy; some were associated with specific pathogens, and for others, the causes were uncertain.[2–4] Bacterial pneumonia is characterized by the abrupt onset of fever, chills, and purulent sputum, and it usually responds to β-lactam antibiotics.[5] Atypical pneumonia has few of these features. It has an insidious onset, nonproductive cough, and no response to β-lactam antibiotics. In the past 50 years, specific etiologic agents have been identified, and antimicrobial therapy has been developed for many of them. It remains clinically useful to differentiate the syndrome of atypical pneumonia from that caused by "typical" bacteria.

## HISTORY

In the late 1800s, influenza and ornithosis (ie, psittacosis) were the first diseases associated with what is now recognized as atypical pneumonia.[3] By the 1930s, diagnostic methods for the identification of influenza, ornithosis, and Q fever were available. In 1934, Gallagher described 16 cases of bronchopneumonia occurring at a boys' preparatory school that were not thought to be caused by streptococcal or mycobacterial infection.[1] In 1938, Reimann described 8 cases of lower respiratory tract infection and coined the term "atypical pneumonia."[2] During the next

several years, there were numerous reports of similar illnesses in schools, colleges, military camps, and health care settings.[3, 6–16] In 1942, because of the numerous outbreaks and epidemics in different parts of the United States, the Director of the Commission on Pneumonia prepared a definition of primary atypical pneumonia (PAP) for the Surgeon General to differentiate this group of diseases from other kinds of pneumonia.[17]

In 1943, it was reported that cold agglutinins developed in the sera of some patients with atypical pneumonia, and subsequently, cold agglutinins were seen in approximately two thirds of patients in one series of PAP.[18–20] In 1944, Eaton and colleagues isolated from the sputa of PAP patients a filterable agent that caused pneumonic lesions in cotton rats and hamsters.[21] During the next decade, investigations continued into the cause and treatment of PAP. Adenovirus was isolated from minced adenoid tissues by Rowe and colleagues in 1953, and investigations of the clinical significance of this virus began.[22, 23] A few years later, Liu demonstrated the Eaton agent in chick embryo lung using an indirect immunofluorescence stain.[24] Chanock and colleagues adapted the Eaton agent to grow in monkey kidney tissue culture and made inocula that were used in human challenge studies to fulfill the Koch postulates.[25–27] At about the same time, this agent was grown on a solid medium and identified as a mycoplasma.[28] In 1963, the agent was named *Mycoplasma pneumoniae*.[29]

Despite the characterization of *M. pneumoniae* and adenoviruses, atypical pneumonia with no identifiable cause continued to occur.[30] It was not until an epidemic of pneumonia occurred at a convention of the American Legion in Philadelphia in 1976 that a new pathogen was identified.[31, 32] McDade isolated a fastidious gram-negative organism, later named *Legionella pneumophila*, from the lung tissue of patients who died of the pneumonia.[32] Subsequent studies delineated the role of this bacterium as a cause of pneumonia (see Chap. 26).

The spectrum of diseases caused by chlamydiae was elucidated during the 1970s. The description of pneumonitis due to *Chlamydia trachomatis* in an infant in 1975 led to a search for disease caused by this agent in children and adults.[33, 34] In 1981, Komaroff and coworkers described 7 patients with definite or suggestive serologic evidence of recent chlamydial infection and pneumonia. None of these patients had other pathogens identified, and it was thought that *C. trachomatis* was responsible for the infections.[34] In 1985, Saikku and colleagues described an epidemic in Finland of mild pneumonia in which serologic responses to a non-*C. trachomatis* strain, TW-183, were demonstrated.[35] One year later, Grayston and associates reported the isolation of chlamydiae from several University of Washington students with acute respiratory disease.[36] They initially thought that these isolates represented a variant of *Chlamydia psittaci*, and they proposed the name "TWAR strain," after the first two isolates (TW-183 and AR-39).[36] Subsequent investigations suggested that at least some of the infections described by Komaroff and coworkers were caused by this strain.[37] Later morphologic and nucleic acid homology studies with this organism led to its designation as a new species, *Chlamydia pneumoniae*.[38–40] Since that time, *C. pneumoniae* has been recognized as a major cause of pneumonia and other respiratory diseases.[41, 42]

Although new pathogens that cause pneumonia have been discovered and characterized during the past several decades, a significant number of pneumonias have no identified etiologic agent. Improved diagnostic techniques may identify known pathogens as the cause of some of these undiagnosed pneumonias, but previously unknown agents probably await discovery.

## EPIDEMIOLOGY

Many pathogens cause the atypical pneumonia syndrome, as do some noninfectious agents. The common and less common infectious causes are shown in Table 27–1. Fungi, viruses, mycobacteriae, legionellae, rickettsiae, and other bacteria are discussed elsewhere in this book in more detail. Several of the less common causes of atypical pneumonia associated with animal, insect, or environmental exposures should be suspected in the appropriate epidemiologic setting.[43] In certain situations, noninfectious causes such as hypersensitivity pneumonitis and inhalation of noxious gases, fumes, or metallic compounds must be considered.[44] Typical bacterial pneumonia, such as that caused by *Streptococcus pneumoniae*, may occasionally present with signs and symptoms characteristic of an atypical pneumonia.[45] The remainder of this chapter concentrates on the epidemiology, clinical characteristics, diagnosis, and treatment of pneumonia caused by *M. pneumoniae, C. pneumoniae,* and *C. psittaci.*

*M. pneumoniae* has been recognized as a significant cause of community-acquired pneumonia for more than 25 years, and more recently, the importance of *C. pneumoniae* has been recognized.[46–53] Table 27–2 shows the percentage of community-acquired pneumonias in hospitalized patients caused by these two pathogens compared with other common bacterial and viral agents as reported in several studies.[54–67, 67a] None of these studies differentiated typical and

Table 27–1. **Infectious Causes of Atypical Pneumonia in Adults**

**Common Causes**
*Mycoplasma pneumoniae*
*Chlamydia pneumoniae*
*Legionella* spp.
Influenza virus types A and B

**Less Common Causes**
*Chlamydia psittaci*
*Coxiella burnetii*
Adenovirus
Respiratory syncytial virus
Parainfluenza virus types 1–3
*Histoplasma capsulatum*
*Coccidiodes immitis*
*Blastomyces dermatiditis*
*Cryptococcus neoformans*
*Mycobacterium* sp.

**Rare Causes**
*Francisella tularensis*
*Bacillus anthracis*
*Yersinia pestis*
*Brucella* spp.
*Rickettsia rickettsii*
*Pasturella multocida*
Cytomegalovirus
Rhinovirus

atypical pneumonia syndromes. It is evident that *S. pneumoniae* has been the principal cause of pneumonia in hospitalized patients and that in some geographic areas *Legionella* spp. have been common.[58, 60] In other areas, *Legionella* spp. were rarely the cause of pneumonia.[57, 63] *M. pneumoniae* has generally accounted for 5% to 10% of pneumonias in hospitalized patients (see Table 27–2). However, because patients with *M. pneumoniae* pneumonia are hospitalized less frequently than those with other types of pneumonia, *M. pneumoniae* is a more common cause of pneumonia than hospital-based series suggest. In a 12-year community survey in Seattle, Foy and coworkers found that 15% of all pneumonias were caused by *M. pneumoniae*.[49] Only 2% of these persons were hospitalized, compared with 16% of all patients with pneumonia. In this survey, epidemics occurred every 4 to 8 years. There was no seasonal variation in the occurrence of *M. pneumoniae* infection or pneumonia, as was seen with other etiologic agents. During the summer, as many as 50% of pneumonia cases were caused by *M. pneumoniae*. School-aged children and young adults were most commonly affected.[49]

*M. pneumoniae* is not highly contagious. It appears to be transmitted during the acute disease, with no cases of late transmission documented from persons who shed the organism for up to 5 months.[48] Infection usually is brought into a family by a school-aged child, and although spread among family members is slow, it is often extensive, with as many as 90% of household members becoming infected.[68, 69] Close contact appears to be required for the spread of infection, because family members and playmates of infected persons were more likely to become infected than were their classmates.[48] The incubation period is 2 to 3 weeks. Outbreaks have been seen in other settings in which close contact is likely to occur: in university dormitories, military barracks, and prisons.[42] However, point-source outbreaks have been documented, demonstrating

Table 27–2. **Atypical Pneumonia Agents Compared With** *Streptococcus pneumoniae* **as Causes of Community-Acquired Pneumonia in Hospitalized Patients**

| Investigation | Percentage of Patients With Specific Etiologic Agents | | | | | |
| --- | --- | --- | --- | --- | --- | --- |
| | *Mycoplasma pneumoniae* | *Chlamydia* spp.* | *Legionella* spp. | *Coxiella burnetii* | *Viruses*† | *Streptococcus pneumoniae* |
| USA, 1969–1970[54] | 4 | ND‡ | ND | ND | 5 | 53 |
| UK, 1974–1980[55] | 14 | 1 | 1 | 3 | 15 | 12 |
| UK, 1979–1982[56] | 0 | ND | 1 | ND | 6 | 50 |
| Finland, 1980–1981[57] | 2 | 9 | <1 | <1 | 7 | 26 |
| UK, 1980–1981[58] | 2 | 6 | 15 | 1 | 9 | 76 |
| South Africa, 1980[59] | 9 | ND | ND | ND | 9 | 22 |
| France, 1982–1983[60] | 9 | 3 | 11 | 1 | 4 | 12 |
| Sweden, 1982–1983[61] | 5 | 1 | 3 | ND | 10 | 47 |
| Canada, 1981–1987[62] | 7 | ND | 3 | 4 | 12 | 9 |
| UK, 1984–1985[63] | 1 | 1 | <1 | 0 | 13 | 36 |
| Sweden, ?[64] | 14 | 2 | 1 | ND | 10 | 54 |
| USA, 1986–1987[65] | 2 | 6 | 7 | ND | ND | 15 |
| Sweden, 1987[66] | 10 | 1 | 4 | ND | 16 | 37 |
| New Zealand, 1988[67] | 18 | 2 | 4 | ND | 11 | 33 |
| Spain, 1990–1991[67a] | 10 | 25 | 4 | 0 | 14 | 15 |

*Combines data for *C. pneumoniae, C. psittaci,* and *C. trachomatis.*
†Influenza virus types A and B were the most commonly identified viruses.
‡Not done.

that a short, intense exposure is sufficient for transmission of infection.[70–72] Table 27–3 summarizes the epidemiology of *M. pneumoniae* pneumonia and contrasts it to that of several other pathogens that cause atypical pneumonia.

*Chlamydia* spp. have been a common cause of pneumonia in hospitalized patients, causing 1% to 9% of cases (see Table 27–2); *C. pneumoniae* has been responsible for up to 10% of outpatient-treated pneumonias.[52] In many of the studies of hospitalized patients, the diagnosis of chlamydial infection was made serologically. Although many of the early studies assumed these infections were caused by *C. psittaci,* most of the infections were probably caused by *C. pneumoniae. C. pneumoniae* infections have occurred throughout the year without seasonal periodicity.[52] Serologic studies suggest that epidemics of infection occur every 4 to 6 years and last 1 to 2 years.[52, 53]

The mode of transmission of *C. pneumoniae* is unknown; respiratory secretions and aerosols may play a role as they do with other respiratory pathogens.[53] The lack of an association between *C. pneumoniae* antibody titers and the number of lifetime sexual partners suggests that infection is not sexually transmitted.[73] The inability to demonstrate an animal reservoir suggests that transmission is from person to person.[53] The incubation period is unknown but is probably several days to weeks. The mean interval between primary infections and secondary cases among contacts in the Danish ornithosis study was 31 days.[52] The spread of infection is slow, taking 5 to 8 months to move through groups of military trainees.[74] Serologic studies suggest that infection is uncommon among children younger than 5 years of age and then rapidly increases during the next 10 years of life.[75] Infection rates approach 10 per 100 person-years for children between the ages of 5 and 14 years and are somewhat lower for adults.[76] Among military trainees, approximately 10% of those with *C. pneumoniae* infection had pneumonia.[74] Pneumonia has been more common with primary infection than with reinfection.[76a] In a longitudinal study from Seattle, Grayston reported the highest incidence of *C. pneumoniae* pneumonia in elderly patients.[76b]

*C. psittaci* occurs sporadically and is a less common cause of community-acquired pneumonia than are *M. pneumoniae* or *C. pneumoniae.* Although it occurs worldwide, *C. psittaci* is more common in developed countries where chickens, ducks, and turkeys are bred for human consumption and psittacine and related birds are kept as pets.[77] In the United States, 100 to 200 cases were reported annually to the Centers for Disease Control between 1978 and 1989.[78] More than one half of these patients have pet birds, although outbreaks of disease have occurred in poultry plant workers.[79, 80] Those at greatest risk of acquiring infection are bird owners or fanciers, pet shop employees, and pigeon fanciers.[77] Other persons who have contact with birds or their excreta are also at risk of acquiring the disease. Psittacine birds are the most common source of infection, but nonpsittacine species may also transmit the disease.[81] This has led some investigators to suggest that ornithosis is a more appropriate term than psittacosis.[82]

*C. psittaci* may be transmitted by aerosol, by direct handling of infected bird tissues, or by mouth-to-beak intimacies.[79, 82] Rarely, bird bites transmit the disease.[82] Person-to-person transmission is rare but has been reported.[83] Only brief exposure to an area where an infected bird has been is necessary for disease transmission, and this may explain the inability to identify an avian source of infection in as many as one third of cases.[79, 84] The incubation period is 1 to 2 weeks.[77] Infections are most common between the ages of 30 and 60 years.[77, 85]

## CLINICAL MANIFESTATIONS

Atypical pneumonia is characterized by the insidious onset of fever, nonproductive cough, and headache; and the causative pathogen cannot be determined using clinical signs and symptoms (Table 27–4). Persons with *M. pneumoniae* infection usually have upper respiratory tract symptoms followed by lower respiratory tract symptoms. *M. pneumoniae* pneumonia occasionally has an abrupt on-

Table 27–3. **Epidemiology of Atypical Pneumonia**

| Epidemiologic Feature | *Mycoplasma pneumoniae* | *Chlamydia pneumoniae* | *Chlamydia psittaci* | *Legionella* spp. | *Coxiella burnetii* |
|---|---|---|---|---|---|
| Occurrence | All year | All year | Sporadic | Peaks late summer to early fall | Sporadic |
| Incubation period | 2–3 wk | Unknown (probably weeks) | 1–2 wk | 2–10 d | 2–6 wk |
| Peak age | 5–20 y | Older adults | 30–60 y | >60 y | 15–64 y |
| Infectivity | Low | Low | High | High | High |
| Transmission | Respiratory secretions; aerosol | Unknown | Aerosol | Uncertain (aerosol, aspiration, direct inoculation) | Aerosol; raw milk ingestion; blood transfusion |
| Person-to-person spread | Yes | Yes | Rare | No | Rare |
| Underlying diseases | | | | Smoking, chronic obstructive pulmonary disease, immunosuppression | |
| Environmental or animal exposure | No | No | Birds | Contaminated water distribution systems | Contaminated dust from infected animals (eg, goats, sheep, cattle, cats) |

set.[42, 46, 48, 50, 68, 86] A sore throat is the initial symptom in many cases; hoarseness may occur within a few days. The cough is nonproductive, constant, and often worse at night. Headache and fever are common but are not as severe as with ornithosis and Q fever. On physical examination, rales are often the only abnormality detected.

*C. pneumoniae* infection usually starts with a sore throat; hoarseness occurs in some cases. Symptoms of pneumonia, if they develop, occur gradually. Cough often begins after a week of other symptoms.[35, 36, 41, 52, 53, 83] Rhonchi and rales are common findings on physical examination.

Unlike *M. pneumoniae* and *C. pneumoniae* pneumonias, ornithosis often begins suddenly with chills and high fever, but it may have a gradual onset over several days.[79, 84, 85] A persistent, nonproductive cough is common. Dyspnea is present only if extensive pulmonary disease occurs. Sore throat and epistaxis have been reported in a few cases and

are usually mild. Rarely, persons with *C. psittaci* pneumonia complain of hemoptysis. Headache with ornithosis is often severe and may be the chief complaint. A relative bradycardia can be detected in approximately one third of infected patients. Physical examination may reveal fever, rales, and occasionally, pharyngeal erythema. Alterations in mental status have been reported at the end of the first week of infection, especially in those who have hypoxemia. Pleural friction rubs may be detected.

Two forms of *Legionella* infections are Pontiac fever and pneumonia. Pontiac fever is a nonspecific febrile illness with no localizing pulmonary findings.[30, 31] The pneumonia associated with *Legionella* infection may have a wide range of associated symptoms, which often include fever, malaise, and a cough that becomes mildly productive after the first few days. In 25% to 50% of cases, diarrhea has been reported. In a small percentage of patients, nausea, vomiting,

Table 27–4. **Clinical Features of Atypical Pneumonia in Adults**

| | Agent | | | | |
|---|---|---|---|---|---|
| Characteristics | Mycoplasma pneumoniae | Chlamydia pneumoniae | Chlamydia psittaci | Legionella spp. | Coxiella burnetii |
| *Symptoms* | | | | | |
| Cough | + * | + | + | + | + |
| Mental confusion | ± | − | ± | + | − |
| Headache | + | − | + | + | + |
| Myalgias | + | ± | + | + | + |
| Ear pain | ± | − | − | − | − |
| Meningismus | − | − | + | − | − |
| Pleuritic pain | ± | − | − | + | − |
| Abdominal pain | − | − | − | ± | − |
| Diarrhea | ± | − | − | + | − |
| *Signs* | | | | | |
| Fever | + | + | + | + | + |
| Rash | Erythema multiforme | − | Horder spots | Pretibial | − |
| Pharyngitis | + | + | ± | − | − |
| Hemoptysis | − | − | ± | + | − |
| Lobar consolidation | ± | ± | ± | ± | ± |
| Cardiac involvement | ± | ± | ± | − | ± |
| Splenomegaly | − | − | + | − | − |
| Relative bradycardia | − | − | + | + | − |

*Key: −, not present; ±, occasionally reported; +, commonly reported.

and abdominal pain occur. Headache and altered mental status are common. In a few cases, hilar adenopathy is found. Rales and evidence of pulmonary consolidation are commonly found on physical examination. Hypotension has been reported in 15% to 20% of patients with severe *Legionella* infection. On laboratory examination, the finding of hyponatremia is more commonly associated with *Legionella* than with any other atypical pneumonia agent.

Q fever, or *Coxiella burnetii* infection, has a wide range of clinical presentations. There are three pneumonia syndromes: atypical pneumonia, rapidly progressive pneumonia, and febrile illness with evidence of pneumonia found incidentally.[87-89] Cough occurs in fewer than 30% of patients with Q fever, but fever is a universal finding. As with ornithosis, severe headache is a common finding. Fatigue and chills are associated with nausea and vomiting in half of the patients. Inspiratory rales are the major physical examination finding of pneumonia.

A specific radiologic diagnosis of atypical pneumonia is rarely possible. Although patchy alveolar or reticular infiltrates are the rule, each common pathogen causing the atypical pneumonia syndrome can produce a lobar infiltrate such as that associated with typical, or bacterial, pneumonia.[79, 85, 90-95] *M. pneumoniae, C. pneumoniae,* and *C. psittaci* organisms have caused radiographic abnormalities out of proportion to the physical examination findings. *M. pneumoniae* has a predilection for the lower lobes; small pleural effusions have been reported in 30% of patients, but large effusions are rare.[96] Unusual roentgenographic findings associated with *M. pneumoniae* have included pneumatoceles, hilar adenopathy, mediastinal mass, and diffuse interstitial fibrosis.[97, 98] The radiographic pattern observed with *C. pneumoniae* is similar to that of *M. pneumoniae,* with segmental pneumonitis a common finding. Pleural effusion has been described with *C. pneumoniae* pneumonia.[99] *C. psittaci* may cause segmental pneumonitis, bilateral infiltrates, or lobar consolidation. Small pleural effusions have been reported in psittacosis.[79] *Legionella* and *C. burnetii* pneumonias have radiographic patterns similar to those seen with other atypical pneumonias. Pleural effusions and hilar adenopathy have been reported in each.[100, 101]

The resolution of common pneumonias has been studied by several investigators (Table 27–5).[102-108] In a study of the radiographic resolution of *S. pneumoniae* pneumonia, Jay and colleagues demonstrated resolution of consolidation on serial chest roentgenograms by 8 to 10 weeks.[105] Roentgenographic abnormalities of bacteremic patients older than 50 years of age resolved more slowly than those of younger patients. Deterioration in roentgenographic findings after initiation of antibiotic therapy is found in pneumococcal and *Legionella* pneumonia. Of all bacterial pneumonias, *Legionella* pneumonias appear to resolve most slowly, with approximately 50% of patients having clear radiographs by 10 weeks.[106, 108] Progression after institution of antibiotic treatment is rare in *M. pneumoniae* pneumonia; roentgenographic resolution is complete in approximately 90% of patients by 8 weeks.[109] In *C. psittaci* pneumonia, speed of resolution is between that of *M. pneumoniae* and *Legionella* pneumonias. Little definitive information is available on the radiographic resolution of *C. pneumoniae* pneumonias; it is likely that resolution is similar to that described for *M. pneumoniae* pneumonia.

The pathogens associated with atypical pneumonia may cause more severe disease in certain hosts. Although less likely to occur in elderly persons, *M. pneumoniae* and *Legionella* infection may be more severe in this age group.[86, 109, 110] The unusual severity of *M. pneumoniae* infection in children with sickle cell disease has been documented.[112] Patients with chronic obstructive pulmonary disease appear to be more severely affected by *M. pneumoniae, C. pneumoniae,* and *Legionella* infections than normal hosts.[111, 113, 114] With the exception of *Legionella,* atypical pneumonia agents rarely cause pneumonia in transplant recipients and cancer patients.[115-117] No increased frequency of atypical pneumonias has been observed in patients with acquired immunodeficiency syndrome.[118]

Atypical pneumonia pathogens have caused pulmonary and extrapulmonary complications (Tables 27–6 through 27–8). The pulmonary complications of *M. pneumoniae* can include empyema, chronic pulmonary fibrosis, or bronchiolitis obliterans.[42, 119-121] Although residual pulmonary abnormalities are rarely associated with other atypical pneumonias, bronchospasm and sarcoidosis have been associated with *C. pneumoniae* infection.[41, 122, 123] Sinusitis

**Table 27–5. Rates of Resolution of Pneumonia Caused by Various Microorganisms**

| Reference | Microbe | No. of Patients | Mean Age (Years) | Patients With Complete Clearing (%) | | | |
|---|---|---|---|---|---|---|---|
| | | | | 2 Weeks | 4 Weeks | 8 Weeks | 12 Weeks |
| | *Streptococcus pneumoniae* | | | | | | |
| 105 | Bacteremic (<50 y) | 36 | NR* | 20 | 60 | 81 | 94 |
| 105 | (≥50 y) | 36 | NR | 6 | 25 | 59 | 75 |
| 106 | | 19 | 61 | 5 | 15 | 35 | 60 |
| 107 | | 69 | NR | NR | 66 | NR | NR |
| 106 | Nonbacteremic | 53 | 47 | 12 | 28 | 70 | 80 |
| 107 | | 289 | NR | NR | 86 | NR | NR |
| 106 | *Mycoplasma pneumoniae* | 37 | 30 | 30 | 50 | 85 | 90 |
| 109 | | 60 | 33 | NR | 40 | 96 | NR |
| 106 | *Chlamydia psittaci* | 10 | 46 | 30 | 50 | 60 | NR |
| 110 | | 29 | 27 | 7 | 52 | 83 | NR |
| 106 | *Legionella* spp. | 42 | 51 | 5 | 12 | 30 | 55 |
| 108 | | 21 | 60 | NR | NR | 29 | NR |

*Not reported.

Modified from Kirtland SH, Winterbauer RH. Slowly resolving, chronic, and recurrent pneumonia. Clin Chest Med 12:303–318, 1991.

Table 27–6. **Extrapulmonary Complications of** *Mycoplasma pneumoniae*

| System | Manifestation |
|---|---|
| Hematologic | Hemolytic anemia |
| Neurologic | Meningoencephalitis, transverse myelitis, brachial plexus neuropathy, mononeuritis multiplex, Guillain-Barré syndrome, sensorineural hearing loss |
| Cardiovascular | Dysrhythmias, ST-T wave changes on electrocardiogram, pericardial effusion, dilated cardiomyopathy |
| Rheumatologic | Arthritis |
| Gastrointestinal | Hepatosplenomegaly (rare), pancreatitis (rare) |
| Renal | Glomeurulonephritis (rare) |
| Dermatologic | Stevens-Johnson syndrome, erythema multiforme, erythema nodosum |

and sinus tenderness are common with *M. pneumoniae* and *C. pneumoniae* infections.[111]

Skin rashes are most commonly seen with *M. pneumoniae* infections. These may be maculopapular, vesicular, or urticarial.[124–126] Erythema multiforme and erythema nodosum have also been reported; the former is associated with respiratory symptoms.[127–130] With ornithosis, Horder spots resembling the rose spots of typhoid fever have been reported.[79] *C. pneumoniae* infection, *Legionella* infection, and Q fever are not reported to have exanthems.

Cardiac involvement has been reported for each of the common atypical pneumonia agents. Dysrhythmias, ST-T wave electrocardiographic changes, pericardial effusions, and heart failure secondary to dilated cardiomyopathy have been reported with *M. pneumoniae* infections.[131–133] Myopericarditis has also been reported with *C. pneumoniae*, *C. psittaci*, and *Legionella* infections.[134–136] Endocarditis has been reported with *C. pneumoniae*, *C. psittaci*, and *Legionella* infections and with Q fever.[137–145] Coronary artery disease and acute myocardial infarction have been associated with serologic evidence of *C. pneumoniae* infection and the organism has been found in atheromatous plaques.[146, 146a]

Central nervous system complications including meningoencephalitis have been reported with *M. pneumoniae* and *C. psittaci* infections and with Q fever.[85, 147–152] Among hospitalized patients with *M. pneumoniae* infections, as many as 10% had one of several neurologic conditions.[110] Approximately 20% of patients with neurologic manifestations and serologic evidence of recent *M. pneumoniae* infection exhibit no respiratory symptoms. Uncommon neurologic complications of *M. pneumoniae* infection include transverse myelitis, peripheral and cranial polyradiculitis, cerebellar ataxia, acute psychosis, and hemiplegia.[110]

Hemolytic anemia, although usually not clinically significant, has been severe enough to cause the death of patients

Table 27–7. **Extrapulmonary Complications of** *Chlamydia pneumoniae*

| System | Manifestation |
|---|---|
| Cardiovascular | Myopericarditis, endocarditis, coronary artery disease, myocardial infarction |
| Gastrointestinal | Abdominal pain and diarrhea |

Table 27–8. **Extrapulmonary Complications of** *Chlamydia psittaci*

| System | Manifestation |
|---|---|
| Hematologic | Hemolytic anemia, disseminated intravascular coagulation |
| Neurologic | Meningoencephalitis |
| Cardiovascular | Myopericarditis, culture-negative endocarditis |
| Rheumatologic | Reactive arthritis |
| Gastrointestinal | Hepatic granuloma |
| Renal | Rhabdomyolysis |
| Dermatologic | Erythema nodosum |

with *M. pneumoniae* infections.[153] Hemolytic anemia is usually associated with IgM cold agglutinin antibodies, which reach their maximum titer after 2 to 3 weeks of illness.[154] Similar cold agglutinin-positive hemolysis has been reported with *Legionella* and adenovirus infections. The hemolytic anemias reported with *C. psittaci* infection and Q fever are not associated with cold agglutinins.[155]

Other uncommon extrapulmonary complications seen with atypical pneumonias include arthritis (eg, *M. pneumoniae*, *C. psittaci*), hepatitis (eg, *C. psittaci*, *C. burnetti*), pancreatitis (eg, *M. pneumoniae*, *Legionella*), disseminated intravascular coagulation (eg, *C. psittaci*, *Legionella*), and rhabdomyolysis (eg, *C. psittaci*, *Legionella*). Death from atypical pneumonia caused by *Mycoplasma* or *Chlamydia* is rare and usually occurs in the presence of other complications. Mortality rates of 1% to 5% have been reported for patients infected with *C. psittaci*.[85] Death from *Legionella* infection may occur in as many as 50% of nosocomial infections but is uncommon in community-acquired infections. Death from Q fever occurs primarily in patients with associated endocarditis.[140]

## DIAGNOSIS

The diagnostic methods for identifying the specific etiologic agents associated with atypical pneumonia include culture, antigen and nucleic acid detection, and serologic methods. Table 27–9 lists some of the diagnostic methods available for detecting *M. pneumoniae*, *C. pneumoniae*, and *C. psittaci*.

*M. pneumoniae* may be identified by culture, but even with optimal culture conditions, recovery rates are low, and results are not available for 1 to 3 weeks.[86, 156] The best specimens for culture are sputa and throat washings, although the organism may also be recovered from pharyngeal swabs.[110, 150] Specimens should be transported to the laboratory immediately after collection in SP4 transport medium for prompt inoculation.[86] SP4 medium is optimal for the isolation of the *M. pneumoniae*.[86, 157, 158] Specimens may be inoculated onto agar plates or into diphasic media (ie, broth over agar). In two comparative trials, the use of diphasic media was reported to be more sensitive, although both methods should be used for maximal yields.[86, 110, 156, 159] Cultures require 5 to 21 days to become positive. The ability of *Mycoplasma* colonies to hemadsorb or hemolyze guinea pig erythrocytes has been used for preliminary identification.[160] However, *Mycobacterium genitalium*, a closely related species that shares antigens with *M. pneumoniae*,

Table 27–9. **Methods for the Diagnosis of** *Mycoplasma pneumoniae,* *Chlamydia pneumoniae,* **and** *Chlamydia psittaci* **Infections**

| Method | *Mycoplasma pneumoniae* | *Chlamydia pneumoniae* | *Chlamydia psittaci* |
|---|---|---|---|
| Culture | G* | R | R† |
| Antigen detection | | | |
|   Fluorescent antibody stain (direct or indirect) | I | I‡ | |
|   Enzyme immunoassay | I | I‡ | I‡ |
| Nucleic acid detection | | | |
|   Hybridization | G | | |
|   Polymerase chain reaction | I | I | I |
| Serology | | | |
|   Complement fixation | S, R | R‡ | S, R‡ |
|   Enzyme immunoassay | G | I | |
|   Microimmunofluorescence | | S, R | |
|   Other methods | G, R | | |

*G, generally available; I, investigational; R, reference or specialty laboratory; S, standard diagnostic method.
†Laboratory hazard.
‡Commercially available but fails to differentiate species, and sensitivity and specificity data are unavailable.

also has this property.[161, 162] Definitive identification depends on the organism's reaction with specific antiserum.[86, 110]

Methods to rapidly detect *M. pneumoniae* organisms in clinical specimens are being developed, and some are now available. Antigen detection using enzyme immunoassays (EIA) and indirect immunofluorescence have been described and may have utility in the future, but these tests are not widely available.[163–167] A method of nucleic acid detection using a species-specific probe to *M. pneumoniae* ribosomal RNA is commercially available. This test has had a sensitivity of 75% to 100% and a specificity of 85% to 98% when culture results are optimal.[165, 168–171] The principal advantage of this method is that results are rapidly available; the major disadvantage is that radioisotopes are used in the detection system. The detection of *M. pneumoniae*-specific DNA using the polymerase chain reaction (PCR) has been reported, but the general application of this method requires further technologic development and clinical testing.[172, 173, 173a]

Serologic tests are the most common way of diagnosing *M. pneumoniae* infection. Cold agglutinins occur in a large number of cases of atypical pneumonia. A test for cold agglutinins is readily available and has been used presumptively to diagnose *M. pneumoniae* infection.[50, 110] A rapid bedside test for cold agglutinins can be performed and is positive at titers of 1:64 or higher.[174] However, as few as 21.5% of cold agglutinin-positive atypical pneumonias can be proven to be a result of *M. pneumoniae* infection.[175] When titers are 1:128 or higher, the percentage increases, but it may still be as low as 50%. Between 33% and 76% of patients with *M. pneumoniae* pneumonia develop cold agglutinins, although they are present more commonly in severely ill patients.[110, 150] Cold agglutinins also have been demonstrated in infections caused by *Legionella, C. psittaci,* respiratory syncytial virus, influenza virus, parainfluenza virus, adenovirus, rubella, and Epstein-Barr virus.[110, 176–178]

Complement fixation has been the standard serologic method used to diagnose *M. pneumoniae* infections.[179] A fourfold rise in titers between acute and convalescent sera is considered diagnostic of recent infection. Titers begin to rise 1 week after infection and peak at 3 to 4 weeks. Al-

though complement fixation has been the gold standard for the serologic diagnosis of *M. pneumoniae* infection, its sensitivity has been reported to be as low as 50% in culture-confirmed cases.[156, 163] Complement fixation measures antibody to glycolipid antigens, and false-positive rises in titers have been observed in bacterial meningitis and acute pancreatitis.[179, 180] Other methods used in the diagnosis of *M. pneumoniae* infection include metabolic inhibition, mycoplasmacidal tests, radioimmunoprecipitation, indirect immunofluorescence, hemagglutination, and EIA.[119, 160, 181–191] Of these tests, the EIA shows the most promise because of its sensitivity and ease of performance. IgM antibodies begin to appear approximately 1 week after infection and are often present at the time of hospitalization.[119, 190, 191] The test is more sensitive in patients younger than 20 years of age, and higher titers are seen in this age group.[189–191] However, EIA-IgG antibodies crossreactive with other mycoplasmal species exist in sera of noninfected persons, causing concern about false-positive reactions.[192] To circumvent this problem, assays using a defined antigen (ie, adherence or P1 protein or short peptides from the P1 protein) are being developed.[193–195] Although crossreactivity with *M. genitalium* remains an issue, these assays have great potential for the early diagnosis of *M. pneumoniae* infection.[196]

The optimal method for identifying *C. pneumoniae* infection is still being defined. Increasing numbers of studies are being reported in which the organism has been isolated in cell cultures.[36, 101, 197–199] The organism may be grown in the yolk sac of embryonated chicken eggs or in HeLa cell cultures.[200] Positive cultures are identified by fluorescent antibody staining of intracellular inclusions.[36] A more sensitive cell line (HL) and modifications in the culture medium have improved the growth of *C. pneumoniae* in cell cultures.[201–203] However, clinical specimens should be processed rapidly, because the organisms quickly become nonviable at room temperature (ie, 1% viable after 24 hours).[204]

Antigen detection methods have been used to identify *C. pneumoniae.* In one series, direct fluorescent antibody staining using *C. pneumoniae*-specific antibodies identified four of six culture-positive specimens; however, specimen processing may affect results.[36, 205] Commercially available EIAs that detect genus-specific antigens have been successful in identifying *C. pneumoniae* in clinical specimens.[197, 206, 207]

These assays do not differentiate *C. pneumoniae* from *C. psittaci* or *C. trachomatis.* DNA amplification using PCR to differentiate the human chlamydial species has also been proposed.[208, 209, 209a] The sensitivity and utility of such tests must be determined.

Serologic methods have been the most common methods used to diagnose *C. pneumoniae* infections. Chlamydial complement fixation antibodies appear first, but they may be absent in as many as 30% of patients.[210] The detection of microimmunofluorescent (MIF) antibodies has been the principal diagnostic serologic method used. This method requires the use of *C. pneumoniae* organisms as antigen. Grayston and colleagues have defined the following as diagnostic of recent infection: a fourfold rise in MIF antibody titer; a single IgM MIF antibody titer of 1:16 or greater, or a single IgG MIF antibody titer of 1:512 or greater.[52] In primary infection, these antibodies appear late, with diagnostic titers of IgM MIF antibodies appearing 3 to 4 weeks after the onset of illness and diagnostic titers of IgG MIF antibodies at 6 to 8 weeks. In reinfection, IgM antibodies may not be detected, and IgG titers may rise quickly to a high titer.[52] There are antigenic differences (possibly different serotypes) between isolates of *C. pneumoniae,* and this may affect the titer of antibody measured.[210] *C. pneumoniae*-specific antigens have been demonstrated, making the development of an EIA possible.[211] An EIA using detergent-treated elementary bodies to measure past exposure to *C. pneumoniae* also has been described.[212]

The diagnosis of *C. psittaci* infection is usually made serologically. Although it can be cultured, it is a laboratory hazard, with deaths in laboratory workers having been reported.[213] Detection of *C. psittaci* using a *Chlamydia* genus-specific EIA and direct fluorescent antibody staining has been reported, and detection of DNA using PCR has been suggested.[208, 209a, 214, 215a] Measurement of complement fixation antibody is the principal method for diagnosis, with a fourfold rise or a single titer of 1:16 or greater suggesting recent infection.[200] These changes may also be seen in *C. pneumoniae* and *C. trachomatis* infections; therefore, epidemiologic information also is useful diagnostically.

For the diagnosis of *Legionella* infection, see Chapter 26.

## TREATMENT

Because identification of the causative agent of atypical pneumonia is usually made retrospectively, the selection of an antimicrobial agent must be made on clinical grounds. In vitro studies of the treatment of *Chlamydia, Mycoplasma,* and *Legionella* infections have demonstrated excellent results with tetracyclines, macrolides, and quinolones but not with penicillins or cephalosporins.[216–225] Few in vitro or in vivo studies have been performed with *C. psittaci,* although this organism has been shown to be sensitive to tetracycline.[226–228] The few published controlled clinical efficacy trials looked at *M. pneumoniae* infections and showed increased speed of resolution of fever, cough, and radiographic changes after 10 to 14 days of tetracycline or erythromycin.[229–231] Relapses after therapy with tetracycline have occurred in a few cases of *M. pneumoniae* and *C. psittaci* infection.[226, 232] Although *M. pneumoniae* can persist in the respiratory tract despite antibiotic treatment, chronic carriage in ornithosis is rare. Failure to respond to appropriate antibiotic therapy has also been reported.[233]

The new macrolide antibiotics, clarithromycin, azithromycin, and roxithromycin, are among the most active antimicrobial agents against typical and atypical pneumonia pathogens.[234] The pharmacokinetics of these macrolide antibiotics allow for once- or twice-daily oral dosing.[235] They have high concentrations in tissue relative to serum and in monocytes and macrophages.[234] The initial clinical studies with clarithromycin (500 mg orally twice daily), azithromycin (500 mg orally each day), and roxithromycin (150 mg orally twice daily) demonstrated greater than 90% cure rates of community-acquired pneumonias.[234–239] Few significant side effects have been reported in early trials. If additional studies of more severely ill patients support the excellent results of early clinical trials, one or more of these macrolide antibiotics will become the treatment of choice for atypical pneumonias and for many common bacterial pneumonias.

## REFERENCES

1. Gallagher JR: Bronchopneumonia in adolescence. Yale J Biol Med 7:23–40, 1934.
2. Reimann HA: An acute infection of the respiratory tract with atypical pneumonia: A disease entity probably caused by a titratable virus. JAMA 111:2377–2384, 1938.
3. Finland M, Dingle JH: Virus pneumonias. I. Pneumonias associated with known nonbacterial agents: Influenza, psittacosis and Q fever. N Engl J Med 227:342–350, 1942.
4. Dingle JH, Finland M: Virus pneumonias. II. Primary atypical pneumonias of unknown etiology. N Engl J Med 227:378–385, 1942.
5. Cotton EM, Strampfer MJ, Cunha BA: *Legionella* and *Mycoplasma* pneumonia—A community hospital experience with atypical pneumonia. Clin Chest Med 8:441–453, 1987.
6. Maxfield JR Jr: Atypical pneumonia with leukopenia. Tex State J Med 35:340–346, 1939.
7. Smiley DR, Showacre ED, Lee WF, et al: Acute interstitial pneumonitis: A new disease entity. JAMA 112:1901–1904, 1939.
8. Rainey WG, Burbidge JR: Acute pneumonitis or atypical pneumonia. J Lancet 59:101–104, 1939.
9. Kneeland Y Jr, Smetana HF: Current bronchopneumonia of unusual character and undetermined etiology. Bull Johns Hopkins Hosp 67:229–267, 1940.
10. Longcope WT: Bronchopneumonia of unknown etiology (variety X). A report of thirty-two cases with two deaths. Bull Johns Hopkins Hosp 67:268–305, 1940.
11. Murray ME Jr: Atypical bronchopneumonia of unknown etiology: Possibly due to a filterable virus. N Engl J Med 222:565–573, 1940.
12. Gallagher JR: Acute pneumonitis: A report of 87 cases among adolescents. Yale J Biol Med 13:663–678, 1941.
13. McKinlay CA, Cowan DW: Acute respiratory infections including lobar pneumonia and atypical pneumonia in a young adult group. J Lancet 61:125–133, 1941.
14. Reimann HA, Havens WP: An epidemic disease of the respiratory tract. Arch Intern Med 65:138–150, 1941.
15. Daniels WB: Bronchopneumonia of unknown etiology in a girls' school. Am J Med Sci 203:263–276, 1942.
16. Marmion BP: Eaton agent—science and scientific acceptance: A historical commentary. Rev Infect Dis 12:338–353, 1990.
17. Official statements: Primary atypical pneumonia, etiology unknown. War Med 2:330–333, 1942.
18. Peterson OL, Ham TH, Finland M: Cold agglutinins (auto-haemagglutinins) in primary atypical pneumonias. Science 97:167, 1943.
19. Turner JC: Development of cold agglutinins in atypical pneumonia. Nature 151:419–420, 1943.
20. Finland M, Peterson OL, Allen HE, et al: Cold agglutinins. I. Occurrence of cold isohaemagglutinins in various conditions. J Clin Invest 24:451–457, 1945.
21. Eaton MD, Meiklejohn G, van Herick W: Studies on the etiology of

primary atypical pneumonia: A filterable agent transmissible to cotton rats, hamsters and chick embryos. J Exp Med 79:649–668, 1944.

22. Rowe WP, Huebner RJ, Gillmore LK, et al: Isolation of a cytopathogenic agent from human adenoids undergoing spontaneous degeneration in tissue culture. Proc Soc Exp Biol Med 84:570–573, 1953.

23. Hilleman MR, Werner JH: Recovery of a new agent from patients with acute respiratory illness. Proc Soc Exp Biol Med 85:183–188, 1954.

24. Liu C: Studies on primary atypical pneumonia. I. Localization, isolation and cultivation of a virus in chick embryos. J Exp Med 106:455–467, 1957.

25. Chanock RM, Fox HH, James WD, et al: Growth of laboratory and naturally occurring strains of Eaton agent in monkey kidney tissue culture. Proc Soc Exp Biol Med 105:371–375, 1960.

26. Chanock RM, Rifkind D, Kravetz HM, et al: Respiratory disease in volunteers infected with Eaton agent: A preliminary report. Proc Natl Acad Sci U S A 47:887–890, 1961.

27. Rifkind D, Chanock RM, Kravetz H, et al: Ear involvement (myringitis) and primary atypical pneumonia following inoculation of volunteers with Eaton Agent. Am Rev Respir Dis 85:479–489, 1962.

28. Chanock RM, Hayflick L, Barile MF: Growth on artificial medium of an agent associated with atypical pneumonia and its identification as a PPLO. Proc Natl Acad Sci U S A 48:41–49, 1961.

29. Chanock RM, Dienes L, Eaton MD, et al: *Mycoplasma pneumoniae:* Proposed nomenclature for atypical pneumonia organism (Eaton agent). Science 140:662, 1963.

30. Thacker SB, Bennet JV, Tsai T, et al: An outbreak in 1965 of severe respiratory illness caused by legionnaires' disease bacterium. J Infect Dis 238:512–519, 1978.

31. Fraser DW, Tsai T, Orenstein W, et al: Legionnaires' disease: Description of an epidemic of pneumonia. N Engl J Med 297:1183–1197, 1977.

32. McDade JE, Shepard DD, Fraser DW, et al: Legionnaires' disease: Isolation of a bacterium and demonstration of its role in other respiratory disease. N Engl J Med 297:1197–1203, 1977.

33. Schachter J, Lum L, Gooding CA, et al: Pneumonitis following inclusion blennorrhea. J Pediatr 87:779–780, 1975.

34. Komaroff AL, Aronson MD, Schachter J: *Chlamydia trachomatis* infection in adults with community-acquired pneumonia. JAMA 245:1319–1322, 1981.

35. Saikku P, Wang SP, Kleemola M, et al: An epidemic of mild pneumonia due to an unusual strain of *Chlamydia psittaci.* J Infect Dis 151:832–839, 1985.

36. Grayston JT, Kuo CC, Wang SP, et al: A new *Chlamydia psittaci* strain, TWAR, isolated in acute respiratory tract infections. N Engl J Med 315:161–168, 1986.

37. Schachter J: Human *Chlamydia psittaci* infection. *In* Oriel JD, Ridgway G, Schachter J, et al (eds): Chlamydial Infections: Proceeding of the Sixth International Symposium on Human Chlamydial Infections. Cambridge, England, Cambridge University Press, 1986:311–320.

38. Chi EY, Kuo CC, Grayston JT: Unique ultrastructure in the elementary body of *Chlamydia* sp. strain TWAR. J Bacteriol 169:3757–3763, 1987.

39. Campbell LA, Kuo CC, Grayston JT: Characterization of the new *Chlamydia* agent, TWAR, as a unique organism by restriction endonuclease analysis and DNA-DNA hybridization. J Clin Microbiol 25:1911–1916, 1987.

40. Grayston JT, Kuo CC, Campbell LA, et al: *Chlamydia pneumoniae* sp. nov. for *Chlamydia* strain TWAR. Int J Syst Bacteriol 39:88–90, 1989.

41. Grayston JT, Wang SP, Kuo CC, et al: Current knowledge on *Chlamydia pneumoniae,* strain TWAR, an important cause of pneumonia and other acute respiratory diseases. Eur J Clin Microbiol Dis 8:191–202, 1989.

42. Atmar RL, Greenberg SB: Pneumonia caused by *Mycoplasma pneumoniae* and the TWAR agent. Semin Respir Infect 4:19–31, 1989.

43. Weinberg AN: Respiratory infections transmitted from animals. Infect Dis Clin North Am 5:649–661, 1991.

44. Casey KR: Atypical pneumonia and environmental factors. Where have you been and what have you done? Clin Chest Med 12:285–302, 1991.

45. Luby JP: Southwestern Internal Medicine Conference: Pneumonias in adults due to mycoplasma, chlamydiae, and viruses. Am J Med Sci 294:45–64, 1987.

46. Alexander ER, Foy HM, Kenny GE, et al: Pneumonia due to *Mycoplasma pneumoniae.* Its incidence in the membership of a co-operative medical group. N Engl J Med 275:131–136, 1966.

47. Mufson MA, Chang V, Gill V, et al: The role of viruses, mycoplasmas and bacteria in acute pneumonia in civilian adults. Am J Epidemiol 86:526–544, 1967.

48. Foy HM, Kenny GE, McMahan R, et al: *Mycoplasma pneumoniae* in the community. Am J Epidemiol 93:55–67, 1971.

49. Foy HM, Kenny GE, Cooney MK, et al: Long-term epidemiology of infections with *Mycoplasma pneumoniae.* J Infect Dis 139:681–687, 1979.

50. Luby JP: Pneumonia caused by *Mycoplasma pneumoniae* infection. Clin Chest Med 12:237–244, 1991.

51. Grayston JT, Diwan VK, Cooney M, et al: Community- and hospital-acquired pneumonia associated with Chlamydia TWAR infection demonstrated serologically. Arch Intern Med 149:169–173, 1989.

52. Grayston JT, Campbell LA, Kuo CC, et al: A new respiratory tract pathogen: *Chlamydia pneumoniae* strain TWAR. J Infect Dis 161:618–625, 1990.

53. Thom DH, Grayston JT: Infections with *Chlamydia pneumoniae* strain TWAR. Clin Chest Med 12:245–256, 1991.

54. Dorff GJ, Rytel MW, Farmer SG, et al: Etiologies and characteristic features of pneumonias in a municipal hospital. Am J Med Sci 266:349–358, 1973.

55. White RJ, Blainey AD, Harrison KJ, et al: Causes of pneumonia presenting to a district general hospital. Thorax 36:566–570, 1981.

56. McNabb WR, Shanson DC, Williams TDM, et al: Adult community-acquired pneumonia in central London. J R Soc Med 77:550–555, 1984.

57. Kerttula Y, Leinonen M, Koskela M, et al: The aetiology of pneumonia. Application of bacterial serology and basic laboratory methods. J Infect 14:21–30, 1987.

58. MacFarlane JT, Finch RG, Ward MJ, et al: Hospital study of adult community-acquired pneumonia. Lancet 2:255–258, 1982.

59. Prout S, Potgieter PD, Forder AA, et al: Acute community-acquired pneumonias. S Afr Med J 64:443–446, 1983.

60. Bornstein N, Fleurette J, Bebear C, et al: Bacteriological and serological diagnosis of community-acquired acute pneumonia, especially legionnaire's disease: Multicentric prospective study of 274 hospitalized patients. Zentralbl Baktiol Hyg 264:93–101, 1987.

61. Holmberg H: Aetiology of community-acquired pneumonia in hospital treated patients. Scand J Infect Dis 19:491–501, 1987.

62. Marrie TJ, Durant H, Yates L: Community-acquired pneumonia requiring hospitalization: 5-year prospective study. Rev Infect Dis 11:586–599, 1989.

63. Woodhead MA, MacFarlane JT, McCracken JS, et al: Prospective study of the aetiology and outcome of pneumonia in the community. Lancet 1:671–674, 1987.

64. Berntsson E, Blomberg J, Lagergard T, et al: Etiology of community-acquired pneumonia in patients requiring hospitalization. Eur J Clin Microbiol 4:268–272, 1985.

65. Fang GD, Fine M, Orloff J, et al: New and emerging etiologies for community-acquired pneumonia with implications for therapy: A prospective multicenter study of 359 cases. Medicine (Baltimore) 69:307–316, 1990.

66. Ortqvist A, Jedlund A, Grillner L, et al: Aetiology, outcome and prognostic factors in community-acquired pneumonia requiring hospitalization. Eur Respir J 3:1105–1113, 1990.

67. Karalus NC, Cursons RT, Leng RA, et al: Community acquired pneumonia: Aetiology and prognostic index evaluation. Thorax 46:413–418, 1991.

67a. Almirall J, Morato I, Riera F, et al: Incidence of community-acquired pneumonia and *Chlamydia pneumoniae* infection: A prospective multicentre study. Eur Resp J 6:14–18, 1993.

68. Foy HM, Grayston JT, Kenny GE, et al: Epidemiology of *Mycoplasma pneumoniae* infection in families. JAMA 197:859–867, 1966.

69. Balassanian N, Robbins FC: *Mycoplasma pneumoniae* infection in families. N Engl J Med 277:719–725, 1967.

70. Evatt BL, Dowdle WR, Johnson M Jr, et al: Epidemic mycoplasma pneumonia. N Engl J Med 285:374–378, 1971.

71. Sande MA, Gadot F, Wenzel RP: Point source epidemic of *Mycoplasma pneumoniae* infection in a prosthodontics laboratory. Am Rev Respir Dis 112:213–217, 1975.

72. Broome CV, LaVentrue M, Kaye HS, et al: An explosive outbreak of *Mycoplasma pneumoniae* infection in a summer camp. Pediatrics 66:884–888, 1980.

73. Li D, Daling JR, Wang SP, et al: Evidence that *Chlamydia pneumoniae,* strain TWAR, is not sexually transmitted. J Infect Dis 160:328–331, 1989.

74. Kleemola M, Saikku P, Visakorpi R, et al: Epidemics of pneumonia caused by TWAR, a new *Chlamydia* organism, in military trainees in Finland. J Infect Dis 157:230–236, 1988.

75. Wang SP, Grayston JT: Population prevalence antibody to *Chlamydia pneumoniae,* strain TWAR. *In* Bowie WR, Caldwell HD, Jones RP, et al (eds): Chlamydial Infections: Proceedings of the Seventh International Symposium on Human Chlamydial Infections. New York, Cambridge University Press, 1990:402–405.

76. Aldous MB, Wang SP, Foy HM, et al: *Chlamydia pneumoniae,* strain TWAR, infection in Seattle children and their families, 1965–1979. *In* Bowie WR, Caldwell HD, Jones RP, et al (eds): Chlamydial Infections: Proceedings of the Seventh International Symposium on Human Chlamydial Infections. New York, Cambridge University Press, 1990:437–440.

76a. Ekman M-J, Grayston JT, Visakorpi R, et al: An epidemic of infections due to *Chlamydia pneumoniae* in military conscripts. Clin Infect Dis 17:420–425, 1993.

76b. Grayston JT: Infections caused by *Chlamydia pneumoniae* strain TWAR. Clin Infect Dis 15:757–763, 1992.

77. Williams LP: Review of the epidemiology of chlamydiosis in the United States. J Am Vet Med Assoc 195:1518–1521, 1989.

78. Centers for Disease Control: Summary of notifiable diseases, United States, 1989. MMWR 38:53–55, 1990.

79. Schaffner W: *Chlamydia psittaci* (psittacosis). *In* Mandell GL, Douglas RG Jr, Bennett JE: Principles and Practice of Infectious Diseases. New York, Churchill Livingstone, 1990:1440–1443.

80. Hedberg K, White KE, Forfang JC, et al: An outbreak of psittacosis in Minnesota turkey industry workers: Implications for modes of transmission and control. Am J Epidemiol 130:569–577, 1989.

81. Potter ME, Kaufmann AK, Plikaytis BD: Psittacosis in the United States, 1979. CDC Surveillance Summaries. MMWR 32(suppl 1SS):27SS–31SS, 1983.

82. MacFarlane JT, Macrae AD: Psittacosis. Br Med Bull 39:163–167, 1983.

83. Meyer KF: The ecology of psittacosis and ornithosis. Medicine (Baltimore) 21:175–206, 1942.

84. Crosse BA: Psittacosis: A clinical review. J Infect 21:251–259, 1990.

85. Yung AP, Grayson ML: Psittacosis—a review of 135 cases. Med J Aust 148:228–233, 1988.

86. Cassell GH: *Mycoplasma pneumoniae.* Infect Med 8 (suppl A):23–28, 1991.

87. Marrie TJ: Q fever pneumonia. Med Grand Rounds 3:354–365, 1985.

88. Spelman DW: Q fever: A study of 111 consecutive cases. Med J Aust 1:547–553, 1982.

89. Sawyer LA, Fishbein DB, McDade JE: Q fever: Current concepts. Rev Infect Dis 9:935–946, 1991.

90. Cameron DC, Borthwick RN, Philip T: The radiographic patterns of acute mycoplasma pneumonitis. Clin Radiol 28:173–180, 1977.

91. Cockcroft DW, Stilwell GA: Lobar pneumonia caused by *Mycoplasma pneumoniae.* Can Med Assoc J 124:1463–1468, 1981.

92. Strutman HR, Rettig PJ, Reyes S: *Chlamydia trachomatis* as a cause of pneumonitis and pleural effusion. J Pediatr 104:588–591, 1984.

93. Edelman RR, Hann LE, Simon M: *Chlamydia trachomatis* pneumonia in adults: Radiographic appearance. Radiology 152:279–282, 1984.

94. Dietrich PA, Johnson RD, Fairbank JT, et al: The chest radiograph in legionnaires' disease. Radiology 127:577–582, 1978.

95. Gordon JD, McKeen AD, Marrie TJ, et al: The radiographic features of epidemic and sporadic Q fever pneumonia. Can Assoc Radiol J 35:293–296, 1984.

96. Fine NL, Smith LR, Sheedy PF: Frequency of pleural effusions in *Mycoplasma* and viral pneumonias. N Engl J Med 283:790–793, 1970.

97. Demos TC, Studlo JD, Puczynski M: *Mycoplasma* pneumonia: Presentation as a mediastinal mass. Am J Radiol 143:981–982, 1984.

98. Kaufman JM, Cuvelier CA, van der Straeten M: Mycoplasma pneumonia with fulminant evolution into diffuse interstitial fibrosis. Thorax 35:140–144, 1980.

99. Augenbraun MH, Roblin PM, Mandel LJ, et al: *Chlamydia pneumoniae* pneumonia with pleural effusion: Diagnosis by culture. Am J Med 91:437–438, 1991.

100. Kroboth FJ, Yu VL, Reddy SC, et al: Clinicoradiographic correlation with the extent of Legionnaire's disease. Am J Roentgenol 141:263–268, 1983.

101. Janower ML, Weiss EB: Mycoplasmal, viral and rickettsial pneumonias. Semin Roentgenol 15:25–34, 1980.

102. Kirtland SH, Winterbauer RH: Slowly resolving, chronic, and recurrent pneumonia. Clin Chest Med 12:303–318, 1991.

103. Jay SJ, Johanson WJ, Pierce AK: The radiographic resolution of *Streptococcus pneumoniae* pneumonia. N Engl J Med 293:798–801, 1975.

104. MacFarlane JT, Miller AC, Smith WH, et al: Comparative radiographic features of community-acquired legionnaires' disease, pneumococcal pneumonia, mycoplasma pneumonia, and psittacosis. Thorax 39:28–33, 1984.

105. Van Metre T Jr: Pneumococcal pneumonia treated with antibiotics: The prognostic significance of certain clinical findings. N Engl J Med 251:1048–1052, 1954.

106. Fairbank JT, Mamourian AC, Dietrich PA, et al: The chest radiograph in legionnaires' disease. Radiology 147:33–34, 1983.

107. Finnegan OL, Fowkes SJ, White RJ: Radiographic appearances of *Mycoplasma* pneumonia. Thorax 36:469–472, 1981.

108. Stenstrom JR, Jansson E, Wager O: Ornithosis pneumonia with special reference to roentgenological lung findings. Acta Med Scand 171:349–356, 1962.

109. Yu VL: *Legionella pneumophila* and related species. Infect Med 8(suppl A):29–35, 1991.

110. Couch RB: *Mycoplasma pneumoniae* (primary atypical pneumonia). *In* Mandell GL, Douglas RG Jr, Bennett JE (eds): Principles and Practice of Infectious Diseases. New York, Churchill Livingstone, 1990:1446–1458.

111. Bates JH: *Chlamydia pneumoniae.* Infect Med 8 (suppl A):18–22, 1991.

112. Shulman ST, Bartlett J, Clyde WA Jr, et al: The unusual severity of mycoplasmal pneumonia in children with sickle-cell disease. N Engl J Med 287:164–167, 1972.

113. Westerberg SC, Smith CB, Renzetti AD: *Mycoplasma* infections in patients with chronic obstructive pulmonary disease. J Infect Dis 127:491–497, 1973.

114. Smith CB, Golden CA, Kanner RE, et al: Association of viral and *Mycoplasma pneumoniae* infections with acute respiratory illness in patients with chronic obstructive pulmonary diseases. Am Rev Respir Dis 121:225–232, 1980.

115. Hofflin JM, Potasman T, Baldwin JC, et al: Infectious complications in heart transplant recipients receiving cyclosporine and corticosteroids. Ann Intern Med 106:209–216, 1987.

116. Kugler JW, Armitage JO, Helms CM, et al: Nosocomial legionnaires' disease. Occurrence in recipients of bone marrow transplants. Am J Med 74:281–288, 1983.

117. Fuller J, Levinson MM, Kline JR, et al: Legionnaires' disease after heart transplantation. Ann Thorac Surg 39:308–311, 1985.

118. Witt DJ, Craven DE, McCabe WR: Bacterial infections in adult patients with the acquired immune deficiency syndrome (AIDS) and AIDS-related complex. Am J Med 82:900–906, 1987.

119. Ali NJ, Sillis M, Andrews BE, et al: The clinical spectrum and diagnosis of *Mycoplasma pneumoniae* infection. Q J Med 58:241–251, 1986.

120. Koletsky RJ, Weinstein AJ: Fulminant *Mycoplasma pneumoniae* infection. Report of a fatal case, and a review of the literature. Am Rev Respir Dis 122:491–496, 1980.

121. Tablan OC, Reyes MP: Chronic interstitial pulmonary fibrosis following *Mycoplasma pneumoniae* pneumonia. Am J Med 79:268–270, 1985.

122. Groenhagen-Riska C, Saikku P, Riska H, et al: Antibodies to TWAR—a novel type of chlamydia—in sarcoidosis. *In* Grassi C, Rizzato G, Pozzi E (eds): Sarcoidosis and other Granulomatous Disorders. Amsterdam, Elsevier Science Publishers, 1988:297–301.

123. Hahn DL, Dodge RW, Golubjatnikov R: Association of *Chlamydia pneumoniae* (strain TWAR) infection with wheezing, asthmatic bronchitis, and adult-onset asthma. JAMA 266:225–230, 1991.

124. Lascari AD, Garfunkel JM, Mauro DG: Varicella-like rash associated with *Mycoplasma* infection. Am J Dis Child 128:254–255, 1974.

125. Teisch JA, Shapiro L, Walzer RA: Vesiculopustular eruption with *Mycoplasma* infection. JAMA 211:1694–1696, 1970.

126. Cherry JD, Hurwitz ES, Welliver RC: *Mycoplasma pneumoniae* infections and exanthems. J Pediatr 87:369–373, 1975.

127. Kalb RE, Grossman ME, Neu HC: Stevens-Johnson syndrome due

to *Mycoplasma pneumoniae* in an adult. Am J Med 79:541–544, 1985.

128. Stutman HR: Stevens-Johnson syndrome and *Mycoplasma pneumoniae:* Evidence for cutaneous infection. J Pediatr 111:845–847, 1987.

129. Lyell A, Gordon AM, Dick HM, et al: Mycoplasmas and erythema multiforme. Lancet 2:1116–1118, 1967.

130. Lyell A, Gordon AM, Dick HM, et al: The role of *Mycoplasma pneumoniae* infection in erythema multiforme. Proc R Soc Med 61:1330–1331, 1968.

131. Sands MG, Satz JE, Turner WE, et al: Pericarditis and perimyocarditis associated with active *Mycoplasma pneumoniae* infection. Ann Intern Med 86:544–548, 1977.

132. Sands MJ, Rosenthal R: Progressive heart failure and death associated with *Mycoplasma pneumoniae* pneumonia. Chest 81:763–765, 1982.

133. Ponka A: Carditis associated with *Mycoplasma pneumoniae* infection. Acta Med Scand 206:77–86, 1979.

134. Grayston JT: *Chlamydiae pneumoniae,* strain TWAR. Chest 64–669, 1989.

135. Dymock JW, Larson JM, MacLennan WJ, et al: Myocarditis associated with psittacosis. Br J Clin Pract 25:240–242, 1971.

136. Devriendt J, Staroukine M, Schils E, et al: Legionellosis and "torsades de pointes." Acta Cardiol 45:329–333, 1990.

137. Jariwalla AG, Davies BH, White J: Infective endocarditis complicating psittacosis: Response to rifampin. Br Med J 280:155, 1980.

138. Jones RB, Priest JB, Kuo C: Subacute chlamydial endocarditis. JAMA 247:655–658, 1982.

139. Tompkins LS, Roessler BJ, Redd SC, et al: *Legionella* prosthetic-valve endocarditis. N Engl J Med 18:530–535, 1988.

140. Grist NR: Q fever endocarditis. Am Heart J 75:846–849, 1968.

141. Tobin MJ, Cahill N, Gearty G, et al: Q fever endocarditis. Am J Med 72:396–400, 1982.

142. Kimbrough RC II, Ormsbee RA, Peacock M: Q fever endocarditis in the United States. Ann Intern Med 91:400–402, 1979.

143. Applefeld MM, Bellingsley LN, Tucker HG, et al: Q fever endocarditis: A case occurring in the United States. Am Heart J 93:669–670, 1977.

144. Raoult D, Etienne J, Massip P, et al: Q fever endocarditis in the south of France. J Infect Dis 155:570–573, 1987.

145. Marrie TJ, Harczy M, Mann OE, et al: Culture-negative endocarditis probably due to *Chlamydia pneumoniae.* J Infect Dis 161:127–129, 1990.

146. Saikku P, Leinonen M, Mattila K, et al: Serological evidence of an association of a novel chlamydia, TWAR, with chronic coronary heart disease and acute myocardial infarction. Lancet 2:983–986, 1988.

146a. Kuo C-C, Shor A, Campbell LA, et al: Demonstration of *Chlamydia pneumoniae* in atherosclerotic lesions of coronary arteries. J Infect Dis 167:841–849, 1993.

147. Bayer AS, Galpin JE, Theofilopoulos AN, et al: Neurologic disease associated with *Mycoplasma pneumoniae* pneumonitis. Demonstration of viable *Mycoplasma pneumoniae* in cerebrospinal fluid and blood by radioisotopic and immunofluorescent tissue culture techniques. Ann Intern Med 94:15–20, 1981.

148. Dorff B, Lind K: Two fatal cases of meningoencephalitis associated with *Mycoplasma pneumoniae* infection. Scand J Infect Dis 8:49–51, 1976.

149. Murray H, Tuazon C: Atypical pneumonias. Med Clin North Am 64:507–527, 1980.

150. Murray HW, Masur H, Senterfit LB, et al: The protean manifestations of *Mycoplasma pneumoniae* infection in adults. Am J Med 58:229–242, 1975.

151. Harrell GT: Rickettsial involvement of the central nervous system. Med Clin North Am 37:395–422, 1953.

152. Gomez-Aranda R, Diaz JKP, Acebol MR, et al: Computed tomographic brain scan findings in Q fever encephalitis. Neuroradiology 26:329–332, 1984.

153. Turtzo DF, Ghatak PK: Acute hemolytic anemia with *Mycoplasma pneumoniae* pneumonia. JAMA 236:1140–1141, 1976.

154. Feizi T: Cold agglutinins, the direct Coombs' test and serum immunoglobulins in *Mycoplasma pneumoniae* infection. Ann N Y Acad Sci 143:801–812, 1967.

155. Cardellach F, Font J, Agusti AGN, et al: Q fever and hemolytic anemia. J Infect Dis 148:769, 1983.

156. Kenny GE, Kaiser GG, Cooney MK, et al: Diagnosis of *Mycoplasma pneumoniae* pneumonia: Sensitivities and specificities of serology

with lipid antigen and isolation of the organism on soy peptone medium for identification of infections. J Clin Microbiol 28:2087–2093, 1990.

157. Tully JG, Rose DL, Whitcomb RF, et al: Enhanced isolation of *Mycoplasma pneumoniae* from throat washings with a newly modified culture medium. J Infect Dis 139:478–482, 1979.

158. Senterfit LB: Laboratory diagnosis of *Mycoplasma* infections. Isr J Med Sci 20:905–907, 1984.

159. Craven RB, Wenzel RP, Calhoun AM, et al: Comparison of the sensitivity of two methods for isolation of *Mycoplasma pneumoniae.* J Clin Microbiol 4:225–226, 1976.

160. Clyde WA Jr, Senterfit LB: Laboratory diagnosis of mycoplasma infections. *In* Razin S, Barile MF (eds): The Mycoplasma IV: Mycoplasma Toxicity. San Diego, Academic Press, 1985:391–402.

161. Lind K, Lindhardt BO, Schutten HJ, et al: Serological cross-reactions between *Mycoplasma genitalium* and *Mycoplasma pneumoniae.* J Clin Microbiol 20:1036–1043, 1984.

162. Baseman JB, Dallo SF, Tully JG, et al: Isolation and characterization of *Mycoplasma genitalium* strains from the human respiratory tract. J Clin Microbiol 26:2266–2269, 1988.

163. Kohler RB: Antigen detection for the rapid diagnosis of *Mycoplasma* and *Legionella* pneumonia. Diagn Microbiol Infect Dis 4:47S–59S, 1986.

164. Kok TW, Varkanis G, Marmion BP, et al: Laboratory diagnosis of *Mycoplasma pneumoniae* infection. 1. Direct detection of antigen in respiratory exudates by enzyme immunoassay. Epidemiol Infect 101:669–684, 1988.

165. Harris R, Marmion BP, Varkanis G, et al: Laboratory diagnosis of *Mycoplasma pneumoniae* infection. 2. Comparison of methods for the direct detection of specific antigen or nucleic acid sequences in respiratory exudates. Epidemiol Infect 101:685–694, 1988.

166. Hers JF, Masurel N: Infection with *Mycoplasma pneumoniae* in civilians in the Netherlands. Ann N Y Acad Sci 143:447–460, 1967.

167. Hirai Y, Shiode J, Masayoshi T, et al: Application of an indirect immunofluorescence test for detection of *Mycoplasma pneumoniae* in respiratory exudates. J Clin Microbiol 29:2007–2012, 1991.

168. Dular R, Kajioka R, Kasatiya S: Comparison of Gen-Probe commercial kit and culture technique for the diagnosis of *Mycoplasma pneumoniae* infection. J Clin Microbiol 26:1068–1069, 1988.

169. Tilton RC, Dias F, Kidd H, et al: DNA probe versus culture for detection of *Mycoplasma pneumoniae* in clinical specimens. Diagn Microbiol Infect Dis 10:109–112, 1988.

170. Hata D, Kuze F, Mochizuki Y, et al: Evaluation of DNA probe test for rapid diagnosis of *Mycoplasma pneumoniae* infections. J Pediatr 116:273–276, 1990.

171. Kleemola SRM, Karjalainen JE, Raty RKH: Rapid diagnosis of *Mycoplasma pneumoniae* infection: Clinical evaluation of a commercial probe test. J Infect Dis 162:70–75, 1990.

172. Bernet C, Garret M, DeBarbeyrac B, et al: Detection of *Mycoplasma pneumoniae* by using the polymerase chain reaction. J Clin Microbiol 27:2492–2496, 1989.

173. DeMatteis M, Quillard M, Lamotte F, et al: Rapid diagnosis of *Mycoplasma pneumoniae* infection: Evaluation of the polymerase chain reaction (PCR). *In* Program and Abstracts of the 31st Interscience Conference on Antimicrobial Agents and Chemotherapy, September 29–October 2, 1991, Chicago. [Abstract 1084] Washington, DC: American Society for Microbiology, 1991:279.

173a. Luneberg E, Jensen JS, Frosch M: Detection of *Mycoplasma pneumoniae* by polymerase chain reaction and nonradioactive hybridization in microtiter plates. J Clin Microbiol 31:1088–1094, 1993.

174. Griffin JP: Rapid screening for cold agglutinins in pneumonia. Ann Intern Med 70:701–705, 1969.

175. Griffin JP, Crawford YE: *Mycoplasma pneumoniae* in primary atypical pneumonia. JAMA 193:1011–1016, 1965.

176. King JW, May JS: Cold agglutinin disease in a patient with legionnaires' disease. Arch Intern Med 140:1537–1539, 1980.

177. Sussman SJ, Magoffin RL, Lennette EH, et al: Cold agglutinins, Eaton agent, and respiratory infections of children. Pediatrics 38:571–577, 1966.

178. Timmerman R, Bieger R: Haemolytic anemia due to cold agglutinins caused by psittacosis. Neth J Med 34:306–309, 1989.

179. Ponka A: The occurrence and clinical picture of serologically verified *Mycoplasma pneumoniae* infections with emphasis on central nervous system, cardiac and joint manifestations. Ann Clin Res 11(suppl 24):1–60, 1979.

180. Kleemola M, Kayhty H: Increase in titers of antibodies to *Myco-*

*plasma pneumoniae* in patients with purulent meningitis. J Infect Dis 146:284–288, 1982.

181. Brunner H, Horswood RL, Chanock RM: More sensitive methods for detection of antibody to *Mycoplasma pneumoniae*. J Infect Dis 127(suppl):S52–S55, 1973.

182. Carter JB, Carter SL: Acute-phase, indirect fluorescent antibody procedure for diagnosis of *Mycoplasma pneumoniae* infection. Ann Clin Lab Sci 13:150–155, 1983.

183. Rousseau SA, Tettmar RE: The serological diagnosis of *Mycoplasma pneumoniae* infection: A comparison of complement fixation, haemagglutination and immunofluorescence. J Hyg Camb 95:345–352, 1985.

184. Hossain A, Bakir TMF, Ramia S: Serological diagnosis of *Mycoplasma pneumoniae* infections. Trop Geogr Med 37:250–257, 1985.

185. Kok TW, Marmion BP, Varkanis G, et al: Laboratory diagnosis of *Mycoplasma pneumoniae* infection. 3. Detection of IgM antibodies to *M. pneumoniae* by a modified indirect haemagglutination test. Epidemiol Infect 103:613–623, 1989.

186. Hirschberg L, Krook A, Pettersson CA, et al: Enzyme-linked immunosorbent assay for detection of *Mycoplasma pneumoniae* specific immunoglobulin M. Eur J Clin Microbiol Infect Dis 7:420–423, 1988.

187. Lee SH, Charoenying S, Brennan T, et al: Comparative studies of three serologic methods for the measurement of *Mycoplasma pneumoniae* antibodies. Am J Clin Pathol 92:342–347, 1989.

188. Wreghitt TG, Sillis M: An investigation of the *Mycoplasma pneumoniae* infections in Cambridge in 1983 using mu-capture enzyme-linked immunosorbent assay (ELISA), indirect immunofluorescence (IF) and complement fixation (CF) tests. Isr J Med Sci 23:704–708, 1987.

189. Moule JH, Caul EO, Wreghitt TG: The specific IgM response to *Mycoplasma pneumoniae* infection: Interpretation and application to early diagnosis. Epidemiol Infect 99:685–692, 1987.

190. Vikefors T, Brodin G, Grandien M, et al: Detection of specific IgM antibodies for the diagnosis of *Mycoplasma pneumoniae* infections: A clinical evaluation. Scand J Infect Dis 20:601–610, 1988.

191. Echevarria JM, Leon P, Balfagon, et al: Diagnosis of *Mycoplasma pneumoniae* infection by microparticle agglutination and antibody-capture enzyme-immunoassay. Eur J Clin Microbiol Dis 9:217–220, 1990.

192. Sasaki T, Bonissol C, Stoiljkovic B, et al: Demonstration of cross-reactive antibodies to mycoplasmas in human sera by ELISA and immunoblotting. Microbiol Immunol 31:639–648, 1987.

193. Jacobs E, Fuchte K, Bredt W: A 168-kilodalton protein of *Mycoplasma pneumoniae* used as antigen in a dot enzyme-linked immunosorbent assay. Eur J Clin Microbiol 5:435–440, 1986.

194. Jacobs E, Buchholz A, Kleinmann B, et al: Use of adherence protein of *Mycoplasma pneumoniae* as antigen for enzyme-linked immunosorbent assay (ELISA). Isr J Med Sci 23:709–712, 1987.

195. Hirschberg L, Holme T, Krook A: Human antibody response to the major adhesin of *Mycoplasma pneumoniae*: Increase in titers against synthetic peptides in patients with pneumonia. APMIS 99:515–520, 1991.

196. Morrison-Plummer J, Lazzell A, Baseman JB: Shared epitopes between *Mycoplasma pneumoniae* major adhesin protein P1 and a 140-kilodalton protein of *Mycoplasma genitalium*. Infect Immun 55:49–56, 1987.

197. Chirgwin K, Roblin PM, Gelling M, et al: Infection with *Chlamydia pneumoniae* in Brooklyn. J Infect Dis 163:757–761, 1991.

198. Campbell JF, Barnes RC, Kozarsky PE, et al: Culture-confirmed pneumonia due to *Chlamydia pneumoniae*. J Infect Dis 164:411–413, 1991.

199. Hammerschlag MR, Chirgwin K, Roblin PM, et al: Persistent infection with *Chlamydia pneumoniae* following acute respiratory illness. Clin Infect Dis 14:178–182, 1992.

200. Barnes RC: Laboratory diagnosis of human chlamydial infections. Clin Microbiol Rev 2:119–136, 1989.

201. Cles LD, Stamm WE: Use of HL cells for improved isolation and passage of *Chlamydia pneumoniae*. J Clin Microbiol 28:938–940, 1990.

202. Kuo CC, Grayston JT: Amino acid requirements for growth of *Chlamydia pneumoniae* in cell cultures: Growth enhancement by lysine or methionine depletion. J Clin Microbiol 28:1098–1100, 1990.

203. Kuo CC, Grayston JT: A sensitive cell line, HL cells, for isolation and propagation of *Chlamydia pneumoniae* strain TWAR. J Infect Dis 162:755–758, 1990.

204. Wang SP, Grayston JT: Microimmunofluorescence serological studies with the TWAR organism. *In* Oriel D, Ridgway G, Schachter J, et al (eds): Chlamydial Infections: Proceedings of the Sixth International Symposium on Human Chlamydial Infections. Cambridge, Cambridge University Press, 1986:329–332.

205. Wang SP, Grayston JT: *Chlamydia pneumoniae* elementary body antigenic reactivity with fluorescent antibody is destroyed by methanol. J Clin Microbiol 29:1539–1541, 1991.

206. Sillis M, White P: Rapid identification of *Chlamydia psittaci* and TWAR *(C. pneumoniae)* in sputum samples using an amplified enzyme immunoassay. J Clin Pathol 43:260, 1990.

207. Sillis M, White PMB: Rapid diagnosis of psittacosis. Lancet 335:726, 1990.

208. Holland SM, Gaydos CA, Quinn TC: Detection and differentiation of *Chlamydia trachomatis, Chlamydia psittaci*, and *Chlamydia pneumoniae* by DNA amplification. J Infect Dis 162:984–987, 1990.

209. Campbell LA, Melgosa MP, Hamilton DJ, et al: Detection of *Chlamydia pneumoniae* by polymerase chain reaction. J Clin Microbiol 30:434–439, 1992.

209a. Tong CYW, Sillis M: Detection of *Chlamydia pneumoniae* and *Chlamydia psittaci* in sputum samples by PCR. J Clin Pathol 46:313–317, 1993.

210. Black CM, Johnson JE, Farshy CE, et al: Antigenic variation among strains of *Chlamydia pneumoniae*. J Clin Microbiol 29:1312–1316, 1991.

211. Campbell LA, Kuo CC, Wang SP, et al: Serological response to *Chlamydia pneumoniae* infection. J Clin Microbiol 28:1261–1264, 1990.

212. Ladany S, Black CM, Farshy CE, et al: Enzyme immunoassay to determine exposure to *Chlamydia pneumoniae* (strain TWAR). J Clin Microbiol 27:2778–2783, 1989.

213. Isaacs D: Psittacosis. Br Med J 289:510–511, 1984.

214. Riordan T, Lewin I, Oliver MY: Rapid diagnosis of psittacosis. Lancet 335:471, 1990.

215. Kaltenboeck B, Kousoulas KG, Storz J: Detection and strain differentiation of *Chlamydia psittaci* by a two-step polymerase chain reaction. J Clin Microbiol 29:1969–1975, 1991.

215a. Oldach DW, Gaydos CA, Mundy LM, et al: Rapid diagnosis of *Chlamydia psittaci* pneumonia. Clin Infect Dis 17:338–343, 1993.

216. Jao RL, Finland M: Susceptibility of *Mycoplasma pneumoniae* to 21 antibiotics in vitro. Am J Med Sci 253:639–650, 1967.

217. Niitu Y, Kubota H, Hasegawa S, et al: Susceptibility of *Mycoplasma pneumoniae* to antibiotics in vitro. Jpn J Microbiol 18:149–155, 1974.

218. Rettig PJ, Rollerson WJ, Marks MI: In vitro activity of six fluoroquinolones against *C. trachomatis. In* Oriel JD, Ridgway G, Schachter J, et al (eds): Chlamydial Infections: Proceeding of the Sixth International Symposium on Human Chlamydial Infections. Cambridge, England, Cambridge University Press, 1986:528–531.

219. Chirgwin K, Roblin PM, Hammerschlag MR: In vitro susceptibilities of *Chlamydia pneumoniae* (*Chlamydia* sp. strain TWAR). Antimicrob Agents Chemother 33:1634–1635, 1989.

220. Cooper MA, Baldwin D, Matthews RS, et al: In-vitro susceptibility of *Chlamydia pneumoniae* (TWAR) to seven antibiotics. J Antimicrob Chemother 28:407–413, 1991.

221. Kuo CC, Grayston JT: In vitro drug susceptibility of *Chlamydia* sp. strain TWAR. Antimicrob Agents Chemother 32:257–258, 1988.

222. Hooper TL, Gould FK, Swinburn CR, et al: Ciprofloxacin: A preferred treatment for *Legionella* infections in patients receiving cyclosporin A. J Antimicrob Chemother 22:952–953, 1988.

223. Unertl KE, Lenhart FP, Forst H, et al: Brief report: Ciprofloxacin in the treatment of legionellosis in critically ill patients including those cases unresponsive to erythromycin. Am J Med 87(suppl 5A):128S–131S, 1989.

224. Barry AL, Jones RN, Thornsberry C: In vitro activities of azithromycin (CP 62,993), clarithromycin (A-56268; TE-031), erythromycin, roxithromycin, and clindamycin. Antimicrob Agents Chemother 32:752–754, 1988.

225. Edelstein PH, Edelstein MAC: In vitro activity of azithromycin against clinical isolates of *Legionella* species. Antimicrob Agents Chemother 35:180–181, 1991.

226. Mardh PA, Lowing C: Treatment of chlamydial infections. Scand J Infect Dis 68(suppl):23–30, 1990.

227. Orfila J, Haider F, Thomas D: Activity of spiramycin against *Chlamydia*, in vitro and in vivo. J Antimicrob Chemother 22(suppl B):73–76, 1988.

228. Pechere JC, Auckenthaler R: In vitro activity of roxithromycin against respiratory and skin pathogens. J Antimicrob Chemother 20(suppl B):1–5, 1987.

229. Shames JM, George RB, Holliday WB, et al: Comparison of antibiotics in the treatment of mycoplasmal pneumonia. Arch Intern Med 125:680–684, 1970.

230. Sabato AR, Martin AJ, Marmion BP, et al: Acute illness, antibiotics and subsequent pulmonary function. Arch Dis Child 59:1034–1037, 1984.

231. Axelrod J, Meyers BR, Hirschman SZ: 7-Chlorolincomycin therapy of pulmonary infections due to *Mycoplasma pneumoniae.* Antimicrob Agents Chemother 2:499–501, 1972.

232. Smith CB, Friedewald WT, Chanock RM: Shedding of *Mycoplasma pneumoniae* after tetracycline and erythromycin therapy. N Engl J Med 276:1172–1175, 1967.

233. Ford MJ, Brunton WAT, Millar J, et al: Mycoplasma pneumonia: Failure of erythromycin therapy. Scott Med J 25:126–128, 1980.

234. Ball AP: Therapeutic considerations for the management of respiratory tract infections. The role of new macrolides and fluoroquinolones. Infect Med 8(suppl A):7–17, 1991.

235. O'Neill SJ, Millar ED, Coles SJ, et al: Safety and efficacy of clarithromycin in the treatment of acute mild to moderate respiratory tract infections. Ir Med J 84:33–35, 1991.

236. Schonwald S, Skerk V, Petricevic I, et al: Comparison of three-day and five-day courses of azithromycin in the treatment of atypical pneumonia. Eur J Clin Microbiol Infect Dis 10:877–880, 1991.

237. Peterslund NA, Hanninen P, Schreiner A, et al: Roxithromycin in the treatment of pneumonia. J Antimicrob Chemother 23:737–741, 1989.

238. Fernandez-MacLoughlin GJ, Lanoel JL, Stamboulian D, et al: Roxithromycin in the treatment of atypical pneumonia. Br J Clin Pract 42:(suppl 55):92–93, 1987.

239. Chien S-M, Pichotta P, Siepman N, et al: Treatment of community-acquired pneumonia: A multicenter, double-blind, randomized study comparing clarithromycin with erythromycin. Chest 103:697–701, 1993.

# Anaerobic Pleuropulmonary Infections: Aspiration, Pneumonia, Abscess, and Empyema

JEFFREY K. GRIFFITHS and DAVID R. SNYDMAN

Anaerobic lung infections have been recognized by physicians since the time of Hippocrates. Despite the advances in medical therapy and technology of the last three decades, anaerobic bacteria are common pathogens of the lower respiratory tract, and they remain an important clinical entity.

Four classic entities are recognized in anaerobic pleuropulmonary infections: aspiration pneumonia, necrotizing pneumonia, lung abscess, and empyema. Most result from the aspiration of oropharyngeal contents into the lung. There is strong and persuasive evidence that transfer of the oral flora into the lung during aspiration often leads to pneumonia caused by anaerobic bacteria and then to abscess and empyema. Persons who develop these classic syndromes are usually those at risk for aspiration. The inoculum of anaerobic bacteria is often provided by the microflora of the mouth, particularly from the gingival crevices. These clinical entities may be thought of as a progression, with aspiration pneumonia the milieu from which abscess and empyema may develop as part of the natural history of untreated anaerobic pleuropulmonary infection.

Changes in clinical medicine have resulted in a shift in the spectrum of disease and in the microbiologic mixture seen in these frequently polymicrobial infections. Outpatient-acquired aspiration disease has a somewhat different flora than hospital-acquired aspiration syndrome, with anaerobic bacteria playing a major part in both settings. The pathophysiology of anaerobic aspiration pneumonia has served as a constructive model for understanding other

pneumonias in which soilage of the lung parenchyma through aspiration is a common mechanism.

Enough is now understood about these syndromes that empiric therapy is often warranted in typical presentations of community-acquired disease. In these circumstances, oral therapy alone usually yields a gratifying resolution of the illness. Confirmatory culture of the pathogens can be problematic, and in this chapter, we delineate some of the difficulties in diagnosis and in treatment. A significant minority of patients with anaerobic lung infections require surgical and medical treatment, and we describe the controversies in their management.

This group of infections remains a problematic entity despite the potency of modern antimicrobial therapy; in an era of immunosuppression, heroic preservation of life, and invasive technologies, new clinical syndromes involving anaerobic lung pathogens may emerge. Our goals in this chapter are to review what is known about anaerobic lung infections, to illustrate guiding principles of clinical practice using actual cases, attendant with their diagnostic pitfalls, and to point out directions for future study.

## HISTORY

Infections of the lung, including anaerobic infections such as anaerobic empyema, have been recognized since classic times. To quote the Hippocratic physicians on the treatment of pulmonary abscesses and empyema:

If as a result of treatment, the pus does not break through, one should not be surprised, for it often breaks into the body, and the patient seems to be better, because the pus has passed from a narrow space to a larger one. As time goes on, the fever becomes more severe, coughing begins, the side begins to pain, the patient cannot lie any more on the healthy side but only on the diseased side; the feet and eyes swell. When the fifteenth day after the rupture has appeared, prepare a warm bath, sit him upon a stool, which is not wobbly, someone should hold his hands, and then shake him by the shoulders and listen to where the noise is heard. And right at this place—preferably on the left—make an incision; then it produces death more rarely. . . . When empyemata are opened by the cautery or by the knife, and the pus flows pure and white, the patient survives, but if it is mixed with blood, muddy and foul smelling, he will die.[1]

Anaerobic bacteria were first identified in foul pleural fluid from empyemas in 1899 and 1904.[2, 3] Because of the similarities between the isolated bacteria and those previously isolated from the oropharynx, the investigators suggested that these infections were secondary to aspiration of oral flora into the lungs. They postulated that this aspiration and a pulmonic infection preceded the development of empyema. D.T. Smith, in the 1920s, was able to experimentally produce pneumonia and abscess of the lung in anesthetized animals through aspiration of "fusospirochetal" organisms. He demonstrated the need for a mixture of anaerobic oral flora to produce typical infections; pure cultures failed to cause pathology.[4–7] Moreover, a degree of anesthesia was necessary; intact clearance mechanisms prevented the successful induction of infection.

We now understand more about the organisms, the pathology, and the epidemiology of these often anaerobic pleuropulmonary infections, but the central concepts have stood the test of time. Events in this process include aspiration, often in a patient with impaired conciousness; localized pneumonia; cavitation; and empyema formation. In 1934, King and Lord observed that 65% of the 210 patients they reviewed had had a tonsillectomy or surgery on the head and neck.[8] In those days, tonsillectomies were performed with the patient upright, the cuffed endotracheal tube had yet to be invented, and anaesthesiology was not yet a specialty. Although empyema may be caused by many organisms carried hematogenously from elsewhere in the body or through local extension of pneumonia into the pleural space, many cases arise because of infections that proceed through the steps outlined previously.

Another advance in the management of these infections was the concept of early drainage of an abscess. In the preantibiotic era of the 1930s, it was recognized that conservative medical management of lung abscess and empyema often failed, as did surgery in the chronic stage of the disease; in either case, the mortality rate was about 30%, with great morbidity among the survivors.[9] Neuhof and Touroff, in an heretical article on surgical therapy, argued for the early drainage of acute putrid abscesses, using a single-stage drainage procedure.[10] By 1945, they had treated 172 cases with a mortality rate of only 2.3%,[11] pointing out the great benefit that drainage alone could provide. This was a remarkable advance in the treatment of

acute lung abscesses. As pointed out by E.W. Wilkins, because of the current era of highly immunodeficient and chronic illnesses, drainage techniques such as this may have a resurgence in popularity,[12] because many patients are too ill to tolerate lobectomy as definitive extirpitive surgery if an abscess cannot be controlled by medical therapy alone.

With the advent of antibiotics, the mortality rate from empyema fell, and the focus shifted from surgical to medical treatment. From 1943 to 1956, the rate of admissions of patients with lung abscesses at the Massachusetts General Hospital fell from 10 to 11 per 10,000 admissions to 1 to 2, a tenfold decline.[13] Finland and Barnes[14] reviewed the transition from the preantibiotic era to the antibiotic era by reviewing cases from 12 selected years from 1935 to 1972. After the transition, the mortality rate fell, and there was a marked decline in the proportion of patients younger than 50 years of age. In this older population, death was common among those with other serious underlying diseases.

The bacteriologic facilities of the time did not allow identification of many anaerobic pathogens: *Streptococcus pneumoniae*, hemolytic streptococci, and *Staphylococcus aureus* were the most common isolates cultured from pleural fluid during 1935. *S. aureus* was the most common isolate cultured from 1955 to 1965, when it was replaced by aerobic gram-negative rods and enterococci. This latter microbiologic group, commonly seen in nosocomial infections and complicated surgical cases, was not seen in community-acquired cases, in which anaerobes were commonly found. In 1973, Weese and colleagues published a review of 122 cases of empyema occurring during four decades at the University of Iowa.[15] They also reported an initial drop in mortality during the immediate period after the introduction of antimicrobials, followed by a disturbing increase in mortality associated with increasing age, severity of underlying disease, polymicrobial infections, and infection with nosocomial gram-negative organisms. They saw a rise and then fall in the frequency of *S. aureus* as the major isolated pathogen, and they noticed the rarity of *S. pneumoniae* as an isolate from empyemas after the introduction of antimicrobials. They did not report on any anaerobic pathogens.

Research into the causes of anaerobic lung infections and empyema declined after the introduction of antimicrobials, despite the fact that the most common form of pulmonary abscess was a "nonspecific" infection with no identifiable aerobic organisms. Penicillin was clearly the drug of choice, although the reasons for its efficacy were unclear. A 1961 paper by Fifer and associates stated,

Culture of sputum frequently yields only ordinary flora which are not usually considered pathogenic, and it is not clearly understood why microorganisms of low virulence should cause an acute suppurative pneumonitis with liquefaction necrosis. The presence of other unidentified microorganisms has been proposed but not proved.[16]

In an extraordinarily fertile period of research in the early 1970s, it became clear that multiple anaerobic organisms were present in most empyema infections. Bartlett, Gorbach, Finegold, and coworkers published a series of articles defining the major role of anaerobes in empyema.[17–21] Their findings were confirmed by others,[22] and therapy for anaerobes in empyema has become part of standard medical and surgical practice.[23]

Another pattern of disease is recognized. As treatment for aspiration-related pulmonary infections has increasingly included excellent anaerobic therapy, the clinical spectrum of *evident* disease has shifted to the aged, the hospitalized, and the immunosuppressed, and complicating malignancy of the lung or other sites is common.[24] Isolated organisms from empyemas increasingly contain highly resistant gram-negative enteric organisms and yeast in addition to the "expected" anaerobes and *S. aureus*. The astute clinician must examine the patient, analyze the epidemiologic circumstances, and carefully gauge the ability of the patient to withstand surgical therapy if needed.

## EPIDEMIOLOGY AND RISK FACTORS

In the experience of Bartlett and others, only 10% to 15% of persons with anaerobic lung abscesses have no obvious predisposition to aspiration or periodontal disease.[25] These are the two most important factors in the development of anaerobic lung infections. Other routes of infection include hematogenous spread from another site, (eg, pelvic thrombophlebitis) or transdiaphragmatic spread from a subdiaphragmatic location, but these are rare. Other conditions thought to be risk factors for anaerobic lung disease include lung carcinomas, bronchiectasis, insulin-dependent diabetes mellitus, and pulmonary infarction. Chronic obstructive pulmonary disease and immunosuppression with steroids do not appear to be risk factors.[26]

### Aspiration

Although normal persons aspirate during sleep,[27, 28] there is no evidence this aspiration of alkaline saliva is of clinical importance. In contrast, some conditions increase the frequency, character, and volume of aspirated fluid until the normal defenses are overwhelmed.

Persons who have altered consciousness, dysphagia with esophageal dysfunction, gastroesophageal reflux, degenerative or acute neurologic diseases, or breaching of the usual structural defenses of the trachea are at risk of aspiration and of aspiration pneumonia (Table 28–1). An impaired gag or cough reflex can occur because of head trauma, a neurologic event such as a stroke, or drug or alcohol ingestion. Aspiration frequently occurs during seizures or during anesthesia.

The specifics of the risk of aspiration usually determine the "usual" patient seen at a particular institution. One typical patient is the alcoholic with poor dentition and gingivitis who aspirates during an alcohol-induced stupor or a bout of vomiting. In communities where alcoholism is common, this presentation is frequently seen. Another typical patient is one who has seizures and who aspirates during one of them. Another is a patient who has a difficult intubation during general anesthesia and who aspirates during the intubation before protection of the airway is secured. Before cuffed endotracheal tubes were available, tonsillectomies were done in the upright, awake patient; in one older

**Table 28–1. Risk Factors for Development of Anaerobic or Mixed Aerobic-Anaerobic Pleuropulmonary Infections**

**Aspiration**
Aspiration during episode of decreased consciousness
  Seizures
  Anesthesia
  Insulin-treated diabetes mellitus
  Drug ingestion (eg, alcohol, heroin, barbiturates)
  Cardiopulmonary arrest
  Metabolic encephalopathy
  Cerebrovascular accident
  Degenerative neurologic diseases (eg, Parkinson disease, multiple
    sclerosis) with a decreased cough reflex
Aspiration secondary to gastrointestinal dysfunction
  Vomiting
  Insulin-treated diabetes mellitus
  Esophageal dysfunction or obstruction
  Impaired emptying of the stomach
  Intestinal obstruction or dysfunction
Aspiration after disruption of usual mechanical barriers
  Endotracheal intubation
  Nasogastric or orogastric tubes
  Tracheostomy
  Incompetence of the glottic structures because of associated diseases
    (eg, malignancy, neurologic paralysis)
**Bacterial Inoculum**
Periodontal disease, with increased numbers of anaerobic organisms
Colonization of the oropharynx, esophagus, or stomach with synergistic
  aerobic organisms (eg, enteric gram-negative rods, *Staphylococcus*
  *aureus*)
**Obstruction**
Bronchogenic carcinoma; rarely, foreign bodies, pulmonary
  malformations

series, 65% of lung abscesses were seen in patients who had had a tonsillectomy or surgery on the head or neck.[29]

An impaired gag reflex or cough reflex may be seen in those after a neurologic event such as a stroke or trauma and in those with a degenerative disorder such as multiple sclerosis or Parkinson disease. It is common for neurologically affected patients to have frequent pneumonias, many of which are anaerobic; pneumonia is a common final illness for many of them.

### Periodontal Disease

The second major predisposing factor in the development of anaerobic lung infections is periodontal disease. In the gingival crevice, between the tooth and the gum tissue, an anaerobic environment prevails that is similar to that of the colon. As in the colon, the flora is overwhelmingly anaerobic, and the density of organisms attains astounding levels, as high as $10^{12}$ per gram of tissue.[30, 31] Normal saliva from a healthy mouth contains about $10^8$ anaerobes per milliliter, but saliva from one with gingivitis may have $10^{11}$/mL.[32] In patients with periodontal disease, far greater numbers of anaerobic bacteria are present in the oropharynx than in people without periodontal illness. This inoculum effect explains the increased chance of infection with anaerobes if aspiration occurs. In the preantibiotic era, the frequent association of lung abscess with infections of the gum, teeth, and tonsils was often recorded.[13]

Periodontal disease is so common in those with anaerobic infections of the lung that a necrotizing pneumonia (ie, gangrene of the lung, usually anaerobic) in the edentulous patient should suggest another predisposing factor, such as the endobronchial obstruction caused by a bronchogenic carcinoma. The old saying that "lung abscess does not occur in the edentulous person" is not true, but in those with periodontal disease, there is a clear increase in the relative risk of anaerobic lung infections. In a study from Honolulu by Pohlson and associates,[24] 15 of 89 patients had lung malignancies, and in Finegold and Bartlett's study from Los Angeles, 7 of 100 had bronchogenic carcinomas.[33] Similarly, obstruction of the bronchial tree by congenital anomaly or by the growth of an endobronchial lesion, such as a carcinoma, is a recognized risk factor for the development of aerobic and anaerobic pneumonia. Bacterial infection is common if obstruction persists for more than a week.[34–37]

In retrospective series of lung abscesses complicating lung cancers, it does not appear that the use of steroids appreciably increases the frequency of lung abscess, nor does it shorten survival in those who develop lung abscess while undergoing chemotherapy for small cell carcinoma.[38]

### Incidence

It is unknown how frequently anaerobic infections occur. In numerous reports from the preantibiotic era, primary lung abscess was diagnosed in 10.5 to 38.3 per 10,000 patients; after the widespread introduction of penicillin, the hospital-based incidence dropped by approximately one order of magnitude.[8, 13, 39–41] It has been suggested that the widespread prophylactic or coincident use of penicillin aborted the successful development of infection in many patients who aspirated; the current clinical practice is to treat suspected cases of aspiration pneumonia as soon as possible to prevent the development of major sequelae.

Bartlett attempted to estimate the frequency of anaerobic bacterial lung infections from published studies of community-acquired pneumonia, hospital-acquired pneumonia, pulmonary abscess, aspiration pneumonia, and empyema.[23] In several carefully conducted studies, anaerobes were found second only to *S. pneumoniae* as etiologic agents in community-acquired bacterial pneumonia, with perhaps a fifth to a third of patients having significant growth of anaerobes from transtracheal aspirates or protected brush bronchoscopy specimens.[42, 43] Among those with nosocomial pneumonias, approximately one third of patients had anaerobic bacteria contributing to their disease; among those with syndromes that were classic for the involvement of anaerobic bacteria (eg, lung abscess, foul empyema), the percentage climbed to 50% to 100%.[23]

### Pathophysiology and Risk of Infection

Anaerobic lung infections can occur by inoculation of the lung parenchyma through aspiration of oropharyngeal fluid, hematogenous spread from a distant source, trauma, or transdiaphragmatic spread. Aspiration of an inoculum from the oropharynx is by far the most common mechanism. The frequency, volume, and character of the aspirate appears to determine the risk of development of an anaerobic infection.

A common sequence in the evolution of anaerobic infection is aspiration and subsequent necrotizing pneumonitis of the bronchioles of a bronchopulmonary segment, with spread to the adjacent parenchyma and abscess formation in the next 7 to 10 days. Pathologic findings usually include a confluent bronchopneumonia, with extensive hemorrhage and abscess formation. Within necrotic tissue may be found microabscesses, and if the area is of sufficient size, a radiologically apparent lung abscess may be seen. Abscesses may be single, multiple, or multilocular, but they reflect an overall process. Single segments, lobes, or even the whole lung may become involved. Variants of this common sequence are discussed later.

Chemical injury to the lung after an acidic aspiration may allow aspirated oral flora to flourish.[44] It appears that the pH of the aspirated fluid and the volume, are important in the development of an acid pneumonitis, thought often to precede anaerobic aspiration pneumonia.[45–52] Acid pneumonitis does not occur under experimental conditions unless the pH of the aspirate is 2.5 or less, and in animals an inoculum of 1 mL/kg or more usually is necessary. A clinically significant volume of aspirate is 25 mL, based on animal models of acid aspiration pneumonitis in which the aspirate has a pH of 2.5 or less. Chemical (acid) pneumonitis injures the lung and predisposes it to subsequent bacterial infection.

Small inocula or those with a pH above 2.5 may not induce the inflammatory changes seen with acid aspiration that are thought to be conducive to infection. An astonishing range of substances have iatrogenically been introduced into the lung without subsequent pneumonitis or infection. One elderly gentleman had 850 mL of an enteral feeding solution instilled into his right lower lobe after improper placement of a feeding tube but had neither an exudative reaction nor any evidence of an infection.

The pathologic changes seen rapidly after acid aspiration in animals include atelectasis, peribronchial hemorrhage, pulmonary edema, and death of bronchial epithelial cells, followed by an intense polymorphonuclear cell and fibrin alveolar exudate. Hyaline membrane formation is seen within 48 hours.[53] Because the acidic pH of gastric contents is lethal to most bacteria, viable bacteria may not be introduced into the site of a chemical pneumonitis at the time of the original aspiration but after the injury has occurred. There are few studies that evaluated the frequency of superinfection (eg, with oral anaerobes or hospital nosocomial organisms) in those who have acid aspiration pneumonitis. In Bynum and Pierce's retrospective review of 50 cases of *significant* aspiration, 12% developed adult respiratory distress syndrome and died; 62% had rapid clearing of the infiltrates; and 26% developed new or growing infiltrates (eg, pneumonia) and fever after initial improvement.[54]

In hospitalized patients who have had the acid barrier of the stomach neutralized (eg, antacids, $H_2$-antagonists, age), colonization of the oropharynx and stomach with aerobic gram-negative organisms occurs frequently. This is thought to be a reservoir of organisms for those who develop hospital-acquired aspiration pneumonia with gram-negative organisms, demonstrating that an acid pH is not *necessary* for the development of aspiration pneumonia, although it is conducive. The prevalence of gram-negative bacteria in the oropharynx ranges from 2%[55] to 9%[56] in nonhospitalized healthy people; in contrast, 45% of patients were colonized with gram-negatives after 4 days of residence in an intensive care unit.[55] In several studies, prophylactic treatment with antacids or histamine type 2 blockers has been associated with an increased risk of nosocomial pneumonia with gram-negative bacteria in hospitalized patients.[57–59] Inglis and group have shown a relationship between gastric aspirate pH, gastroduodenal dysfunction, and gastric bacterial overgrowth in 15 mechanically ventilated patients.[17a] The prevention of hospital-acquired pneumonia in critically ill patients has proved difficult when the trachea's protected environment is broached by mechanical ventilation and gastric acidity allows colonization.[17b]

Particulate matter within an aspirate may predispose the patient to infection in two ways: as a contaminated foreign object and by obstruction of the airways. Anaerobic bacteria from the oropharynx appear to be the usual pathogens after an acute obstruction, based on reports and animal studies.[60]

Aspirated material generally settles as gravity dictates: in the recumbent patient, into the superior segments of the lower lobe and into the posterior segments of the upper lobe.[61] The right side is affected twice as commonly as the left, probably because of the asymmetry of the tracheal branching, with greater angulation of the left main stem bronchus and the more direct path into the right lung. In the upright person, the basilar segments of the lower lobes are most dependent. In Fifer and colleagues' report in 1961,[16] 31 of 55 patients had a period of unconsciousness before the development of lung abscess, and 42 of the 56 abscesses were in the right lung. Schweppe and coworkers found, in reviewing the Massachusetts General Hospital's experience from 1943 to 1956, 108 (73%) of 148 abscesses in the right chest.[13] As surgical procedures with the patient in a sitting position (eg, tonsillectomy, tooth extraction) have become less common, the incidence of lower lobe abscess (especially of the basilar segments) has decreased markedly.[41]

## BACTERIAL PATHOGENS OF ASPIRATION AND ABSCESS

A polymicrobial flora is usually found in infection after oropharyngeal or gastric aspiration. In these cases, anaerobes are found in 60% to 85%, and aerobic organisms are found in about half. Over 200 species of anaerobic bacteria are found in the oral cavity. Species that are well represented in clinical studies or which are pathogenic in animal models include anaerobic streptococci such as the *Peptostreptococcus* spp., *Fusobacterium nucleatum*, the *Prevotella melanogenicus* (formerly *Bacteroides melanogenicus*) group of organisms and the *Bacteroides fragilis* and *Porphyromonia* group of organisms (Table 28–2).[23, 62] The first three have been labeled "the big three" of anaerobic pleuropulmonary infection, and a relative predominance of one organism over another is not thought to have any clinical consequence. A variety of other organisms identified in early studies have been consolidated into these groups, and many anaerobic streptococci have been reclassified as microaerophilic or aerobic streptococci, such as in the transformation of *Peptostreptococcus intermedius* into *Streptococcus intermedius*.

**Table 28–2. Anaerobic Bacteria Associated With Anaerobic or Mixed Aerobic-Anaerobic Pleuropulmonary Infections**

**Major Pathogens**
*Peptostreptococcus* species*
*Fusobacterium nucleatum, F. necrophorum*
*Prevotella melaninogenicus* (formerly *Bacteroides melaninogenicus*) group organisms (form black or pigmented colonies)
*Porphyromonas* (formerly *Bacteroides*) species: *P. asaccharolyticus, P. endodontalis, P. gingivalis*
**Variable Incidence but of Concern**
*Bacteroides fragilis, B. thetaiotaomicron*, and group resistance to penicillin G, other penicillins, cephalosporins, and clindamycin increasing and common
**Frequently Found but of Uncertain Pathogenicity**
*Veillonella* species (differentiated only by DNA hybridization)

*Several aerotolerant *Peptostreptococcus* species have been reclassified as *Streptococcus* species, such as *S. intermedius, S. parvulus, S. constellatus*, and *S. morbillorum*.

Although *B. fragilis* was found in 15% to 20% of patients in studies from two decades ago[63, 64] and although penicillin-resistant *B. fragilis* involvement has been known to lead to treatment failure,[65] the extent of the role *B. fragilis* plays in these infections remains unclear. *B. fragilis* is not a part of the normal oral flora, unlike a number of other *Bacteroides* species. Some studies have found a frequency that is lower, 5% or less, in cases of lung abscess, empyema, and aspiration pneumonia.[66, 67] Because the major danger in *Bacteroides* involvement is penicillin resistance, it is not at all reassuring to know that in at least 10% to 15% of anaerobic lung disease isolates, other penicillin-resistant anaerobic organisms can be found.[23, 68] In some series, up to 40% of *Fusobacterium* isolates and 60% of non-*fragilis Bacteroides* species have been demonstrated to produce a penicillinase.[69]

In studies of children with anaerobic pleuropulmonary infections, the distribution and resistance patterns of isolates have been similar to that in adults.[70–72]

Hospital-acquired aspiration pneumonia is often complicated by the presence of gram-negative enteric bacteria. Colonization of the oropharynx with gram-negative enteric bacteria is unusual in normal humans and correlates with the severity of other underlying illnesses.[56] These bacteria include *Escherichia coli, Klebsiella pneumoniae, Pseudomonas aeruginosa, Enterobacter cloacae, Citrobacter freundii, Acinetobacter lwoffi*, and *Eikenella corrodens*. Other bacteria frequently found in hospital-acquired aspiration include *S. aureus, Enterococcus faecalis, S. pneumoniae, S. intermedius, Haemophilus influenzae, H. parainfluenzae*, and a variety of oral streptococci, such as *S. morbillorum, S. constellatus*, and *S. salivarius*.

The following are key points:

Aspiration-related pleuropulmonary infections are usually polymicrobial, and anaerobes play a dominant role.

In persons at risk for upper respiratory tract or proximal gut colonization with unusual organisms, the organisms are found in the flora of those with aspiration syndromes. For example, hospitalized patients and alcoholics[73] are at risk of disease with enteric and nosocomial gram-negative rods or *S. aureus*.

It is unclear whether each of the organisms in a polymicrobial anaerobic infection is pathogenic when occurring alone.

Because of the difficulty in culturing anaerobes and in obtaining adequate samples, the clinician must assume the presence of anaerobes in aspiration pneumonia and associated infections. Sputum culture isolates should be regarded with suspicion and may mislead the clinician.

## DIAGNOSIS AND INFECTIOUS MANIFESTATIONS

### Diagnostic Techniques

Techniques that are appropriate for obtaining specimens for anaerobic culture include aspiration of empyema fluid, transthoracic needle biopsies, transtracheal needle aspiration, and protected brush bronchoscopy aspiration (Table 28–3). Expectorated sputum is contaminated by the bacteria of the upper airway, and blind reliance on the result of a sputum culture for this group of infections is an error of judgment. The clinician must presume anaerobes are present and recognize that microbiology laboratories will (appropriately) not culture sputum for anaerobes. Putrid sputum, an hallmark of anaerobic infection, is seen in perhaps half of those with anaerobic empyema or lung abscess. Transtracheal aspiration is rarely performed, and the other methods are invasive. Because adequate microbiologic samples are not commonly obtained, the presence of anaerobic bacteria must be assumed. Correlate blood cultures are usually found only if an anaerobic lung infection is of hematogenous origin. Many laboratories do not speciate anaerobic isolates, and the initial Gram stain of a clinically appropriate specimen is often crucial because it shows the typical morphology of anaerobes and other bacteria.

Transtracheal aspiration has been the technique most thoroughly described in the literature. The specificity of the technique should be high, because any bacteria cultured from below the vocal chords is probably the authentic, causative pathogen in pneumonia or other bacterial diseases. In those with chronic bronchitis, bronchiectasis, or pulmonary neoplasm or in those undergoing frequent tracheal suction, nonpathogenic organisms—usually aerobic—may be isolated and confuse issues of causality. Clinicians frequently see neurologically devastated, chronically ventilated patients who have asymptomatic chronic colonization of the trachea with highly resistant enteric gram-negative bacilli or *S. aureus* without evident pulmonary disease. In unskilled hands, transtracheal aspiration may lead to hemorrhagic complications, and this has diminished its popularity.

Special mention should be made of protected brush bronchoscopy techniques. Bronchoscopes are routinely contaminated by oral flora during passage through the oropharynx, and protection of the collection system is necessary if representative cultures of the infected lung are to be obtained with a bronchoscope. A wire brush inside a telescoping dual catheter system with occlusion of the catheter distal to the brush is used. The occluding plug, usually made of polyethylene glycol, is pushed out during collection, and the specimen brush collects 1 to 10 μL of fluid. The pneumonic fluid is transported to the laboratory in 1 mL of Ringer's lactate and is cultured quantitatively. Rigid adherence to scrupulous technique is crucial, and prior antimicrobial therapy may decrease the sensitivity of the examination.[74] Bacterial counts in pneumonia usually are in the range of $10^6$ to $10^8$/mL using this technique.[75] Because of the dilutions made, a bacterial growth of $10^3$ or more colony forming units per milliliter of Ringer's lactate is the lowest count that indicates a significant growth; the physician may feel more confident with higher counts. Bronchoalveolar lavage, a technique in which saline is instilled into a segment of the lung and then aspirated for culture, has not been studied as extensively as the protected brush technique.

In most studies, bronchoalveolar lavage, protected specimen brush culture, and endotracheal aspiration are roughly comparable techniques. Marquette and coworkers in France found the overall diagnostic accuracy of endotracheal aspiration about the same as that of protected specimen brush culture;[76] Roger-Moreau and colleagues in Bordeaux found that bronchoalveolar lavage may be superior to protected specimen brush culture if direct microscopic examination of lavage fluid showed more than 3% of aspirated cells to contain intracellular bacteria.[76a] Torres and group in Barcelona compared all three techniques and found that endotracheal aspiration and protected specimen brush culture had specificities of 85% and bronchoalveolar lavage had specificities of 78% for pneumonia, and that bronchoalveolar lavage had a higher rate of false-positive results in their hands.[76b]

The interpretation of marginal specimens is important. The clinical laboratory at Duke University has published guidelines that allowed them to reject poor quality endotracheal suction aspirates (41% of all submitted) and save $66,000 per year in laboratory charges.[76c] Another group found that when protected specimen brush colony counts are borderline, either the passage of time without antibiotics or another brushing resolved the issue.[76d]

Transthoracic aspiration of empyema or transthoracic needle biopsy may cause pneumothorax, pyothorax, or hemothorax; the technique is probably best done with ultra-

**Table 28–3. Diagnostic Techniques for Culturing Organisms in Anaerobic and Mixed Aerobic-Anaerobic Pleuropulmonary Infections**

| Technique | Comments |
|---|---|
| Sputum culture | Worthless and misleading |
| Gas chromatography | Uses fermentation products or fatty acid bacterial components to identify specific bacterial "signatures," still a research tool |
| Sputum odor, Gram stain | Can be helpful, especially if odor foul and mixed "oral" organisms seen |
| Transtracheal aspiration | A "gold standard" technique, although results must be interpreted with caution for a patient whose trachea may be colonized, and hemorrhagic complications can occur |
| Protected brush bronchoscopy | A gold standard tool, especially helpful in those without prior antimicrobial therapy, and gaining in popularity |
| Transthoracic biopsy or transthoracic aspiration | Perhaps the highest culture yield of all; relatively few reports in the literature; can lead to pneumothorax, pyothorax, or hemothorax |

sound or computed tomography (CT) guidance for most accurate insertion. In a series from Spain, Pena and colleagues[67] sampled abscesses in 50 consecutive patients through percutaneous aspiration with a 22-gauge needle under fluoroscopic guidance at their university, tertiary-care, referral hospital. Initial therapy was intravenous clindamycin plus tobramycin in those without foul sputum. Pneumothorax occurred as the sole complication in 7 patients (14%), requiring chest tube placement in 5 patients (10%). Nine of the 50 samples were sterile, one grew unsuspected *M. tuberculosis,* and of the remaining 40, culture results led to a significant change in therapy for 23 patients. In most of these 23, organisms resistant to clindamycin or tobramycin were found. For persons with hospital-acquired infection, giant lung abscess, severe presentation, or persistent toxicity, percutaneous lung aspiration may be a useful diagnostic method.

For patients with severe disease who are too ill to undergo surgery, transthoracic drainage of abscess or empyema may be lifesaving. This is discussed in the section on therapy.

It is important to transport specimens rapidly to the microbiology laboratory for proper analysis; exposure to an aerobic milieu suppresses or prevents culture of anaerobes. Although numerous commercial systems for anaerobic transport exist, the clinician may confidently transport tissue or aspirated pus in a sealed syringe without air.

## Clinical Presentations

In patients in whom classic anaerobic infection occurs, an insidious process begins in which tissue necrosis may occur 1 or several weeks after the initial incident. In several natural history studies predating the antimicrobial era, necrosis occurred 8 to 14 days after the onset of pneumonitis.[20, 21, 77] This process is usually peripheral. In contrast to this anaerobic suppurative necrosis, the pneumonia caused by aerobic organisms is generally more acute in onset, and lung necrosis develops later in the course of the illness. With the exception of *K. pneumoniae, P. aeruginosa, S. aureus,* and some of the streptococci, few aerobic pathogens have such a marked propensity for causing lung necrosis in pure culture. Mixed infections containing anaerobes and aerobes tend to act more like anaerobic infections and can be quite necrotic.

As a clinical correlate of this time course, expectoration of foul sputum is rare in the prenecrosis period, although mild hemoptysis may be seen; after cavitation occurs, putrid expectoration becomes a common finding in 40% to 75% of cases.[78]

Because the segmental areas of the lung are prone to soilage by aspiration, it is not surprising that the pleural space is often involved by the infection. In a radiologic review of 69 bacteriologically proven anaerobic infections, Landay and coworkers found that 30% of the patients had radiographically evident disease in the pleura alone, 20% had a mixture of pleural and parenchymal disease, and 50% had parenchymal disease alone. Over half had abscess at presentation, and many of the others developed cavities despite antimicrobial therapy. The pleural disease was invariably empyema, which progressed rapidly.[79]

A clinical correlate of this predilection for the pleura is the symptom of pleuritis, seen in about half of patients.[21, 80] About half have findings of pneumonia on auscultation.

A virulent variant of aspiration pneumonia is anaerobic pneumonitis, in which indolence, tissue necrosis, and putrid discharge are absent. In some reports, this constitutes half of the hospital-acquired aspiration-related infections; a complex microflora is present, and anaerobes, enteric nosocomial gram-negative bacilli, and *S. aureus* are found in over half of these patients. It is impossible to clinically differentiate this variant from ''typical'' pneumonia caused by pathogens such as *S. pneumoniae.*

Another variant is chronic destructive pneumonia.[81] The disease course usually is altered by the indiscriminate use of antimicrobials over weeks to months. Unlike the normal-appearing lung tissue around many anaerobic lung abscesses, chronic destructive pneumonia may involve bronchial and parenchymal tissue adjacent to an abscess or microabscesses. Pathologically, involved tissue is fibrotic and shrunken, often studded with microabscesses, and bronchiectasis is commonly seen. Le Roux and others have advanced the theory that this disease may be more common in Africa because of associated malnutrition, iron overload, intermittent antibiotic use, and prior tuberculosis in the population.[82]

Solitary lung abscess is not a common presentation. Defined as a cavity 2 cm or larger on roentgenographic examination, lung abscess is usually found in a single lobe of the lung (Fig. 28–1). Necrotizing pneumonia is characterized by multiple small cavitary lesions within an area of pneumonia. Experienced clinicians have estimated that a minimum of 1 to 2 weeks passes from the initial aspiration event to the development of lung abscess. In general, patients with lung abscess have a median symptomatic period of 2 weeks before evaluation; some have had symptoms for months before seeking medical attention, and about half have lost weight.[23] The location of abscesses is similar to the location of dependent aspiration inocula. Weight loss and malaise are indicative of the catabolic process associated with chronic infection. Little information is available on the mechanisms of these changes, the degree of weight loss, or the metabolic parameters that accompany chronic abscess or empyema.

Empyema is pus in the pleural space. An area of lung parenchyma adjacent to the pleura is first involved, and the nearby pleural cavity becomes infected secondarily. Empyema often complicates anaerobic abscess or necrotizing pneumonia.

The pleura consists of thin fibroelastic sheets with a single, flat endothelial layer. Adjacent is a connective tissue layer containing nutritional blood vessels and lymphatics. With pleural involvement during infection, there is swelling of the connective tissue layer between the fibroelastic sheets, and an exudate forms in the pleural cavity. The fibroelastic layers often resist the further spread of the infection. Fibrin is deposited, more on the parietal than the visceral surface, and eventually this becomes vascularized during the process of organization. These exudative reactions may seal the borders of an empyema or fix the underlying lung to the overlying thoracic cage. In time, empyematous or abscess fluid may drain through fistulas; bronchopulmonary fistulas are common in chronic disease,

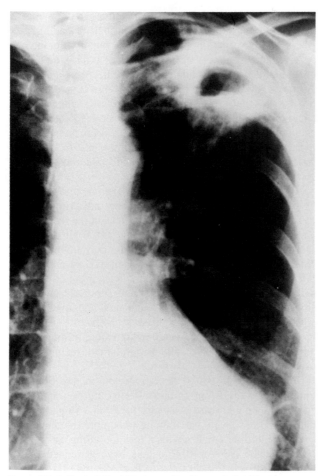

**Figure 28–1.** Typical "putrid abscess" with an air-fluid level was associated with insidious weight loss, foul sputum, and low-grade fever in a middle-aged man, 6 weeks after an aspiration. It resolved with oral clindamycin therapy. (Courtesy of Mark Drapkin, M.D., Newton-Wellesley Hospital, Newton, MA.)

with bronchopleural or bronchocutaneous (ie, empyema necessitans or fistula) fistulas less so.

## Radiologic Evaluation

A lung abscess contains destroyed, necrotic lung parenchyma surrounded by and stabilized by inflamed lung. After the necrotic debris is able to drain, usually through a bronchus, air overlies residual pus and creates an air-fluid level. Abscesses are usually spherical or oval. An empyema instead conforms to the contours of the pleural space and may be mobile as the patient changes position. Adjacent lung may or may not be involved; if it is not, it is often compressed. The contours of the area are triangular or fusiform. If air is trapped in an empyema, it may suggest a bronchopleural fistula or, less commonly, a pleurocutaneous fistula. Friedman and Hellekant[83] evaluated more than 30 cases of empyema and lung abscess complicated by bronchopleural fistula and concluded that abscesses and empyema with air-fluid levels could usually be differentiated by conventional radiography. With empyema, the frontal views usually show a wide air-fluid level, but on a lateral view, the anteroposterior diameter is narrow. Abscesses tend to

be spherical and farther from the ribs, and the air-fluid level size is similar on both anteroposterior and lateral films.

Schachter and coworkers[84] evaluated 48 patients with suppurative lung infection and concluded that four criteria are useful in differentiating empyema with bronchopleural fistula from lung abscess: prior pleural effusion on earlier radiographs, extension of the air-fluid level to the chest wall, a tapering border of the air-fluid collection, and extension of the air-fluid collection across the fissure lines.

The use of CT scans to visualize the thoracic contents has proven helpful when standard radiography was not diagnostic. CT helps to define the interface between the lung parenchyma and the pleural space if the infection is near the thoracic wall, and it can define the shape of an infected area if both are involved. On CT scans, abscesses are spherical or oval and do not change position with motion. An empyema retains the triangular or crescenteric shape seen on regular radiographs and may shift as the patient shifts. The interface with the lung wall is usually acutely defined with an abscess or obtuse and tapering in empyema as the pleural space becomes inflamed.

The lung parenchyma surrounding an abscess is often involved, and the interface between the abscess cavity and the adjacent lung is indistinct. Bronchi and pulmonary vessels extend to the abscess and are usually not bowed away or displaced by the abscess. In contrast, the walls of an empyema are usually defined by the pleura and appear thin and uniform. As the pleural space fills, it compresses the underlying lung parenchyma beneath it, and bronchi and pulmonary vessels are displaced away from their usual path.[85]

Stark and coworkers[86] reviewed 70 inflammatory lesions in 63 patients with lung abscess or empyema, excluding 17 patients with necrotic lung tumors or malignant pleural effusions. They found that the CT scans were 100% accurate for case diagnosis and that for 47% of their series additional information was obtained by CT that was not available by conventional radiography. For 34%, CT more accurately defined the extent of disease. In their retrospective series, the most reliable features for the differential diagnosis of lung abscess and empyema were wall characteristics, pleural separation, and lung compression. They found size, shape, and the angle of the chest wall defined by conventional radiographs less helpful, "though also best assessed by CT."[86]

We recommend the use of CT if conventional radiographs do not satisfy the clinician in defining the full extent of the disease or if abscess and empyema cannot be confidently differentiated. Because abscesses are usually treated medically and empyema is treated surgically and medically, this differentiation is important. Although no large prospective comparison of conventional radiography with CT has been reported, the value of CT in these circumstances as an adjunct to radiographs cannot be underestimated.

## TREATMENT

### Medical Therapy

Initial therapy of apiration pneumonia, anaerobic pneumonia, and lung abscess should be medical in all but the

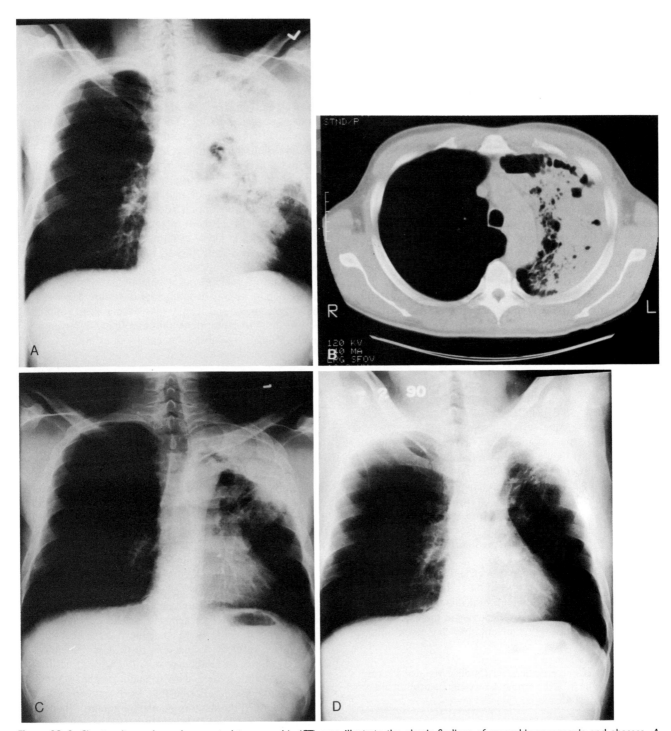

**Figure 28–2.** Chest radiographs and computed tomographic (CT) scan illustrate the classic findings of anaerobic pneumonia and abscess. *A,* Complete consolidation of the left upper lobe with multiple abscesses and air-fluid levels can be seen in a middle-aged man after aspiration. *B,* CT scan shows air space consolidation and air bronchograms, indicative of pneumonia and multiple air-filled cavities peripherally. A large air-fluid level can be seen anteriorly near the midline, indicating a large anterior abscess cavity. Notice the lack of displacement of pulmonary tissue by the infection, suggesting that there is no empyema. *C* and *D,* Resolving disease 2 and 4.5 months after presentation and prolonged treatment with oral penicillin. After therapy, a pleural apical ''cap'' of scar tissue was the only detectable residuum of the infection.

sickest patients. However, empyema requires the drainage of entrapped fluid, with rare exceptions. Initial tube thoracostomy is rarely indicated, except for acutely draining an abscess of pus in a severely ill patient.

The widespread availability of penicillin after World War II revolutionized the therapy of lung abscess and empyema.

Penicillin, because of its excellent activity against several oral anaerobes and *S. pneumoniae,* quickly became recognized as the therapy of choice for primary lung abscess (Fig. 28–2). Tetracyclines were found to be an adequate alternative for penicillin-allergic patients. Metronidazole had a disappointing record in treating these infections, and it should not be used as sole therapy for anaerobic pleuropulmonary infections. Only about 50% of patients respond to metronidazole, presumably because of the contributing role of microaerophilic and aerobic streptococci in these polymicrobial infections.[87, 88] The combination of penicillin and metronidazole, both inexpensive and oral, has theoretical appeal, although experience is limited.[89] We cannot recommend this combination until confirmatory studies are available.

Clindamycin has gained popularity for treating these infections, based on a relatively small number of trials in which it proved equal to or better than penicillin.[90, 91] A worrisome trend has been the development of widespread penicillin resistance in the anaerobic population found in pleuropulmonary infections, accounting for the potential advantage clindamycin enjoys.

Many other antimicrobials have excellent anaerobic activity and, although expensive, are reasonable alternatives to clindamycin and penicillin. These include ampicillin-sulbactam, imipenem, ticarcillin-clavulanate, and amoxicillin-clavulanic acid. Because ceftizoxime has poor anaerobic activity using certain testing methodologies but much better activity using broth microdilution techniques, its place remains uncertain.[92] We recommend the use of clindamycin or amoxicillin-clavulanate (Augmentin) for oral therapy in typical cases and reservation of other agents or combinations for cases of hospital-acquired aspiration pneumonia with gram-negative bacillary or staphylococcal involvement. Because of the serious nature of gram-negative or *Staphylococcus* pneumonia, these organisms warrant specific treatment if they are found or probable. Drugs such as ampicillin-sulbactam or ticarcillin-clavulanate may be extremely useful if nosocomial organisms and anaerobes are present. Table 28–4 lists our recommendations for therapy. Although we do not recommend the use of tetracyclines, we recognize that their use may be attractive in clinical situations in which cost is a predominant concern, as in developing countries.

If penicillin is used, many physicians recommend doses of 12 million U each day (2 million U intravenously every 4 hours) for an adult, although oral therapy (3 g daily, at 750 mg every 6 hours) was efficacious in the experience of Weiss.[93] For adults, clindamycin may be given intravenously at a dose of 1800 mg per day (600 mg every 8 hours) or 300 mg orally three or four times each day. Because of the perceived risk of pseudomembranous colitis in those who take clindamycin, many clinicians treat anaerobic aspiration pneumonia with penicillin, using clindamycin in cases of treatment failure. The relative merits of this approach are unclear. The literature increasingly reports instances of penicillin failure and of penicillinase-producing anaerobic organisms; we do not think that penicillin should be used as initial presumptive treatment.

In the experience of those who have treated hundreds of cases of anaerobic infection, radiographic progression in the first 7 to 14 days of therapy is common and not an indication that initial antimicrobial therapy is deficient. Perhaps 85% to 90% of these infections respond well to antimicrobial therapy. Other criteria, such as the fever curve, are useful in assessing the adequacy of therapy; the response to antibiotic treatment is similar in anaerobic pneumonitis and in pneumococcal pneumonia (see Fig. 28–2). After cavitary lesions or empyema develops, fever resolution is prolonged, and it may take longer than a month to resolve despite appropriate antimicrobials. Empyema demands drainage, but abscess generally does not.

## Surgical Therapy

In the preantibiotic era, surgery became the therapy of choice for lung abscess and empyema. With the development of potent antimicrobial agents, the need for surgery has decreased but has not been obviated. In a few patients, medical therapy is doomed to failure and is only adjunctive to surgical treatment. In a 1987 review, Bartlett pooled 2439 cases of pulmonary abscess reported in the world's literature from 1946 to 1985 and arrived at an estimate of 10% to 12% requiring surgical intervention, usually lobectomy.[23] Indications for surgical therapy of abscess include failure to respond to medical treatment, hemorrhage, and an associated neoplasm. Surgical resection of dead lung tissue in cases of pulmonary gangrene can be lifesaving. Surgical resection is the widely accepted surgical "gold standard" in those who do not respond adequately to medical therapy.

Adequate surgical drainage is critical in patients with empyema. Early in the course of the disease, free-flowing exudate may be drained with frequent needle aspirations, but this circumstance is unusual. Most patients with empyema require thoracotomy tube drainage. Inadequate drainage of pleural or subdiaphragmatic infections has been associated with poor outcomes,[77, 81] and proper drainage should not be delayed after the diagnosis of empyema has been made.

Percutaneous drainage of refractory lung abscesses has been reported for a variety of circumstances.[94–99] Often these abscesses are peripheral and adjacent inflammation has extended to the pleural surfaces, allowing formation of a pleural symphysis. Before the use of antibiotics, surgeons created a pleural symphysis by resecting a short segment of a rib overlying the abscess by subperiosteal excision and inserting an irritant such as a strip of gauze into the incision. In 4 or 5 days, a tube could be inserted into the underlying abscess with less danger of pneumothorax. With

**Table 28–4. Recommendations for Empiric Medical Therapy of Anaerobic or Mixed Aerobic-Anaerobic Pleuropulmonary Infections**

| Treatment | Dosage |
|---|---|
| Clindamycin | 300 mg PO q 6–8 h; 600–900 mg IV q 6–8 h Add aminoglycoside or other agent, (eg, fluoroquinolone) active against gram-negative enteric organisms and *S. aureus* if nosocomial infection or colonization likely, as for hospital-acquired aspiration pneumonia |
| Suggested alternatives | |
|   Amoxicillin-clavulanate | 500 mg PO thrice daily |
|   Ampicillin-sulbactam | 1.5–3.0 g IV q 6 h |
|   Ticarcillin-clavulanate | 3.1 g IV q 6–8 h |
| Penicillin* | 3 g PO daily divided q 6 h; 12–24 million U IV divided q 4 h |

*Inexpensive alternative that may be appropriate in specific cases.

Table 28–5. **Percutaneous or Catheter Drainage of Lung Abscesses in Adults or Children Not Responsive to Medical Management**

| Investigation | No. of Patients | Reasons for Drainage* | Outcomes |
|---|---|---|---|
| Weissberg, 1984[102] | 7 | Severe sepsis despite 2–4 wk of antibiotics | 7 of 7 survived |
| Yellin et al, 1985[99] | 10 | | 7 of 10 cured after 22–40 d of antibiotics before drainage<br>3 of 10 with malignancy required eventual lobectomy; 1 died 1 mo after surgery, other 2 cured of infection and malignancy |
| Mengoli, 1985[103] | 3 | Giant abscesses (≥8 cm) not responsive to medical management | 3 of 3 cured |
| Lorenzo et al, 1985[104] | 3 | Failure to respond to medical management | 3 of 3 cured with needle aspiration |
| Snow et al, 1985[105] | 3 | Sepsis | 3 of 3 cured; only 1 clearly anaerobic |
| Rice et al, 1987[101] | 14 | Sepsis (11), abscess under tension (7), failure to wean from ventilator (4), soiling of contralateral lung (4) | 11 of 14 discharged from hospital, only 1 of 3 deaths from abscess |
| Parker et al, 1987[106] | 6 | Failure to respond to medical therapy | 5 of 6 promptly responded to small catheter drainage; sixth improved after antibiotic modified |
| Schmitt et al, 1988[107] | 3 | Inability to maintain drainage by bronchoscopy | 3 cured with placement through the nares of catheter into abscess cavity |
| Cuestas et al, 1989[108] | 2 | Progressive abscess and pneumonia in young infants | 2 of 2 cured |
| Ball et al, 1989[109] | 7 | Esophageal perforation with extrapulmonary abscess (4), large lung abscesses (3) | 4 of 4 with esophageal perforations healed, 3 of 3 with intrapulmonary abscess healed |
| van Sonnenberg et al, 1991[110] | 19 | Sepsis despite antibiotics | 19 of 19 cured by CT-guided catheter drainage; hemothorax in 1 patient without pleural syndesis |

*Tube drainage unless otherwise specified.

the advent of immunosuppressive therapies and an increased population of ill people (eg, those with advanced chronic lung disease) who cannot tolerate major surgery such as lobectomy, these techniques may enjoy a resurgence.[100] Eleven reports on percutaneous drainage are reviewed in Table 28–5; although the reasons for drainage varied, 73 of 77 reported patients left the hospital alive.

## REFERENCES

1. Hippocrates: [Quotation] In Major's Classic Descriptions of Disease. Springfield, IL, CC Thomas, 1965.
2. Rendu, Rist E: Étude clinique et bactériologique de trois cas de pleurésie putride. Bull Soc Hop Paris 16:133–150, 1899.
3. Guillemot L, Halle J, Rist E: Recherches bactériologiques et expérimentales sur les pleurésies putrides. Arch Med Exp Anat Pathol 16:571, 1904.
4. Smith DT: Experimental aspiratory abscess. Arch Surg 14:231, 1927.
5. Smith DT: Fusospirochetal disease of the lungs, its bacteriology, pathology and experimental reproduction. Am Rev Tuberc 16:584, 1927.
6. Smith DT: Fuso-spirochetal diseases of the lungs. Tubercle 9:480, 1928.
7. Smith DT: Fuso-spirochetal disease of the lungs produced with cultures from Vincent's angina. J Infect Dis 46:303, 1930.
8. King DS, Lord FT: Certain aspects of pulmonary abscess from analysis of 210 cases. Ann Intern Med 8:468–474, 1934.
9. Allen CI, Blackman JF: Treatment of lung abscess, with report of 100 consecutive cases. J Thorac Surg 6:156, 1936.
10. Neuhof H, Touroff AS: Acute putrid abscess of the lung: Principles of operative treatment. Surg Gynecol Obstet 63:353, 1936.
11. Neuhof H: Acute putrid abscess of the lung. Gynecol Obstet Surg 80:351, 1945.
12. Wilkins EW: Classics in thoracic surgery: Acute putrid abscess of the lung. Ann Thorac Surg 44:560–561, 1987.
13. Schweppe HI, Knowles JH, Kane L: Lung abscess: An analysis of the Massachusetts General Hospital cases from 1943 through 1956. N Engl J Med 265:1039–1043, 1961.
14. Finland M, Barnes MW: Changing ecology of acute bacterial empyema: Occurrence and mortality at Boston City Hospital during 12 selected years from 1935 to 1972. J Infect Dis 137:274–291, 1978.
15. Weese WC, Shindler ER, Smith AM, Rabinovich S: Empyema of the thorax then and now. Arch Intern Med 131:516–520, 1973.
16. Fifer WR, Husebye K, Chedister C, Miller M: Primary lung abscess. Analysis of therapy and results in 55 cases. Arch Intern Med 107:100–112, 1961.
17. Bartlett JG, Gorbach SL, Thadepalli H, Finegold SM: Bacteriology of empyema. Lancet 1:338–340, 1974.
17a. Inglis TJ, Sproat LJ, Sherratt MJ, et al: Gastroduodenal dysfunction as a cause of gastric bacterial overgrowth in patients undergoing mechanical ventilation of the lungs. Br J Anaesth 68:499–502, 1992.
17b. Hamer DH, Barza M: Prevention of hospital-acquired pneumonia in critically ill patients. Antimicrob Agents Chemother 37:931–939, 1993.
18. Bartlett JG, Gorbach SL, Tally FP, Finegold SM: Bacteriology and treatment of primary lung abscess. Am Rev Respir Dis 109:510–518, 1974.
19. Bartlett JG, Finegold SM: Anaerobic pleuropulmonary infections. Medicine (Baltimore) 51:413–450, 1972.
20. Bartlett JG, Gorbach SL: Critical review: The triple threat of aspiration pneumonia. Chest 68:560–566, 1975.
21. Bartlett JG, Finegold SM: State of the art: Anaerobic infections of the lung and pleural space. Am Rev Respir Dis 110:56–77, 1974.
22. Sullivan KM, O'Toole RD, Fisher RH, Sullivan KN: Anaerobic empyema thoracis: The role of anaerobes in 226 cases of culture-proven empyemas. Arch Intern Med 131:521–527, 1973.
23. Bartlett JG: Anaerobic bacterial infections of the lung. Chest 91:901–909, 1987.
24. Pohlson EC, McNamara JJ, Char C, Kurata L: Lung abscess: A changing pattern of the disease. Am J Surg 150:97–101, 1985.
25. Bartlett J. Lung abscess and necrotizing pneumonia. In Gorbach SL, Bartlett J, Blacklow N (eds): Infectious Diseases. Philadelphia, WB Saunders, 1992:518–521.
26. Hill MK, Sanders CV: Anaerobic disease of the lung. Infect Dis Clin North Am 5:453–466, 1991.
27. Amberson JB: Aspiration bronchopneumonia. Int Clin 3:126–138, 1937.
28. Huxley EJ, Viroslav J, Gray WRT, et al: Pharyngeal aspiration in normal adults and patients with depressed consciousness. Am J Med 64:546, 1978.

29. King DS, Lord FT: Certain aspects of pulmonary abscess from analysis of 210 cases. Ann Intern Med 8:468–474, 1934.

30. Slots J: Microflora in the healthy gingival sulcus in man. Scand J Dent Res 85:247–254, 1977.

31. Socransky SS: Microbiology of periodontal disease: Present status and future considerations. J Periodontol 48:497–504, 1977.

32. Lassche WJ: Anaerobic Bacteria: Role in Disease. Springfield, IL, CC Thomas, 1974:409–434.

33. Finegold SM, Bartlett JG: Anaerobic pleuropulmonary infections. Cleve Clinic Q 42:101–111, 1975.

34. Clerf LH: Foreign bodies in the air and food passages. Surg Gynecol Obstet 70:328, 1940.

35. Hedblom CA: Foreign bodies of dental origin in a bronchus pulmonary complication. Ann Surg 87:184, 1963.

36. Kim IG, Brummitt WM, Humphry A, et al: Foreign body in the airway: A review of 202 cases. Laryngoscope 83:347, 1973.

37. Abdulmajid OA, Ebeid AM, Motaweh MM, Kleibo S: Aspirated foreign bodies in the tracheobronchial tree: Report of 250 cases. Thorax 31:635, 1976.

38. Hansen SW, Aabo K, Osterlind K: Lung abscess in small cell carcinoma of the lung during chemotherapy and corticosteroids: An analysis of 276 patients. Eur J Respir Dis 68:7–11, 1986.

39. Sweet RH: Lung abscess: Analysis of Massachusetts General Hospital cases from 1933 through 1937. Surg Gynecol Obstet 70:1011–1021, 1940.

40. Lord FT: Certain aspects of pulmonary abscess, from analysis of 227 cases. Boston Med Soc J 192:785–788, 1925.

41. Sweet RH: Analysis of Massachusetts General Hospital cases of lung abscess from 1938 through 1942. Surg Gynecol Obstet 80:568–574, 1945.

42. Ries K, Levison ME, Kaye D: Transtracheal aspiration in pulmonary infection. Arch Intern Med 133:453–458, 1974.

43. Pollack HM, Hawkins EL, Bonner JR, Sparkman T, Bass JB Jr: Diagnosis of bacterial pulmonary infections with quantitative protected catheter cultures obtained during bronchoscopy. J Clin Microbiol 17:255–259, 1983.

44. Johanson WG Jr, Jay SJ, Pierce AK: Bacterial growth in vivo. An important determinant of the pulmonary clearance of *Diplococcus pneumoniae* in rats. J Clin Invest 53:1320–1325, 1974.

45. Scott DB: Mendelson's syndrome. Br J Anesthesiol 50:977, 1978.

46. Toung TJ, Bordos D, Benson DW, et al: Aspiration pneumonia: Experimental evaluation of albumin and steroid therapy. Ann Surg 183:179, 1976.

47. Wolfe JE, Bone RC, Ruth WE: Effects of corticosteroids in the treatment of patients with gastric aspiration. Am J Med 63:719, 1977.

48. Chapman RL Jr, Downs JB, Modell JH, et al: The ineffectiveness of steroid therapy in treating aspiration of hydrochloric acid. Arch Surg 108:858, 1974.

49. Fisk RL, Symes JF, Aldridge LL, et al: The pathophysiology and experimental therapy of acid pneumonitis in ex vivo lungs. Chest 57:364, 1970.

50. Halmagyi DJF: Lung changes and incidence of respiration arrest in rats after aspiration of sea and fresh water. J Appl Physiol 16:41, 1961.

51. Teabeaut J II: Aspiration of gastric contents: An experimental study. Am J Pathol 28:51, 1952.

52. Toung TJ, Cameron JL, Kimera T, et al: Aspiration pneumonia: Treatment with osmotically active agents. Surgery 89:588, 1981.

53. Greenfield LJ, Singleton RP, McCaffree DR, et al: Pulmonary effects of experimental graded aspiration of hydrochloric acid. Ann Surg 170:74, 1969.

54. Bynum LJ, Pierce AK: Pulmonary aspiration of gastric contents. Am Rev Respir Dis 114:1129, 1976.

55. Johanson WG, Pierce AK, Sanford JP: Changing pharyngeal bacterial flora of hospitalized patients: Emergence of gram-negative bacilli. N Engl J Med 281:1137–1140, 1969.

56. Valenti WM, Trudell RG, Bentley DW: Factors predisposing to oropharyngeal colonization with gram-negative bacilli in the aged. N Engl J Med 298:1108–1111, 1978.

57. DuMoulin GC, Paterson DG, Hedley-Whyte J, Lisbon A: Aspiration of gastric bacteria in antacid-treated patients: A frequent cause of postoperative colonisation of the airway. Lancet 1:242–245, 1982.

58. Eddleston JM, Vohra A, Scott P, et al: A comparison of the frequency of stress ulceration and secondary pneumonia in sucralfate-or ranitidine-treated intensive care unit patients. Crit Care Med 19:1491–1496, 1991.

59. Kappstein I, Schulgen G, Friedrich T, et al: Incidence of pneumonia in mechanically ventilated patients treated with sucralfate or cimetidine as prophylaxis for stress bleeding: Bacterial colonization of the stomach. Am J Med 91(suppl 2A):125S–131S, 1991.

60. Lansing AM, Jamieson WG: Mechanisms of fever in pulmonary atelectasis. Arch Surg 87:184, 1963.

61. Brock RC: Lung Abscess. Springfield, IL, CC Thomas, 1952.

62. Kannangara DW, Thadepalli H, Bach VT, Webb D: Animal model for anaerobic lung abscess. Infect Immun 31:592–597, 1981.

63. Bartlett JG, Gorbach SL, Tally F, Finegold S: Bacteriology and treatment of primary lung abscess. Am Rev Respir Dis 109:510–518, 1974.

64. Lorber B, Swenson RM: Bacteriology of aspiration pneumonia. A prospective study of community and hospital acquired cases. Ann Intern Med 81:329–331, 1974.

65. Thadepalli H, Kannangara DW, Bach VT: Penicillin failure in the treatment of *Bacteroides fragilis* lung abscess. Chemotherapy 29:289–293, 1983.

66. Neild JE, Eykyn SJ, Phillips I: Lung abscess and empyema. Q J Med 57:875–882, 1985.

67. Pena N, Munoz F, Vargas J, Alfageme I, Umbria S, Florez C: Yield of percutaneous needle lung aspiration in lung abscess. Chest 97:69–74, 1990.

68. Guidol F, Manresa F, Pallares R, et al: Clindamycin v. penicillin for anaerobic lung infections. High rate of penicillin failures associated with penicillin-resistant *Bacteroides melanogenicus.* Arch Intern Med 150:2525–2529, 1990.

69. Appelbaum PC, Spangler SK, Jacobs MR: Beta-lactamase production and susceptibilities to amoxicillin, amoxicillin-clavulanate, ticarcillin, ticarcillin-clavulanate, cefoxitin, imipenem and metronidazole of 320 non-*Bacteroides fragilis Bacteroides* isolates and 129 fusobacteria from 28 U.S. centers. Antimicrob Agents Chemother 34:1546, 1990.

70. Shanks GD, Berman JD: Anaerobic pulmonary abscesses. Clin Pediatr 25:520–522, 1986.

71. Brook I, Finegold SM: Bacteriology of aspiration pneumonia in children. Pediatrics 65:1115–1120, 1980.

72. Brook I, Finegold SM: Bacteriology and therapy of lung abscesses in children. J Pediatr 94:10–12, 1979.

73. Bombalaski JS, Phair JP: Alcohol, immunosuppression, and the lung. Arch Intern Med 142:2073, 1982.

74. Broughton WA, Middleton RM, Kirkpatrick MB, Bass JB Jr: Bronchoscopic protected specimen brush and bronchoalveolar lavage in the diagnosis of bacterial pneumonia. Infect Dis Clin North Am 5:437–452, 1991.

75. Wimberley N, Faling LJ, Bartlett JG: A fiberoptic bronchoscopy technique to obtain uncontaminated lower airway secretions for bacterial culture. Am Rev Respir Dis 119:337, 1979.

76. Marquette CH, Georges H, Wallet F, et al: Diagnostic efficiency of endotracheal aspirates with quantitative bacterial cultures in intubated patients with suspected pneumonia. Comparison with the protected specimen brush. Am Rev Respir Dis 148:138–144, 1993.

76a. Roger-Moreau I, de Barbeyrac B, Ducoudre M, et al: Evaluation of bronchoalveolar lavage for the diagnosis of bacterial pneumonia in ventilated patients. Ann Biol Clin 50:587–591, 1992.

76b. Torres A, Martos A, Puig de la Bellacase A, et al: Specificity of endotracheal aspiration, protected specimen brush, and bronchoalveolar lavage in mechanically ventilated patients. Am Rev Respir Dis 147:952–957, 1993.

76c. Morris AJ, Tanner DC, Reller LB: Rejection criteria for endotracheal aspirates from adults. J Clin Microbiol 31:1027–1029, 1993.

76d. Dreyfuss D, Mier L, Le Bourdelles G, et al: Clinical significance of borderline quantitative protected brush specimen culture results. Am Rev Respir Dis 147:946–951, 1993.

77. Kline BS, Berger SS: Pulmonary abscess and pulmonary gangrene. Analysis of ninety cases observed in ten years. Arch Intern Med 56:753–772, 1935.

78. Gorbach SL, Bartlett JG: Anaerobic infections. N Engl J Med 290:1237, 1974.

79. Landay MJ, Christensen EE, Bynum LJ, et al: Anaerobic pleural and pulmonary infections. Am J Roentgenol 134:233, 1980.

80. Gopalakrishna KV, Lerner PI: Primary lung abscess. Analysis of 66 cases. Cleve Clin Q 42:3, 1975.

81. Cameron EWJ, Appelbaum PC, et al: Characteristics and management of chronic destructive pneumonia. Thorax 35:340, 1980.
82. Le Roux BT, Mohlala ML, Odell JA, Whitton ID: Suppurative Diseases of the Lung and Pleural Space. Part 1: Empyema Thoracis and Lung Abscess. Chicago, Year Book Medical Publishers, 1986:44–49.
83. Friedman PJ, Hellekant CAG: Radiologic recognition of bronchopleural fistula. Radiology 124:289–295, 1977.
84. Schachter EN, Kreisman H, Putnam C: Diagnostic problems in suppurative lung disease. Arch Intern Med 136:167–171, 1976.
85. Williford ME, Godwin JD: Computed tomography of lung abscess and empyema. Radiol Clin North Am 21:575–583, 1983.
86. Stark DD, Federle MP, Goodman PC, Podrasky AE, Webb WR: Differentiating lung abscess and empyema: Radiography and computed tomography. Am J Radiol 141:163–167, 1983.
87. Sanders CV, Hanna BJ, Lewis AB: Metronidazole in the treatment of anaerobic infections. Am Rev Respir Dis 120:337, 1979.
88. Perlino CA: Metronidazole vs clindamycin treatment of anaerobic pulmonary infection. Arch Intern Med 141:1424, 1981.
89. Eykyn SJ: The therapeutic use of metronidazole in anaerobic infection: Six years' experience in a London hospital. Surgery 93:209, 1983.
90. Levison ME, Mangura CT, Lorber B, et al: Clindamycin compared with penicillin for the treatment of anaerobic lung abscess. Ann Intern Med 98:466–471, 1983.
91. Gudiol F, Manresa F, Pallares R, et al: Clindamycin v. penicillin for anaerobic lung infections. High rate of penicillin failures associates with penicillin-resistant *Bacteroides melanogenicus*. Arch Intern Med 150:2525–2529, 1990.
92. Cucharal GJ, Snydman DR, McDermott L, et al: Antimicrobial susceptibility patterns of the *Bacteroides fragilis* group in the United States, 1989. Clin Ther 14:122–136, 1992.
93. Weiss W: Oral antibiotic therapy of acute primary lung abscess: Comparison of penicillin and tetracycline. Curr Ther Res 12:154, 1970.
94. Cameron EWJ, Whitton ID: Percutaneous drainage in the treatment of *Klebsiella pneumoniae* lung abscess. Thorax 32:673, 1977.
95. Morris JF, Okies JE: Enterococcal lung abscess: Medical and surgical therapy. Chest 65:688, 1974.
96. Vainrub B, Musher DM, Guinn GA, et al: Percutaneous drainage of lung abscess. Am Rev Respir Dis 117:153, 1978.
97. Keller FS, Rosch J, Barker AF, Dotter CT: Percutaneous interventional catheter therapy for lesions of the chest and lungs. Chest 81:407, 1982.
98. Adebonojo SA, Grillo IA, Osinowo O, Adebo OA: Suppurative diseases of the lung and pleura: A continuing challenge in developing countries. Ann Thorac Surg 33:40–47, 1982.
99. Yellin A, Yellin EO, Lieberman Y: Percutaneous tube drainage: The treatment of choice for refractory lung abscess. Ann Thorac Surg, 39:266–270, 1985.
100. Baker RB: The treatment of lung abscess—current concepts. [Editorial] Chest 87:709–710, 1987.
101. Rice TW, Ginsberg RJ, Todd TR: Tube drainage of lung abscess. Ann Thoracic Surg 44:356–359, 1987.
102. Weissberg B: Percutaneous drainage of lung abscess. J Thorac Cardiovasc Surg 87:308–312, 1984.
103. Mengoli L: Giant lung abscess treated by tube thoracostomy. J Thorac Cardiovasc Surg 90:186–194, 1985.
104. Lorenzo RL, Bradford BF, Black J, Smith CD: Lung abscesses in children: Diagnostic and therapeutic needle aspiration. Radiology 157:79–80, 1985.
105. Snow N, Lucas A, Horrigan TP: Utility of pneumonotomy in the treatment of cavitary lung disease. Chest 87:731–734, 1985.
106. Parker LA, Melton JW, Delany DJ, Yankaskas BC: Percutaneous small bore catheter drainage in the management of lung abscesses. Chest 92:213–218, 1987.
107. Schmitt GS, Ohar JM, Kanter KR, Naunheim KS: Indwelling transbronchial catheter drainage of pulmonary abscess. Ann Thorac Surg 45:43–47, 1988.
108. Cuestas RA, Kienzle GD, Armstrong JD: Percutaneous drainage of lung abscesses in infants. Pediatr Infect Dis J 8:390–392, 1989.
109. Ball WS Jr, Bisset GS 3rd, Towbin RB: Percutaneous drainage of chest abscesses in children. Radiology 171:431–434, 1989.
110. van Sonnenberg E, D'Agostino HB, Casola G, et al: Lung abscess: CT-guided drainage. Radiology 178:347–351, 1991.

# CHAPTER 29

# Community-Acquired Gram-Negative Pneumonias

## HOI HO and ABRAHAM VERGHESE

Aerobic gram-negative organisms have become the most important causes of nosocomial pneumonia. For this reason, much of the literature about gram-negative pneumonia describes infection acquired in hospital settings. Aerobic gram-negative bacillary pneumonias cause a small percentage of all community-acquired pneumonias. *Branhamella (Moraxella) catarrhalis, Legionella* infections, and *Haemophilus influenzae,* all important causes of community-acquired pneumonia resulting from gram-negative organisms, are discussed elsewhere in this book, as are the rare pneumonias associated with tularemia, plague, and melioidosis.

The history of aerobic gram-negative pneumonia is short. Although *Klebsiella* pneumonia had been known for a long time, the description of aerobic gram-negative bacillary pneumonia caused by other enteric organisms emerged in the 1960s, after Jay Sanford and his colleagues at the University of Texas Southwestern Medical School and Tillotson and Lerner at Wayne State University began to describe patients with this syndrome. The observations in the two cities were different: the cases from Texas seemed to be nosocomial, but those from Michigan were community-acquired.[1] Since then, concomitant with the development of more invasive surgery and more potent chemotherapy, gram-negative enteric pneumonia has become synonymous with nosocomial pneumonia and often with pneumonia among patients in intensive care units.

The exact proportion of community-acquired pneumonias caused by gram-negative aerobic bacteria varies from study to study and reflects the method of diagnosis and the location of the study. In some estimates, it is as high as 20%,[2] but in a study from England,[3] *Escherichia coli* accounted for 0.8% of all pneumonias, and no other aerobic gram-negative bacillary organisms were encountered. In the

same study, legionnaires disease accounted for 15% of all community-acquired pneumonias. The picture of community-acquired and nosocomial pneumonia in North America has changed since the early descriptions of Sanford, Tillotson, and Lerner.[1] These changes seem to be related to the aging of the population, a trend to treat many illnesses in the outpatient setting, and an increasing list of antibiotics and other medications that can interfere with host defenses.

A prospective multicenter study[4] of 359 cases of community-acquired pneumonia provides excellent data from a mix of hospitals (eg, veterans hospital, community hospital, university hospital) in Pittsburgh. Aerobic gram-negative rods caused 5.9% of all cases and were ranked fifth behind *Streptococcus pneumoniae, H. influenzae, Legionella* species, and *Chlamydia* pneumonia. Aerobic gram-negative bacilli were relatively uncommon as a group: *Pseudomonas aeruginosa* (7 patients), *E. coli* (4), *Klebsiella* species (3), *Enterobacter cloacae* (2), *Acinetobacter* spp. (1), *Proteus mirabilis* (1), *Providencia* spp. (1), *Pasteurella multocida* (1), and *Acinetobacter* or *Serratia* spp. (1). No seasonal variation was seen for these types of pneumonia. Immunosuppression and malignancy were no more common in this subgroup than in the general population, although patients with gram-negative pneumonia were more likely to have an underlying disease (88.2%) than patients in other subgroups. Prior antibiotic therapy, often mentioned as an important predisposing factor in gram-negative infection, affected 6 of 21 patients with gram-negative community-acquired infection. The percentage of aerobic gram-negative pneumonias among nursing home patients was 10.9%, which was double the incidence among patients not in nursing homes.

It appears from the previously described study, from our experience, and from the general experience of other infec-

**Table 29–1. Enteric Gram-Negative Organisms Causing Community-Acquired Pneumonia**

| Organism | Epidemiology | Clinical Features | X-ray Appearance | Treatment |
|---|---|---|---|---|
| *Klebsiella pneumoniae* | In the past, alcoholics, men, diabetics | In the past, currant jelly sputum, patient critically ill | In the past, bulging fissures | Second- or third-generation cephalosporin |
| *Acinetobacter* | Welders, foundry workers, smokers | Acute onset, shock, hypoxemia; bacteremia common | Unilateral with rapid progression to bilateral | Aminoglycoside, ceftazidime |
| *Escherichia coli* | Urinary or abdominal source; older patients | Not distinctive | Lobar consolidation or patchy broncho-pneumonia | Imipenem Third-generation cephalosporin |
| *Proteus, Serratia, Pseudomonas* | Not distinctive; prior antibiotics and humidifiers may predispose | Not distinctive | Not distinctive | As for nosocomial cases |

tious disease practitioners with an interest in pneumonia (Berk SL, Marrie TJ, Rivera M: personal communication) that the classic descriptions of aerobic gram-negative pneumonia (eg, bulging fissures in *Klebsiella* pneumonia) are no longer common. For instance, alcoholism—a predisposing factor mentioned in all textbooks in the context of *Klebsiella* pneumonia acquired in the community—was a factor for only 1 of 3 patients with *Klebsiella* infection in the Pittsburgh study.[4]

## PATHOPHYSIOLOGY

Knowledge of the epidemiology of gram-negative enteric organisms is useful in postulating the mechanisms by which community-acquired pneumonia occurs with these organisms.

The respiratory tract is vulnerable to infection by aspiration of oropharyngeal organisms,[5] which can overcome local pulmonary defenses and produce pneumonia. However, the oropharynx of the healthy host is typically resistant to colonization by enteric organisms. This resistance is a function of good health.[6, 7] The elegant studies of Valenti and Phair[8, 9] have shown that colonization by enteric organisms occurs as a function of the degree of debility in hospitalized patients. Among healthy hospital personnel, oropharyngeal colonization by gram-negative enteric organisms is rare. Presumably, there is a set of patients in the community who have some of the characteristics of the debilitated hospital patient and may be colonized with potential enteric pathogens. This is particularly true of the nursing home patient. The predisposition of the alcoholic to *Klebsiella* or other gram-negative infections may be related to debility and colonization of the oropharynx by this organism.

Bacteremic spread of gram-negative organisms to the respiratory tree from other sites of infection has been well described, especially from urinary tract. This mechanism appears important for *E. coli* pneumonia.[9a] As the population ages, more men and women with symptomatic or asymptomatic bacteriuria are living in the community.

The aerosol spread of gram-negative pneumonia in the hospital setting has become uncommon because of the precautions and preventive measures instituted in most respiratory therapy units. However, more persons are using respiratory therapy equipment in their homes, and they may

not always follow the same guidelines for cleaning and changing tubes as are recommended in the hospital.

The remainder of this chapter focuses on *Klebsiella pneumoniae, Acinetobacter, E. coli, P. aeruginosa, Proteus,* and *Serratia,* with a brief mention of some of the other pathogens. In many instances, the descriptions from older papers may not be representative of modern clinical experience, and the manifestations of diseases as encountered in this decade are emphasized. Features of each entity are summarized in Table 29–1.

## *KLEBSIELLA PNEUMONIAE* PNEUMONIA

In 1882, Friedlander[10] described what he believed was the causative organism of lobar pneumonia; his findings were based on an autopsy study of 8 patients with acute pneumonia. However, it was soon shown that the pneumococcus and not *Klebsiella* was the main cause of lobar pneumonia, and *Klebsiella* was relegated to the role of secondary invader. A series of reports, particularly that of Solomon, established that the organism was a true pathogen. The incidence of infection with *Klebsiella* showed an increase with the advent of antibiotics,[11] although in the last decade, it seemed again to be less common than reported.

## Clinical Features

The following clinical features are based on early reports of patients primarily from the community. The report of Solomon is particularly detailed and instructive and a reminder to the reader that the disease now rarely takes this form. Men tended to predominate in these reports, and most infections tended to occur in older persons.[12–16] There are several reports suggesting that *Klebsiella* may be an important etiologic agent in nursing homes. Garb and coworkers[17] found *Klebsiella* to be the etiologic agent in 14 (40%) of 35 elderly nursing home residents with pneumonia. Nicolle and colleagues[18] found *Klebsiella* in 63% of patients from whom sputum was obtained, but they did not think it to be more than a colonizer in most patients. Other nursing home studies have suggested that the pneumococcus may be more common. As always with studies of pneumonia, difficulty in differentiating colonization from infection may obscure the true incidence of infection. Alcoholism has long been considered an important preexisting disease[14–16] except possibly in black populations.[19, 20] Chronic lung disease and diabetes mellitus are common underlying conditions mentioned in older series.[21, 22]

The onset of illness is described in the older literature as occurring suddenly and with pleuritic chest pain. Rigors occur in 60% of patients. Blood-tinged sputum is consistently mentioned in many reports; in the "typical" presentation, it is a brick red mixture of sputum and blood that is extremely tenacious and, in its most extreme form, may resemble currant jelly. Solomon wrote that it was "as if the blood and the mucus had been whipped together into a uniform emulsion. In appearance it resembles chocolate pudding, though of a redder hue." According to Solomon, the typical "pneumonic" sputum is "the color of prune juice and is more viscid and ropy, resembling taffy rather than an emulsion."[14]

The patient with the typical syndrome in the past was often quite ill, with fever, dyspnea, and cyanosis. Frank signs of consolidation were present, and involvement of more than one lobe occurred in two thirds of patients. A quarter of these patients had positive blood cultures. The outcome in the early years of experience with this organism was often fatal, and it is worth abstracting from the clinical description by Solomon in 1937: "The clinical course was generally fulminating. Thirty-one of the thirty-two patients died, a mortality rate of approximately 97 percent. Death occurred from the second to the sixteenth day, the average day of death being between the sixth and the seventh day of illness, fatal termination being usually preceded by pulmonary edema."[14]

The radiographic features alone are not sufficiently distinctive to allow *Klebsiella* to be diagnosed with any confidence. Lobar consolidation and lung abscess formation can occur. The "bulging fissure" occurs with more frequency than in other pneumonias.[23] Rapidly progressing necrotizing pneumonia occurs in as many as half of the surviving patients.[24] Complications include the development of pericarditis, meningitis, gastroenteritis, and empyema.[13, 14, 19] Lerner[2] described a chronic, thick-walled, unclosing cavity as a complication of *Klebsiella* infection.

## Diagnosis

The classic clinical picture seems uncommon today, and therefore this disease must be diagnosed by demonstrating the organism on Gram stain and culture of specimens from a patient with a new infiltrate seen on the chest radiograph and with fever and other clinical signs of infection. This disorder must be suspected in the alcoholic or diabetic presenting with tenacious sputum and a dense consolidation. Every effort must be made to obtain sputum in these cases. Typically, the organism appears as a large gram-negative rod, with a refractive zone around it that suggests the presence of a capsule. It grows readily on usual laboratory isolation media for sputum; colonies are characteristically slimy and gray. The methods of diagnosis and the attendant controversies are discussed elsewhere in this book.

## Treatment

The mortality rate for classic *Klebsiella* pneumonia was 51% to 97%.[13, 14, 20] The mortality in the present era is unknown. The cephalosporins are remarkably active against *Klebsiella*. This organism and its syndromes of infection may represent the one true indication for cephalosporins, a setting in which they are the drugs of choice. With increasing use of ceftazidime therapy for multiresistant *Acinetobacter* infections, however, a nosocomial outbreak of *Klebsiella* infections resistant to most third-generation cephalosporins has been reported.[25] Some representative minimal inhibitory concentrations for first-, second-, and third-generation cephalosporins against *Klebsiella* are shown in Table 29–2.[26] It is common practice in treating the seriously ill patient with gram-negative bacillary infection to add a second drug. No evidence exists that this is necessary or even desirable, because the danger of antagonism instead of synergy is real.

## *ACINETOBACTER* PNEUMONIA

*Acinetobacter* is still not a common cause of pneumonia, accounting for only 2 of 359 cases of community-acquired pneumonia in the study by Fang and associates,[4] but notably accounting for 1 of 28 bacteremic patients. *Acinetobacter* species are ubiquitous, nonfermentative, gram-negative bacilli. Previous designations—*Bacterium anitratum, Herellea vaginicola, Achromobacter anitratus, Mima polymorpha*—are a source of confusion. The last name refers to the ability of this small, gram-negative rod to be confused on Gram stain with other organisms, particularly *Neisseria* in cerebrospinal fluid and *H. influenzae* in sputum.

*Acinetobacter* can be isolated from 100% of soil and water samples. It can be found on the skin of 25% of healthy, ambulatory adults, and it is the most common gram-negative organism persistently carried on the skin of adults. Of the two species of *Acinetobacter, lwoffi* has the greatest predilection for the urinary tract, and *anitratus* is isolated from all other sites. Transient colonization of the oropharynx has also been described in 7% of healthy adults.[27]

Rudin and others reviewed their experience with 6 bacteremic cases and reviewed the descriptions in the literature of an additional 6 cases.[28] The 12 patients had a median age of 50 years, and most were men. Alcoholism seemed

Table 29–2. **Susceptibility of *Klebsiella pneumoniae* to Cephalosporins**

| Cephalosporin | Minimal Inhibitory Concentration 90s ($\mu$g/mL) |
|---|---|
| First generation | |
| Cefazolin | 6.0 |
| Second generation | |
| Cefuroxime | 4.0 |
| Cefoxitin | 8.0 |
| Third generation | |
| Ceftazidime | 0.5 |
| Cefoperazone | 4.0 |
| Cefotaxime | 0.25 |

to be the most common underlying disease. The typical presentation was that of an acute pneumonia with fever, pleuritic pain, cough, and shortness of breath for 3 days. All patients were considered seriously ill. Eight patients were hypoxemic, and 7 eventually developed shock. The radiographic picture was unilateral, showing a tendency to progress to bilateral involvement shortly after admission. Pleural effusion appeared to be common (5 of 12 patients), and the organism was recovered on culture. The mortality rate was 43%, and all 5 patients who died had a fulminant course. Inappropriate antibiotic use was associated with death.

*Acinetobacter* pneumonia was also reported in 3 welders in a foundry; all cases were caused by *Acinetobacter* var *anitratus* serotype 7J. Two of the men died, and the autopsy showed pneumoconiosis of dust mixed with iron particles in the lungs. It appears that chronic exposure to such particles may be a predisposing factor to this pneumonia.[29]

A report by Barnes and coworkers[30] describes an unusual experience with pneumonia in general and with *Acinetobacter* in particular. Pneumonia appears to be a common entity in New Guinea, and the researchers were able to identify 5 patients, by a combination of percutaneous lung aspirates and blood cultures in the course of 1 year. The median age was 35 years, and 4 of the 5 patients were smokers or had chronic lung disease. The radiographic pattern was predominantly one of lobar consolidation, and 1 patient developed "bulging fissure." The organism is resistant to penicillin, and both patients who received penicillin alone died; the 3 patients who survived had received gentamicin in addition to penicillin.

A single report of chronic *Acinetobacter* pneumonia[31] with chest wall invasion in a heavy smoker raises the possibility that this organism can cause chronic disease with chest wall involvement in the manner more typical of *Actinomyces*.

## *ESCHERICHIA COLI* PNEUMONIA

Tillotson and Lerner[9a] described 20 patients with *E. coli* pneumonia in 1967. They described the disease as being primarily community acquired (19 of 20 cases). *E. coli* was recovered from the blood of 8 of 18 patients, the pleural fluid of 6 of 7 patients, and the urine of 8 of 13 patients tested. From this report emerged the concept that *E. coli* pneumonia was the result of bacterial seeding of the lung from a gastrointestinal or genitourinary source; 8 patients in the series were thought to have a source in the kidney. The infiltrates were primarily in the lower lobe, often with metapneumonic empyemas.

Berk and colleagues,[32] almost 15 years later, described a series of well-documented *E. coli* pneumonias in elderly men. They found 8 of their 17 patients to have community-acquired infection; the presence of the K1 capsular polysaccharide seemed to correlate with community acquisition of pneumonia. The average age of patients was in the early 1970s—an older age group than in Tillotson and Lerner's series—and all patients had some underlying disease. In contrast to the series by Tillotson and Lerner, chest radiographs showed patchy bronchopneumonias in most patients, with consolidation a less common feature. Two patients

with non-K1 disease developed cavitation of the lungs. Six patients had a history of underlying urinary tract disease. The study confirmed the report of Tillotson and Lerner of an association with a gastrointestinal or urinary source.

Jonas and Cunha[33] reviewed 9 cases of bacteremic *E. coli* pneumonia and found their patients to have a mean age of 67 years. The lobar picture on the chest radiograph was similar to that described by Tillotson and Lerner. The fatal outcome of 8 of the 9 patients suggests that this is a disease with a high mortality rate. Clinical suspicion should be aroused when a patient with a known genitourinary source or abdominal source of infection then develops a pulmonary infiltrate.

## *PROTEUS* PNEUMONIA

The organisms of the genus *Proteus* are ubiquitous and can be isolated from human feces, manure, and sewage. Even though all three strains of the genus *Proteus* are human pathogens, *P. mirabilis* is the most commonly identified organism in pulmonary infections compared with *P. vulgaris* and *P. (Morganella) morganii*.[34]

In 1894, *P. vulgaris* was first reported by Reed as the etiologic agent in a case of pneumonia.[35] Most lower respiratory tract infections caused by *Proteus* are nosocomial infections.[36] Like other enteric bacteria, this organism is still a rare cause of community-acquired pneumonia. Fang and associates identified 1 case (0.3%) of *Proteus* pneumonia in 359 cases of community-acquired pneumonia.[4] Similarly, in a prospective study, Woodhead found only 1 case (0.4%) of *Proteus* pneumonia in 238 episodes of lower respiratory tract infection.[37]

The comprehensive 1968 report of Tillotson and Lerner is one of the few available descriptions of community-acquired *Proteus* pneumonia.[38] In this study, during a 30-month surveillance of pneumonia caused by gram-negative bacilli at the Detroit General Hospital, 6 (7.3%) of 82 patients were found to have *Proteus* pneumonia. The mean age of patients was 59, and there was a predominance of black men among the patients. They all had chronic lung diseases, and most were alcoholics. Antibiotic administration before admission was not reported for any of the 6 patients. Most of these patients had bronchitic complaints, with sudden worsening of respiratory symptoms a few days before hospitalization. Chills, fever, dyspnea, tenacious yellow sputum, and pleuritic chest pain were frequently present. Physical examination revealed signs of pulmonary consolidation and of tracheal deviation to the affected site in most of the patients with upper lobe pneumonia.

The radiographically demonstrated infiltrates involved the dependent regions of both lower lobes, with multiple, small cavitations described.[39] In some patients, these progressed to larger cavities. Pneumatocele formation was rare but was reported in a few patients.[40, 41] Pleural effusion or empyema was observed in approximately one third of the patients with *Proteus* pneumonia.[35, 39] This complication is thought to be less frequent than that caused by *E. coli* (40%) or *Pseudomonas* (80%).[2] Because *P. vulgaris* and *P. mirabilis* have urease enzymes and can split urea to form ammonia, body fluid infected with these organisms may have an elevated pH. In patients with *Proteus* empyema, this finding does not preclude the indication for thoracotomy, which often expects a low pH of the pleural fluid.[42, 43] The predominant pathologic feature of *Proteus* pneumonia is multiple lung cavitations, in which the cavities are irregularly interspersed within the diseased lung.[39]

The mortality rate was 17% in Tillotson and Lerner's study and 75% in the report by Unger and associates. This striking difference is probably related to the nosocomial setting of the second group.

## *SERRATIA* PNEUMONIA

*Serratia* is a motile, aerobic, gram-negative bacillus, a member of the division *Klebsiella-Enterobacter-Serratia*. There are three species in the *Serratia* group: *S. marcescens, S. liquefaciens,* and *S. rubidaea.*

Once considered a harmless saprophyte, *S. marcescens* is now recognized as an important pathogen of nosocomial infections in general and of bacteremic gram-negative pneumonia in particular.[44–47] Although contaminated saline solutions from nebulizers or respiratory equipment have been associated with hospital infections, they have not been linked to community-acquired *Serratia* pneumonia. *Serratia* is rarely isolated from oropharyngeal secretions in the alcoholic or diabetic.[48, 49] However, these organisms may colonize the upper airways of elderly nursing home residents, especially those who have previously received antibiotics.[5, 50]

Community-acquired *Serratia* pneumonia remains a rare clinical entity. Fang and associates[4] had only 1 patient (0.3%) with *Serratia* pneumonia of 359 cases of community-acquired pneumonia. However, in another study of 17 patients with community-acquired, gram-negative pneumonia documented by transtracheal aspirates, Karnad found 2 cases (12%) of *Serratia* pneumonia.[36] Metz reported a series of 5 patients with *Serratia* pneumonia, all presenting a typical picture of bacterial pneumonia with fever, chills, and productive cough.[46] Only 1 patient had hemoptysis. Although pseudohemoptysis was mentioned in isolated case reports,[51] it was absent in this series of patients, despite the fact that three of five isolates were pigmented *Serratia* strains.

Chest radiographs frequently showed patchy bronchial pneumonia,[44] with diffuse bilateral infiltrates occurring in more than half of the cases. Lung abscesses were not observed in Metz's series, but they were reported for 5 of 18 patients in Balikian's study.[44]

Pleural effusion was found in more than one third of the patients, and the pleural fluid could be hemorrhagic.[46] The common pathologic finding was focal bronchial pneumonia with multiple microabscesses.[46]

The mortality rate of *Serratia* pneumonia is high (approaching 80%), and this is probably related to the underlying diseases (eg, cardiovascular disease, malignancy, multiple organ failure) and to the multiple antibiotic resistance of *Serratia*. Treatment of this infection is the same as for nosocomial pneumonia.

## *PSEUDOMONAS AERUGINOSA* PNEUMONIA

*P. aeruginosa* is dealt with in more detail in the section on nosocomial pneumonia. It is primarily found in patients

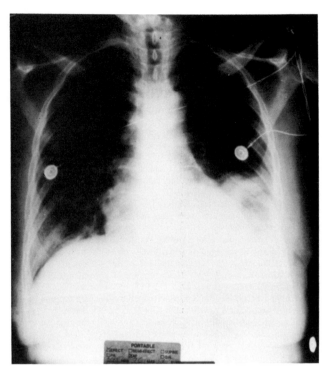

**Figure 29–1.** Patient with a left lower lobe infiltrate and bacteremic *Pseudomonas aeruginosa* pneumonia.

with compromised host defense systems (eg, neutropenia, mechanical ventilation, burns, cystic fibrosis). In the survey from Pittsburgh,[4] *Pseudomonas* accounted for 7 (1.9%) of 359 cases of community-acquired pneumonia. In the 1966 paper by Tillotson and Lerner,[9a] *P. aeruginosa* pneumonia was reported to be more common in summer or autumn. The mortality rate for *Pseudomonas* pneumonia in this series was higher (72%) than for other gram-negative organisms, and at autopsy, a striking acute hepatitis with polymorphonuclear leukocytic infiltrates was described in 2 fatal cases. Walled-off loci of dense collections of neutrophils were also described. In a case of community-acquired *P. aeruginosa* pneumonia associated with the use of a humidifier at home,[52] the patient had a long history of asthma. He had a left lower lobe infiltrate with a small pleural effusion, and cultures of sputum, pleural fluid, and blood all grew the organism. The humidifier, which was extremely dirty, grew the same strain of *P. aeruginosa*. Other cases of community-acquired infection that have been reported in the literature have been associated with cystic fibrosis, severe combined immunodeficiency syndrome, and chronic granulomatous disease.

Treatment of *P. aeruginosa* pneumonia is the same as for nosocomial cases.

Figure 29–1 shows a chest radiograph of an intravenous drug user who presented with fulminant community-acquired *P. aeruginosa* pneumonia.

## REFERENCES

1. Lerner AM: Gram-negative bacillary pneumonias. *In* Weinstein L, Fields BN (eds): Seminars in Infectious Disease, vol 5. New York, Thieme-Stratton, 1983:159–170.

2. Lerner AM: The gram-negative bacillary pneumonias. Dis Mon 27:1, 1980.

3. Macfarlane JT, Finch RG, Ward MJ, Macrae AD: Hospital study of adult community-acquired pneumonia. Lancet 2:255–258, 1982.

4. Fang GD, Fine M, Orloff J, et al: New and emerging etiologies for community acquired pneumonia with implications for therapy. A prospective multicenter study of 359 cases. Medicine (Baltimore) 69:307–316, 1990.

5. Verghese A, Berk SL: Bacterial pneumonia in the elderly. Medicine (Baltimore) 62:271–285, 1983.

6. Johanson WG Jr, Woods DE, Chaudhuri T: Association of respiratory tract colonization with adherence of gram-negative bacilli to epithelial cells. J Infect Dis 139:667–273, 1979.

7. Johanson WG Jr, Higuchi JH, Chaudhuri TR, et al: Bacterial adherence to epithelial cells in bacillary colonization of the respiratory tract. Am Rev Respir Dis 121:55, 1980.

8. Valenti WM, Trudell RG, Bentley DW: Factors predisposing to oropharyngeal colonization with gram-negative bacilli in the aged. N Engl J Med 298:1108, 1978.

9. Phair JP, Kauffman CA, Bjornson A: Investigation of host defense mechanisms in the aged as determinants of nosocomial colonization and pneumonia. J Reticuloendothel Soc 23:397, 1978.

9a. Tillotson JR, Lerner AM: Characteristics of pneumonias caused by *Escherichia coli*. N Engl J Med 277:115–122, 1967.

10. Friedlander C: Ueber die Schizomyceten bei der acuten fibrosen Pneumonie. Arch Pathol Anat Physiol Klin Med 87:319, 1882.

11. Pierce AK, Sanford JP: State of the art: Aerobic gram-negative bacillary pneumonias. Am Rev Respir Dis 110:647–658, 1974.

12. Edmondson EB, Sanford JP: The *Klebsiella-Enterobacter (Aerobacter)-Serratia* group. A clinical and bacteriological evaluation. Medicine (Baltimore) 46:323, 1967.

13. Hyde L, Hyde B: Primary Friedlander pneumonia. Am J Med Sci 205:660, 1943.

14. Solomon S: Primary Friedlander pneumonia. JAMA 108:937, 1937.

15. Limson BM, Romansky MJ, Shea JG: An evaluation of twenty-two patients with acute and chronic pulmonary infection with Friedlander's bacillus. Ann Intern Med 44:1070–1081, 1956.

16. Manfredi F, Daly WJ, Behnke RH: Clinical observations of acute Friedlander pneumonia. Ann Intern Med 58:642–653, 1963.

17. Garb JL, Brown RB, Garb JR, et al: Differences in etiology of pneumonias in nursing home and community patients. JAMA 240:2169–2172, 1978.

18. Nicolle LE, McIntyre M, Zacharias H, et al: Twelve-month surveillance of infections in institutionalized elderly men. J Am Geriatr Soc 32:513–519, 1984.

19. Bullowa JGM, Chess J, Friedman NB: Pneumonia due to *Bacillus friedlanderi*. Arch Intern Med 60:735, 1937.

20. Weiss W, Eisenberg GM, Alexander JD Jr, Flippin HF: *Klebsiella* pulmonary disease. Am J Med Sci 228:148–155, 1954.

21. Wylie RH, Kirschner PA: Friedlander's pneumonia. Am Rev Tuberc 61:465, 1950.

22. Holmes BR: Friedlander's pneumonia. Am J Roentgenol 75:728–747, 1956.

23. Felson B, Rosenberg LS, Hamburger M Jr: Roentgen findings in acute Friedlander's pneumonia. Radiology 53:559–565, 1949.

24. Kirby WMM, Coleman DH: Antibiotic therapy of Friedlander's pneumonia. Am J Med 11:179–187, 1951.·

25. Meyer KS, Urban C, Eagan JA, Berger BJ, Rahal JJ: Nosocomial outbreak of *Klebsiella* infection resistant to late-generation cephalosporins. Ann Intern Med 119:353–358, 1993.

26. Donowitz GR, Mandell GL: Cephalosporins. *In* Mandell GL, Douglas RG, Bennett JE (eds): Principles and Practice of Infectious Diseases. New York, Churchill Livingstone, 1990:246.

27. Rosenthal S, Tager IB: Prevalence of gram-negative rods in the normal pharyngeal flora. Ann Intern Med 83:355–357, 1975.

28. Rudin ML, Michael JR, Huxley EJ: Community acquired acinetobacter pneumonia Am J Med 67:39–43, 1979.

29. Cordes LG, Brink EW, Checko PJ, et al: A cluster of *Acinetobacter* pneumonia in foundry workers. Ann Intern Med 95:688–693, 1981.

30. Barnes DJ, Naraqi S, Igo JD: Community acquired *Acinetobacter* pneumonia in adults in Papua New Guinea. Rev Infect Dis 10:636–639, 1988.

31. Suchyta MR, Peters JI, Black RD: Case report: Chronic *Acinetobacter calcoaceticus* var *anitratus* pneumonia. Am J Med Sci 294:117–119, 1987.

32. Berk SL, Neumann P, Holtsclaw S, Smith JK: *Escherichia coli* pneumonia in the elderly. With reference to the role of K1 capsular polysaccharide antigen. Am J Med 72:899–902, 1982.

33. Jonas M, Cunha BA: Bacteremic *Escherichia coli* pneumonia. Arch Intern Med 142:2157–2159, 1982.

34. Adler JL, Burke JP, Martin DF, et al: *Proteus* infections in a general hospital. I. Biochemical characteristics and antibiotic susceptibility of the organisms. Ann Intern Med 75:517–530, 1971.

35. Reed W: Association of *Proteus vulgaris* and *Diplococcus lanceolatus* in a case of croupous pneumonia. Johns Hopkins Hosp Bull 5:24, 1894.

36. Karnad A, Alvarez S, Berk SL: Pneumonia caused by gram-negative bacilli. Am J Med 79:61–67, 1985.

37. Woodhead MA, Macfarlane JT, McCracken JS: Prospective study of the aetiology and outcome of pneumonia in the community. Lancet 1:671–674, 1987.

38. Tillotson JR, Lerner AM: Characteristics of pneumonia caused by *Bacillus proteus*. Ann Intern Med 68:287, 1968.

39. Unger JD, Rose HD, Unger GF: Gram-negative pneumonia. Radiology 107:283–291, 1973.

40. Lysy J, Werezberger A, Globus M, et al: Pneumatocele formation in a patient with *Proteus mirabilis* pneumonia. Postgrad Med 61:255, 1985.

41. Thapa BR, Kumar L, Mitra SK: *Proteus mirabilis* pneumonia with giant pneumatocele. Indian J Pediatr 54:593–597, 1987.

42. Isenstein D, Honig E: *Proteus vulgaris* empyema and increased pleural fluid pH. Chest 97:511, 1990.

43. Pine JR, Hollman JL: Elevated pleural fluid pH in *Proteus mirabilis* empyema. Chest 84:109–111, 1983.

44. Balikian JP, Herman PG, Godleski JJ: *Serratia* pneumonia. Radiology 137:309–311, 1980.

45. Yu VL: *Serratia marcescens*: Historical perspective and clinical review. N Engl J Med 300:887–893, 1979.

46. Meltz DJ, Grieco MH: Characteristics of *Serratia marcescens* pneumonia. Arch Intern Med 132:359–364, 1973.

47. Wilkowske CJ, Washington JA, Martin WJ, Ritts RE: *Serratia marcescens*: Biochemical characteristics, antibiotic susceptibility patterns, and clinical significance. JAMA 214:2157–2162, 1970.

48. Fuxench-Lopez Z: Pharyngeal flora in ambulatory alcoholic patients: prevalence of gram-negative bacilli. Arch Intern Med 138:1815–1816, 1978.

49. Mackowiak PA, Martin RM, Smith JW: The role of bacterial interference in the increased prevalence of oropharyngeal gram-negative bacilli among alcoholics and diabetics. Am Rev Respir Dis 120:589–593, 1979.

50. Tillotson JR, Finland M: Bacterial colonization and clinical superinfection of the respiratory tract complicating antibiotic treatment of pneumonia. J Infect Dis 119:597–624, 1969.

51. Robinson W, Wooley PB: Pseudohemoptysis due to *Chromobacterium prodigiosum*. Lancet 1:819, 1957.

52. Harris AA, Goodman L, Levin S: Community acquired *Pseudomonas aeruginosa* pneumonia associated with the use of a home humidifier. West J Med 141:521–523, 1984.

# CHAPTER 30

# Pseudomonal Infections of the Lung

MARC M. DUNN

## PSEUDOMONAS AERUGINOSA

### Bacteriology

*Pseudomonas aeruginosa* is a motile, gram-negative, aerobic rod. It belongs to the family Pseudomoniae along with *Pseudomonas cepacia,* another bacterial species pathogenic for humans. It has minimal specific growth conditions and grows in a variety of media, but *P. aeruginosa* does not ferment sugar. Usually an obligate aerobe, this organism can grow anaerobically if nitrates are available, its growth requirements are so minimal that it is capable of growing in distilled water, and it is hardy enough to grow in the presence of some disinfectants.[1] Genetic recombination occurs through conjugation, transduction, and transformation.[1] Although it grows optimally at 37° to 42°C, it may also grow at temperatures between 20° and 37°C.[2] Approximately half of the strains produce pyocyanin, a pigment that is relatively specific for *P. aeruginosa.*

Mucoid strains of *P. aeruginosa* are prevalent in cystic fibrosis (CF), and the production of this material is phage-dependent and easily lost in culture.[3] Gene activation for alginate production partially depends on high osmolarity, a condition affecting the airways of CF patients, and may predispose to colonization with these *Pseudomonas* variants. This mucoid or alginate substance is a polyanionic, heteropolymeric polysaccharide composed of mannuronic and glucuronic acids, and it covers microcolonies of *P. aeruginosa* in the airways of CF patients. Other strains of *P. aeruginosa* found in the sputum of CF patients frequently have unusual traits, including serum sensitivity and rough colony formation.[4–7] Rough strains lack the extensive O side chain moiety of the lipopolysaccharide molecule.

### Epidemiology

*P. aeruginosa* is a ubiquitous resident in the hospital and in the outside environment. Moisture is a requirement for its growth. It has been isolated from soil, animals, plants, and water, and in the hospital environment, it has been identified in respiratory therapy equipment, disinfectants, sinks, mops, flowers, and vegetables.

Colonization of the respiratory tract in humans depends on the clinical setting. The throats of only 0% to 6% of healthy persons are colonized by gram-negative bacteria.[8] Several factors place specific subgroups of patients at risk for pulmonary colonization and infection with *P. aeruginosa,* including CF, bronchiectasis, certain malignancies, neutropenia, glucocorticoid therapy, use of broad-spectrum antibiotics, and use of respiratory therapy equipment.[2] Nebulizers are particularly likely to harbor gram-negative bacteria,[9] but with greater attention to the sterility of respiratory therapy equipment, there has been a decrease in the incidence of gram-negative nosocomial pneumonia from this source.

Most respiratory infections with *P. aeruginosa* are nosocomially acquired, with the exception of those involving CF patients. Within the hospital, *P. aeruginosa* is the most common bacterial cause of pneumonia,[10] reflecting this organism's hardiness and ability to capitalize on breakdowns in human antimicrobial defenses.

### Pathogenesis

The success of *P. aeruginosa* as a respiratory pathogen depends on alterations in host defenses and the bacteria's ability to adapt itself to diverse environmental conditions.

Lower respiratory tract infections caused by *P. aeruginosa* can be acquired through several routes: hematogenous, aerosol, direct inoculation from medical personnel into an endotracheal tube, or aspiration from the oropharynx. In all of these instances, alteration or evasion of the usual defense mechanisms occurs. Hematogenously acquired infection usually follows a high degree of inoculum seeding of the bloodstream in the immunocompromised patient. Pneumonia acquired through aerosol transmission is usually the result of contamination of respiratory therapy equipment, including ventilators, used by relatively immunocompromised patients. These patients frequently have underlying chronic illnesses and iatrogenic compromise of pulmonary defenses, such as placement of endotracheal tubes and administration of broad-spectrum antibiotics.

Endotracheal tubes may predispose patients to *Pseudomonas* pulmonary infections by damaging the respiratory epithelium near the distal end of the tube. A biofilm consisting of bacteria accumulates on the inner surface of endotracheal tubes.[11] Contaminated material can then be detached during mechanical ventilation. This is a time-related phenomenon; the biofilm accumulation increases with longer tube placement.

The more common pathogenic sequence for the development of *Pseudomonas* pneumonia in nonintubated patients without CF is colonization of the oropharynx followed by aspiration of contaminated secretions. This sequence depends on complex alterations in host defenses and specific contributions from *P. aeruginosa* that result in clinical infection.

Colonization of the oropharynx is a process that occurs after alteration of the adherence properties of the airway epithelium[12] or loss of the epithelial lining as a precondition for surface growth of *Pseudomonas* organisms. Increased adherence of *P. aeruginosa* to the oropharyngeal respiratory epithelium appears to follow the loss of fibronectin from the surface of these cells, although this concept has been challenged.[13, 14] This loss appears to be the result of increased salivary protease activity in the upper airway.[15]

A variety of clinical conditions increase the likelihood of *Pseudomonas* colonization of the upper airways. These include altered mental status, hypotension, acidosis, azotemia, and alteration in the leukocyte count.[9] Airway intubation is also associated with an increased frequency of gram-negative adherence to tracheal cells[16] and with colonization of the respiratory tract, especially the lower tract.[17] Increased adherence to tracheal epithelial cells is particularly likely in poorly nourished patients with tracheostomies.[18] *P. aeruginosa* has relatively poor avidity for unaltered epithelium, although it can adhere to normal tracheal ciliated epithelial cells. It is likely that most instances of colonization are preceded by alterations or damage to the upper respiratory tract epithelium. It appears that mechanical trauma during intubation may result in denudation of the epithelial surface and exposure of a distinct receptor that is partially carbohydrate in nature.[19] In this setting, adherence is followed by rapid growth in situ.

The exact nature of the receptor for *P. aeruginosa* in the upper respiratory tract epithelium remains unclear. *Pseudomonas* organisms bind to glycosphingolipids including gangliotriaosylceramide and gangliotetraosylceramide.[20, 21] Some strains of *Pseudomonas* also bind to sialic acids or lactosylceramide residues.[21] Different receptor components may be involved in different cells or stages of cellular differentiation.

The most likely mechanism of *Pseudomonas* adherence to the respiratory epithelium is through bacterial pili,[22–24] although many other adhesins probably exist. The pili are located on the pole of the bacterium and appear to confer intracellular survival advantages to bacteria possessing them.[20] Other components, including exoenzyme S, of the bacterial surface probably augment binding to epithelial cell surfaces.[25] The properties of motility may be important, at least initially, in *Pseudomonas* adherence. Most *Pseudomonas* strains contain flagella at the time of colonization, and this may increase contact with epithelial cells.[26, 27]

The early events in the pathogenesis of *P. aeruginosa* respiratory tract infections in CF patients are similar to the events in nosocomial pneumonia. However, the interactions between *P. aeruginosa* and the airway are more complex because of additional factors, including the mucoid exopolysaccharide of *Pseudomonas* and the augmentation of an airway lectin. It also appears that there is increased binding of *P. aeruginosa* to CF epithelium compared with normal epithelium. This may be caused by increased receptor density on CF epithelial cells. There may also be qualitative differences in receptors between CF and normal cells.[28]

The colonizing strains of *P. aeruginosa* in CF patients are predominantly mucoid. The mucoid exopolysaccharide (ie, alginate) may offer a selective advantage to the organism by augmenting the binding of these bacteria to the upper airway surface.[23] Mucoexopolysaccharide adheres to the epithelial membrane,[23, 29] but alginate and pili adhere to airway mucins.[30–33] *N*-acetylneuraminic acid and *N*-acetylglucosamine are among the components of mucin that adhere to *P. aeruginosa*.

The lungs of patients with CF are coated extracellularly and intracellularly with a heparin lectin that adheres to alginate.[34] This lectin is also present in normal lungs, but it is more prominent in patients with CF. The increased avidity of mucoid *Pseudomonas* for the airway epithelium in CF patients may add to its pathogenicity. However, the binding to airway mucus or secretions has the potential for beneficial or detrimental effects. If mucociliary clearance is unimpaired, this binding may hasten the clearance of *Pseudomonas*. However, if mucociliary flow is impaired, as in CF, adherence to airway secretions may increase the local bacterial population. Airway mucins or *Pseudomonas* exopolysaccharide may also coat the bacteria, making them less susceptible to normal host defense mechanisms. Mucin has other properties that may enhance *Pseudomonas'* ability to colonize the airways of the CF patient. For example, several of the amino acids in mucin are chemotactic for *P. aeruginosa*,[35] and mucin can serve as a source of nutrition, providing nitrogen and carbon for the bacteria.[35]

*P. aeruginosa* produces a number of substances that contribute to its virulence in the lung. Perhaps the best characterized of these substances is exotoxin A. Exotoxin A inhibits protein synthesis in a manner similar to diphtheria toxin, by inhibiting the enzymatic transfer of the adenine diphosphate ribosyl moiety of NAD to mammalian elongation factor 2.[36, 37] Most clinical strains of *P. aeruginosa* produce and release exotoxin A,[38] and cellular cytotoxicity induced by exotoxin A has been demonstrated in vitro. Exotoxin A has been demonstrated to be a virulence factor in animal models of acute and chronic *Pseudomonas* pneumonia.[39, 40] Exoenzyme S is another protease with properties similar to those of exotoxin A,[41] and its role as a virulence factor in experimental *Pseudomonas* pneumonia has also been demonstrated.

Other *Pseudomonas* products can be grouped according to category and include proteases, cytotoxins, hemolysins, and pigments. The proteases include elastase and alkaline protease. *Pseudomonas* elastase is a metalloproteinase with elastolytic and collagenolytic properties, able to degrade human lung elastin,[42] laminin, and types III and IV collagen.[43] This probably results in the noticeable tissue destruction seen with *Pseudomonas* pneumonia[44–46] and may increase the propensity for systemic invasion with this organism. *Pseudomonas* elastase can also degrade bronchial mucus inhibitor, $\alpha_1$-protease inhibitor, and $\alpha_2$-macroglobulin.[29] In this way, it may augment the autolytic activity of phagocytic proteases. *Pseudomonas* elastase may also cleave IgG, resulting in ineffectual binding of intact IgG to phagocyte Fc receptors.[47] This effect and its ability to cleave complement components C3 and C5 result in impairment of the local immune response directed against *P. aeruginosa* and may contribute to the persistence of this organism in CF airways.[29] The tenacity of the organism is aided by the ability of its elastase to disrupt respiratory cilia.[48] This results in immobility of respiratory secretions and promotes colonization by *Pseudomonas*. Alkaline protease is less well studied but appears to share some of the properties of elastase.[36, 43, 44]

*P. aeruginosa* produces at least three hemolysins. Phospholipase C is a heat labile protein that acts on phosphatidylcholine,[36] a compound that comprises approximately 75% of surfactant. Phospholipase C may alter the physiologic characteristics of lung units during *Pseudomonas* pneumonia. Phospholipase C hydrolyzes other phospholipids into diacylglycerol and phosphorylcholine.[1] These phospholipids, including phosphatidylcholine, lysophosphatidylcholine, and sphingomyelin, occur in cell membranes, and degradation of these components may result in alteration of cellular function. Rhamnolipid, a hemolytic glycolipid, also produces ciliostasis and cell membrane damage, as well as having mucus-secretagogue properties.[49] Cytotoxin, a 25-kd protein, is cytotoxic for most cells and can induce pulmonary edema and elevated pulmonary artery pressure in isolated lung models.[45, 50]

*P. aeruginosa* produces several pigments with biologic properties that may add to bacterial virulence, including pyocyanin, pyoverdin, and hydroxyphenazine. Pyocyanin and 1-hydroxyphenazine are cilioinhibitory in vitro.[49, 51] Pyocyanin may also have antibiotic activity favoring the growth of *Pseudomonas* rather than other bacteria in some circumstances.[1, 2, 52] Pyocyanin and 1-hydroxyphenazine may also augment certain neutrophilic functions, including superoxide production and lysozyme release, but decrease the release of lipoxygenase products.

The combined effect of these products may include inhibition of the mucociliary, phagocytic, and inflammatory properties of the lung. In the appropriate setting, this may help *Pseudomonas* to persist in the bronchiectatic lung, in association with CF, or in overwhelming infection, with dissemination in acute *Pseudomonas* pneumonia.

## Infectious Manifestations

### Pathology

*P. aeruginosa* is among the bacteria that cause necrosis of the lung. Microscopic foci of necrosis and alveolar hemorrhage are observed in acute infections,[36, 53] and the alveolar septa may be destroyed or fragmented. In well-developed infections, microabscesses form, and the inflammatory cells consist of monocytes and lymphocytes. There is a prominent vascular component in well-developed pneumonia, with colonies of gram-negative bacteria in the septa and walls of small arteries and veins, and vasculitis, with necrosis and scarring, can be found in the wall of the vessel. This is also associated with cytolysis of all vascular wall components, but there is a surprisingly small inflammatory component within the vessel.

Early pathologic events are distinct from the stage of advanced pneumonia, with an early and pronounced neutrophilic alveolitis after aerosol or intrabronchial challenge with *P. aeruginosa* in animal models.[54, 55] Complement, especially C5a, is at least partially responsible for the recruitment of these neutrophils to the lung.[56] Furthermore, these cells are crucial for pulmonary defense against *P. aeruginosa*.[57] The mononuclear infiltrate probably follows the initial acute neutrophilic alveolitis of *Pseudomonas* pneumonia.

The bronchial lesion in CF is characterized by peribronchial inflammation and inflammation within the lumen.[58] Ciliary loss within the airway is evident, as is goblet cell hyperplasia, but the alveoli are relatively spared. Other findings include bronchiectasis, mucopurulent plugging, and epithelial metaplasia.[59]

### Physiology

Information about the physiologic changes occurring during *Pseudomonas* pneumonia has been largely derived from animal studies. Models of acute bilateral pneumonia demonstrate loss of lung volume, including decreased functional residual capacity and total lung capacity.[60] Compliance decreases but is related to the decreased lung volumes. Hypoxemia is routine because of considerable shunting and ventilation-perfusion mismatch,[60, 61] and this is further accentuated by some component of paresis of hypoxic vasoconstriction. If the animals become septic, the expected hemodynamics of increased cardiac index, decreased systemic vascular resistance, and decreased systemic arterial pressure ensue. Chronic models of *Pseudomonas* pneumonia are associated with decreased hypoxic vasoreactivity and with elevations of pulmonary arterial pressure as the infection becomes established.[62] The abnormal pulmonary vasoreactivity appears to be related to prostaglandin production.

### Clinical Features

Pneumonia caused by *P. aeruginosa* shares features with that caused by a number of other gram-negative bacilli. It is a more common etiologic agent for pneumonia than the other members of its family, however, and is one of the most common organisms responsible for nosocomial pneumonia.[63, 64] The organism commonly preys on immunocompromised persons, including those with leukemia and solid malignancies,[65] and those with other underlying illnesses such as alcoholism, heart disease, renal disease, or diabetes mellitus and those on corticosteroid therapy.[9]

There are no specific hallmarks of *Pseudomonas* pneumonia. Associated symptoms and signs include apprehension, confusion, and cyanosis,[9] and as with other bacterial pneumonias, fever, chills, tachypnea, and dyspnea are common. Cough usually produces purulent sputum. An alteration of diurnal temperature patterns, with a peak in the morning, has been described.[9, 53]

The chest roentgenogram is nonspecific; descriptions have included patchy infiltrates, diffuse bronchopneumonia, and nodular infiltrates.[53, 66] The necrotizing and vasocentric properties of the organism may account for some radiographic features. Nodules may increase in size, combine, and form abscesses. *Pseudomonas* pneumonia is usually multilobar and frequently involves the lower lobes.[9] There is no evidence that nosocomial pneumonia due to *P. aeruginosa* is radiologically distinct from that caused by other bacteria. Pleural effusions are common, and empyema formation has also been associated with *Pseudomonas* pneumonia, but the frequency with which this occurs is unknown.

Even within the realm of nosocomial or gram-negative bacterial pneumonia, *P. aeruginosa* is particularly virulent, partially because of some of the exoproducts mentioned earlier. Mortality rates of approximately 70% have been reported,[62, 65] and because the illness is frequently fulminant, there is little time for antibiotic therapy to take effect. Findings associated with mortality include azotemia, abnormal hepatic function, leukopenia, and bacteremia.[53, 63, 66] In particular, bacteremia or a peripheral leukocyte count of less than 4000/mm$^3$ is associated with almost uniform fatality.

The usual *Pseudomonas* lower respiratory tract infection in CF patients is indolent, unlike the acute pneumonia described earlier. The mortality rate associated with a single episode of a *Pseudomonas* pulmonary infection is low. It is often difficult to differentiate colonization, acute bronchitis, and pneumonia in these patients. A quarter of affected children are colonized before their first year of life, and 50% to 70% are colonized by 7 years of age.[63, 67] Intermittent colonization by *P. aeruginosa* precedes the chronic colonization that is so common in those with CF. The strains of *P. aeruginosa* colonizing the airways of CF patients usually revert to mucoid forms.

The clinical effects of *P. aeruginosa* in CF patients can be divided into those resulting from acute infection and those producing long-term effects. Acute exacerbations are frequently characterized by increasing sputum production, tachypnea, progressive dyspnea, or rales.[68] These episodes rarely result in more fulminant pneumonia. Recurrent infections and chronic carriage of *P. aeruginosa* result in long-term clinical deterioration. The long-term prognosis of CF patients is worse if their disease is associated with early colonization by *Pseudomonas*, which causes more rapid pulmonary function deterioration.[69, 70] The prognosis is also worse with high and progressively increasing serum levels of precipitins to *Pseudomonas* (which suggest a higher bacterial burden),[70] high or rising antibody titers to *Pseudomonas* proteases,[71] or the transition from colonization by a nonmucoid to a mucoid *Pseudomonas* variant.[29] *P. aerugi-*

*nosa* is responsible for acute infections in the CF patient and is intimately related to the chronic destruction that occurs in CF airways.

## Treatment

Treatment of acute pneumonia caused by *P. aeruginosa* requires antibiotics and supportive care. Generally, two antibiotics with antipseudomonal activity are given parenterally. The use of two antipseudomonal antibiotics for patients with *Pseudomonas* pneumonia and bacteremia has been associated with a significant improvement in survival compared with a single agent. This trend has persisted in patients with *Pseudomonas* who were neutropenic.[72] Aminoglycosides and antipseudomonal penicillins have been used, but a variety of agents of other classes are available. Antibiotic selection should be based on in vitro sensitivities of the isolated strain of *P. aeruginosa*. However, there is some question about any relation between in vitro antibiotic sensitivity of *P. aeruginosa* and survival of the patient. Combination therapy with two antibiotics remains the preferred approach.

The therapeutic approach to *Pseudomonas* infections in CF patients is more complex and controversial. Clinical pneumonia should be treated in the same manner as pneumonia in patients without CF. However, most antibiotics have a decreased half-life in CF patients, and higher doses are usually required for bactericidal serum levels to be achieved.[73] Guidelines for the treatment of exacerbations of chronic bronchiectasis are more problematic. There are at least three possible goals that have been addressed when approaching such exacerbations: eradication of infection, short-term improvement of symptoms, and long-term alteration of prognosis with aggressive treatment of exacerbations. Most physicians agree that eradication of *Pseudomonas* from the sputum of CF patients can, at best, occur for only a short period after the respiratory tract has been colonized.[74] The difficulty in eradicating bacteria may partially be caused by the antibiotic inhibitory effects of alginate.[71] There is also a poor correlation between the clinical and the bacteriologic responses to antibiotics in some studies.[74–78] Other studies show an association between decreased sputum bacterial density and clinical status for some patients. A reasonable goal in patients with CF who are treated with antibiotics is probably symptomatic improvement rather than eradication of infection. Objective response can further be assessed by a decrease in the granulocyte count, increase in weight, decrease in temperature, and decrease in sputum bacterial density.[70]

The risk of an early, aggressive approach to exacerbations of respiratory infection caused by *Pseudomonas* is selection for antibiotic-resistant strains of bacteria. Although this problem is not inconsequential, the true activities of antibiotics in this setting are complex. Clinical response or lack of response to antibiotics does not necessarily correlate with the in vitro sensitivity of the strain of *P. aeruginosa* isolated. A variety of explanations for this phenomenon have been described. It is not uncommon for more than one strain of *P. aeruginosa* to be present in the sputum.[68] Each of these strains may have a unique sensitivity profile, causing a lack of response despite appropriate antibiotic sensitivity to a single isolated organism. A good clinical response may follow administration of an antibiotic with suboptimal efficacy in vitro against a particular strain of *Pseudomonas*. One proposed explanation for this is inhibition of expression of a variety of *Pseudomonas* exoproducts by subinhibitory concentrations of some antibiotics.[75, 78] Decreased exoproduct activity can immediately diminish the pathologic consequences of the infection. In addition, it may interrupt a self-perpetuating cycle in which increased tissue destruction leads to improvement of the bacterial growth conditions, eventually resulting in further bacterial growth.

The long-term prognosis for CF patients may be improved with aggressive therapy for *Pseudomonas* infections, although this remains controversial. Some studies have demonstrated short-term improvement in pulmonary function parameters[67, 70, 79, 80] in cases in which antibiotics led to a reduction in the quantity of sputum *P. aeruginosa*, and this approach may improve lung function in CF patients more than bronchodilators and chest physiotherapy alone.[81] However, these studies frequently suffer from being uncontrolled, or they have used historical controls,[82] and long-term data are rarely available.[83]

Other approaches include home antibiotic and aerosol antibiotic therapy.[79] The rationale for home antibiotic therapy is that it is less costly and may decrease cross-colonization with resistant organisms spread in the hospital setting.[84, 85] This form of therapy has become technically feasible only with the advent of chronic indwelling intravenous catheters.

The clinical experience with aerosolized antibiotics is vast. Putative positive effects have included a decrement in *Pseudomonas* colonization,[79, 87] improvement in pulmonary function,[80, 86, 87] weight gain,[83] and decreased number of admissions to the hospital.[88] Antibiotic toxicity is minimized because serum antibiotic levels are usually negligible. These studies have usually employed aminoglycosides, including tobramycin, gentamycin, and amikacin.[80, 84, 87–89] Other studies have shown no benefit, and the potential problems with this form of therapy include the emergence of resistant organisms, because *Pseudomonas* is rarely eliminated.[74, 85] Well-controlled studies aimed at assessing clear-cut, long-term clinical effects with this approach are needed.

Other experimental approaches have been directed at the immune and inflammatory aspects of *Pseudomonas* lung infections. There are many studies that demonstrate the efficacy of passive or active immunization in limited experimental models.[89–91] The efficacy of active or passive immunization in normal, immunocompromised, or CF patients is less clear.[92–97] Antigenic heterogeneity among pathogenic strains and the lack of a clear common opsonic antigen are among the difficulties in vaccine design for *P. aeruginosa*. Attempts at discovering and immunizing against common antigens remain experimental.[98, 99] Immunization against lipopolysaccharide does not confer opsonic protection in experimental models.[100, 101] It is also possible that elicited anti-*Pseudomonas* antibodies may contribute to the pulmonary pathology of CF. This may occur through the formation of immune complexes that subsequently induce a local inflammatory response. A significant amount of the damage caused by *Pseudomonas* infections is probably the result of inflammatory cells and their products. This has provided

the rationale for animal studies that have modified the inflammatory infiltrate with cyclogenase inhibitors and assessed the outcome. In general, salutary effects have been seen in these studies.[102–104] Similar approaches have not been attempted in human studies.

## PSEUDOMONAS CEPACIA

*P. cepacia* belongs to the family Pseudomoniae. It was first described as a pulmonary pathogen in CF patients in the 1980s,[105] and the prevalence of this organism in CF patients appears to be increasing.[106] Like *P. aeruginosa*, it is a hardy organism that has been isolated from aerosol antibiotic solutions, anesthetics, distilled water, intravenous solutions, and disinfectants,[105] but nosocomial transmission has been poorly documented. Clinical isolates of *P. cepacia* are aerobic, nonfermenting, and oxidize glucose, and they are resistant to multiple antibiotics. Possible virulence factors include a protease and lipase produced by this organism,[107] although it produces neither alginate nor an elastase.[108]

The adherence characteristics of *P. cepacia* have been less clearly delineated than those of *P. aeruginosa*. However, it is likely that *P. cepacia* adheres to mucin and epithelial cells. The mucin receptor is probably carbohydrate in nature,[109] but there is some controversy regarding the receptor for *P. cepacia* on epithelial cells and particularly whether this is a receptor shared with *P. aeruginosa*.[107] The actions of *P. aeruginosa* exoproducts on epithelial cells may result in increased adherence of *P. cepacia* to these cells.[107] In this manner, colonization of the airways with *P. aeruginosa* may increase the likelihood of subsequent *P. cepacia* colonization. *P. cepacia* probably adheres to epithelial cells in part by fimbriae[110] that have at least some antigen homology with pili from *P. aeruginosa*.

Several risk factors have been identified for *P. cepacia* colonization in CF patients, including older age, female sex, previous aerosol antibiotic therapy, and a more severe stage of CF.[111] Person-to-person transmission has also been suspected.[108]

Three different clinical profiles follow *P. cepacia* colonization:[106, 109] no change in the patient's clinical status, a slow, sustained clinical deterioration, or a much more rapid deterioration. Accompanying findings may include pneumonia, elevated erythrocyte sedimentation rate, decline in pulmonary function, and some cases of blood culture positivity. The pathologic picture in the fulminant form is one of necrotizing pneumonia and microabscess formation.[106] Women and more severely impaired CF patients have poorer survival rates than do other patients colonized with *P. cepacia*.

It is likely that this microorganism will continue to cause clinical illness in CF patients. Greater knowledge about its virulence, adherence factors, and treatment strategies is likely to be forthcoming.

## REFERENCES

1. Holby N: *Pseudomonas aeruginosa* infection in cystic fibrosis: Relationship between mucoid strains of *Pseudomonas aeruginosa* and

the humoral immune response. Acta Pathol Microbiol Scand B 82:551–558, 1974.

2. Morrison AJ, Wenzel RP: Epidemiology of infections due to *Pseudomonas aeruginosa*. Rev Infect Dis 6:S627–S642, 1984.

3. Vasil ML: *Pseudomonas aeruginosa*: Biology, mechanisms of virulence, epidemiology. J Pediatr 108:800–805, 1986.

4. Hancock REW, Mutharia LM, Chan L, Darveau RP, Speert DP, Pier GB: *Pseudomonas aeruginosa* isolates from patients with cystic fibrosis: A class of serum sensitive, nontypable strains deficient in lipopolysaccharide O side chains. Infect Immun 42:170–177, 1983.

5. Hoiby N, Olling S: *Pseudomonas aeruginosa* infection in cystic fibrosis. Bactericidal effect of serum from normal individuals and patients with cystic fibrosis on *P. aeruginosa* strains from patients with cystic fibrosis and other diseases. Acta Pathol Microbiol Scand C 85:107–114, 1977.

6. Schiller NL, Hatch RA: The serum sensitivity, colonial morphology, serogroup specificity, and outer membrane protein profile of *Pseudomonas aeruginosa* strains isolated from several clinical sites. Diagn Microbiol Infect Dis 1:145–157, 1983.

7. Thomassen MJ, Demko CA: Serum bactericidal effect on *Pseudomonas aeruginosa* isolates from cystic fibrosis patients. Infect Immun 33:512–518, 1983.

8. Pollack M: *Pseudomonas aeruginosa. In* Mandell GL, Douglas RG, Bennett JE (eds): Principles and Practice of Infectious Diseases, ed. 3. New York, Churchill Livingstone, 1990:1673–1691.

9. Pierce AK, Sanford JP: Aerobic gram-negative bacillary pneumonias. Am Rev Respir Dis 110:647–656, 1974.

10. Craven DE, Steges KA, Barder TW: Preventing nosocomial pneumonia: State of the art and perspectives for the 1990s. Am J Med 91:44S–53S, 1991.

11. Inglis TJ, Millar MR, Gareth Jones J, Robinson DA: Tracheal tube biofilm as a source of bacterial colonization of the lung. J Clin Microbiol 27:2014–2018, 1989.

12. Higuchi JH, Johanson WG: The relationship between adherence of *Pseudomonas aeruginosa* to upper respiratory cells in vitro and susceptibility to colonization in vivo. J Lab Clin Med 95:698–704, 1980.

13. Mason CM, Bawden RE, Pierce AK, Dal Nogarde AR: Fibronectin is not detectable on the intact buccal epithelial surface of normal rats or humans. Am J Respir Cell Mol Biol 3:563–570, 1990.

14. Plotkowski MC, Chevillard M, Pierrot D, et al: Differential adhesion of *Pseudomonas aeruginosa* to human respiratory epithelial cells in primary culture. J Clin Invest 87:2018–2028, 1991.

15. Woods DE, Straus DC, Johanson WG, Bass JE: Role of salivary protease activity in adherence of gram-negative bacilli to mammalian buccal epithelial cells in vivo. J Clin Invest 68:1435–1440, 1981.

16. Ramphal R, Small PM, Shands JW, Fischlschweiger W, Small PA: Adherence of *Pseudomonas aeruginosa* to tracheal cells injured by influenza infection or by endotracheal intubation. Infect Immun 27:614–619, 1980.

17. Niederman MS, Ferranti RD, Ziegler A, Merrill WW, Reynolds HY: Respiratory infections complicating long term tracheostomy. Chest 85:39–44, 1984.

18. Niederman MS, Merrill WW, Ferranti RD, Pagano KM, Palmer LB, Reynolds HY: Nutritional status and bacterial binding in the lower respiratory tract in patients with chronic tracheostomy. Ann Intern Med 100:795–800, 1989.

19. Yamaguchi T, Yamada H: Role of mechanical injury on airway surface in the pathogenesis of *Pseudomonas aeruginosa*. Am Rev Respir Dis 144:1147–1152, 1991.

20. Baker N, Hansson GC, Leffler H, Riise G, Svanborg-Eden C: Glycosphingolipid receptors for *Pseudomonas aeruginosa*. Infect Immun 58:2361–2366, 1990.

21. Krivan HC, Ginsburg V, Roberts DD: *Pseudomonas aeruginosa* and *Pseudomonas cepacia* isolated from cystic fibrosis patients bind specifically to gangliotetraosylceramide (asialo GM1) and gangliotriaosylceramide (asialo GM2). Arch Biochem Biophys 260:493–496, 1988.

22. Woods DE, Straus DC, Johanson WG, Berry VK, Bass JA: Role of pili in adherence of *Pseudomonas aeruginosa* to mammalian buccal epithelial cells. Infect Immun 29:1146–1151, 1980.

23. Hata JS, Fick RB: Airway adherence of *Pseudomonas aeruginosa*: Mucoexopolysaccharide binding to human and bovine airway proteins. J Lab Clin Med 117:410–422, 1991.

24. Doig P, Todd T, Sastry PA, et al: Role of pili in adhesion of *Pseudomonas aeruginosa* to human respiratory epithelial cells. Infect Immun 56:1641–1646, 1988.

25. Baker NR, Minor V, Deal C, Shahrabadi MS, Simpson DA, Woods DE: *Pseudomonas aeruginosa* exoenzyme S is an adhesin. Infect Immun 59:2859–2863, 1991.

26. Saiman L, Ishimoto K, Lory S, Prince A: The effect of piliation and exoproduct expression on the adherence of *Pseudomonas aeruginosa* to respiratory epithelial monolayers. J Infect Dis 161:541–548, 1990.

27. Luzer MA, Thomassen MJ, Montie TC: Flagella and motility alterations in *Pseudomonas aeruginosa* strains from patients with cystic fibrosis: Relationship to patient clinical condition. Infect Immun 58:577–582, 1985.

28. Saiman L, Cacalano G, Gruenert D, Prince A: Comparison of adherence of *Pseudomonas aeruginosa* to respiratory epithelial cells from cystic fibrosis patients and healthy subjects. Infect Immun 60:2808–2814, 1992.

29. Fick RB: Pathogenesis of the *Pseudomonas* lung lesion in cystic fibrosis. Chest 96:158–164, 1989.

30. Chi E, Mehl T, Nunn D, Lory S: Interaction of *Pseudomonas aeruginosa* with A549 pneumocyte cells. Infect Immun 59:822–828, 1991.

31. Ramphal R, Guay C, Pier GB: *Pseudomonas aeruginosa* adhesins for tracheobronchial mucin. Infect Immun 55:600–603, 1987.

32. Ramphal R, Pyle M: Evidence for mucins and sialic acid as receptors for *Pseudomonas aeruginosa* in the lower respiratory tract. Infect Immun 41:339–344, 1983.

33. Vishawath S, Ramphal R: Tracheobronchial mucin receptor for *Pseudomonas aeruginosa*: Predominance of amino sugars in binding sites. Infect Immun 48:331–335, 1985.

34. Ceri H, Hwang WS, Rabin H: Structure, secretion, and bacterial specificity of an endogenous lectin from cystic fibrosis lung. Am J Respir Cell Mol Biol 5:51–55, 1991.

35. Nelson JW, Tredgett MW, Sheehan JK, Thornton DJ, Notman D, Govan JRW: Mucinophilic and chemotactic properties of *Pseudomonas aeruginosa* in relation to pulmonary colonization in cystic fibrosis. Infect Immun 58:1489–1495, 1990.

36. Woods DE, Sokol PA: Role of *Pseudomonas aeruginosa* extracellular enzymes in lung disease. Clin Invest Med 9:108–112, 1986.

37. Iglewski BH, Liu P, Kabat K: Mechanism of action of *Pseudomonas aeruginosa* exotoxin A: Adenine diphosphate ribosylation of elongation factor 2. Infect Immun 15:138–144, 1977.

38. Pollack M, Taylor NJ: Exotoxin production by clinical strains of *Pseudomonas aeruginosa*. Infect Immun 15:676, 1977.

39. Woods DE, Cryz SJ, Freedman RL, Iglewski BH: Contribution of toxin A and elastase to virulence of *Pseudomonas aeruginosa* in chronic lung infections in rats. Infect Immun 36:1223–1228, 1982.

40. Blackwood L, Stone RM, Iglewski BH, Pennington JE: Evaluation of *Pseudomonas aeruginosa* exotoxin A and elastase as virulence factors in acute lung infections. Infect Immun 39:198–201, 1983.

41. Iglewski BH, Sadoff J, Bjorn MJ, Maxwell ES: *Pseudomonas aeruginosa* exoenzyme S: An adenosine diphosphate ribosyltransferase distinct from toxin A. Proc Natl Acad Sci USA 75:3211–3215, 1978.

42. Hemdaoui A, Wund-Bisseret F, Bieth JG: Fast solubilization of human lung elastin by *Pseudomonas aeruginosa* elastase. Am Rev Respir Dis 135:860–863, 1987.

43. Heck LW, Morihara K, Mahal WB, Miller EJ: Specific cleavage of human type III and IV collagens by *Pseudomonas aeruginosa* elastase. Infect Immun 51:115–117, 1986.

44. Amitani R, Wilson R, Rutman A, et al: Effects of human neutrophil elastase and *Pseudomonas aeruginosa* proteinases on human respiratory epithelium. Am J Respir Cell Mol Biol 4:26–32, 1991.

45. Grimminger F, Walmrath D, Walter H, Lutz F, Seeger W: Induction of vascular injury by *Pseudomonas aeruginosa* cytotoxin in rabbit lungs is associated with the generation of different leukotrienes and hydroxyeicosatetranoic acids. J Infect Dis 163:362–370, 1991.

46. Bruce MC, Poncz L, Klinger JD, Stern RC, Tomachefski JF, Dearborn DG: Biochemical and pathologic evidence for proteolytic destruction of lung connective tissue in cystic fibrosis. Am Rev Respir Dis 132:529–535, 1985.

47. Bainbridge T, Fick RB: Functional importance of cystic fibrosis immunoglobulin G fragments generated by *Pseudomonas aeruginosa* elastase. J Lab Clin Med 114:728–733, 1989.

48. Angley ST, Hasten AJ, Kreppers F, Higgins ML: Disruption of respiratory cilia by proteases including those of *Pseudomonas aeruginosa*. Infect Immun 54:379–385, 1986.

49. Read RC, Roberts P, Munro N, et al: Effect of *Pseudomonas aeruginosa* rhamnolipids on mucociliary transport and ciliary beating. J Appl Physiol 72:2271–2277, 1992.

50. Seeger W, Walmrath D, Neuhof H, Lutz F: Pulmonary microvascular injury induced by *Pseudomonas aeruginosa* cytotoxin in isolated rabbit lungs. Infect Immun 52:846–852, 1986.

51. Wilson R, Sykes DA, Watson D, Rutman A, Taylor GW, Cole PJ: Measurement of *Pseudomonas aeruginosa* phenazine pigments in sputum and assessment of their contribution to sputum sol toxicity for respiratory epithelium. Infect Immun 56:2515–2517, 1988.

52. Ras GJ, Anderson R, Taylor GW, et al: Proinflammatory interactions of pyocyanin and 1-hydroxyphenazine with human neutrophils in vitro. J Infect Dis 162:178–185, 1990.

53. Tillotson JR, Lerner AM: Characteristics of nonbacteremic *Pseudomonas* pneumonia. Ann Intern Med 68:295–307, 1968.

54. Toews GB, Gross GN, Pierce AK: The relationship of inoculum size to lung bacterial clearance and phagocytic cell response. Am Rev Respir Dis 120:559–566, 1979.

55. Rehm SR, Gross GN, Pierce AK: Early bacterial clearance from murine lungs: Species dependent phagocyte response. J Clin Invest 66:194–199, 1980.

56. Larsen GL, Mitchell BC, Harper TB, Henson PM: The pulmonary response in C5 sufficient and deficient mice to *Pseudomonas aeruginosa*. Am Rev Respir Dis 126:306–311, 1982.

57. Dunn MM, Kamp DW: Pulmonary clearance of *Pseudomonas aeruginosa* in neutropenic mice: Effects of systemic immunization. Am Rev Respir Dis 135:1294–1299, 1987.

58. Thomassen MJ, Demko CA, Doershuk CF: Cystic fibrosis: A review of pulmonary infections and interventions. Pediatr Pulmonol 3:334–351, 1987.

59. Bedrossian CW, Greenberg SD, Singer DB, Hansen JJ, Rosenberg JS: The lung in cystic fibrosis. A quantitative study including prevalence of pathologic findings among different age groups. Hum Pathol 2:195–204, 1976.

60. Hanly P, Light RB: Lung mechanics, gas exchange, pulmonary perfusion, and hemodynamics in a canine model of acute *Pseudomonas* pneumonia. Lung 165:305–322, 1987.

61. Mustard RA, Fisher J, Hayman S, et al: Cardiopulmonary responses to *Pseudomonas* septicemia in swine: An improved model of the adult respiratory distress syndrome. Lab Anim Sci 39:37–43, 1989.

62. Graham LM, Vasil A, Vasil ML, Voelkel NF, Stenmark KR: Decreased pulmonary vasoreactivity in an animal model of chronic *Pseudomonas* pneumonia. Am Rev Respir Dis 142:221–229, 1990.

63. Jimenez P, Torres A, Rodriguez-Roisin R, et al: Incidence and etiology of pneumonia acquired during mechanical ventilation. Crit Care Med 17:882–885, 1989.

64. Stevens RM, Teres D, Skillman JJ, Feingold DS: Pneumonia in an intensive care unit. Arch Intern Med 134:106–110, 1974.

65. Pennington JE, Reynolds HY, Carbone PP: *Pseudomonas* pneumonia: A retrospective study of 36 cases. Am J Med 55:155–160, 1973.

66. Tillotson JR, Lerner AM: Pneumonias caused by gram-negative bacilli. Medicine (Baltimore) 45:65–76, 1966.

67. Kerem E, Corey M, Gold R, Levison H: Pulmonary function and clinical course in patients with cystic fibrosis after pulmonary colonization with *Pseudomonas aeruginosa*. J Pediatr 116:714–719, 1990.

68. Nelson JD: Management of acute pulmonary exacerbations in cystic fibrosis: A critical appraisal. J Pediatr 106:1030–1033, 1985.

69. Hoiby N: Microbiology of lung infections in cystic fibrosis patients. Acta Paediatr Scand Suppl 301:33–54, 1982.

70. Smith AL, Ramsey B, Redding G, Haas J: Endobronchial infection in cystic fibrosis. Acta Paediatr Scand Suppl 363:31–36, 1989.

71. Hoiby N, Koch C: *Pseudomonas aeruginosa* infection in cystic fibrosis and its management. Thorax 45:881–884, 1990.

72. Hilf M, Yu VH, Sharp J, Zuravleff JJ, Korvick JA, Muder RR: Antibiotic therapy for *Pseudomonas aeruginosa* bacteremia: Outcome correlations in a prospective study of 200 patients. Am J Med 87:540–545, 1989.

73. Neijens HJ: Strategies and perspectives in treatment of respiratory infections. Acta Paediatr Scand Suppl 363:66–73, 1989.

74. MacLusky I, Levison H, Gold R, McLaughlin FJ: Inhaled antibiotics in cystic fibrosis: Is there a therapeutic effect? J Pediatr 108:861–865, 1986.

75. Grimwood K, To M, Rabin HR, Woods DE: Subinhibitory antibiotics reduce *Pseudomonas aeruginosa* tissue injury in the rat lung. J Antimicrob Chemother 24:937–945, 1989.

76. Matsen JM, Bosso JA: The use of aztreonam in the cystic fibrosis patient. Pediatr Infect Dis J 8:S117–S119, 1989.

77. Stephens D, Garey N, Isles A, Levison H, Gold R: Efficacy of inhaled tobramycin in the treatment of pulmonary exacerbations in children with cystic fibrosis. Pediatr Infect Dis J 2:209–211, 1983.

78. LeVatte MA, Woods DE, Shahrabadi MS, Semple R, Sokol PA: Subinhibitory concentrations of tetracycline inhibit surface expression of the *Pseudomonas aeruginosa* ferripyochelin binding protein in vivo. J Antimicrob Chemother 26:215–225, 1990.

79. Schaad UB, Wedgwood-Krucko J, Suter S, Kraemer R: Efficacy of inhaled amikacin as adjunct to intravenous combination therapy (ceftazidime and amikacin) in cystic fibrosis. J Pediatr 111:599–605, 1987.

80. MacLusky IB, Gold R, Corey M, Levison H: Long-term effects of inhaled tobramycin in patients with cystic fibrosis colonized with *Pseudomonas aeruginosa*. Pediatr Pulmonol 7:42–48, 1989.

81. Regelman WE, Elliott GR, Warwicke WJ, Clawson C: Reduction of sputum *Pseudomonas aeruginosa* density by antibiotics improves lung function in cystic fibrosis more than do bronchodilators and chest physiotherapy alone. Am Rev Respir Dis 141:914–921, 1990.

82. Szaff M, Holby N, Flensborg EW: Frequent antibiotic therapy improves survival of cystic fibrosis patients with chronic *Pseudomonas aeruginosa* infection. Acta Paediatr Scand 72:651–657, 1983.

83. Smith AL, Ramsey BW, Hedges DL, et al: Safety of aerosol tobramycin administration for 3 months to patients with cystic fibrosis. Pediatr Pulmonol 7:265–271, 1989.

84. Kuzemko JA: Home treatment of pulmonary infections in cystic fibrosis. Chest 94:162S–165S, 1988.

85. Fick RB, Stillwell PC: Controversies in the management of pulmonary disease due to cystic fibrosis. Chest 95:1319–1326, 1989.

86. Hodson ME, Penketh ARL, Batten JC: Aerosol carbenicillin and gentamicin therapy of *Pseudomonas aeruginosa* infection in patients with cystic fibrosis. Lancet 2:1137–1139, 1981.

87. Ramsey BW, Dorkin HL, Eisenberg JD, et al: Efficacy of aerosolized tobramycin in patients with cystic fibrosis. N Engl J Med 328:1740–1746, 1993.

88. Stead RJ, Hodson ME, Batten JC: Inhaled ceftazidime compared with gentamicin and carbenicillin in older patients with cystic fibrosis infected with *Pseudomonas aeruginosa*. Br J Dis Chest 81:272–279, 1987.

89. Zweerink HJ, Detolla LJ, Gammon MC, Hutchison CF, Puckett JM, Sigal NH: A human monoclonal antibody that protects mice against *Pseudomonas*-induced pneumonia. J Infect Dis 162:254–257, 1990.

90. Collins MS, Edwards A, Roby RE, Mehton NS, Ladehoff D: *Pseudomonas* immune globulin therapy improves survival in experimental *Pseudomonas aeruginosa* bacteremic pneumonia. Antibiot Chemother 42:184–192, 1989.

91. Schrieber JR, Pier GB, Grout M, Nixon K, Patawaran M: Induction of opsonic antibodies to *Pseudomonas aeruginosa* mucoid exopolysaccharide by an anti-idiotypic monoclonal antibody. J Infect Dis 164:507–514, 1991.

92. Winnie GB, Cowan RG, Wade NA: Intravenous immune globulin treatment of pulmonary exacerbations in cystic fibrosis. J Pediatr 114:309–314, 1989.

93. Saravolatz LD, Markowitz N, Collins MS, Bogdanoff D, Pennington JE: Safety, pharmacokinetics, and functional activity of human anti-*Pseudomonas aeruginosa* monoclonal antibodies in septic and nonseptic patients. J Infect Dis 164:803–806, 1991.

94. Van Wye JE, Collins MS, Baylor M, et al: *Pseudomonas* hyperimmune globulin passive immunotherapy for pulmonary exacerbations in cystic fibrosis. Pediatr Pulmonol 9:7–18, 1990.

95. Langford DT, Hiller J: Prospective, controlled study of a polyvalent *pseudomonas* vaccine in cystic fibrosis—three year results. Arch Dis Child 59:1131–1134, 1984.

96. Haghbin M, Armstrong D, Murphy ML: Controlled prospective trial of *Pseudomonas aeruginosa* vaccine in children with acute leukemia. Cancer 32:761–766, 1973.

97. Pennington JE, Reynolds HY, Wood RE, Robinson RA, Levine AS: Use of a *Pseudomonas aeruginosa* vaccine in patients with acute leukemia and cystic fibrosis. Am J Med 58:629–636, 1975.

98. Gilleland HE, Parker MG, Matthews JM, Berg RD: Use of a purified outer membrane protein F (porin) preparation of *Pseudomonas aeruginosa* as a protective vaccine in mice. Infect Immun 44:49–54, 1984.

99. Gilleland HE, Gilleland LB, Matthews-Greer JM: Outer membrane protein F preparation of *Pseudomonas aeruginosa* as a vaccine

against chronic pulmonary infection with heterologous immunotype strains in a rat model. Infect Immun 56:1017–1022, 1988.

100. Pennington JE, Menkes E: Type specific vs. cross-protective vaccination for gram-negative bacterial pneumonia. J Infect Dis 144:599–603, 1981.

101. Pennington JE, Hickey WF, Blackwood LL, Arnaut MA: Active immunization with lipopolysaccharide *Pseudomonas* antigen for chronic *Pseudomonas* bronchopneumonia in guinea pigs. J Clin Invest 68:1140–1148, 1981.

102. Konstan MW, Vargo KM, Davis PB: Ibuprofen attenuates the inflammatory response to *Pseudomonas aeruginosa* in a rat model of chronic pulmonary infection. Am Rev Respir Dis 141:186–192, 1990.

103. Sordelli DO, Cerquetti MC, Fontan PA, Meiss RP: Piroxicam treatment protects mice from lethal pulmonary challenge with *Pseudomonas aeruginosa*. J Infect Dis 159:232–238, 1989.

104. Sordelli DO, Cerquetti MC, Fontan PA, Garcia VE: *Pseudomonas aeruginosa* pneumonia. Treatment with nonsteroidal anti-inflammatory agents to prevent lung tissue damage. Antibiot Chemother 42:247–253, 1989.

105. Isles A, MacLusky I, Corey M, et al: *Pseudomonas cepacia* infection in cystic fibrosis: An emerging problem. J Pediatr 104:206, 1984.

106. Tomashefski JF, Thomassen MJ, Bruce MC, Goldberg HI, Konstan MW, Stern RC: *Pseudomonas cepacia* associated pneumonia in cystic fibrosis. Arch Pathol Lab Med 112:166–172, 1988.

107. Saiman L, Cacalano G, Prince A: *Pseudomonas cepacia* adherence to respiratory epithelial cells is enhanced by *Pseudomonas aeruginosa*. Infect Immun 58:2578–2584, 1990.

108. *Pseudomonas cepacia*—more than a harmless commensal. Lancet 139:1385–1386, 1992.

109. Sajjan US, Corey M, Karmali A, Forstner JF: Binding of *Pseudomonas cepacia* to normal human intestinal mucin and respiratory mucin from patients with cystic fibrosis. J Clin Invest 89:648–656, 1992.

110. Kuehn M, Lent K, Haas J, Hagenzieker J, Cervin M, Smith AL: Fimbriation of *Pseudomonas cepacia*. Infect Immun 60:2002–2007, 1992.

111. Tablan OC, Martone WJ, Doershuk CF, et al: Colonization of the respiratory tract with *Pseudomonas cepacia* in cystic fibrosis: Risk factors and outcomes. Chest 91:527–532, 1987.

# CHAPTER 31

# Group B Streptococcal and Other Nonpneumococcal Streptococcal Pneumonia

STEVEN L. BERK

Group B β-hemolytic streptococci (eg, *Streptococcus agalactiae*) have been recognized as important pathogens in neonatal sepsis and postpartum fever in women for the past 30 years. The neonate is prone to group B β-hemolytic streptoccocal (GBS) bacteremia and pneumonia. Infants with GBS pneumonia present with jaundice, lethargy, and grunting respirations. Neonates with pneumonia are always in respiratory distress, with tachypnea and cyanosis.[1] A chest radiograph has the same patterns as those of hyaline membrane disease. GBS infection is also a serious problem for adults other than pregnant women.[2–13a] This chapter reviews the clinical features of GBS pneumonia in adults.

## GROUP B β-HEMOLYTIC STREPTOCOCCAL PNEUMONIA

### Microbiology

Group B streptococci are facultative diplococci. They characteristically form a narrow zone of β-hemolysis on sheep blood agar, although some strains are nonhemolytic. Definitive methods of identification require hyperimmune group-specific antisera that detect the group B antigen. Several commercial kits offer sensitive and specific identification. Some laboratories use presumptive biochemical methods of identification, such as hydrolysis of sodium hippurate and bile esculin or resistance to bacitracin. More than 98% of group B streptococci produce an extracellular protein, CAMP factor, which can be used to rapidly identify group B streptococci.[14]

Group B streptococci have two cell wall carbohydrate antigens. One is common to all group B streptococci (ie, C substance). The other is type specific and has five subtypes: Ia, Ib, Ic, II, and III. Neonates at risk for type III invasive disease are those with low levels of antibody to this capsular antigen.[15] Most infants with late-onset pneumonia and meningitis have type III strains. The serotypes in adult infection have not been well characterized.

A sputum Gram stain often suggests β-hemolytic pneumonia (Fig. 31–1). The smear reveals gram-positive cocci in chains. Diplococcal forms are not characteristic.

### Epidemiology

Schwartz and coworkers[16] studied the incidence of invasive GBS disease in adults. As part of a Centers for Disease Control (CDC) study, laboratory records from 37 acute care hospitals in a seven-county Atlanta health district were reviewed. Infection occurred in 56 men and nonpregnant women. The incidence of GBS infection was 3.0 per 100,000 men and 1.5 per 100,000 women. Pneumonia was the third most common cause of GBS infection in the series, representing 11% of cases. Although group B streptococci have been described as a cause of nosocomial and community-acquired pneumonia in adults, the overall importance of these pathogens has not been well defined. Fang and colleagues,[17] in a prospective multicenter study of community-acquired pneumonia, found only 4 of 359 cases to be caused by group B streptococci. In 1 year at our 512-bed Veterans Administration Medical Center, group B

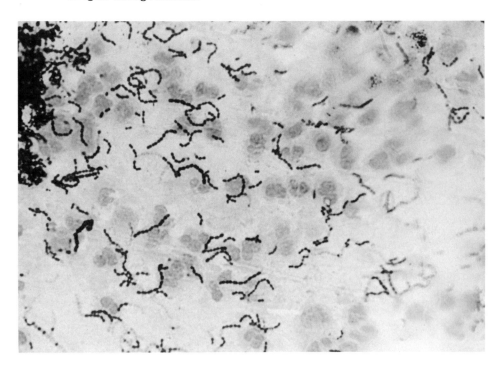

**Figure 31–1.** Gram-stained smear from a patient with group B streptococcal pneumonia.

streptococci were isolated from the sputum of 35 patients, 10 of whom had definite evidence of pneumonia.[18]

## Predisposing Factors

GBS pneumonia has been reported most commonly in elderly, debilitated patients (Table 31–1). The patients with GBS bacteremic pneumonia reported by Duma[10] and Lerner[19] were in their late fifties and sixties. Gallagher and Watanakunakorn[2] reported cases of GBS bacteremic pneumonia in a community hospital, all of which occurred in patients older than 70 years of age. Verghese and coworkers[6] reported 7 patients with GBS pneumonia who had a mean age of 78 years. Ekenna and colleagues,[18] reporting from the same institution, found the average age of patients with GBS isolated from sputum to be 68.1 years, compared with 56 years for all other types of β-hemolytic streptococci ($P<.02$).

Diabetes mellitus is an important underlying disease in GBS pneumonia and infection. In the CDC study of GBS bacteremia in adults, diabetes mellitus was the most frequent underlying condition, occurring in 29% of patients. Bayer and colleagues[4] found diabetes mellitus in 71% of patients with GBS pneumonia, and Gallagher and Watanakunakorn[2] found a rate of 40% in a similar patient population. Verghese[6] and Ekenna[18] reported a 29% and 27% incidence, respectively, of underlying DM. George and Savage[7] reported a case of fatal GBS empyema in an insulin-dependent diabetic.

An interesting association between neurologic disease and GBS pneumonia has been observed by several investigators. In the series of patients reported by Verghese and associates, 6 of 7 patients with pneumonia had cerebrovascular disease and dementia. Dworzack and coworkers also noticed a high incidence of neurologic disease in their veteran patients with GBS pneumonia.[20] Ekenna and associates found that 57% of patients with GBS in sputum had cere-

brovascular disease, compared with 21% who had other β-hemolytic streptococci in sputum. The significance of this association with neurologic impairment is not clear but may represent predisposition to aspiration and to prior antibiotic therapy.

## Clinical Features

GBS pneumonia has been described in bacteremic patients and in patients who were diagnosed by transtracheal aspiration (TTA). These patients tend to be more ill than pneumonia patients diagnosed by expectorated sputum. Patients have been described as tachycardic and tachypneic with an average temperature of 39°C, and leukocyte counts are usually elevated above 15,000/mm³. The mortality rate is estimated at 50% to 100%, but the severity of underlying disease is difficult to separate from pneumonia as the lethal event. The organism is often found with copathogens, particularly *Staphylococcus aureus*.[3] Both organisms have been isolated from TTA and blood cultures.[2, 3] In one study using expectorated sputum for diagnosis, *S. aureus* was cultured along with group B streptococci from 12 of 35 patients. *S. aureus* was found with other β-hemolytic streptococci in only 2 of 34 ($P<.01$). Necrotizing pneumonia has been reported (Fig. 31–2).[3]

Unlike pneumonia caused by group A β-hemolytic strep-

**Table 31–1. Predisposing Factors for Group B Streptococcal Pneumonia**

| |
|---|
| Extremes of age (ie, neonates, elderly) |
| Diabetes mellitus |
| Neurologic impairment |
|     Dementia |
|     Cerebrovascular disease |
| Malignancy |
| Tube feeding |

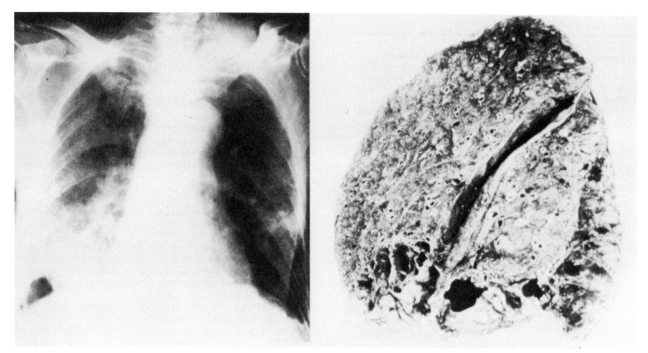

**Figure 31–2.** Chest x-ray film and autopsy specimen show necrotizing group B streptococcal pneumonia. (From Verghese A, Berk SL, Boelen LJ, et al: Group B streptococcal pneumonia in the elderly. Arch Intern Med 142:1642–1645, 1982. Copyright 1982, American Medical Association.)

tococci, pneumonia with group B organisms rarely causes empyema. George and Savage[7] reported a case of GBS pneumonia and empyema in an insulin-dependent diabetic patient and found 7 additional cases of GBS empyema in the literature.

There are no data on the seasonality of GBS pneumonia or on coexisting viral infections. The frequent association of GBS disease and *S. aureus* infection and of *S. aureus* infection and influenza suggest that influenza may be a predisposing factor, particularly in the very elderly, debilitated patients in whom GBS pneumonia is most likely to occur. Jones, Menna, and Wennerstrom[21] reported a lethal synergism induced in mice by influenza A virus and type Ia group B streptococci. Jones and Menna[22] found a 120-fold increase in the adherence of type Ia GBS to mouse tracheal tissue in vivo with influenza A coinfection.

### Antibiotic Therapy

Because of the toxic clinical picture of many patients, the severity of their underlying disease, and the high mortality rate, treatment with aggressive antibiotic therapy and close monitoring are recommended. GBS organisms are always sensitive to penicillin in vitro, and high-dose penicillin is the recommended treatment. Higher doses of penicillin than those given for group A infection may be necessary, because the minimum inhibitory concentrations (MICs) of penicillin are fourfold to tenfold greater for group B than for group A organisms.[23, 24] Parenteral therapy for 10 to 14 days appears to be prudent, although few clinical data are available for this recommendation. The importance of penicillin-tolerant strains in pneumonia is also unknown. Patients who are doing poorly on penicillin

should have analysis performed for MICs and for minimum bactericidal concentrations.

Imipenem has good in vitro activity against the GBS organisms,[25] as do vancomycin and first-generation cephalosporins. Ciprofloxacin has moderate in vitro activity but probably should not be considered a drug of choice because of its broad-spectrum activity.[26]

Because mixed infection with *S. aureus* or gram-negative bacilli is common, the initial therapy may have to cover a broad spectrum of pathogens until the results of blood and sputum cultures become available.

### OTHER NONPNEUMOCOCCAL STREPTOCOCCAL PNEUMONIAS

Group A β-hemolytic streptococcal pneumonias have become an infrequent cause of lower respiratory infection. Epidemics have been described among military recruits.[27] The disease often occurred after influenza. About one third of patients had symptoms of streptococcal pharyngitis. Bisno described clinical features of dyspnea, pleuritic chest pain, and hemoptysis. Empyema occurred in 30% to 40% of patients.[28] Fang and colleagues[17] found no cases of group A streptococci in their series on community-acquired pneumonia.

Group C streptococcal pneumonia has been discussed in a review by Stamm and Cobbs.[29] The clinical features were similar to those seen in group A pneumonia; upper respiratory symptoms occurred, and empyema was common. Vartian and coworkers found group G streptococci caused pneumonia in patients with underlying malignancies.[30]

Sarkar and associates[31] reported 3 cases of primary *Streptococcus viridans* pneumonia in previously healthy adults. The diagnosis was made on the basis of sputum Gram stain

Table 31–2. **Enterococcal Pneumonia in Series of Enterococcal Bacteremia**

| Investigation | Cases of Pneumonia | Cases of Bacteremia | Comments |
|---|---|---|---|
| Garrison et al[34] | 4 | 114 | All 4 patients died |
| Bryan et al[35] | 9 | 190 | 67% mortality rate in Veterans Administration and community hospitals |
| Barrall et al[36] | 1 | 73 | Surgical series |
| Maki and Agger[37] | 1 | 153 | |
| Malone et al[38] | 4 | 55 | 3 of 4 pneumonias were nosocomial; 50% mortality rate |
| Rimailho et al[39] | 3 | 35 | Protected brush used |
| Gullberg et al[40] | 5 | 75 | 4 of 5 patients using mechanical ventilators |

and positive blood cultures. The clinical features suggested pneumonia. Because the organism is part of normal throat flora, further studies are required to support its role as a respiratory pathogen.

## Enterococcal Pneumonia

*Enterococcus fecalis* (formerly called *Streptococcus fecalis*) is a group D streptococcal organism well appreciated as a pathogen in endocarditis, urinary tract infection, and intraabdominal processes. The incidence of nosocomial enterococcal infections has increased over the past 10 years, in part because of superinfection related to therapy with third-generation cephalosporins.[32]

Berk and colleagues[33] described 2 patients with enterococcal pneumonia documented by TTA. Both were older veterans who were receiving enteral hyperalimentation and broad-spectrum antibiotic therapy. Although there have been no other papers on enterococcal pneumonia, several series of patients with enterococcal bacteremia have revealed the lower respiratory tract to be a source of infection. Table 31–2 summarizes these studies. A total of 27 cases of bacteremic enterococcal pneumonia have been reported. Patients tended to be elderly, and pneumonia was almost always hospital acquired. Clinical characteristics of these pneumonias were not reported. About half of all patients with enterococcal bacteremia had been receiving cephalosporin therapy.

*E. fecalis* shows tolerance to the effect of ampicillin and penicillin. For serious infections in which a bactericidal effect is necessary, an aminoglycoside should be added to penicillin or vancomycin. Whether such bactericidal activity is necessary in the treatment of pneumonia is unknown. High-grade resistance to aminoglycosides is increasingly reported. Each aminoglycoside should be studied separately, because high-grade resistance may occur to one aminoglycoside and not another. *E. fecalis* is susceptible to imipenem and ciprofloxacin, and these antibiotics may be useful in pneumonia, particularly if there is high-grade aminoglycoside resistance.

## REFERENCES

1. Baker CJ: Group B streptococcal infections in neonates. Pediatr Rev 1:5–15, 1979.
2. Gallagher PG, Watanakunakorn C: Group B streptococcal bacteremia in a community teaching hospital. Am J Med 78:795–800, 1985.
3. Verghese A, Mireault K, Arbeit RD: Group B streptococal bacteremia in men. Rev Infect Dis 8:912–917, 1986.
4. Bayer AS, Chow AW, Anthony BF, et al: Serious infections in adults due to group B streptococci. Am J Med 61:498–503, 1976.
5. Roberts FJ: Group A and group B beta hemolytic streptococcal bacteremia. Rev Infect Dis 10:228–229, 1988.
6. Verghese A, Berk SL, Boelen LJ, et al: Group B streptococcal pneumonia in the elderly. Arch Intern Med 142:1642–1645, 1982.
7. George AL Jr, Savage AM: Fatal group B streptococcal empyema in an adult. South Med J 80:1436–1438, 1987.
8. Gallagher PG, Watanakunakorn C: Group B streptococcal endocarditis: Report of seven cases and review of the literature, 1962–1985. Rev Infect Dis 8:175–188, 1986.
9. Backes RJ, Wilson WR, Geraci JE: Group B streptococcal infective endocarditis. Arch Intern Med 145:693–696, 1985.
10. Duma RJ, Weinberg AN, Merdrek RF, et al: Streptococcal infection. A bacteriologic and clinical study of streptococcal bacteremia. Medicine (Baltimore) 48:87–127, 1969.
11. Small CB, Slater IN, Lowy FD, et al: Group B streptococcal arthritis in adults. Am J Med 76:367–375, 1984.
12. Pischel KD, Weisman MH, Cone RO: Unique features of group B streptococcal arthritis in adults. Arch Intern Med 145:97–102, 1985.
13. Ridgeway NA, Perlman PE, Verghese A: Epiglottic abscess due to group B *Streptococcus*. Ann Otol Rhinol Laryngol 93:277–278, 1984.
13a. Farley MM, Harvey RC, Stull T, et al: A population based assessment of invasive disease due to group B *Streptococcus* in nonpregnant adults. N Engl J Med 328:1807–1811, 1993.
14. Ratner HB, Weeks IS, Stratton CW: Evaluation of Spot-CAMP test for identification of group B streptococci. J Clin Microbiol 24:296–297, 1986.
15. Baker CJ, Kasper DL: Correlation of maternal antibody deficiency with susceptibility to neonatal group B streptococcal infection. N Engl J Med 294:753–756, 1976.
16. Schwartz B, Schuchat A, Oxtoby M, et al: Invasive group B streptococcal disease in adults. JAMA 266:1112–1114, 1991.
17. Fang G, Fine M, Orloff J, et al: New and emerging etiologies for community-acquired pneumonia with implications for therapy. A prospective multicenter study of 359 cases. Medicine (Baltimore) 69:307–316, 1990.
18. Ekenna O, Verghese A, Karnad A, et al: Isolation of beta-hemolytic streptococci from the respiratory tract: Serotypic distribution and clinical significance. Am J Med Sci 295:94–191, 1988.
19. Lerner PI, Gropulakrishna KV, Wolinsky E: Group B *Streptococcus* (*S. agalactiae*) bacteremia in adults: Analysis of 32 cases and review of the literature. Medicine (Baltimore) 56:457–473, 1977.
20. Dworzack DL, Hodges GR, Barnes WG: Group B streptococcal infections in adult males. Am J Med Sci 277:67–73, 1979.
21. Jones WT, Menna JH, Wennerstrom DE: Lethal synergism induced in mice by influenza type A virus and type Ia group B streptococci. Infect Immun 41:618–623, 1983.
22. Jones WT, Menna JH: Influenza type A virus-mediated adherence of type Ia group B streptococci to mouse tracheal tissue in vivo. Infect Immun 38:791–794, 1982.
23. Baker CJ: Group B streptococcal infections. Adv Intern Med 25:475–501, 1980.
24. Edwards MS, Baker CJ: *Streptococcus agalactiae* (group B streptococcus). *In* Mandell GL, Douglas RG Jr, Bennett JE (eds): Principles and Practice of Infectious Diseases, ed 3. New York, Churchill Livingstone, 1990:1554–1563.
25. Kim KS: Antimicrobial susceptibility of GBS. Antibiot Chemother 35:83–89, 1985.
26. Folston KBI: Susceptibility of group B and group G streptococci to newer antimicrobial agents. Eur J Clin Microbiol 5:534–536, 1986.
27. Basiliere JL, Bistrong HW, Spence WF: Streptococcal pneumonia: Recent outbreaks in military recruit populations. Am J Med 44:580–589, 1968.
28. Bisno AL: *Streptococcus pyogenes*. *In* Mandell GL, Douglas RG Jr, Bennett JE (eds): Principles and Practice of Infectious Diseases, ed 3. New York, Churchill Livingstone 1990:1527.

29. Stamm AM, Cobbs CG: Group C streptococcal pneumonia: Report of a fatal case and review of the literature. Rev Infect Dis 2:889–898, 1980.

30. Vartian C, Lerner PI, Shlaes DM, Gopalkrishna KV: Infections due to Lancefield group G streptococci. Medicine (Baltimore) 64:75–88, 1985.

31. Sarkar TK, Murarka RS, Gilardi GL: Primary *Streptococcus viridans* pneumonia. Chest 96:831–832, 1989.

32. Yu VL: Enterococcal superinfection and colonization after therapy with moxalactam, a new broad spectrum antibiotic. Ann Intern Med 94:784–785, 1981.

33. Berk SL, Verghese A, Holtsclaw SA, et al: Enterococcal pneumonia: Occurrence in patients receiving broad spectrum antibiotic regimens and enteral feeding. Am J Med 74:153–154, 1983.

34. Garrison RN, Fry DE, Berberich S, et al: Enterococcal bacteremia: Clinical implications and determinants of death. Ann Surg 196:43–47, 1982.

35. Bryan CS, Reynolds KL, Brown JJ: Mortality associated with enterococcal bacteremia. Surg Gynecol Obstet 160:557–561, 1983.

36. Barrall DT, Kenney PR, Slotman GJ, et al: Enterococcal bacteremia in surgical patients. Arch Surg 120:57–59, 1985.

37. Maki DG, Agger WA: Enterococcal bacteremia: Clinical features, the risk of endocarditis and management. Medicine (Baltimore) 67:248–264, 1988.

38. Malone DA, Wagner RA, Myers JP, et al: Enterococcal bacteremia in two large community teaching hospitals. Am J Med 81:601–606, 1981.

39. Rimailho A, Lampl E, Riou B, et al: Enterococcal bacteremia in a medical intensive care unit. Crit Care Med 16:126–129, 1988.

40. Gullberg RM, Homann SR, Phair JP: Enterococcal bacteremia: Analysis of 75 episodes. Rev Infect Dis 2:80–85, 1989.

# CHAPTER 32

# *Moraxella (Branhamella) catarrhalis* Pneumonia

JAMES MYERS and STEVEN L. BERK

*Moraxella (Branhamella) catarrhalis*, once considered a harmless commensal of the upper respiratory tract, is now a well-documented cause of infection in humans. There are several lines of evidence to support the organism's role in human disease. Increasing numbers of reports have documented *M. catarrhalis* infection by isolating the organism from pure culture of blood. More than 25 such cases are documented in the literature.[1-3]

Purulent secretions have been aspirated from patients with clinical disease and shown to grow *M. catarrhalis* in pure culture. These data include isolates from tympanocentesis in patients with otitis media,[4, 5] maxillary sinus aspiration in patients with acute sinusitis,[6] and joint aspiration in patients with acute arthritis.[7, 8] Transtracheal aspiration has been useful in documenting the role of *M. catarrhalis* in acute bacterial pneumonia.[9-18]

Measurements of specific antibody or changes in the bactericidal activity of acute and convalescent sera have suggested the development of infection in symptomatic patients.[19-21] Patients with clinical *M. catarrhalis* pulmonary infection have improved with treatment.[22] The patients with *M. catarrhalis* in sputum are more likely to have clinical symptoms than those with noncatarrhalis *Neisseria* species in sputum.[23] With the pathogenicity of the organism generally accepted, studies of virulence, immune response, epidemiology, and antibiotic therapy were initiated.

## HISTORY

*M. catarrhalis* has been recognized as a respiratory pathogen since 1881, but there has been a long history of debate about its commensal on virulent status. The history of the organism, from *Micrococcus catarrhalis*, as it was referred to by German investigators, to *Neisseria catarrhalis, Branhamella catarrhalis*, and *Moraxella catarrhalis*, has been reviewed by Berk.[24] Ghon and Pfeiffer[25] and other German clinicians suspected its role in respiratory infection because of its isolation from purulent sputum and its appearance on sputum smears and autopsy tissue. There was little interest in the organism in the United States at that time. An intriguing exception was Sir William Osler who, shortly before his death from pneumonia, wrote, ''No fever since the 16th but cough persists with an occasional paroxysm—bouts as bad as senile whooping cough. One night they nearly blew my candle out. No 3 pneumococcus with *M. catarrhalis.*''[26]

The organism became appreciated as a commensal in the United States partly because of the work of Gordon,[27] who showed that what was then called *N. catarrhalis* did not cause cold symptoms and could be found as oral flora in patients with and without upper respiratory symptoms. As observed by Wallace and Musher, our appreciation of *M. catarrhalis* as a pathogen occurred in much the same way as our awareness of *Haemophilus* influenza.

In many respects, the evolution of our understanding of *B. catarrhalis* from that of an unimportant commensal microorganism to a not uncommon pulmonary pathogen mimics the story of nontypeable *Hemophilus* influenza. Although known and recognized by microbiologists for at least 50 years, both organisms tended to be regarded as colonizing or commensal bacteria by clinicians, who generally ignored their presence in bronchopulmonary secretions of patients with chronic pulmonary disease, the usual setting in which they were isolated. Clinical interest in both species has grown dramatically, thanks to the use of new diagnostic techniques such as transtracheal aspiration and better microbiologic techniques, both of which have facilitated the recognition of these organisms and, in turn, have stimulated the search for them in the appropriate clinical setting.[27]

## MICROBIOLOGY

*M. catarrhalis* is a gram-negative diplococcus that resembles *Neisseria gonorrhoeae* or *Neisseria meningitidis* on smear. The organism can be resistant to decolorization, and occasionally, this leads to confusion with *Staphylococcus aureus* or other gram-positive cocci. *M. catarrhalis* is not found in clusters like *S. aureus*; rather, the flat sides of the organism abut each other, looking more like the organisms of the genus *Neisseria.*

*M. catarrhalis* colonies on blood agar are circular, grayish white, nonhemolytic, and opaque. They usually are 2 to 3 mm in diameter. A useful characteristic of the organism is the ability of the organism to remain intact when pushed over the surface of the agar by a wire loop. This ''hockey puck'' phenomenon can be a preliminary aid in differentiating this organism from other respiratory tract flora.[28]

*M. catarrhalis* does not ferment the simple sugars glucose, maltose, sucrose, or lactose. *Neisseria flavescens* shares this fermentation pattern but is differentiated from *M. catarrhalis* by its inability to produce DNase or reduce nitrate.

Other useful characteristics of *M. catarrhalis* include the hydrolysis of tributyrin and aminopeptidase substrates. Weiner and Penha describe the value of Bacto TB hydrolysis reagent (Difco, Tween 80) as an alternative to DNase testing or tributyrin hydrolysis. Hydrolysis of the Tween 80 reagent causes a color change from amber to pink-red after overnight incubation.[29]

Jonsson and associates[30] studied the reliability of routine diagnostic tests for the identification of *Moraxella* in sputum. They found that a test for DNA hydrolysis was critical for accurate separation of *M. catarrhalis* from other *Neisseria* species. Selective media for *M. catarrhalis* have been developed to increase culture sensitivity and for use in surveillance studies.[31, 32]

Vaneechoutte and colleagues[31] added sodium acetazolamide to selective media containing vancomycin, trimethoprim, and amphotericin B. Incubation of inoculated media in air reduced the growth of *Neisseria* species, which produce carbonic anhydrase. This enzyme is not made by *M. catarrhalis.*

Soto and colleagues[33] looked for phenotypic differences among 27 isolates of *M. catarrhalis* from patients who were thought to have colonization or respiratory infection with the organism. Significant correlation existed between serum resistance and susceptibility to trypsin or the ability to agglutinate human erythrocytes.

Disease-causing isolates of *M. catarrhalis* were more often (43%) serum resistant than colonizing strains, but bacteremic strains were no more serum resistant than nonbacteremic strains in patients with pneumonia.[34]

The outer membrane proteins (OMPs) of *M. catarrhalis* have been purified by sucrose density centrifugation. Murphy[35] compared the OMPs of 50 strains from several sources and identified eight major proteins. The patterns were strikingly similar. The lipopolysaccharide (LPS) of *M. catarrhalis* appears to be unique to this organism. It lacks the long repeating units that characterize the enteric gramnegative organisms. The LPS consists of a lipid A moiety and a seven-residue oligosaccharide region.[6, 36] Further investigation may show whether enough antigenic diversity exists in OMPs or LPS to develop a typing system similar to that used with the gonococci.

Patterson applied restriction endonuclease typing to investigate a hospital outbreak of *M. catarrhalis* infection.[37] Phenotypic characteristics may also be useful in typing *M. catarrhalis.* Phenotypic differences need to be correlated with OMP and restriction endonuclease data in order to better understand the pathogenesis of this organism.[37a]

## HOST RESPONSE

Patients with antibody deficiencies may be more susceptible to *M. catarrhalis* infections.[38, 39] Immunity is probably acquired during childhood for most persons. Antibody responses to *M. catarrhalis* infection have been studied using complement fixation, immunodiffusion, an enzyme-linked immunoassay (EIA), an immunofluorescent assay, and serum bactericidal assay. Chapman and associates[21] used a bactericidal assay in patients with *M. catarrhalis* pneumonia or tracheobronchitis and found that 32% and 90% of acute and convalescent sera showed bactericidal activity against *M. catarrhalis*, respectively.

Chi and coworkers[20] developed an EIA using a *Branhamella* antigen, P-protein, to compare antibody levels of patients infected with *M. catarrhalis* with those in normal controls. Acute-phase titers to P-protein were found to be relatively increased in those infected. Antibody titers of convalescent sera increased over those of acute-phase sera in 46% of pneumonia patients and 50% of tracheobronchitis patients.

A serologic diagnosis has limited usefulness because antibodies are detected in samples from many healthy control patients, and consistent rises in antibody titer do not always occur in the convalescent phase of infection.

## *MORAXELLA CATARRHALIS* PNEUMONIA

### Epidemiology

Most patients with *M. catarrhalis* respiratory infections have an underlying illness, usually chronic obstructive pulmonary disease.[9] *M. catarrhalis* pneumonia has also been reported in patients with acquired immunodeficiency syndrome.[40] A retrospective comparison of *M. catarrhalis*, *Streptococcus pneumoniae*, and *Haemophilus influenzae* pneumonia at our institution found no difference between the three groups in regard to underlying disease.[41]

### Oropharyngeal Colonization

*M. catarrhalis* often colonizes the nasopharynx of children and adults. The incidence of colonization varies from study to study and may depend on the patient population and season of the year.

Vaneechoutte,[31] using a selective medium, found the organism in 50% of children studied. We have not found the organism to be a common colonizer of nursing home patients or those in a Veterans Administration Medical Center (VAMC) hospital intermediate care unit. Japanese investigators found that colonization was more likely to occur during winter months[42] and in patients with chronic lung disease.[43]

Sarubbi and colleagues[44] found *M. catarrhalis* respiratory infection to be more common during winter months at a VAMC and suggested influenza or other viral infections may be a contributing factor (Fig. 32–1).

## Clinical Characteristics

Hager and associates[9] reviewed the clinical characteristics of 429 cases of *M. catarrhalis* respiratory infections from the literature. The mean age of patients was 64.8 years. Seventy-seven percent of patients were cigarette smokers, and 84% of 422 patients had underlying cardiopulmonary disease. Cough, sputum production, and low-grade fever characterized acute bronchitis in these patients. Patients with pneumonia also had low-grade fever (mean 38.4°C) and modestly elevated leukocyte counts (mean, 12,800/mm³). High fever, pleuritic chest pain, and bacteremia were unusual. Necrotizing pneumonia did not occur. The overall mortality rate was 7%. Figure 32–2 shows the underlying cardiopulmonary diseases in patients with *M. catarrhalis* pneumonia.

Wright and colleagues described the clinical characteristics of 42 cases of *M. catarrhalis* pneumonia.[45] As in other studies, the patients were elderly (55% >65 years of age) and had severe underlying obstructive lung disease. Many patients were malnourished and had low serum albumin values. Only 57% of patients had a temperature greater than 100°F. The mean leukocyte count was 15,000/mm³. Chest radiographs were variable, showing consolidation (43%) and bibasilar interstitial patterns. *M. catarrhalis* infection is often easily diagnosed by Gram stain smear of expectorated sputum (Fig. 32–3). Table 32–1 compares the clinical and laboratory findings from the Wright and Hager studies.

Myers and coworkers[41] retrospectively compared *M. catarrhalis* pneumonia with that caused by *S. pneumoniae* or *H. influenzae*. Patients with pneumococcal pneumonia were more likely to be bacteremic than those who had *H. influenzae* or *M. catarrhalis* infection. No other differences in clinical or laboratory features were apparent in the three groups. The average length of stay, need for assisted ventilation or oxygen therapy, and frequency of consolidation seen on chest radiographs did not differ among the groups.

*Moraxella* pneumonia is increasingly affecting children and neonates.[45–48] Many such patients have been in intensive care units or on mechanical ventilation, but some have been previously healthy.

## Antibiotic Susceptibility and β-Lactamase Production

The in vitro susceptibility of *M. catarrhalis* to old and new antibiotics has been well studied.[49–52] Most *M. catarrhalis* isolates now produce β-lactamase. Wallace and colleagues[53, 54] have documented that the production of β-lactamase by *M. catarrhalis* is a relatively new phenomenon. Enzyme-producing strains were first reported from Europe in the late 1970s.[55] Wallace and associates found the first β-lactamase–producing strains in the United States to have occurred at about the same time.[54] In a study of 378 *M. catarrhalis* isolates from 15 medical centers in the United States, 84% of strains were found to produce β-lactamase.[56]

The β-lactamases of *M. catarrhalis* are called BRO-1 and BRO-2. Isolates with BRO-1 have higher minimum inhibitory concentrations (MICs) than those producing BRO-2. Table 32–2 compares the BRO-1 and BRO-2 enzymes.[54] These enzymes are strongly membrane-associated.[54] Clinically, they confer resistance only to penicillin

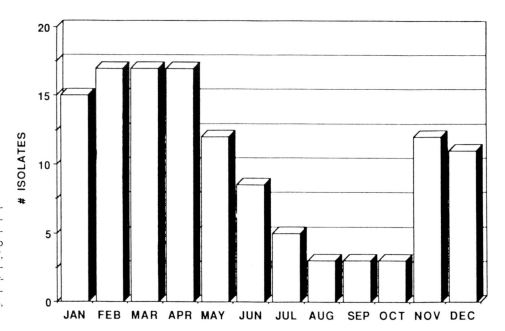

**Figure 32–1.** Average monthly isolation of *M. catarrhalis* at the Veterans Administration Medical Center, Johnson City, TN, from 1986 to 1989. (From Sarubbi FA, Myers JW, Williams JJ, et al: Respiratory infections caused by *Branhamella catarrhalis*. Selected epidemiologic features. Am J Med 88(suppl 5A):10S, 1990.)

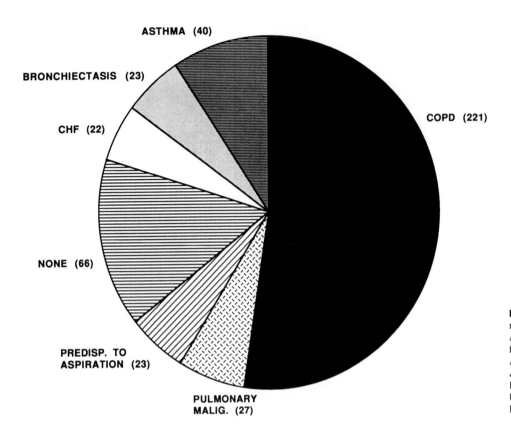

**Figure 32–2.** Underlying cardiopulmonary disease in 422 cases of *Moraxella catarrhalis* respiratory infection. (From Hager H, Verghese A, Alvarez S, et al: *Branhamella catarrhalis* respiratory infections. Rev Infect Dis 9:1140–1149, 1987. The University of Chicago Press, publisher.)

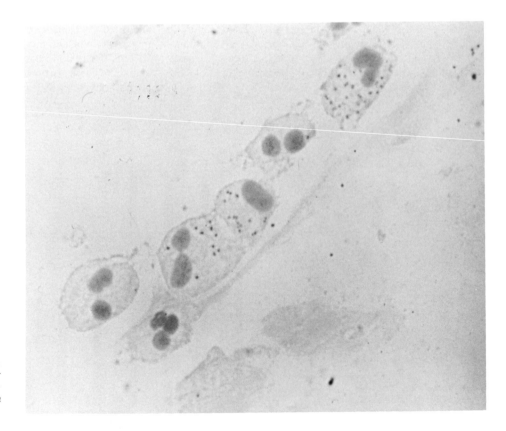

**Figure 32–3.** A sputum Gram stain shows many polymorphonuclear leukocytes and intracellular gram-negative diplococci of *Moraxella catarrhalis*.

Table 32–1. **Clinical and Laboratory Findings for**
*Moraxella catarrhalis* **Pneumonia**

| Clinical Description | Wright et al[45] | Hager et al[9] |
|---|---|---|
| Mean age (y) | 64 (15.2 ± SD) | 65 |
| Current smokers (%) | 52 | 65 |
| Chronic obstructive lung disease (%) | 52 | 64 |
| Cancer (%) | 29 | 19 (31/166) |
| Nonconsolidative infiltrates on x-ray (%) | 38 | 37 |
| β-Lactamase positive (%) | 67 | 53 |
| Mean peak temperature (°C) | 38.1 | 38.4 |
| (°F) | 100.6 | 101.1 |
| Range peak temperature (°C) | 37.0–39.7 | 37.5–40.1 |
| Mean peak leukocyte count (cells/mm³) | 15,000 | 12,800 |
| Hospital mortality (%) | 21 | 7 |
| Three months mortality (%) | 45 | Not given |

Modified from Wright PW, Wallace RJ Jr, Shepherd JR: A descriptive study of 42 cases of *Branhamella catarrhalis* pneumonia. Am J Med 88(suppl 5A):7S, 1990.

and ampicillin. From 1976 to 1977, these two enzymes appeared globally in this species.[51] *Moraxella lacunata* and *Moraxella nonliquefaciens* acquired these enzymes at approximately the same time.

Most β-lactamase–producing strains have MICs of 2.0 μg/mL or less to ampicillin.[54] These organisms would usually be called susceptible by the National Committee for Clinical Laboratory Standards. The MIC breakpoints for *Moraxella* are now such that strains with an MIC of less than 0.25 μg/mL are considered susceptible, and those of more than 0.5 μg/mL are resistant.

The MIC ranges for 19 antibiotics are shown in Table 32–3. Tetracycline resistance was first reported in 1983. Up to 43% of *M. catarrhalis* may be resistant in some areas.[58] Resistance has also been reported to erythromycin.[54] Common β-lactamase inhibitors inhibit BRO-1 and BRO-2.[57] No clear-cut drug of choice exists for *M. catarrhalis*. The empiric use of penicillin or ampicillin to treat respiratory infections in chronic lung disease patients is not a good choice in view of *M. catarrhalis* resistance.

The seasonal occurrence of *M. catarrhalis* pneumonia, documented in several distinct geographic areas, may be an important clue to pathogenesis of infection. As a first step, coinfection with agents such as influenza must be assessed.

## PNEUMONIA CAUSED BY OTHER *NEISSERIA* SPECIES

*N. meningitidis* has been reported in outbreaks of pneumonia since 1919.[59] It is possible that the organism was

Table 32–2. **BRO Enzymes in *Moraxella catarrhalis***

BRO-1 (Ravasio) present in 90% strains United States, Belgium
BRO-2 (1908) present in remaining 10%
Both enzymes have the same substrate and inhibitor profile
BRO-1 production is two to three times that of BRO-2
Isolates with BRO-1 have higher MICs than those with BRO-2

Modified from Wallace RJ Jr, Nash DP, Steingrube MS: Antibiotic susceptibilities and drug resistance in *Moraxella (Branhamella) catarrhalis*. Am J Med 88(suppl 5A):49S, 1990.

Table 32–3. **Susceptibility Patterns of *Moraxella catarrhalis* to Antimicrobial Agents**

| Antibiotic | MIC Values (μg/mL)* | | |
|---|---|---|---|
| | *MIC Range* | *MIC₅₀* | *MIC₉₀* |
| Penicillin G | <0.125–16.0 | 2.0 | 8.0 |
| Ampicillin | <0.125–4.0 | 0.25 | 1.0 |
| Methicillin | <0.25–16.0 | 2.0 | 16.0 |
| Ticarcillin | <0.5–16.0 | 1.0 | 8.0 |
| Piperacillin | <0.125–0.25 | <0.125 | 0.125 |
| Amoxicillin plus clavulanic acid | <0.06–0.25 | <0.06 | 0.25 |
| Clindamycin | 0.125–2.0 | 1.0 | 1.0 |
| Erythromycin | <0.06–0.25 | 0.125 | 0.25 |
| Vancomycin | <0.5–64 | 16.0 | 32.0 |
| Cephalothin | <0.5–8.0 | 4.0 | 4.0 |
| Cefamandole | 0.25–4.0 | 2.0 | 4.0 |
| Cefoxitin | <0.06–0.25 | 0.125 | 0.125 |
| Cefuroxime | 0.125–1.0 | 0.5 | 1.0 |
| Cefotaxime | <0.125–0.5 | 0.25 | 0.5 |
| Cefoperazone | <0.125–2.0 | 0.25 | 1.0 |
| Ceftazidime | <0.06–0.125 | <0.06 | <0.06 |
| Trimethoprim-sulfamethoxazole | <0.25–4.75/ 0.25–4.75 | <0.25/4.75 | <0.25/4.75 |
| Tetracycline | <0.06–0.25 | 0.125 | 0.125 |
| Chloramphenicol | 0.25–0.50 | 0.50 | 0.50 |

*MIC, minimal inhibitory concentration. Values for trimethoprim and sulfamethoxazole are separated by a slash.

Modified from Hager H, Verghese A, Alvarez S, et al: *Branhamella catarrhalis* respiratory infections. Rev Infect Dis 9:1140–1149, 1987. The University of Chicago Press, publisher.

mistaken for *M. catarrhalis* in some early studies. Koppes and colleagues[60] documented an outbreak among military recruits using transtracheal aspiration. Sixty-eight cases were diagnosed, and all patients survived. Most had upper and lower respiratory symptoms. An outbreak in a nursing home was associated with influenza.[61] Kerttula,[62] in a study in Finland, found 6 of 162 cases of pneumonia to be caused by *N. meningitidis*.

Gilrane and associates[63] reported 2 patients with *Neisseria sicca* pneumonia. Both were diagnosed by sheathed bronchoscopy, and both patients did well. The investigators found an additional case reported in the literature.[64] Thorsteinsson and colleagues[65] reported a patient with *Neisseria mucosa* empyema that developed after surgery.

## REFERENCES

1. Wallace MR, Oldfield EC III: *Moraxella (Branhamella) catarrhalis* bacteremia. Arch Intern Med 150:1332–1334, 1990.
2. Cimolai N, Adderley RI: *Branhamella catarrhalis* bacteremia in children. Acta Paediatr Scand 78:465–468, 1989.
3. Choo PW, Gantz NM: *Branhamella catarrhalis* pneumonia with bacteremia. South Med J 82:1317–1318, 1989.
4. Shurin PA, Marchant CD, Kim CH, et al: Emergence of *Branhamella catarrhalis* as important agents of acute otitis media. Pediatr Infect Dis 2:34–38, 1983.
5. Van Hare GFP, Shurin C, Marchant D, et al: Acute otitis media caused by *Branhamella catarrhalis*: Biology and therapy. Rev Infect Dis 9:16–27, 1987.
6. Wald ED, Milmoe GJ, Bowen AD, et al: Acute maxillary sinusitis in children. N Engl J Med 304:749–754, 1981.
7. Craig DB, Wehrle PA: *Branhamella catarrhalis* septic arthritis. J Rheumatol 10:985–986, 1983.
8. Izraeli S, Flasterstein B, Shamir R, et al: *Branhamella catarrhalis* as a cause of suppurative arthritis. Pediatr Infect Dis J 8:256–257, 1989.

9. Hager H, Verghese A, Alvarez S, et al: *Branhamella catarrhalis* respiratory infections. Rev Infect Dis 9:1140–1149, 1987.

10. West M, Berk SL, Smith JK: *Branhamella catarrhalis* pneumonia. South Med J 75:1021–1023, 1982.

11. Slevin NJ, Aitken J, Thornley PE: Clinical and microbiological features of *Branhamella catarrhalis* bronchopulmonary infections. Lancet 1:782–783, 1984.

12. Louie MH, Gabay EL, Mathisen GE, et al: *Branhamella catarrhalis* pneumonia. West J Med 138:47–49, 1983.

13. Ninane G, Joly J, Kraytman M: Bronchopulmonary infection due to *Branhamella catarrhalis*: 11 cases assessed by transtracheal puncture. Br Med J 1:276–278, 1978.

14. Ninane G, Joly J, Kraytman M, et al: Bronchopulmonary infection due to beta-lactamase producing *Branhamella catarrhalis* treated with amoxicillin-clavulanic acid. [Letter] Lancet 2:257, 1978.

15. Aitken JM, Thornlee PE: Isolation of *Branhamella catarrhalis* from sputum and tracheal aspirate. J Clin Microbiol 18:1262–1263, 1983.

16. Srinivasan G, Ralf MJ, Templeton WC, et al: *Branhamella catarrhalis* pneumonia: Report of two cases and review of the literature. Am Rev Respir Dis 123:553–555, 1981.

17. Doern GV, Miller MJ, Winn RE: *Branhamella (Neisseria) catarrhalis* systemic disease in humans. Arch Intern Med 141:1690–1692, 1981.

18. Thornley PE, Aitken J, Drennam CJ, et al: *Branhamella catarrhalis* infection of the lower respiratory tract: Reliable diagnosis by sputum examination. Br Med J 285:1537–1538, 1982.

19. Borson JE, Axelsson A, Holm SE: Studies on *Branhamella catarrhalis (Neisseria catarrhalis)* with special reference to maxillary sinusitis. Scand J Infect Dis 8:151–155, 1976.

20. Chi DS, Verghese A, Moore C, et al: Antibody response to P-protein in patients with *Branhamella catarrhalis* infections. Am J Med 88:25S–27S, 1990.

21. Chapman S, Musher DM, Jonsson S: Development of bactericidal antibody during *Branhamella catarrhalis* infection. J Infect Dis 151:878–882, 1985.

22. Nicotra B, Rivera M, Luman JI, et al: *Branhamella catarrhalis* as a lower respiratory tract pathogen in patients with chronic lung disease. Arch Intern Med 146:890–893, 1986.

23. Yuen KY, Seto WH, Ong SG: The significance of *Branhamella catarrhalis* in bronchopulmonary infection—a case-control study. J Infect Dis 19:251–256, 1991.

24. Berk SL: From *Micrococcus* to *Moraxella*. The reemergence of *Branhamella catarrhalis*. Arch Intern Med 150:2254–2257, 1990.

25. Ghon A, Pfeiffer H: Der Mikrococcus catarrhalis. (R. Pfeiffer) als Krankheitserreger. Z Klin Med 44:263–281, 1902.

26. Cushing H: The Life of Sir William Osler. Oxford, England, Clarendon Press, 1925:672.

27. Gordon JE: The gram-negative cocci in colds and influenza. J Infect Dis 29:463–494, 1921.

28. Shurin PA, Marchant CD, Kim CH, et al: Emergence of beta-lactamase–producing strains of *Branhamella catarrhalis* as important agents of acute otitis media. Pediatr Infect Dis J 2:34–38, 1983.

29. Weiner M, Penha PD: Evaluation of Bacto TB hydrolysis reagent (Tween 80) for the identification of *Branhamella catarrhalis*. J Clin Microbiol 1:126–127, 1990.

30. Jonsson I, Eriksson B, Krook A: Minimal criteria for identification of *Moraxella (Branhamella) catarrhalis*. Karolinska Institute, Roslagstull's Hospital, Stockholm, Sweden. APMIS 10:954–956, 1990.

31. Vaneechoutte M, Verschraegen G, Claeys G, et al: Selective medium for *Branhamella catarrhalis* with acetazolamide as a specific inhibitor of *Neisseria* spp. J Clin Microbiol 26:2544–2548, 1988.

32. Soto-Hernandez JL, Nunley D, Holtsclaw-Berk S, et al: Selective medium with DNase test agar and a modified toluidine blue O technique for primary isolation of *Branhamella catarrhalis* in sputum. J Clin Microbiol 26:405–408, 1988.

33. Soto-Hernandez JL, Holtsclaw-Berk S, Harvill LM, et al: Phenotypic characteristics of *Branhamella catarrhalis* strains. J Clin Microbiol 26:405–408, 1988.

34. Jordan KL, Berk SH, Berk SL: A comparison of serum bactericidal activity and phenotypic characteristics of bacteremic, pneumonia-causing strains, and colonizing strains of *Branhamella catarrhalis*. Am J Med 88(suppl 5A):28S–32S, 1990.

35. Murphy TF, Loeb MR: Isolation of the outer membrane of *Branhamella catarrhalis*. Microb Pathog 6:159–174, 1989.

36. Johnson KG, McDonald IJ, Perry MB: Studies on the cellular and free lipopolysaccharides from *Branhamella catarrhalis*. Can J Med 22:460–467, 1976.

37. Patterson JE, Patterson TF, Farrel P, et al: Evaluation of restriction endonuclease analysis as an epidemiologic typing system for *Branhamella catarrhalis*. J Clin Microbiol 27:944–946, 1989.

37a. Hulminen ME, MacIver I, Latmer JL, et al: A major outer membrane protein of *Moraxella catarrhalis* is a target for antibodies that enhance pulmonary clearance of the pathogen in an animal model. Infect Immun 61:2003–2010, 1993.

38. Karnad A, Alvarez S, Berk SL: *Branhamella catarrhalis* pneumonia in patients with immunoglobulin abnormalities. South Med J 79:1360–1362, 1986.

39. McNeely DJ, Kitchens CS, Kluge RM: Fatal *Neisseria (Branhamella) catarrhalis* pneumonia in an immunodeficient host. Am Rev Respir Dis 114:399–402, 1976.

40. Polsky B, Gold JWM, Whimbey E, et al: Bacterial pneumonia in patients with AIDS. Ann Intern Med 104:38–41, 1986.

41. Myers JW, Kalbfleisch J, Sarubbi FA: *Moraxella catarrhalis* pneumonia: A comparative study with pneumonias due to *S. pneumoniae* and *H. influenzae*. Presented at the American College of Chest Physicians' 56th Annual Scientific Assembly, Toronto, Canada, October, 1990.

42. Mbaki N, Rikitomi N, Nagatake T, Matsumoto K: Correlation between *Branhamella catarrhalis* adherence to oropharyngeal cells and seasonal incidence of lower respiratory tract infections. Tohoku J Exp Med 153:111–121, 1987.

43. Rikitomi N, Mbaki N, Nagatake T, et al: Adherence of *Branhamella catarrhalis* to human pharyngeal cells: Relationship between adherence in vitro and chronic respiratory infections. Nippon Kyobu Shikkan Gakkai Zasshi 24:633–638, 1986.

44. Sarubbi FA, Myers JW, Williams JJ, et al: Respiratory infections caused by *Branhamella catarrhalis*. Selected epidemiologic features. Am J Med 88(suppl 5A):9S–14S, 1990.

45. Wright PW, Wallace RJ Jr, Shepherd JR: A descriptive study of 42 cases of *Branhamella catarrhalis* pneumonia. Am J Med 88(suppl 5A):2S–8S, 1990.

46. Ohlsson A, Bailey T: Neonatal pneumonia caused by *Branhamella catarrhalis*. Scand J Infect Dis 17:225–228, 1985.

47. Moreno Galdo A, Ferrer MA, Aizpurua Galdeano P, et al: *Branhamella catarrhalis*: Its respiratory pathogenicity in childhood. An Esp Pediatr 33:135–139, 1990.

48. Dyson C, Poonyth HD, Watkinson M, et al: Life threatening *Branhamella catarrhalis* pneumonia in young infants. J Infect Dis 21:305–307, 1990.

49. Alvarez S, Jones M, Holtsclaw-Berk S, et al: In vitro susceptibilities and β-lactamase production of 53 clinical isolates of *Branhamella catarrhalis*. Antimicrob Agents Chemother 27:646–647, 1985.

50. Sweeney KG, Verghese A, Needham CA: In vitro susceptibilities of isolates from patients with *Branhamella catarrhalis* pneumonia compared with those of colonizing strains. Antimicrob Agents Chemother 27:499–502, 1985.

51. Ahmad F, McLeod DT, Croughan MJ, et al: Antimicrobial susceptibility of *Branhamella catarrhalis* isolates from bronchopulmonary infections. Antimicrob Agents Chemother 26:424–425, 1984.

52. Doern GV, Jones RN: Antimicrobial susceptibility testing of *Haemophilus influenzae, Branhamella catarrhalis*, and *Neisseria gonorrhoeae*. Antimicrob Agents Chemother 32:1747–1753, 1988.

53. Wallace RJ Jr, Steingrube VA, Nash DR, et al: BRO β-lactamases of *Branhamella catarrhalis* and *Moraxella* subgenus *Moraxella*, including evidence for chromosomal β-lactamase transfer by conjugation in *B. catarrhalis, M. nonliquefaciens* and *M. lacunata*. Antimicrob Agents Chemother 33:1845–1854, 1989.

54. Wallace RJ Jr, Nash DP, Steingrube MS: Antibiotic susceptibilities and drug resistance in *Moraxella (Branhamella) catarrhalis*. Am J Med 88(suppl 5A):46S–50S, 1990.

55. Percival A, Corkill JE, Rowlands J, et al: Pathogenicity of and beta-lactamase production by *Branhamella (Neisseria) catarrhalis*. Lancet 2:1175, 1977.

56. Jorgenssen JH, Maher LA, Howell AW, et al: National surveillance of antimicrobial resistance among respiratory isolates of *Haemophilus influenzae, Branhamella catarrhalis* and *Streptococcus pneumoniae*. [Abstract 1289] Presented at the 29th Interscience Conference on Antimicrobial Agents and Chemotherapy, American Society for Microbiology, Washington, DC, 1989.

57. Catlin BW: *Branhamella catarrhalis*: An organism gaining respect as a pathogen. Clin Microbiol Rev 3:293–320, 1990.

58. Kallings I: Sensitivity of *Branhamella catarrhalis* to oral antibiotics. Drugs 31(suppl 3):17–22, 1986.

59. Holm ML, Davison WC, Emmons VB: *Meningococcus* pneumonia: I. The occurrence of post-influenzal pneumonia in which *Diplococcus intracellularis* meningitidis was isolated from observation at Camp Coetquidon. Bull Johns Hopkins Hosp 30:324–329, 1919.

60. Koppes GM, Ellenbogen C, Gebhart RJ: Group Y meningococcal disease in United States Air Force recruits. Am J Med 62:661–666, 1977.

61. Young LS, LaForce FM, Head JJ, et al: A simultaneous outbreak of meningococcal and influenza infection. N Engl J Med 287:5–9, 1972.

62. Kerttula Y, Leinonen M, Koskela M, et al: The aetiology of pneumonia. Application of bacterial serology and basic laboratory methods. J Infect 14:21–30, 1987.

63. Gilrane T, Tracy JD, Greenlee RM, et al: *Neisseria sicca* pneumonia. Report of two cases and review of the literature. Am J Med 78:1038–1040, 1985.

64. Alcid DV: *Neisseria sicca* pneumonia. Chest 77:123–124, 1980.

65. Thorsteinsson SB, Minuth JN, Musher DM: Postpneumonectomy empyema due to *Neisseria mucosa*. Am J Clin Pathol 64:534, 1975.

# CHAPTER 33

# Fungal Diseases of the Lung

PHILIP C. JOHNSON, SCOTT F. DAVIES, and GEORGE A. SAROSI

Community-acquired fungal diseases occur almost exclusively in the New World. North America is truly the home of histoplasmosis and blastomycosis. Coccidioidomycosis occurs in North America and to a lesser extent in South America. Paracoccidioidomycosis, another community-acquired fungal disease, occurs exclusively in South and Central America. Although histoplasmosis and blastomycosis are occasionally diagnosed on other continents, the major endemic areas for all these fungi are in the Western hemisphere.

All four endemic mycoses share certain characteristics. The causative organisms exist in nature in their saprophytic form. Under appropriate conditions of climate and temperature, spores are formed. If the sites are disturbed, the spores become airborne, producing an infecting aerosol. If a mammal is close to the site when the infective aerosol is formed, infection may occur. After inhalation into mammalian lungs, the saprophytic forms of these fungi change to a parasitic form. This characteristic is referred to as dimorphism. *Histoplasma capsulatum, Blastomyces dermatitidis*, and *Paracoccidioides brasiliensis* convert to a parasitic yeast form at 37°C (ie, thermal dimorphism), and the spores of *Coccidioides immitis* convert to the spherule form in tissue (ie, tissue dimorphism).

Because *P. brasiliensis* occurs outside the United States, the major focus of this discussion is the great endemic mycoses of North America—histoplasmosis, blastomycosis, and coccidioidomycosis. Their respective endemic areas are large and have been defined by the use of skin tests for *H. capsulatum*[1] and *C. immitis*[2] and by tabulation of patients for *B. dermatitidis*.[3] Blastomycosis and histoplasmosis are endemic in the midwest and south-central United States, but blastomycosis extends farther north.[4] The endemic area for coccidioidomycosis includes the southwest United States and adjacent areas of Mexico.

*Cryptococcus neoformans* is a soil-dwelling, encapsulated yeast that causes disease in normal and immunosuppressed hosts. This organism is not dimorphic; the saprophytic and parasitic phases are simple yeasts. *C. neoformans* is widely distributed in nature, and disease due to the fungus has been recognized throughout the world.

The dimorphic fungi and *C. neoformans* share certain important characteristics. The portal of entry for all is the lung. In the alveolus, conversion to the parasitic phase enhances resistance to polymorphonuclear phagocytes (PMNs). After the fungi are in their parasitic form, they cannot be killed by immigrating PMNs.[5] The *Cryptococcus* organism does not have a parasitic form, but its thick polysaccharide capsule is antiphagocytic.[6] Elimination of all these fungi depends on intact T-cell–mediated immunity. With the advent of specific T-cell immunity, the infection can be contained. Most immunologically intact persons can effectively deal with these infections. Any diminution of T-cell activity allows progression, and there is epidemiologic evidence that dormant organisms within the mammalian host may reactivate when intercurrent illness or therapy depresses T-cell–mediated immunity. This behavior is similar to the epidemiology of *Mycobacterium tuberculosis*. All five fungal organisms should be viewed as T-cell opportunists, although data for *P. brasiliensis* are scanty.

The common dimorphic fungus, *Sporothrix schenckii*, is primarily acquired by subcutaneous inoculation of the infecting particles. Patients with lung disease, presumably acquired by inhalation, have been reported. These pulmonary infections are rare and are not discussed in this chapter.

## HISTOPLASMOSIS

Histoplasmosis was first recognized at autopsy by Samuel Darling, a U.S. pathologist working in Panama.[7] Perhaps because he was looking for leishmaniasis, he thought that his patients had a protozoan infection. Because of the histopathologic appearance (now recognized as an artifact), he thought that the organism was encapsulated, and he named it *Histoplasma capsulatum*. By 1912, DeRocha-Lima speculated that the organism was a fungus, but the name, more suitable for a protozoan, stayed.

Darling's original observation was almost forgotten by 1927, when C.J. Watson, working as a pathology resident, described a similar case, also at autopsy, in a native of Minnesota.[8] The next advance in knowledge about histoplasmosis was made in 1934 by Dodd and Tompkins at Vanderbilt University. They observed intracellular organisms in the circulating phagocytes of a child dying of an unknown febrile illness with features including severe anemia and hepatosplenomegaly.[9] After the death of the child, DeMonbreum isolated the organism from postmortem material by inoculating organ filtrates into laboratory animals. He confirmed DeRocha-Lima's hypothesis that the organism was a fungus.[10] He also demonstrated the thermal dimorphism of the fungus. After a series of publications from the Vanderbilt group, additional patients with widely disseminated histoplasmosis were recognized, but the disease remained a great curiosity, and the prevailing wisdom stated that histoplasmosis was a rare and highly lethal infection.

This perception changed when Christie and Peterson used DeMonbreum's original isolate to produce a skin test antigen, histoplasmin. They began skin test surveys, first concentrating on patients in the Nashville area with pulmonary calcification and negative tuberculin skin tests. Most had a positive histoplasmin skin test. They correctly surmised that these positive skin test reactions were immunologic footprints of a benign, self-limited form of histoplasmosis.[11] Their observations were quickly confirmed by Palmer of the United States Public Health Service.[12] Histoplasmosis moved from the ranks of medical curiosity to be recognized as an extremely common and almost universally benign illness.

Emmons and his associates were able to recover the fungus from soil.[13] The epidemiology of histoplasmosis became clear. The organism grows in microfoci of nitrogen-enriched soil. If these microfoci are disturbed, an infectious aerosol is formed. Mammals coming in contact with the airborne spores can be infected.

An extensive skin test survey by the U.S. Public Health Service showed high skin test reactivity throughout the south-central United States.[14] On the basis of this skin test survey, the best estimates are that more than 50 million people in this area have been infected with the fungus and perhaps as many as 500,000 new cases occur annually.

Because the organism requires organic nitrogen for growth, areas heavily contaminated with bird droppings serve as excellent foci. During the 1950s and 1960s, most outbreaks were traced to abandoned chicken houses. Most epidemics now occur in urban centers, where treed areas frequented by gregarious blackbirds are the sites for fungal growth.[15] The organism also exists in caves, where bat droppings serve as the source of organic nitrogen.

Virtually all modern outbreaks have occurred in urban areas on the fringe of an endemic area where few cases of histoplasmosis had previously been recognized. From Mason City, Iowa,[16] to Montreal, Canada, to Indianapolis, Indiana,[17] this has held true. The usual precipitating event is heavy construction activity, creating the infecting aerosol. The potential exists for successful decontamination; this was done in Mason City with a topical 3% solution of formaldehyde.[18]

## Pathogenesis

The portal of entry for *H. capsulatum* is the lung. After inhalation, some spores elude nonspecific pulmonary defenses and reach the alveoli. Conversion to the parasitic yeast phase begins immediately. The yeast multiply by binary fission. The primary cellular response to the infection includes PMNs, followed by the rapid accumulation of macrophages. Neutrophils are unable to kill the yeast. Macrophages ingest the yeast, but in their preimmune state, they cannot kill them; the yeast continue to grow within the macrophages until the development of specific T-cell–mediated immunity. During the preimmune phase, the yeast actively multiply within macrophages and disseminate throughout the body. Metastatic foci are established in tissues rich in reticuloendothelial (RE) cells, such as liver, spleen, lymph nodes, and bone marrow.

Intracellular proliferation of the fungus continues until the development of T-cell immunity, which checks the further advance of the illness. With the specific immunity response, immune lymphocytes move into the lung and other infected organs. These lymphocytes then "arm" the macrophages, which improves their ability to sequester and kill the fungus. Granulomas form, and depending on the intensity of the inflammatory process, a central necrosis develops that is indistinguishable from that seen in tuberculosis. Areas of caseation necrosis occur in the lung and at all metastatic sites. Healing occurs by fibrosis, which encapsulates the necrotic material, which may calcify. Calcification occurs more frequently in younger persons. The lung calcifications are sometimes similar to the classic Ghon complex and mistakenly ascribed to remote tuberculosis.[19] Because necrosis may occur in extrapulmonary lesions, similar calcification may be seen in the liver and spleen.

## Clinical Manifestations

After inhalation of the fungus, most normal persons have few or no symptoms. If symptoms develop, they are so nonspecific that sporadically occurring infections are almost never diagnosed. Most of our understanding of benign, self-limited histoplasmosis comes from the careful study of outbreaks in which groups of infected patients can be identified. Respiratory symptoms are most common. Because the symptoms vary with the size of the infecting dose, they are often severe if the infection is acquired in a closed space but trivial if the infection is acquired in an open area. Most early outbreaks were cases of infection acquired indoors, and the frequency of highly symptomatic cases was quite high.[20] In community-wide outbreaks, symptomatic disease occurred less frequently. Symptoms, even trivial ones, are recognized in fewer than 50% of the patients involved in large, open-air outbreaks. Asymptomatic patients are usually identified by serologic studies.

The incubation time for acute histoplasmosis is 9 to 17 days. In 1982, we studied an outbreak for which the time of exposure was known within 2 hours. In this outbreak, the mean incubation time was 14 days, with a very sharp and narrow peak.[21] Goodwin had previously calculated, on the basis of other reports, that 14 days should be the mean incubation time.[22]

Symptomatic patients with histoplasmosis have an illness that resembles influenza. The onset is abrupt, with fever, chills, and substernal chest pain. A nonproductive cough may develop. Headache is common, and arthralgias and myalgias are frequent.[22] Although respiratory complaints are extremely common, serious interference with gas exchange is uncommon. However, with a large infecting dose, rapid progression of illness may lead to the adult respiratory distress syndrome (ARDS).

Even in symptomatic patients, the chest roentgenogram may be negative. More often, the initial chest radiograph shows single or multiple areas of pneumonitis, usually in the lower lung fields, presumably because of their better ventilation. Another hallmark of acute histoplasmosis is the rapid involvement of the draining lymph nodes. Hilar adenopathy is common and ipsilateral. If the characteristic pulmonary infiltrate and hilar lymph node complex is seen in appropriate epidemiologic circumstances, the diagnosis is relatively easy. However, hilar adenopathy may exist without parenchymal infiltrates, and parenchymal infiltrates are not always associated with hilar adenopathy. Moreover, completely asymptomatic persons may have infiltrates or hilar nodes. If these findings are discovered accidentally on routine chest roentgenograms, invasive diagnostic tests are often done, but these can sometimes be avoided if histoplasmosis is considered and diagnosed serologically.

The disease usually lasts 1 to 3 weeks. In some cases, the chest radiograph clears. In other cases, the primary parenchymal infiltrate fails to resolve. It undergoes necrosis, rounds off, and is contained by fibrous tissue. These rounded, densely fibrotic lesions present as "coin" lesions that are hard to differentiate from bronchogenic carcinoma. In the absence of calcification, the only way to establish the benign nature of these nodules is to resect them. After calcification occurs, the differential diagnosis is easier. Dense central calcification with subsequent ring calcification around the periphery is typical of a benign lesion. Calcification may also involve the hilar nodes, as in tuberculosis (Fig. 33–1). Foci of calcification in histoplasmosis tend to be larger; they have been described as "mulberry" calcifications (Fig. 33–2). After a large infecting dose, many small, punctate areas of calcification may occur on the chest radiograph (ie, "buckshot" calcification). These are characteristic of healed primary histoplasmosis (Fig. 33–3).[22]

The issue of possible reinfection in histoplasmosis is extremely confusing. It is virtually impossible to reinfect an animal that has recovered from primary infection.[23] However, circumstantial evidence suggests that reinfection may occur among humans.[24] Skin test reactivity to histoplasmin in any cohort wanes with advancing age.[25] Goodwin has proposed that some patients in highly endemic areas maintain a positive skin test by repeated exposure to the organism, refreshing immunologic memory.[1, 22] Histoplasmosis reinfection remains unproven.

The physical examination during the acute phase of histoplasmosis is usually negative. Hepatosplenomegaly suggests disseminated disease.[26] However, there are several striking syndromes that occur with acute histoplasmosis. The best described is the arthralgia, erythema nodosum, and erythema multiforme complex.[27] Although arthralgias are common during the acute phase of the illness and may be severe enough to interfere with walking, they usually resolve rapidly. Occasionally, severe arthralgias are associated with the erythema multiforme and erythema nodosum. These are recognized in a few patients during epidemics, and they frequently serve as evidence that histoplasmosis is the cause of the outbreak. These "allergic" skin manifestations occur most frequently in Caucasian women and may occur without other manifestations of histoplasmosis. Incidence is estimated at 1 in 200 infections.[15]

Pericarditis may complicate the course of acute histoplasmosis. It has been thought of as a great rarity, but, during a large outbreak in Indianapolis, pericarditis was a relatively common complication of acute histoplasmosis. Forty-five (6.3%) of 712 patients had pericarditis. The pericardial effusions are usually sterile and are not thought to be secondary to direct involvement of the pericardium by the organism.[28]

Enlarged intrathoracic lymph nodes (ie, mediastinal granuloma) frequently impinge on adjacent mediastinal structures. Involvement of the peritracheal nodes may cause irritating cough or dyspnea. Pressure on the esophagus may lead to dysphagia. Enlarged nodes adjacent to the superior vena cava may obstruct it and cause edema of the head and upper extremities. In some patients, the "middle lobe syndrome" may occur secondary to impingement on the middle lobe bronchus. Large nodes in strategic places can be resected, but the back wall of the nodal mass is left behind and not dissected off the adjacent structure. Surgery may improve the symptoms, but the natural history tends to be benign with gradual improvement.

One of the most feared complications of histoplasmosis is the development of exuberant mediastinal fibrosis, which can entrap vital mediastinal structures and lead to severe functional derangement. Bronchi, pulmonary arteries, and pulmonary veins may be entrapped, causing pulmonary hypertension and death from cor pulmonale (Fig. 33–4). Diffuse mediastinal fibrosis does not respond to drug therapy, and surgery is also unsuccessful.[29] It is a different disorder from mediastinal granuloma, in which individual lymph nodes are enlarged.

If primary histoplasmosis occurs in patients with structurally abnormal lungs, the clinical picture is different. In smokers with centrilobular emphysema of the upper lung zones, the primary infection often involves these upper zones.[30] Areas of centrilobular emphysema are outlined by the infiltrate, mimicking cavities and leading to confusion with reinfection tuberculosis.[31] Most of these patients recover uneventfully, with slow clearing of the chest radiograph (Fig. 33–5).[32] Approximately 20% develop a progressive and destructive upper lobe disease closely mimicking tuberculosis (Fig. 33–6).[31, 33] Such patients were first recognized in tuberculosis sanatoria, where they had been admitted under the mistaken assumption that they suffered from tuberculosis rather than histoplasmosis.[34]

The clinical manifestations of acute, self-limited upper lobe histoplasmosis in smokers with emphysema are similar to those of acute histoplasmosis in normal hosts.[31] In con-

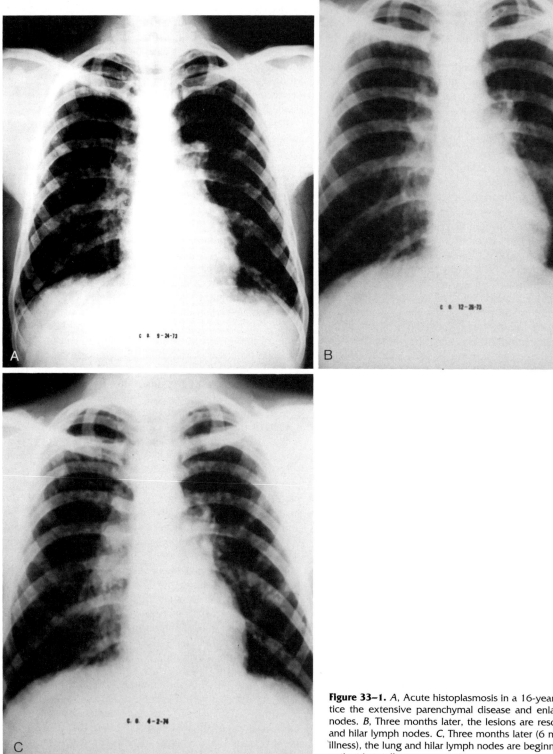

**Figure 33–1.** *A,* Acute histoplasmosis in a 16-year-old student. Notice the extensive parenchymal disease and enlarged hilar lymph nodes. *B,* Three months later, the lesions are resolving in the lung and hilar lymph nodes. *C,* Three months later (6 months after acute illness), the lung and hilar lymph nodes are beginning to calcify. The patient is totally asymptomatic.

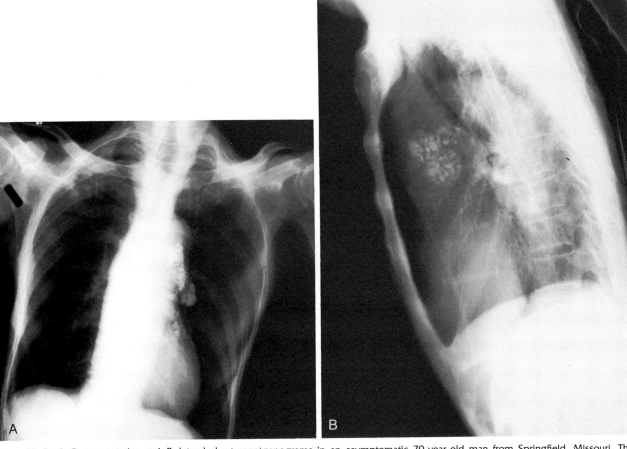

**Figure 33–2.** *A*, Posteroanterior and *B*, lateral chest roentgenograms in an asymptomatic 79-year-old man from Springfield, Missouri. The tuberculin skin test was negative, and the histoplasmin skin test was 28 mm and necrotic. Notice the extensive, large, "mulberry" calcifications.

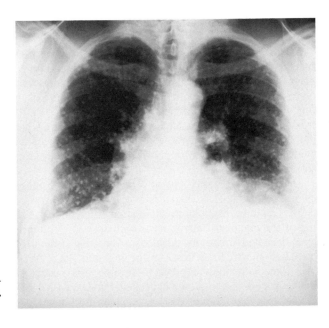

**Figure 33–3.** Incidental finding of multiple calcified granulomas in a 54-year-old man from Nashville, Tennessee. The PPD skin test was negative, and the histoplasmin skin test was positive.

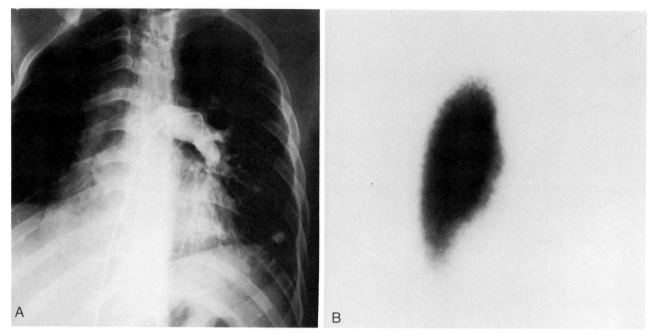

**Figure 33–4.** *A*, Pulmonary angiograph in a patient with breathlessness. Notice the complete lack of perfusion of the right lung. *B*, Posterior view of a perfusion lung scan of the same patient. An open biopsy showed dense fibrosis with occasional *Histoplasma capsulatum* yeasts.

trast, symptoms of progressive pulmonary disease involving the upper zones resemble those of tuberculosis, with low-grade fever, anorexia, and weight loss. There is usually a progressive cough and production of mucopurulent sputum. Night sweats occur but are usually not as severe as in tuberculosis.[33]

Progressive pulmonary histoplasmosis is sometimes called chronic pulmonary histoplasmosis or chronic cavitary histoplasmosis. The radiographic findings are identical to those of adult reinfection tuberculosis, and great care is necessary to differentiate these two illnesses.[31, 33]

### Progressive Disseminated Histoplasmosis

After the acute infection, but before establishment of the specific T-cell–mediated immunologic response, the fungus gains access to the circulation through the hilar lymph nodes. It is likely that extrapulmonary dissemination of the fungus occurs in most patients. Evidence for this comes from careful postmortem studies in Cincinnati, Ohio, where more than 70% of patients who died of other causes had evidence of healed histoplasma granulomas in their spleens.[19]

The circulating yeast cells of *H. capsulatum* are phagocytosed by cells of the fixed RE system. After ingestion, there is rapid intracellular multiplication of the fungus. Killing of the organism cannot occur until specific T-lymphocyte–mediated immunity develops. After this occurs, the "armed" macrophage destroys the ingested fungi. When T-cell–mediated immunity fails to develop or is inadequate, the yeast continue to grow unchecked. Parasitized RE cells die, and the multiplying yeast are released. Additional macrophages are recruited to phagocytose the extracellular yeast, which continue to multiply within the next macro-

phage that ingests them. In persons with inadequate T-cell–mediated immunity, whether induced by drugs or by an underlying illness, a severe, progressive systemic illness develops that eventually kills the patient. This illness is referred to as progressive disseminated histoplasmosis (PDH).[26] The term "progressive" is important, because disseminated histoplasmosis without progression occurs in most cases of acute histoplasma infection.[22, 35]

Patients with PDH have high fever and anorexia, and it is a rapidly progressive, wasting illness. Respiratory symptoms may or may not be prominent; they are absent in about one third of patients. Physical examination reveals a febrile and ill patient. Hepatosplenomegaly frequently occurs. Mucocutaneous ulcers may develop.[26] The laboratory evaluation shows pancytopenia, abnormal liver function test results, and occasionally the finding of disseminated intravascular coagulation. The initial chest radiogram may show a variety of patterns, ranging from normal to a classic miliary pattern. The bone marrow, the easiest place to sample the RE system, shows collections of macrophages filled with intracellular yeasts with or without necrosis. In many patients, there is little evidence of granuloma formation.[36] Before the common use of immunosuppressive cytotoxic and glucocorticoid therapy, this form of histoplasmosis was seen primarily in young children and was referred to as the "infantile" form of the disease.[26] With the advent of the human immunodeficiency virus (HIV) pandemic, most patients with this form of illness are HIV-positive.[37, 38] Patients with Hodgkin disease may develop PDH, even before therapy (Fig. 33–7).[39]

The clinical onset of PDH often is closely related to the onset of an immunosuppressing illness or the initiation of immunosuppressive therapy, most commonly glucocorticoids.[40] This temporal association gives credence to the theory that reactivation of previously healed and dormant

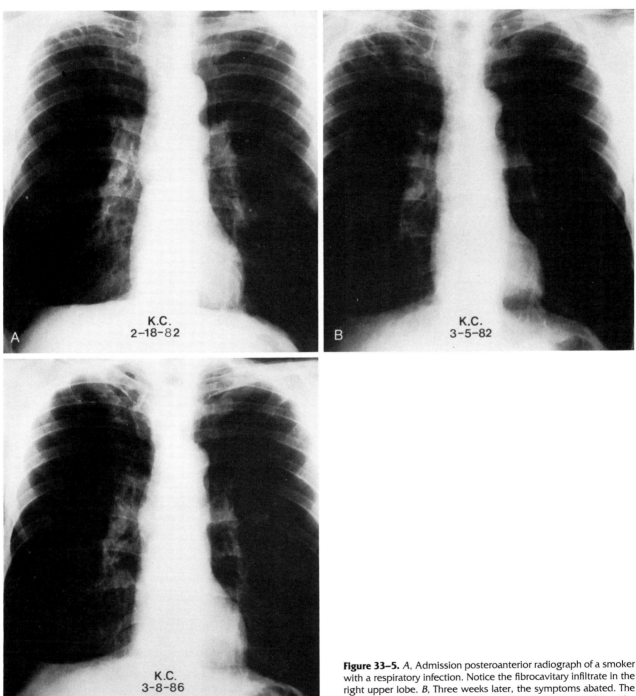

**Figure 33–5.** *A*, Admission posteroanterior radiograph of a smoker with a respiratory infection. Notice the fibrocavitary infiltrate in the right upper lobe. *B*, Three weeks later, the symptoms abated. The *Histoplasma* yeast phase titer was 1:32. *C*, Four years later, the infiltrate has cleared. The patient was not treated with antifungal therapy.

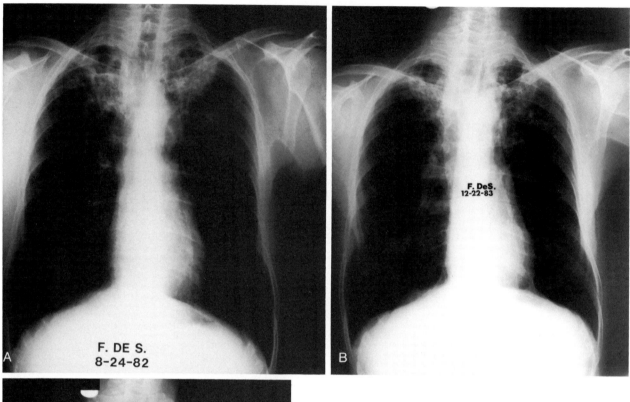

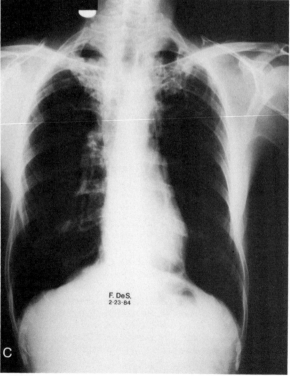

**Figure 33–6.** *A,* Admission chest radiograph of a 45-year-old man with established chronic obstructive pulmonary disease. Bilateral apical fibrocavitary disease was revealed, and multiple sputum cultures were positive for *H. capsulatum. B,* After more than 1 year of treatment with ketoconazole, the radiograph improved, but the sputum culture was still positive for the fungus. *C,* After 2.0 g of amphotericin B, the chest radiograph improved further, and the sputum no longer grew *H. capsulatum.*

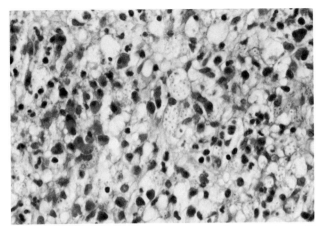

**Figure 33–7.** Bone marrow biopsy specimen from a patient with Hodgkin disease and progressive disseminated histoplasmosis. Notice the large number of small yeasts within parasitized macrophages and the lack of granuloma formation. It is unusual to see the organisms without special stains (H&E stain; original magnification × 1000).

histoplasmosis may be the mechanism of infection for some patients with PDH. This is best demonstrated by HIV-infected patients who, after many years of residence in non-endemic areas, develop PDH under pressure of diminished CD4 lymphocyte counts.[37] On the east coast of the United States, most of these patients have come from the Caribbean basin, an area endemic for *H. capsulatum*.[41] On the west coast, most patients have come from the midwestern United States.

There is ample evidence that primary infections in immunosuppressed persons rapidly disseminate. In a community-wide outbreak of histoplasmosis in Indianapolis, Indiana, most patients who developed PDH were immunocompromised.[42] An astonishing one fourth or more of HIV-infected patients developed PDH during a subsequent outbreak.[38]

Some patients with PDH have a milder and more chronic illness. Careful evaluation of these patients after recovery reveals no obvious T-cell dysfunction. It is tempting to speculate that these persons may have had a transient T-cell dysfunction, possibly from an acute viral illness, but this hypothesis is unproven.[26] Some patients develop a chronic wasting disease similar to chronic tuberculosis. The main clinical findings are weight loss and low-grade fever. Mucocutaneous junction and mucosal ulcers may be seen in the mouth, pharynx, or rectum and on the glans penis. Extensive granulomatous involvement of the adrenal glands may destroy them and cause Addison disease. Histopathologic examination of involved tissues shows well-formed epithelioid granulomas with few organisms visible (Fig. 33–8).[26, 43]

Involvement of the central nervous system (CNS) by *H. capsulatum* is rare and may present as a space-occupying lesion (eg, intracranial histoplasmoma) or as chronic meningitis.[44] Endovascular infections may involve the valvular endocardium and abdominal aortic aneurysms.[45]

## Diagnosis

As for all infectious diseases, the most important test is culture of the organism from biologic material. However,

because productive cough is uncommon in patients with acute histoplasmosis, cultural recovery of the organism during acute histoplasmosis is uncommon.[22] Direct examination of respiratory secretions using 10% potassium hydroxide (KOH) is seldom helpful because of the small size of the organism and its usual location within cells. In contrast, patients with blastomycosis and coccidioidomycosis have purulent secretions. Sputum cultures are often positive, and characteristic large organisms are easily identified in KOH-digested sputum.[46]

Patients presenting with the chronic upper lobe cavitary form of the disease usually have positive sputum cultures. The organism can easily survive transport to reference laboratories. Multiple sputum cultures must be done, because shedding of the organism is intermittent. Our custom is to obtain six consecutive morning sputum specimens. In patients who cannot produce adequate sputum, sputum can be induced with 10% NaCl nebulization before proceeding to fiberoptic bronchoscopy. Bronchoscopic specimens include bronchoalveolar lavage, brushing, and transbronchial biopsies.

In extremely ill patients with suspected PDH, the fastest way to make the diagnosis is to sample the RE system. Bone marrow biopsy is the best and safest method (see Fig. 33–7).[36] Liver biopsy also samples the RE system but has more risk, especially if there is thrombocytopenia (see Fig. 33–8). Since the availability of the lysis centrifugation system, blood cultures have become more useful,[35] especially in HIV-infected patients in whom the density of circulating organisms is high. In one series, 91% of HIV-infected patients with subsequently proven PDH had positive blood cultures.[38]

Culture recovery of the organism is seldom difficult, but it is time consuming. The rate of growth depends on inoculum size—the larger the inoculum, the more rapid is the growth. It is helpful if the physician informs the laboratory that histoplasmosis is suspected. Often, a tentative diagnosis may be suggested much earlier. When the mycelia begin to grow, large tuberculate conidiospores can be seen that suggest *H. capsulatum*. All biopsied material should be examined by special stains. For rapid diagnosis, the use of

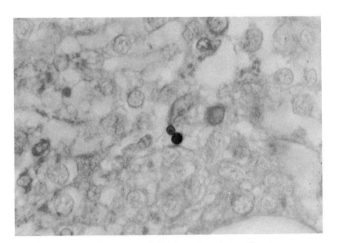

**Figure 33–8.** Liver biopsy specimen from a patient without any apparent T-cell dysfunction and progressive disseminated histoplasmosis. Notice the organisms in the Kupffer cell (methenamine silver stain; original magnification × 1000).

a supravital stain such as a Giemsa stain is recommended. Because the organisms are frequently intracellular, PDH can sometimes be diagnosed by examining the buffy coat of the peripheral blood after supravital staining (Fig. 33–9).[47] The laboratory must be alerted that a fungus is suspected. Tissue sections stained by standard hematoxylin and eosin stain seldom reveal the organism.[47] If a fungus is suspected, other special stains can be used to enhance diagnostic accuracy. The periodic acid-Schiff (PAS) stain preserves morphology. Standard silver stains also demonstrate the organisms.

## Immunologic Testing

Intradermal skin testing with 0.1 mL of histoplasmin has been used extensively in epidemiologic studies. Because positive reactions are long lasting, skin testing is less useful for individual diagnoses. A positive skin test, even if there is an active pulmonary infiltrate, is not diagnostic of current histoplasmosis. It is more likely that the pulmonary infiltrate is caused by another infection and the positive skin test is a relic of remote histoplasmosis. This skin test is useless for diagnosis in highly endemic areas, where by age 18 virtually everyone has a positive histoplasma skin test.[48] Most patients with PDH have a negative skin test reaction because the infection is causing a specific T-cell defect or because an underlying disease is depressing cell-mediated immunity.[43] A positive skin test reaction does not prove current histoplasmosis, and a negative skin test reaction does not rule it out. The histoplasmin skin test should be used as an epidemiologic tool only and not for diagnosis of individual infections.[48]

Serologic tests are extremely important in the diagnosis and management of histoplasmosis. There are three available tests: complement fixation (CF), immunodiffusion (ID), and a newer radioimmunoassay (RIA).

The standard is the CF test. The test becomes positive between 3 and 6 weeks after infection and remains positive for months to years. A single titer of 1:32 to the yeast-phase antigen or a fourfold titer rise in the presence of a compatible clinical illness suggests histoplasmosis. Regrettably, CF test results are negative for about 30% of patients

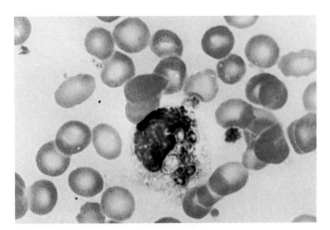

**Figure 33–9.** Multiple yeasts of *H. capsulatum* within a phagocyte in the peripheral blood in an HIV-infected patient (Wright stain; original magnification × 1000).

with acute histoplasmosis and for as many as 50% of the patients with PDH. Many patients with chronic upper lobe pulmonary histoplasmosis have titers lower than 1:8.[48]

The ID test for precipitating antibodies to the H and M antigens of *H. capsulatum* identifies only 50% of the patients with acute symptomatic histoplasmosis and does not become positive for 4 to 6 weeks after exposure.[48]

Wheat introduced the RIA into clinical practice, measuring diagnostic levels in about 80% of his patients. However, the test is less specific than ID or high-titer CF.[49]

These three serologic tests measure antibodies produced against the fungus. The tests are reasonably well standardized; the main problem is lack of timeliness. Several weeks may pass before serodiagnostic tests become positive. By the time a firm diagnosis is established, most patients have recovered.[48]

Wheat introduced a newer approach for diagnosing histoplasmosis—he measures fungal antigens. Although the specificity is very good, the sensitivity remains poor in acute histoplasmosis, in chronic cavitary histoplasmosis, and in some patients with PDH who are only moderately immunosuppressed.[50] Antigen testing is most valuable in HIV-infected patients because of the increased density of organisms. Wheat reported that histoplasma polysaccharide antigen (HPA) was positive in urine from 70 to 72 patients with PDH complicating HIV infection.[38] The test was also useful for following the course of treatment[48] and for predicting relapses.[51]

## Treatment

Most patients with acute histoplasmosis are not aware of the infection or have a rapidly evolving, self-limited illness. For a few patients with overwhelming pulmonary infections leading to gas exchange problems, amphotericin B (AMB) is the drug of choice. Although anecdotal reports suggest that a total dose of 500 mg of AMB may be effective, this reduced dose has not been compared with a full course of AMB.[52]

Progressive upper lobe cavitary disease can be treated with 400 mg per day of ketoconazole, which may be increased in a stepwise fashion to 800 mg per day, if necessary.[53] Alternately, AMB (35 mg/kg total dose) administered over 12 to 16 weeks provides excellent results.[54]

All patients with PDH must be treated promptly and aggressively. Our custom has been to initiate treatment with AMB and to aim for a total dose of 40 mg/kg.[43] Some patients with more chronic cases of PDH have been treated with ketoconazole.[53] Although this form of therapy may be effective in stable patients, the slow onset of action of ketoconazole precludes its use in most patients with PDH. Itraconazole is somewhat more effective than ketoconazole but is not equivalent to AMB.

AMB is highly effective in the treatment of PDH. Relapses are uncommon after a full course of AMB, even in classically immunosuppressed patients, including organ transplant recipients and patients receiving chronic prednisone therapy. However, HIV-infected patients with PDH frequently relapse (Fig. 33–10) and require long-term suppressive therapy.[47] After completion of an initial 1 g of AMB, weekly or biweekly infusion of 50 to 80 mg AMB

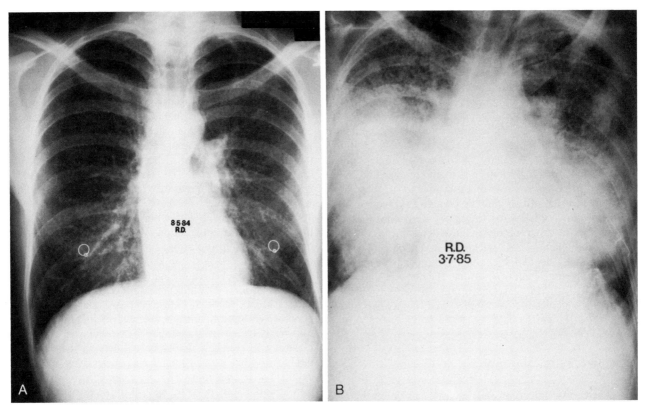

**Figure 33–10.** *A*, Admission chest radiograph of a patient infected with HIV. Notice the innumerable 2- to 3-mm lesions. There was marked improvement with amphotericin B therapy. *B*, Suppressive therapy with ketoconazole failed, and he was next seen moribund. (Reprinted with permission from Johnson PC, Sarosi GA, Septimus EJ, Satterwhite TK: Progressive disseminated histoplasmosis in patients with acquired immune deficiency syndrome: A report of 12 cases and a literature review. Semin Respir Infect 1:1–8, 1986.)

reduces the incidence of relapse.[55] Suppressive therapy with ketoconazole is not effective.[47] Itraconazole, a new triazole, is highly effective in preventing relapse after completion of primary AMB therapy of PDH in HIV-infected patients.[56] The drug may also be effective as primary therapy. The usual daily dose is 200 mg. The dose can be increased if necessary to 200 mg twice daily.

AMB and the oral imidazole compounds are the main effective therapies for fungal diseases. AMB is the only broad-spectrum fungicidal antibiotic. The agent is highly effective but does have potentially serious side effects. Renal tubular toxicity is almost universal and is dose dependent, leading to renal potassium wasting. The most feared complication of AMB is a dose-dependent decrease in renal function.[57] To prevent this, careful weekly monitoring of renal function is mandatory. The dose should be reduced if the creatinine level reaches 2.0 mg/dL and should be temporarily stopped if the creatinine level reaches 3.0 mg/dL. Saline loading before AMB infusion helps to reduce nephrotoxicity. Loss of potassium in the urine is extremely common. All patients who receive AMB should be treated with supplemental potassium.

Many AMB infusions induce fever and chills, which are not dangerous but are quite bothersome. This febrile response can be blunted by premedication with 600 mg of aspirin and 50 mg of diphenhydramine (Benadryl) 15 to 30 minutes before the start of the infusion. Reduction of infusion time from the customary 4 to 6 hours to 90 minutes also can reduce the length and severity of febrile reactions. If pretreatment with aspirin is inadequate, codeine in a dose

of 60 mg or meperidine (Demerol) in a dose of 50 to 75 mg is even more effective to block AMB reactions. Most patients have febrile reactions early in the course of treatment, but these reactions diminish in severity and frequency as treatment continues. To reduce the incidence of phlebitis at the site of peripheral intravenous lines, 25 mg of hydrocortisone hemisuccinate can be mixed with the infusion. This is not necessary if the infusion is given in a central line.

Many authorities recommend the use of a test dose of 1 mg. We have not followed this practice because true anaphylaxis is almost never seen. It is also customary to begin AMB administration at smaller doses and proceed to the desired full dose. However, there is only limited evidence that this method reduces the incidence of AMB reactions or reduces toxicity. Nevertheless, our practice has been to start infusion in stable, adult patients at 10 mg daily and advance by 10-mg daily increments until the desired full dose, usually 50 mg, is reached. After the patient is afebrile, we switch to a Monday, Wednesday, and Friday schedule, which can be given on an outpatient basis. We never exceed a 50-mg single dose in stable patients, but we have occasionally given much larger doses (1–1.5 mg/kg), especially in life-threatening situations to patients with underlying hematologic neoplasms.

In 1980, a new treatment era began with the availability of ketoconazole, an orally administered azole compound. Subsequently, fluconazole, a triazole compound, was released. The second triazole compound, itraconazole, was released in 1992.[58] Because ketoconazole has been used the longest, the clinical experience is more extensive than with the newer drugs. Although it is effective, ketoconazole is not equal in effectiveness to AMB.[53] It should not be used in life-threatening situations. Fluconazole, which is more water soluble and has many fewer side effects, has emerged as the drug of choice for long-term suppressive therapy of cryptococcal meningitis complicating AIDS. Itraconazole is the drug of choice for mild to moderate cases of blastomycosis and will probably replace ketoconazole for treatment of some forms of histoplasmosis.[58]

The gastrointestinal toxicity of the azoles limits their dosage. Daily administration of ketoconazole should not exceed 800 mg. Itraconazole given at 200 to 400 mg per day has fewer side effects than ketoconazole. Fluconazole at 400 mg per day has little toxicity.[59] Ketoconazole can interfere with testosterone biosynthesis, causing loss of libido in young men.[60] These effects are reversible.

Ketoconazole and, to a lesser degree, itraconazole require gastric acidity for absorption so that $H_2$-blockers and antacids (often given for gastrointestinal side effects) block absorption. Fluconazole is rapidly and completely absorbed.

## BLASTOMYCOSIS

Blastomycosis is the only endemic mycosis that was first described in the United States. Gilchrist, from Johns Hopkins University, recognized the first case in 1894 and subsequently found 1 more patient.[61] He thought the causative organism was a protozoan, a mistake also made by Darling in discussing histoplasmosis[7] and by Wernicke in describing coccidioidomycosis.[62] However, Gilchrist quickly refuted his own theory about causation. He isolated the organism, recognized it as a fungus, and fulfilled Koch's postulates by infecting a dog with the isolated organism.[63] Additional patients with blastomycosis soon were identified, especially from Chicago, and for a while blastomycosis was known as ''the Chicago disease.'' Advances in understanding the disease were slow, and although new cases were reported, no new insight about the pathogenesis of the disease emerged. In 1939, Martin and Smith reviewed all the available published material and proposed a synthesis, but regrettably, they added to the confusion. They separated the pulmonary and cutaneous forms of the disease, proposing that the former was acquired by inhalation and the latter by inoculation.[64] This artificial separation persisted for an additional 12 years. In 1951, Schwarz and Baum disproved the artificial separation by showing that cutaneous disease was caused by hematogenous spread after a primary pulmonary infection. Even if the cutaneous disease appeared to be isolated, many patients had had a previous pulmonary process.[65] Almost all cases are acquired by inhalation, with the only exceptions a few cases of inoculation disease, usually from surgical or pathologic accidents[66, 67] or rarely from animal bites[68] or from sexual intercourse.[69]

Attempts to elucidate the epidemiology of blastomycosis have been less successful. Methods that were useful in the epidemiologic investigation of histoplasmosis have been less so when applied to blastomycosis. All attempts to produce a reliable and reproducible skin test antigen have

failed.[4] Nationwide surveys of skin test sensitivity, so helpful in histoplasmosis, cannot be done. As a result, the endemic area of blastomycosis cannot be defined with any degree of certainty, and it is only inferred from the origin of reported cases.[3] The apparent endemic area includes the south and east United States and most of the Midwest, extending west to the Minnesota and North Dakota border, going straight south to include Louisiana and the eastern edge of Texas. The endemic area extends north and west into Canada.[70] The apparent endemic area for blastomycosis overlaps the area known to be endemic for *Histoplasma*.[1] Only the northwest limits (ie, northern Wisconsin and Minnesota and adjacent areas of Canada) are not coendemic with *Histoplasma*.

Many patients with active blastomycosis have a negative blastomycin skin test reaction. Many of these same patients have a positive histoplasmin skin test reaction. One logical interpretation is that crossreactions are common and *Blastomyces* does not elicit an appropriate delayed hypersensitivity reaction.[71] We think an alternate explanation is possible. Most reported blastomycosis patients with a nonreactive blastomycin skin test have disseminated blastomycosis or severe pulmonary blastomycosis. A positive blastomycin skin test would be unlikely in these sick patients. Most of these patients also have lived in an area coendemic for histoplasmosis. Because *Histoplasma* infection is almost universal by age 18 in many of these areas, it is not surprising that many of the patients had a positive histoplasmin skin test reaction in the face of active blastomycosis.[48]

Evidence that the blastomycin skin test is better than previously thought has emerged from two epidemic investigations. We investigated an outbreak in 1972 in Big Fork, Minnesota, where 18 of 21 exposed persons had evidence of blastomycosis. Big Fork, in northern Minnesota, is well beyond the recognized endemic area for histoplasmosis. Twelve patients had abnormal chest radiographs, and 4 of these 12 had positive sputum cultures. Ten of 12, including all 4 with positive cultures, had positive blastomycin skin test reactions, using a skin test antigen that has been in existence since the 1940s. More importantly, 6 additional patients with a positive exposure history and a negative chest radiograph also demonstrated a positive skin test reaction to blastomycin. Of the 21 patients, 16 had positive blastomycin skin test reactions, and only 2 patients with abnormal chest radiographs did not. The remaining 3 patients apparently were not infected. Only 1 of the 21 patients had a positive histoplasmin skin test, effectively invalidating the old concept that crossreactions to histoplasmin skin test antigen are common among patients with blastomycosis.

The study of this outbreak documented that the blastomycin skin test was surprisingly sensitive in acute pulmonary blastomycosis.[72] In this cohort, skin test results were not confused by background histoplasmin sensitivity. The 16 patients with positive blastomycin skin tests were retested 3 years later, and only 5 still had a 5-mm reaction.[73] This suggests that the blastomycin skin test is quite sensitive but the reaction decays quickly. Patients with old exposures to the fungus may not maintain skin test positivity. The alternate explanation for the low skin test positivity rate in endemic areas is that blastomycosis is uncommon, especially compared with histoplasmosis.

New information about the epidemiology of blastomycosis has come from Klein and associates; they investigated the largest point-source outbreak to date, which occurred in the summer of 1984 in Eagle River in northern Wisconsin. This part of Wisconsin is outside the endemic area for histoplasmosis. Of the total of 48 proven or probable cases, 19 of 46 tested had positive skin test results. Fifteen of 17 subjects with positive skin test results and 18 additional subjects with negative results demonstrated positive in vitro lymphocyte transformation to a blastomycete antigen (ie, laboratory counterpart of a positive skin test). All subjects had negative histoplasmin skin test results. The investigators recovered the fungus from a beaver lodge.[74] Cultural identification from soil had not been accomplished in previous outbreaks.[72]

These two outbreaks helped clarify the epidemiology of blastomycosis. *B. dermatitidis* is a soil-dwelling fungus spread by aerosol formation. Many infected persons develop a positive blastomycin skin test reaction or its in vitro correlate. Epidemics can occur when microfoci of fungal growth are disturbed.

Other mammals are susceptible to the disease. Dogs in rural areas commonly develop severe disease. Canine blastomycosis is well recognized by the veterinary medical community.[75] If veterinarians are encountering dogs with blastomycosis, human cases are probably occurring in the same community.

Careful study of point-source outbreaks suggests that asymptomatic blastomycosis may occur. Most persons infected with *H. capsulatum* and *C. immitis* have positive skin test reactions without any clinical illness. Because of the lack of a good blastomycin skin test, asymptomatic, subclinical blastomycosis resulting only in skin test conversion has not been recognized. During the study of the Big Fork epidemic, several patients with abnormal radiographs and positive blastomycin skin test results had no symptoms.[76] It is almost certain that some patients with previous *Blastomyces* infection did not develop clinically detectable disease. Similar patients were identified during the investigation of the Eagle River outbreak.[74]

To further confirm the presence of asymptomatic infections, Vaaler and his associates showed that forestry workers from northern Minnesota but not forestry workers from nonendemic areas of Washington State had in vitro lymphocyte reactivity to a *Blastomyces* antigen without any history of clinical illness.[77] These studies suggest that many *Blastomyces* infections are asymptomatic. Symptomatic patients may be the minority, as is the case with histoplasmosis and coccidioidomycosis.

## Pathogenesis

At ambient temperatures, the fungus grows in nature as an aerial mycelium. Rising soil temperature favors growth, and rain on the day of exposure enhances the release of fungal spores.[74] If the site is disturbed, small (2–5 μm) infecting conidia become airborne, and an infectious aerosol is formed. When these spores are inhaled by humans or other mammals, some may elude nonspecific lung defenses and reach the alveoli.

The initial inflammatory response is predominantly by PMNs. PMNs can destroy the conidia, but they are unable to kill the parasitic yeast form.[5] During the first few days, the nature of the inflammatory exudate[78] changes, and macrophages move in. The macrophages ingest the spores but are unable to kill them until specific T-cell–mediated immunity develops. With the development of T-cell–mediated immunity, the now "armed" macrophages can kill the ingested yeasts. Eventually granuloma formation and healing takes place. This process is similar to and different from that observed in histoplasmosis. Both infections begin as a PMN-rich inflammatory exudate, but the PMNs disappear during the later phases of infection in histoplasmosis. PMNs never leave the inflammatory exudate in blastomycosis. Although the relative proportion of PMNs varies among patients, there is always a mixed pyogranulomatous exudate. In some instances, the PMN component is so predominant that the histopathology mimics bacterial infection.

If blastomycosis involves the skin and other squamous epithelial sites, such as the oropharynx, hyperplasia occurs with exaggerated downward growth of the rete pegs. Between these finger-like projections are microabscesses.[4] The markedly hyperplastic response of squamous epithelium to infection by *Blastomyces* organisms can lead to confusion with and occasional misdiagnosis as malignancy. The presence of the organisms within microabscesses, which is best confirmed by the use of special stains, proves blastomycosis. Careful examination of the cell nuclei shows benign uniformity, unlike the marked variation seen in a neoplasm. Tragic errors have been made when a mistaken diagnosis of malignancy is followed by radical surgery or radiation therapy.

Unlike histoplasmosis, in which extrapulmonary dissemination during the preimmune phase of the infection is universal,[1] the exact frequency of extrapulmonary spread in blastomycosis is unknown. In some instances, extrapulmonary dissemination does occur. The involved organs, in decreasing order of frequency, are the skin, bone, genitourinary system, and meninges; virtually all other organs may be involved.[4]

## Clinical Manifestations

In most primary blastomycotic infections, the portal of entry is the lung.[74, 76] Only rare cases of direct inoculation into subcutaneous tissues have been documented.[66, 67] After inhalation, the mean incubation time is approximately 45 days.[74]

The acute disease resembles bacterial pneumonia. The onset of symptoms is abrupt, with high fever and chills followed by a cough that rapidly becomes productive of purulent sputum.[76] Arthralgias and myalgias may occur, but they are not as common as they are in histoplasmosis. Pleuritic chest pain also occurs.

Most patients with acute pulmonary blastomycosis have been diagnosed during epidemics. More frequent sporadic cases of pulmonary blastomycosis usually present as subacute or even chronic illness. Symptoms include low-grade fever, cough productive of mucopurulent sputum, and weight loss. Clinicians often initially suspect bronchogenic neoplasm or tuberculosis.[71, 79, 80]

The results of physical examination are often negative during acute pulmonary blastomycosis. Erythema nodosum may accompany the onset of the pulmonary disease, although it occurs less frequently than with the other endemic mycoses.[81, 82] Direct involvement of the skin may occur early or late, and the skin must be examined carefully. The usual areas of skin involvement are the face, hands, and legs. Initial laboratory examination usually shows few abnormalities, but an elevated leukocyte count with a left shift may be observed.

The chest roentgenographic findings vary. In the epidemic form, the disease is usually bilateral and involves predominantly the lower lung fields, mimicking closely the other endemic mycoses (Fig. 33–11). In patients with subacute disease, lesions vary from single or multiple, round densities to segmental and even lobar consolidation. Perihilar infiltrates are common,[83] and they are more common on the right side. On the lateral film, there is a mass-like infiltrate in the apical posterior segment of the right lower lobe. On the posteroanterior film, this infiltrate projects over the right hilum. This presentation mimics bronchogenic carcinoma (Fig. 33–12). Cavitation is uncommon, and hilar adenopathy is less frequent than in histoplasmosis or coccidioidomycosis. Calcification from pulmonary blastomycosis has been reported but is evidently rare. In more than 140 patients, we have never seen a calcified blastomycotic lesion.

Extrapulmonary dissemination of the fungus usually occurs early, during the symptomatic phase of the illness. The distant skin or bone lesion may be the only manifestation of disease, because the primary pulmonary process has already healed. In other cases, when the patient is tested for a cutaneous or bony lesion, a routine chest radiograph shows a totally asymptomatic pulmonary lesion, which proves to be *Blastomyces*. It is clear why early investigators had so much trouble understanding the ''isolated'' form of cutaneous disease. There is now ample evidence that the characteristic cutaneous ulcer in blastomycosis always represents dissemination from a central focus.[84] We and others have documented cases in which initial pulmonary infection resolved spontaneously without a diagnosis but recurred as symptomatic extrapulmonary disseminated blastomycosis months to years later.[84] Careful retrospective evaluation of bronchoscopic material, obtained to rule out cancer, showed characteristic *Blastomyces* yeast on the Papanicolaou-stained slides (Fig. 33–13).[85]

Patients with blastomycosis have no obvious immune defects. Nevertheless, in patients with demonstrable T-cell defects, such as organ transplant recipients or patients receiving high doses of glucocorticoids, *Blastomyces* behaves as an opportunist. The pace of the illness is often more rapid and the involvement is more extensive than in normal hosts.[86] A small number of HIV-infected patients have developed severe blastomycosis while significantly T-cell depleted from their HIV infection. In these patients, the disease is usually widespread, involving multiple sites.[87]

## Diagnosis

The quickest and simplest way to establish the diagnosis of blastomycosis is to examine sputum or aspirated pus after digestion by 10% KOH. Under reduced light, the organisms are readily seen as large (8–20 μm), single budding yeasts with a broad neck of attachment between the two cells. The doubly refractile nature of the wall becomes apparent on varying the focus, and multiple nuclei are visible (Fig. 33–14).[4] Another quick and reliable test is examination of respiratory secretions using the Papanicolaou technique. The fungi are large, dark pink- to red-staining organisms, with the characteristic budding and doubly refractile cell wall clearly visible (see Fig. 33–13). The main difficulty with the Papanicolaou smear is that cytotechnologists are trained to look for malignancy rather than for infection, and it is relatively easy to overlook the organisms unless the cytotechnician specifically looks for them.[46]

Many patients are diagnosed by histopathologic examination of biopsied or resected specimens. In rare instances, the standard hematoxylin and eosin stain may show the fungus, although special stains usually are needed. Most laboratories use one of several modifications of the silver stain or the PAS stain. The PAS stain better preserves morphologic detail.[4]

Isolation and identification of the organism by the mycology laboratory is not difficult, but it is time consuming. Depending on the inoculum size, growth may occur as early as 5 to 7 days after exposure. If inoculum size is small, it may take as long as 30 days to grow the fungus. Until recently, positive identification of the fungus required conversion of the mycelial isolate to the yeast phase and then back again to the mycelial phase. With exoantigen testing, final identification can be made as soon as there is moderate growth on the culture plate, sometimes within 5 days.

There is no commercially available skin test antigen. In vitro transformation of antigen-stimulated lymphocytes is an excellent test to measure cell-mediated immune response, but it is available only in a single research laboratory.[88] With newer, more purified antigens, a skin test may be developed.

Serologic tests are available: complement fixation, agar gel double diffusion, and an enzyme immunoassay. None of these tests has a high enough sensitivity to be reliable. Specificity is moderately good, and positive test results should prompt further investigation.[48, 89] However, a negative test result does not rule out blastomycosis. In our series of more than 140 patients, no patient was first diagnosed by serology.

## Blastomycosis Complicating Infection With Human Immunodeficiency Virus

Because intact T-cell function is essential for recovery from the primary infection, it is not surprising that HIV-infected patients can have severe, progressive disease. Although blastomycosis is an uncommon infection and is limited geographically, a handful of coinfections with HIV have been reported. The illness is similar to that in noncompromised hosts, but it is more severe. Extensive extrapulmonary dissemination, including meningitis, is more common.[87]

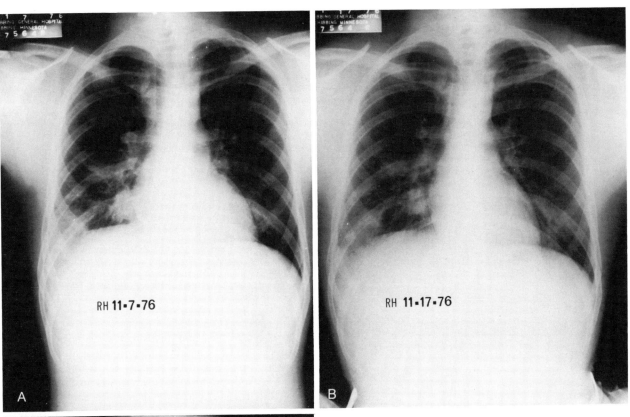

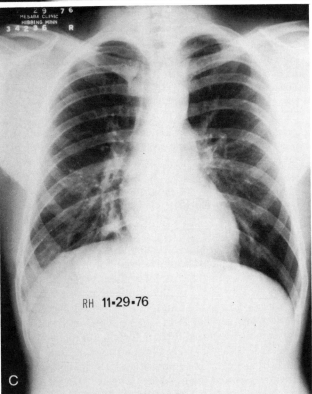

**Figure 33–11.** *A,* An admission chest radiograph of a 21-year-old man with blastomycosis shows bilateral lower zone infiltrates. A sputum KOH preparation showed *Blastomyces dermatitidis. B,* Ten days later, the symptoms resolved without antifungal chemotherapy. Notice the more nodular nature of these lesions. *C,* Three weeks after presentation, the nodules are resolving.

## Treatment

Several controversies surround the treatment of blastomycosis. The first is whether all patients with documented blastomycosis require treatment.

Many patients with pulmonary blastomycosis who present during an epidemic, including some who are quite ill, recover spontaneously. This was documented in the outbreaks in Big Fork, Minnesota,[76] and Eagle River, Wisconsin.[74] All untreated patients recovered without specific ther-

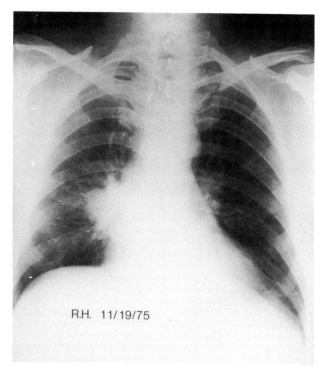

**Figure 33–12.** Posteroanterior radiograph of a 63-year-old heavy smoker with blood-tinged purulent sputum. Bronchoscopy showed no endobronchial lesion. No KOH preparation was performed. Right lower lobe and right middle lobe resection showed blastomycosis.

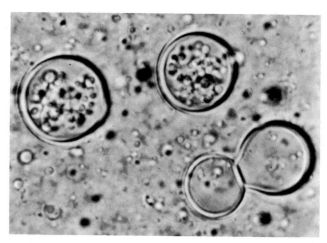

**Figure 33–14.** Sputum after 10% KOH digestion. Notice the characteristic large, single budding yeast with doubly refractile walls (original magnification × 1000). (Reprinted with permission from Sarosi GA, Davies SF: Blastomycosis. State of the art. Am Rev Respir Dis 120:911–938, 1979.)

apy and have remained well for many years. Moreover, we have followed a carefully selected group of patients with sporadic blastomycosis limited to the lung who were not critically ill when the diagnosis was made or whose more severe illness was already resolving by the time the diagnosis was made. Of 39 patients followed for as long as two decades, only 1 patient has relapsed.[89]

The concept of self-limited blastomycosis is well established. We think that some stable patients with acute infection limited to the lungs may be followed without treatment if there is careful follow-up. If the pulmonary disease progresses or there is extrapulmonary spread, we initiate anti-

fungal treatment. Many investigators do not consider our approach acceptable and recommend that all patients with blastomycosis should be treated. Their argument may be valid. If we had had an acceptable, low-toxicity alternative to AMB in 1972, when we recognized and followed self-limited blastomycosis in Big Fork, Minnesota, we would have used it. Our respect for the potential toxicity of AMB influenced us to observe without therapy the spontaneous resolution of the disease. Seriously ill patients, especially patients whose ventilatory status is compromised, must be treated immediately with AMB.[4] Patients with pulmonary blastomycosis who have had a chronic illness with weight loss, resembling tuberculosis, usually fail to improve under observation and require therapy.[90]

Extrapulmonary blastomycosis always requires treatment. In life-threatening situations[4] or if the meninges are involved, AMB therapy is mandatory. It is given to a total cumulative dose of 2 g.[91] In patients with subacute forms of illness who do not have meningitis, ketoconazole has been used (Fig. 33–15).[53, 92] The starting dose is 400 mg, which can be increased in 200 mg increments, as needed, to a maximum of 800 mg. Excellent results have been reported by various investigators using ketoconazole.[92]

Itraconazole has been released for use in the United States. Early work, especially by the Mycoses Study Group, shows that this drug is highly effective for blastomycosis. The usual dose is 200 mg per day, with a maximum dose of 400 mg per day.[58] In our opinion, itraconazole (200 mg/d) is the preferred therapy for mild to moderate pulmonary and extrapulmonary blastomycosis, excluding meningitis. Blastomycosis complicating HIV infection should always be treated with AMB, whether the meninges are involved or not.[87] After stabilization of the disease, oral suppressive therapy with itraconazole should be given.

## COCCIDIOIDOMYCOSIS

### History and Epidemiology

Coccidioidomycosis was the first of the three major endemic mycoses to be recognized. Initially, Posadas[93] and

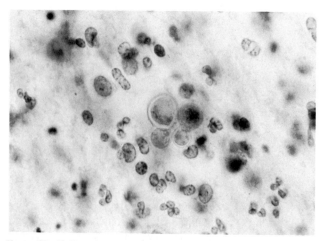

**Figure 33–13.** Bronchoalveolar material shows the characteristic large, single budding yeasts of *B. dermatitidis* (Papanicolaou stain; original magnification × 1000).

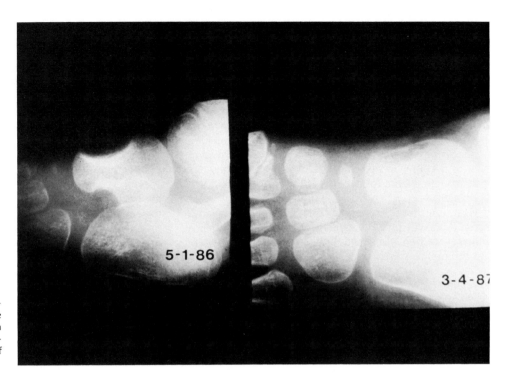

**Figure 33–15.** Blastomycosis involving the talus of a child. Notice the sclerotic margin of the lesion *(left)*. After 10 months of ketoconazole therapy, there is evidence of healing.

Wernicke[62] thought they had discovered a new protozoan infection, but the fungal cause of the disease was clearly established by 1896.[94] Shortly afterward, it became obvious that the disease was much more common in central California than in Argentina. Because there were no immunodiagnostic tests, only the most severe cases were recognized. For many years, most reports dealt with the severe form of the disease, referring to it as coccidioidal granuloma, but no one described less severe infections. By 1930, practitioners in the San Joaquin Valley in California had recognized several self-limited syndromes, which included a nonspecific febrile illness (ie, valley fever), acute polyarthritis (ie, desert rheumatism), and erythema nodosum (ie, the bumps). All of these syndromes were manifestations of primary coccidioidomycosis. Even if severe, they were usually self-limited.

Dickson[95] and Dickson and Gifford[96] first described primary pulmonary coccidioidomycosis, also a benign illness. By carefully studying a laboratory accident, they were able to prove that valley fever and the bumps were acute manifestations of coccidioidomycosis acquired by inhalation.

World War II increased our knowledge of coccidioidomycosis, largely from the work of C.E. Smith. He did extensive epidemiologic studies on the large numbers of recruits brought to the San Joaquin Valley and to central Arizona for flight training. Most persons whose coccidioidomycosis skin test converted from negative to positive had no symptoms. Most symptomatic patients had a nonspecific febrile illness or a self-limited respiratory illness. Only a few had erythema nodosum or the polyarthralgia syndrome. Recruits who entered training with positive skin test results were protected and did not become ill. Only a few documented new infections progressed to dissemination.[2] Infections seemed to be related to disturbance of the soil; most occurred in dry, dusty conditions. The rate of infection diminished during the cold and wet rainy season. After

construction activities on the bases slowed, the grass began to grow, sidewalks were finished, and the frequency of new infections decreased markedly.[97]

The Army required a complete postmortem examination of all soldiers who died.[98] This policy provided useful information on the fatal form of coccidioidomycosis. Different racial groups had different degrees of risk. Blacks had a higher incidence of disseminated disease than Caucasians, even though the risk of infection, as measured by skin test conversion, was not significantly different. A racial difference in risk of dissemination was subsequently confirmed in the study of the great windstorm in California in 1979.[99]

The known endemic region for coccidioidomycosis includes the desert areas of the southwestern United States and contiguous areas in northern Mexico. In the United States, the endemic area extends from western Texas to the coastal range in California, and there are a few isolated microfoci in Los Angeles County. The fungus is endemic in Argentina and a few other places where appropriate desert conditions (eg, lower Sonoran life zone) are found. The fungus grows as an aerial mycelium, composed of septate hyphae. Mature hyphae have arthrospores alternating with empty cells. These mycelia break easily, and the arthrospores become airborne. They are small, thick walled, and barrel shaped, about 2 to 5 μm long.[2]

## Pathogenesis

Aerosolized spores can be inhaled. A few organisms may elude the nonspecific lung defenses and reach the alveoli. Germination begins, and the arthrospores convert to the tissue phase of the fungus, becoming spherules. These large structures are 10 to 80 μm in diameter. Further reproduction occurs by formation of endospores within the spherule. After the spherule matures, it ruptures, and the endospores are released. Each endospore can develop into a new giant spherule.

The initial inflammatory response is neutrophilic. Macrophages also increase in number. The macrophages phagocytose the arthrospores and present antigens to specific T lymphocytes, which then multiply. These T cells recruit and arm more macrophages, completing the cell-mediated immune response. Histopathologically, coccidioidomycosis is a mixed pyogenic and granulomatous infection, more similar to blastomycosis than to histoplasmosis. Development of T-cell–mediated immunity and its histopathologic correlate, granuloma formation, is important for control of the infection.

Most infections are asymptomatic or mildly symptomatic. Although proof is lacking, it appears that in most primary infections the fungus remains localized in the lung and the draining hilar lymph nodes. Bloodborne dissemination occurs occasionally, with involvement of virtually all organs.

## Clinical Manifestations

The usual portal of entry is the lung. Rarely, the organism may be directly inoculated subcutaneously, usually during a surgical or pathologic accident. The cardinal clinical manifestation of the disease is an area of pneumonia. A pulmonary infiltrate is common, even among asymptomatic patients detected by skin test conversion. Symptomatic disease ranges from a mild respiratory illness to rapidly progressive ARDS. Symptoms are highly variable. Most patients have fever, cough, and pleuritic chest pain (Fig. 33–16). Pleuritic chest pain can be severe and is frequently incapacitating.[100] Headaches frequently accompany the acute illness, causing concern because of the potential for meningitis. Spread to the meninges can occur early during the clinical illness. If headache is severe or unrelenting or if there is any evidence of meningeal irrita-

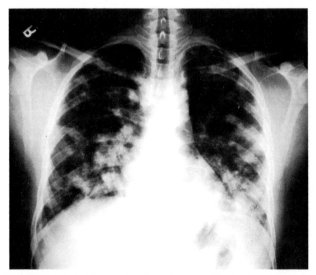

**Figure 33–16.** A 19-year-old Hispanic man with pleuritic chest pain and extensive bilateral infiltrates. The serum IgM antibody for coccidioidomycosis was found to be positive by immunodiffusion.

tion, a lumbar puncture should be performed immediately to exclude coccidioidomycotic meningitis.

A nonspecific, "toxic" rash occurs in as many as 50% of the patients with acute infection. This figure was derived from the study of a single outbreak; among sporadic cases, the frequency is much lower.[101] The rash is erythematous and is slightly raised but not quite papular. It usually occurs early during the illness, about the same time that the skin test becomes positive. Because coccidioidomycosis frequently occurs during the hot summer months, the rash is frequently misdiagnosed as a heat rash. The "allergic" or specific skin manifestations of primary coccidioidomycosis are erythema nodosum and, less commonly, erythema multiforme. These striking findings also occur about the same time as skin test conversion. For many years, the appearance of erythema nodosum was thought to be a highly favorable prognostic sign, portending spontaneous recovery. We now know, however, that some cases of erythema nodosum progress to life-threatening illness. Erythema nodosum occurs most commonly in adult Caucasian women.[102]

About three fourths of the patients with symptomatic primary pulmonary coccidioidomycosis have abnormal chest radiographs. The abnormality usually is a single area of pneumonitis with or without enlargement of the draining hilar lymph nodes. Isolated hilar adenopathy may occur with no obvious infiltrate.[103]

The usual clinical course of the primary illness is rapid improvement. After 6 to 8 weeks, the chest radiograph has cleared and symptoms have abated. For a few patients, symptoms and roentgenographic abnormalities may persist beyond 6 to 8 weeks, a condition referred to as persistent pulmonary coccidioidomycosis. The patchy pulmonary infiltrate may gradually harden and round off, producing a coin lesion, which is common in the endemic area. Coin lesions are different in coccidioidomycosis from those in histoplasmosis. In histoplasmosis, they are healing granulomas, but in coccidioidomycosis, they are abscesses undergoing resolution.[104] Needle biopsy of *Histoplasma* granulomas rarely shows the organism; needle biopsy of coccidioidomycotic lesions usually does.

There is necrotic material in the center of these rounded lesions, and expectoration of this semisolid material frequently creates a cavity. The hallmark of chronic, persistent coccidioidomycosis is the presence of a thin-walled cavity evolving from a solid pulmonary lesion (Fig. 33–17).[105] Most cavities are asymptomatic, and the only common complaint is occasional bouts of hemoptysis. Established cavities remain stable for long periods, and there is seldom a need for medical intervention. Approximately 50% of cavities smaller than 4 cm in diameter close within 2 years.[106]

Even though the cavitary lesions are usually benign, several complications can occur. The lesions may enlarge, migrate subpleurally, and eventually rupture into the pleural space, leading to a pneumohemothorax or pyopneumothorax (Fig. 33–18). This is a life-threatening complication, and prompt diagnosis and treatment are important.[104, 107] Hemoptysis is a frequent complication of coccidioidal cavities; although it is sometimes alarming, it is seldom life-threatening. These cavities occasionally develop fungus balls, usually caused by *Aspergillus* species or rarely by *C.*

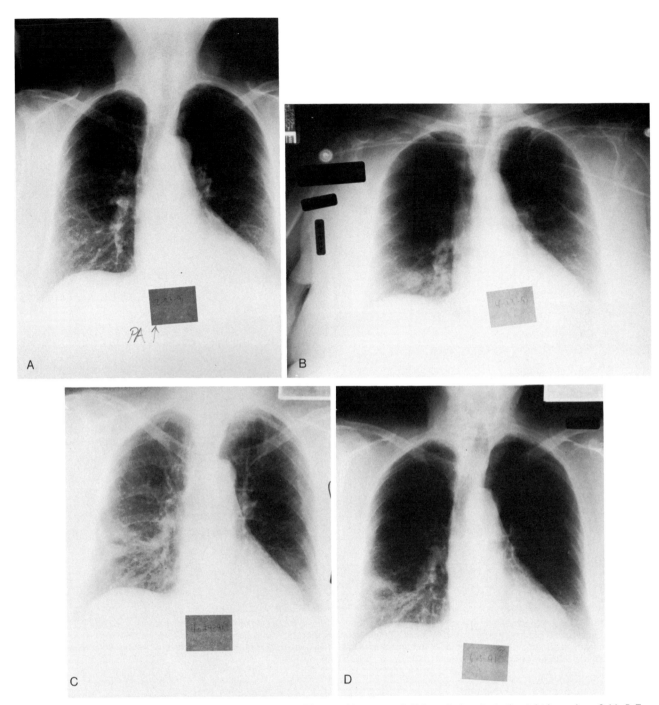

**Figure 33–17.** Changing appearance of a thin-walled cavity in a 70-year-old woman. *A,* Thin-walled cavity in the right lower lung field. *B,* Two months later, a solid coin lesion is seen. *C,* One day later, part of the coin lesion is expectorated, leaving a partially evacuated abscess. *D,* Six weeks later, the contents of the cavity are diminished further.

*immitis.* Bacterial superinfection of the cavities may also occur.

If primary pulmonary coccidioidomycosis fails to resolve and instead progresses within the chest, the condition is called progressive primary coccidioidomycosis. Symptoms include fever and cough, and the prognosis is quite poor. Many of these patients have underlying immune defects or belong to racial groups with a higher incidence of severe disease. The chest radiograph usually shows progression of the parenchymal infiltrate, but the radiographic finding is not diagnostic.

Rarely, pulmonary coccidioidomycosis presents with a tuberculosis-like picture, slowly progressive, with low-grade fever, night sweats, cough, weight loss, and occasional hemoptysis. The chest radiograph resembles that for the adult form of reinfection tuberculosis. The usual patient is older, and the disease progresses slowly (Fig. 33–19). Treatment is necessary to prevent further pulmonary destruction.[108]

## Disseminated Coccidioidomycosis

In most patients, the primary coccidioidomycotic infection is restricted to the lungs and resolves spontaneously.

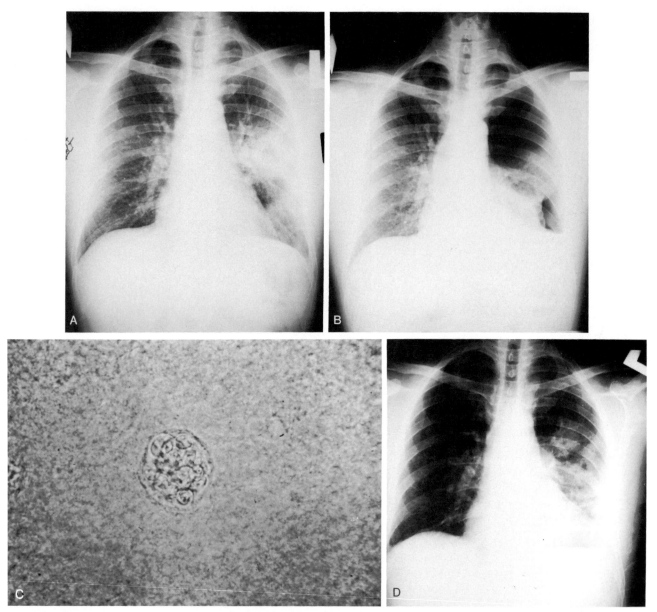

**Figure 33–18.** *A,* Thick-walled cavity in the left mid-lung in a 45-year-old man. The tentative diagnosis is coccidioidomycosis. *B,* Five days later the patient experienced sudden chest pain and dyspnea. The chest radiograph shows a collapsed lung with an air-fluid level. *C,* Giant spherule from the pleural fluid. *D,* After chest tube removal, the bronchopleural fistula appears closed. Notice the elevated left hemidiaphragm secondary to partial obliteration of the pleural space. Patient continues to receive amphotericin B.

Occasionally, the pulmonary infection progresses. Although a few patients die of coccidioidomycosis limited to the lung, most recover or stabilize. In a few patients, the fungus leaves the lung and disseminates widely throughout the body. Unlike histoplasmosis, in which extrapulmonary dissemination is the rule, the actual frequency of dissemination in coccidioidomycosis is unknown.

Disseminated disease occurs primarily in persons receiving glucocorticoid or cytotoxic therapy,[109] organ transplant recipients,[110] and HIV-infected patients in advanced stages of their disease.[111] Risk factors include T-cell immunosuppression, race, and sex. Disseminated disease is far more likely to occur in blacks and Native Americans than in whites.[112, 113] Male sex further increases the risk of dissemination. Diabetes mellitus has long been thought to increase

the risk of dissemination, but solid data supporting this general impression are lacking. Very young or very old persons are more likely to develop disseminated coccidioidomycosis. Pregnancy has long been thought to lead to an increased risk of dissemination, but recent data cast some doubt on this observation.[114] Nevertheless, many experts feel that coccidioidomycosis occurring during the third trimester of pregnancy is a potentially severe illness with high risk for dissemination and requires prompt treatment.

The temporal relation of dissemination to the primary infection is seldom established. Most authorities think that dissemination tends to occur early during the course of the disease.[112] In many patients, however, the appearance of disseminated disease is the first sign that the patient is suffering from coccidioidomycosis. It is possible that in

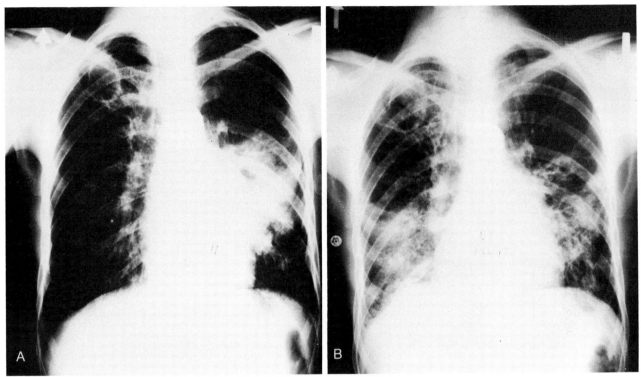

**Figure 33–19.** *A,* Large, right, apical, thin-walled cavity and dense left-sided infiltrate in a 48-year-old homeless man. The sputum culture yielded *Coccidioides immitis.* The patient refused treatment. *B,* Thirteen months later, the thin-walled cavity is slightly enlarged, the left-sided infiltrate appears less dense with apparent cavitation, and the right lower lobe is involved. The sputum is still positive for *C. immitis.* The patient again refused treatment.

these persons an asymptomatic primary pulmonary infection resolved without any symptoms, preceding eventual dissemination by an unknown interval.

*C. immitis* can disseminate to any organ of the body, but the skin is the most common site of dissemination. Single or multiple sites may be involved, and its gross appearance is not diagnostic. Presentations vary from trivial lesions resembling folliculitis to large, draining pustules and ulcers. Skin lesions may heal spontaneously or follow a rapidly progressive course with enlargement and destruction of underlying tissues. In addition to the dermis, subcutaneous tissues are frequently involved. Subcutaneous abscesses often are associated with sinus tracts to the skin. These drain thick, yellow pus loaded with spherules.

Bone is the next most common site of involvement. Involvement of many bones may be part of a widespread disseminated illness. On the other extreme, a single bony lesion may represent the entire extent of disease. The vertebrae are most frequently involved, followed by the skull and long bones. Infection of virtually every bone in the body has been documented. The radiographic appearance of coccidioidomycotic osteomyelitis is similar to that of other forms of chronic osteomyelitis, including tuberculosis and blastomycosis. Osteomyelitis of the spine usually narrows the disk space and causes sclerosis of the two adjacent vertebrae. The vertebral lesions resemble tuberculosis radiographically, but actual gibbus formation is unusual.[115] With vertebral involvement, there may be large paraspinous abscesses that sometimes compromise the spinal cord.[116] Paraspinous abscesses should be drained. Because bony lesions are common, every patient with coccidioidomycosis

should have a bone scan to search for asymptomatic bony lesions. This is particularly true for patients about to undergo therapy. If asymptomatic skeletal lesions are not recognized before initiation of therapy, their appearance during therapy may be misconstrued as evidence of therapeutic failure.

Joint involvement may be the result of hematogenous dissemination to the joint or dissemination from an adjacent bony structure. The knees and ankles are most frequently involved. Even though there is clinical evidence of chronic arthritis, the actual organism is seldom recognized in the fluid by smear or culture. Most patients require synovial biopsy for accurate diagnosis.

The genitourinary system is not a frequent site of dissemination, but coccidiouria is fairly common and should be looked for in all patients suspected of having coccidioidomycosis. The presence of *C. immitis* in the urine does not prove disseminated disease, but in one report, urine cultures were positive for *C. immitis* in 7 of 29 patients with pulmonary disease. Two of the 7 patients with positive urine cultures were not treated, and the disease resolved spontaneously.[117]

Involvement of the meninges is the most dreaded complication of coccidioidomycosis. Meningeal involvement occurs in approximately one third of the patients with disseminated coccidioidomycosis. These patients often have no other evidence of coccidioidomycosis. Coccidioidomycotic meningitis is a chronic illness and seldom has the dramatic clinical findings of acute bacterial meningitis. The usual manifestations are the onset of headache and minimal alteration of higher cortical functions.[118, 119] Many patients

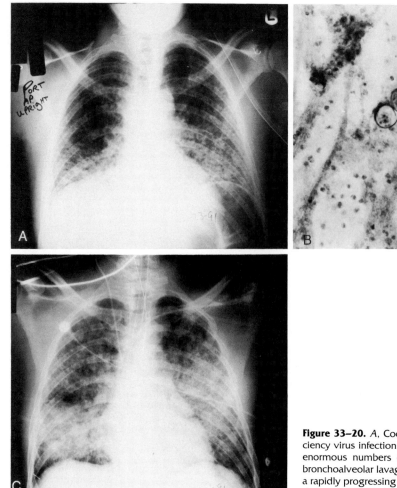

**Figure 33–20.** *A,* Coccidioidomycosis complicating a human immunodeficiency virus infection in a 33-year-old intravenous drug abuser. Notice the enormous numbers of 2- to 8-mm nodules. *B,* Papanicolaou smear of bronchoalveolar lavage fluid shows two giant spherules. *C,* Four days later, a rapidly progressing infiltrate resulted in ventilatory failure despite aggressive amphotericin B treatment. The patient died the next day.

with meningitis are diagnosed only because a lumbar puncture done for routine evaluation of a patient with disseminated disease reveals cerebral spinal fluid (CSF) pleocytosis.

Coccidioidomycotic meningitis is a disease of the base of the brain, which explains most of its clinical behavior. During disease progression, a thick, plastic exudate at the base of the brain obstructs the aqueduct of Sylvius and the foramina of the fourth ventricle, leading to obstructing hydrocephalus. This complication occurs gradually and should be suspected if the patient's mental status deteriorates suddenly. In patients who are deteriorating, signs of intracranial hypertension, including papilledema, are frequently seen. Examination of the CSF shows the characteristic manifestations of chronic meningitis: a mononuclear cell pleocytosis with only occasional polymorphonuclear leukocytes, increased protein, and decreased glucose levels. Many investigators mention CSF eosinophilia as an important finding, but in our experience, it is uncommon. Nevertheless, if eosinophils are seen in the CSF of a patient with chronic meningitis, that finding suggests coccidioidomycosis as the cause.

Coccidioidomycosis in HIV-infected patients follows a variable course, depending on the timing of the infection relative to the course of the HIV infection. Patients who become infected when their CD4 counts are normal or near

normal develop an illness similar to that seen in the general population.[111] However, if the CD4 count falls to 200 or below, a severe, rapidly progressive, disseminated disease develops. The patient has high fever, weight loss, and dyspnea. Physical examination frequently shows evidence of extensive pneumonitis. Hepatosplenomegaly may occur. Laboratory examination usually reveals hypoxemia, and the chest radiograph shows diffuse micronodular to macronodular infiltrates (Fig. 33–20) that are frequently mistaken for the more common *Pneumocystis carinii* pneumonia in this population. Meningeal involvement is common; approximately 25% of patients with the reticulonodular form of disseminated coccidioidomycosis have concomitant meningitis.

## Diagnosis

### Direct Smear and Cultures

Direct examination of expectorated sputum, bronchoscopic specimens, or aspirated pus is the best method for diagnosing the infection. For expectorated sputum and bronchoalveolar lavage specimens, the best preparation appears to be the Papanicolaou stain (see Fig. 33–20*B*). Digestion by 10% KOH can also be used. From a single published comparative study, it appears that the Papanicolaou stain has approximately twice the sensitivity of KOH digestion.[120]

Histopathologic examination of tissue biopsies is helpful. If fully mature, unruptured giant spherules are seen, the diagnosis is certain. Unfortunately, intact spherules are uncommon in histopathologic preparations. If only endospores are seen, speciation of the fungus is more difficult. Giant spherules are revealed by standard hematoxylin and eosin stain and with special stains. Special stains, including the silver stain and the PAS stain, are especially useful if only endospores are visible.

Recovery of the fungus in culture is not difficult. Extreme caution must be used in handling the specimen, because there is a high risk of infecting susceptible laboratory workers. The following guidelines are important:

1. Never place biologic material suspected of harboring *C. immitis* in a flat Petri dish; opening the dish may create an infecting aerosol.
2. All work on suspected colonies must be under a safety hood.
3. Before any work is performed on the organisms, the mycelial mat should be wetted to avoid aerosol formation.

Because of the extreme biohazard represented by *C. immitis*, many laboratories have simplified their identification procedures. Exotoxin assay is performed on the supernates of liquid mycelial-phase cultures. Expert laboratories using exoantigen testing can confirm coccidioidomycosis in 5 to 7 working days.[121]

If traditional laboratory methods are used, the mycelial isolate should be further confirmed by animal inoculation or slide cultures. Both techniques are hazardous to laboratory personnel.

### Serology

Serologic tests have remained the cornerstone of diagnosing coccidioidomycosis. Largely because of the pioneering work of C.E. Smith, serology in coccidioidomycosis is extremely helpful for diagnosis and for prognosis.

The tube precipitin (TP) test detects IgM antibodies and is used to diagnose early infection. As many as 90% of symptomatic patients have positive IgM TP test results by the end of the third week. Thereafter, the frequency of positive results decreases, and the test results are negative by 3 to 6 months. The TP test is highly specific: a positive test means a recent infection with *C. immitis*.[2] The TP test is not 100% sensitive, and for mild infection, the test result is often negative.

A newer method for the measurement of IgM antibodies is the latex particle agglutination (LPA) test. Its main advantage is its simplicity, which allows it to be performed in less experienced community hospital laboratories.[122] The LPA test is more sensitive than the TP test but has many more false-positive results. This test cannot be used to examine CSF. Most laboratories use a well-standardized coccidioidomycosis immunodiffusion test for IgM. Sensitivity and specificity are similar to the old TP test, which remains available only in a few highly specialized laboratories.

The most important serodiagnostic test remains the CF test. CF antibodies are IgG antibodies. They appear later than the IgM class antibodies. CF activity begins in 6 to 8 weeks and persists for many months. Although this test is highly specific, it is less sensitive, especially in patients with mild infections and in patients whose only evidence of infection is skin test conversion. Nevertheless, CF testing remains extremely important for management of patients with coccidioidomycosis. High or rising titers are associated with a poor prognosis, but no specific titer guarantees a good or bad outcome in a specific patient.[123]

Few reports in the medical literature have been as misunderstood as Smith's work on the coccidioidomycosis CF test.[123] He performed almost 40,000 CF tests and showed that many patients with high titers had disseminated disease or infection that was about to disseminate. However, not all patients with disseminated disease had high titers, nor did all patients with high titers have disseminated disease. Any patient whose CF titer is rising under observation or whose previously stable CF titer begins to rise after therapy should be evaluated carefully to seek evidence of disseminated disease. To complicate matters further, most laboratories use a CF test that is different from the one used by Smith and still used by Pappagianis at University of California–Davis.[122] A high titer was 1:32 in Smith's assay, but it is different (usually higher) in other assays.

The immunodiffusion test for IgG antibody is readily available and has the approximate sensitivity and specificity of the more cumbersome CF test. RIA and enzyme immunoassays are being developed.[124] As in histoplasmosis, extreme sensitivity may be accompanied by reduced specificity.

### Skin Testing

There are two highly specific skin test antigens in use: coccidioidin, which is a filtrate of the mycelial growth of the fungus, and spherulin, which is prepared from spherules. Both antigens are injected in the same manner as in the tuberculin skin test (ie, 0.1 mL is injected intradermally). Induration is measured at 48 hours. A 5-mm induration is a positive test result. In preliminary studies, it appeared that spherulin had the greater sensitivity, but in day-to-day clinical evaluation of symptomatic patients, both skin tests have roughly equal sensitivity.[125] Both tests are reasonably specific, although there is approximately a 10% crossreactivity with the histoplasmin skin test.[126]

As with the histoplasmin skin test, the main value of the coccidioidin skin test is epidemiologic. Because the test is long lasting, a positive skin test reaction may result from a recent or remote infection. The utility for individual case diagnosis is limited. Many patients with clinical coccidioidomycosis do not have a positive skin test. As many as 50% of patients with disseminated coccidioidomycosis have negative skin test results, as is the case with progressive disseminated histoplasmosis and disseminated tuberculosis. As many as 10% of patients with proven coccidioidomycotic pulmonary cavities or abscesses also fail to develop a positive skin test reading. After skin test reactivity is acquired, it appears to persist for a long time, perhaps for life. In endemic areas, where the diagnosis of pulmonary coccidioidomycosis is likely to be considered, a positive result cannot be assumed to be causally related to the acute clinical illness being evaluated, unless the patient was known to have a negative reaction to the skin test in the recent past. Crossreaction with histoplasmin does occur, creating a considerable problem in west Texas, where the known endemic areas for both diseases overlap.

If a previously negative skin test result converts to positive, it proves a recent coccidioidomycotic infection. If a patient with extensive disease has a positive reaction that later becomes negative, it is likely that there is impending or actual dissemination.

## Treatment

Most patients with acute coccidioidomycosis require no specific treatment, and most never come to medical attention. In these patients, the infection is asymptomatic or produces such minimal symptoms that a physician's counsel is not sought. Most patients with diagnosed mild or moderately symptomatic disease require no treatment, but after the diagnosis is established, careful clinical and serologic evaluation is necessary to identify patients in whom the disease is likely to progress.

Disseminated disease is most likely to develop in blacks and Hispanics,[112, 113] perhaps in patients with diabetes, and especially in patients who are immunosuppressed.[109–111] Many investigators think that all acute infections in these patients should be treated to prevent dissemination. Although no controlled studies have been performed, many authorities recommend brief courses of AMB, ranging from 500 to 2000 mg.[127]

If symptomatic pulmonary disease persists for 6 weeks, spontaneous clearing is less likely. Patients with persistent disease may also be given AMB to approximately the same total dose to reduce the risk of local progression and to prevent dissemination. In current practice in the endemic area, many high-risk patients with acute infection and many patients with persistent disease are given oral fluconazole therapy for various periods without proof of efficacy. Before the availability of fluconazole, ketoconazole was used in the same way, especially for patients with persistent coccidioidomycosis. Many patients had clinical improvement, but the relapse rate after cessation of therapy was as high as 50%.[128] No controlled studies have evaluated these agents prospectively, nor has there been any comparison of the two oral agents or of the azoles and AMB.

Occasionally, patients present with a long history of chronic, slowly progressive pulmonary illness. This chronic, low-grade but destructive tuberculosis-like disease requires treatment. Treatment may be AMB, to a total dose of 2000 to 3000 mg,[108] or fluconazole. Neither form of treatment has been carefully evaluated.

The characteristic thin-walled cavitary lesion of coccidioidomycosis usually does not require treatment. About 50% of lesions smaller than 4 cm in diameter resolve within 2 years under observation. If cavities persist beyond 2 years, if they enlarge or migrate subpleurally, or if hemoptysis is annoying, treatment seems reasonable. AMB and the oral azoles have been used, but there has been no careful evaluation of efficacy. Similarly, pulmonary nodules (ie, blocked cavities or coccidioidal abscesses) can be observed

initially, but many lesions are removed surgically to rule out bronchogenic cancer. If the lesions are resected incidentally (under the assumption that they are cancer), some authorities suggest postoperative treatment with AMB. The need for this treatment is not established. If the pleural space is contaminated during surgery, most authorities agree that treatment is necessary.[107] The optimal total dose and the required duration of therapy are unknown. Early anecdotal experience suggested that 500 mg of intravenous AMB given preoperatively and postoperatively helps to provide a therapeutic umbrella. Although this practice is common and seems reasonable, it has not been evaluated.

Disseminated coccidioidomycosis requires rapid and aggressive treatment. AMB remains the treatment of choice, although AMB therapy in this disease is not as effective as it is in histoplasmosis and blastomycosis. The standard total dose of AMB in coccidioidomycosis is between 2500 and 3000 mg, administered over several months.[102] If the clinical disease fails to respond, much larger total doses are given by extending the therapy. Our practice has been to treat patients with up to 50 mg of AMB daily until their condition stabilizes or improves. Then we give 50 mg three times weekly on an outpatient basis.

Disseminated coccidioidomycosis in AIDS is a therapeutic challenge. The disease progresses rapidly. In our series, 49% of the patients died within 3 months. In such a rapidly progressive disease, only AMB should be used. Some patients do respond to AMB. After stabilization of the clinical illness, it is reasonable to switch to oral fluconazole ($\geq$400 mg/d). All patients in our series who survived more than 1 year had received a minimum of 1 g of AMB and continuous suppressive therapy with an oral azole.

Coccidioidomycotic meningitis is also a major therapeutic challenge. Standard therapy includes systemic AMB (2500–3000 mg) plus intensive and long-term intrathecal AMB therapy.[102, 118] To accomplish intrathecal treatment, a reservoir is placed in one of the lateral ventricles.[129] The diaphragm of the reservoir is placed subcutaneously just below the hairline to avoid staphylococcal superinfection. Intraventricular AMB in doses between 0.25 and 1 mg is injected two or three times weekly, until the symptoms and CSF pleocytosis improves. After clinical improvement and diminished CSF pleocytosis, the frequency of intrathecal injections is gradually reduced from twice weekly, to weekly, to every other week, and to monthly treatment. Many authorities think the patient should receive continuous monthly infusions for life. Even with this method of treatment, relapses are common. With careful management, the patient may be maintained in a good clinical state for a long time, even a decade or more.

Fluconazole is an acceptable alternative for treatment of meningeal coccidioidomycosis, even in HIV-infected patients. Cure of the disease should not be expected, but many patients are maintained in good functional state and can lead essentially normal lives. Our practice is to use fluconazole in stable patients without focal neurologic findings or ventricular dilatation. All other patients should still receive AMB as primary therapy.

The treatment of coccidioidomycosis remains a difficult clinical problem. None of the standard antifungal agents is highly effective, and the clinical response is not predictable. Each patient's treatment must be individualized.

# CRYPTOCOCCOSIS

*C. neoformans* is a truly cosmopolitan yeast that has been isolated on all continents. Most isolations from nature have come from soil heavily contaminated by bird droppings, especially pigeon droppings. In nature and in the human host, the organism is a yeast with a carbohydrate capsule. It is 4 to 8 μm in diameter. It is likely that small, capsule-poor organisms are the infecting particles.[130] After entering the human host, the capsule is reconstituted. *C. neoformans* is the only encapsulated yeast that infects man.

## Pathogenesis

As with the dimorphic fungi, the portal of entry is the lung. Once in the alveoli, the large capsule reappears, and the fungus multiplies by binary fission. The large capsule is antiphagocytic. Nonencapsulated cryptococcal species are easily ingested and destroyed by neutrophils, but *C. neoformans* organisms with their large capsules resist phagocytosis.[6] Within the neutrophil, killing of the organism is accomplished by oxidative and nonoxidative pathways. Patients with chronic granulomatous disease lack effective oxidative metabolism in their neutrophils and kill cryptococci poorly.

After *C. neoformans* gains a foothold in the mammalian lung, T-cell–mediated immunity is required for adequate handling of the organism. This was recognized in the preantibiotic era, when many patients with Hodgkin disease suffered from cryptococcal meningitis.[131] Since the advent of the HIV pandemic, the importance of intact T-cell–mediated immunity has been confirmed.[132] Cryptococcus disease is the most common fungal disease complicating HIV infection.

In the normal lung, granuloma formation checks further fungal growth.[133] Extrapulmonary spread of the organism during the preimmune phase of self-limited pulmonary infection is probably common, as it is in histoplasmosis.

In patients with suppressed T-cell–mediated immunity, granuloma formation does not occur, and growth continues. At surgery or postmortem examination, large masses of cryptococci are seen without any evidence of tissue reaction, producing large gelatinous masses. The most important feature of the pathogenesis of cryptococcal disease is its remarkable tropism for the CNS. Cryptococcal meningitis is the most commonly recognized form of the illness.

## Clinical Manifestations

Isolated pulmonary disease is uncommon, even though the lung is the portal of entry. Campbell, in his classic review of cryptococcal pulmonary disease in 1966, identified only 101 cases of cryptococcal disease restricted to the lung.[134] Although no large review has been published since then, isolated pulmonary disease (ie, without extrapulmonary spread) is still uncommon.

Some patients have no pulmonary symptoms and present with an abnormality discovered on a routine chest radiograph. Symptomatic patients have fever, chest pain, and cough, usually of modest intensity.[135] Asymptomatic pulmonary cryptococcal infection may be common. Fifty percent to 75% of patients with cryptococcal meningitis (excluding those with AIDS) have normal chest radiographs and no history of pneumonia.[136]

The findings of the chest radiograph are highly variable, including size and location of infiltrates. Infiltrates may be single or multiple, and the disease is often confused with other pulmonary infections or neoplasms. Primary tuberculosis may be suspected if there is a peripheral infiltrate with ipsilateral hilar adenopathy.[137] Occasionally, patients exhibit masses as large as 10 cm in diameter, mimicking cancer.

Most patients diagnosed with pulmonary or CNS cryptococcosis have abnormal cell-mediated immunity. However, immunologically intact persons can also develop cryptococcosis, although the pulmonary disease usually is self-limited. The natural history of cryptococcal pulmonary infection in immunocompromised patients is dissemination.[135]

Involvement of the CNS is the most clinically significant form of cryptococcal infection. The severity of symptoms ranges from asymptomatic meningitis to focal neurologic findings to coma.[138, 139] The tempo of the CNS involvement is also highly variable; extremely long life has been reported with proven cryptococcal meningitis, but the disease may also kill within a few days of onset. In some persons, there may be no meningeal signs despite fulminant meningitis.

## Diagnosis

*C. neoformans* grows readily on routine laboratory media. However, a positive sputum culture, even in the presence of radiographic abnormality, must be interpreted carefully. The organism frequently colonizes airways. Most susceptible are patients with chronic bronchitis and immunosuppressed patients who are at high risk for dissemination.[140] Non-*neoformans* cryptococci are frequently isolated in the laboratory, and only biochemical tests can separate these commensals from *C. neoformans*. With rare exceptions, CNS isolations are *C. neoformans*, and a positive CSF culture indicates clinically significant meningitis.

In histopathologic sections, the organism appears as a budding yeast. In standard hematoxylin and eosin-stained sections, the unstained capsule appears as a halo surrounding the yeast. A silver stain shows the organism but not the capsule. The mucicarmine stain colors the carbohydrate capsule bright red.

The CSF shows a mononuclear cell pleocytosis. The leukocyte count is highly variable and may be less than 5/mm³ or even zero. The protein concentration is usually elevated, and the glucose level is reduced, occasionally to very low levels. The oldest test for cryptococcal meningitis is the India ink preparation, positive in 70% of HIV-infected patients but less sensitive in other patients. The best single test for cryptococcal meningitis is the LPA test for measuring cryptococcal antigen, which is positive for 90% to 95% of patients with cryptococcal meningitis.[132] Cryptococcal antigen can also be measured in serum. The serum test result is likely to be negative for cryptococcal meningitis in nonimmunocompromised hosts. In HIV-infected patients with cryptococcal disease, the serum test is positive for very high titers, usually higher than simultaneous CSF titers.[132] If carefully performed with adequate controls, the test has almost no false-positive results.[141]

Other extrapulmonary sites of involvement by the cryptococci include the skin, bones, and prostate. Unless there is evidence of direct local inoculation (ie, chancre, draining lymph node), all forms of cutaneous cryptococcal disease should be assumed to represent dissemination from a central focus, usually the meninges or the lungs.[142]

## Treatment

A positive sputum culture should be interpreted with a degree of skepticism. Even if the chest radiograph is abnormal, there are several possible explanations. The organism may be a contaminant, a colonizer, or the cause of a self-limited pneumonia. After treatment for routine bacterial pathogens, a period of watchful waiting is indicated, provided a lumbar puncture shows no evidence of cryptococcal meningitis.

If the patient is immunosuppressed, especially by HIV infection, treatment should be given if *C. neoformans* is isolated from any site. All patients must have a lumbar puncture, even if there are no symptoms of CNS disease.

Treatment of cryptococcal pulmonary disease is not based on carefully performed prospective studies. Treatment recommendations are based on the large experience with cryptococcal meningitis, on anecdotes, and on opinions. Treatment options for meningitis include AMB alone to a total dose of 1 to 2 g[138] or a combination of AMB (0.3–0.6 mg/kg daily) with 5-flucytosine (5-FC) (150 mg/kg/d) for a minimum of 6 weeks.[143] Even shorter treatment courses have been effective for patients with cryptococcal meningitis who were not immunosuppressed and were not transplant recipients. Great care is necessary when using 5-FC. The drug accumulates rapidly, especially if renal function is reduced. If the serum level is high (>100 µg/mL), 5-FC is toxic to bone marrow. If a rapid turnaround time for 5-FC levels cannot be assured, we do not use this agent.

Treatment of cryptococcal disease in AIDS is a different problem. Relapses are almost universal after apparently successful treatment.[132] To induce a remission, AMB with or without 5-FC should be used and continued until there are at least two negative spinal fluid cultures.[144] After this apparent sterilization of the CNS, fluconazole suppression therapy should be given for the rest of the patient's life. Fluconazole (200 mg/d) is more successful as suppressive therapy than AMB and is the preferred therapy.[145]

There are ongoing studies to try to improve treatment. One study uses higher initial doses of AMB and a faster switch to fluconazole. Fluconazole alone appears to be an effective treatment for primary cryptococcal meningitis, but there may be excess early deaths.[144] Primary fluconazole therapy, even in clinical studies, should be used only in neurologically intact patients.

Risk factors for a poor outcome despite adequate treatment include HIV infection,[132, 145] lymphoreticular malignancy, glucocorticoid therapy, high opening pressure on the initial lumbar puncture, a CNS leukocyte count of less than 20 cells/mm³, a positive India ink smear, the isolation of

the fungus from an extraneural site, and a cryptococcal antigen titer of 1:32 or greater.[146]

Treatment of isolated cryptococcal pulmonary infections in nonimmunosuppressed patients may not be necessary, because the natural history is spontaneous improvement.[135] However, the risk of meningeal dissemination, although low, does exist. Because fluconazole is a nontoxic oral agent, treatment with this agent may be reasonable for all patients with cryptococcal pneumonia.

## REFERENCES

1. Goodwin RA Jr, DesPrez RM: Histoplasmosis: State of the art. Am Rev Respir Dis 117:929–956, 1978.
2. Drutz DJ, Catanzaro A: Coccidioidomycosis: State of the art. Part I. Am Rev Respir Dis 117:559–585, 1978.
3. Furcolow ML, Chick EW, Busey JD, Menges RW: Prevalence and incidence studies of human and canine blastomycosis I: Cases in the United States 1895–1968. Am Rev Respir Dis 102:60–67, 1970.
4. Sarosi GA, Davies SF: Blastomycosis: State of the art. Am Rev Respir Dis 120:911–938, 1979.
5. Schaffner A, Davis CE, Schaffner T, Markert M, Douglas H, Braude AI: In vitro susceptibility of fungi to killing by neutrophil granulocytes discriminates between primary pathogenicity and opportunism. J Clin Invest 78:511–524, 1986.
6. Bulmer GS, Sans MDF: *Cryptococcus neoformans* II: Phagocytosis by human leukocytes. J Bacteriol 94:1480–1483, 1967.
7. Darling ST: A protozoan general infection producing pseudotubercles in the lungs and focal necrosis in the liver, spleen and lymph nodes. JAMA 46:1283–1285, 1986.
8. Riley WA, Watson CJ: Histoplasmosis of Darling with report of a case originating in Minnesota. Am J Trop Med 6:271–282, 1926.
9. Dodd K, Tompkins EH: Case of histoplasmosis of Darling in an infant. Am J Trop Health 14:127–134, 1934.
10. De-Monbreum WA: The cultivation and cultural characteristics of Darling's *Histoplasma capsulatum*. Am J Trop Med 14:93–126, 1934.
11. Christie A, Peterson JC: Pulmonary calcifications in negative reactors to tuberculin. Am J Public Health 35:1131–1145, 1945.
12. Palmer CE: Nontuberculous pulmonary calcification. Public Health Rep 60:513–521, 1945.
13. Emmons CW, Morlan HB, Hill EL: Isolation of *Histoplasma capsulatum* from soil. Public Health Rep 64:892–896, 1949.
14. Edwards LD, Acquaviva FA, Livesay VT, et al: An atlas of sensitivity to tuberculin, PPD-B, and histoplasmin in the United States. Am Rev Respir Dis 90(suppl):1–132, 1969.
15. Sarosi GA, Parker JD, Tosh FE: Histoplasmosis outbreaks: Their patterns. *In* Balows A (ed): Histoplasmosis. Proceedings of the Second National Conference. Springfield, IL, Charles C Thomas, 1971:123–128.
16. D'Alessio DJ, Heeren RH, Hendricks SL, Ogilvie P, Furcolow ML: A starling roost as the source of urban epidemic histoplasmosis in an area of low incidence. Am Rev Respir Dis 932:725–731, 1965.
17. Wheat LJ, Slama TG, Eitzen HE, Kohler RB, French MLV, Biesecker JD: A large outbreak of histoplasmosis: Clinical features. Ann Intern Med 94:331–337, 1981.
18. U.S. Department of Health, Education and Welfare: Histoplasmosis control: Decontamination of bird roosts, chicken houses and other sources (No. 00–3021). Atlanta, GA, Centers for Disease Control, 1977.
19. Straub M, Schwarz J: Healed primary complex in histoplasmosis. Am J Clin Pathol 25:727–738, 1955.
20. Feller AE, Furcolow ML, Larsh HW, Langmuir AD, Dingle JH: Outbreak of an unusual form of pneumonia at Camp Gruber, Oklahoma, in 1944. Follow-up studies implicating *H. capsulatum* as the etiologic agent. Am J Med 21:184–192, 1956.
21. Davies SF: Serodiagnosis of histoplasmosis. Semin Respir Infect 1:9–15, 1986.
22. Goodwin RA Jr, Loyd JE, DesPrez RM: Histoplasmosis in normal hosts. Medicine (Baltimore) 60:231–266, 1981.
23. Procknow JJ: Reinfection histoplasmosis. *In* Balows A (ed): Histo-

plasmosis. Proceedings of the Second National Conference. Springfield, IL, Charles C Thomas, 1971:252–259.

24. Tosh FE: Reinfection histoplasmosis. *In* Balows A (ed): Histoplasmosis. Proceedings of the Second National Conference. Springfield, IL, Charles C Thomas, 1971:260–267.

25. Zeidberg LD, Dillin A, Glass RS: Some factors in the epidemiology of histoplasmin sensitivity in Williamson County, Tennessee. Am J Public Health 41:80–81, 1951.

26. Goodman RA Jr, Shapiro JL, Thurman GH, et al: Disseminated histoplasmosis: Clinical and pathologic correlations. Medicine (Baltimore) 59:1–33, 1980.

27. Medeiros AA, Marty SD, Tosh FE, Chin TDY: Erythema nodosum and erythema multiforme as clinical manifestations of histoplasmosis in community outbreak. N Engl J Med 274:415–420, 1966.

28. Wheat LJ, Stein L, Corya BC, et al: Pericarditis as a manifestation of histoplasmosis during two large urban outbreaks. Medicine (Baltimore) 62:110–118, 1983.

29. Goodwin RA Jr, Nickell JD, DesPrez RM: Mediastinal fibrosis complicating healed primary histoplasmosis and tuberculosis. Medicine (Baltimore) 51:227–246, 1972.

30. Tosh FE, Doto IL, D'Alessio DJ, Medeiros AA, Hendricks SL, Chin TDY: The second of two epidemics of histoplasmosis resulting from work on the same starling roost. Am Rev Respir Dis 94:406–414, 1966.

31. Davies SF, Sarosi GA: Acute cavitary histoplasmosis. Chest 73:103–105, 1978.

32. Goodwin RA Jr, Snell JD, Hubbard WW, et al: Early chronic pulmonary histoplasmosis. Am Rev Respir Dis 93:47–51, 1966.

33. Goodwin RA Jr, Owens FT, Snell JD, et al: Chronic pulmonary histoplasmosis. Medicine (Baltimore) 55:413–452, 1976.

34. Bunnell IL, Furcolow ML: A report of ten proved cases of histoplasmosis. US Public Health Rep 63:299–316, 1948.

35. Paya CU, Roberts GN, Cockerill FR III: Transient fungemia in acute pulmonary histoplasmosis: Detection by new blood-culturing techniques. J Infect Dis 156:313–315, 1987.

36. Davies SF, McKenna RW, Sarosi GA: Trephine biopsy of the bone marrow in disseminated histoplasmosis. Am J Med 67:617–622, 1979.

37. Johnson PC, Hamill RJ, Sarosi GA: Clinical review: Progressive disseminated histoplasmosis in the AIDS patient. Semin Respir Infect 4:139–446, 1989.

38. Wheat LJ, Connolly-Stringfield PA, Baker RL, et al: Disseminated histoplasmosis in the acquired immunodeficiency syndrome: Clinical findings, diagnosis and treatment, and review of the literature. Medicine (Baltimore) 69:361–374, 1990.

39. Tompsett R, Portera LA: Histoplasmosis: Twenty year experience in a general hospital. Trans Am Clin Climatol Assoc 87:214–223, 1975.

40. Davies SF, Khan M, Sarosi GA: Disseminated histoplasmosis in immunologically suppressed patients. Am J Med 64:94–100, 1978.

41. Salzman SH, Smith RL, Aranda CP: Histoplasmosis in patients at risk for the acquired immunodeficiency syndrome in a nonendemic setting. Chest 93:916–921, 1988.

42. Wheat LJ, Slama TG, Norton JA, et al: Risk factors for disseminated or fatal histoplasmosis. Ann Intern Med 96:159–163, 1982.

43. Sarosi GA, Voth DW, Dahl BA, Doto IL, Tosh FE: Disseminated histoplasmosis: Results of long-term follow-up. Ann Intern Med 75:511–516, 1971.

44. Anaissi E, Fainstein V, Samo T, Bodey GP, Sarosi GA: Central nervous system histoplasmosis. Am J Med 84:215–217, 1988.

45. Harris RL, Lawrie GM, Wheeler TM, et al: Successful management of *Histoplasma capsulatum* infection of an abdominal aortic aneurysm. Vasc Surg 1:40–44, 1986.

46. Sanders JS, Sarosi GA, Nollet DJ, Thompson JL: Exfoliative cytology in the rapid diagnosis of pulmonary blastomycosis. Chest 72:193–196, 1977.

47. Sarosi GA, Johnson PC: Disseminated histoplasmosis in patients infected with human immunodeficiency virus. Clin Infect Dis 14(suppl 1):60–67, 1992.

48. Davies SF, Sarosi GA: Role of serodiagnostic tests and skin tests in the diagnosis of fungal disease. Clin Chest Med 8:135–146, 1987.

49. Wheat LJ, Kohler RB, French MLV, et al: Immunoglobulin M and G histoplasma antibody response in histoplasmosis. Am Rev Respir Dis 128:65–70, 1983.

50. Wheat LJ, Kohler RB, Tewari RP: Diagnosis of disseminated histoplasmosis by detection of *Histoplasma capsulatum* antigen in serum and urine specimens. N Engl J Med 314:83–88, 1986.

51. Wheat LJ, Connolly-Stringfield P, Blair R, Connolly K, Garringer T, Katz BP: Histoplasmosis relapse in patients with AIDS: Detection using *Histoplasma capsulatum* variety *capsulatum* antigen levels. Ann Intern Med 115:936–941, 1991.

52. Naylor BA: Low dose amphotericin B therapy for acute pulmonary histoplasmosis. Chest 71:404–406, 1977.

53. Mycosis Study Group: Treatment of blastomycosis and histoplasmosis with ketoconazole. Ann Intern Med 103:861–873, 1985.

54. Parker JD, Sarosi GA, Doto IL, Bailey RE, Tosh FE: Treatment of chronic pulmonary histoplasmosis. N Engl J Med 283:225–229, 1970.

55. McKinsey DS, Gupta MR, Riddler SA, et al: Long-term amphotericin B therapy for disseminated histoplasmosis in patients with the acquired immunodeficiency syndrome (AIDS). Ann Intern Med 75:511–516, 1971.

56. Wheat J, Hafner R, Wulfsohn M, Spencer P, Squires K, Powderly W, et al: Prevention of relapse of histoplasmosis with itraconazole in patients with THA-acquired immunodeficiency syndrome. Ann Intern Med 118:610–616, 1993.

57. Butler WT, Bennett JE, Aling DW: Nephrotoxicity of amphotericin B. Early and late effects in 81 patients. Ann Intern Med 6:175–187, 1964.

58. Dismukes WE, Bradsher RW Jr, Cloud GC, et al: Itraconazole therapy for blastomycosis and histoplasmosis. Am J Med 93:489–497, 1992.

59. Saag MS, Dismukes WE: Azole antifungal agents: Emphasis on new triazoles. Antimicrob Agents Chemother 32:1–8, 1988.

60. Pont A, Graybill JR, Craven PC, et al: High-dose ketoconazole therapy and adrenal and testicular function in humans. Arch Intern Med 144:2150–2153, 1984.

61. Gilchrist TC: Protozoan dermatitis. J Cutan Gen Dis 12:496–499, 1894.

62. Wernicke E: Über einen Protozoenbefunde bei Mycosis fungoides. Zentralbl Bakt 12:859–861, 1892.

63. Gilchrist TC, Stokes WR: Case of pseudolupus vulgaris caused by blastomycosis. J Exp Med 3:53–78, 1898.

64. Martin DS, Smith DT: Blastomycosis II. A report of thirteen new cases. Am Rev Tuberc 39:488–515, 1939.

65. Schwarz J, Baum GL: Blastomycosis. Am J Clin Pathol 11:999–1029, 1951.

66. Larsh HW, Schwarz J: Accidental inoculation blastomycosis. Cutis 19:334–337, 1977.

67. Larson DM, Eckman MR, Alber RL, et al: Primary cutaneous (inoculation) blastomycosis: An occupation hazard to pathologists. Am J Clin Pathol 79:253–255, 1983.

68. Jaspers RH: Transmission of blastomycosis from animals to man. J Am Vet Med Assoc 164:8, 1974.

69. Farber ER, Leahy MD, Meadows TR: Endometrial blastomycosis acquired by sexual contact. Obstet Gynecol 32:195–199, 1968.

70. Kepron MD, Schoemperlen B, Hershfield ES, Zylak CJ, Cherniak RM: North American blastomycosis in central Canada. Can Med Assoc J 106:243–246, 1972.

71. Witorsch P, Utz JP: North American blastomycosis. A study of 40 patients. Medicine (Baltimore) 47:169–200, 1968.

72. Tosh FE, Hammerman KJ, Weeks RJ, Sarosi GA: A common source of epidemic North American blastomycosis. Am Rev Respir Dis 109:525–529, 1974.

73. Sarosi GA, King RA: Apparent diminution of the blastomycin skin test: Follow-up of an epidemic of blastomycosis. Am Rev Respir Dis 116:785–788, 1977.

74. Klein BS, Vergeront JM, Weeks RJ, et al: Isolation of *Blastomyces dermatitidis* in soil associated with a large outbreak of blastomycosis in Wisconsin. N Engl J Med 314:529–534, 1986.

75. Sarosi GA, Eckman MR, Davies SF, et al: Canine blastomycosis as a harbinger of human disease. Ann Intern Med 91:733–735, 1979.

76. Sarosi GA, Hammerman KJ, Tosh FE, Kronenberg RS: Clinical features of acute pulmonary blastomycosis. N Engl J Med 290:540–543, 1974.

77. Vaaler AK, Bradsher RW, Davies SF: Evidence of subclinical blastomycosis in forestry workers in northern Minnesota and northern Wisconsin. Am J Med 89:470–476, 1990.

78. Schwarz J, Salfelder K: Blastomycosis. A review of 152 cases. Curr Top Pathol 65:165, 1977.

79. Abernathy RS: Clinical manifestations of pulmonary blastomycosis. Ann Intern Med 51:707–727, 1959.

80. Kunkel WM Jr, Weed LA, McDonald Jr, Clagett OT: North Ameri-

can blastomycosis: Gilchrist's disease. A clinicopathologic study of 90 cases. Surg Gynecol Obstet 99:1–26, 1954.

81. Smith JR Jr, Harris JS, Conant NF, et al: An epidemic of North American blastomycosis. JAMA 158:641–645, 1951.

82. Miller DD, Davies SF, Sarosi GA: Erythema nodosum and blastomycosis. Arch Intern Med 142:1839, 1982.

83. Laskey WL, Sarosi GA: The radiologic appearance of pulmonary blastomycosis. Radiology 126:351–357, 1978.

84. Sarosi GA, Davies SF, Phillips JR: Self-limited blastomycosis: A report of 39 cases. Semin Respir Infect 1:40–44, 1986.

85. Laskey WL, Sarosi GA: Endogenous reactivation in blastomycosis. Ann Intern Med 88:50–52, 1978.

86. Davies SF, Sarosi GA: Clinical manifestations and management of blastomycosis in the compromised patient. In Warnock DW, Richardson MD (eds): Fungal Infection in the Compromised Patient, ed 2. New York, Wiley & Sons, 1991:215–229.

87. Pappas PG, Pottage JC, Powderly WG, et al: Blastomycosis in patients with the acquired immunodeficiency syndrome. Ann Intern Med 116:847–853, 1992.

88. Bradsher RW: Development of specific immunity in patients with pulmonary or extrapulmonary blastomycosis. Am Rev Respir Dis 129:430–434, 1984.

89. Klein BS, Vergeront JM, Kaufman L, et al: Serological tests for blastomycosis: Assessment during a large point-source outbreak in Wisconsin. J Infect Dis 155:262–268, 1987.

90. Parker JD, Doto IL, Tosh FE: A decade of experience with blastomycosis and its treatment with amphotericin B. Am Rev Respir Dis 99:895–902, 1969.

91. Kravitz GE, Davies SF, Eckman MR, Sarosi GA: Chronic blastomycotic meningitis. Am J Med 71:501–505, 1981.

92. Bradsher RW, Rice DC, Abernathy RS: Ketoconazole therapy for endemic blastomycosis. Ann Intern Med 103:872–875, 1985.

93. Posadas A: Un nuevo caso de micosis fungoides con psorospermias. Ann Circ Med Argent 15:585–597, 1892.

94. Rixford E, Gilchrist TC: Two cases of protozoan (coccidioidal) infection of the skin and other organs. Johns Hopkins Hosp Rep 1:209–265, 1896.

95. Dickson EC: Coccidioidomycosis—the preliminary acute infection with fungus coccidioides. JAMA 111:1362–1365, 1938.

96. Dickson EC, Gifford MA: Coccidioides infection (coccidioidomycosis) II. The primary type of infection. Arch Intern Med 62:858–871, 1938.

97. Smith CE, Beard RR, Rosenberger HG, et al: Effect of season and dust control on coccidioidomycosis. JAMA 132:833–839, 1946.

98. Forbus WD, Bestebreurtje AM: Coccidioidomycosis. A study of 95 cases of the disseminated type with special reference to the pathogenesis of the disease. Milit Surg 99:653–719, 1946.

99. Flynn NM, Hoeprich PD, Kawachi MM, et al: An unusual outbreak of windborne coccidioidomycosis. N Engl J Med 301:358–361, 1979.

100. Goldstein DM, McDonald JB: Primary pulmonary coccidioidomycosis. Follow-up of 75 cases with 10 more cases from a new endemic area. JAMA 124:557–561, 1944.

101. Werner SB, Pappagianis D, Heindl I, Mickel A: An epidemic of coccidioidomycosis among archeology students in Northern California. N Engl J Med 286:507–512, 1972.

102. Drutz DJ, Catanzaro A: Coccidioidomycosis. State of the art. Part II. Am Rev Respir Dis 177:727–771, 1978.

103. Bayer AS: Fungal pneumonias, pulmonary coccidioidal syndromes (part I). Chest 79:575–583, 1981.

104. Bayer AS: Fungal pneumonias, pulmonary coccidioidal syndromes (part II). Chest 79:686–691, 1981.

105. Winn WA: A long-term study of 300 patients with cavitary abscess lesions of the lung of coccidioidal origin. Dis Chest 54(suppl 1):12–16, 1968.

106. Hyde L: Coccidioidal pulmonary cavitation. Dis Chest 54(suppl 1):17–21, 1968.

107. Cunningham RT, Einstein H: Coccidioidal pulmonary cavities with rupture. J Thorac Cardiovasc Surg 84:172–177, 1982.

108. Sarosi GA, Parker JD, Doto IL, Tosh FE: Chronic pulmonary coccidioidomycosis. N Engl J Med 283:325–329, 1970.

109. Deresinski SC, Stevens DA: Coccidioidomycosis in compromised hosts: Experience at Stanford University Hospital. Medicine (Baltimore) 54:377–395, 1975.

110. Cohen IM, Galgiani JN, Potter D, Ogden DA: Coccidioidomycosis in renal replacement therapy. Arch Intern Med 142:489–494, 1982.

111. Fish DG, Ampel NM, Galgiani JN, et al: Coccidioidomycosis during human immunodeficiency virus infection. A review of 77 patients. Medicine (Baltimore) 60:384–391, 1990.

112. Smith CE, Beard RR, Whiting EG, et al: Varieties of coccidioidal infection in relation to the epidemiology and control of the disease. Am J Public Health 36:1394–1402, 1946.

113. Pappagianis D, Lindsay S, Beall S, et al: Ethnic background and the clinical course of coccidioidomycosis. [Letter] Am Rev Respir Dis 120:959–961, 1979.

114. Catanzaro A: Pulmonary mycosis in pregnant women. Chest 86:145–185, 1984.

115. Dalinka MK, Greendyke WH: The spinal manifestations of coccidioidomycosis. J Can Assoc Radiol 22:93–99, 1971.

116. Dalinka MK, Dinnenberg S, Greendyke WH, Hopkins R: Roentgenographic features of osseous coccidioidomycosis and differential diagnosis. J Bone Joint Surg [Am] 53A:1157–1164, 1971.

117. DeFelice R, Wieden MA, Galgiani JN: The incidence and implications of coccidioidouria. Am Rev Respir Dis 125:49–52, 1982.

118. Winn WA: Coccidioidal meningitis: A follow-up report. In Ajello L (ed): Coccidioidomycosis. Tucson, University of Arizona Press, 1966:55–61.

119. Bouze E, Dreyer JS, Hewitt WL, Meyer RD: Coccidioidal meningitis. An analysis of thirty-one cases and review of the literature. Medicine (Baltimore) 60:139–172, 1981.

120. Warlick MA, Quan SF, Sobonya RE: Rapid diagnosis of pulmonary coccidioidomycosis. Cytologic vs. potassium hydroxide preparation. Arch Intern Med 143:723–725, 1983.

121. Standard PG, Kaufman L: Immunological procedure for the rapid and specific identification of Coccidioides immitis cultures. J Clin Microbiol 5:149–153, 1977.

122. Pappagianis D, Krasnow RI, Beall S: False-positive reactions of cerebrospinal fluid and diluted sera with the coccidioidal latex-agglutination test. Am J Clin Pathol 66:916–921, 1976.

123. Smith CE, Saito MT, Beard RR, Kepp RM, Clark RW, Eddie BM: Serologic tests in the diagnosis and prognosis of coccidioidomycosis. Am J Hyg 52:1–21, 1950.

124. Catanzaro A, Flatauer F: Detection of serum antibodies in coccidioidomycosis by solid-phase radioimmunoassay. J Infect Dis 147:32–39, 1983.

125. Sarosi GA, Catanzaro A, Daniel TM, et al: Clinical usefulness of skin testing in histoplasmosis, coccidioidomycosis and blastomycosis: Official statement of the American Thoracic Society. Am Rev Respir Dis 138:1081–1082, 1988.

126. Levine HB, Restrepo MA, Ten Eyck DR, Stevens DA: Spherulin and coccidioidin: Cross-reactions in dermal sensitivity to histoplasmin and paracoccidioidin. Am J Epidemiol 101:515–522, 1975.

127. Sarosi GA, Bates JH, Bradsher RW, et al: Chemotherapy of the pulmonary mycoses: Official statement of The American Thoracic Society. Am Rev Respir Dis 138:1078–1081, 1988.

128. Galgiani JN, Stevens DA, Graybill JR, et al: Ketoconazole therapy of progressive coccidioidomycosis. Comparison of 400 and 800 mg doses and observations at higher doses. Am J Med 84:603–610, 1988.

129. Diamond RD, Bennett JE: A subcutaneous reservoir for intrathecal therapy of fungal meningitis. N Engl J Med 288:186–188, 1973.

130. Powell KE, Dahl BA, Weeks RJ, Tosh ED: Airborne Cryptococcus neoformans: Particles from pigeon excreta compatible with alveolar deposition. J Infect Dis 125:412–415, 1972.

131. Collins UP, Gellhorn A, Trimble JR: The coincidence of cryptococcosis and disease of the reticuloendothelial and lymphatic systems. Cancer 4:883–889, 1951.

132. Chuck SL, Sande MA: Infections with Cryptococcus neoformans in the acquired immunodeficiency syndrome. N Engl J Med 321:794–799, 1989.

133. Salyer WR, Salyer DC, Baker RD: Primary complex of cryptococcus and pulmonary lymph nodes. J Infect Dis 130:74–77, 1974.

134. Campbell GD: Primary pulmonary cryptococcosis. Am Rev Respir Dis 94:236–243, 1966.

135. Kerkering TM, Duma RD, Shadomy S: The evolution of pulmonary cryptococcosis. Ann Intern Med 94:611–616, 1981.

136. Lewis JI, Rabinovich SH: The wide spectrum of cryptococcal infections. Am J Med 53:315–322, 1972.

137. Baker RD: The primary pulmonary lymph node complex of cryptococcosis. Am J Clin Pathol 65:83–92, 1976.

138. Sarosi GA, Parker JD, Doto IL, Tosh FE: Amphotericin B in cryptococcal meningitis. Ann Intern Med 71:1079–1087, 1969.

139. Mangham D, Gerding DN, Sarosi GA: Fungal meningitis manifesting as hydrocephalus. Arch Intern Med 143:728–731, 1983.
140. Hammerman KJ, Powell KE, Christianson CS, et al: Pulmonary cryptococcosis: Clinical forms and treatment. Am Rev Respir Dis 108:1116–1123, 1973.
141. Bennett JE, Bailey JW: Control for rheumatoid factor in the latex test for cryptococcosis. Am J Clin Pathol 56:360–365, 1971.
142. Sarosi GA, Silberfarb PM, Tosh FE: Cutaneous cryptococcosis. A sentinel of disseminated disease. Arch Dermatol 104:1–3, 1971.
143. Bennett JE, Dismukes WE, Duma RJ, et al: A comparison of amphotericin B alone and combined with flucytosine in the treatment of cryptococcal meningitis. N Engl J Med 301:126–131, 1979.
144. Saag MS, Powderly WG, Cloud GA, et al: Comparison of amphotericin B with fluconazole in the treatment of acute AIDS-associated cryptococcal meningitis. N Engl J Med 326:83–89, 1992.
145. Powderly WG, Saag MS, Cloud GA, et al: Controlled trial of fluconazole or amphotericin B to prevent relapse of cryptococcal meningitis in patients with the acquired immunodeficiency syndrome. N Engl J Med 326:793–798, 1992.
146. Diamond RD, Bennett JE: Prognostic factors in cryptococcal meningitis. Ann Intern Med 80:176–181, 1974.

# CHAPTER 34

# Nocardiosis*

GREGORY A. FILICE

Pulmonary nocardiosis is an indolent process caused by the aerobic actinomycete, *Nocardia asteroides*, or less commonly, by other species of *Nocardia*. In about half of the cases of pulmonary nocardiosis, infection disseminates to brain, skin, bone, and other organs. Manifestations of disseminated disease may be the presenting complaints, and pulmonary disease may be asymptomatic or unapparent.

The term nocardiosis is used in this chapter to refer to pulmonary or disseminated nocardiosis. These syndromes are usually parts of the same pathophysiologic process. *Nocardia* infection is also associated with other syndromes, including cellulitis, lymphocutaneous syndrome, mycetoma, and eye infections.

## MICROBIOLOGY

*Nocardia* is a genus in the family Nocardiaceae, order Actinomycetales. Because the taxonomy of Actinomycetales is complex and incomplete, the nomenclature has changed frequently. Bergey's Manual[1] lists nine *Nocardia* species, but only three are well-documented pathogens of humans: *N. asteroides, N. brasiliensis*, and *N. otitidiscaviarum* (formerly *N. caviae*). *Nocardia farcinica* and *Nocardia nova* are species of uncertain or controversial status that have been associated with disease in humans and that may be worth differentiating from *N. asteroides* because of differences in antimicrobial susceptibilities.[2–4] *Nocardia transvalensis* has been associated with disseminated infection in 3 patients with host defense defects and with mycetoma in 4 patients.[5] *Actinomadura madurae, Actinomadura pelletierii*, and *Streptomyces somaliensis* are related pathogens that cause actinomycetoma. Nocardiaceae are definitively differentiated from other Actinomycetales by the composition of their cell walls, phospholipids, and fatty acids.[1]

Nocardiae are gram-positive, partially acid-fast, crooked, nonmotile, aerobic rods. They are approximately 1 μm wide. As they grow, the bacilli divide by binary fission, but the individual cells remain attached to one another and form long, branching filaments. Under conditions unfavorable for growth, the filaments break up into bacillary or coccoid forms.

*Nocardia* species are common, worldwide inhabitants of soil, where they contribute to decay of organic matter. These bacteria do not regularly colonize animals, but they are an economically important pathogen in bovine mastitis, and nocardial disease has been described in a variety of other mammals and birds. Because the usual habitat of *Nocardia* species is soil and because nocardiae form aerial mycelia, it is thought that pulmonary nocardiosis occurs after inhalation of fragmented mycelia.

## EPIDEMIOLOGY

Nocardiosis has a worldwide distribution. It was estimated[6] in 1974 that between 500 and 1000 cases of *Nocardia* infection were diagnosed annually in the United States, 85% of them pulmonary or systemic. The disease usually occurs in adults, and males are affected twice as often as females. There is no well documented seasonality or association with particular occupations.

Nocardiosis occurs in apparently healthy people, but the risk is greater in those with one or more risk factors.[7] People with deficient cell-mediated immunity, especially those with lymphoma and those who have received transplants, are at increased risk.[8, 9] Nocardiosis has been reported in numerous persons with the acquired immunodeficiency syndrome (AIDS),[10–12] although it is not as common as some other opportunistic infections in this group. Nocardiosis has also been associated with pulmonary alveolar proteinosis,[13] tuberculosis,[14] and chronic granulomatous dis-

*All material in this chapter is in the public domain, with the exception of any borrowed figures or tables.

ease.[15] Nocardiosis has also been reported frequently in people with chronic obstructive pulmonary disease, alcoholism, or diabetes mellitus, but a definite association is harder to prove for these diseases because they are so common.

Mycetoma is found mainly in tropical and subtropical regions. Most cases have been reported from Mexico, Central and South America, Africa, and India. The few cases reported in the United States occurred predominantly in southern regions.[16] Mycetoma may be caused by one of several actinomycetes, and it is often referred to as actinomycetoma. Several fungi are associated with mycetoma, which may be called eumycetoma. Botryomycosis is a closely related disease caused by bacteria not included in Actinomycetales, most commonly *Staphylococcus aureus* or *Pseudomonas aeruginosa*. Mycetomas usually occur on extremities; mycetoma of the foot is sometimes referred to as "madura foot." Mycetoma can also occur on the posterior part of the neck or on the upper back and may penetrate to thoracic structures. The clinical syndrome is similar regardless of the causative microorganism, but there are striking differences in the distribution of organisms that cause the mycetoma syndrome in different regions.

The most important risk factor for mycetoma is frequent contact with soil or vegetable matter. For example, infections on the back and neck often occur in laborers who carry straw, wood, or burlap bags, and mycetomas on feet occur in people who work outdoors without shoes or with sandals. Most cases tend to occur in male unskilled laborers in the third to fifth decades of life.

Four outbreaks of nocardiosis have been reported. In one,[17] 7 cases occurred among patients in a renal dialysis unit. The mechanism of spread was not identified. In the second,[18] a cluster of subcutaneous abscesses occurred in patients who received subcutaneous injections of contaminated solutions. In the third,[19] a cluster of 3 cases occurred among patients at a cancer hospital. One of these 3 patients had a laryngeal lesion, and a second, who had been in contact with the first, came down with pulmonary nocardiosis 10 days later. In the fourth outbreak,[20] 2 renal transplant recipients developed nocardiosis within weeks of each other, and their organisms were similar but not identical. Except for the circumstances of the second[18] and third[19] outbreaks, there is no evidence for person-to-person spread.

## PATHOGENESIS

The characteristic histologic feature of *Nocardia* infection is an abscess extensively infiltrated with neutrophils. There is often extensive necrosis. Granulation tissue usually surrounds the lesions, but extensive fibrosis or encapsulation is usually not observed. Rarely, there is extensive fibrosis approaching that seen in actinomycosis, but granules do not appear in pus draining from lesions. In the lungs, there are usually multiple abscesses, which may become confluent. In other organs, the distribution of abscesses is variable. Microcolonies are occasionally observed in histologic preparations but almost never in discharges from lesions.

Pulmonary infection disseminates in half of the cases. The most common sites, in order of decreasing frequency, are brain, skin and supporting structures, and kidneys.[7]

Dense encapsulation is unusual. Sinus tracts exiting through the skin are common. Daughter lesions often occur in the central nervous system, and brain abscesses tend to burrow into the ventricles or out into the subarachnoid space. Rarely, epithelioid granulomas are observed in the central nervous system.

The pathologic characteristics of mycetoma depend on the etiologic agent. In mycetoma caused by actinomycetes, there is suppurative inflammation with sinus tract formation. There are many granules composed of dense masses of bacterial filaments. The filaments radiate outward from the center of the granule. Inflammatory cells, chiefly neutrophils, line up around the periphery. The tips of the nocardial filaments may expand slightly at their ends, but they usually do not exhibit the marked clubbing characteristic of the ends of filaments of granules in actinomycosis. In eumycetoma, the initial histologic appearance is also suppurative, but later lesions are characterized by epithelioid granulomas and multinucleated giant cells. Fungal hyphae are much broader and stain differently than actinomycotic filaments.

Circumstantial evidence indicates that people are exposed to nocardial hyphae frequently but usually do not become ill. Neutrophils inhibit the organisms,[21] although they do not kill them as efficiently as they do more common bacterial pathogens.[22] Cell-mediated immunity is also important for adequate control,[23–25] probably in concert with neutrophils.[25] In vitro, activated macrophages inhibit and kill nocardiae, but resident, nonactivated macrophages do not.[24, 26] T lymphocytes have also been shown to kill nocardiae.[27]

The mechanisms by which phagocytes inhibit or kill nocardiae are not completely worked out. These bacteria are extraordinarily resistant to products of the phagocytic respiratory burst.[22, 28, 29] However, the fact that patients with chronic granulomatous disease are unusually susceptible to *Nocardia* infections suggests that the respiratory burst does have some importance. Inhibition of nocardiae by neutrophils is attributable to lysozyme and other cationic proteins.[21]

## CLINICAL MANIFESTATIONS

### Pulmonary Disease

*N. asteroides* infection typically presents as a subacute pneumonia; symptoms have usually been present for 1 to several weeks. The disease may be more acute in immunosuppressed patients. Cough is prominent and often produces small amounts of sputum, typically thick and purulent. Fever, anorexia, weight loss, and malaise are common. Dyspnea, pleuritic pain, and hemoptysis are less common. Tracheitis and bronchitis are uncommon manifestations of nocardiosis.

Remissions and exacerbations lasting for days or weeks are common. Because pulmonary nocardiosis is often indolent and because symptoms are nondescript, patients may be only superficially evaluated when they first present. Several short courses of oral antimicrobial therapy may be prescribed before a physician recognizes that the illness is unusual and makes serious attempts to establish a specific diagnosis.

Roentgenographic patterns of pulmonary nocardiosis vary.[30] Infiltrates (Figs. 34–1*B, C* and 34–2) and nodules (Fig. 34–3) are common. Infiltrates may be of any size and are usually of moderate or greater density. Cavitation is common (see Fig. 34–2), and empyema develops in one third of these patients.

The clinical appearance may suggest anaerobic lung abscess, but the sputum is not malodorous in nocardiosis. Nodules and cavitation may suggest malignancy. The clinical appearance may resemble pulmonary tuberculosis or one of several fungal pneumonias, but volume loss and fibrosis are usually less prominent with nocardiosis.

Pulmonary nocardiosis may spread directly from the lungs to involve adjacent tissue. Pericarditis,[7] mediastinitis,[7] and the superior vena cava syndrome[31] have been reported. Direct spread through the chest wall occurs in fewer than 10% of patients, much less commonly than in actinomycosis.

*Nocardia* species are sometimes isolated from patients without apparent nocardial disease who appear to be colonized.[32, 33] Many of these colonized patients have underlying pulmonary disease. A positive sputum culture in the presence of symptoms and signs of pulmonary infection is indicative of *Nocardia* pneumonia. In the absence of clinical evidence of pneumonia, the presence of nocardiae on Gram stain and the ability to isolate nocardiae in multiple cultures are factors suggesting an increased likelihood of nocardial disease. A positive sputum culture in an immunosuppressed patient usually reflects disease and not colonization.

### Extrapulmonary Disease

In one half of all cases of pulmonary nocardiosis, there is disease outside the lungs.[34] One fifth of patients with disseminated disease present only with disease outside the lungs, which is assumed to have spread hematogenously from an asymptomatic or healed pulmonary focus.

Central nervous system disease is the most common manifestation of disseminated disease and occurs in one fourth of all cases of pulmonary nocardiosis. There usually

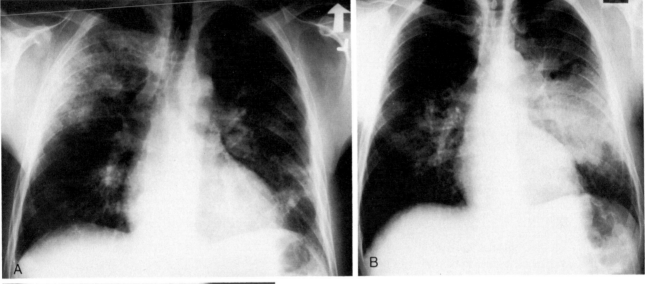

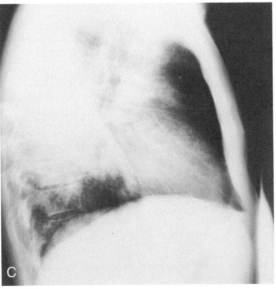

**Figure 34–1.** Pulmonary nocardiosis in a patient with underlying pulmonary alveolar proteinosis. *A,* In July 1989, this infiltrate was thought to represent bacterial pneumonia, and the patient was treated with a short course of antibiotics. *B* and *C,* In September 1991, bronchoscopy yielded *Nocardia asteroides* and a voluminous lipid content in the macrophages and extracellular fluid, leading to the diagnoses of pulmonary alveolar proteinosis and nocardia pneumonia.

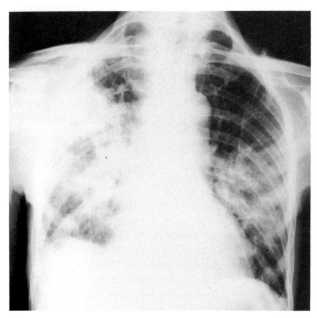

**Figure 34–2.** Pulmonary nocardiosis. Patchy infiltrates are seen bilaterally. A large cavity occupies the right upper lobe.

are one or more supratentorial brain abscesses, often multiloculated. The principal symptoms and signs of headache, nausea, vomiting, and depressed consciousness are typical of bacterial brain abscess in general, except that nocardial brain abscesses tend to be more indolent. Abscesses elsewhere in the central nervous system are much less common. Meningitis without apparent brain abscess is rare.[35] The diagnosis of meningitis is difficult to make because the organism is not easily recovered from cerebrospinal fluid.

Other common sites of dissemination are the skin and subcutaneous tissues, kidneys, bone, and muscle; however, dissemination to almost every organ has occurred. Peritonitis and endocarditis have been reported. Typically, disease spreads only to a handful of sites, but cases with widespread dissemination have been reported. The typical manifestation of disseminated disease is a subacute or chronic abscess. Abscesses tend to be firm with little or no fluctuation. Fistulas from deep abscesses draining small amounts of pus are common. Nocardial abscesses do not result in as much fibrosis or fistula formation as actinomycotic abscesses.

Infection from transcutaneous inoculation usually takes one of three forms: cellulitis, a lymphocutaneous form, or mycetoma. In the United States, cellulitis is most common, followed by the lymphocutaneous form and by actinomycetoma. Cellulitis usually begins 1 to 3 weeks after a recognized breach of the skin. Often, there has been obvious contamination of the wound with soil. A subacute cellulitis with pain, swelling, erythema, and warmth develops over days or a few weeks. The lesions are usually firm and nonfluctuant. The process may progress to involve underlying muscles, tendons, bones, and joints.[35a] Dissemination is rare.[36] In cold climates, most cases are associated with *N. asteroides*; in warmer climates, *N. brasiliensis* is more common.[37, 38]

The lymphocutaneous form is also called lymphangitic, or sporotrichoid. There is typically a pyodermatous lesion

at the site of inoculation.[37] The lesions often have areas of crusting, drainage, and central ulceration. The drainage may be purulent or honey colored. There are nodular lesions along lymphatics that drain the primary lesion. The lymphangitic form closely resembles lymphocutaneous sporotrichosis. Most cases of the lymphocutaneous syndrome are associated with *N. brasiliensis* instead of *N. asteroides*.

A mycetoma usually begins with a nodular swelling of the affected area.[16, 39] There may be a history of local trauma. The nodule breaks down and drains, and gradually, a fistula appears. Soon, the fistula is accompanied by others. The fistulas tend to come and go, with new ones forming as old ones disappear. The discharge is serous or purulent and may be bloody. The discharge often contains granules 0.1 to 2 mm in diameter that are masses of mycelia. Granules of *Nocardia* species are usually white. Those of other organisms can be shades of red, yellow, brown, or black. The lesions spread slowly along fascial planes to involve adjacent areas of skin, subcutaneous tissue, and bone. Over months to years, there is extensive deformation of the affected part. The most common location for mycetoma is on the feet or lower legs, followed by the hands, the back, and rarely, other parts of the body. Lesions involving soft tissues are only mildly painful. Pain is greater if lesions affect bones or joints. Systemic symptoms are absent or minimal. Mycetoma rarely disseminates, and lesions on the hands and feet usually cause only local disability, but lesions on the head, neck, and trunk can invade locally to involve deep organs and lead to severe disability or death.

*Nocardia* species, usually *N. asteroides*, are uncommon causes of subacute keratitis.[40] The infection usually occurs after trauma to the eye. Nocardial infection of lacrimal glands has been reported.[7] Disease involving deeper structures in the eye occasionally complicates disseminated nocardiosis.[41, 42]

## DIAGNOSIS

Examination of sputum for gram-positive, branching, filamentous organisms is the first step in the evaluation of

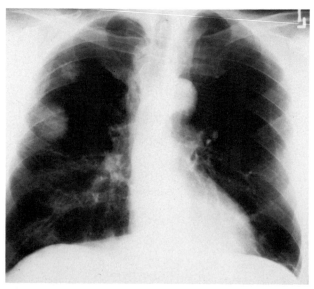

**Figure 34–3.** Pulmonary nocardiosis. Numerous nodules are seen without cavitation.

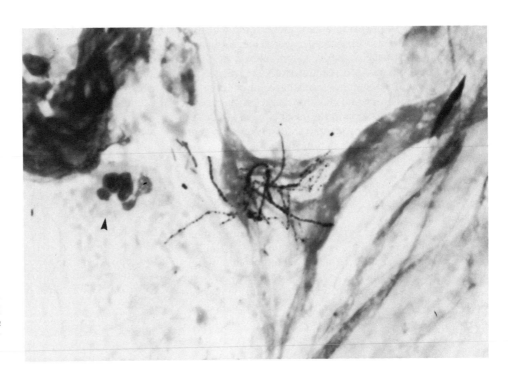

**Figure 34–4.** A Gram stain of expectorated sputum demonstrated the typical filaments of *Nocardia asteroides.* The arrowhead indicates a nearby neutrophil (bar = 10 μm).

pulmonary nocardiosis. Sputum smears from well-documented cases often fail to yield the organism. Some samples with negative smears yield the organism in culture, but cultures grow slowly, and it is often inappropriate to wait long enough for growth. If sputum smears do not yield the diagnosis in a suspect case and the diagnosis is not apparent by other means, more invasive procedures should be performed to make the diagnosis. Transtracheal aspiration, bronchoscopy, needle aspiration, and open lung biopsy have been used. The choice among these procedures depends on the location and nature of the lesions, the seriousness and tempo of the illness, and the expertise available for the more invasive procedures. Samples should be sent for Gram stain, modified acid-fast stain, and cultured specifically for *Nocardia* species.

Nocardiae have a unique propensity to produce cellulitis in the tissues overlying the cricothyroid membrane after transtracheal aspiration,[43, 44] and other procedures should be used if nocardiosis is strongly suspected. Cellulitis in this location has promptly responded to appropriate therapy.

All patients with nocardial pneumonia should carefully be evaluated for disseminated disease. Lesions elsewhere may be asymptomatic and occult. Computed tomography of the head with and without radiographic contrast medium should be done if there are signs or symptoms suggesting brain involvement.

If there is evidence suggesting disseminated disease, appropriate specimens should be obtained. The results of routine blood cultures are usually negative, but if biphasic culture bottles are inoculated and incubated aerobically for as long as 30 days, nocardiae can be isolated from blood.[45] If clinical findings indicate that cerebrospinal fluid or urine should be cultured, these specimens should be concentrated first. For cellulitis or sporotrichoid skin infections, smears of purulent material should be examined and cultures made. However, the results of smears and cultures of this material are often negative, and biopsies are then necessary. For

mycetoma, an effort should be made to find granules in the discharge. They should be washed in saline, examined microscopically, and cultured.[46] The color of the granule and the microscopic appearance often lead to a relatively firm diagnosis before cultures become positive.

On Gram stain, nocardiae are thin, crooked, branching filaments (Fig. 34–4). They are weakly to strongly gram-positive and appear beaded. Most nocardiae in clinical specimens are acid-fast if a weak acid is used for decolorization, as with the modified Kinyoun, Ziehl-Neelsen, or Fite-Faraco methods. They usually lose their acid-fast characteristics in laboratory culture. Ordinarily, *Actinomyces* and *Streptomyces* are gram-positive but not acid-fast. With some acid-fast staining methods, such as the Putt modification of the Ziehl-Neelsen method,[47] *Actinomyces* may retain the carbolfuchsin dye and appear to be acid-fast. Such stains should not be used to differentiate *Nocardia* from *Actinomyces. Nocardia* organisms may take up silver stains.

The laboratory should be alerted if *Nocardia* is suspected so that the likelihood of culturing it is maximized. Nocardiae grow readily on most nonselective laboratory media, but the growth rate is slower than for most bacterial pathogens. Colonies usually take 2 to 14 days to appear. The characteristic colonial morphology may not appear for as long as 4 weeks. There may be heavy growth of other flora before *Nocardia* appears, and nocardial colonies may only be apparent through the bottom of the plate. Nocardiae grow readily on nonselective mycobacterial and fungal media, but they may not survive sputum digestion procedures.

In difficult cases, paraffin baiting can be employed because nocardiae are among the few aerobic microorganisms that can use paraffin as a carbon source. Solid paraffin is placed on the surface of the agar after inoculation, and the paraffin just above the surface of the agar is observed for nocardial growth.[48]

Colonies are typically hard and wrinkled. They may produce orange, red, pink, peach, yellow, cream, or purple pigments. Some strains form a dark greenish-brown, soluble pigment that diffuses into the agar. Nocardiae form aerial hyphae that usually impart a dry, velvety, or chalky appearance to colonies. Most strains exude a characteristic earthy odor, but other soil organisms have similar odors.

Colonial morphology and staining characteristics are the best guides to identification in the usual clinical laboratory. Definitive identification of aerobic actinomycetes to genus and species level is complex and incompletely worked out. The commonly performed biochemical tests listed in Table 34–1 can be used to presumptively differentiate *Nocardia* from other species, but the usual clinical laboratory should refer suspect isolates to a reference laboratory for definitive identification.

Several presumptive tests for diagnosis of nocardiosis have been studied, including tests for antibodies[49–52] and for nocardial metabolites in serum or cerebrospinal fluid.[53] None is ready for clinical use at this time. With some serologic tests, false-positive reactions occur in persons with other actinomycete infections. Attempts to define specific antigens may circumvent this problem.[51]

## THERAPY

Soon after they became available, sulfonamides were established as the drugs of choice for treating nocardiosis. If used in adequate doses for adequate periods, they are usually highly successful.[54] In recent series, the case-fatality ratios of patients treated with sulfonamides were less than 5%, although there have been well-documented failures.[55] Antimicrobial susceptibility testing of *Nocardia* species has not been developed to a point at which clinical relevance is assured, and choices of antimicrobials should be based on published clinical experience.

Many patients have been treated with the combination of sulfamethoxazole and trimethoprim (co-trimoxazole) with success similar to that obtained with sulfonamides alone.[37, 38] Failures have been observed with co-trimoxazole,[56] just as they have with sulfonamides alone. Controlled trials comparing sulfonamide therapy with the combination have not been done. In vitro, there is evidence that the combination is synergistic under some conditions but not others.[57] The effect of the combination on *Nocardia* depends on the sulfamethoxazole-trimethoprim ratio,[57]

which changes in the body during therapy. The addition of trimethoprim to the sulfonamide clearly increases the risk of toxicity, especially in patients who have received myelotoxic chemotherapy.[38] Whether sulfamethoxazole and trimethoprim should be used in place of sulfonamides alone is unknown.

Among the sulfonamides, sulfadiazine[33] and sulfisoxazole[54] have been widely and successfully used. Good results have been achieved with 4 to 12 g per day in four to six divided doses. In difficult cases, sulfonamide levels should be measured and dosages should be adjusted to keep serum levels between 100 and 150 μg/mL. The physician should specify for the laboratory which sulfonamide is to be measured. The published experience with co-trimoxazole has been with commercial preparations that combine one part trimethoprim with five parts sulfamethoxazole. Good results have been achieved with 5 to 20 mg/kg per day of trimethoprim and 25 to 100 mg/kg per day of sulfamethoxazole in two to three divided doses.

Many other orally administered antimicrobials have been used, but there is considerably less experience with these agents. Minocycline is the best established alternative drug,[58, 59] and it should be given in doses of 100 to 200 mg twice daily. There is little clinical evidence that other tetracyclines are reliably effective. Chloramphenicol,[34] cycloserine,[34] and ampicillin[45] have appeared effective in some cases. These antimicrobials frequently have been used in combination with others, often sulfonamides, and it has been difficult to sort out the effects of the individual drugs. The recommended doses for chloramphenicol are 1 g four times each day; for cycloserine, 250 mg three times each day; and for ampicillin, 1 g four times each day. Ampicillin and erythromycin (500–750 mg four times each day) may be effective if used together[33, 58]; erythromycin has only rarely been effective if used alone.[4]

Among parenterally administered drugs, amikacin has been used most extensively and seems effective.[60] Amikacin should be given in doses of 5 to 7.5 mg/kg every 12 hours. Serum levels should be monitored with prolonged therapy, in patients with diminished renal function, or in the elderly. More extensive, earlier experience with streptomycin has been disappointing. The limited experience with newer β-lactam antibiotics suggests that they may be helpful alone[12, 60a] or in combination with other antimicrobials.[10, 11, 61]

There is evidence that *N. asteroides* and *N. brasiliensis*

Table 34–1. **Presumptive Identification of *Nocardia* and *Streptomyces***

| Property | *Nocardia asteroides* | *Nocardia brasiliensis* | *Nocardia otitidiscaviarum* | *Streptomyces* Species |
|---|---|---|---|---|
| Acid fastness | ±* | ± | ± | − |
| Decomposition of | | | | |
| Casein | − | + | − | + |
| Hypoxanthine | − | + | + | ± |
| Xanthine | − | − | + | ± |
| Tyrosine | − | + | ± | + |
| Nitrate from nitrite | + | + | + | ± |
| Acid formed from | | | | |
| Arabinose | − | − | ± | ± |
| Inositol | − | + | + | |

*Abbreviations: +, positive in >90% of strains; −, negative in >90% of strains; ±, variable.

Adapted from Lechevalier HA: Nocardioform actinomycetes. *In* Williams ST, Sharpe ME, Holt JG (eds): Bergey's Manual of Systematic Bacteriology, vol 4. Baltimore, Williams & Wilkins, 1989:2348–2361.

produce β-lactamases and that β-lactamase inhibitors enhance susceptibility of many strains to penicillin antibiotics.[62, 63] Reports on use of the combination of amoxicillin and clavulanic acid for treatment are emerging.[64, 65] In one case, the combination was used with amikacin, and in the other case, resistance to amoxicillin and clavulanic acid developed.[64] The clinical usefulness of β-lactamase inhibitors in therapy of nocardiosis remains unproven.

In vitro tests of susceptibility of *Nocardia* species to antimicrobials are of uncertain clinical value. The methods are not standardized, and the variable results depend on the methods used.[66] The results obtained from in vitro tests have not correlated with the results of treatment of human infection. Susceptibility testing of *Nocardia* species should not be used routinely to guide therapy. In cases in which the clinically proven antimicrobials fail or cannot be used, susceptibility testing may be used to guide the choice of alternative agents, but this should be considered experimental. To help with such a choice, the results of in vitro susceptibility tests for certain agents are presented in Table 34–2. The agents were selected because they have appeared useful on clinical grounds or because they appeared quite active in vitro. Most studies have found that sulfonamides, most aminoglycosides, minocycline, fusidic acid, and some newly developed β-lactam antibiotics are active against most strains.

*N. asteroides* is a heterogeneous taxon, and some reports suggest that strains can be divided into subgroups with different antimicrobial susceptibilities and biochemical characteristics.[3, 4] The clinical relevance of these differences is unclear, but further research may demonstrate that biochemical identification and antimicrobial susceptibility testing has important clinical implications.

In many reported cases, multiple antimicrobials (other than the previously discussed combinations of co-trimoxazole or amoxicillin and clavulanic acid) have been used to treat nocardiosis. The combination often has included a sulfonamide or minocycline. Whether therapy with two or more agents is better than therapy with a single agent is not known. Because therapy with multiple drugs increases the risk of toxicity, therapy for nocardiosis with two or more agents should be considered experimental.

Surgery is used in treating nocardiosis as it is for other infectious diseases. Empyemas should be drained. Lung abscesses usually respond to antimicrobial therapy alone, and excision is rarely required. Abscesses outside the chest or central nervous system should be drained. Antimicrobial therapy alone usually suffices for nocardial mycetoma. Drainage of deep lesions and excision of heavily involved tissue may facilitate healing of nocardial mycetoma, but structure and function should be preserved whenever possible.

Some nocardial brain abscesses should be treated surgically by aspiration, excision, or drainage. The choice among these techniques depends on the individual circumstances.[66] Surgery should be performed if the diagnosis is unclear, if an abscess is large and accessible, or if an abscess fails to respond to chemotherapy. For small abscesses, for abscesses in inaccessible places, or for abscesses in areas where surgical treatment would have unacceptable neurologic consequences, chemotherapy should be attempted first. Neurosurgical consultation is important for proper decision making and monitoring. In cases managed with chemotherapy alone, results should be carefully monitored with repeated computed tomography.

Certain kinds of immunosuppressive therapy markedly increase the risk of nocardiosis. It is not clear whether successful therapy is less likely if immunosuppressive therapy is continued during the treatment of nocardiosis. Many patients with transplanted organs have continued to take immunosuppressive medication out of necessity and have responded well to antinocardial therapy.[54] Immunosuppressive therapy should be continued if it is necessary for treatment of an underlying disease or to prevent rejection of a transplanted organ. In other cases, it seems prudent to reduce or eliminate immunosuppressive therapy.

*Nocardia* infections tend to relapse, and long courses of antimicrobial therapy are necessary. For nonimmunosuppressed patients, treatment of pulmonary nocardiosis or systemic nocardiosis outside the central nervous system should be continued for 6 to 12 months. Ordinarily, treatment of central nervous system nocardiosis should be continued for 1 year. If all apparent disease has been excised, and this is confirmed by computed tomography or magnetic resonance imaging, the duration of therapy might be reduced to 6 months. For immunosuppressed patients, treatment of pulmonary or systemic nocardiosis should be continued for 1 year. For a few patients, much longer periods of therapy

Table 34–2. **Antimicrobial Susceptibilities of *Nocardia* Species**

| Antimicrobial | Minimum Inhibitory Concentration (μg/mL) | | | Moderately Susceptible Breakpoint (μg/mL) | Susceptible (%) |
| --- | --- | --- | --- | --- | --- |
| | *Range* | *50%* | *90%* | | |
| Sulfamethoxazole[67] | ≤1–16 | 2 | 8 | 32 | 100 |
| Minocycline[67] | ≤0.5–>8 | 2 | 8 | 8 | 100 |
| Doxycycline[69] | 2–32 | 4 | 32 | 8 | Unavailable |
| Erythromycin[67] | ≤0.25–>8 | >8 | >8 | 4 | 22 |
| Amikacin[67] | ≤0.25–>32 | 0.5 | 1 | 32 | 95 |
| Gentamicin[67] | 1–>32 | 4 | >32 | 8 | 67 |
| Cefotaxime[68] | ≤0.5–>32 | 2 | >32 | 16 | 71 |
| Ceftizoxime[68] | <0.5–>32 | 8 | >32 | 16 | 63 |
| Ceftriaxone[67] | ≤0.5–>64 | 4 | >64 | 32 | 82 |
| Imipenem[67] | <0.5–>32 | 1 | 16 | 8 | 88 |
| Fusidic acid[68] | ≤0.5–>32 | 8 | 16 | ≤8 | 85 |
| Ampicillin[67] | 0.5–>32 | >32 | >32 | 16 | 40 |
| Ciprofloxacin[67] | ≤0.25–≥4 | ≥4 | ≥4 | 2 | 29 |

have been required.[54, 55, 70] If nocardial disease is unusually extensive or if the response to therapy is slow, these recommendations should be exceeded.

Patients with cellulitis or the lymphocutaneous syndrome should be treated for 2 months if infection is limited to soft tissues and 4 months if bone is involved. Some patients with extensive disease have required longer durations of therapy.[71] There are few data on the duration of therapy for immunosuppressed patients with local disease.[38] Because local inoculation nocardiosis has disseminated, and immunosuppressed patients with other forms of nocardiosis tend to relapse, it seems prudent to treat local inoculation nocardiosis in immunosuppressed people for longer periods. Therapy of mycetoma with *Nocardia* species should be continued for 6 to 12 months after clinical cure. Relapses of nocardial mycetoma are common, and longer durations may be necessary.

Nocardial keratitis should be treated with sulfonamides administered orally and topically until the infection appears cured.[40] After this time, oral therapy alone should be continued for 2 to 4 months.

Before sulfonamides became available, pulmonary and systemic nocardiosis infections were almost always fatal. Sulfonamides improved the prognosis, but a review of all cases reported from 1945 to 1968 found that 61% of patients had died.[72] In a review of all treated patients reported from 1948 to 1975, the mortality rate was 21%.[73] In the latter review, the mortality rate depended on the site of disease. In patients with disease limited to the lungs, the mortality rate was 7.6%, but the mortality rate for patients with brain abscess was 48%. In series marked by early recognition and prompt treatment of nocardiosis, mortality rates have been less than 5%.[54, 55] Central nervous system disease has been uncommon in these recent series, perhaps because early treatment prevented it.

Improvement is usually noticeable after 3 to 5 days of treatment, and continued improvement is the rule if the diagnosis is made early in the disease. Sometimes, disease progresses or relapses during therapy. Patients should be followed carefully for at least 6 months after therapy has ended. Any child with nocardiosis and no known cause of immunosuppression should have tests performed to determine the adequacy of the child's phagocytic respiratory burst to exclude chronic granulomatous disease.

## REFERENCES

1. Lechevalier HA: Nocardioform actinomycetes. *In* Williams ST, Sharpe ME, Holt JG (eds): Bergey's Manual of Systematic Bacteriology, vol 4. Baltimore, Williams & Wilkins, 1989:2348.
2. Tsakamura M, Ohta M: *Nocardia farcinica* as a pathogen of lung infection. Microbiol Immunol 24:237, 1980.
3. Wallace RJ Jr, Tsukamura M, Brown BA, et al: Cefotaxime-resistant *Nocardia asteroides* strains are isolates of the controversial species *Nocardia farcinica*. J Clin Microbiol 28:2726, 1990.
4. Wallace RJ Jr, Brown BA, Tsukamura M, et al: Clinical and laboratory features of *Nocardia nova*. J Clin Microbiol 29:2407, 1991.
5. McNeil MM, Brown JM, Magruder CH, et al: Disseminated *Nocardia transvalensis* infection: An unusual opportunistic pathogen in severely immunocompromised patients. J Infect Dis 165:175, 1992.
6. Beaman BL, Burnside J, Edwards B, et al: Nocardial infections in the United States, 1972–1974. J Infect Dis 134:286, 1976.
7. Palmer DL, Harvey RL, Wheeler JK: Diagnostic and therapeutic considerations in *Nocardia asteroides* infection. Medicine (Baltimore) 53:391, 1974.
8. Berkey P, Bodey GP: Nocardial infection in patients with neoplastic disease. Rev Infect Dis 11:407, 1989.
9. Wilson JP, Turner HR, Kirchner KA, et al: Nocardial infections in renal transplant recipients. Medicine (Baltimore) 68:38, 1989.
10. Kim J, Minamoto GY, Greico MH: Nocardial infection as a complication of AIDS: Report of six cases and review. Rev Infect Dis 13:624, 1991.
11. Kim J, Minamoto GY, Hoy CD, et al: Presumptive cerebral *Nocardia asteroides* infection in AIDS: Treatment with ceftriaxone and minocycline. Am J Med 90:656, 1991.
12. Telzak EE, Hii J, Polsky B, et al: *Nocardia* infection in the acquired immunodeficiency syndrome. Diagn Microbiol Infect Dis 12:517, 1989.
13. Andriole VT, Ballas M, Wilson GL: The association of nocardiosis and pulmonary alveolar proteinosis. A case study. Ann Intern Med 60:266, 1964.
14. Stein L, Estrellado RE, Judd JM: Nocardiosis and tuberculosis. Report of a case of coexistent pulmonary tuberculosis and extrapulmonary nocardiosis. J Thorac Cardiovasc Surg 43:314, 1962.
15. Idriss ZH, Cunningham RJ, Wilfert CM: Nocardiosis in children: Report of three cases and review of the literature. Pediatrics 55:479, 1975.
16. Tight RR, Bartlett MS: Actinomycetoma in the United States. Rev Infect Dis 3:1139, 1981.
17. Lovett IS, Houang ET, Burge S, et al: An outbreak of *Nocardia asteroides* infection in a renal transplant unit. Q J Med 50:123, 1981.
18. Centers for Disease Control: Cutaneous nocardiosis in cancer patients receiving immunotherapy injections—Bahamas. MMWR 33:471, 1984.
19. Cox F, Hughes WT: Contagious and other aspects of nocardiosis in the compromised host. Pediatrics 55:135, 1975.
20. Baddour LM, Baselski VS, Herr MJ, et al: Nocardiosis in recipients of renal transplants: Evidence for nosocomial acquisition. Am J Infect Control 14:214, 1986.
21. Filice GA: Inhibition of *Nocardia asteroides* by neutrophils. J Infect Dis 151:47, 1985.
22. Filice GA, Beaman BL, Krick JA, et al: Effects of human neutrophils and monocytes on *Nocardia asteroides*: Failure of killing despite occurrence of the oxidative metabolic burst. J Infect Dis 142:432, 1980.
23. Krick JA, Remington JS: Resistance to infection with *Nocardia asteroides*. J Infect Dis 131:665, 1975.
24. Beaman BL: Interaction of *Nocardia asteroides* at different phases of growth with in vitro-maintained macrophages obtained from the lungs of normal and immunized mice. Infect Immun 26:355, 1979.
25. Filice GA, Niewoehner DE: Contribution of neutrophils and cell-mediated immunity to control of *Nocardia asteroides* in murine lungs. J Infect Dis 156:113, 1987.
26. Filice GA, Beaman BL, Remington JS: Effects of activated macrophages on *Nocardia asteroides*. Infect Immun 27:643, 1980.
27. Deem R, Doughty FA, Beaman BL: Immunologically specific direct T lymphocyte-mediated killing of *Nocardia asteroides*. J Immunol 130:2401, 1983.
28. Filice GA: Resistance of *Nocardia asteroides* to oxygen-dependent killing by neutrophils. J Infect Dis 148:861, 1983.
29. Beaman BL, Scates SM, Moring SE, et al: Purification and properties of a unique superoxide dismutase from *Nocardia asteroides*. J Biol Chem 258:91, 1983.
30. Grossman CB, Bragg DG, Armstrong D: Roentgen manifestations of pulmonary nocardiosis. Radiology 96:325, 1970.
31. Chapman JR, Walesby RK: *Nocardia asteroides* causing vena caval obstruction. Br J Dis Chest 75:99, 1981.
32. Young LS, Armstrong D, Blevins A, et al: *Nocardia asteroides* infection complicating neoplastic disease. Am J Med 50:356, 1970.
33. Frazier AR, Rosenow EC III, Roberts GD: Nocardiosis. A review of 25 cases occurring during 24 months. Mayo Clin Proc 50:657, 1975.
34. Neu HC, Silva M, Hazen E, et al: Necrotizing nocardial pneumonia. Ann Intern Med 66:274, 1967.
35. Bross JE, Gordon G: Nocardial meningitis: Case reports and review. Rev Infect Dis 13:160, 1991.
35a. Freiberg AA, Herzenberg JE, Sangeorzan JA: Thorn synovitis of the knee joint with *Nocardia* pyarthrosis. Clin Orthop Rel Res 287:233, 1993.
36. Kahn FW, Gornick CC, Tofte RW: Primary cutaneous *Nocardia asteroides* infection with dissemination. Am J Med 70:859, 1981.

37. Satterwhite TK, Wallace RJ Jr: Primary cutaneous nocardiosis. JAMA 242:333, 1979.
38. Wallace RJ Jr, Septimus EJ, Williams TW Jr, et al: Use of trimethoprim-sulfamethoxazole for treatment of infections due to *Nocardia*. Rev Infect Dis 4:315, 1982.
39. Green WO Jr, Adams TE: Mycetoma in the United States. A review and report of seven additional cases. Am J Clin Pathol 42:75, 1964.
40. Hirst LW, Harrison GK, Merz WG, et al: *Nocardia asteroides* keratitis. Br J Ophthalmol 63:449, 1979.
41. Jampol LM, Strauch BS, Albert DM: Intraocular nocardiosis. Am J Ophthalmol 67:568, 1973.
42. Knouse MC, Lorber B: Early diagnosis of *Nocardia asteroides* endophthalmitis by retinal biopsy: Case report and review. Rev Infect Dis 3:393, 1990.
43. Goldman AL, Light L: Anterior cervical infections: Complications of transtracheal aspirations. Am Rev Respir Dis 111:707, 1975.
44. Deresinski SC, Stevens DA: Am Rev Respir Dis 111:708, 1975.
45. Roberts GD, Brewer NS, Hermans PE: Diagnosis of nocardiosis by blood culture. Mayo Clin Proc 49:293, 1974.
46. Venugopal TV, Venugopal PV: Mycetoma. *In* Braude AI, Davis CE, Fierer J (eds): Medical Microbiology and Infectious Diseases. Philadelphia, WB Saunders, 1981:1762.
47. Robboy SJ, Vickery AL: Tinctorial and morphologic properties distinguishing actinomycosis and nocardiosis. N Engl J Med 282:593, 1970.
48. Mishra SK, Randhawa HS, Sandu RS: Observations on paraffin baiting as a laboratory diagnostic procedure in nocardiosis. Mycopathologia 51:147, 1973.
49. Shainhouse JZ, Pier AC, Stevens DA: Complement fixation antibody test for human nocardiosis. J Clin Microbiol 8:516, 1978.
50. Blumer SO, Kaufman L: Microimmunodiffusion test for nocardiosis. J Clin Microbiol 10:308, 1979.
51. Sugar AM, Schoolnik GK, Stevens DA: Antibody response in human nocardiosis: Identification of two immunodominant culture filtrate antigens derived from *Nocardia asteroides*. J Infect Dis 151:895, 1985.
51a. Angeles AM, Sugar AM: Rapid diagnosis of nocardiosis with an enzyme immunoassay. J Infect Dis 155:292, 1987.
52. Boiron P, Provost F: Enzyme immunoassay on whole *Nocardia asteroides* cells for human nocardiosis. Serodiagn Immunother Infect Dis 2:445, 1988.
53. Brooks JB, Kasin JV, Fast DM, et al: Detection of metabolites by frequency-pulsed electron capture gas-liquid chromatography in serum and cerebrospinal fluid of a patient with *Nocardia* infection. J Clin Microbiol 25:445, 1987.
54. Simpson GL, Stinson EB, Egger MJ, et al: Nocardial infections in the immunocompromised host: A detailed study in a defined population. Rev Infect Dis 3:492, 1981.
55. Smego RA, Moeller MB, Gallis HA: Trimethoprim-sulfamethoxazole therapy for *Nocardia* infections. Arch Intern Med 143:711, 1983.
56. Geiseler PJ, Check F, Lamothe F, et al: Failure of trimethoprim/sulfamethoxazole in invasive *Nocardia asteroides* infection. Arch Intern Med 139:355, 1979.
57. Bennett JE, Jennings NE: Factors influencing susceptibility of *Nocardia* species to trimethoprim-sulfamethoxazole. Antimicrob Agents Chemother 13:624, 1978.
58. Bach MC, Monaco AP, Finland M: Pulmonary nocardiosis. Therapy with minocycline and with erythromycin plus ampicillin. JAMA 224:1378, 1973.
59. Peterson EA, Nash ML, Mammana RB, et al: Minocycline treatment of pulmonary nocardiosis. JAMA 250:930, 1983.
60. Goldstein FW, Hautefort B, Acar JF: Amikacin-containing regimens for treatment of nocardiosis in immunocompromised patients. Eur J Clin Microbiol Infect Dis 6:198, 1987.
60a. Lo W, Rolston KVI: Use of imipenem in the treatment of pulmonary nocardiosis. Chest 103:951, 1993.
61. Fried J, Hinthorn D, Ralstin J, et al: Cure of brain abscess caused by *Nocardia asteroides* resistant to multiple antibiotics. South Med J 81:412, 1988.
62. Kitzis MD, Gutmann L, Acar JF: In vitro susceptibility of *Nocardia asteroides* to 21 beta-lactam antibiotics, in combination with three β-lactamase inhibitors, and its relationship to the β-lactamase content. J Antimicrob Chemother 15:23, 1985.
63. Wallace RJ Jr, Nash DR, Johnson WK, et al: β-Lactam resistance in *Nocardia brasiliensis* is mediated by β-lactamase and reversed in the presence of clavulanic acid. J Infect Dis 156:959, 1987.
64. Steingrube VA, Wallace RJ Jr, Brown BA, et al: Acquired resistance of *Nocardia brasiliensis* to clavulanic acid related to a change in β-lactamase following therapy with amoxicillin-clavulanic acid. Antimicrob Agents Chemother 35:524, 1991.
65. Stasiecki P, Diehl V, Vlaho M, et al: New effective therapy of systemic infection with *Nocardia asteroides*. Dtsch Med Wochenschr 110:1733, 1985.
66. Filice GA, Simpson GL: Management of *Nocardia* infections. *In* Remington JS, Swartz MN (eds): Current Clinical Topics in Infectious Diseases, vol 5. New York, McGraw-Hill, 1984:49.
67. Wallace RJ, Steele LC, Sumter G, et al: Antimicrobial susceptibility patterns of *Nocardia asteroides*. Antimicrob Agents Chemother 32:1776, 1988.
68. Southern PM, Kutscher AE, Ragsdale R, et al: Susceptibility in vitro of *Nocardia* species to antimicrobial agents. Diagn Microbiol Infect Dis 8:119, 1987.
69. Gutmann L, Goldstein FW, Kitzis MD, et al: Susceptibility of *Nocardia asteroides* to 46 antibiotics, including 22 β-lactams. Antimicrob Agents Chemother 23:248, 1983.
70. Stropes L, Bartlett M, White A: Multiple recurrences of nocardial pneumonia. Am J Med Sci 280:119, 1980.
71. Vasarinsh P: Primary cutaneous nocardiosis. Arch Dermatol 98:489, 1968.
72. Presant CA, Wiernik PH, Serpick AA: Factors affecting survival in nocardiosis. Am Rev Respir Dis 108:1444, 1973.
73. Geiseler PJ, Andersen BR: Results of therapy in systemic nocardiosis. Am J Med Sci 278:188, 1979.

# CHAPTER 35

# Actinomycosis*

GREGORY A. FILICE

Pulmonary actinomycosis is a characteristic, indolent disease that is usually caused by *Actinomyces israelii* and related bacteria. Cervicofacial and abdominal actinomycosis are distinctive syndromes with similar clinical and microbiologic features. Occasionally, other species of *Actinomyces* and the related bacterium, *Arachnia propionica*, are isolated in cases that are otherwise typical of actinomycosis. Clinically, these cases are almost indistinguishable from cases associated with *A. israelii*. Occasionally, *Actinomyces* species or *A. propionica* are isolated from patients with other infectious syndromes.[1] Without the typical clinical features of actinomycosis, these cases can be treated like other infections associated with upper respiratory anaerobic bacteria.

## EPIDEMIOLOGY AND PREVENTION

Actinomycosis has been known since the nineteenth century[2, 3] and was more common earlier in this century. As dental health in the developed world has improved, actinomycosis has become uncommon. The disease occurs worldwide. Males are affected more often than females,[4] and actinomycosis can affect any age group. The incidence is not precisely known; the disease is uncommon but not rare. Tooth decay and gingival diseases predispose to cervicofacial and thoracic actinomycosis, and maintenance of good oral hygiene prevents these diseases.

## MICROBIOLOGY

*Actinomyces* is a bacterial genus in the family Actinomycetaceae, order Actinomycetales. Other *Actinomyces*

species associated with human actinomycosis include *A. naeslundii,*[5] *A. viscosus,*[6] and *A. meyeri.*[7] *A. propionica* has also been implicated in human actinomycosis.[8] *Actinomyces bovis* and *Actinomyces suis* cause analogous diseases in cattle and pigs, respectively.

*Actinomyces* are gram-positive, non–acid-fast, nonmotile, and strict or facultative anaerobes. *A. israelii* grows in branching, crooked filaments approximately 0.3 to 0.5 μm wide. The filaments consist of bacilli joined end to end that vary in length up to approximately 50 μm. Under unfavorable conditions, the filaments break up into coccoid and bacillary forms. *Actinomyces* organisms do not form spores. The morphologies of the various species associated with the actinomycosis syndromes are similar, but not identical.

Pathogenic species of *Actinomyces* and *Arachnia* inhabit anaerobic niches in the mouth, including gingival crevices, plaque, and tonsilar crypts. Their numbers are increased in some patients with gingivitis or peridontitis.[9] These bacteria are swallowed and pass through the gastrointestinal tract, but they are not recognized in the established gastrointestinal flora.

## PATHOGENESIS

*Actinomyces* are unable to invade healthy tissues. Cervicofacial actinomycosis occurs in people with periodontal disease because of unhealthy supporting tissues and because of large numbers of the causative bacteria. Trauma with inoculation of oral secretions into devitalized tissue may lead to actinomycosis. The infection may remain localized to the tissues surrounding the oral cavity or may extend to involve nearby structures. Actinomycotic infec-

---

tions are not confined by tissue planes, and fistulas or abscesses are present in many cases, often at some distance from primary lesions. Cervicofacial infections may descend through the neck into the mediastinum.

People with carious teeth or periodontal disease are predisposed to thoracic actinomycosis.[10] Aspiration of infective material is probably the inciting event in most cases, but spread from oral lesions through the lymphatics or the bloodstream may also occur. Mediastinal actinomycosis may follow extension from a cervicofacial lesion or from the lungs.[4]

Other syndromes include abdominal actinomycosis, uterine colonization or disease, and disseminated infection. Abdominal actinomycosis occurs after the intestinal mucosa has been interrupted and organisms passing through the gastrointestinal tract escape into tissues. The disease is indolent, with nonspecific symptoms and signs. Liver involvement is common. Eventually, fistulas track into other body cavities, including the thoracic cavity,[4] or to the exterior, and this may be an important clue to the diagnosis. Uterine infection is commonly associated with foreign bodies, especially intrauterine contraceptive devices. Disseminated infection results from hematogenous spread.[4] People with disseminated malignancy seem to have a predilection for disseminated actinomycosis.[11]

The lesions of actinomycosis often contain other bacteria, sometimes referred to as concomitant bacteria. The concomitant bacteria often are part of the oral or gastrointestinal flora with *Actinomyces*. The relationship between one such bacterium, *Actinobacillus actinomycetemcomitans*, and actinomycosis is so close that isolation of *A. actinomycetemcomitans* from a tissue infection should prompt a careful search for *Actinomyces*. Some investigators[12] think that other bacteria are indispensable for actinomycosis to develop and that, if cultures yield only *Actinomyces*, these other bacteria have been missed. Others think that *Actinomyces* are sufficient.

In tissues, *Actinomyces* bacteria tend to grow in dense microcolonies that may reach 4 mm in diameter (Fig. 35–1). Hyphae at the periphery of a microcolony may form ''clubs'' that consist of mycelia embedded in a mucopolysaccharide matrix containing substantial amounts of $Ca_3(PO_4)_2$. Typically, neutrophils line up around the periphery of the microcolony, but the colony itself contains few host cells. These colonies are often discharged in pus and are then called sulfur granules or grains because of their yellow color. The yellow color is not from sulfur; their sulfur content is low.

## PATHOLOGY

The typical lesion is an abscess surrounded by intense fibrosis.[4, 13] Pus is usually white or yellow and has no distinctive odor. Malodorous pus suggests the presence of other anaerobic organisms, possibly causing combined infection with *Actinomyces*. Fistulas are common, especially in late infections. In lungs, consolidation can occur without roentgenologically apparent abscesses. Abscesses are filled with neutrophils and a few scattered granules. They are surrounded by dense fibrosis and often foamy macrophages. Plasma cells and lymphocytes are found in the periphery of

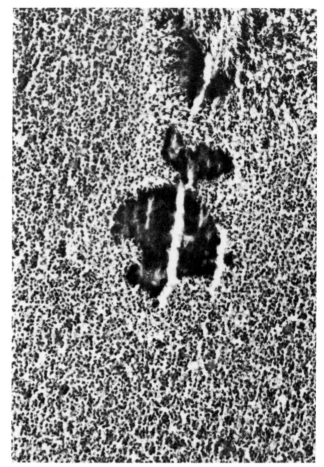

**Figure 35–1.** Hepatic actinomycosis. An extensive purulent infiltrate effaced the normal hepatic architecture, and granules were found within the infiltrate.

lesions. Giant cells are uncommon, and epithelioid granulomas are rare.

## CLINICAL MANIFESTATIONS

### Pulmonary Involvement

Pulmonary actinomycosis begins insidiously with cough, sputum production, fever, and weight loss. Hemoptysis or pleuritic pain occurs in some patients. Symptoms may be surprisingly mild for the extent of pulmonary disease. Occasionally, patients with pulmonary disease have no symptoms referable to the chest and present with manifestations of disease elsewhere.[14] Anemia and leukocytosis with a predominance of neutrophils are common hematologic findings. Fistulas may track from pulmonary lesions through the chest wall, although this is less common than in earlier decades.[15] Empyema and mediastinal involvement are common. Mediastinal involvement may result from lung or cervicofacial disease. Pericarditis,[4, 16] the superior vena cava syndrome,[17, 18] and involvement of other mediastinal structures[4, 11, 13, 16, 17, 19] have been reported.

Certain roentgenographic features are characteristic. Infiltrates tend to be dense (Fig. 35–2) and often suggest lung cancer (Fig. 35–3).[10, 11, 20, 21] The diagnosis is often made

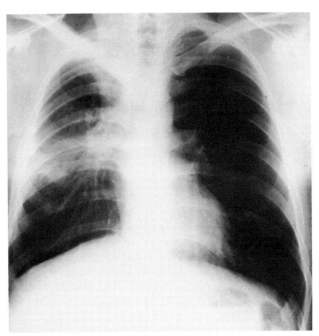

**Figure 35–2.** Pulmonary actinomycosis. Extensive, irregularly distributed infiltrates were found in the right lung.

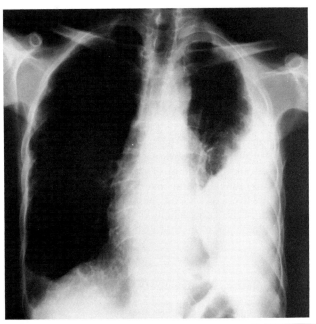

**Figure 35–4.** Pulmonary actinomycosis. Infiltration and an extensive empyema are seen in the left chest.

unexpectedly in the course of surgery[10, 11] or irradiation[20] for presumed cancer. Actinomycosis can complicate bronchogenic carcinoma and lead to diagnostic confusion.[22] Empyema is common (Fig. 35–4). An open bronchus leading into a lesion should suggest actinomycosis or another al-

veolar process rather than an obstructing bronchial carcinoma. Cavities are observed in almost 50% of the cases and are usually small. Because of the lack of regard for anatomic barriers, actinomycosis may involve multiple lobes by spread through interlobar fissures.[21] Other patterns include fibronodular (Fig. 35–5), cavitary, or alveolar infiltrates (see Fig. 35–2).[4, 20, 21] Occasionally, the erosion of a blood vessel results in miliary disease.

Rib involvement typically produces extensive periosteal reaction, which has been called "wavy periostitis."[21] Roentgenographs may also demonstrate involvement of other thoracic bones, including those of the shoulder girdle,

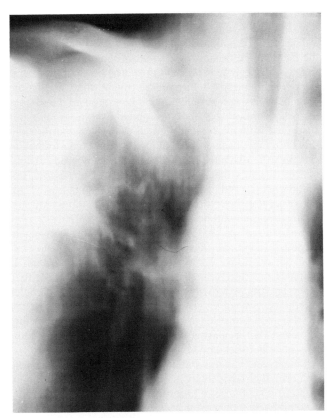

**Figure 35–3.** Pulmonary actinomycosis. There is a peripheral infiltrate with central adenopathy, which suggested a diagnosis of carcinoma.

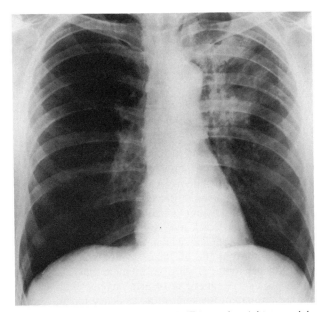

**Figure 35–5.** Pulmonary actinomycosis. This patchy, right upper lobe infiltrate suggested tuberculosis. Cavities were not observed.

the sternum, and thoracic vertebrae. The vertebral involvement is characteristic, with the vertebrae appearing mottled because of parallel processes of resorption and new bone formation.[21] Spread to adjacent vertebrae and intervertebral disk space narrowing are distinctly unusual with actinomycosis, although they are common with pyogenic and tuberculous osteomyelitis.

Because of the indolent nature of actinomycosis and because sputum cultures are not helpful, the diagnosis is often made after some delay. It is often made at the time of surgery or after spread of disease to other structures. Other diseases in the differential diagnosis include tuberculosis, nocardiosis, fungal pneumonia, and carcinoma. Occasionally, actinomycosis and tuberculosis coexist or occur sequentially in the same patient.[4, 21] In advanced cases, clubbing, pulmonary osteoarthropathy, or amyloidosis may occur.[4]

## Extrapulmonary Involvement

### Cervicofacial Disease

The typical presentation of cervicofacial actinomycosis is that of an indolent swelling.[11, 23] The degree of pain ranges from none to moderate. Lesions are typically indurated and occasionally fluctuant. There may be a distinctive bluish discoloration to the skin. In advanced cases, fistulas develop, and induration becomes prominent, often with a ''woody'' character. Actinomycosis uncommonly presents as an acute, poorly localized, severely painful cellulitis. Poor conditions of the teeth and supporting structures are usually preceding conditions. Often, jaw pain, tooth pain, or dental manipulation is reported by the patient.

The most common location for cervicofacial disease is along the lower border of the mandible, especially near the angle. Trismus may occur from irritation of the temporomandibular joint. Maxillary infection is rare and tends to present as a localized abscess, usually periapical or gingival. Infection may present in any other location in or near the mouth, including the salivary glands, tongue, pharynx, larynx, palate, paranasal sinuses, lacrimal glands, neck, or scalp. Meningitis or brain abscess may result from extension into the central nervous system. The infection tends to spread contiguously, and regional lymph node swelling is uncommon. Osteomyelitis may occur with roentgenographic features typical of bacterial osteomyelitis.

### Abdominal Disease

Abdominal actinomycosis is usually extremely indolent. Complaints tend to be nonspecific, and the diagnosis has often been delayed months or even years. Common locations include the liver,[23a] the ileocecal region, the pelvis, and the perianal region. Fistulas from infected foci are common and may track long distances before finding their way to the surface. The availability of computed tomography has improved the diagnosis of abdominal actinomycosis. Images typically show an irregular mass that crosses tissue planes.[24] Magnetic resonance imaging findings have not been reported. Because of the tendency for fibrosis and delayed diagnosis, most infections are characterized by extensive scarring, often with bowel obstruction. The differ-

ential diagnosis includes cancer, tuberculosis, other granulomatous diseases, and amebiasis.

### Disseminated Disease

Although uncommon, disseminated disease may result from any form of actinomycosis,[11, 14, 25] and a variety of sites may be involved. The lesions are indolent like actinomycosis in other sites. They tend to drain, and the presence of granules in the drainage is an important diagnostic clue. Endocarditis has been reported.[25a]

### Pelvic Disease in Females

Involvement of pelvic organs can occur as a result of spread of abdominal disease or of invasion through the female genital tract. The latter is facilitated by the presence of a foreign body, typically a pessary in decades past and intrauterine contraceptive devices (IUDs) more recently. Colonization of the uterus occurs uncommonly in women with IUDs. These women are usually asymptomatic, and the *Actinomyces* are usually observed on Papanicolaou smears. Superficial endometritis with or without symptoms occurs in some women with *Actinomyces* colonization.[26] Rarely, the infection invades the uterus extensively and spreads to nearby structures.

*Actinomyces* are implicated occasionally in lacrimal canaliculitis, in which they tend to form concretions.[27] The infection is not invasive.

## DIAGNOSIS

Diagnosis of pulmonary actinomycosis is complicated by the fact that the organisms are part of the upper respiratory flora. In suspected cases, sputum should be examined carefully for granules. Although rarely found, they suggest the diagnosis. Suspect particles should be examined microscopically to confirm that they are actinomycotic granules. If suspected actinomycosis is limited to the lungs, aspiration, bronchoscopy, or open lung biopsy should be performed to establish the diagnosis. The value of bronchoscopy is limited by the fact that lesions are usually parenchymal, not intrabronchial, and specimens may be contaminated by upper respiratory secretions.[28] Transbronchial biopsy of suspicious areas should be performed.

Disease outside the chest may offer a more convenient diagnostic approach. The presence of granules in secretions from an otherwise compatible lesion is a strong clue. If granules are not immediately apparent in drainage, they often are trapped in a gauze dressing. Suspect particles should be placed in water or 10% potassium hydroxide (KOH) and examined for the presence of typical branching mycelia. The organisms can be cultured from granules if they have not succumbed to oxygen exposure.

Smears and cultures should be made from involved tissue or normally sterile body secretions. Material for culture should be kept strictly anaerobic and inoculated promptly, preferably at the bedside. Specimens should be obtained before antimicrobial therapy is given if possible. If smears and cultures are negative, a biopsy is required to establish

**Table 35–1. Presumptive Identification of Bacteria Associated With Actinomycosis and Related Bacteria**

| Property | Actinomyces israelii | Actinomyces odontolyticus | Actinomyces naeslundii | Actinomyces viscosus | Actinomyces meyeri | Arachnia propionica | Proprionibacterium acnes | Bifidobacterium adolescentis | Rothia dentocariosus |
|---|---|---|---|---|---|---|---|---|---|
| Catalase | – * | – | – | + | – | – | + | – | + |
| Nitrite from nitrate | +(–) | +(–) | + | + | –(+) | + | + | – | + |
| Nitrogen from nitrite | – | – | – | ± | NR | NR | NR | – | + |
| Hydrolysis of | | | | | | | | | |
| Casein | – | – | – | – | NR | – | + | – | – |
| Gelatin | – | – | – | – | – | – | + | – | – |
| Starch | – | – | – | + | – | – | – | + | – |
| Acid from | | | | | | | | | |
| Starch | – | – | – | A, ± | A | – | – | A | – |
| Mannitol | A | – | – | – | – | A | A (–) | A | – |
| Xylose | A | A | – | – | A (–) | – | – | A | – |
| Rabinose | A, ± | – (A) | – | A, ± | – (A) | – | A | A | – |
| Oxygen tolerance | Anaer | Fac anaer | Fac anaer | Fac anaer | Anaer | Fac anaer | Anaer | Anaer | Fac anaer |
| Production of propionic acid | – | – | – | – | – | + | + | – | – |

*Abbreviations: +, positive reaction; –, negative reaction; ± variable; A, acid formed but no gas; Anaer, anaerobic; Fac anaer, facultatively anaerobic; ( ), occurs in a minority of strains; NR, not reported.

Data from Pine L: *Actinomyces* and microaerophilic actinomycetes. *In* Braude AI, Davis CE, Fierer J (eds): Medical Microbiology and Infectious Diseases. Philadelphia, WB Saunders, 1981:448–467; Sutter VL, Citron DM, Finegold SM: Wadsworth Anaerobic Bacteriology Manual. St. Louis, CV Mosby, 1980; Virginia Polytechnic Institute: Anaerobe Laboratory Manual, ed 4. Blacksburg, Virginia, Virginia Polytechnic Institute, 1977.

the diagnosis. Blood should be cultured anaerobically. Positive results are rare, but they confirm the diagnosis.

In tissues or secretions, *Actinomyces* organisms are long, branching filaments, often intertwined. Filaments are usually gram positive, but with age and under certain conditions, they may appear gram-negative. The filaments typically appear beaded, and gram-positive segments interspersed with gram-negative ones may give the impression of many bacilli or cocci lined up end to end. On Gram stain, *Actinomyces* are indistinguishable from *Nocardia* (see Fig. 34–4). *Actinomyces* filaments can also be seen in KOH preparations. They are not acid fast; the presence of acid-fast organisms should suggest *Mycobacterium* or *Nocardia*. *Actinomyces* take up silver and periodic acid-Schiff stains.

For isolation in culture, specimens should be inoculated onto brain-heart infusion agar with and without whole defibrinated blood (eg, rabbit, sheep, horse) and into *Actinomyces* broth or fluid thioglycolate broth.[29] Cultures should be incubated in the presence of carbon dioxide aerobically and anaerobically. Commercial preparations of thioglycolate broth vary in composition and in their ability to support the growth of *Actinomyces*. Thioglycolate broth should contain cysteine and phosphate. The higher the glucose content, the better the growth, and for optimal results, thioglycolate medium should be fortified with 0.2% sterile rabbit serum just before use.

The agar surface can be examined after 24 to 48 hours by transmitted or reflected light for colonial morphology. *A. israelii* typically produces small "mycelial" or "spider" colonies that contain a central mass of bacteria with hyphae radiating outward onto the agar surface.[29] Other species produce round, entire microcolonies. Eventually the colonies can become quite irregular, and they are often described as resembling a raspberry or molar tooth. There

may be mild α-hemolysis. In broth, light, flaky colonies resembling suspended bread crumbs appear near the bottom of the tube.

*Actinomyces* and related organisms are almost all catalase negative; the important exception is *A. viscosus*. This test is useful for separating *Actinomyces* species from other organisms that may resemble them, particularly *Rothia dentocariosus* and *Propionibacterium acnes*. A catalase-positive actinomycete isolated from clinical material should suggest one of these species or a member of the typically aerobic genuses, *Nocardia*, *Mycobacterium*, and *Streptomyces*. Other biochemical characteristics useful for differentiation appear in Table 35–1. Fluorescein-conjugated antibody preparations have been used for speciation,[30] but the reagents are not widely available. Serologic tests have not proved useful for diagnosis.[31]

## THERAPY

Penicillin is the drug of choice for treatment of actinomycosis.[4, 11, 32, 33] In severe cases, penicillin should be given intravenously in high doses, 10 to 20 million units per day for several days or weeks. Then, therapy should be continued with oral penicillin in maximal tolerated doses. For milder cases, treatment can be initiated with shorter courses of intravenous therapy followed by oral therapy or with oral therapy alone.[34, 35] Probenecid should be given early in therapy and in more difficult cases to delay the secretion of penicillin. Tetracycline[17] and clindamycin[35–37] have also been used with good results. Sulfadiazine, erythromycin, and chloramphenicol have been used successfully in small numbers of cases.[33] The dosages of these other drugs are not well established.

In vitro tests have been used to determine susceptibility of *Actinomyces* to antimicrobials in limited studies.[38, 39] The slow growth and oxygen intolerance make testing difficult, and methods are not standardized. The ability of these tests to predict clinical response has not been demonstrated, but in difficult cases the results of such tests can guide alternative therapy. Susceptibilities of the different species causing actinomycotic syndromes are close enough that they can be considered together.[39] Penicillin, erythromycin, cephaloridine, minocycline, rifampin, and clindamycin are very active.[39] Organisms are inhibited by achievable concentrations of cephalothin, ampicillin, lincomycin, tetracycline, doxycycline, and chloramphenicol. A few strains are susceptible to sulfamethoxazole. Metronidazole is ineffective.

Other bacteria frequently accompany *Actinomyces* in tissue and may contribute to the pathogenesis of the disease. The antimicrobial susceptibilities of the wide range of organisms that have been isolated do not always correspond with those of *Actinomyces*.[40] It usually has not been necessary to add additional antimicrobial therapy to treat these associated organisms. They may be important for the pathogenesis, but *Actinomyces* are essential, and antimicrobial agents active against *Actinomyces* usually cure the disease.

Surgery should be used to drain abscesses and relieve obstruction. In earlier decades, there was some enthusiasm for radical excision of fistulas. With high-dose, prolonged antimicrobial therapy, surgery is seldom necessary.

Therapy should be continued for 6 to 12 months, because actinomycosis has a marked tendency to relapse. The exact duration should depend on the extent of the disease and the response to treatment. Longer durations of treatment should be used for central nervous system disease.

Women who have had pelvic disease with *Actinomyces* should not use IUDs. The approach to women who have IUDs and positive smears or cultures for *Actinomyces* is controversial.[41] Some physicians remove the device whether or not the women have symptoms. The women at least should be advised of the very small risk of actinomycosis and instructed to seek medical attention immediately if symptoms or signs of endometritis develop. If women with IUDs and microbiologic evidence of *Actinomyces* colonization have symptoms, the conservative approach is to remove the IUD and substitute another form of birth control. If the woman desires to keep the IUD, antimicrobial therapy against *Actinomyces* with careful follow-up is an alternative.

In cases of lacrimal canaliculitis from *Actinomyces*, a combination of removal of the concretions and topical antibiotics is curative.

The prognosis of actinomycosis varies with the site of disease. Before the antimicrobial era, it was estimated[15] that fewer than 20% of patients with thoracic disease survived. About 30% of patients with abdominal disease survived, but more than 95% of patients with cervicofacial disease survived. Current estimates are imprecise, but the prognosis is decidedly better with appropriate antimicrobial therapy. If the disease is recognized and treated early, death should not result from actinomycosis.[11]

## REFERENCES

1. Harrison RN, Thomas DJB: Acute actinomycotic empyema. Thorax 34:406, 1979.
2. Israel J: Neue Beobachtungen auf dem Gebiete der Mykosen des Menschen. Arch Pathol Anat Physiol Klin Med 126:15, 1878.
3. Richtsmeier WJ, Johns ME: Actinomycosis of the head and neck. Crit Rev Clin Lab Sci 11:175, 1979.
4. Bates M, Cruickshank G: Thoracic actinomycosis. Thorax 12:99, 1957.
5. Coleman RM, Georg LK, Rozzell AR: *Actinomyces naeslundii* as an agent in human actinomycosis. Appl Microbiol 18:420, 1969.
6. Radford BL, Ryan WJ: Isolation of *Actinomyces viscosus* from two patients with clinical infections. J Clin Pathol 30:518, 1977.
7. Rose HD, Varkey B, Kutty CPK: Thoracic actinomycosis caused by *Actinomyces meyeri*. Am Rev Respir Dis 125:251, 1982.
8. Brock DW, Georg LK, Brown JM, Hicklin MD: Actinomycosis caused by *Arachnia propionica*. Report of 11 cases. Am J Clin Pathol 59:66, 1973.
9. Socransky SS: Microbiology of periodontal disease—present status and future considerations. J Periodontal 48:497, 1977.
10. McQuarrie DG, Hall WH: Actinomycosis of the lung and chest wall. Surgery 64:905, 1968.
11. Weese WC, Smith IM: A study of 57 cases of actinomycosis over a 36-year period. Arch Intern Med 135:1562, 1975.
12. Pulverer G, Schaal KP: Human actinomycosis. Drugs Exp Clin Res 10:187, 1984.
13. Brown JR: Human actinomycosis. A study of 181 subjects. Hum Pathol 4:319, 1973.
14. Webb AK, Howell R, Hickman JA: Thoracic actinomycosis presenting with peripheral skin lesions. Thorax 33:818, 1978.
15. Cope Z: Actinomycosis. London, Oxford University Press, 1938.
16. Dutton WP, Inclan AP: Cardiac actinomycosis. Dis Chest 54:463, 1968.
17. Martin WJ, Nichols DR, Wellman WE, Weed LA: Disseminated actinomycosis treated with tetracycline. Arch Intern Med 97:252, 1956.
18. Prather JR, Eastridge CE, Hughes FA, McCaughan JJ: Actinomycosis of the thorax. Diagnosis and treatment. Ann Thorac Surg 9:307, 1970.
19. Slutzker AD, Claypool WD: Pericardial actinomycosis with cardiac tamponade from a contiguous thoracic lesion. Thorax 44:442, 1989.
20. Balikian JP, Cheng TH, Costello P, German PG: Pulmonary actinomycosis. A report of three cases. Diagn Radiol 128:613, 1978.
21. Flynn MW, Felson F: The roentgen manifestations of thoracic actinomycosis. Am J Roentgenol 110:707, 1970.
22. Slade PR, Slesser BV, Southgate J: Thoracic actinomycosis. Thorax 28:73, 1973.
23. Bartels LJ, Vrabec DP: Cervicofacial actinomycosis. Arch Otolaryngol 104:705, 1978.
23a. Muyamoto MI, Fang FC: Pyogenic liver abscess involving *Actinomyces:* Case report and review. Clin Infect Dis 16:303, 1993.
24. Shaw HR, Williamson MR, Boyd CM, Balachandran S, Angtuaco TL, McConnell JR: CT findings in abdominal actinomycosis. J Comput Assist Tomogr 11:466, 1987.
25. Butas CA, Read SE, Coleman RE, Abramovitch H: Disseminated actinomycosis. Can Med Assoc J 103:1069, 1970.
25a. Lam S, Samraj J, Rahman S, Hilton E: Primary actinomycotic endocarditis: Case report and review. Clin Infect Dis 16:481, 1993.
26. Luff RD, Gupta PK, Spence MR, Frost JK: Pelvic actinomycosis and the intrauterine contraceptive device. A cyto-histomorphologic study. Am J Clin Pathol 69:581, 1978.
27. Pine L, Hardin H, Turner L: Actinomycotic lacrimal canaliculitis. Am J Ophthalmol 49:1278, 1960.
28. Kinnear WJM, MacFarlane JT: A survey of thoracic actinomycosis. Respir Med 84:57, 1990.
29. Pine L: *Actinomyces* and microaerophilic actinomycetes. *In* Braude AI, Davis CE, Fierer J (eds): Medical Microbiology and Infectious Diseases. Philadelphia, WB Saunders, 1981:448.
30. Gerencser MA, Slack JM: Serological identification of *Actinomyces* using fluorescent antibody techniques. J Dent Res 55:A184, 1976.
31. Georg L, Coleman RM, Brown JM: Evaluation of an agar gel precipitin test for the serodiagnosis of actinomycosis. J Immunol 100:1288, 1968.
32. Harvey JC, Cantrell JR, Fisher AM: Actinomycosis: Its recognition and treatment. Ann Intern Med 46:868, 1957.
33. Peabody JW, Seabury JH: Actinomycosis and nocardiosis. A review of basic differences in therapy. Am J Med 28:99, 1960.
34. Nelson JD, Hermann DW: Oral penicillin therapy for thoracic actinomycosis. Pediatr Infect Dis 5:594, 1986.
35. Badgett JT, Adams G: Mandibular actinomycosis treated with oral clindamycin. Pediatr Infect Dis J 6:221, 1987.

36. Rose HD, Rytel MW: Actinomycosis treated with clindamycin. JAMA 221:1052, 1972.

37. Fass RJ, Scholand JF, Hodges GR, Saslaw S: Clindamycin in the treatment of serious anaerobic infections. Ann Intern Med 78:853, 1973.

38. Blake GC: Sensitivities of colonies and suspensions of *Actinomyces israelii* to penicillins, tetracyclines and erythromycin. Br Med J 1:145, 1964.

39. Lerner PI: Susceptibility of pathogenic actinomycetes to antimicrobial compounds. Antimicrob Agents Chemother 5:302, 1974.

40. Hoffler U, Niederau W, Pulverer G: Susceptibility of *Bacterium actinomycetemcomitans* to 45 antibiotics. Antimicrob Agents Chemother 17:943, 1980.

41. Gupta PK, Woodruff JD: *Actinomyces* in vaginal smears. JAMA 247:1175, 1982.

# CHAPTER 36

# Pneumonic Forms of Bacterial Zoonosis: Plague, Anthrax, and Tularemia

RICHARD J. WALLACE, Jr.

## PULMONARY INVOLVEMENT WITH ZOONOSES

Zoonoses are diseases of animals that can be transmitted to humans. Some are transmitted indirectly through an arthropod vector (eg, rodent fleas for *Yersinia pestis*, ticks, horse flies, fleas for *Francisella tularensis*), some by direct contact with infected animals or body fluids or tissues (eg, rabbits for *F. tularensis*, wool or hides for *Bacillus anthracis*), and some rarely through human-to-human transmission (eg, pneumonic plague). Although these diseases can be acquired in the home, they usually occur as a consequence of travel to a highly endemic area or recreational and outside work activities that bring a person in contact with the disease.

Most zoonotic diseases occur infrequently, and recognition often is delayed. They may not even be considered if a specific organ system, such as the lung, is involved.

This chapter discusses three bacterial zoonoses: plague, anthrax, and tularemia, with an emphasis on the pulmonary manifestations and presentations of each of these diseases.

## PLAGUE

Plague is a bacterial disease of enormous historical interest because of its impact on medieval Europe.[1] Modern control of the urban rat population, which was the major reservoir for plague in medieval times, has dramatically diminished the clinical significance of the disease in cities and urban areas. In the United States, fewer than 20 cases per year are reported to the Centers for Disease Control (Fig. 36–1).[2]

The etiologic agent of plague is *Y. pestis*, a small, aerobic, gram-negative rod. The major reservoir for plague in the United States is small rodents in the southwestern states from Texas to California.[1, 2] Periodically, these animals are killed off by the plague bacillus, and the fleas leave the dead host to seek a live one, which occasionally is a human. Because most of these fleas are host specific, they rarely bite humans even if they are the only hosts available. The most common clinical disease is bubonic plague, a disease of large suppurative lymph nodes that drain the site of primary skin inoculation.

Pulmonary plague is a relatively rare event and may be primary or secondary. The most common is secondary pneumonic disease, which results from septicemia and hematogenous spread from infected lymph nodes. This complication occurs in only 5% to 15% of cases of bubonic plague,[1, 3] and because of its rarity it can be difficult to diagnose if the major clinical symptoms are respiratory.

A much rarer form of disease is primary pneumonic plague, in which infected droplets are inhaled from an animal or from a human with secondary plague pneumonia. This type of disease occurs after exposure to sick cats and dogs. Human-to-human transmission of plague has not been reported in the United States in more than 50 years.

The radiographic features of plague are nonspecific.[4] They usually show alveolar infiltrates that are unilateral or bilateral. A unique feature for bacterial pneumonia is the frequent presence of hilar or mediastinal adenopathy. Sputum Gram stains usually show gram-negative rods, and sputum cultures grow *Y. pestis*.

The diagnosis of plague pneumonia depends on a high

**PLAGUE — In humans, by year, United States, 1955–1990**

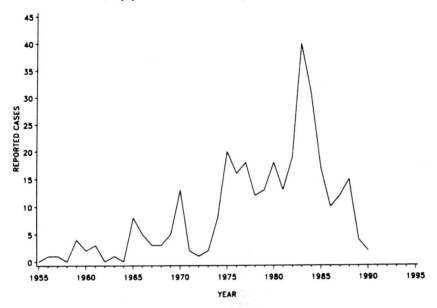

**Figure 36–1.** Cases of plague reported in the United States between 1955 and 1990. (From Graphs and maps for selected notifiable diseases in the United States. MMWR 39(53):35, 1991.)

index of suspicion. The disease is active primarily in the summer months in the southwestern states of New Mexico and Arizona in persons with outdoor activities or possible exposure to infected felines or rodents. Patients with plague almost never are aware of the flea bite itself. The organism is readily grown from blood cultures and is readily seen on Gram stain and grown from infected lymph node specimens. A fluorescent antibody stain is available for direct secretion staining.

The treatment of choice for plague pneumonia is streptomycin. Alternative agents are tetracyclines or chloramphenicol. The penicillins and cephalosporins usually are ineffective and should not be used in therapy. Plague is readily treatable if correctly diagnosed, with an overall mortality rate of 20% in the chemotherapeutic era.

## ANTHRAX

Anthrax is a zoonotic disease of major historical significance microbiologically, because the etiologic agent, *B. anthracis*, was the first bacterial pathogen to be grown in a culture media from infected tissues by Koch in 1876 and was the model used in the development of Koch's postulates.[5] The causative agent is an aerobic, spore-forming, gram-positive rod. The organism and its spores are commonly present on imported raw animal fibers, including goat hair, goat skins, and wool. In some areas of the world, agricultural sources such as infected cattle are also a major source of the organism.

Human anthrax takes a variety of clinical forms, with cutaneous infection (ie, malignant pustule) caused by local inoculation being responsible for 95% of the disease reported in the United States.[5] Anthrax pneumonia usually does not result from inhalation of infectious spores. The organism is usually deposited in the upper airway or tracheobronchial tree, but without evident alveolar disease. The organism spreads through the lymphatics, with resultant, often massive, hilar and mediastinal adenopathy.

Anthrax is a relatively rare disease in the United States, with fewer than 10 cases reported to the Centers for Disease Control in Atlanta during the past decade.[6] All of these cases were occupationally acquired by persons in industrial (eg, processing of wool or goat hair) or agricultural settings.

*B. anthracis* is susceptible to penicillin, and early disease is relatively easily treated. The organism produces several virulent toxins, allowing far advanced disease to progress despite antimicrobial therapy.

## TULAREMIA

Tularemia is a bacterial disease produced by a small, fastidious, gram-negative bacillus currently known as *F. tularensis*. The name honors Edward Francis, who did much of the early bacteriologic and epidemiologic studies with the organism, and Tulare County in California, where the disease was first discovered among ground squirrels.[7]

The disease is endemic in many areas of the world, but in the United States, it is localized in the south central states of Texas, Arkansas, Oklahoma, Missouri, Illinois, Virginia, and Tennessee (Fig. 36–2). Approximately 200 cases of disease per year are reported (Fig. 36–3). The major reservoir of disease is the tick, which can transmit infection transovarially so that each new generation of ticks carries the organism, probably in the feces. Although ticks and, less commonly, deer flies are the major vectors, more than 100 wild animals and nine domestic species can become infected and transmit the disease.[8] High-risk exposure includes a history of a tick bite or of handling of rabbits (ie, rabbit fever) or squirrels. Human disease related to ticks is at its peak during the summer months (Fig. 36–4).

Two subtypes of *F. tularensis* have been recognized. Type A is thought to be common in rabbits and transmitted by tick bites, and type B is associated with infected rodents and is transmitted by exposure to contaminated water.[8]

Pneumonia is a relatively common presentation of tula-

## TULAREMIA — Reported cases, by county, United States, 1990

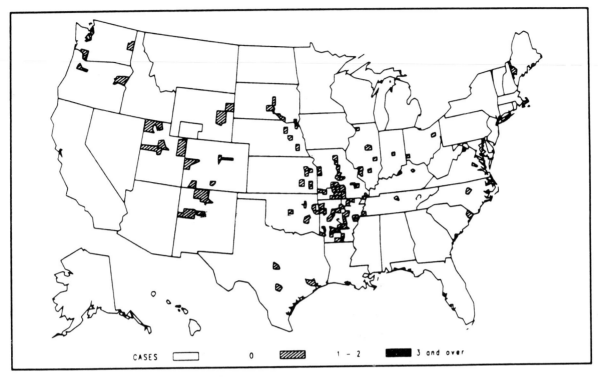

Note: Two cases reported in Alaska.

**Figure 36–2.** Geographic distribution of cases of tularemia in the United States reported to the Centers for Disease Control in 1990. (From Graphs and maps for selected notifiable diseases in the United States. MMWR 39(53):48, 1991.)

remia.[7] Most cases present as a secondary manifestation of the classic ulceroglandular disease that results from the usual tick bite or exposure to an infected rabbit. Not all cases do, however, and in endemic areas, cases of pneumonia are seen with no cutaneous or lymph node disease.

It is estimated that pneumonia secondary to hematogenous dissemination occurs in approximately 10% of patients with ulceroglandular disease and 30% to 80% of patients with the typhoidal form of the disease. Rarely, pneumonia can occur from inhalation of infected aerosols, usually while

## TULAREMIA — By year, United States, 1955–1990

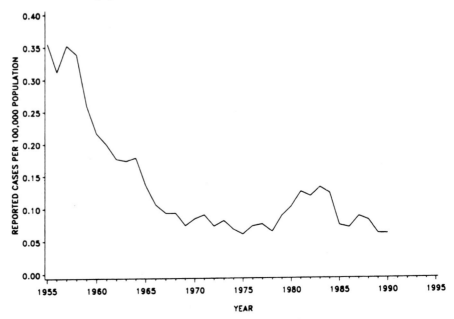

**Figure 36–3.** Annual incidence of cases of tularemia reported in the United States between 1955 and 1990. (From Graphs and maps for selected notifiable diseases in the United States. MMWR 39(53):48, 1991.)

### Month of onset for human tularemia by exposure -- Texas, 1980-1989

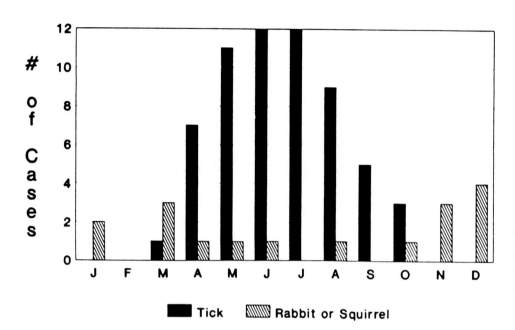

■ **Tick**   ▨ **Rabbit or Squirrel**

**Figure 36–4.** Monthly cases of tularemia in Texas related to type of exposure. (From Jeffery Taylor, MPH, Infectious Disease Epidemiology and Surveillance Program, Texas Department of Health. Tularemia. Texas Preventable Disease News 51(6):2, 1991.)

cleaning or manipulating infected rabbits. The radiographic features of tularemia pneumonia are variable and nonspecific.[9] They usually show alveolar infiltrates without cavitation. The organisms are rarely seen on Gram stains of sputum or pleural fluid, and the leukocyte count may not be elevated. Diagnostically, the disease is often thought of as an atypical pneumonia.

The diagnosis of tularemia pneumonia should be suspected for anyone who presents with pneumonia in the summer months who has an outdoor exposure, especially if they have a history of a recent tick bite, or who has been cleaning or handling wild rabbits. The absence of these findings should not exclude this diagnosis. An ulcerative skin lesion at a possible site of a tick bite with or without related suppurative lymphadenopathy should alert the examiner to the diagnosis. The organism can be grown from skin lesions, lymph nodes, and sputum on specialized media that contain cysteine. The organism has been readily grown on enriched gonococcal (gc) chocolate agar or *Legionella* media (eg, charcoal-yeast extract, CYE agar) with prolonged incubation.[8] The organism can also be grown from most blood culture systems. Because of its contagiousness in the laboratory, great care should be taken in handling infected tissues or working with cultures. Serologic analysis for tularemia is readily available, although clinical correlation is required, because nonspecific agglutinin titers greater than 1:80 occur in patients with no evidence of infection or disease.[10]

The treatment of choice for tularemia pneumonia and other forms of tularemia is streptomycin. Doses depend on patient's size, age, and calculated creatinine clearance, as for any aminoglycoside. For young patients with normal body weights and renal function, a dose of 1.0 g twice daily has been recommended. In vitro studies have shown *F.*

*tularensis* to be resistant to essentially all β-lactams, but it exhibits low minimal inhibitory concentrations for all aminoglycosides and for tetracyclines and chloramphenicol.[11] Gentamicin has been used successfully for treating tularemia pneumonia,[12] and this aminoglycoside and tobramycin produce serum levels that can be monitored. For diagnosed tularemia, the mortality rate is 1% to 5%.

### REFERENCES

1. Reed WP, Palmer DL, Williams RC Jr, Kisch AL: Bubonic plague in the southwestern United States. Medicine (Baltimore) 49:465–486, 1970.
2. Kaufman AF, Boyce JM, Martone WJ: From the Centers for Disease Control—Trends in human plague in the United States. J Infect Dis 141:522–524, 1980.
3. Crook LD, Tempest B: Plague—A clinical review of 27 cases. Arch Intern Med 152:1253–1256, 1992.
4. Alsofrom DJ, Mettler FA, Mann JM: Radiographic manifestations of plague in New Mexico, 1975–1980. Radiology 139:561–565, 1981.
5. Brachman PS: Anthrax. Ann NY Acad Sci 174:577–582, 1970.
6. Human cutaneous anthrax—North Carolina, 1987. MMWR 37:413–414, 1988.
7. Dienst FT Jr: Tularemia—A perusal of three hundred thirty-nine cases. J La State Med Soc 115:114–126, 1963.
8. Evans ME: *Francisella tularensis*. Infect Control 6:381–383, 1985.
9. Overholt EL, Tiggert WD: Roentgenographic manifestations of pulmonary tularemia. Radiology 74:758–764, 1960.
10. Gelfand MS, Slade W, Abolnik IZ: Tularemia serology: Differentiating true-positive and false-positive titers. Infect Dis Clin Pract 1:105–108, 1991.
11. Baker CN, Hollis DG, Thornsberry C: Antimicrobial susceptibility of *Francisella tularensis* with a modified Mueller-Hinton broth. J Clin Microbiol 22:212–215, 1985.
12. Mason WL, Eigelsbach HT, Little SF, Bates JH: Treatment of tularemia, including pulmonary tularemia, with gentamicin. Am Rev Respir Dis 121:39–45, 1980.

# CHAPTER 37

# Pneumocystis carinii

PAUL E. ZIMMERMAN and WILLIAM J. MARTIN II

*Pneumocystis carinii*, a once obscure pathogen, has been recognized as a cause of pneumonia in humans since 1942, when Van der Meer and Brug demonstrated the organism in the lungs of infants and an adult.[1] *P. carinii* was later determined to be the cause of infantile epidemic interstitial plasma cell pneumonia, which was prevalent in the orphanages of Europe after World War II, where conditions of overcrowding and malnutrition flourished. In the United States, since the mid-1950s, *P. carinii* pneumonia has often been the sentinel infection revealing a congenital or acquired childhood immunodeficiency, or it has been the result of immune suppression caused by lymphoreticular or hematologic malignancies, organ transplantation, or drugs, particularly corticosteroids or cyclosporine.[2–4] Since the early 1980s, the incidence of *P. carinii* pneumonia has exploded, paralleling the spread of human immunodeficiency virus (HIV) infection. *P. carinii* has again emerged as a diagnostic indicator, this time for the acquired immunodeficiency syndrome (AIDS). *P. carinii* pneumonia represents the AIDS-defining infection in more than 60% of the HIV-positive patients who progress to develop AIDS.[5] Currently, HIV-infected persons represent the population with the greatest incidence of *P. carinii* pneumonia, and *P. carinii* pneumonia is the most frequent cause of life-threatening infection in patients with AIDS.

The common variable in each of these patient populations is the profound impairment of cell-mediated immunity, suggesting that the integrity of the T-lymphocyte response is essential in host defense against *Pneumocystis* pneumonia. Direct evidence supporting the importance of T lymphocytes in the development of *Pneumocystis* pneumonia has come from depletion and reconstitution experiments in animal models.[6, 7] Reduced T-lymphocyte numbers and impaired function are well recognized in HIV infection. The most crucial cell population in the T-lymphocyte component of host defense are the CD4+ (helper T) lymphocytes. The risk of *Pneumocystis* pneumonia in HIV-infected patients closely correlates with the number of circulating CD4+ cells, to the extent that a fall in the CD4+ cell count to less than 200 cells/mm³ is a harbinger for the development of *P. carinii* pneumonia.[8]

## EPIDEMIOLOGY

*P. carinii* is distributed worldwide and is found in a wide variety of animals and in humans. Immunologic studies suggest a heterogeneity of *P. carinii* strains between species. If *P. carinii* chromosomes are compared using pulsed-field gel electrophoresis, clear intraspecies and interspecies differences are found to exist.[9]

*P. carinii* has traditionally been classified as a protozoan. This probably occurred because of its historic misidentification as a trypanosome by Chagas in 1909,[10] and its response to antiprotozoal chemotherapeutic agents (eg, pentamidine isethionate, trimethoprim-sulfamethoxazole). The first clue that *P. carinii* might not be a protozoan occurred with the recognition that the protozoan enzymes dihydrofolate reductase and thymidylate synthase occur on the same polypeptide chain. These two enzymes in *P. carinii* are neither physically nor genetically linked.[11] Analysis of the small subunit of *P. carinii* ribosomal RNA, a ubiquitous and highly conserved ribosomal subunit in eukaryotes, demonstrated that *P. carinii* is more closely related to the fungi than to protozoa.[12, 13] *P. carinii* is thought to be most closely related phylogenetically to the Ascomycetes (yeast) group of fungi.[14] The cyst wall of *P. carinii* is similar in morphology and chemical composition, containing an abundance of β-1,3-glucans, to the cell wall of some yeasts, such as *Saccharomyces cerevisiae*.[15]

The life cycle of *P. carinii* is not delineated, but two forms of *P. carinii* are consistently identified in vivo and in vitro. The trophozoite form exists as a small, 1- to 4-μm, thin-walled organism with a single nucleus. The cyst form is larger, 5 to 8 μm, and contains 4 to 8 daughter forms, known as sporozoites or intracystic bodies, within a thick-walled cyst.[16] Replication of the organism may occur by sexual and/or asexual reproduction. Sexual reproduction probably occurs after conjugation of two trophozoite forms. The nuclear material undergoes mitosis, producing as many as eight separate nuclei, which mature into the sporozoites contained within the mature cyst. After excystation, a new generation of trophozoite forms is produced. Asexual reproduction may occur through binary fission or budding of the trophozoite form.[17]

The infective form of the organism remains unknown. The probable link of *P. carinii* to the fungi suggests the possibility that a yet unidentified stage (eg, spores) may be involved in transmission of infection.[18] This would be analogous to the transmission of disease caused by the fungus *Histoplasma capsulatum*. The yeast form of *H. capsulatum* exists only in the host; the infective particles responsible for transmission of disease are the microconidia, which exist entirely outside the host. Alternatively, the small (1–4 μm) size of the trophozoite form is ideal for aerosol transmission and deposition into the alveolar air spaces, the primary site of disease.[19] Animal studies have demonstrated that *P. carinii* pneumonia can successfully be transmitted through the air, directly from the environment or from animal to animal.[20] Transmission from food, water, feces, or soil has not been demonstrated.[20, 21] Indirect evidence for person-to-person transmission of *P. carinii* has been observed in outbreaks of *P. carinii* pneumonia in children living in orphanages after World War II and, more recently, in adult and pediatric patients in transplant centers and cancer hospitals.[22, 23] In all of these cases, successful transmission has occurred in immunocompromised patients. Even though direct evidence for transmission from person to person is not available, some experts recommend that immunocompromised patients be isolated from active cases of *P. carinii* pneumonia.[24]

*Pneumocystis* pneumonia is only rarely encountered in immunologically competent hosts.[25] Infection is so infrequent in normal hosts as to suggest that these patients had some type of undetected immune impairment. Whether pneumonia caused by *P. carinii* in the immunocompromised person results from primary infection, activation of a latent infection, or an opportunistic reinfection has not been determined. Primary infection seems unlikely, because it is estimated that approximately 75% of all children already have serologic evidence of an asymptomatic infection by 4 years of age.[26, 27] Studies using corticosteroids to induce spontaneous *P. carinii* pneumonia in rats suggest that disease in animals represents a reactivation of a latent infection.[28] In patients with impairment of cellular immunity, successful reinfection may occur after exposure to this ubiquitous organism.

## PATHOGENESIS

The most crucial element in host defense against *Pneumocystis* pneumonia is the cell-mediated arm of immunity: the CD4+ lymphocytes. Regardless of the source of infection, after immunity becomes impaired beyond a critical level, primary infection or reactivation of *P. carinii* is likely to occur.

With rare exceptions, infection with *P. carinii* is limited to the lungs[29, 30] and is characterized by an alveolar filling process. Extrapulmonary spread usually is limited to hilar or mediastinal lymph nodes, retroperitoneal lymph nodes, or the spleen. Less common sites of spread include the bone marrow, adrenal glands, gastrointestinal tract, thyroid gland, and the eyes. In only half of all cases with extrapulmonary spread of *P. carinii* are the lungs concomitantly involved.[31]

Corticosteroid-immunosuppressed rats have been used extensively to characterize the histopathology of *P. carinii* pneumonia. Initial infection is thought to first involve accumulation of single or small clusters of *P. carinii* organisms in the peribronchial intraalveolar spaces, with preservation of the alveolar architecture.[7, 32] The alveolar lining fluid layer is thickened, and the alveolar macrophages become vacuolated with increased numbers of cytoplasmic lamellar inclusion bodies. Initially, there is no host inflammatory response.[32]

As the pneumonia progresses, *P. carinii* organisms spread to adjacent alveoli and ultimately to the whole lung. *P. carinii* organisms appear to attach selectively to type I alveolar epithelial cells (Fig. 37–1).[33, 34] This is followed by type I cell degeneration and necrosis, with subsequent type II cell reparative hyperplasia. The mechanism of attachment appears not to involve extracellular organelles or membrane fusion.[33–35] *P. carinii* attachment to cultured lung cells is mediated by the extracellular matrix protein fibronectin.[36] Type I pneumocytes express a fibronectin receptor, but type II cells do not; this may explain the apparent selectivity of *P. carinii* for the type I cell.

After the organism is firmly anchored to the alveolar epithelium, lung cell injury occurs in the absence of host inflammatory changes. This is observed ultrastructurally as subepithelial bleb formation and cytoplasmic vacuolation of the type I pneumocyte. The subepithelial bleb increases in size, eventually separating the type I cell from the basal lamina, leaving behind a denuded basement membrane. Endothelial cells also show focal intracellular and subcellular vacuolization; however, complete detachment of the endothelium from the basement membrane is not observed.[35] These ultrastructural changes suggest that, as a result of a primary epithelial cell injury induced by *P. carinii*, there is an increased permeability of the alveolar-capillary membrane, resulting in the transudation of fluid from the vascular space into the alveoli.[35] One possible mechanism for this epithelial injury is the release of proteolytic enzymes from *P. carinii* as the trophozoites detach and move from the alveolar epithelium into the alveolar spaces.[37] In the advanced stages of the pneumonia, as cellular destruction proceeds, the pulmonary interstitium becomes infiltrated with mononuclear inflammatory cells, and the alveoli become consolidated with a foamy, amorphous, eosinophilic material and widespread inflammation (Fig. 37–2). The interstitium is replaced with focal areas of fibrosis.[38] Rarely, a granulomatous replacement of the interstitium is found.[39] If left untreated, death from respiratory failure occurs.

A noncellular eosinophilic material, observed by light microscopy, fills the alveolar spaces and encases the *P. carinii* organisms. This material is a mixture of surfactant-like lipoproteinaceous material, degenerating host and par-

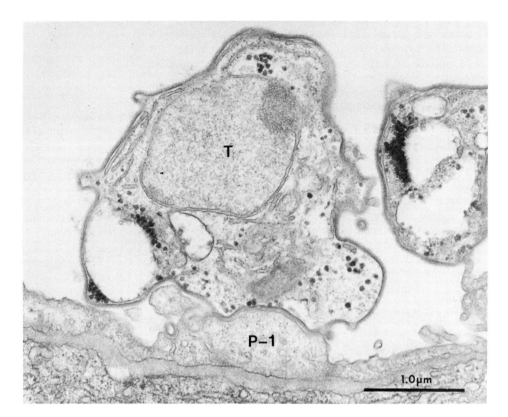

**Figure 37–1.** The electron micrograph demonstrates selective attachment of a *Pneumocystis carinii* trophozoite *(T)* to a type I alveolar epithelial cell *(P-1)*. The cell membranes of the trophozoite form and the type 1 pneumocyte are closely apposed without evidence of membrane fusion.

asite membranes, and serum proteins, not unlike the substance seen in the alveolar filling process in primary pulmonary alveolar proteinosis.[35, 40] *P. carinii* is a recognized cause of secondary pulmonary alveolar proteinosis.[41] *P. carinii* organisms firmly associate with desaturated phosphatidylcholine, the predominate phospholipid in alveolar surfactant.[42] *P. carinii* also bind surfactant protein A,[43] a surfactant-associated protein known to inhibit secretion and

enhance uptake of phospholipids by type II alveolar epithelial cells in vitro.[44] Surfactant protein A levels are increased in *Pneumocystis* pneumonia,[45] possibly as a direct result of the type II pneumocyte hyperplasia or indirectly as a result of the sequestering of available free surfactant protein A in the alveolar lining layer by *P. carinii*, resulting in a relative overproduction of this surfactant apoprotein. *P. carinii* binding to surfactant protein A may disrupt surfactant ho-

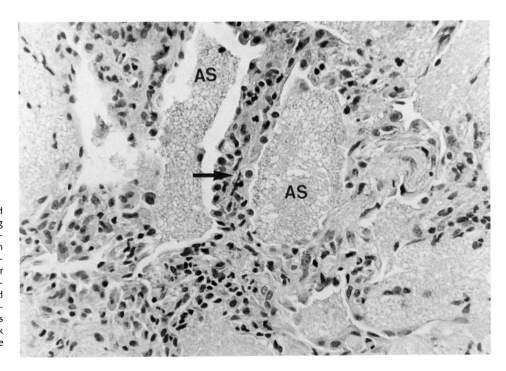

**Figure 37–2.** Hematoxylin and eosin stain of a transbronchial lung biopsy demonstrates the typical alveolar filling process observed in *P. carinii* pneumonia (original magnification × 400). The alveolar septa are thickened *(arrow)*. Alveolar type II cell hyperplasia and minimal mononuclear inflammation are seen. The alveolar spaces *(AS)* are filled with a lacy network of periodic acid-Schiff–positive acellular material.

meostasis and disorganize the alveolar surfactant film. This increases alveolar surface tension, with consequent alveolar edema and instability. This may partially explain the atelectasis and loss of lung compliance observed with *Pneumocystis* pneumonia. The interaction of *P. carinii* with this abundant lipoproteinaceous material probably contributes to the hypoxemia observed in *P. carinii* pneumonia.

## CLINICAL FEATURES

The symptoms reported by patients with *P. carinii* pneumonia are similar to those found in other ''atypical'' or nonbacterial pneumonias.[46] *P. carinii* pneumonia presents with a more insidious behavior in patients with AIDS than in patients with other types of immunosuppression. Patients with AIDS typically have less fever and a longer duration of symptoms than patients with non–AIDS-related *P. carinii* pneumonia.[47] In both groups, cough, fever, and dyspnea are the most frequently reported symptoms (Table 37–1). Dyspnea may be quite mild, especially in patients with AIDS. In the appropriate setting, a subtle increase in dyspnea on exertion in an HIV-positive or AIDS patient warrants further investigation. Cough is typically nonproductive. Cough productive of purulent sputum should suggest an alternative diagnosis or a bacterial coinfection. Other less common symptoms include hemoptysis, pleuritic chest pain, chills, sweats, fatigue, and anorexia.[47–49] *P. carinii* pneumonia in patients receiving aerosolized pentamidine prophylaxis presents with similar symptoms.[50]

Physical findings are nonspecific. The physical examination often reveals fever, tachypnea, and tachycardia. Auscultation of the chest may reveal inspiratory crackles or, rarely, wheezes, but the chest examination may be normal in half of the patients.[48] The remainder of the physical examination offers no further clues to the diagnosis of *Pneumocystis* pneumonia, other than the findings of the primary disease, which may suggest underlying immune suppression. As with other atypical pneumonias, the examination findings are often less severe than the chest roentgenogram or pulmonary function studies suggest.

Table 37–1. **Clinical Features of *Pneumocystis carinii* Pneumonia at Presentation in HIV-related and Non–HIV-related Immunosuppression**

| Clinical Features | HIV-related Immunosuppression | Non–HIV-related Immunosuppression |
|---|---|---|
| Symptoms (%) | | |
| Fever | 81 | 87 |
| Cough | 81 | 71 |
| Shortness of breath | 68 | 66 |
| Chills | 26 | 26 |
| Sputum | 23 | 21 |
| Chest pain | 23 | 24 |
| Median duration of symptoms* (days) | 28 (1–270)† | 5 (1–42)† |

*$P < .01$.
†Numbers in parentheses are the range.
Reproduced, with permission, from Kovacs JA, Hiemenz JW, Macher AM, et al: *Pneumocystis carinii* pneumonia: A comparison between patients with acquired immunodeficiency syndrome and patients with other immunodeficiencies. Ann Intern Med 1984; 100:663–671.

## COMPLICATIONS

Complications associated with *P. carinii* pneumonia include spontaneous pneumothorax in 6% to 9% of cases,[51, 52] systemic dissemination of the *P. carinii* infection, respiratory failure, and concomitant viral, fungal, or bacterial infections.

The systemic dissemination of *P. carinii* organisms, which has been observed in AIDS and non-AIDS patients, may in part be related to the use of inhaled pentamidine prophylaxis; however, not all patients with extrapulmonary spread of *P. carinii* have received aerosolized pentamidine prophylaxis.[31]

In AIDS patients, approximately one third of those with *Pneumocystis* pneumonia have a coinfection found at bronchoscopy. Coinfections with cytomegalovirus (CMV) and *Mycobacterium avium-intracellulare* occur most commonly.[53] The short-term and long-term survival of patients with *P. carinii* alone or *P. carinii* plus CMV at bronchoscopy are similar whether specific anti-CMV therapy is provided or not.[54] Aspergillomas developing in remanent cavities as a consequence of a prior lung infection with *P. carinii* have been reported.[55]

The most serious complication of *P. carinii* pneumonia is the development of acute respiratory failure. Hypoxemia is found invariably in cases of *Pneumocystis* pneumonia, and an estimated 5% to 30% of these patients develop respiratory failure.[56] A high mortality rate is observed among patients whose pneumonia progresses to respiratory failure and who require endotracheal intubation and mechanical ventilation. Patients with AIDS and *P. carinii* pneumonia are significantly less hypoxemic on room air than patients with non-AIDS *Pneumocystis* pneumonia.[47, 57] Despite this higher observed $PaO_2$, AIDS patients with *P. carinii* pneumonia have a significantly greater number of organisms in their lungs than patients with *Pneumocystis* pneumonia who are immunosuppressed from other causes.[57] The disparity in the arterial oxygen tensions observed between the two groups does not depend on the organism load in the lung. However, patients with *P. carinii* pneumonia and AIDS generally have fewer neutrophils recovered from their alveolar spaces by bronchoalveolar lavage (BAL) compared with patients without AIDS.[57] An increased recovery of neutrophils from the lung by BAL positively correlates with the degree of impaired oxygenation that is found in *P. carinii* pneumonia.[57, 58] It appears that the host inflammatory response is a more important cause of the observed hypoxemia than is the overall organism burden in the lung.

BAL neutrophilia is a reliable predictor for the development of respiratory failure.[57, 59] If respiratory failure occurs, most of these patients will die despite intubation and mechanical ventilation. The best prognostic indicator for survival is the level of oxygenation at the time of diagnosis.[60, 61] Predictors of poor clinical outcome include longer duration of symptoms before diagnosis, requirement for mechanical ventilation that is not temporally associated with diagnostic bronchoscopy, failure of the serum lactate dehydrogenase (LDH) concentration to diminish during the first week after initiation of specific anti-*Pneumocystis* therapy, and a low serum albumin concentration.[60–63] The survival rate associated with respiratory failure, which once approached 0%, has improved to approximately 40%.[61, 64]

## DIAGNOSTIC APPROACH

There is no single noninvasive laboratory test that is pathognomonic for *P. carinii* infection, except for the direct visualization of *P. carinii* in the pulmonary secretions. Chest roentgenograms reveal parenchymal infiltrates in more than 90% of cases. Particularly early in the course of the disease, the chest roentgenogram is normal in 5% of patients.[51, 65] The roentgenographic appearance of *Pneumocystis* pneumonia in AIDS and non-AIDS patients has been described as a bilateral perihilar reticulonodular infiltrate (Fig. 37–3). The infiltrate appears as an interstitial infiltrate in 75% of the cases, with the remainder appearing as an alveolar or a combined interstitial-alveolar process.[51] Air bronchograms are commonly seen in the basal segments, particularly in advanced cases of disease.

In AIDS patients with *P. carinii* pneumonia, the lung is diffusely involved in approximately half the cases at the time of diagnosis. If localized infiltrates occur, the lower lung fields are more commonly involved than the upper and middle lung fields. A localized segmental infiltrate or lobar consolidation suggests bacterial pneumonia.[49] Unilateral involvement is seen in approximately 5% of such patients.[51] Other roentgenographic abnormalities associated with *Pneumocystis* pneumonia include pneumothorax, cavities, thin-walled cysts or pneumatoceles, abscesses, honeycombed parenchymal changes, bilateral hilar adenopathy, and pleural effusion. The presence of pleural effusion in *P. carinii* pneumonia suggests the concomitant occurrence of pulmonary Kaposi sarcoma.[49] Patients receiving inhaled aerosolized pentamidine have increased reports of atypical infiltrates, particularly upper lobe or peripheral infiltrates,

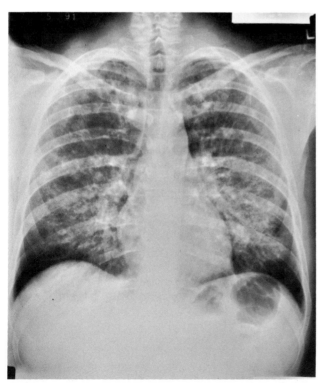

**Figure 37–3.** Roentgenographic appearance of *P. carinii* pneumonia. The posteroanterior film demonstrates a typical perihilar and diffuse interstitial and alveolar infiltrate.

pneumothoraces, and hilar or mediastinal adenopathy.[50] With the increasing incidence of this disease, there is no "typical" roentgenographic pattern of *Pneumocystis* pneumonia.

With institution of anti-*Pneumocystis* therapy, roentgenographic improvement is seen at the end of 1 week in 17% of patients. After 2 months, complete resolution of the roentgenographic changes is seen in 33% of patients.[51]

Routine laboratory studies, a complete blood count with differential, and blood chemistries are nonspecific. The leukocyte count typically is not elevated in *Pneumocystis* pneumonia. The lymphopenia is not significantly different in AIDS and non-AIDS *P. carinii* pneumonia.[47] A peripheral eosinophilia is an uncommon occurrence but has been reported, predominantly in children.[66]

Blood chemistries show an elevation in the serum LDH activity in more than 90% of patients with *Pneumocystis* pneumonia.[63, 67] There is no significant difference in the degree of elevation in the serum LDH concentration in patients with AIDS and those with non-AIDS *P. carinii* pneumonia. The serum LDH activity appears to parallel disease activity. As the pneumonitis resolves with treatment, the LDH concentration decreases, but in pneumonia not responding to therapy, the LDH level rises.[63] A rise in the LDH level heralds the relapse of pneumonia.[68] For HIV-infected patients with bilateral interstitial infiltrates, an elevated serum LDH concentration likely indicates *P. carinii* pneumonia, and a normal LDH concentration supports the absence of disease.[69, 70] For those with kidney or liver disease, the serum LDH concentration becomes less useful.

Arterial blood gas analysis in *P. carinii* pneumonia has only a moderate diagnostic sensitivity and a very low specificity. Patients with AIDS-related *P. carinii* pneumonia are more likely to have a room air PaO$_2$ of 80 mm Hg or higher than patients without AIDS.[47] An elevated (A-a) O$_2$ gradient is a common finding; however, it may be normal in as many as 24% of patients.[69] The (A-a) O$_2$ gradient is widened less in AIDS than in non-AIDS *P. carinii* pneumonia.

Pulmonary function tests, including simple spirometry and lung volumes, inconsistently show a mild restrictive pattern and are not useful in the diagnosis of *Pneumocystis* pneumonia. The resting diffusing capacity is a sensitive indicator for the presence of *Pneumocystis*, and the value is abnormal in almost 100% of patients.[51, 71, 72] However, because of this high sensitivity, it lacks specificity and is frequently abnormal in asymptomatic or symptomatic non–*Pneumocystis*-related pulmonary processes in patients with HIV infection.[73] An even more sensitive test with a high negative predictive value is the demonstration of an incremental increase in the (A-a) O$_2$ gradient induced by simple exercise.[71]

Gallium 67 lung scanning is a highly sensitive (>90%) test for the detection of *P. carinii* pneumonia and most commonly shows an intense and diffuse uptake pattern in the lungs. However, because of the propensity for AIDS patients to harbor other infections in their lungs, it has a low specificity.[74, 75] If a grading system is used to quantify the intensity of uptake, the specificity of [67]Ga scanning for *Pneumocystis* pneumonia increases to greater than 90%.[74] Diffuse bilateral uptake of [67]Ga into the lungs is typically not seen if the patient has been receiving aerosolized pentamidine.[76] Localized pulmonary uptake suggests bacterial pneumonia, and intrathoracic lymph node involvement sug-

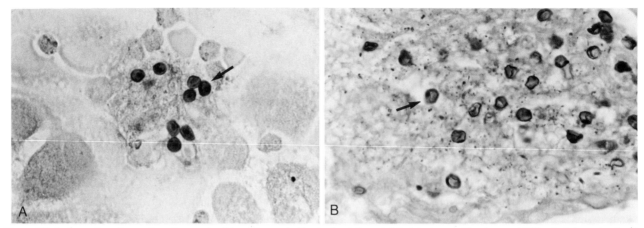

**Figure 37–4.** Gomori methenamine silver stain of bronchoscopically obtained *P. carinii* (original magnification × 1000). *A,* A bronchoalveolar specimen demonstrates *P. carinii* cysts, and the characteristic "hat shape" or "smiling faces" are seen *(arrow). B,* A transbronchial biopsy demonstrates numerous cysts in the alveolar space.

gests *M. avium-intracellulare* infection or lymphoma.[75] In an AIDS patient with an abnormal chest roentgenogram and a negative [67]Ga scan, a noninflammatory process such as pulmonary Kaposi sarcoma is likely.[75] [67]Ga scans are most useful in the screening of symptomatic patients with normal chest roentgenograms and pulmonary function studies who are at increased risk for *Pneumocystis* pneumonia.

Despite the high sensitivities of the tests providing indirect evidence for the presence of *P. carinii* pneumonia, a definitive diagnosis cannot be made unless *P. carinii* organisms are seen in the pulmonary secretions. Traditionally, the organism has been identified using a cyst wall stain such as the toluidine blue O or Gomori methenamine silver stains. The Giemsa stain or Diff-Quik, a modified Wright-Giemsa stain, has been used to identify the trophozoite forms and intracystic sporozoite forms in pulmonary secretions.

The least expensive and noninvasive method for identifying *P. carinii* in pulmonary secretions is the collection and staining of an induced sputum specimen. Before 1986, the use of expectorated sputum for the identification of *Pneumocystis* organisms in non-AIDS immunosuppressed hosts was rarely successful.[2] However, as a result of the AIDS epidemic, new techniques for the rapid and noninvasive diagnosis of *P. carinii* pneumonia have become available. Consequently, examination of induced sputum obtained from non-AIDS patients has a much higher sensitivity and specificity than previously reported and is positive in most patients with *Pneumocystis* pneumonia.[77]

The successful use of induced sputum for the diagnosis of *P. carinii* pneumonia is tedious and requires specialized clinical laboratory expertise to obtain reproducible and reliable results. In laboratories with specialized expertise in the examination of induced sputum for *P. carinii*, a modified Giemsa or Gomori methenamine silver stain correctly identifies more than 55% of *P. carinii* cases in AIDS patients later found to have *P. carinii* pneumonia.[78] The sensitivity of this test can be improved if the sputum is first liquefied and concentrated with dithiothreitol and by sedimentation before staining.[79] Newer direct and indirect immunofluorescence techniques using monoclonal antibodies to *P. carinii* have much higher sensitivities (92%–97%) and

no reported false-positive results.[80, 81] The sensitivity of induced sputum for identifying *P. carinii* pneumonia in AIDS patients receiving aerosolized pentamidine is similar to that of patients not receiving prophylaxis.[82] Unfortunately, the sensitivity of an induced sputum is not high enough to confidently exclude the diagnosis of *P. carinii* pneumonia if a negative smear is obtained.

In the case of repeatedly negative sputum smears, a more invasive diagnostic procedure is required. Transthoracic or transtracheal needle aspiration techniques have been tried but are no more sensitive than the currently available induced sputum techniques and carry a significantly greater risk of morbidity.[2, 46] These techniques are not recommended for routine diagnostic testing. Nonbronchoscopic lung lavage using a blindly placed tracheal catheter has been successfully used in the diagnosis of *P. carinii* pneumonia. This technique has a sensitivity and specificity of 87% and 100%, respectively, approaching that obtained by BAL.[83] This may be an attractive alternative to bronchoscopy and BAL in endotracheally intubated patients.[84]

If the results of sputum analysis and nonbronchoscopic lavage are negative, flexible fiberoptic bronchoscopy is the procedure of choice. BAL and transbronchial lung biopsy are highly sensitive and specific techniques for identifying *P. carinii* infections in a variety of immunocompromised hosts (Fig. 37–4).[85–88] The diagnostic sensitivity of combined BAL and transbronchial biopsy for identifying *P. carinii* is 100%, and the sensitivity of each test alone is approximately 97%.[86, 89] Because of the increased risk of hemorrhage and pneumothorax associated with transbronchial biopsy, it is recommended that patients with AIDS have bronchoscopy with BAL alone performed first. If nondiagnostic, lavage can be repeated and combined with transbronchial biopsy. In patients who are receiving inhaled pentamidine prophylaxis, the diagnostic yield of BAL alone has been reported to be lower (62%), and both BAL and transbronchial biopsy were recommended to be performed initially.[76]

Because of the high diagnostic yield and low morbidity associated with bronchoscopy using BAL with or without transbronchial biopsy, open lung biopsy is rarely indicated. Open lung biopsy for the diagnosis of *P. carinii* pneumonia should be reserved for those situations in which a high index of suspicion for *P. carinii* exists and BAL and transbronchial biopsy have been repeatedly nondiagnostic. The sensitivity of open lung biopsy is not significantly greater than that of combined BAL and transbronchial biopsy.[53]

The clinician's decision to choose a particular diagnostic approach must balance the probability that a test will obtain an accurate diagnosis with the cost and morbidity associated with that test. Failure to correctly identify cases of isolated or combined infection, malignancy, cytotoxic drug reaction, or progression of the primary disease may delay effective therapy and increase the morbidity and cost of medical care. For example, in hospitals with small numbers of patients with AIDS, sputum analysis for *P. carinii* pneumonia has been notoriously inaccurate, but in major endemic areas, sputum analysis is often the diagnostic method of choice. The clinician must consider the experience of the technical service in obtaining the sputum sample and the skill of the laboratory in identifying the organisms. In AIDS patients with evidence of lung infection, sputum samples can easily be obtained; if not diagnostic, bronchoscopy with BAL can be performed quickly.

## TREATMENT

Most therapeutic agents available for the prophylaxis and treatment of *P. carinii* pneumonia belong to the aromatic diamidine and folate antagonist classes of drugs (Table 37–2). Pentamidine isethionate, an effective antiprotozoal antibiotic, was initially the drug of choice in the treatment of *P. carinii* pneumonia in non-AIDS immunocompromised patients.[46, 90] Pentamidine, despite its therapeutic efficacy, has numerous undesirable side defects. Pain, swelling, and sterile abscess formation occur commonly at the site of intramuscular injection. Significant hypotension may occur after a single intramuscular dose or after rapid intravenous infusions; mild to life-threatening hypoglycemia in 6% to 9% of patients may occur during or shortly after drug administration. Insulin-requiring diabetes mellitus has developed as a consequence of pentamidine administration. Other adverse drug effects include thrombophlebitis, localized or generalized urticarial skin eruptions, reversible acute renal failure, azotemia, hepatic transaminase elevation, neutropenia, thrombocytopenia, fever, hypocalcemia, mental status changes, and life-threatening ventricular arrhythmias.[90]

In the mid-1970s, trimethoprim-sulfamethoxazole was found to be as efficacious as pentamidine for the treatment of *Pneumocystis* pneumonia.[91, 92] In the AIDS and non-AIDS immunosuppressed patient populations, the incidence of adverse reactions to pentamidine is greater than 70%.[93] However, in non-AIDS patients receiving trimethoprim-sulfamethoxazole for *P. carinii* pneumonia, the incidence of adverse reactions is less than 10%.[92, 93] Most reactions are minor and include gastrointestinal upset and rash. Trimethoprim-sulfamethoxazole is the preferred drug for treatment of *P. carinii* pneumonia in this group of patients.

AIDS patients with *Pneumocystis* pneumonia have a greater incidence of toxic and "allergic" drug reactions when treated with trimethoprim-sulfamethoxazole than they do with pentamidine.[94] Trimethoprim-sulfamethoxazole in AIDS patients is associated with adverse reactions in 50% to 80% of patients, with toxic reactions serious enough to require a change of therapy to another drug in 50%.[94, 95] Rash, fever, neutropenia, and hepatic transaminase elevation are the most commonly reported toxicities in AIDS patients.[94] Despite the apparent predisposition of AIDS patients to sulfonamide reactions, trimethoprim-sulfamethoxazole has been shown to be significantly more effective and to have fewer serious reactions than intravenous pentamidine.[95]

A 21-day course of intravenous or oral trimethoprim-sulfamethoxazole (20 mg/kg/d and 100 mg/kg/d, respectively), given in four divided doses, is the preferred therapy for *P. carinii* pneumonia in AIDS and non-AIDS patients. A 21-day course of intravenous pentamidine isethionate (4 mg/kg/d) is the alternate choice. Because of the high incidence of adverse side effects with both drugs, a reduced dose of trimethoprim-sulfamethoxazole (15 mg/kg/d and 75 mg/kg/d, respectively) or pentamidine (3 mg/kg/d) appears to improve patient tolerance without compromising efficacy.[95]

Despite the apparent success of trimethoprim-sulfamethoxazole and pentamidine in the treatment of *P. carinii* pneumonia, failure to respond to treatment occurs in 20% to 30% of patients,[93] and different treatment regimens are being investigated.

**Table 37–2. Recommended Antimicrobial Agents and Alternatives for the Treatment of *Pneumocystis carinii* Pneumonia**

| Agent | Route | Dose |
|---|---|---|
| Conventional treatment | | |
| Trimethoprim* | IV or PO | 20 mg/kg/d in four divided doses |
| Plus sulfamethoxazole† | IV or PO | 100 mg/kg/d in four divided doses |
| Pentamidine isethionate‡ | IM or IV | 4 mg/kg/d single dose |
| Investigational treatment | | |
| Trimethoprim* | IV or PO | 20 mg/kg/d in four divided doses |
| Plus dapsone† | PO | 100 mg/kg/d single dose |
| Primaquine§ | PO | 30 mg/d single dose |
| Plus clindamycin§ | IV or PO | 3600 mg/d in four divided doses |
| Trimetrexate* | IV | 30 mg/m²/d single dose |
| Plus leucovorin | IV or PO | 20 mg/m²/d q 6 h |

*Dihydrofolate reductase inhibitor.
†Para-aminobenzoic acid–dihydrofolate pathway inhibitor.
‡Aromatic diamidine.
§Other mechanism of action.

Trimethoprim alone has no discernible effect on *P. carinii* infection.[94] Similarly, isolated treatment with the sulfone dapsone has poor efficacy in the treatment of *P. carinii* pneumonia.[96] However, the combination of trimethoprim and dapsone (20 mg/kg/d in four divided doses and 100 mg/d as a single dose, respectively) has been demonstrated in uncontrolled trials to be as effective as trimethoprim-sulfamethoxazole but with fewer associated toxic effects.[97] Seventy per cent of patients who experience adverse reactions to trimethoprim-sulfamethoxazole are able to tolerate trimethoprim-dapsone.[93]

The use of the antimalarial drug primaquine alone or the lincosamine clindamycin alone was ineffective in the treatment of *P. carinii* pneumonia. Small clinical trials have revealed a synergy between the two drugs, demonstrating the clindamycin-primaquine combination to be an effective treatment for *P. carinii* pneumonia.[98, 99] This combination does not include a sulfone or sulfonamide, and intravenous clindamycin (3600 mg/d in four divided doses) plus oral primaquine (30 mg/d as a single dose) has fewer adverse drug reactions in HIV-infected patients than the standard dose of trimethoprim-sulfamethoxazole.[99] As with dapsone, primaquine therapy has a significant risk of methemoglobinemia and hemolysis in glucose-6-phosphate–deficient patients.

Trimetrexate and piritrexim are potent inhibitors of mammalian and microbial dihydrofolate reductase. Leucovorin is a charged folate analog that requires an active transport system to enter into cells. Mammalian cells possess this transport system, but *Pneumocystis* does not; a trimetrexate-leucovorin combination therefore can be selectively toxic to *P. carinii* organisms. Treatment success rates using intravenous trimetrexate (30 mg/m² as a single dose) and intravenous or oral leucovorin (20 mg/m² every 6 hours) are lower than those achieved with trimethoprim-sulfamethoxazole, and patients treated with trimetrexate and leucovorin have a high incidence of relapse.[100]

Aerosolized pentamidine, effective in the primary and secondary prophylaxis of *P. carinii* pneumonia,[101, 102] has not been demonstrated to be an effective treatment alternative for *P. carinii* pneumonia. This is true despite the ability of aerosolization to achieve significantly higher pentamidine concentrations in the bronchoalveolar secretions compared with intravenously administered pentamidine.

Despite the increasing armamentarium for the treatment of *P. carinii* pneumonia, a significant number of patients receiving optimal anti-*P. carinii* therapy progress to respiratory failure, and the mortality rate remains high. The adjuvant use of corticosteroids with specific anti-*Pneumocystis* therapy has reduced the risk of respiratory failure and death among patients with AIDS and moderate to severe *P. carinii* pneumonia.[103–105] The use of corticosteroids has reduced the incidence of drug toxicity, reduced the severity and duration of hypoxemia that frequently occurs early after initiation of anti-*Pneumocystis* therapy, and accelerated the rate of recovery as measured by oxygen saturations, serum LDH concentrations, vital signs, and exercise tolerance.[104, 105]

It is paradoxic that corticosteroids, which are used to induce latent *P. carinii* pneumonia in laboratory animals, appear to have a beneficial impact on the course of *P. carinii* pneumonia in HIV-infected patients. The mechanism of the improvement has not been delineated.

Adjunctive corticosteroid treatment should be administered to any adult or adolescent with documented or suspected HIV infection and documented or suspected *P. carinii* pneumonia if at the time of presentation the room air Pao₂ is less than 70 mm Hg or the (A-a) O₂ gradient is greater than 35 mm Hg. Corticosteroid treatment should be initiated concomitantly with specific anti-*P. carinii* therapy and continued throughout the duration of therapy. The recommended dose of prednisone or prednisolone is in the range of 40 mg every 12 hours to 60 mg every 24 hours for the first 5 to 7 days of treatment, followed by a dose tapering to zero by day 21.[106]

The effects of a tapering 3-week course of steroids on the relapse rate of *P. carinii* pneumonia or the predisposition to or augmentation of concomitant opportunistic infections is not known. In reports of steroid use during only the initial week of treatment, there is no demonstration of increased incidence of opportunistic infection or relapse of *P. carinii* pneumonia.[107]

## PROPHYLAXIS

The risk of primary *P. carinii* pneumonia is directly proportional to the degree of immunosuppression. For AIDS patients, *P. carinii* pneumonia prophylaxis should be started if the CD4⁺ lymphocyte count falls below 200/mm³ or below 20% of the total lymphocyte count.[108] The relapse rate for *P. carinii* infection among AIDS patients is greater than 50% at 6 months,[102] but relapse occurs in only 10% to 20% of patients immunosuppressed from other causes per year.[46] The increased incidence of relapse in AIDS patients may be related to their progressive immunosuppression and to the failure to sterilize the lung with therapy. In AIDS patients, repeat bronchoscopy after specific anti-*P. carinii* treatment reveals persistent organisms; this is a rare finding in non-AIDS patients treated for *P. carinii* pneumonia.[38, 109, 110]

Antibiotic prophylaxis for *Pneumocystis* pneumonia in HIV infection is discussed in Chapter 50. In non–HIV-related immunodeficiency, trimethoprim-sulfamethoxazole is well tolerated and effective for primary and secondary *P. carinii* pneumonia prophylaxis when administered orally 2 to 3 consecutive days per week or on alternate days.[111]

## REFERENCES

1. Van der Meer G, Brug SL: Infection par *Pneumocystis* chez l'homme et chez les animaux. Ann Soc Belg Med Trop 22:301, 1942.
2. Walzer PD, Perl DP, Krogstad DS, et al: *Pneumocystis carinii* pneumonia in the United States. Epidemiologic, diagnostic, and clinical features. Ann Intern med 80:83, 1974.
3. Hughes WT: *Pneumocystis carinii* pneumonia. Chest 85:810, 1984.
4. Hughes WT, Smith B: Provocation of infection due to *Pneumocystis carinii* by cyclosporin A. J Infect Dis 145:767, 1982.
5. Hopewell PC: *Pneumocystis carinii* pneumonia: Diagnosis. J Infect Dis 157:1115, 1988.
6. Harmsen AG, Stankiewicz M: Requirement for CD4⁺ cells in resistance to *Pneumocystis carinii* pneumonia in mice. J Exp Med 172:937, 1990.
7. Shellito J, Suzara VV, Blumenfeld W, et al: A new model of *Pneumocystis carinii* infection in mice selectively depleted of helper T lymphocytes. J Clin Invest 85:1686, 1990.
8. Masur H, Ognibene FP, Yarchoan R, et al: CD4 counts as predictors

of opportunistic pneumonias in human immunodeficiency virus (HIV) infection. Ann Intern Med 111:223, 1989.

9. Hong S-T, Steele PE, Cushion MT, et al: *Pneumocystis carinii* karyotypes. J Clin Microbiol 28:1785, 1990.

10. Chagas C: Nova tripanozomiaze humana. Mem Instit Oswaldo Cruz 1:159, 1909.

11. Edman U, Edman JC, Lundgren B, et al: Isolation and expression of the *Pneumocystis carinii* thymidylate synthase gene. Proc Natl Acad Sci USA 86:6503, 1989.

12. Edman JC, Kovacs JA, Masur H, et al: Ribosomal RNA sequence shows *Pneumocystis carinii* to be a member of the fungi. Nature 334:519, 1988.

13. Stringer SL, Stringer JR, Blase MA, et al: *Pneumocystis carinii*: Sequence from ribosomal RNA implies a close relationship with fungi. Exp Parasitol 68:450, 1989.

14. Masur H, Lane HC, Kovacs JA, et al: *Pneumocystis* pneumonia: From bench to clinic. Ann Intern Med 111:813, 1989.

15. Matsumoto Y, Matsuda S, Tegoshi T: Yeast glucan in the cyst wall of *Pneumocystis carinii*. J Protozool 36:21S, 1989.

16. Cushion MT, Ruffolo JJ, Walzer PD: Analysis of the developmental stages of *Pneumocystis carinii*, in vitro. Lab Invest 58:324, 1988.

17. Vavra J, Kucera K: *Pneumocystis carinii delanoe*, its ultrastructure and ultrastructural affinities. J Protozool 17:463, 1970.

18. Walzer PD: *Pneumocystis carinii*—new clinical spectrum? [Editorial] N Engl J Med 324:263, 1991.

19. Murray JF: Deposition of particles and vapors. *In* Murray JF (ed): The Normal Lung. Philadelphia, WB Saunders, 1986:316.

20. Hughes WT: Natural mode of acquisition for de novo infection with *Pneumocystis carinii*. J Infect Dis 145:842, 1982.

21. Hughes WT, Bartley DL, Smith BM: A natural source of infection due to *Pneumocystis carinii*. J Infect Dis 147:595, 1983.

22. Singer C, Armstrong D, Rosen PP, et al: *Pneumocystis carinii* pneumonia: A cluster of eleven cases. Ann Intern Med 82:772, 1975.

23. Ruebush TK II, Weinstein RA, Baehner RL, et al: An outbreak of *Pneumocystis* pneumonia in children with acute lymphocytic leukemia. Am J Dis Child 132:143, 1978.

24. Giron JA, Martinex S, Walzer PD: Should patients with *Pneumocystis carinii* be isolated? [Letter] Lancet 2:46, 1982.

25. Jacobs JL, Libby DM, Winters RA, et al: A cluster of *Pneumocystis carinii* pneumonia in adults without predisposing illnesses. N Engl J Med 324:246, 1991.

26. Meuwissen JHET, Taber I, Leeuwenberg ADEM, et al: Parasitologic and serologic observations of infection with *Pneumocystis* in humans. J Infect Dis 136:43, 1977.

27. Pifer LL, Hughes WT, Stagno S, et al: *Pneumocystis carinii* infection: Evidence for high prevalence in normal and immunosuppressed children. Pediatrics 61:35, 1978.

28. Frenkel JK, Good JT, Schultz JA: Latent *Pneumocystis carinii* infection in rats, relapse and chemotherapy. Lab Invest 15:1559, 1966.

29. Henderson DW, Humeniuk V, Meadows R, et al: *Pneumocystis carinii* pneumonia with vascular and lymph node involvement. Pathology 6:235, 1974.

30. Unger PD, Rosenblum M, Krown SE: Disseminated *Pneumocystis carinii* infection in a patient with acquired immunodeficiency syndrome. Hum Pathol 19:113, 1988.

31. Cohen OJ, Stoeckle MY: Extrapulmonary *Pneumocystis carinii* infections in the acquired immunodeficiency syndrome. Arch Intern Med 151:1205, 1991.

32. Lankin PN, Minda M, Pietra GG, et al: Alveolar response to experimental *Pneumocystis carinii* pneumonia in the rat. Am J Pathol 99:561, 1980.

33. Henshaw NG, Carson JL, Collier AM: Ultrastructural observations of *Pneumocystis carinii* attachment to rat lung. J Infect Dis 151:181, 1985.

34. Yoneda K, Walzer PD: Interaction of *Pneumocystis carinii* with host lungs: An ultrastructural study. Infect Immun 29:692, 1980.

35. Yoneda K, Walzer PD: Mechanism of pulmonary alveolar injury in experimental *Pneumocystis carinii* pneumonia in the rat. Br J Exp Pathol 62:339, 1981.

36. Pottratz ST, Martin WJ II: Role of fibronectin in *Pneumocystis carinii* attachment to cultured lung cells. J Clin Invest 85:351, 1990.

37. Breite WM, Bailey AM, Kachel DL, et al: *Pneumocystis carinii* contain a serine proteinase capable of degrading fibronectin. [Abstract] Clin Res 39:728a, 1991.

38. DeLorenzo LJ, Maguire GP, Wormser GP, et al: Persistence of *Pneumocystis carinii* pneumonia in the acquired immunodeficiency syndrome: Evaluation of therapy by follow-up transbronchial lung biopsy. Chest 88:79, 1985.

39. Blumenfeld W, Basgoz N, Owen WF, et al: Granulomatous pulmonary lesions in patients with the acquired immunodeficiency syndrome (AIDS) and *Pneumocystis carinii* infection. Ann Intern Med 109:505, 1988.

40. Rosen SH, Castleman B, Liebow AA: Pulmonary alveolar proteinosis. N Engl J Med 258:1123, 1958.

41. Van Nheiu JT, Vojtek A-M, Bernaudin J-F, et al: Pulmonary alveolar proteinosis associated with *Pneumocystis carinii*. Chest 98:801, 1991.

42. Pesanti EL: Phospholipid profile of *Pneumocystis carinii* and its interaction with alveolar type II epithelial cells. Infect Immun 55:736, 1987.

43. Zimmerman PE, Voelker DR, McCormack FX, et al: The 120 kD surface glycoprotein of *Pneumocystis carinii* is a ligand for surfactant protein A. J Clin Invest 86:143, 1992.

44. Kuroki Y, Mason RJ, Voelker DR: Pulmonary surfactant apoprotein A: Structure and modulation of surfactant secretion by rat alveolar type II cells. J Biol Chem 263:3388, 1988.

45. Phelps DS, Rose RM: Increased recovery of surfactant protein A in AIDS-related pneumonia. Am Rev Respir Dis 143:1072, 1991.

46. Petersen C, Slutkin G, Mills J: Parasitic infections. *In* Murray JF, Nadel JA (eds): Textbook of Respiratory Medicine. Philadelphia, WB Saunders, 1988:950.

47. Kovacs JA, Hiemenz JW, Macher AM, et al: *Pneumocystis carinii* pneumonia: A comparison between patients with acquired immunodeficiency syndrome and patients with other immunodeficiencies. Ann Intern Med 100:663, 1984.

48. Peters SG, Prakash UB: *Pneumocystis carinii* pneumonia: Review of 53 cases. Am J Med 82:73, 1973.

49. Stover DE, White DA, Romano PA, et al: Spectrum of pulmonary disease associated with the acquired immune deficiency syndrome. Am J Med 78:429, 1985.

50. Edelstein H, McCabe RE: Atypical presentations of *Pneumocystis carinii* pneumonia in patients receiving inhaled pentamidine prophylaxis. Chest 98:1366, 1990.

51. DeLorenzo LJ, Huang CT, Maguire GP, et al: Roentgenographic patterns of *Pneumocystis carinii* pneumonia in 104 patients with AIDS. Chest 91:323, 1987.

52. McClellan MD, Miller SB, Parsons PE, et al: Pneumothorax with *Pneumocystis carinii* pneumonia in AIDS. Chest 100:1224, 1991.

53. Murray JF, Felton CP, Garay SM, et al: Pulmonary complications of the acquired immunodeficiency syndrome: Report of a National Heart, Lung, and Blood Institute workshop. N Engl J Med 310:1682, 1984.

54. Bower M, Simon BE, Nelson MR, et al: The significance of the detection of cytomegalovirus in the bronchoalveolar lavage fluid in AIDS patients with pneumonia. AIDS 4:317, 1990.

55. Torrents C, Alvarez-Castells A, de Vera PV, et al: Postpneumocystis aspergilloma in AIDS: CT features. J Comput Assist Tomogr 15:304, 1991.

56. Masur H, Meier P, McCutchan JA, et al: Consensus statement on the use of corticosteroids as adjunctive therapy for *Pneumocystis* pneumonia in the acquired immunodeficiency syndrome. N Engl J Med 323:1500, 1990.

57. Limper AH, Offord KP, Smith TF, et al: *Pneumocystis carinii* pneumonia: Differences in lung parasite number and inflammation in patients with and without AIDS. Am Rev Respir Dis 140:1204, 1989.

58. Smith RL, El Sadr WM, Lewis ML: Correlation of bronchoalveolar lavage cell populations with clinical severity of *Pneumocystis carinii* pneumonia. Chest 92:60, 1988.

59. Mason GR, Hashimoto CH, Dickman PS, et al: Prognostic implications of bronchoalveolar lavage neutrophilia in patients with *Pneumocystis carinii* pneumonia and AIDS. Am Rev Respir Dis 139:1336, 1989.

60. Brenner M, Ognibene FP, Lack EE, et al: Prognostic factors and life expectancy of patients with acquired immunodeficiency syndrome and *Pneumocystis carinii* pneumonia. Am Rev Respir Dis 136:1199, 1987.

61. El Sadr W, Simberkoff MS: Survival and prognostic factors in severe *Pneumocystis carinii* pneumonia requiring mechanical ventilation. Am Rev Respir Dis 137:1264, 1987.

62. Wachter RM, Russi MB, Bloch DA, et al: *Pneumocystis carinii* pneumonia and respiratory failure in AIDS. Am Rev Respir Dis 143:251, 1991.

63. Zaman MK, White DA: Serum lactate dehydrogenase levels and *Pneumocystis carinii* pneumonia. Am Rev Respir Dis 137:796, 1988.

64. Friedman Y, Franklin C, Rackow EC, et al: Improved survival in patients with AIDS, *Pneumocystis carinii* pneumonia, and severe respiratory failure. Chest 96:862, 1989.

65. Gedroyc WMW, Reidy JF: The early chest radiograph changes of *Pneumocystis* pneumonia. Clin Radiol 36:331, 1985.

66. Pattison N, Wright T, Herrod HG, et al: *Pneumocystis carinii* pneumonitis, eosinophilia and hypogammaglobulinemia. Pediatr Infect Dis J 6:293, 1987.

67. Kagawa FT, Kirsh CM, Yenokida GG, et al: Serum lactate dehydrogenase activity in patients with AIDS and *Pneumocystis carinii* pneumonia. Chest 94:1031, 1988.

68. Silverman BA, Rubinstein A: Serum lactate dehydrogenase levels in adults and children with acquired immune deficiency syndrome (AIDS) and AIDS-related complex: Possible indicator of B cell lymphoproliferation and disease activity. Am J Med 78:728, 1985.

69. O'Brien RF: In search of shortcuts: Definitive and indirect tests in the diagnosis of *Pneumocystis carinii* pneumonia in AIDS. Am Rev Respir Dis 139:1324, 1989.

70. Boudes P: Practical utility of lactate dehydrogenase in the diagnosis of human immunodeficiency virus-related *Pneumocystis carinii* pneumonia. Arch Intern Med 151:198, 1991.

71. Stover DE, Greeno RA, Gagliardi AJ: The use of a simple exercise test for the diagnosis of *Pneumocystis carinii* pneumonia in patients with AIDS. Am Rev Respir Dis 139:1343, 1989.

72. Nisam M, Wong S, Fallat RJ: Pulse oximetry and diffusing capacity in AIDS patients with *Pneumocystis carinii* pneumonia. Chest 92:134s, 1987.

73. Shaw RJ, Roussak C, Forster SM, et al: Lung function abnormalities in patients infected with the human immunodeficiency virus with and without overt pneumonitis. Thorax 43:436, 1988.

74. Coleman DL, Hattner RS, Luce JM, et al: Correlation between gallium lung scans and fiberoptic bronchoscopy in patients with suspected *Pneumocystis carinii* pneumonia and the acquired immune deficiency syndrome. Am Rev Respir Dis 130:1166, 1984.

75. Kramer EL, Sanger JJ, Garay SM, et al: Gallium-67 scans of the chest in patients with acquired immunodeficiency syndrome. J Nucl Med 28:1107, 1987.

76. Jules-Elysee KM, Stover DE, Zaman MB, et al: Aerosolized pentamidine: Effect on diagnosis and presentation of *Pneumocystis carinii* pneumonia. Ann Intern Med 112:750, 1990.

77. Masur H, Gill VJ, Ognibene FP, et al: Diagnosis of *Pneumocystis* pneumonia by induced sputum technique in patients without the acquired immunodeficiency syndrome. Ann Intern Med 109:755, 1988.

78. Pitchenik AE, Ganjei P, Torres A, et al: Sputum examination for the diagnosis of *Pneumocystis carinii* pneumonia in the acquired immunodeficiency syndrome. Am Rev Respir Dis 133:226, 1986.

79. Zaman MK, Wooten OJ, Suprahmanya B, et al: Rapid noninvasive diagnosis of *Pneumocystis carinii* from induced liquefied sputum. Ann Intern Med 109:7, 1988.

80. Kovacs JA, Ng VL, Masur H, et al: Diagnosis of *Pneumocystis carinii* pneumonia: Improved detection in sputum with use of monoclonal antibodies. N Engl J Med 318:589, 1988.

81. Cregan P, Yamamoto A, Lum A, et al: Comparison of four methods for rapid detection of *Pneumocystis carinii* in respiratory specimens. J Clin Microbiol 28:2432, 1990.

82. Metersky ML, Catanzaro A: Diagnostic approach to *Pneumocystis carinii* pneumonia in the setting of prophylactic aerosolized pentamidine. Chest 100:1345, 1991.

83. Martin WR, Albertson TE, Siegel B: Tracheal catheters in patients with acquired immunodeficiency syndrome for the diagnosis of *Pneumocystis carinii* pneumonia. Chest 98:29, 1990.

84. Caughey G, Wong H, Gamsu G, et al: Nonbronchoscopic bronchoalveolar lavage for the diagnosis of *Pneumocystis carinii* pneumonia in the acquired immunodeficiency syndrome. Chest 88:659, 1985.

85. Coleman DL, Dodek PM, Luce JM, et al: Diagnostic utility of fiberoptic bronchoscopy in patients with *Pneumocystis carinii* pneumonia and the acquired immune deficiency syndrome. Am Rev Respir Dis 128:795, 1983.

86. Broaddus C, Dake MD, Stulbarg MS, et al: Bronchoalveolar lavage and transbronchial biopsy for the diagnosis of pulmonary infections in the acquired immunodeficiency syndrome. Ann Intern Med 102:747, 1985.

87. Ellis JH: Transbronchial lung biopsy via the fiberoptic bronchoscope. Chest 68:524, 1975.

88. Kelley J, Landis JN, Davis GS, et al: Diagnosis of pneumonia due to *Pneumocystis* by subsegmental pulmonary lavage via the fiberoptic bronchoscope. Chest 74:24, 1978.

89. Golden JA, Hollander H, Stulbarg MS, et al: Bronchoalveolar lavage as the exclusive diagnostic modality for *Pneumocystis carinii* pneumonia. Chest 90:18, 1986.

90. Pearson RD, Hewlett EL: Pentamidine for the treatment of *Pneumocystis carinii* pneumonia and other protozoal diseases. Ann Intern Med 103:782, 1985.

91. Hughes WT, McNabb PC, Makres TD, et al: Efficacy of trimethoprim and sulfamethoxazole in the prevention and treatment of *Pneumocystis carinii* pneumonia. Antimicrob Agents Chemother 5:289, 1974.

92. Hughes WT, Feldman S, Chaudhary SC, et al: Comparison of pentamidine isethionate and trimethoprim sulfamethoxazole in the treatment of *Pneumocystis carinii* pneumonia. J Pediatr 92:285, 1978.

93. Hughes WT: Prevention and treatment of *Pneumocystis carinii* pneumonia. Annu Rev Med 42:287, 1991.

94. Gordin FM, Simon GL, Wofsy CB, et al: Adverse reactions to trimethoprim-sulfamethoxazole in patients with the acquired immunodeficiency syndrome. Ann Intern Med 100:495, 1984.

95. Sattler FR, Cowan R, Nielsen DM, et al: Trimethoprim-sulfamethoxazole compared with pentamidine for treatment of *Pneumocystis carinii* pneumonia in the acquired immunodeficiency syndrome. Ann Intern Med 109:280, 1988.

96. Mills J, Leoung G, Medina I, et al: Dapsone treatment of *Pneumocystis carinii* pneumonia in the acquired immunodeficiency syndrome. Antimicrob Agents Chemother 32:1057, 1988.

97. Leoung GS, Mills J, Hopewell PC, et al: Dapsone-trimethoprim for *Pneumocystis carinii* pneumonia in the acquired immunodeficiency syndrome. Ann Intern Med 105:45, 1986.

98. Kay R, DuBois RE: Clindamycin/primaquine therapy and secondary prophylaxis against *Pneumocystis carinii* pneumonia in patients with AIDS. South Med J 83:403, 1990.

99. Ruf B, Rohde I, Pohle HD: Efficacy of clindamycin/primaquine (C-P) vs trimethoprim/sulfamethoxazole (TMP/SMZ) in acute treatment of *Pneumocystis carinii* pneumonia (PCP). Am Rev Respir Dis 141:A154, 1990.

100. Allegra CJ, Chabner BA, Tuazon CU, et al: Trimetrexate for the treatment of *Pneumocystis carinii* pneumonia in patients with the acquired immunodeficiency syndrome. N Engl J Med 317:978, 1987.

101. Hirschel B, Lazzarin A, Chopard P, et al: A controlled study of inhaled pentamidine for primary prevention of *Pneumocystis carinii* pneumonia. N Engl J Med 324:1079, 1991.

102. Montaner JSG, Lawson LM, Gervais A, et al: Aerosol pentamidine for secondary prophylaxis of AIDS-related *Pneumocystis carinii* pneumonia. Ann Intern Med 114:948, 1991.

103. Bossette SA, Sattler FR, Chiu J, et al: Controlled trial of early adjunctive treatment with corticosteroids for *Pneumocystis carinii* pneumonia in the acquired immunodeficiency syndrome. N Engl J Med 323:1451, 1990.

104. Walmsley S, Salit IE, Brunton J: The possible role of corticosteroid therapy for *Pneumocystis carinii* pneumonia in the acquired immunodeficiency syndrome (AIDS). J Acquir Immune Defic Syndr 1:354, 1988.

105. Montaner JSG, Lawson LM, Levitt N, et al: Corticosteroids prevent early deterioration in patients with moderately severe *Pneumocystis carinii* pneumonia and the acquired immunodeficiency syndrome (AIDS). Ann Intern Med 113:14, 1990.

106. Koraks JA, Masur H: Are corticosteroids beneficial as adjunctive therapy for *Pneumocystis* pneumonia in AIDS? Ann Intern Med 113:1, 1990.

107. Lambertus MW, Goetz MB: Complications of corticosteroid therapy in patients with acquired immunodeficiency syndrome and *Pneumocystis carinii* pneumonia. Chest 98:38, 1990.

108. Centers for Disease Control: Guidelines for prophylaxis against *Pneumocystis carinii* pneumonia for persons infected with human immunodeficiency virus. MMWR 38(suppl 5):1, 1989.

109. Shelhamer JH, Ognibene FP, Macher AM, et al: Persistence of *Pneumocystis carinii* in lung tissue of acquired immunodeficiency syndrome patients treated for *Pneumocystis* pneumonia. Am Rev Respir Dis 130:1161, 1984.

110. Ruskin J: Newer developments in diagnosis and treatment of *Pneumocystis* infections. *In* Remington JS, Swartz MN (eds): Current Clinical Topics in Infectious Diseases. New York, McGraw-Hill International, 1986:194.

111. Wormser GP, Horowitz HW, Duncanson FP, et al: Low-dose intermittent trimethoprim-sulfamethoxazole for prevention of *Pneumocystis carinii* pneumonia in patients with human immunodeficiency virus infection. Arch Intern Med 151:688, 1991.

# CHAPTER 38

# Tuberculosis

JEFFREY GLASSROTH

The genus *Mycobacterium* contains numerous species, of which *Mycobacterium tuberculosis* is the most virulent. Worldwide, it is estimated that 1 billion persons are infected with *M. tuberculosis*, that there are as many as 16 million cases of disease each year, and that about 3 million persons die each year of their disease.[1] For many years, the situation in the United States and much of the developed world belied these figures. New cases of tuberculosis (TB) declined throughout the United States, and it was even anticipated that TB might be eradicated early in the next century. However, a variety of geopolitical, socioeconomic, and biologic conditions have contributed to reversal of the decline in TB in the United States. Moreover, many of these new cases of disease present special problems in diagnosis and treatment that did not exist as recently as a decade ago.

## PATHOBIOLOGY OF TUBERCULOSIS

*M. tuberculosis* is invariably transmitted through infected respiratory secretions known as droplet nucleii. These particles, particularly those about 1 to 5 μm in diameter, are readily produced when an infectious patient with respiratory TB coughs or speaks.[2] Infected droplet nuclei may be inhaled by contacts of the source case. If they are inhaled by a previously uninfected, "naive" host, a series of events, some poorly understood, ensue. Tubercle bacilli probably multiply, unimpeded by specific immunity. A period of asymptomatic lymphohematogenous spread probably occurs in which mycobacteria translocate to many organs, creating the potential for later extrapulmonary disease. At the same time, mycobacterial antigens are processed by the host immune system, with initial stages probably involving subsets of T lymphocytes known as γ-δ T cells and macrophages. Over a period of weeks, specific immunity involving helper T lymphocytes develops. These events result in the containment of the primary infection and the prevention of subsequent disease.

Associated with the development of specific immunity is the development of skin test reactivity to antigens such as tuberculin, which are derived from *M. tuberculosis*. Skin test reactivity serves as a convenient marker for infection by the organism. It is generally thought that most TB results from progression of the primary infection or from reactivation after some period (often years) of quiescence after the initial infection. The host immune response to the tubercle bacillus is probably responsible for a substantial amount of the tissue damage occurring in cases of active disease. Approximately 10% of persons infected with *M. tuberculosis* develop TB, about half in the first 1 to 2 years after infection. Although it is relatively easy to appreciate why persons with defects of cellular immunity such as those resulting from infection with the human immunodeficiency virus (HIV) might not effectively contain tubercle bacilli after infection, it is less clear why other, ostensibly healthy persons, progress to active disease.

## EPIDEMIOLOGY

Although all population groups have some risk of TB, that risk is not equally distributed (Table 38–1). In the United States, a substantial proportion of TB cases continue to arise from a pool of 8 to 10 million previously (remotely) infected persons. However, recent trends suggest that an increasing proportion of patients were more recently infected. If the age of TB patients is considered by racial groupings, blacks and Hispanics between the ages of 25 and 44 years have had an increase of more than 25% in TB cases between 1986 and 1988. In contrast, the rate for non-Hispanic whites of the same age increased only 0.5% during those years.

Table 38–1. **Estimated Relative Risk of Tuberculosis**

| Factor | Relative Risk* |
|---|---|
| Living in the United States | 1.0 |
| Nonhispanic white, living in the community | 0.58 |
| Minority groups (U.S. born) | 4.8–10.1 |
| Foreign born | 13.1 |
| HIV-infected person | 11.0 |
| Prison inmate | 3.9–11.6 |
| Nursing home resident | 1.8–5.7 |

*An annual tuberculosis case rate of 9.5 per 100,000 is assumed for all persons living in the United States (ie, relative risk = 1.0). Available data for specified subgroups are then compared with that rate to develop the estimates of relative risk.

The age shift in tuberculosis is also related to the fact that about 25% of TB cases in the United States now occur among foreign-born persons, who tend to be younger. The period of greatest risk is within the first 1 to 2 years of arrival in the United States, with 55% of the TB in foreign-born persons occurring during that period. Not all groups are equally at risk, and the risk of members of a particular group reflects the prevalence of TB in their country of origin. Immigrants from Central and South America, the Caribbean, Africa, and Southeast Asia appear to have the highest TB risk. Persons infected with HIV tend to be young and also appear to be quite sensitive to infection with *M. tuberculosis.* After infection, they appear to progress to active disease at a rate of at least 7% to 8% per year.[3] The entire progression may occur within days or weeks of the initial infection.[4] This represents an extraordinarily rapid pace and a serious challenge to TB control programs.

Institutionalized persons appear to be at increased risk of TB. Several elegant studies indicated that TB risk may be increased severalfold among nursing home residents.[5, 6] Similar data from the nation's penal system indicate that at least some prisons also constitute an environment where TB occurs with increased frequency and from which it may reenter the general population.[7] Although it is difficult to define the precise magnitude of the problem, it appears that homeless persons may represent a growing proportion of the TB patients diagnosed in some areas of the United States.[8] Shelters, urban missions, and other facilities serving homeless persons should be included on the list of institutional settings worthy of special attention for purposes of TB control.

## CLINICAL PRESENTATION

Tuberculosis is a disease with protean clinical manifestations, and its occurrence in HIV-coinfected persons has increased the frequency with which hitherto "unusual" forms of TB are encountered. Overall, about 83% of TB patients in the United States have pulmonary disease, and the remainder have extrapulmonary disease with or without a pulmonary component. Among HIV-coinfected persons, this association is drastically altered and may even be reversed. In one report of 132 HIV-coinfected persons, 62% had extrapulmonary disease with or without a pulmonary component, and 38% had only pulmonary disease.[9] Although the location of the TB did not appear to correlate with stage of the HIV infection in that study, most experienced clinicians perceive that TB tends to be more "typical" in anatomic involvement, cavitation, and other features when encountered early in the course of HIV infection than when diagnosed during later stages.

The traditional teaching about pulmonary disease has been that TB involves primarily the upper lobe and superior segments of the lower lobes, often with cavitation.[10] However, there are many exceptions to this generalization. In a study performed in the pre-HIV era, Khan and colleagues reported a series of 88 patients with pulmonary TB seen in the Boston area. One third of these patients had atypical radiographic presentations of their disease. These included manifestations of primary infection with adenopathy and effusion, lower lung field disease, miliary disease, and single or multiple nodules (ie, tuberculoma).[11] Others have reported similar findings and have observed a particular propensity for alcoholics, diabetics, and pregnant women to develop tuberculosis involving the lower lung fields.[12] Generalized infiltrates and the adult respiratory distress syndrome have also been associated with TB.[13]

With the advent of HIV infection, previously unusual radiographic manifestations of TB are being encountered with increasing frequency. Pitchenik and Robinson in Florida compared the radiographic findings for 17 TB patients with AIDS with the findings for 30 TB patients who did not have AIDS. The TB/AIDS patients were significantly more likely to have adenopathy, lower lung field infiltrates, or diffuse interstitial infiltrates than the patients without AIDS. Conversely, two thirds of the non-AIDS patients had cavitation, but none of the TB/AIDS patients did.[14] Several TB/AIDS patients had normal chest x-ray films despite bacteriologically confirmed pulmonary TB. It should be emphasized that the TB/AIDS patients had advanced HIV infection as evidenced by their history of a prior AIDS-defining illness. Presumably, HIV-infected persons with less advanced infections and relatively preserved immunity may be expected to present more frequently with typical radiographic disease. However, clinicians must consider TB as a possible diagnosis with virtually any radiographic abnormality and, in some cases, even when the chest radiograph is normal.

Extrapulmonary disease accounts for about 17% of the tuberculosis diagnosed in the United States. Although any organ system may be involved, the sites most commonly seen, in declining order of frequency, are the lymph nodes, pleura, genitourinary tract, and the bones and joints. Meningeal TB accounts for about 1% of cases. Disease in any of these areas may present with localized symptoms, such as pain, swelling, or dysfunction of the involved organ, or as a constitutional process with less specific symptoms and signs. Among HIV-infected persons, extrapulmonary TB is especially frequent.[15, 16] The presentation of extrapulmonary TB in AIDS patients is similar in many respects to its presentation in more intact hosts. Because patients with HIV infection, particularly those with advanced infection, may have other comorbidities, it is relatively easy to attribute nonspecific or constitutional symptoms of TB to other conditions. Although the host response in these patients may be limited and cavitation, for example, is less common, the bacillary load is usually great in these patients. Blood, urine, or stool cultures positive for TB are far more common among AIDS patients than among non-AIDS patients.[17]

Table 38–2. **Available Diagnostic Tests**

| Test | Speed | Application Directly to Clinical Specimen | Relative Sensitivity | Relative Specificity |
|------|-------|------|------|------|
| AFB stain | Minutes | Yes | + | + |
| Conventional culture | Weeks–minutes | Yes | + + | + + + |
| Radiometric culture | Days–weeks | Yes | + + | + + + |
| Antigen detection | Weeks | No | + + | + + |
| HPLC | Weeks | No | + + | + + + |
| Nucleic acid probes | Weeks (require growing culture) | No | + + + | + + + |
| PCR + nucleic acid probes | Days | Yes | + + + | + + + |

AFB, acid-fast bacillus; HPLC, high-performance liquid chromatography; PCR, polymerase chain reaction.

Other groups seem to be particularly disposed to extrapulmonary disease. This includes intravenous drug users, even in the absence of HIV infection,[18] and patients undergoing maintenance hemodialysis.[19, 20] Organ transplantation is an increasingly common procedure. The most carefully studied group with respect to TB acquired after transplantation is renal transplant recipients. These patients appear to be at increased risk for TB, and the disease is extrapulmonary in as many as two thirds of cases, with disseminated disease accounting for much of the extrapulmonary disease.[21] Recipients of other types of transplants, who receive similar levels of immunosuppression, can be expected to have a similar clinical experience.

## APPROACH TO DIAGNOSIS

Until recently, the tools available for diagnosing TB had changed little from the earlier part of the century. Conventional culture techniques, often taking many weeks to complete, represented the ''gold standard'' of diagnosis. Staining for acid-fast bacilli (AFB) was a more rapid albeit less specific tool. Other studies, including the x-ray film and tuberculin skin test, provided circumstantial evidence that TB might be present.[22] Despite major developments in diagnostic technology, many of the classic diagnostic tools remain useful and will continue to play a role in the evaluation of the TB patient.

TB often produces nonspecific abnormalities in body fluids. For example, the blood may show a variety of cytopenias, monocytosis or lymphocytosis, and rarely demonstrate findings consistent with disseminated intravascular coagulation.[23, 24] Serum calcium is occasionally elevated, probably because of enhanced vitamin D metabolism by activated monocytes and macrophages.

If TB involves extrapulmonary sites, other, somewhat stereotypic abnormalities may be observed. Elevation of protein and reduction of glucose concentration may be observed in pleural, cerebrospinal, peritoneal, and joint fluids if TB involves these sites. Leukocytosis frequently occurs, initially with polymorphonuclear leukocytes (PMNs) predominating for the first several days. In joint effusions, PMNs tend to remain predominant, but in other fluids, lymphocytes usually become the most common cell. In pleural fluid, mesothelial cells are usually a common finding but account for fewer than 2% of cells if tuberculosis is the cause of effusion.[25]

Involvement of the genitourinary tract classically produces ''sterile'' pyuria, although microscopic hematuria and a reduced urine pH may also occur. These findings should prompt a urine culture for TB. Even in the presence of a normal urine sediment, urine cultures from patients with TB may be positive for *M. tuberculosis*. The rate of culture positivity approaches 20% among patients with disseminated disease.[26] Because of the relative frequency of extrapulmonary and disseminated TB among HIV-coinfected patients, urine culture for mycobacteria may be particularly useful.[17]

Conventional culture techniques use a variety of media, but these usually are egg-potato based (eg, Löwenstein-Jensen) or agar based (eg, Middlebrook 7H-11). Specimens must be prepared before culture. This includes an important digestion-decontamination step for specimens that are usually not sterile (eg, sputum). If growth occurs, speciation is performed by means of a series of physical and biochemical tests. Regardless of the initial handling of the specimen, it usually requires 3 to 6 weeks longer for the clinician to receive confirmation of a positive culture for *M. tuberculosis*. Conventional cultures are highly specific and have a sensitivity that is perhaps one log order greater than AFB smear. Cultures also permit the performance of drug susceptibility testing. Their major drawbacks are the time required for their completion (Table 38–2) and the need for a moderately sophisticated laboratory.

Classic staining for AFB is a rapid and relatively easy procedure requiring minimal equipment to perform. Variations on the traditional (eg, Ziehl-Neelsen) AFB stain are the fluorochrome stains such as auramine and rhodamine. Fluorochrome-stained specimens require a more sophisticated laboratory and a bright light (fluorescence) microscope. Their major advantage is enabling the microscopist to screen slides quickly for acid-fast material that stands out against the dark, nonfluorescent background on the slide. Because of a tendency for more frequent false-positive results with fluorochrome stains, positive slide results should be confirmed by conventional AFB staining techniques. AFB staining techniques have several advantages over other tests (see Table 38–2), including low cost and speed. The smear result, particularly in untreated patients, provides a measure of infectiousness because patients who are smear and culture positive appear far more infectious than those who are smear negative and culture positive.[27] Major drawbacks include the fact that these stains are not able to differentiate *M. tuberculosis* from other species of mycobacteria or other acid-fast genuses such as *Nocardia* and the relative insensitivity of these techniques. Smears are estimated to require about $10^4$ organisms/mm$^3$ of specimen to reliably produce a positive result.

A biopsy and histologic examination of involved tissues may be helpful in selected patients. Depending on the pattern that is found and whether acid-fast organisms are identified, the histologic findings may be ''highly suggestive'' of TB. In some situations, such as HIV-infection, there may be minimal tissue reaction even though AFB are abundant. Involvement of tissues that do not communicate externally often requires a biopsy to facilitate a diagnosis. For example, isolated pleural or peritoneal disease or interstitial involvement of the lung as it occurs in miliary TB are settings in which a biopsy may be helpful. Transbronchial biopsy may contribute to a diagnosis in as many as 85% of patients with a miliary pattern on their chest radiographs.[28] Transbronchial biopsy may also be useful in expediting a diagnosis of pulmonary TB in patients with more typical chest radiographic patterns but negative sputum smears. Although histologic analysis is helpful, the culture results of these biopsies are often negative.[29] Given the disseminated nature of miliary disease, extrapulmonary sites should also be considered for biopsy if that diagnosis is entertained.

The liver and bone marrow may be involved with miliary disease and may yield diagnostic information in 40% to 60% of patients. In this setting, a liver biopsy, although more invasive, seems to have a somewhat higher yield, with as many as 91% of specimens in one study showing granulomas (half with caseation) and 40% providing a positive culture. In contrast, bone marrow biopsy yielded granulomas, most noncaseating, in about half the patients and positive cultures for *M. tuberculosis* in only 25% of the patients.[30]

Newer innovations have accelerated the speed with which cultures can be grown and speciated and offer the potential for substantial additional progress. Radiometric culture systems are now used extensively. These systems incorporate a radiolabeled substrate such as $^{14}$C-palmitic acid into the culture media. As mycobacteria metabolize the substrate, radiolabeled $^{14}CO_2$ is released. This label can be detected well in advance of visible growth, which is the endpoint for conventional systems. By applying NAP (*p*-nitro-α-acetylamino-β-hydroxypropiophenone), which inhibits the growth of *M. tuberculosis* but not nontuberculous mycobacteria, tubercle bacilli can be differentiated from other species of mycobacteria. Radiometric assays are at least as sensitive as conventional cultures and provide identification of mycobacteria in about 1 week. Specimens with high concentrations of mycobacterial growth may produce a positive radiometric culture in as little as 3 days.[31] These culture systems can also be adapted for drug susceptibility testing of many antituberculosis agents with a similar savings in time. These systems are technically sophisticated and costly, making them most appropriate for relatively large microbiology laboratories. As these systems are further refined, alternative, nonradioactive endpoints will probably be used, making rapid culture systems even more attractive.

Nucleic acid probes have been used extensively for identifying other organisms and are now available for evaluating mycobacteria growing in culture. Nucleic acid probes use DNA (cDNA) or RNA (cRNA) that are complementary to unique portions of the nucleic acid within a particular species of mycobacteria. If the appropriate nucleic acid sequences are present in sufficient amounts within the sample, the cDNA or cRNA hybridizes with the native nucleic acid, producing a measurable signal endpoint. Although these systems are highly specific,[32] they require a high concentration of mycobacteria and related nucleic acid to obtain a positive result. Even using cRNA probes that hybridize with relatively abundant ribosomal RNA, as many as $10^5$ or $10^6$ mycobacteria must be present. This means that a growing culture must be obtained before the probe is applied. Although the actual probing can be rapidly accomplished, culture growth requires weeks for completion. Combining the probe with a radiometric culture system expedites the process further but still requires at least 1 week.[33]

Other technologies may permit even more rapid identification of mycobacteria. The polymerase chain reaction (PCR) may be used to amplify the amount of DNA in a clinical specimen. Over a number of cycles, taking only hours to complete, PCR can multiply the portion of nucleic acid that is of interest by several log orders of magnitude. This technology has been successfully applied to specimens such as sputum and has allowed accurate identification of mycobacteria in these specimens within 48 hours.[34]

A variety of chromatographic procedures, including gas-liquid chromatography and high-performance liquid chromatography, have been used to identify unique lipid moieties in mycobacteria. Although these techniques are rapid, they require special technological skills and high concentrations of mycobacteria to produce good results. Chromatography also requires growing cultures for at least several weeks.

Restriction fragment length polymorphism is an elegant new tool that has been used epidemiologically to provide DNA ''fingerprints.''[4] Highly specific enzymes (ie, endonucleases) cleave off fragments of DNA, providing the fingerprint. Comparing the fingerprints from one specimen with another can determine whether the strains of mycobacteria are the same or different. In this way, multiple isolates from different patients may be traced to a single source case.

Serologic testing for antibody to mycobacterial antigens and direct identification of antigens themselves produce only moderate degrees of sensitivity and specificity in currently available systems. The identification of additional epitopes could make these tests more appropriate for general use.[35]

Despite much progress in the area of diagnostics, there are many situations in which a diagnosis of TB is deferred or cannot be confirmed. In such a situation, the managing clinician should consider empiric treatment. Response to the therapeutic trial may help to establish the diagnosis. Therapy should not be withheld if clinical suspicion for this diagnosis is high but the diagnosis has not been confirmed.

## TREATMENT

### General Considerations

*M. tuberculosis* is a slowly growing organism, and because most of the agents used to treat the disease require a metabolically active organism, treatment has traditionally been prolonged. Even without prior drug exposure, spontaneous drug-resistant mycobacteria occur somewhat predictably and in relation to the number of organisms present. For example, there are likely to be some organisms that are spontaneously resistant to isoniazid (INH) in a tuberculous focus containing $10^5$ or more bacilli, a number frequently encountered clinically. Similar frequencies may be calculated for other drugs. The likelihood of spontaneous resistance to multiple drugs is the product of the probability of resistance to each individual agent. Use of multiple drugs greatly reduces the likelihood of emergence of a resistant strain. Treatment regimens for TB have been characterized by the use of multiple drugs given over prolonged periods.

Based on the work of Grosset and others, the concept of subpopulations of tubercle bacilli has emerged.[36] This view holds that in a patient with TB, tubercle bacilli occur in various numbers in three compartments. There is a large population of extracellular, metabolically active organisms existing, for example, in a tuberculous cavity. The other two populations are thought to be much smaller and to contain organisms that are multiplying more slowly or only intermittently, one within monocytes and macrophages and one extracellularly within the tuberculous caseum. It is thought that the first large group is responsible for the patient's infectiousness (ie, if the disease is within the respiratory tract), and because of the large number of organisms in this compartment, it is a source of potential drug resistance if an inadequate drug regimen is prescribed. The slowly multiplying populations, also called "persisters," represent groups that must be eliminated to secure a lasting cure of the disease.

The various antituberculosis drugs are not equally effective against all these populations. INH and, to a lesser extent, rifampin, streptomycin, and ethambutol are especially effective against the metabolically active extracellular group of organisms.[37] Rifampin appears uniquely active against the slowly growing extracellular population,[38] and pyrazinamide (PZA), in experimental systems, seems especially useful against the population of intracellular tubercle bacilli.[39] These and other antimycobacterial agents are described in Table 38–3.

Several studies have confirmed that treatment duration can be substantially reduced with excellent results by using regimens containing drugs that are especially active against one or another of these populations. In a landmark study conducted by the British Thoracic and Tuberculosis Association, it was demonstrated that a regimen containing INH and rifampin given for 9 months and supplemented by streptomycin or ethambutol during the first 2 months of therapy produced cure rates in patients with extensive pulmonary TB as high as those produced by a similar regimen given for a standard duration of 18 months.[40] Using the same regimens but for only 6 months in patients with less extensive pulmonary disease produced an unacceptably high relapse or failure rate of 5.6%. Subsequent studies confirmed these results and proved that the supplemental use of streptomycin or ethambutol was unnecessary if the tubercle bacilli were fully sensitive to INH and rifampin. After an initial period of daily treatment, it is possible to provide therapy on an intermittent basis, such as twice weekly, for 9 months and achieve cure rates of about 95%.[41] Intermittent regimens are particularly important because they make directly supervised treatment of potentially non-

Table 38–3. **Drugs for the Management of Tuberculosis**

| Drug | Daily Therapy | Twice Weekly Therapy |
|---|---|---|
| **Major** | | |
| Isoniazid | 5–20 mg/kg to 300 mg | 20–40 mg/kg |
| Rifampin | 10–20 mg/kg to 600 mg | 10–20 mg/kg |
| **Major Adjuncts** | | |
| Pyrazinamide | 25–30 mg/kg to 2 g | 50–70 mg/kg |
| Ethambutol | 15–25 mg/kg | 50 mg/kg |
| Streptomycin | 15–20 mg/kg to 1 g | 25–30 mg/kg |
| **Minor** | | |
| Ethionamide | 15–30 mg/kg to 1 g | 1 g |
| Cycloserine | 10–20 mg/kg to 1 g | 1 g |
| Kanamycin | 15–30 mg/kg to 1 g | 1 g |
| Capreomycin | 15–30 mg/kg to 1 g | 1 g |
| Amikacin | 7.5–10 mg/kg | |
| Para-aminosalicylic acid | 150 mg/kg to 12 g | 12 g |
| Thiacetazone* | 2 mg/kg to 150 mg | |
| **New or Experimental** | | |
| Fluoroquinolones | Optimal dosing and suitability for | |
| Clofazamine | intermittent therapy are undefined | |
| Amoxicillin-clavulanate | | |

*Not available in the United States.

compliant patients more practical. When PZA is added to a rifampin and INH-containing regimen for the first 2 months of treatment, a total duration of therapy of 6 months can achieve cure rates for pulmonary TB of greater than 98%.[42] This 6-month regimen can also be administered intermittently with good results.[43]

Although most studies of short-course chemotherapy have involved patients with pulmonary TB, Dutt and colleagues have reported results with INH and rifampin used for 9 months to treat patients with various forms of extrapulmonary disease. With the exception of several treatment failures involving patients with tuberculous osteomyelitis, 9 months of INH and rifampin produced excellent results, even in cases of miliary and meningeal disease.[44] It is presumed that the addition of PZA to this regimen for the first 2 months would constitute an effective 6-month therapy regimen for extrapulmonary disease, and the work of Cohn and colleagues supports that conclusion.[43]

INH and rifampin form the cornerstone of all short-course regimens. The addition of PZA for the first 2 months permits a reduction in total treatment time from 9 to 6 months. The substitution of other drugs or resistance to one or more of these agents usually requires a more protracted period of drug treatment.

The use of these 6- and 9-month short-course treatment regimens has several advantages over the formerly standard 18- to 24-month regimens. Chief among these is the increased likelihood that patients will comply with treatment. Short-course regimens also tend to be cheaper because fewer total visits and tests are required. Because patients receive medication for a much briefer time, there is less chance for drug reactions or toxicity to occur.

It appears unlikely that further substantial reductions in treatment can be attained using currently available drugs without incurring unacceptable increases in relapses and treatment failures. Even if multiple drugs including INH, rifampin, and PZA are given for 4 months to patients with pulmonary disease, early relapse or failure rates usually exceed 7%.[45] This emphasizes the relatively limited margin for noncompliance that the shorter-duration regimens probably have.

### Selecting a Therapeutic Regimen

The 6- to 9-month regimens are preferred. This assumes that patients' organisms are sensitive to INH and rifampin and that no contraindication exists to the use of a particular drug or drug combination in a regimen. Because adherence to a regimen can almost never be ensured, directly observed therapy should be provided whenever possible. Drug susceptibility is becoming a problem in many locales. Reports have appeared from several areas around the United States describing multidrug-resistant TB, particularly among HIV-coinfected persons.[46, 47] Resistance to INH and rifampin has been common among these patients. These reports emphasize the need for clinicians to be aware of drug resistance patterns in the areas where they practice. At least two drugs to which a patient's organism are presumed to be sensitive should be prescribed. Drug susceptibility testing should be obtained on the initial isolate to guide subsequent adjustments in therapy. In areas where a rate of primary resistance to INH is not documented to be less than 4%, ethambutol or streptomycin should be added to the initial regimen.[47a] This agent can be dropped after sensitivity to the other drugs being used is confirmed. Because it appears to have relatively limited impact on the large population of metabolically active extracellular tubercle bacilli from which resistance is thought to emerge, PZA may not be suitable as a companion drug for purposes of preventing resistance. It is now common to use INH, rifampin, PZA, and ethambutol as initial therapy because primary drug resistance to INH or rifampin generally cannot be excluded.

Patients who were previously treated for TB and who failed treatment or relapsed present a special problem in management. Many of these patients acquired secondary resistance to one or more of the drugs they previously received. The likelihood of secondary resistance is in part related to the length of time that drugs were taken previously. The probability of resistance increases sharply if previous therapy was taken for more than 1 month, and it attains a level of more than 70% among patients previously treated for more than 24 months.[48] Clinicians should consider this when selecting a retreatment regimen. As with suspected primary resistance, these patients should receive at least two new drugs to which their organism is believed sensitive. Alternatively, if the patient is not critically ill and the likelihood of secondary resistance is deemed small (eg, only a brief period of prior therapy), the same regimen as was previously used may be prescribed again. Drug susceptibility testing is essential for these patients, because the results are used to modify treatment. If extensive resistance to the commonly used first-line drugs is encountered, less effective and generally more toxic *minor* agents must be employed (see Table 38–3). This usually precludes short-course chemotherapy, necessitating a more protracted course of treatment. If organisms are resistant to *major and minor* agents, experimental treatments may be attempted using some traditional agents to which the tubercle bacilli may be partially sensitive and adding various combinations

of agents such as fluoroquinolone and one of the macrolides.[48a] The results of such regimens are likely to be inferior to those obtained with standard treatment. Surgery may be useful in selected patients.[48a] The use of adjunctive measures to reduce transmission of these difficult-to-treat organisms, particularly the use of ultraviolet lights, should be reinforced in settings where these bacilli are likely to be encountered.[49]

The selection of treatment for tuberculosis in HIV-coinfected persons may be approached in much the same way as when treating immunocompetent patients. TB in HIV-infected persons appears to respond well to standard regimens, with sputum and culture conversion of pulmonary cases occurring at about the same rate as persons without HIV infection. This is true regardless of the stage of HIV infection. The treatment failure rate for HIV-infected patients treated with 9 months of INH and rifampin for drug-sensitive TB is low and similar to that encountered when treating other drug-susceptible patients.[9] HIV-coinfected patients do appear to have an increased incidence of adverse drug reactions and must be carefully monitored during treatment. Reaction to thiacetazone, an antituberculosis agent not available in the United States but used extensively elsewhere, seems to be a particular problem because of its frequent association with Stevens-Johnson syndrome in HIV-coinfected patients. This drug should not be used in HIV-coinfected patients. Despite the generally favorable response to TB treatment of HIV-coinfected patients, there is an impression among many clinicians that TB/HIV patients may deteriorate and die sooner than other persons at a comparable stage of HIV infection but without concomitant TB. Further study of this association appears warranted.

The treatment of TB during pregnancy and in the postpartum period requires special consideration. Most first-line drugs, including rifampin and ethambutol, appear to be well tolerated by pregnant women and their babies.[50] Pyridoxine (vitamin $B_6$) should be provided to pregnant women to prevent peripheral neuropathy.[51] There has been some concern that INH-associated hepatitis, including severe forms, may be increased in the immediate postpartum period.[52] The magnitude of the increase is not well defined, but it is reasonable to monitor liver function closely when INH is used in this setting. Little is known about the safety of PZA in pregnancy, and it is probably best to avoid this drug during that period. Streptomycin is known to be teratogenic and should not be given to pregnant women. Because rifampin and INH are excreted in breast milk, some clinicians suggest having breast-feeding mothers take these medications immediately after a feeding. The next feeding can be provided to the baby by bottle. This approach greatly reduces the amount of medication the infant receives. The baby must not receive a therapeutic amount of medication through the mother's milk. If the baby of a tuberculous mother also requires treatment for tuberculosis, this must be provided directly to the infant.[50]

### Monitoring Therapy and Encouraging Compliance

In addition to following the therapeutic response, follow-up care should be directed toward encouraging and monitoring compliance and detecting adverse reactions to the drugs prescribed.[53] Patient contact should be made at regular intervals, usually not less frequently than once each month. For pulmonary disease, sputum should be monitored, if possible, to confirm smear and culture conversion. Smear conversion is a useful index of therapeutic response and an indication of reduced infection. Culture conversion confirms a therapeutic response. Patients whose sputum culture does not convert to negative after about 3 months of therapy should be reassessed for drug resistance. Culture conversion also can be used to monitor the therapeutic response of extrapulmonary disease if specimens are readily available. Screening for adverse reactions is accomplished primarily by obtaining an interval history and by examination focused on symptoms or signs that may indicate a drug-related problem. This approach is complemented by the use of laboratory testing to evaluate the findings of the initial screening and to assess routinely patients thought to be at increased risk for a particular drug toxicity.

Interactions with the patients should be used to encourage and assess compliance with treatment. If problems are identified, an effort should be made to discover and eliminate obstacles to compliance. If there is still concern about noncompliance, consideration should be given to providing directly supervised twice-weekly therapy. Baseline liver function tests, a complete blood count, and platelet count, serum creatinine levels, and uric acid levels (if PZA is used) provide references for later comparison and identify persons at potential risk for toxicity. Visual acuity and color vision testing are helpful when ethambutol is prescribed. Patients at increased risk of hepatotoxicity, including those with underlying liver disease or chronic alcohol ingestion should have tests repeated periodically. Those at particular risk for other known toxicities of the agents prescribed, such as patients with a history of hyperuricemia receiving PZA or patients with underlying ocular disease or receiving relatively high doses of ethambutol (eg, 25 mg/kg/d), should have the relevant test repeated periodically to guide adjustments in therapy. Routine laboratory testing, beyond the baseline assessment, is unnecessary for most other patients.

## PREVENTION

TB is a preventable disease. Prompt and effective treatment of potentially infectious TB patients limits the transmission of infection to susceptible hosts. However, additional opportunities for prevention are available, including the vaccination of uninfected persons, provision of medication to uninfected persons exposed to potentially infectious patients (ie, primary prophylaxis), and provision of medication to persons who are infected but not yet ill with TB (ie, secondary prevention).

Vaccination against TB with vaccines prepared from various strains of the bacillus Calmette-Guérin (BCG) has been employed in many areas of the world for years. Studies of the degree of protection against TB conferred by BCG vaccination have yielded results ranging from 0 (no protection) found in studies conducted in the southeastern United States by the Public Health Service,[54] to 80% reduction in TB cases observed in a British study.[55] The reasons for this wide variation in efficacy are uncertain, but a review of the methods and statistical aspects of several large BCG trials concluded that BCG is likely to confer some protection.[56] Moreover, the vaccine is likely to be particularly useful in preventing the most aggressive forms of TB, such as disseminated disease.

Why not rely on BCG vaccination as the principal tool of TB prevention? First is the problem of efficacy; BCG is not completely effective and in some settings may be only marginally effective. More important is the fact that BCG probably confers no benefit to persons who have already been infected by *M. tuberculosis* as judged by a positive tuberculin skin test. In the United States, where most cases of TB arise from a pool of approximately 10 million previously infected persons, BCG would not be expected to have a major impact. Because BCG vaccination may cause conversion of the tuberculin skin test, vaccination creates the problem of determining if a positive skin test results from a virulent infection or from vaccination. BCG vaccine uses live attenuated bacilli, and infections, both local and disseminated, resulting from BCG have been reported.[51, 57, 58] Vaccination is contraindicated for persons with compromised immunity. Although theoretically desirable, BCG vaccination has many practical limitations, particularly in developed countries. Current recommendations for BCG relegate its use to uninfected, immunocompetent persons who are continuously exposed to potentially infectious TB cases and in circumstances in which other preventive measures are unavailable (eg, multidrug resistant TB) or likely to fail (eg, noncompliance).[59]

In the United States, TB prevention has relied heavily on the use of INH prophylaxis. This approach derives from the landmark results of several large U.S. Public Health Service studies and others, which indicated that INH, given as a single agent to persons who are likely to be infected with *M. tuberculosis* could reduce their risk of developing TB by 70% or more.[60] This protective effect appears to last beyond the period of treatment and is presumably lifelong.[61] Based on these results, INH prophylaxis became widely used to reduce the risk of TB among persons with positive tuberculin skin tests. A few years later, the potential risks of INH, particularly hepatitis, became better appreciated. An important prospective study demonstrated that the risk of hepatitis associated with INH increased with age and, to some extent, with alcohol consumption.[62] Among persons younger than 35 years of age, INH-associated hepatitis is uncommon, but it increases to a peak incidence of about 2.3% among persons 55 years of age and then decreases somewhat among persons older than 70 years of age.[62] Based on these observations and the fact that the risk of TB is not equal among all persons with a reaction to a tuberculin skin test, risk-benefit analyses have been performed to define the characteristics of persons who are likely to derive the greatest reduction in TB risk by taking INH despite the risk of developing hepatitis.[63]

Several guidelines for the use of INH preventive therapy have been developed (Table 38–4). With the intent of providing INH preventive therapy to those most likely to benefit from it, these guidelines incorporate the risk of developing TB, the personal and public health implications of TB (ie, risk and epidemiologic groups), and the hepatitis risk (ie, age less or greater than 35 years). The sensitivity and specificity of the skin test for detecting a tuberculous

Table 38–4. **Guidelines for Isoniazid Preventive Therapy**

| Risk Group | Age Group | |
|---|---|---|
| | *<35 Years* | *>35 Years* |
| High-grade risk factor (recent TB contact, HIV coinfected, stable abnormal chest radiograph)* | All ages 5 TU PPD reaction ≥ 5 mm† | |
| Low-grade risk factor | All ages 5 TU PPD reaction ≥ 10 mm | |
| No high-risk factors/high-incidence group (eg, foreign born, medically underserved, jail or nursing home resident) | Treat if PPD reaction ≥ 10 mm | Do not treat |
| No risk factors/low-incidence group | Treat if PPD reaction ≥ 15 mm | Do not treat |

*TB, tuberculosis; HIV, human immunodeficiency virus.

†Reactions are to 5 tuberculin units (TU) of purified protein derivative (PPD). Reaction size refers to the degree of induration.

Modified from Centers for Disease Control: The use of preventive therapy for tuberculous infection in the United States. Recommendations of the Advisory Committee for Elimination of Tuberculosis. MMWR 39(RR-8):9, 1990.

infection is adjusted by varying the cutoff used to define a positive reaction. Before beginning preventive therapy with INH, the possibility of active disease should be eliminated by means of a careful history, physical examination, and chest x-ray film. Any abnormality consistent with active TB should be evaluated and preventive therapy deferred until the evaluation is completed. In situations in which active disease is likely, particularly if the patient is ill or considered potentially infectious because of a positive sputum AFB smear, it is usually advisable to begin therapy for active disease with two or more drugs. If active TB is later excluded by culture results or other information, preventive therapy with INH alone can be continued. Treatment of active disease with INH alone carries the risk of selecting out INH-resistant tubercle bacilli.

Candidates for preventive therapy should be screened for contraindications to INH, prior therapy or potential drug interactions, and alcohol use. If preventive therapy is begun, it should be monitored at about monthly intervals. Persons receiving INH should be encouraged to take their medications, and they should be questioned about symptoms suggestive of side effects, particularly hepatitis or neuritis. They should be encouraged to report immediately any symptoms if they occur between visits. The use of laboratory testing to monitor for hepatitis is controversial. Elevations of serum transaminase levels occur in 10% to 20% of people taking INH.[64, 65] In most cases, these abnormalities resolve even if the medication is continued. However, progressive abnormalities of liver function can occur, as can fatal hepatitis.[66] Routine testing of liver function does increase the cost of providing preventive therapy and may cause discontinuation of treatment in some persons who may ultimately have an uneventful course of therapy and benefit from treatment. However, periodic testing of liver function may provide some additional margin of safety,[65] although this has not been rigorously tested. Liver function tests should be obtained promptly to evaluate any symptoms or signs suggestive of hepatitis.

Providing INH preventive therapy for more than 1 year

appears to provide no added benefit.[67] Most patients given prophylaxis are thought to derive the most benefit available to them in the first 6 months of treatment,[68] and it appears that this treatment constitutes the best therapeutic program.[6] Although several regimens using multiple drugs for briefer periods show promise,[69, 70] none has been proven effective.

In some instances, it is useful to provide primary prophylaxis, in which INH is given to someone who is not thought to be infected with *M. tuberculosis* but who has a continuing exposure to a potentially infectious carrier. In these situations, INH can be provided to the contact until the source case is rendered noninfectious or the exposure is otherwise interrupted. When used in this way, INH is protective only while it is taken. Any subsequent infection or exposure by the person receiving primary prophylaxis requires additional intervention.

The management of TB infections during pregnancy is another important situation. Pregnancy and the postpartum period may represent times of increased risk for reactivation of infection. Ideally, this risk would be reduced by the provision of INH prophylaxis whenever a positive tuberculin skin test is identified in a pregnant woman. This approach must be tempered by the potential risks that INH might have for the fetus, the newborn breast-fed infant, or the mother. These issues have been reviewed elsewhere.[50] Although INH does not seem to have an adverse effect on the developing fetus, preventive therapy should be deferred until after delivery to coincide with the period of greatest reactivation risk. However, if a newly acquired infection by the mother is documented, INH should be started after the first trimester.[71] Although the amount of INH excreted in the breast milk does not provide a therapeutic dose of medication to the baby, some drug is ingested.[72] To minimize this, the mother can be instructed to take her INH immediately after a feeding of the infant and to provide a bottle for the infant's next meal.[72] There is some concern that postpartum women, particularly Hispanic women, may be at increased risk of INH-associated hepatitis.[52] Until further information is available, particular attention should be given to monitoring for hepatic toxicity in this setting.

An especially difficult situation is preventive treatment of persons infected by INH-resistant tubercle bacilli. Although only INH has been proven effective as a prophylactic agent, many experienced clinicians believe that other drugs, particularly rifampin, are equally effective. A decision analysis using the Delphi technique suggests that as the probability of infection with an INH-resistant organism increases, use of a rifampin-containing regimen becomes the preferred approach to prophylaxis.[73] Even less information is available to guide treatment if infection occurs with an organism resistant to multiple drugs including INH and rifampin. Other drugs such as PZA and agents that are not traditionally used for the management of *M. tuberculosis*, such as fluoroquinolones, may be considered in these situations.

TB remains an important clinical and public health problem. The HIV epidemic, the emergence of drug-resistant strains of tubercle bacilli, and a variety of other epidemiologic and social factors have greatly complicated the management of TB. Nonetheless, scientific and technologic advances have provided the potential for continued progress in controlling this disease.

# REFERENCES

1. Murray CJL, Styblo K, Rouillon A: Tuberculosis in developing countries: Burden, intervention and cost. Bull Int Union Tuberc Lung Dis 65:6, 1990.
2. Loudon RG, Roberts RM: Droplet expulsion from the respiratory tract. Am Rev Respir Dis 95:435, 1967.
3. Selwyn PA, Hartel D, Lewis VA, et al: A prospective study of the risk of tuberculosis among intravenous drug users with immunodeficiency virus infection. N Engl J Med 320:545, 1989.
4. Daley CL, Small PM, Schecter GF, et al: An outbreak of tuberculosis with accelerated progression among persons infected with the human immunodeficiency virus—an analysis using restriction-fragment length polymorphism. N Engl J Med 326:231, 1992.
5. Centers for Disease Control: Prevention and control of tuberculosis in facilities providing long-term care to the elderly. Recommendations of the Advisory Committee for Elimination of Tuberculosis. MMWR 39:7, 1990.
6. Stead WW, Lofgren JP, Warren E, Thomas C: Tuberculosis as an endemic and nosocomial infection among the elderly in nursing homes. N Engl J Med 312:1483, 1985.
7. Braun MM, Truman BI, Maguire B: Increasing incidence of tuberculosis in prison inmate population. JAMA 261:393, 1989.
8. Brudney K, Dobkin J: Resurgent tuberculosis in New York City: Human immunodeficiency virus, homelessness and the decline of tuberculosis control programs. Am Rev Respir Dis 144:745, 1991.
9. Small PM, Schecter GF, Goodman PC, Sande MA, Chaisson RE, Hopewell PC: Treatment of tuberculosis in patients with advanced human immunodeficiency virus infection. N Engl J Med 324:289, 1991.
10. Stead WW: Pathogenesis of a first episode of chronic pulmonary tuberculosis in man: Recrudescence of residuals of the primary infection or exogenous reinfection. Am Rev Respir Dis 95:729, 1967.
11. Khan MA, Kovnat DM, Bachus B, Whitcomb ME, Brody JS, Snider GL: Clinical and roentgenographic spectrum of pulmonary tuberculosis in adults. Am J Med 62:31, 1977.
12. Hadlock FT, Park SK, Awe RJ, Rivera M: Unusual radiographic findings in adult pulmonary tuberculosis. AJR 134:1015, 1980.
13. Huseby JS, Hudson LD: Miliary tuberculosis and adult respiratory distress syndrome. Ann Intern Med 85:609, 1976.
14. Pitchenik AE, Robinson HA: The radiographic appearance of tuberculosis in patients with the acquired immune deficiency syndrome (AIDS) and pre-AIDS. Am Rev Respir Dis 131:393, 1985.
15. Suderam G, McDonald RJ, Maniatis T, Oleske J, Reichman LB: Tuberculosis as a manifestation of the acquired immunodeficiency syndrome (AIDS). JAMA 256:362, 1986.
16. Berenguer J, Moreno S, Laguna F, et al: Tuberculous meningitis in patients infected with the human immunodeficiency virus. N Engl J Med 326:668, 1992.
17. Chaisson RE, Schecter GF, Theuer CP, Rutherford GW, Echenberg DF, Hopewell PC: Tuberculosis in patients with the acquired immunodeficiency syndrome: Clinical features, response to therapy and survival. Am Rev Respir Dis 136:570, 1987.
18. Reichman LB, Felton CP, Edsall JR: Drug dependence, a possible new risk factor for tuberculosis disease. Arch Intern Med 139:337, 1979.
19. Lundin AP, Adler AJ, Berlyne GM, Friedman EA: Tuberculosis in patients undergoing maintenance hemodialysis. Am J Med 67:597, 1979.
20. Andrew OT, Schoenfeld P, Hopewell PC, Humphreys MH: Tuberculosis in patients with end stage renal disease. Am J Med 68:59, 1980.
21. Qunibi WY, Al-Sibai MB, Taher S, et al: Mycobacterial infection after renal transplantation—report of 14 cases and review of the literature. Q J Med 77:1039, 1990.
22. American Thoracic Society and Centers for Disease Control: Diagnostic standards and classification of tuberculosis 1990. Am Rev Respir Dis 142:725, 1990.
23. Maartens G, Wilcox PA, Benatar SR: Miliary tuberculosis: Rapid diagnosis, hematologic abnormalities in 109 treated adults. Am J Med 89:291, 1990.
24. Glasser RM, Walker RI, Herion JC: The significance of the blood in patients with tuberculosis. Arch Intern Med 125:691, 1970.
25. Light RW, Erozan YS, Ball WC: Cells in pleural fluid: Their value in differential diagnosis. Arch Intern Med 125:691, 1970.
26. Bentz RR, Dimchoff DG, Nemiroff MJ, Tsang A, Weg JG: The incidence of urine cultures positive for *Mycobacterium tuberculosis* in a general patient population. Am Rev Respir Dis 111:647, 1973.
27. Narain R: Microscopy positive and microscopy negative cases of pulmonary tuberculosis. Am Rev Respir Dis 103:761, 1971.
28. Burke JR, Viroslav J, Bynum LJ: Miliary tuberculosis diagnosed by fiberoptic bronchoscopy and transbronchial biopsy. Tubercle 59:107, 1978.
29. Stenson W, Aranda C, Bevelaqua FA: Transbronchial biopsy culture in pulmonary tuberculosis. Chest 83:883, 1983.
30. Cucin RL, Coleman M, Eckardt JJ, Silver RT: The diagnosis of miliary tuberculosis: Utility of peripheral blood abnormalities, bone marrow and liver needle biopsy. J Chronic Dis 22:355, 1973.
31. Siddiqi SH, Hwangbo CC, Silcox V, Good RC, Snider DE Jr, Middlebrook G: Rapid radiometric methods to detect and differentiate mycobacterium tuberculosis, bovis from other mycobacterial species. Am Rev Respir Dis 130:634, 1984.
32. Drake TA, Hindler JA, Berlin OGW, Brakner DA: Rapid identification of *Mycobacterium avium* in culture using DNA probes. J Clin Microbiol 25:1442, 1989.
33. Ellner PD, Kiehn TE, Cammarata R, Hosmer M: Rapid detection of pathogenic mycobacteria by combining radiometric and nucleic acid probe methods. J Clin Microbiol 26:1349, 1988.
34. Eisenach KD, Sifford MD, Cave MD, Bates JH, Crawford JT: Detection of *Mycobacterium tuberculosis* in sputum samples using a polymerase chain reaction. Am Rev Respir Dis 144:1160, 1991.
35. Daniel TM, DeBanne SM: The serodiagnosis of tuberculosis and other mycobacterial diseases by enzyme-linked immunosorbent assay. Am Rev Respir Dis 135:1137, 1987.
36. Grosset J: Bacteriologic basis of short-course chemotherapy for tuberculosis. Clin Chest Med 1:231, 1980.
37. Jindani A, Aber VR, Edwards EA, Mitchison DA: The early bactericidal activity of drugs in patients with pulmonary tuberculosis. Am Rev Respir Dis 121:939, 1980.
38. Dickinson JM, Mitchison DA: Experimental models to explain the high sterilizing activity of rifampin in the chemotherapy of tuberculosis. Am Rev Respir Dis 123:367, 1981.
39. Mackaness GB: The intracellular activation of pyrazinamide and nicotinamide. Am Rev Tuberc 74:718, 1956.
40. British Thoracic and Tuberculosis Association: Short-course chemotherapy in pulmonary tuberculosis. Lancet 1:119, 1975.
41. Dutt AD, Jones L, Stead WW: Short-course chemotherapy for tuberculosis with largely twice weekly isoniazid-rifampin. Chest 75:441, 1979.
42. Snider DE, Gracyzyk J, Bek E, Rogowski J: Supervised six-months treatment of newly diagnosed pulmonary tuberculosis using isoniazid, rifampin and pyrazinamide with and without streptomycin. Am Rev Respir Dis 130:1091, 1984.
43. Cohn DL, Caitlin BJ, Peterson KL, Judson FN, Sbarbaro JA: A 62 dose, 6 month therapy for pulmonary and extrapulmonary tuberculosis. Ann Intern Med 112:407, 1990.
44. Dutt AK, Moers D, Stead WW: Short-course chemotherapy for extrapulmonary tuberculosis. Nine years' experience. Ann Intern Med 104:7, 1986.
45. Singapore Tuberculosis Service and British Medical Research Council: Long-term followup of a clinical trial of six-month and four-month regimens of chemotherapy in the treatment of pulmonary tuberculosis. Am Rev Respir Dis 133:779, 1986.
46. Chawla PK, Klapper PJ, Kamholz SL, Pollack AH, Heurich AE: Drug-resistant tuberculosis in an urban population including patients at risk for human immunodeficiency virus infection. Am Rev Respir Dis 146:280, 1992.
47. Fischl MA, Uttamchandani RB, Daikos GL, et al: An outbreak of tuberculosis caused by multiple-drug–resistant tubercle bacilli among patients with HIV infection. Ann Intern Med 117:177, 1992.
47a. Centers for Disease Control and Prevention: Initial therapy for tuberculosis in the era of multidrug resistance. Recommendations of the Advisory Council for the Elimination of Tuberculosis. MMWR 42(RR-7). 1, 1993.
48. Costello HD, Caras GJ, Snider DE: Drug resistance among previously treated tuberculosis patients, a brief report. Am Rev Respir Dis 121:313, 1980.
48a. Iseman MD: Treatment of multidrug-resistant tuberculosis. N Engl J Med 329:784, 1993.
49. Iseman MD: A leap of faith. What can we do to curtail intrainstitutional transmission of tuberculosis? Ann Intern Med 117:251, 1992.
50. Hamadeh A, Glassroth J: Tuberculosis and pregnancy. Chest 101:1114, 1992.

51. Snider DE: Pyridoxine supplementation during isoniazid therapy. Tubercle 61:191, 1980.
52. Frank AL, Blinkin NJ, Snider DE, Rokaw WM, Becker S: Isoniazid hepatitis among pregnant and postpartum Hispanic patients. Public Health Rep 104:151, 1989.
53. Barnes PF, Barrows SA: Tuberculosis in the 1990s. Ann Int Med 119:400, 1993.
54. Comstock G, Palmer C: Long-term results of BCG vaccination in the southern United States. Am Rev Respir Dis 93:171, 1966.
55. Great Britain Medical Research Council: BCG and vole bacillus vaccines in the prevention of tuberculosis in adolescence and early life. Br Med J 1:413, 1956.
56. Clemens JD, Chuong JH, Feinstein AR: The BCG controversy. A methodological and statistical reappraisal. JAMA 249:2362, 1983.
57. Mortensson W, Eklof O, Jorulf H: Radiologic aspects of BCG-osteomyelitis in infants and children. Acta Radiol Diagn 17:845, 1976.
58. Centers for Disease Control: Disseminated *Mycobacterium bovis* infection from BCG vaccination of a patient with acquired immunodeficiency syndrome. MMWR 34:227, 1985.
59. Centers for Disease Control: Recommendation of the Immunization Practices Advisory Committee. Use of BCG vaccines in the control of tuberculosis: A joint statement of the ACIP and the Advisory Committee for Elimination of Tuberculosis. MMWR 37:663, 1988.
60. Ferebee SH: Controlled chemoprophylaxis trials in TB. A general review. Adv Tuberc Res 17:28, 1970.
61. Comstock GW, Baum C, Snider DE: Isoniazid prophylaxis among Alaskan Eskimos: A final report of the Bethel isoniazid studies. Am Rev Respir Dis 119:827, 1979.
62. Kopanoff DE, Snider DE, Caras GJ: Isoniazid-related hepatitis: A U.S. Public Health Service cooperative surveillance study. Am Rev Respir Dis 117:991, 1978.
63. Comstock GW, Edwards PQ: The competing risks of tuberculosis and hepatitis for adult tuberculin reactors. Am Rev Respir Dis 111:573, 1975.
64. Bailey WC, Taylor SL, Dascomb HE, Greenberg HB, Ziskind MM: Disturbed hepatic function during isoniazid chemoprophylaxis. Am Rev Respir Dis 107:523, 1973.
65. Byrd RB, Horn BR, Solomon DA, Griggs GA: Toxic effects of isoniazid in tuberculosis chemoprophylaxis. Role of biochemical monitoring in 1,000 patients. JAMA 241:1239, 1979.
66. Snider DE, Caras GJ: Isoniazid-associated hepatitis deaths. A review of available information. Am Rev Respir Dis 145:494, 1992.
67. Comstock GW, Ferebee SH: How much isoniazid is needed for prophylaxis? Am Rev Respir Dis 101:780, 1970.
68. International Union Against Tuberculosis Committee on Prophylaxis: Efficacy of various durations of isoniazid preventive therapy for tuberculosis: Five years of follow-up in the IUAT trial. Bull WHO 60:555, 1982.
69. Centers for Disease Control: The use of preventive therapy for tuberculous infection in the United States. Recommendations of the Advisory Committee for Elimination of Tuberculosis. MMWR 39(RR-8):9, 1990.
70. Lecoeur HF, Truffot-Pernot C, Grosset JH: Experimental short-course preventive therapy of tuberculosis with rifampin and pyrazinamide. Am Rev Respir Dis 140:1189, 1989.
71. American Thoracic Society: Treatment of tuberculosis and tuberculosis infection in adults and children. Am Rev Respir Dis 134:355, 1986.
72. Snider DE, Powell KE: Should women taking antituberculosis drugs breast-feed? Arch Intern Med 144:589, 1984.
73. Koplan JP, Farer LS: Choice of preventive treatment for isoniazid-resistant tuberculous infection. Use of decision analysis and the Delphi technique. JAMA 244:2736, 1980.

# Mycobacteria Other Than
## *Mycobacterium tuberculosis*

RICHARD J. WALLACE, Jr.

Mycobacteria other than those causing tuberculosis are an increasingly recognized cause of chronic lung disease, although in the era of widespread prevalence of infection and disease caused by *Mycobacterium tuberculosis*, these organisms were rarely encountered. If recovered in sputum from a patient, the taxonomy of the organism and its role in disease were generally uncertain. With improved chemotherapy for tuberculosis (TB) and decline in the number of cases of TB in the United States, the number of isolations of these nontuberculous mycobacteria (NTM) began to increase, and attracted more scientific attention.

By the 1950s, most species of NTM had been described, including *M. kansasii*, *M. avium*, *M. intracellulare*, *M. fortuitum*, and *M. scrofulaceum*.[1] A major step forward in the understanding of these organisms was the introduction of the Runyon Classification System, a method devised by Ernest Runyon that divided potentially pathogenic human isolates of the NTM into four groups on the basis of growth rates, colony morphology, and pigmentation. This allowed mycobacterial laboratories to more readily identify individual species of NTM, allowing better characterization of the disease syndromes associated with these organisms. This classification system has been replaced by more complex and sophisticated test methods.

Another milestone in the understanding of lung disease caused by NTM was the publication in 1969 of a map of skin test reactivity within the United States to an *M. avium* complex antigen preparation.[2] This skin test, called PPD-B or the Battey antigen after the Battey State Hospital in Rome, Georgia, where much of the early clinical disease caused by *M. avium* complex was first described, was applied to approximately 275,000 naval recruits who had lived their entire lives in a single county. The subsequent map showed a striking distribution of skin test reactivity that was greatest among recruits from the southeastern and gulf coast states (Fig. 39–1). In these areas, more than 70% of those tested had been infected with *M. avium* complex or an antigenically similar organism, resulting in a strongly positive skin test to PPD-B.

Another milestone in our knowledge of lung disease caused by NTM was an exhaustive review of clinical and laboratory features of these organisms written by Wolinsky and published in 1979.[1] This provided one of the first reference sources for physicians to review the clinical significance of the many species of NTM organisms and the clinical disease syndromes they produced.

At least 10 slowly growing species and seven taxonomic groups of rapidly growing mycobacteria are recognized causes of chronic lung disease (Table 39–1).[3] Most can be readily identified within the laboratory using a variety of biochemical, chromatographic, and molecular biologic techniques. Because single positive sputum cultures that contain small numbers of colonies can occur in the absence of disease (and probably in the absence of infection), sputum cultures alone do not always provide a diagnosis of NTM lung disease. Several investigators have provided diagnostic criteria for NTM.[4] Lung cavitation appeared to be relatively common with *M. avium* complex and *M. kansasii* infections, and this combined with the presence of multiple positive sputum cultures for these organisms made a generally acceptable set of diagnostic criteria for disease. Diagnostic problems occurred for patients with positive sputa for these species who did not have cavitary disease and for organisms such as *Mycobacterium abscessus* (formerly *M. chelonae* subspecies *abscessus*), which rarely cause cavitation.

In 1990, the American Thoracic Society published diagnostic criteria for lung disease caused by NTM that in-

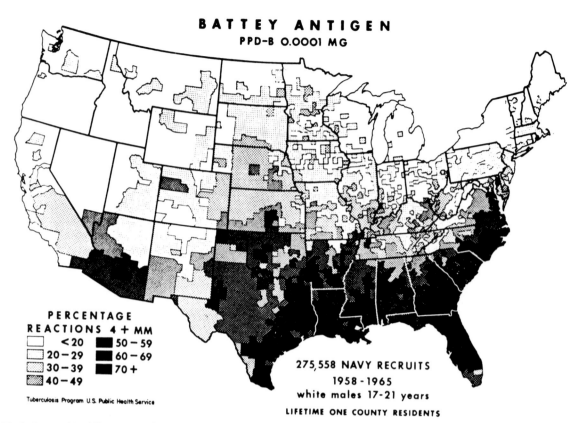

**Figure 39–1.** Geographic differences in skin test reactivity to a *Mycobacterium avium* complex antigen (PPD-B) among 275,000 naval recruits who had lived their entire lives in a single country. (From Edwards LB, Acquaviva FA, Livesay VT, et al: An atlas of sensitivity to tuberculin, PPD-B, and histoplasmin in the United States. Am Rev Respir Dis 99:13, 1969.)

cluded criteria for cavitary and noncavitary diseases.[3] A summary of these criteria is provided in Table 39–2. In general, sputum samples that are smear positive or contain moderate or heavy growth on culture of an NTM are almost always associated with clinical disease and require follow-up regardless of the radiographic picture. Single culture-positive samples that are smear negative should be as-

Table 39–1. **Nontuberculous Mycobacterial Species or Taxonomic Groups That Cause Chronic Lung Infections**

**Frequent Pathogens**
Rapidly growing mycobacteria
    *M. abscessus*
    *M. fortuitum*
Slowly growing mycobacteria
    *M. avium* complex
    *M. kansasii*
    *M. xenopi*
**Infrequent or Rare Pathogens**
Rapidly growing mycobacteria
    *M. peregrinum*
    *M. fortuitum* unnamed third biovariant complex
    *M. chelonae*-like organism (MCLO)
    *M. smegmatis*
Slowly growing mycobacteria
    *M. szulgai*
    *M. simiae*
    *M. shimoidei*
    *M. malmoense*
    *M. asiaticum*
    *M. thermoresistibile*

sessed with the previously mentioned diagnostic criteria in mind.

The incidence and prevalence of NTM lung disease are unknown. Because of the lack of diagnostic criteria for disease and the fact that, unlike TB, disease caused by NTM is not legally reportable, there is no definitive information about the frequency of these diseases. A national survey based on state health department laboratory reports from 1979 through 1980 was done by the Centers for Disease Control.[5] Of the 32,000 isolates assessed, approximately one third were NTM. The most commonly recognized species were *M. avium* complex (61%), *M. fortuitum* complex (19%), and *M. kansasii* (10%). Almost all of the reported isolates were from sputa. A second study done by some of the same investigators for the period 1981 through 1983 showed similar numbers, with an estimated prevalence rate of 1.8 cases of NTM disease per 100,000 persons within the United States.[6] Because disease caused by NTM shows a definite geographic predilection, attack rates vary considerably depending on where one lives. Although subsequent summary data have not been published, some laboratories have informally reported that more than 50% of the currently evaluated mycobacterial species are NTM. Most of this increase appears to be related to *M. avium* complex and the high incidence of disseminated *M. avium* complex disease in patients with acquired immunodeficiency syndrome (AIDS).

Skin test reactivity to soluble TB antigens (ie, PPD-S) has provided reasonable data on the geographic prevalence of infection caused by *M. tuberculosis*. Because commer-

**Table 39–2. Recommended Diagnostic Criteria for Pulmonary Disease Due to Nontuberculous Mycobacteria**

A. Patients with cavitary lung disease
   1. Presence of two or more sputum specimens (or sputum and a bronchial washing) that are acid-fast bacilli smear-positive or result in moderate to heavy growth of NTM on culture
   2. Other reasonable causes for the disease process have been excluded (eg, tuberculosis, fungal disease)
B. Patients with noncavitary lung disease
   1. Presence of two or more sputum specimens (or sputum and a bronchial washing) that are acid-fast bacilli smear-positive or produce moderate to heavy growth on culture
   2. If the isolate is *M. kansasii* or *M. avium* complex, failure of the sputum cultures to clear with bronchial toilet or within 2 weeks of institution of specific mycobacterial drug therapy (although only studied for these two species, criterion is probably valid for other species)
   3. Other reasonable causes of the disease process have been excluded
C. Patients with cavitary or noncavitary lung disease whose sputum evaluation is nondiagnostic or another disease cannot be excluded
   1. Transbronchial or open lung biopsy yields the organism and shows mycobacterial histopathologic features (ie, granulomatous inflammation, with or without acid-fast bacilli); no other criteria needed
   2. Transbronchial or open lung biopsy fails to grow the organism but shows mycobacterial histopathologic features in the absence of a prior history of other granulomatous or mycobacterial disease plus
      a. Presence of two or more positive cultures of sputum or bronchial washings
      b. Other reasonable causes for granulomatous disease have been excluded

From Wallace RJ Jr, O'Brien R, Glassroth J, Raleigh J, Dutt A: Diagnosis and treatment of disease caused by nontuberculous mycobacteria. Am Rev Respir Dis 142:940–953, 1990.

cial skin test antigens to NTM are not available, data of this type for NTM species other than *M. avium* complex have not been compiled.

Susceptibility testing of NTM is more difficult and more controversial than testing for *M. tuberculosis*. Single test concentrations (ie, critical concentrations) were chosen to separate treated from untreated strains of *M. tuberculosis* and provided reasonable predictive values of clinical susceptibility and resistance. These same values have not been useful for *M. avium* complex, because most isolates are resistant to these single-drug concentrations,[7] but combination drug therapy is often clinically and microbiologically successful.[8] The American Thoracic Society recently rec-

ommended that routine susceptibility testing of *M. avium* complex be discontinued,[3] a recommendation that most laboratories have followed. The use of single-drug concentrations chosen for *M. tuberculosis* has some clinical value for species of NTM other than *M. avium* complex, but it is not apparent for all drugs, and this approach has not been subjected to clinical trials. Susceptibility testing to antituberculous drugs is not recommended for the rapidly growing mycobacteria, but isolates are tested against selected antibacterial agents such as imipenem and amikacin.[3] A summary of the percentage of isolates of NTM susceptible to the commonly used antituberculous drugs is given in Table 39–3.

Therapy for lung disease caused by NTM, like susceptibility testing, is more difficult and more controversial than for *M. tuberculosis*. There have been few controlled drug trials (most involving *M. kansasii*)[8–11] and no comparative drug trials. Recommendations for therapy are based primarily on recommendations of the American Thoracic Society published in 1990.[3] They represent a consensus about treatment and, as such, are open to conjecture and criticism about drug choices.[12] The approval of clarithromycin by the Food and Drug Administration in December 1991 provided a new agent that may have a role in the therapy of some or most of these diseases, but clarification awaits the results of clinical studies.

## MYCOBACTERIUM AVIUM COMPLEX

### Clinical Features

*M. avium* complex lung disease is encountered everywhere in the United States, but the area of greatest prevalence appears to be the southeastern and gulf coast states. These are the same areas that showed the highest degree of skin test reactivity to the *M. avium* antigen preparation used to test naval recruits.[2] *M. avium* complex isolates are readily recovered from the water in these areas, and organisms similar to those causing human disease have been recovered from aerosols near these waters.[13, 14]

The classic patient with *M. avium* complex lung disease is white and presents with complaints of cough and sputum production. These patients are typically in their late fifties and sixties and have no history of PPD reactivity or con-

**Table 39–3. Drug Susceptibilities of Nontuberculous Mycobacterial Species Associated With Lung Disease Tested at the Centers for Disease Control Between 1980 and 1984**

| Organism | No. Tested | Percentage of Strains Inhibited at Given Concentrations (μg/mL)* | | | | | | | | | |
|---|---|---|---|---|---|---|---|---|---|---|---|
| | | **INH** 0.2 | **1.0** | **5.0** | **RMP** 1.0 | **EMB** 5.0 | **SM** 2.0 | **10** | **CAP** 10 | **PZA** 25 | **CYCL** 30 | **ETH** 5 |
| *M. avium* complex | 713 | <1 | 1 | 25 | 14 | 13 | 8 | 40 | 9 | <1 | 26 | 5 |
| *M. kansasii* | 71 | 6 | 45 | 92 | 82 | 42 | 11 | 77 | 48 | 2 | 83 | 68 |
| *M. simiae* | 28 | <1 | <1 | 4 | 4 | <1 | <1 | 14 | 4 | <1 | 57 | <1 |
| *M. asiaticum* | 10 | <1 | 10 | 40 | <1 | 20 | <1 | 70 | 20 | <1 | 70 | <1 |
| *M. szulgai* | 23 | 13 | 30 | 61 | 61 | 39 | 39 | 87 | 70 | <1 | 30 | 13 |
| *M. xenopi* | 25 | 64 | 92 | 96 | 92 | 64 | 100 | 100 | 100 | 13 | 72 | 92 |
| *M. malmoense* | 47 | <1 | 2 | 43 | 60 | 21 | 38 | 68 | 47 | 2 | 62 | 53 |
| *M. fortuitum* | 98 | <1 | 1 | 14 | 2 | 3 | 1 | 4 | 49 | <1 | 2 | <1 |
| *M. abscessus* | 170 | <1 | <1 | 1 | <1 | 5 | 2 | 4 | 2 | <1 | <1 | <1 |

*INH, isoniazid; RMP, rifampin; EMB, ethambutol; SM, streptomycin; CAP, capreomycin; PZA, pyrazinamide; CYCL, cycloserine; ETH, ethionamide.

Reprinted by permission of the publisher from Identification and drug susceptibility test results from *Mycobacterium* spp., by Good RC, Silcox VA, Kilburn JO, Plikaytis BC, Clinical Microbiology Newsletter 7:133–136, 1985. Copyright 1985 by Elsevier Science Publishing Co., Inc.

tacts with tuberculosis. Initial studies of *M. avium* complex showed a male predominance, but later studies have shown more females than males. Underlying disorders commonly include cigarette abuse, chronic obstructive lung disease, previous TB, and silicosis.[1, 15, 16] Although *M. avium* complex lung disease is rarely seen in children,[17] it has been encountered in as many as 10% of children with cystic fibrosis living in highly endemic areas. Thirty percent to 50% of adult patients have no readily apparent risk factor or underlying disease.[15] With progression of the disease, fever, weight loss, dyspnea, and fatigue occur. Fever is present less often and is less severe than in patients with TB. Hemoptysis commonly occurs.

The radiographic presentation of *M. avium* complex often is one of two patterns. The most common, seen in approximately two thirds of patients, is upper lobe cavitary disease that exactly mimics TB (Fig. 39–2). Thin-walled cavities are thought to occur more frequently than with TB, but this is of little value when assessing the individual patient. The second pattern is patchy, interstitial disease that radiographically and clinically mimics bronchiectasis (Fig. 39–3). Patients with this form of disease were often assumed to have bronchiectasis with colonization, although most had no antecedent illness that would have explained the bronchiectasis, and almost all patients were smear and culture positive for *M. avium* complex at the first assessment in their disease. Most patients had no radiographic studies (eg, bronchography, computed tomography) to confirm the bronchiectasis, but they were given the diagnosis because the chest radiograph was consistent and because of the history of episodic cough and sputum production. Studies using high-resolution computed tomography of the lungs have shown that multiple small (<5-mm) lung nodules combined with bronchiectasis (almost always in the same lobe of the lung) are highly indicative of *M. avium* complex lung disease.[17a] A good study of the progressive nature of this disease in normal hosts was published by Prince and associates in 1989.[18]

Although disseminated *M. avium* complex disease is common in AIDS, clinically significant lung disease is not. Most patients with disseminated *M. avium* complex disease have positive lung cultures at autopsy but no recognized histopathologic change. Sputum cultures that grow low numbers of *M. avium* complex frequently are seen in AIDS patients with and without disseminated disease. Specific radiographic changes in the lungs of patients with AIDS due to this species have not been described, although interstitial and alveolar infiltrates are evident in some patients.[19] Cavitary disease and upper lobe infiltrates are conspicuously absent.[19] Disseminated *M. avium* complex disease in patients infected with the human immunodeficiency virus (HIV) usually presents late in the patient's HIV illness with fever and weight loss. Typically, patients have CD4 counts of less than 50. Occasionally, diarrhea is a predominant symptom. On physical examination, hepatosplenomegaly is frequently detected. Intraabdominal lymphadenopathy simulating lymphoma may also be present.

## Laboratory Features

*M. avium* complex is readily recognized in the laboratory by acid-fast smear and culture using techniques standardized for TB. The organisms grow well in BACTEC broth and on Middlebrook 7H10 agar, typically producing small, flat, transparent, smooth colonies on agar that are nonpigmented. Their colony morphology readily differentiates them from *M. tuberculosis*. Commercially available nucleic acid probes can identify *M. avium* complex isolates with greater than 99% accuracy in 1 day after the colonies have grown, a technique currently used in most laboratories. *M. avium* and *M. intracellulare* are separate species, but their separation has no clinical value for the patient with lung disease and generally is not done, but specific DNA probes that recognize only *M. avium* or *M. intracellulare* are commercially available.

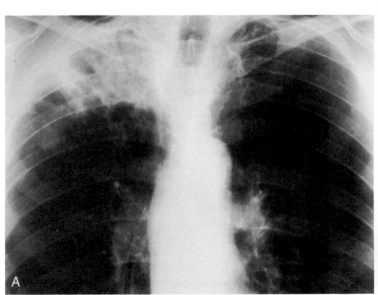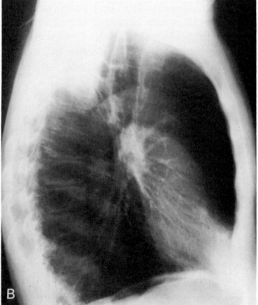

**Figure 39–2.** *A,* The posteroanterior chest radiograph and *B,* lateral chest radiograph demonstrate right upper lobe fibrocavitary disease due to *Mycobacterium avium* complex. Radiographically, the disease is indistinguishable from tuberculosis.

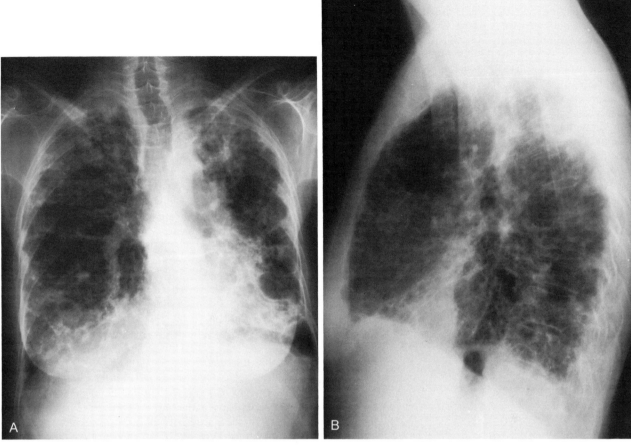

**Figure 39–3.** *A,* Posteroanterior x-ray film and *B,* lateral x-ray film demonstrate far-advanced, end-stage lung disease due to *Mycobacterium avium* complex in a 60-year-old woman.

Routine susceptibility testing of *M. avium* complex using standard *M. tuberculosis* critical concentrations is no longer recommended.[3] Laboratory efforts have centered on the potential usefulness of specific minimum inhibitory concentration (MIC) determinations as a tool to guide drug therapy.[12] Unfortunately, this technique has yet to be used in a clinical trial in which empiric therapy and therapy based on in vitro MICs is compared. Definite acquired drug resistance after therapy has not been documented for *M. avium* complex isolates treated with the traditional antituberculous agents.[3]

**Treatment**

Therapy for *M. avium* complex lung disease is not totally satisfactory, and primary treatment failure and relapse rates are much higher than for treatment of *M. tuberculosis*. The American Thoracic Society[3] recommends a four-drug regimen: isoniazid (300 mg); rifampin (600 mg); ethambutol (25 mg/kg for 2 months, then 15 mg/kg); and streptomycin (0.5–1.0 g five times each week for 8–12 weeks; then 500 mg to 1.0 g two or three times each week for 3 months as tolerated).

Drugs are to be administered for 18 to 24 months, with a minimum of 12 months of culture negativity on therapy.[3] The use of lesser regimens (eg, isoniazid and rifampin) is discouraged because the microbiologic responses are limited, and there is concern that the activity of these drugs may not be as good when subsequently included in the recommended four-drug regimen. The response rate for the four-drug regimen has not been well established, but probably approximates 75%.[8, 20] Relapse rates are unknown. The discontinuation of production of streptomycin in 1991 in the United States made the use of this regimen impossible, but the drug became available again in late 1993. Many physicians used amikacin in place of streptomycin but with a maximum daily dose of 500 mg because of its greater likelihood of toxicity.

After the initiation of therapy, patients should be monitored for potential toxic reactions.[3] Monthly eye examinations for visual acuity and red-green color discrimination should be performed, and patients should be instructed to report immediately any changes in vision. Because of the greater incidence of isoniazid toxicity in older patients, most physicians monitor liver function tests with SGOT determinations for the first 3 months of therapy and thereafter based on clinical symptoms. For patients on aminoglycosides, baseline blood urea nitrogen and serum creatinine levels should be obtained. Periodic monitoring of renal function is recommended for high-risk patients, including patients older than 50 years of age and patients with any impairment of renal function. Baseline hearing tests are also recommended if feasible. Patients should be warned to watch for signs of ototoxicity, including tinnitus, hearing loss, and loss of balance. In stable patients, these may be signs of changing renal function with increasing serum levels. Clinical judgment is required, because serum streptomycin levels are not readily available.

The role of surgery for *M. avium* complex disease has not been established. Because the combination of primary treatment failure and relapses may approach 50%, most physicians currently assess patients with localized disease for surgical resection as part of their therapy. This is especially important for patients who relapse or respond poorly to initial drug therapy. Some studies have suggested that a patient's prognosis is improved if surgery is part of the therapy.[21, 22]

Patients should be followed with monthly sputum examinations until sputum conversion has occurred and then periodically thereafter. For patients who do poorly clinically or who fail to show improvement bacteriologically, other drugs should be considered for therapy. These include ciprofloxacin (750 mg twice daily), cycloserine (250 mg three times daily), and ethionamide (250 mg three times daily).

Clarithromycin and azithromycin are macrolides that appear to have excellent activity in the therapy of disseminated *M. avium* disease in AIDS.[23] Their usefulness and role in the therapy for *M. avium* lung disease has not been defined, but they offer exciting potential for therapy of a difficult disease. Trials of clarithromycin and azithromycin are ongoing. One such study demonstrated that clarithromycin at the 1.0 g twice a day dose used in therapy of AIDS patients results in unacceptable levels of toxicity and discontinuation of the drug (85%) in elderly patients with *M. avium* complex disease. A lower dosage of 500 mg twice a day in the same patients was well tolerated.[23a] In a subsequent controlled trial of clarithromycin at 500 mg twice a day as monotherapy for 4 months in 19 patients with *M. avium* complex lung disease, approximately 60% had sputum converted to negative and another 21% showed significant reductions in sputum positivity.[23b] The efficacy or toxicity of clarithromycin when given in combination with other drugs has yet to be determined.

Another potential therapeutic drug recently made available for the therapy of *M. avium* complex lung disease is rifabutin (formerly LM-427, ansamycin). Rifabutin inhibits most *M. avium* complex isolates at 2 μg/mL,[7] although peak serum levels with doses of 150 mg are less than 0.5 μg/mL. Rifabutin at 300 mg/d has been shown in two randomized clinical trials to prevent (or reduce) disseminated *M. avium* complex disease in AIDS.[23c] Studies using higher doses of rifabutin (450–600 mg) have produced increased survival among AIDS patients with disseminated *M. avium* complex disease with no apparent increase in toxicity compared with the lower doses.[24, 25] The efficacy of rifabutin at these higher doses for *M. avium* complex lung disease must be determined. Preliminary studies suggest that clarithromycin given in combination with high-dose (600 mg/d) rifabutin may increase the toxicity of rifabutin.

## MYCOBACTERIUM KANSASII

### Clinical Features

Because large-scale testing of skin test reactivity to *M. kansasii* antigens has not been performed, the geographic locales of *M. kansasii* are less well known than those of *M. avium* complex. However, based on reports of clinical disease, the organism seems to predominate along the southeastern and southern coastal states and the central plains states. The organism has rarely been recovered from the environment. It has never been found in soil or natural water supplies, but it has been recovered from tap water in cities where *M. kansasii* is endemic.[26] Previous studies in Texas suggested that *M. kansasii* disease is concentrated in urban areas, supporting the possible association between clinical disease and recovery of the organism from potable water supplies.

Clinical pulmonary disease caused by *M. kansasii* is similar to TB. Fever is probably less common than in disease due to *M. tuberculosis*, but other clinical signs, including cough, sputum production, hemoptysis, and weight loss, are relatively common. The disease is most often encountered in white males, although it is encountered in all races in proportion to their presence in the population at large. There appears to be no definite association with alcoholism, but a history of cigarette abuse and chronic lung disease is found for as many as 50% of patients who develop *M. kansasii* lung disease. HIV infection has some association with *M. kansasii* lung disease, although the number of patients reported has been relatively small. Many of these patients have disseminated disease, with involvement of the blood, skin, central nervous system, or gastrointestinal tract as well as the lung.[27, 28]

Radiographic features of *M. kansasii* lung disease in HIV-negative patients are similar to those seen with *M. tuberculosis*. Approximately 80% to 90% of patients have cavitary disease, with a preponderance of involvement of the upper lobes (Fig. 39–4). In HIV-positive patients, cavitary disease appears to be unusual. Most patients have interstitial or alveolar infiltrates, which are frequently bilateral.[27, 28]

### Laboratory Features

*M. kansasii* is regularly seen on acid-fast smears and recovered by culture techniques designed for *M. tuberculosis*. It grows readily in the BACTEC broth and on 7H10

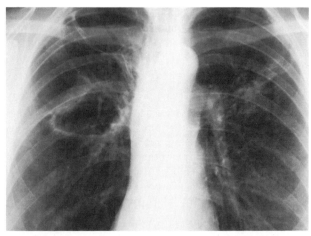

**Figure 39–4.** Two large, thin-walled cavities in the right apex and right upper lobe of a 35-year-old woman with *Mycobacterium kansasii*.

agar or Löwenstein-Jensen agar. The organism typically produces rough, large colonies that turn bright yellow with exposure to light (ie, photochromogen). A species-specific DNA probe for *M. kansasii* has been described and is commercially available. The organism is also identified by biochemical tests and by high-pressure liquid chromatography.[23c] On acid-fast smears, *M. kansasii* typically is a large, long bacillus that shows unusual beading if stained with Ziehl-Neelsen or Kinyoun stains. This often signals the presence of *M. kansasii*.

Traditional proportion method susceptibilities of *M. kansasii* using the single critical concentrations for *M. tuberculosis* are most useful for rifampin and ethambutol. Essentially all untreated strains are susceptible to 1 μg/mL and 5 μg/mL, respectively, of these two drugs. Unfortunately, the single critical concentrations of 1 μg/mL of isoniazid and 2 μg/mL of streptomycin used to separate treated from untreated strains of *M. tuberculosis* are not particularly useful for *M. kansasii*. Because they are close to the exact MIC of most strains, repeated tests from the same isolate may show susceptibility, partial resistance, or resistance when these concentrations are tested. Resistance to isoniazid or streptomycin using these concentrations should be ignored and play no role in deciding therapy. If 5 μg/mL of isoniazid or 10 μg/mL of streptomycin is used as a critical concentration, almost all isolates will be susceptible (see Table 39–3). Because these concentrations are generally useful only for *M. kansasii* and some other species of NTM, few laboratories perform them. *M. kansasii* is resistant to pyrazinamide at all test concentrations in vitro, as are all species of NTM.

Acquired drug resistance to rifampin, isoniazid, and ethambutol after drug therapy has been demonstrated, the latter two by MICs.[29] Additional drugs with in vitro activity against *M. kansasii* at achievable serum levels include ciprofloxacin and ofloxacin, clarithromycin, ethionamide, cycloserine, and sulfonamides.

## Treatment

In the era before rifampin, sputum conversions for *M. kansasii* with regimens containing isoniazid and streptomycin were in the range of 60% to 80%. Surgical resection for localized disease was an important part of therapy. With the introduction of rifampin and ethambutol, this approach to disease management changed dramatically. With rifampin-containing regimens, sputum conversion rates by 4 months are almost 100%. In 180 patients from three studies who were treated with rifampin-containing regimens, all sputum samples converted to negative.[9, 30, 31]

Treatment failure rates and long-term relapse rates appear to be about 1%. Failures appear to be related to the development of resistance to rifampin.

The American Thoracic Society recommendation for treatment of pulmonary disease caused by *M. kansasii* includes isoniazid (300 mg/d), ethambutol (15 mg/kg/d), and rifampin (600 mg/d) for 18 months.[3] For patients who are unable to tolerate isoniazid, a third drug should be used. Possible alternatives include cycloserine, ethionamide, ciprofloxacin, ofloxacin, and clarithromycin. The latter three drugs have substantially less toxicity and are probably preferred.

Short-course regimens such as those used for treating of *M. tuberculosis* are not available for *M. kansasii*. The short-course regimen of isoniazid and rifampin daily for 2 months, followed by twice-weekly doses for 7 months, which was popularized as the Arkansas regimen, is associated with an unacceptable treatment failure rate. Because pyrazinamide has no activity against *M. kansasii*, the treatment regimen recommended by the American Thoracic Society for *M. tuberculosis* (ie, 2 months of pyrazinamide, rifampin, and isoniazid, followed by 4 months of rifampin and isoniazid) is probably not effective for *M. kansasii*. One study of 40 patients by Ahn and colleagues demonstrated that the addition of streptomycin (1 g twice weekly for the first 3 months) to the currently recommended three-drug regimen resulted in a long-term success rate of 97%.[10] A preliminary report of low-dose ethambutol (15 mg/kg) and rifampin given for 9 months has been reported in abstract form from the British Medical Research Council,[11] but the final study with long-term follow-up is not yet available. Until further studies are reported, short-course regimens should generally not be used with *M. kansasii*.

For organisms that have become resistant to rifampin, a regimen that includes a sulfonamide and a daily injectable has proven effective in almost 90% of patients.[29] This regimen consists of daily high-dose isoniazid (900 mg), pyridoxine, ethambutol (25 mg/kg) for the duration of therapy, sulfamethoxazole (1 g twice daily), and streptomycin. The last is usually given five times a week for the first 2 to 3 months, then two or three times per week as tolerated to complete at least 6 months of therapy. The oral portion of the regimen is given until the patient has been culture negative for 12 to 15 months on therapy.[29]

For patients with HIV infection and *M. kansasii*, the treatment regimen recommended by the Centers for Disease Control is the same as for HIV-negative patients. Some researchers have advocated the addition of streptomycin (1 g twice each week for the first 3 months). Therapy should be continued until the patient is culture negative for 15 months. Because the number of patients has been so small, it is unknown if long-term suppressive therapy may be needed in these patients. Initial studies with advanced AIDS and disseminated *M. kansasii* suggested that the latter disease responded poorly or not at all to therapy.[27, 28] Studies that identified patients early in their course of HIV disease and patients with predominantly pulmonary disease have suggested that these patients respond well to therapy in a manner comparable to those with *M. tuberculosis*.

Studies suggest that the newer macrolides, especially clarithromycin, are extremely active against *M. kansasii* in vitro. However, because of the small number of patients encountered annually, attempts to initiate a clinical trial to see if this drug would allow a shorter course of therapy or greatly improve on one of the current drugs have not been done. The one reported clinical trial of treatment of rifampin-resistant *M. kansasii* was done before the development of clarithromycin.[29] It seems likely that this drug can be useful in several settings of *M. kansasii* disease, but there is no clinical experience with it.

## RAPIDLY GROWING MYCOBACTERIA

### Clinical Features

Because of the absence of a large-scale study of skin test reactivity of rapidly growing mycobacterial skin test antigens, the distribution of infection with these organisms within the United States is unknown. However, *M. fortuitum* is readily recovered from soil and water supplies almost everywhere in the United States.[1] The clinical disease that has been reported usually has been along the southeastern and southern coastal states. This is comparable to areas of major activity of *M. avium* complex. Patients who acquire rapidly growing mycobacterial lung disease are typically white, female nonsmokers.[32, 32a] Approximately 40% of patients have an underlying disorder that appears to facilitate development of the mycobacterial disease. Recognized diseases include previously diagnosed and treated mycobacterial lung disease including TB, cystic fibrosis, and gastroesophageal diseases associated with recurrent vomiting (primarily achalasia).[32a] In the remaining 60% of patients with rapidly growing mycobacterial lung disease, no specific abnormality is evident. The average age of the adult patient is approximately 60 years. Most patients who experience the onset of the disease before they reach 40 years of age have one of the definable underlying disorders.[32a]

The usual presenting symptom for patients with rapidly growing mycobacterial lung disease is cough. With time, sputum production, weight loss, malaise, and fever develop in most patients. Hemoptysis occurs, but it appears to be less common than with other mycobacterial lung diseases. In some patients, the clinical illness exactly mimics bronchiectasis.[32, 32a] The patients have episodic cough, sputum production, and low-grade fever that is interspersed with periods of relative well-being and minimal respiratory symptoms. Because of this, some patients with rapidly growing mycobacterial lung disease are given the clinical diagnosis of bronchiectasis and may carry this diagnosis for years before acid-fast (AFB) smears and cultures are done. If the patient has no definable infection or disease that would lead to bronchiectasis, if radiographic studies were not done and this is just a clinical diagnosis, and AFB smears and cultures are positive the first time they are ordered, rapidly growing mycobacterial lung disease should be suspected.

Chest radiographs with rapidly growing mycobacterial lung disease are quite different from those with *M. kansasii* or *M. tuberculosis*.[32] Cavitary disease is produced by the mycobacteria in about 15% of cases.[32a] The organism usually produces a patchy, reticular, nodular, upper lobe infiltrate. Some are scar-like, causing the disease to be overlooked and the radiographic changes ascribed to some previous illness. In patients who have preexisting mycobacterial disease, the infiltrates almost invariably occur in the area of worst lung damage produced by the previous mycobacteria (Figs. 39–5 through 39–7). In patients with achalasia or coexistent exogenous lipoid pneumonia, the infiltrates often have a dense, alveolar character and are bilateral. In patients who have primary lung disease without associated underlying risk factors, bilateral patchy interstitial disease is common.

## Laboratory Features

The rapidly growing mycobacteria are the most difficult of the nontuberculous mycobacteria to be recognized by the

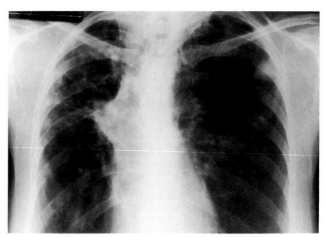

**Figure 39–5.** Residual right upper lobe disease in a patient successfully treated for *Mycobacterium avium* complex lung disease.

standard staining and culture techniques used for *M. tuberculosis*. The organisms do not always stain well with the Ziehl-Neelsen or Kinyoun method and may not be recognized readily with the fluorochrome method. It is common to see a sputum sample which is AFB smear negative but has 4 + growth, suggesting that the organisms were not stainable. Rapidly growing mycobacteria are the most susceptible of the mycobacteria to the decontamination procedures used to remove bacteria from the sample. The organisms are almost completely killed by the use of 4% sodium hydroxide, and historically, recognition of the organism as a pathogen generally occurred only after 1.75% to 2% sodium hydroxide was adopted for decontamination. With prolonged exposure or even standard use of this procedure, it is common to have AFB-positive sputum smears but to grow only four or five colonies on the plates. Quantitation of the amount of rapidly growing mycobacterial organisms present by smear or culture can be difficult and should be assessed carefully.

Although there are six or seven recognized pathogenic groups of rapidly growing mycobacteria, more than 95% of clinical lung disease is caused by two groups. *M. abscessus* is responsible for approximately 85% of isolates, and *M.*

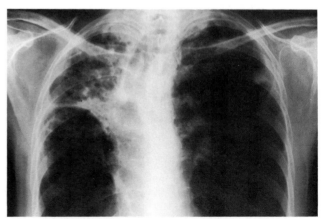

**Figure 39–6.** New right upper lobe infiltrate in the same patient shown in Figure 39–5. Multiple sputum samples were smear and culture positive for *Mycobacterium abscessus*.

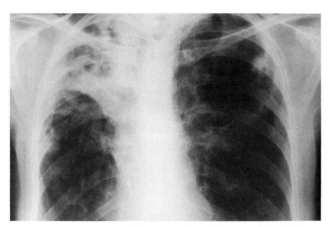

**Figure 39–7.** Progression of disease in the right upper lobe infiltrate that was shown in Figure 39–6 after 1 year.

*fortuitum* (formerly *M. fortuitum* biovariant *fortuitum*) is responsible for another 10% to 12% of isolates.[32a]

According to drug susceptibilities, *M. abscessus* is resistant to all the antituberculous agents (see Table 39–3) and is resistant to almost all oral agents used to treat *M. fortuitum* and *M. abscessus*.[33] About one third of isolates are moderately susceptible to erythromycin,[33] but clinical experience with the use of erythromycin for these organisms has generally been poor. All isolates of *M. abscessus* are susceptible in vitro to low concentrations of clarithromycin.[34] Because clinical trials of this drug have not been performed, it is uncertain if the drug will prove to be efficacious in vivo. *M. abscessus* is usually susceptible to amikacin and cefoxitin,[33] and some isolates are moderately susceptible to imipenem.

Isolates of *M. fortuitum* are much more drug susceptible; essentially all isolates are susceptible in vitro to achievable serum levels of amikacin, cefoxitin, imipenem, sulfonamides, ciprofloxacin, and ofloxacin, and approximately 50% are susceptible to doxycycline and minocycline.[33] Separation of *M. fortuitum* from *M. abscessus* is done fairly readily if at least two laboratory tests (usually iron uptake and nitrate reduction) are used.[35]

**Therapy**

Because isolates of *M. abscessus* are resistant to most oral drugs other than clarithromycin, attempts at cure with drugs in the past for this organism have been unsuccessful. The use of amikacin plus cefoxitin or impenem has usually resulted in clinical and microbiologic improvement, but because the drugs cannot be given long enough, relapse invariably occurs after the drugs are discontinued. The best modality for treatment for *M. abscessus* is surgical resection of the localized area of the lung, with prior drug therapy to try to reduce the organism burden.[32a] Whether clarithromycin can produce a change in this management is unknown, because clinical trials have not been performed. Most patients who have localized disease and who are surgical candidates should undergo a course of injectable therapy followed by surgical resection of diseased tissue.

*M. fortuitum* requires a different approach because it is much more susceptible to drugs. Patients with this disease usually are given amikacin plus imipenem or cefoxitin for 4 to 8 weeks and are then treated with two oral agents until cultures have been negative for approximately 1 year. The success rate with *M. fortuitum* is high, although the number of cases studied is small because it is an infrequent cause of lung disease.

Patients with underlying lipoid pneumonia or achalasia frequently develop a sepsis-like syndrome. These patients have high fevers, have leukocyte counts in excess of 20,000/mm³, and appear moderately ill in a way that is unusual for rapidly growing mycobacterial lung disease. These patients respond to therapy, but the decline in the leukocyte count and temperature often takes 4 to 6 weeks.

## MYCOBACTERIUM XENOPI

Once a rare cause of lung disease, *M. xenopi* is now a relatively common cause of NTM lung disease in several areas outside the United States, including England and Canada.[36] The organism is frequently recovered from tap water, especially hot water, and can be a contaminant in the patient and the laboratory. The organism can also be a cause of nosocomial lung disease, and many of the reported cases have been in clusters with a suggested common source.[37, 38] The clinical disease is similar to other nontuberculous disease in its presentation. The organism is relatively susceptible to drug treatment (see Table 39–3), and therapy with the four-drug regimen used for treating *M. avium* complex is usually successful. Surgery has been used for some patients, especially those who fail initial drug therapy.

## INFREQUENT PATHOGENS

### Mycobacterium szulgai

The slowly growing species of *M. szulgai* has relatively confusing morphologic features in that it is a scotochromogen (ie, forms pigment after growth in the dark) at 37°C but may behave like a photochromogen at 25°C. Approximately 20 cases of lung disease due to *M. szulgai* have been reported.[38, 39] The disease was comparable to chronic tuberculosis and occurred primarily in elderly white men. Therapy with three to four drugs with a regimen comparable to that recommended for *M. avium* complex resulted in clinical and microbiologic improvement.

### Mycobacterium simiae

*M. simiae* is a nonpigmented, slowly growing species that morphologically resembles *M. avium* complex. In the summary of state health department laboratory isolates of NTM from 1981 through 1983 assembled by the Centers for Disease Control,[6] 67 of the isolates (1.2%) were attributed to *M. simiae*. Most primary physicians did not think the organism was causing clinical disease, but multiple positive sputa from patients with chronic lung disease have been reported.[38] *M. simiae* is the most resistant of all the NTM to drug therapy, with most isolates resistant to all drugs tested in vitro, including clarithromycin.

## Mycobacterium malmoense

*M. malmoense* is a species of nonpigmented, slowly growing NTM that was first described as a lung pathogen in 1977 in 4 patients from Malmo, Sweden. Since then, it has been recognized with increasing frequency in patients from Europe, especially Sweden and Great Britain. It has rarely been identified in patients in the United States. The organism grows relatively poorly and can be confused with other slowly growing, nonpigmented NTM. The organism can be recovered from patients in the apparent absence of any lung disease. However, some patients have disease that is similar in character and presentation to that caused by other NTM.[40] The optimal therapy for treatment of this disease is unknown.

## Miscellaneous Species

A few additional species of *Mycobacterium* have caused chronic lung disease,[38] including *M. asiaticum*,[38, 41] *M. shimoidei*,[38] *M. thermoresistibile*,[38] *M. smegmatis*, *M. peregrinum*, *M. fortuitum*, the unnamed third biovariant complex, *M. chelonae*, and the *M. chelonae*-like organisms. The numbers of these cases are too small to allow any characterization of the epidemiology, clinical features, or treatment of the diseases.

## REFERENCES

1. Wolinsky E: Nontuberculous mycobacteria and associated diseases. Am Rev Respir Dis 119:107–159, 1979.
2. Edwards LB, Acquaviva FA, Livesay VT, Cross FW, Palmer CE: An atlas of sensitivity to tuberculin, PPD-B, and histoplasmin in the United States. Am Rev Respir Dis 99:1–132, 1969.
3. Wallace RJ Jr, O'Brien R, Glassroth J, Raleigh J, Dutt A: Diagnosis and treatment of disease caused by nontuberculous mycobacteria. Am Rev Respir Dis 142:940–953, 1990.
4. Ahn CH, McLarty JW, Ahn SS, Ahn SI, Hurst GA: Diagnostic criteria for pulmonary disease caused by *Mycobacterium kansasii* and *Mycobacterium intracellulare*. Am Rev Respir Dis 125:388–391, 1982.
5. Good RC, Snider DE: Isolation of nontuberculous mycobacteria in the United States, 1980. J Infect Dis 146:829–833, 1982.
6. O'Brien RJ, Geiter LJ, Snider DE: The epidemiology of nontuberculous mycobacterial diseases in the United States: Results from a national survey. Am Rev Respir Dis 135:1007–1014, 1987.
7. Woodley CL, Kilburn JO: In vitro susceptibility of *Mycobacterium avium* complex and *Mycobacterium tuberculosis* strains to a spiropiperidyl rifamycin. Am Rev Respir Dis 126:586–587, 1982.
8. Ahn CH, Ahn SS, Anderson RA, Murphy DT, Mammo A: A four-drug regimen for initial treatment of cavitary disease caused by *Mycobacterium avium* complex. Am Rev Respir Dis 134:438–441, 1986.
9. Ahn CH, Lowell JR, Ahn SA, Ahn S, Hurst GA: Chemotherapy for pulmonary disease due to *Mycobacterium kansasii*: Efficacies of some individual drugs. Rev Infect Dis 3:1028–1034, 1981.
10. Ahn CH, Lowell JR, Ahn SS, Ahn SI, Hurst GA: Short-course chemotherapy for pulmonary disease caused by *Mycobacterium kansasii*. Am Rev Respir Dis 128:1048–1050, 1983.
11. Campbell IA: A study of 9-month treatment with rifampicin and ethambutol in pulmonary infection with *M. kansasii*. [Abstract] Bull Union Tuber 61:43, 1986.
12. Heifets LB, Iseman MD: Individualized therapy versus standard regimens in the treatment of *Mycobacterium avium* infections. [Editorial] Am Rev Respir Dis 144:1–2, 1991.
13. Meissner G, Anz W: Sources of *Mycobacterium avium*-complex infection resulting in human disease. Am Rev Respir Dis 116:1057–1064, 1977.
14. Meissner PS, Falkinham JO: Plasmid DNA profiles as epidemiologic markers for clinical and environmental isolates of *Mycobacterium avium*, *Mycobacterium intracellulare*, and *Mycobacterium scrofulaceum*. J Infect Dis 153:325–331, 1986.
15. Rosenweig DY: Pulmonary mycobacterial infections due to *Mycobacterium intracellulare-avium* complex. Chest 75:115–119, 1979.
16. Davidson PT, Khanijo V, Goble M, Mouding TS: Treatment of disease due to *Mycobacterium intracellulare*. Rev Infect Dis 3:1052–1059, 1981.
17. Lincoln EM, Gilbert LA: Disease in children due to mycobacteria other than *Mycobacterium tuberculosis*. Am Rev Respir Dis 105:683–714, 1972.
17a. Swensen SJ, Hartman TE, Williams DE. Computed tomographic diagnosis of *Mycobacterium avium-intracellulare* complex in patients with bronchiectasis. Chest 105:49–52, 1994.
18. Prince DA, Peterson DD, Steiner RM, et al: Infection with *Mycobacterium avium* complex in patients without predisposing conditions. N Engl J Med 321:863–868, 1989.
19. Modilevsky TA, Sattler FR, Barnes PF: Mycobacterial disease in patients with human immunodeficiency virus infection. Arch Intern Med 149:2201–2205, 1989.
20. Seibert AF, Bass JB: Four-drug therapy of pulmonary disease due to *Mycobacterium-avium* complex. [Abstract] The 1989 Annual Meeting of American Thoracic Society, May 14–17, 1989, Cincinnati, Ohio.
21. Corpe RF: Surgical management of pulmonary disease due to *Mycobacterium avium-intracellulare*. Rev Infect Dis 3:1064–1067, 1981.
22. Moran JF, Alexander LG, Staub EW, Young WG, Sealy WC: Long-term results of pulmonary resection for atypical mycobacterial disease. Ann Thorac Surg 35:597–604, 1983.
23. Dautzenberg B, Truffot C, Legris S, et al: Activity of clarithromycin against *Mycobacterium avium* infection in patients with the acquired immune deficiency syndrome. Am Rev Respir Dis 144:564–569, 1991.
23a. Wallace RJ Jr, Brown BA, Griffith DE: Drug intolerance to high-dose clarithromycin among elderly patients. Diagn Microbiol Infect Dis 16:215–221, 1993.
23b. Wallace RJ Jr, Brown BA, Griffith DE, et al: Initial clarithromycin monotherapy for *Mycobacterium avium-intracellulare* complex lung disease. Am J Respir Crit Care Med (in press).
23c. Nightingale SD, Cameron DW, Gordin FM, et al: Two controlled trials of rifabutin prophylaxis against *Mycobacterium avium* complex infection in AIDS. N Engl J Med 329:828–834, 1993.
24. Agins BD, Berman DA, Spicehandler D, El-Sadr W, Simberkoff MS, Rahal JJ: Effect of combined therapy with ansamycin, clofazimine, ethambutol, and isoniazid for *Mycobacterium avium* infection in patients with AIDS. J Infect Dis 159:784–787, 1989.
25. Hoy J, Mijch A, Sandland M, Grayson L, Lucas R, Dwyer B: Quadruple-drug therapy for *Mycobacterium avium-intracellulare* bacteremia in AIDS patients. J Infect Dis 161:801–805, 1990.
26. Steadham JE: High-catalase strains of *Mycobacterium kansasii* isolated from water in Texas. J Clin Microbiol 11:496–498, 1980.
27. Carpenter JL, Parks JM: *Mycobacterium kansasii* infections in patients positive for human immunodeficiency virus. Rev Infect Dis 13:789–796, 1991.
28. Sherer R, Sable R, Sonnenberg M, et al: Disseminated infection with *Mycobacterium kansasii* in the acquired immunodeficiency syndrome. Ann Intern Med 105:710–712, 1986.
29. Ahn CH, Wallace RJ Jr, Steele LC, Murphy DT: Sulfonamide-containing regimens for disease caused by rifampin-resistant *Mycobacterium kansasii*. Am Rev Respir Dis 135:10–16, 1987.
30. Pezzia W, Raleigh JW, Bailey MC, Toth EA, Silverblatt J: Treatment of pulmonary disease due to *Mycobacterium kansasii*: Recent experience with rifampin. Rev Infect Dis 3:1035–1039, 1981.
31. Banks J, Hunter AM, Campbell IA, Jenkins PA, Smith AP: Pulmonary infection with *Mycobacterium kansasii* in Wales, 1970–9: Review of treatment and response. Thorax 38:271–274, 1983.
32. Wallace RJ Jr: The clinical presentation, diagnosis, and therapy of cutaneous and pulmonary infections due to the rapidly growing mycobacteria *M. fortuitum* and *M. chelonae*. Clin Chest Med 10:419–429, 1989.
32a. Griffith DE, Girard WM, Wallace RJ Jr: Clinical features of pulmonary disease caused by rapidly growing mycobacteria. Am Rev Respir Dis 147:1271–1278, 1993.
33. Swenson JM, Wallace RJ Jr, Silcox VA, Thornsberry C: Antimicrobial susceptibility of five subgroups of *Mycobacterium fortuitum* and *Mycobacterium chelonae*. Antimicrob Agents Chemother 28:807–811, 1985.

34. Brown BA, Wallace RJ Jr, Onyi GO, DeRosas V, Wallace RJ III: Activities of four macrolides, including clarithromycin, against *Mycobacterium fortuitum*, *Mycobacterium chelonae*, and *M. chelonae*-like organisms. Antimicrob Agents Chemother 36:180–184, 1992.

35. Silcox VA, Good RC, Floyd MM: Identification of clinically significant *Mycobacterium fortuitum* complex isolates. J Clin Microbiol 14:686–691, 1981.

36. Yates MD, Grange JM, Collins CH: The nature of mycobacterial disease in south east England, 1977–84. J Epidemiol Community Health 40:295–300, 1986.

37. Costrini AM, Mahler DA, Gross WM, Hawkins JE, Yesner R, D'Esopo ND: Clinical and roentgenographic features of nosocomial pulmonary disease due to *Mycobacterium xenopi*. Am Rev Respir Dis 123:104–109, 1981.

38. Wayne LG, Sramek HA: Agents of newly recognized or infrequently encountered mycobacterial diseases. Clin Microbiol Rev 5:1–25, 1992.

39. Maloney JM, Gregg CR, Stephens DS, Manian FA, Rimland D: Infections caused by *Mycobacterium szulgai* in humans. Rev Infect Dis 9:1120–1126, 1987.

40. Alberts WM, Chandler KW, Solomon DA, Goldman AL: Pulmonary disease caused by *Mycobacterium malmoense*. Am Rev Respir Dis 135:1375–1378, 1987.

41. Blacklock ZM: *Mycobacterium asiaticum* as a potential pulmonary pathogen for humans. Am Rev Respir Dis 127:241–244, 1983.

# CHAPTER 40

# Viral Pneumonia in Immunocompetent Adults

THOMAS R. CATE

The syndrome of nonbacterial or atypical pneumonia is characterized by a constellation of findings that include fever and malaise; cough that is often paroxysmal; production of small amounts of sputum with a relative paucity of polymorphonuclear cells (PMNs) and mixed flora on Gram stain; ill-defined, patchy, or diffuse pulmonary infiltrates seen on the chest radiograph; and a peripheral leukocyte count that is low, normal, or modestly elevated with little or no increase in mature PMNs or band forms.

The infectious agents that can produce this syndrome include several viruses and *Chlamydia* species, *Mycoplasma pneumoniae*, and *Coxiella burnetti*; it may also be mimicked by certain other infections, notably legionnaires disease. A presumptive etiologic diagnosis may be possible with knowledge of the patient's age and state of immunocompetence, epidemiologic circumstances, and response to empiric therapy; occasional findings such as a rash or bullous myringitis may provide additional clues. However, a definitive diagnosis often depends on laboratory results that return after the illness has run its course. That situation is changing with the increasing availability of rapid diagnostic techniques, a development prompted by recognition that knowledge of the diagnosis can have important implications for therapeutic and preventive measures. Respiratory viral diseases can be ameliorated by antiviral therapies such as ribavirin for respiratory syncytial virus (RSV) infections of young children and amantadine for influenza A virus infections in persons of all ages.

This chapter focuses on viral pneumonias in immunocompetent adults. Although RSV, parainfluenza viruses, enteroviruses, and rhinoviruses are rarely involved, the most prominent etiologic agents in this setting are the influenza viruses. Influenza viruses are the main topic of this chapter, including a description of the agents, their epidemiology, clinical manifestations, diagnosis, treatment, and prevention. Adenoviruses are also important causes of pneumonia in young children and in adults in special circumstances, and pneumonia is a potentially severe complication of measles and varicella virus infections in adults. Characteristics of the aforementioned viruses and the diseases that they produce are briefly described.

## INFLUENZA

### The Viruses

Influenza viruses belong to the *Orthomyxoviridae* family. They are enveloped, pleomorphic particles about 100 nm in diameter and covered with surface projections.[1–3] Influenza viruses can be subdivided into types A, B, and C on the basis of the essentially stable antigenic specificity of two internal components, nucleoprotein (NP) that is complexed with the segmented RNA genome, and a component of the matrix protein (M1) that lines the undersurface of the virion envelope. Type C influenza viruses differ from types A and B in several ways, including epidemiologic behavior (eg, less severe respiratory illness without seasonality) and structure (eg, single surface glycoprotein versus two for types A and B), and they have been placed in a separate genus. Because the typical winter influenza epidemics during which pneumonia occurs are caused entirely by types A and B, only these influenza virus types are considered in this chapter.

The surface projections from the influenza virus envelope consist of the hemagglutinin (HA) and neuraminidase (NA) glycoproteins. HA attaches to sialic acid-containing structures on the surface of cells, which leads to endocytosis of the virion. If the HA has previously undergone posttranslational cleavage into HA1 and HA2 by an exogenous protease, the lowered pH within the endosome causes a conformational change that uncovers a fusion peptide on HA2. A second component of matrix protein appears to play a critical role in mediating this conformational change, perhaps by serving as an ion channel. Fusion with the endosome membrane permits emptying of the viral genomic material into the cell cytoplasm so that replication can begin. The primary role of NA appears to occur at the other end of the replication cycle. NA can hydrolyze sialic acid residues from cell-surface glycoconjugates and from viral glycoproteins; this prevents aggregation of new virions released from the infected cell and facilitates the spread of infection.

The nucleocapsids of influenza viruses consist of segments of negative-stranded RNA that are each complexed with NP and with three viral polymerases, PA, PB1, and PB2. These ribonucleoprotein (RNP) complexes are transported from the infected cell's cytoplasm to the nucleus, where the viral RNA is transcribed by the polymerases into mRNA. The viral polymerase is unable to initiate viral mRNA synthesis de novo and appropriates fragments of host-cell mRNA to serve as primers. Newly formed viral mRNA then returns to the cytoplasm for translation into viral proteins. Included in the latter are nonstructural proteins, NS1 and NS2, which have uncertain function but accumulate in the nucleus and cytoplasm, respectively, and structural elements that begin nascent viral assembly at the cell membrane. Meanwhile, polymerase activity in the nucleus turns to replication of the viral RNA through production of complementary viral RNA templates that are copied to yield new genomic segments. These, along with newly produced viral NP and polymerases, form RNP complexes that are transported to the virus-modified cell membrane for inclusion into new viruses as they bud from the cell surface. In the process of budding, the new viruses appropriate some of the host-cell membrane for their envelope.

Protection against infection with influenza viruses is mediated by antibody directed primarily against the HA surface glycoprotein.[1–5] Antibodies to NA can reduce the severity of influenza virus infection by interfering with virus release and spread within the infected person. Although antibodies to other viral components are induced during infection, their role in preventing infection is negligible. Cytotoxic T-cell immune responses are also induced during influenza virus infection. Surface glycoproteins of the virions can be targets for these T cells, but they more often have specificity for internal viral components. The major role of cytotoxic T cells is in effecting recovery from influenza virus infection, but T-cell immunity appears to have little or no role in preventing the infection.

A notable characteristic of influenza viruses is the relatively high frequency of antigenic changes in their surface glycoproteins, which renders immunity derived from prior infection or vaccination less effective. Minor antigenic change (ie, drift) occurs in all influenza types and is a result of mutational changes. These mutations are more frequent in RNA than in DNA viruses because of the lack of RNA proofreading enzymes.

Type A influenza viruses also exhibit major antigenic changes (ie, shifts) in one or both of their surface glycoproteins at one- to four-decade intervals; these changes render

immunity directed against earlier versions of the glycoproteins almost totally ineffective. The mechanism involved depends on the segmented nature of the viral genome. Influenza virus types A and B both have eight RNA segments (ie, PB1, PB2, PA, HA, NP, NA, M, NS) that code for at least 10 proteins. If two influenza viruses of the same type infect a cell at the same time, reassortment of the RNA segments occurs during replication, yielding daughter viruses with a mixture of genomic material from the two parents. If the mix provides some advantage to a daughter virus, such as evasion of immunologic defenses or enhanced replication or virulence, proliferation and spread of that daughter virus are favored.

The additional factor that permits periodic formation of ''new'' type A influenza viruses is the existence of numerous mammalian and avian influenza A viruses in nature, a genetic reservoir that is lacking for type B viruses. Most of the animal and avian viruses replicate very poorly or not at all in cells of human origin. But if a person becomes infected at the same time with a ''human'' strain to which he is partially immune and an animal strain with dissimilar surface glycoproteins, a daughter virus having ''internal'' genes favoring growth in human cells and a ''new'' HA or NA may emerge. Swine may be an important intermediate host for reassortment of influenza A viruses, because avian and human strains can infect them. Many influenza A subtypes appear to have originated in the Far East, perhaps because the density of human, swine, and duck populations increases the likelihood of dual infections. About 14 HA and 9 NA subtypes exist in nature, and the number of possible influenza A subtypes classified on the basis of these surface glycoproteins is high. Less easily recognized reassortment of internal genes also increases potential variability in viral virulence, which is determined by the interaction of multiple genes but can be greatly influenced by a point mutation or complete change of a single gene. Apparent limits exist on the number of influenza A viruses that are epidemiologically significant, perhaps because of selective survival of those viruses endowed with genes that operate together most efficiently in the host.

When a new influenza A subtype emerges as a human pathogen, it typically spreads rapidly, unopposed by effective immune defenses, and completely replaces the previous A subtype as a human pathogen. The succession of local epidemics as a new subtype spreads around the world is called a pandemic. Human influenza viruses were first grown in 1933. Since then, an A/H2N2 pandemic strain arose in 1957, and A/H3N2 in 1968. Persons tend to maintain relatively high serum antibody titers against the influenza virus with which they were first infected as a child, a phenomenon known as original antigenic sin. Seroepidemiologic studies of this phenomenon indicate that A/H1N1-like viruses originally recovered from swine were responsible for the devastating 1918 pandemic, and that the pandemics of 1889 and 1900 were probably caused by A/H2N8 and A/H3N8 viruses, respectively. The return of A/H1N1 as a human pathogen in 1977 after an absence of only 20 years created an unusual circumstance; persons in their mid-twenties and older were largely immune, and A/H1N1 viruses have continued to cocirculate with strains of the A/H3N2 subtype rather than displacing the latter.

The complete nomenclature of influenza viruses includes the virus type, the species of animal or bird from which it was recovered, the location where it was recovered, the specimen number assigned at the recovery site, and the year of recovery. For type A influenza viruses, the subtype designations of the HA and NA are also included in parentheses. Examples of some contemporary viruses are A/Chicken/Pennsylvania/1370/83 (H5N2), a lethal poultry virus that necessitated destruction of numerous infected flocks for its eradication, and A/Texas/36/91 (H1N1), A/Beijing/32/92 (H3N2), and B/Panama/45/90, the three virus strains represented in the influenza vaccine prepared for the winter of 1993 to 1994.

## Epidemiology

Influenza outbreaks of varying severity occur annually, typically over a period of 6 to 10 weeks during the winter months in temperate climates.[6, 7] The reason for the winter timing is uncertain but may involve a variety of factors, such as greater congregation of people inside, less fresh air ventilation, and increased survival of influenza viruses at lower humidity. Influenza viruses totally disappear from a given population between outbreaks, only to return the next year after circling the globe in a succession of outbreaks, during which new variants often arise. Although a mixture of influenza virus variants is often detected during localized outbreaks, one variant typically predominates; this is most frequently a type A strain, with type B predominating at intervals of about 2 to 4 years. The proportion of persons affected in a community may be less than 10% during mild outbreaks and 20% or more during severe epidemics in interpandemic eras. Attack rates approaching 50% and occurring over a shorter period (5 to 6 weeks) may be expected with a new pandemic influenza A virus.

The spread of influenza through the community follows a fairly typical pattern, with increases in the number of visits to medical facilities for febrile respiratory disease producing a bell-shaped curve during moderate to severe epidemics.[8] Increases in school absenteeism are frequently the first sign of an influenza epidemic, and school children appear to be important in disseminating the virus by carrying it home to their younger siblings and parents.[9] The peak increases in industrial absenteeism for respiratory disease and in hospitalizations of infants and adults for pneumonia tend to occur during the second half of the outbreak. The excess deaths caused by pneumonia and influenza, which are routinely used to track influenza activity nationally, occur mostly in the later phases of a local epidemic.

The overall attack rates for influenza virus infection are highest in young children and decrease with increasing age.[10, 11] Contributing factors to this decrease may include partial immunity as a result of prior infection with related viruses, particularly with type B and A/H1N1 viruses, and a decreased likelihood of exposure of elderly persons to infected school children. Hospitalizations for severe or complicated influenza follow a different pattern, with peaks at opposite ends of the age spectrum (ie, infants and persons older than 64 years of age).[12, 13] Deaths as a result of influenza follow yet another age-related pattern. Among those hospitalized with the infection, deaths occur in only 1% to 2% of those younger than 45 years of age, but in 10% to 15% of those older than 64 years of age. Excess deaths

from pneumonia related to influenza numbered at least 10,000 during each of 7 influenza epidemics in the period of 1977 through 1988, and more than 40,000 in two of them.[14] Increases in mortality from ischemic cardiovascular disease tend to parallel those for influenza-related pneumonia, thus suggesting that the actual number of deaths precipitated by influenza virus infections during epidemics may be considerably greater than that attributed to influenza pneumonia alone.[15]

An important contributing factor to influenza mortality is the presence of certain chronic diseases, most notably those of the heart and lungs; each increases the risk of death from influenza pneumonia by more than 100-fold during epidemics, and together they increase the risk by 800-fold.[16] Other chronic diseases that increase the risk of influenza mortality to a lesser extent include metabolic diseases such as diabetes mellitus, renal dysfunction, anemia, and immunosuppression. The increased risk of influenza complications in the elderly is caused largely by the presence of one or more of these chronic diseases.

Nursing home residents are at a particularly high risk for explosive influenza outbreaks with devastating consequences. Part of the reason may be the decline in T-cell function that occurs in the very elderly.[17] Also, close confinement of susceptible persons in residential communities can foster explosive outbreaks of infection, even with viruses that have a relatively low potential for spread in the open population.[18] Influenza infection rates approximating 60% and complications leading to hospitalization or death in as many as 40% of those affected have been described in nursing homes.[19]

## Clinical Manifestations

Influenza virus infection often spreads rapidly through a population. Transmission can occur by means of small particle aerosols generated by the cough that is characteristic of the illness[20] and through close contact. Respiratory epithelial cells, from ciliated columnar cells to alveolar pneumocytes, are the primary targets of influenza viruses.[21, 22] Effects of the infection can include sloughing of infected epithelial cells, extravasation of fluid and blood, submucosal inflammation, and alveolar collapse secondary to loss of surfactant. Virus titers in respiratory secretions are usually highest in the first 1 to 3 days of the illness, and isolation attempts typically fail after 5 to 7 days. Although the influenza viruses are rarely found outside the respiratory tract, the infection is associated with prominent systemic symptoms, possibly because of the release of various cytokines. For example, influenza viruses can infect macrophages and greatly augment their production of tumor necrosis factor-α in response to lipopolysaccharide.[23] Facilitation of secondary bacterial infections is responsible for a major part of influenza's severe morbidity and mortality. It seems likely that several different mechanisms are involved, including impaired mucociliary clearance, extravasated fluid that can serve as a nutrient-rich culture medium, impaired macrophage function, and enhanced adherence of bacteria to altered epithelial cells.[24-26]

The symptoms of influenza illness typically begin precipitously after an incubation period of 1 to 4 days and include fever, nonproductive cough, rasping substernal discomfort with cough, headache, mild sore throat, myalgia, malaise, and lethargy.[7, 27] Upper respiratory symptoms such as nasal obstruction and discharge may be present but are often obscured by the cough and systemic symptoms. Physical examination usually reveals an uncomfortable, febrile, coughing patient with flushed skin, mucosal hyperemia, and hypertrophy of pharyngeal lymphoid tissue. The uncomplicated illness typically lasts 3 to 6 days, but cough and lethargy may persist for several more days or weeks.

Pulmonary involvement, at least down to the level of the small airways, is a regular component of uncomplicated influenza. Pulmonary function tests of patients with acute, uncomplicated influenza routinely reveal evidence of small airways dysfunction,[28] increased alveolar-arterial oxygen gradients,[29] and reduced carbon monoxide diffusion gradients,[30] and these changes may take weeks to clear. That these are a direct effect of influenza virus infection in the small airways is suggested by the more rapid recovery if the antiviral agent amantadine is used for treatment of influenza A virus infection.[31] Influenza virus infection can also provoke transient bronchial hyperreactivity, which may precipitate asthma attacks in patients with asthmatic backgrounds, an effect that is not reversed more quickly by amantadine therapy for type A infection.[28]

Pneumonia accounts for most of the more severe morbidity and the mortality that accompany influenza virus epidemics. Detailed descriptions of the various pulmonary syndromes that can occur with influenza virus infection often have been published after arrival of a new pandemic influenza virus. The extreme intensity of these epidemics typically produces a sudden, massive influx of very ill patients. Without planning, this burden can easily overwhelm medical care providers who have managed to avoid the illness or to work through it. Even with the best care, many patients who were productive citizens only days before may die of the complications of the infection.

Four different categories of pneumonia associated with influenza were described by Louria and coworkers after the 1957 to 1958 Asian influenza pandemic caused by A/Jap/305/57-like (H2N2) viruses:[32]

1. Influenza virus infection with physical signs of lower respiratory tract involvement but without alveolar infiltrates detectable by roentgenography
2. Influenza virus infection followed by secondary bacterial pneumonia
3. An acute, rapidly progressive pneumonia apparently produced by influenza virus infection alone
4. Concomitant viral and bacterial pneumonia

Additional groups of investigators described pneumonic complications of influenza during the Asian influenza pandemic and during the subsequent Hong Kong influenza pandemic of 1968 to 1969 caused by A/Aichi/2/68-like (H3N2) viruses,[33–38] and the following descriptions draw on these reports.

The chest radiographs of patients with uncomplicated influenza often exhibit increased interstitial markings associated with peribronchial inflammation, which may be termed "interstitial pneumonia." It can be difficult to ascertain whether some patchy alveolar infiltrate is also present. Radiographs illustrating interstitial influenza pneumonia with what was interpreted as patchy alveolar infiltrates are shown in Figure 40–1. Ten of the 91 patients with pulmonary complications of influenza described by Petersdorf and associates[34] were initially thought to have patchy alveolar infiltrates; upon review, however, they were reclassified as having only tracheobronchitis. When rhonchi from bronchitis and rales that can be caused by small airways and/or alveolar disease are present in a febrile, prostrate patient, the clinician may have difficulty determining whether significant alveolar involvement has occurred.

Pulmonary emboli can enter into the differential diagnosis of influenza. Of the total of 33 patients with pulmonary complications of influenza described by Louria and coworkers,[32] 3 had rhonchi and rales without signs of consolidation on physical examination and without a distinguishable alveolar infiltrate on the chest radiographs. Two of the 3 patients produced small amounts of blood-tinged sputum with their coughing, 2 complained of pleuritic chest pain, and 1 was described as having bilateral friction rubs. This clinical syndrome can simulate pulmonary emboli, and concern about the latter diagnosis may be increased by the perfusion abnormalities that can occur secondary to influenza's patchy involvement of small airways.[39]

The diagnosis of influenza may seem clear if the patient has typical symptoms of fever, headache, cough, mild sore throat, and some nasal congestion preceding the chest complaints and if the illness occurs in the midst of an epidemic, but such illnesses can occur with only a small amount of influenza in the community, and chest symptoms can be the presenting complaint.[39] Employing a test for rapid diagnosis of influenza A virus infection could be rewarding if this infection is recognized as part of the differential diagnosis for pulmonary emboli in the appropriate setting.

The prognosis for full recovery from this type of influenza involvement of the lungs without clear-cut consolidation is good with only supportive care. Early oral amantadine therapy can speed recovery from the small airways disease caused by influenza A virus infection,[31] but whether it can also reduce the probability of progression to more severe complications in patients with underlying high-risk conditions is uncertain. This may be another indication for therapeutic use of amantadine.

Among patients with unequivocal influenza-associated consolidation of the lungs, the most frequent pathogenesis is *localized* secondary bacterial pneumonia occurring a few days after the onset of influenza. The patient has a typical influenza syndrome and seems to be recovering after a few days, only to develop a recurrence of coughing, fever, and production of sputum that is purulent and may become bloody. Shaking chills and localized pleuritic pain may be present. Physical examination typically reveals signs of localized consolidation. A localized, dense, lobular or lobar pneumonia is seen on the chest radiograph, sometimes involving more than one lobe. The leukocyte count is often elevated, and a shift to immature PMN forms is typical. The bacteria seen on the Gram stain of sputum and in culture are often pneumococci, but a variety of organisms can be involved, most notably *Staphylococcus aureus*.

In a series from Grady Memorial Hospital,[38] the proportion of pneumonias caused by pneumococci fell from 61.7% in a nonepidemic period to 48.2% during the influenza A/Hong Kong (H3N2) epidemic of 1968 to 1969, and the proportion associated with *S. aureus* rose from 10.2%

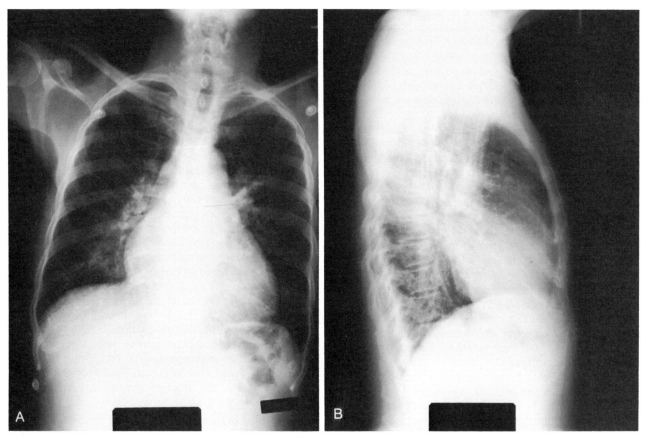

**Figure 40–1.** *A* and *B*, Mild influenza A/H3N2 pneumonia, documented by throat cultures, involving primarily the right lower lobe in a 62-year-old woman. Cultures of sputum for bacteria yielded normal flora and blood cultures were negative. The patient's temperature gradually decreased from a high of 105° F to normal over the next 4 days, with only some increased interstitial markings remaining on the chest roentgenograms.

to 25.9%. The reason for the increased frequency of *S. aureus* pneumonia in association with influenza is uncertain; enhanced adherence of these organisms to the surface of respiratory epithelial cells altered by the viral infection could be a factor.[26] A potential consequence of the increased frequency of *S. aureus* infections is the association of toxic shock syndrome with influenza.[40] These late bacterial pneumonias behave in a fashion similar to those occurring in the absence of influenza, and they typically respond well to appropriate antibacterial therapy. Antivirals do not have a role in their treatment.

A much more ominous situation is the development of *diffuse* pneumonia during the acute phase (first 1–3 days) of influenza illness. The presence of rheumatic valvular disease (especially mitral stenosis), chronic cardiovascular disease, or other conditions that can increase pulmonary vascular congestion, such as the late stages of pregnancy, are important predisposing factors for this complication. These patients present with dyspnea, cyanosis, bloody sputum, high fever, and profound prostration in addition to their other influenza symptoms. The physical examination may reveal diffuse fine rales, coarse bubbly rales, rhonchi, prolonged expiration, or wheezing, sometimes with variation from hour to hour. Diffuse haziness of the chest radiograph may resemble pulmonary edema. This syndrome can be caused by influenza virus alone or by a combined viral and bacterial pneumonia, and it may be difficult to differentiate these causes clinically. The leukocyte count may be

low in both situations, and the patient may be unable to produce sputum from deep within the lung. Witnessing a patient with sputum appearing like red wine as a result of hemolysis of the erythrocytes and absence of the leukocytes but finding multiple staphylococcal microabscesses at autopsy a day later emphasizes the diagnostic difficulty. Staphylococci may have a special propensity for enhancing influenza virus infection in that they can supply a protease to facilitate cleavage of the viral HA, which is necessary for infectivity of the virus.[41]

Although antibacterial agents do not have a role in the management of uncomplicated influenza, their early use in the treatment of diffuse pneumonia complicating influenza may be appropriate while awaiting cultures.[35] Progressive respiratory failure in these patients often necessitates prolonged ventilatory support, which brings with it the frequent complication of secondary bacterial infection; late pneumonia caused by *Pseudomonas aeruginosa* and other opportunists has often been observed in these patients. If early antibacterial therapy is used, it should be as narrowly focused as possible (ie, against pneumococci and staphylococci) in an attempt to reduce the pressure toward secondary infection with multidrug-resistant organisms. It is not clear whether antiviral therapy with oral amantadine provides any benefit to these patients. Anecdotal reports suggest that aerosolized ribavirin can be beneficial,[42] although it is not officially approved for this purpose.

The rate of death with diffuse pneumonia complicating

acute influenza is quite high, 60% to 80%, and is typically a result of respiratory failure or secondary bacterial pneumonia. Among patients who die early, the lungs are grossly hemorrhagic and edematous, resembling liver. Microscopic findings include patchy loss of respiratory epithelial cells, producing lesions ranging from tracheobronchial ulcerations to loss of alveolar lining cells; occasional necrosis of alveolar septae in segments of the lung; submucosal edema, inflammatory cells, and capillary dilatation; and alveoli filled with fluid, erythrocytes, and hemosiderin-ladened macrophages and lined with hyaline membranes in some cases. Inflammation of pleural surfaces is not a component of ''pure'' influenza pneumonia at autopsy, so a definite pleural rub heard over other prominent pulmonary sounds in these patients should suggest bacterial superinfection or some other process. If secondary bacterial pneumonia is present, infiltration of PMNs and microabscess formation often are seen. Those patients who survive have various degrees of permanent impairment of pulmonary function secondary to diffuse pulmonary fibrosis, although it may not interfere with ordinary activities of daily living.[43]

The spectrum of overt pneumonias seen in conjunction with an influenza epidemic includes many that are between the early diffuse and late localized varieties described above. The fourth category of Louria and coworkers,[32] concomitant viral and bacterial pneumonia, included several patients who had a day or so of improvement in the initial influenza syndrome before onset of prominent chest symptoms, who developed sputum that was both bloody and purulent, and who had both diffuse and localized chest findings. Antimicrobial therapy for these patients must focus on the expected bacterial component, and many require ventilatory support. Four of the 9 patients categorized by Louria and coworkers as having combined viral and bacterial pneumonia died. Underlying high-risk conditions are important cofactors in setting the stage for development of these influenza-associated pneumonias and in determining the consequences of the illness.

## Diagnosis

Respiratory viruses other than influenza are typically displaced during an influenza epidemic, and most influenza-like illness in the midst of an epidemic is caused by infection with the circulating influenza virus. Information on the prevalent influenza virus strain is generally available from the Centers for Disease Control or local health authorities, and it is usually not necessary to perform viral diagnostic tests to make decisions about treatment or prophylaxis. However, viral diagnostic tests may be desirable or necessary in certain situations, such as at the beginning of an outbreak to identify the circulating influenza virus; at the beginning or end of an epidemic when other viruses that can cause influenza-like illnesses may be present; during a mild influenza outbreak when other respiratory viruses are not fully displaced; during a mixed influenza A and B outbreak if the issue of whether to use amantadine is being debated (amantadine only works against type A strains); or in confirming the cause of a particularly severe or unusual clinical presentation.[1, 2]

Influenza viruses can readily be cultured from respiratory

secretions during the first 2 to 3 days of illness, with the frequency of isolation then decreasing rapidly over the next 2 to 3 days and usually being negative after a week. Specimens may be sputum, nasopharyngeal wash or aspirate, or nose or throat swabs; they should be placed in or diluted with a carrier medium such as veal infusion broth plus 0.5% bovine serum albumen and maintained on ice during transport to the laboratory. The viruses grow well in primary rhesus monkey kidney cells, in the Madin-Darby canine kidney cell line with addition of trypsin to the medium, and in the allantoic or amniotic cavities of embryonated chicken eggs. Influenza viruses do not produce a characteristic cytopathic effect but may make tissue culture cells appear toxic. Virus is generally recognized in tissue culture by adherence of guinea pig erythrocytes to the surface of infected cells (ie, hemadsorption) and in fluids from embryonated eggs by hemagglutination. Identity of the virus may be established by methods such as immunofluorescence assays on infected cells or hemagglutination inhibition assays on virus-containing fluids using specific antisera. The laboratory typically is able to report positive isolation of an influenza virus within 3 to 4 days for 50% or more of those specimens that ultimately are positive.

Confirmation of influenza virus infection can also be accomplished by demonstrating an increase in the amount of antibody to the virus in a convalescent-phase serum (ie, 2–3 weeks after the onset of illness) compared with the amount in an acute-phase serum. If the patient presents 5 or more days after onset of the illness, this may be the only means for establishing the diagnosis, because virus cultures are likely to be negative. However, it has the disadvantage of providing an answer long after the acute illness has run its course. Methods of testing include a complement fixation (CF) assay against a laboratory virus of the same type as the current epidemic strain (ie, detects antibodies to antigenically stable internal components of the virus), a CF assay against the current epidemic strain (ie, detects antibodies to both internal components and surface antigens), and an HI or neutralizing antibody assay against the current epidemic strain (ie, detects only strain-specific antibodies against surface antigens, primarily the HA). Considerations of cost, complexity, and sensitivity have led most labs to use HI as the standard assay for serodiagnosis of influenza. An HI antibody titer that is four or more times greater in the convalescent than in the acute serum is diagnostic and is found in two thirds or more of patients with recent influenza virus infection. Enzyme-linked immunoassays against isolated HA antigen or whole virus offer greater sensitivity for serodiagnosis but are not routinely available.

If a more rapid diagnosis than can be achieved by culture is clinically desirable, as sometimes may be the case when considering whether to administer amantadine for treatment or prevention of possible influenza A virus infections, tests for detection of viral antigen may be employed. Monoclonal antibodies for immunofluorescent staining of exfoliated cells are commercially available for detection of influenza virus types A and B and other respiratory viruses; the procedure is performed in a few hours and requires some expertise for interpretation. A commercially available enzyme immunoassay membrane test (Directogen Flu-A, Becton Dickinson Microbiology Systems, Cockeysville, MD) employs a monoclonal antibody against type A NP to detect viruses of this type in nasopharyngeal aspirates, washings, or swabs; it can detect an influenza A virus infection within 15 minutes in an office setting, and its sensitivity and specificity are 90% or greater compared with cultures for the virus and IF staining.[44] A variety of other methods for rapid diagnosis are under development or available within specific laboratories.

## Treatment

After infection by an influenza virus has begun in a patient, the major objectives should be to prevent complications such as pneumonia and to avoid transmitting the virus to others, particularly to those with underlying diseases that place them at high risk for complications. Rest is important for both of these objectives, but sedatives are usually unnecessary and may interfere with clearance of secretions, promoting secondary infection. Increased fluid intake is necessary to compensate for losses from fever and to maintain the flow of secretions; a decongestant such as pseudoephedrine may facilitate the latter. Use of an antihistamine may be indicated for excessive secretions in persons with an allergic background, but caution is necessary if amantadine is to be employed therapeutically, because the combination may increase the likelihood of central nervous system (CNS) side effects.[45] If necessary for rest, an antipyretic analgesic such as aspirin, ibuprofen, or acetaminophen may be employed, but only acetaminophen should be used in children because of its documented safety and the association of aspirin with Reye syndrome.

Oral administration of amantadine or its congener, rimantadine, within 48 hours of onset of influenza A virus infection and continuation for 3 to 5 days (1–2 days after major symptoms abate) can shorten the duration of fever and symptoms,[46, 47] and amantadine has been shown to speed recovery from the small airways dysfunction caused by the infection.[31] The CNS side effects sometimes observed during use of amantadine for prophylaxis are usually obscured by symptoms of the illness when it is used therapeutically.

Neither amantadine nor rimantadine has activity against influenza B or any other virus in achievable concentrations, and the clinician should have reasonable evidence of an influenza A virus infection before using one of them therapeutically. Therapy with amantadine or rimantadine may reduce the frequency of the more severe complications of influenza, but this has not been proven, nor has therapeutic benefit after complications have set in.

Although the two antivirals, amantadine and rimantadine, have different pharmacokinetic and toxicity profiles, both inhibit an early step in influenza A virus replication, and cross-resistance can develop during therapy or in vitro. This resistance is associated with a mutation in the viral gene coding for the M2 protein,[48] and it is a potential deterrent to the routine therapeutic use of these medications because resistant virus can be transmitted to others and cause disease. Resistant influenza A viruses have not been detected spreading in the community in the absence of treatment with one of these antivirals.[49] The development of resistance was previously observed during treatment primarily in children, who normally excrete influenza viruses in higher titers and longer than adults because of less cross-reacting immunity from prior infections, but it has also been described in a nursing home outbreak with subsequent spread in the facility.[50] Patients being treated with amantadine or rimantadine should be considered to remain infectious and should be appropriately isolated, particularly from high-risk persons who may depend on one of these antivirals for prophylaxis. Details about the pharmacokinetics and side effects of amantadine, the only one of these two antivirals available commercially, are described later under preventive measures.

Therapy for pneumonia complicating influenza requires the appropriate use of antimicrobials against potential bacterial pathogens, and often requires ventilatory support. In murine models, administration of amantadine or ribavirin by small particle aerosol appears to offer therapeutic benefits later in the course of influenza-related pneumonia than administration by a nonrespiratory route.[51] Ribavirin has an advantage over amantadine in being active against type B and type A influenza in addition to other viruses, and small-particle ribavirin aerosol is approved for treatment of severe RSV infections in infants and young children. Case reports have described the successful use of ribavirin aerosol for therapy of severe influenza[42] and RSV[52] pneumonias in adults, but its use must be considered experimental. The aerosol administration of ribavirin must be carefully monitored in patients requiring assisted ventilation, because the drug deposits in the ventilatory apparatus and can cause malfunction.

## Prevention

The primary means for attempting to prevent influenza virus infections is vaccination.[14] Influenza vaccines are prepared from virus strains grown in embryonated chicken eggs, treated with formalin to render them noninfectious (ie, inactivated), and selectively concentrated to remove all but traces of egg protein. They are trivalent, containing 15 μg of hemagglutinin each from A/H1N1, A/H3N2, and type B strains. The strains to be included each year are updated to represent the most recent variants obtained from worldwide surveillance, but in the United States and Europe, the choices must be made by about the end of the preceding influenza season to allow sufficient time for the manufacturers to prepare and distribute vaccine for use the following autumn. This timing occasionally causes a problem if a new variant or subtype arises in the spring or summer during influenza's continuous passage around the globe, and such an occurrence may necessitate emergency preparation of an additional monovalent vaccine against the new strain.

Two different types of vaccine preparations are available: whole virus, consisting of a suspension of purified virions, and subvirion, containing partially purified surface glycoproteins derived after chemical disruption of the virions. Persons older than 12 years of age react similarly to the two vaccine preparations, but younger children should receive only subvirion vaccine, because whole-virus vaccine is significantly more reactogenic in them. Injection of the vaccine into the deltoid muscle causes local tenderness for 1 to 2 days in up to one third of recipients and local erythema or induration for a few days in some persons. Systemic symptoms such as malaise or myalgia occur in

5% to 10% of recipients, and fever in a smaller proportion; these typically begin within a few hours of vaccination and last 1 to 2 days. Immediate allergic reactions are extremely rare and are presumably caused by traces of egg protein in the vaccine; persons with a history of immediate-type reactions to egg protein should not receive influenza vaccine.

An increased incidence of Guillain-Barré syndrome (GBS) occurred within a few weeks of vaccination against "swine" influenza in 1976 and 1977 (one case per 100,000 recipients). Evaluations of subsequent influenza vaccines have not documented an epidemiologic association with GBS; a small increase in the incidence of GBS was noted among 18- to 64-year-old adults who received influenza vaccine in 1990 and 1991, but it lacked a clear timing relationship to the vaccination and did not occur in older adults.[14] If there is an increased risk of GBS after influenza vaccine, it is very low and considerably less than the risk of severe influenza during an epidemic.

Influenza vaccine should be administered during the autumn months, usually by mid-November, so that antibody titers will be at their peak when influenza epidemics start, typically 1 to 2 months later. Vaccination can reduce influenza attack rates by 70% to 90% among military personnel if a good match exists between vaccine and epidemic strains.[53] Among elderly, high-risk patients, protection against the severe consequences of influenza such as pneumonia and death approaches similar levels,[54, 55] although protection against any influenza-related illness may be only half as good. Nursing home residents can exhibit the phenomenon of herd immunity, with the likelihood of an influenza outbreak in the facility being significantly reduced if 70% or more of the residents have received the vaccine.[56] Protection begins about 2 weeks after vaccination,[57] and though it seemed to last as long as 3 years in one study among school children,[58] protection lasted less than 1 year in another study among nursing home residents.[59] Influenza vaccine should therefore be administered annually to high-risk persons, even if none of the strains included in the vaccine has changed.

Protection resulting from natural infection with an influenza virus is considerably longer-lasting and broader (ie, active against many subsequent variants) than that provided by inactivated virus vaccines. Studies of vaccination programs among children have not yielded evidence of continuing protection of the children by annual vaccination[60] or of protection of the community,[61] unless very high vaccination rates are achieved.[61a] Healthy persons at low risk for severe influenza disease may be better served by being allowed to acquire the natural infection and develop the stronger, more durable immunity that follows. A hope for the future is that developmental, live-attenuated influenza virus vaccines given by nose drops, which seem to be more effective than inactivated vaccines in children, may permit actual control of influenza epidemics.[62]

The primary objective of current influenza vaccine strategy is reduction of the severe morbidity and the mortality associated with influenza epidemics by annual vaccination of those persons at high risk for complications of the infection.[14] These include persons older than 64 years of age, those residing in facilities for care of the chronically infirm, and those with chronic heart or lung disease or other chronic disorders that might impair host defenses, particularly if these underlying problems have necessitated regular

medical care or hospitalization in the preceding year. Optimal delivery of vaccine to such high-risk persons is rarely achieved on a wide scale, and strong arguments can be made for administrative and organizational interventions in clinics and hospitals to enhance delivery.[63, 64] Those who provide care to or live with high-risk persons should also receive vaccine to reduce the likelihood that they will transmit influenza virus.

Influenza vaccine is not contraindicated in pregnancy. Pregnant women should receive influenza vaccine if they have other conditions that place them at high risk for complications, as should any woman who will be in the late third trimester during the influenza season. Other strong candidates for vaccine programs are those who provide essential community services and those in institutional or work settings that would be disrupted by numerous absences.

The only commercially available alternative to influenza vaccine at this time is amantadine. The efficacy of this orally administered medication for prevention of influenza A virus infections is about as great as that of influenza vaccine.[47] It has advantages over vaccine in providing protection that begins within a few hours and in being active against all subtypes and variants of type A viruses, and it does not interfere with antibody responses to vaccine. Disadvantages of amantadine compared with vaccine are the loss of protection shortly after daily dosing is stopped, the absence of protection against influenza B viruses, potential CNS side effects, and higher cost if continued for longer than about 2 weeks. Amantadine is well absorbed after oral administration, has a half-life of 10 to 20 hours, permitting once-daily dosing, and is excreted by the kidneys without being metabolized.[65, 66] The recommended daily dose for healthy persons from 10 to 64 years of age is 200 mg/d, but only 100 mg/d should be given to those 65 years of age and older because of the normal decline in renal function with increasing age. In frail, elderly persons, it may be safer to employ a dose of 1.4 mg/kg/d, not to exceed 100 mg/d.[67] Further reductions in dose are required proportionate to any reductions in creatinine clearance below normal.

Amantadine causes CNS side effects such as insomnia, nervousness, dizziness, and difficulty concentrating in as many as one third of healthy young adults taking 200 mg/d for prophylaxis,[68, 69] but these side effects are usually mild, always disappear after amantadine is stopped, and may abate even if the drug is continued at the same dose. Elderly persons can have more troublesome mood changes, agitation, confusion, and falls.[70, 71] Concomitant medications such as antihistamines, anticholinergics, and psychoactive drugs increase the likelihood of CNS side effects with amantadine[45, 71] and should be avoided if possible. The frequency of side effects increases with higher blood levels of amantadine and may be reduced by taking half doses twice daily. However, about 3 days are required before steady-state serum levels of amantadine are achieved, and it may be desirable to give an initial loading dose if rapid therapeutic or prophylactic effects are needed. If side effects persist, use of half the recommended daily dose may reduce them and still be effective prophylactically,[72, 73] or it may be necessary to discontinue the medication. Persons with seizures should always be given half the usual dose, because amantadine can increase seizure activity in a dose-related fashion.[74] Amantadine has beneficial effects in the treatment of patients with Parkinson disease, and prolonged use in this setting attests to its general safety, but livedo reticularis and edema of the lower extremities may occur.[75]

The recommended uses of amantadine prophylaxis are for control of influenza A outbreaks in institutions such as nursing homes; to provide protection to high-risk persons, their care providers, and other close associates for the 2-week interval before vaccine becomes effective if vaccination has been delayed until the onset of an influenza A epidemic; and to protect the same groups throughout the epidemic if they cannot be vaccinated because of hypersensitivity or if the outbreak is caused by an influenza A variant not covered by the vaccine.[14] If amantadine is used for control of an institutional influenza A outbreak, it should be administered to all residents, regardless of whether they have received vaccine, and it should be administered until the epidemic is essentially over, perhaps for as long as 1 month. Quick recognition and confirmation of an influenza A outbreak in the institution and preapproved orders so that amantadine prophylaxis can be begun rapidly are critical to the success of the program; the effort is worthwhile because it can abort such outbreaks and prevent considerable morbidity and mortality.[70, 74] Residents with respiratory symptoms should be isolated to guard against the possibility of spread of amantadine-resistant viruses.[50]

It is likely that a new influenza A pandemic strain will arise in the next 10 to 20 years, and proper use of a vaccine and an antiviral agent such as amantadine will be extremely important. Hospital planning for a major epidemic also must include considerations such as excluding visitors and personnel with respiratory illness, cohorting patients with such illness and marshalling resources for their management, and closing the institution to nonemergent admissions.[76]

## ADENOVIRUSES

Adenoviruses are nonenveloped, icosahedral, double-stranded DNA viruses that are about 70 nm in diameter.[77–79] The outer protein shell, or capsid, is composed of 240 hexons and 12 pentons at the vertices formed by adjoining sides. Protruding from the pentons are fibers with terminal knobs which serve to attach the virion to cellular receptors. Two genera, *Mastadenovirus* from mammals and *Aviadenovirus* from birds, each have a unique group-specific antigen carried by the penton. Adenoviruses from birds and from lower mammals do not have any known role in human disease. Type-specific neutralizing and hemagglutination-inhibiting antibodies are directed at antigens of the hexon and fiber, respectively.

At least 47 human adenovirus types have been identified,[80] many of which are ''orphans'' with no known disease association. Human adenoviruses are subdivided into subgenera A through G on the basis of antigenic crossreactivity, DNA hybridization characteristics, differential agglutination of erythrocytes from different species, and ability to transform cells of various animal species. Despite the oncogenic potential of some human adenoviruses in animals, no role for these viruses in human malignancy has been identified. Most adenoviruses can infect epithelial

cells of human or monkey origin, producing intranuclear inclusions and cell lysis, but they can also cause persistent, low-grade infection, often in lymphoid tissues. They were first recovered by Rowe in 1953 from surgically removed adenoids.[81] Immunity to adenovirus infections is serotype-specific, and clearance of an established infection appears to depend on the whole gamut of host defense mechanisms, with a major role for cell-mediated immunity. Certain adenovirus gene products may facilitate development of persistent infection by inhibiting lysis of infected cells by tumor necrosis factor,[82] inhibiting the antiviral mechanisms of interferons,[83] and interfering with the natural killer cell[84] and cytotoxic T-cell[85] responses to the infection. As a consequence of these persistent infections, mere recovery of an adenovirus from a throat or stool specimen does not establish a role in any current disease.

Adenoviruses can cause a wide spectrum of disease, including pharyngoconjunctival fever, laryngotracheobronchitis, atypical pneumonia, keratoconjunctivitis, hemorrhagic cystitis, infantile diarrhea and intussusception, meningoencephalitis, and disseminated disease occurring primarily in immunocompromised patients and involving multiple organs including the liver. Different adenovirus serotypes have predilections for causing one or more of the syndromes, depending on the patient's age and immunocompetency.

Adenovirus pneumonia in immunocompetent adults is observed primarily among military recruits and may be caused by infection with serotypes 4, 7, 21, 14, or 3, in approximate decreasing order of frequency; outbreaks of such infections may occur. The characteristic illness is atypical pneumonia. It can be difficult to differentiate clinically from illnesses caused by influenza[86] or by *M. pneumoniae*,[87] although patients with adenovirus atypical pneumonia tend to have higher rates of pharyngitis, hoarseness, and cervical adenitis. Adenovirus pneumonia in children is fatal in 5% to 20% of cases and can result in chronic restrictive or obstructive changes in pulmonary function.[88] In adults, it is usually self-limited, with only occasional bacterial superinfection[89] and rare deaths. Nevertheless, isolated cases of adult respiratory distress syndrome due to adenovirus pneumonia in immunocompetent civilians have been described[90] and have sometimes been fatal.[91] Also, adenovirus type 7 pneumonia complicated by disseminated intravascular coagulation has caused deaths in military recruits.[92] Transmissions of adenovirus infection to health care workers caring for infected patients have been documented with an incubation period of 2 to 18 days (mean, 9 days).[90, 93] Attention should be given to isolation of patients suspected of being infected with an adenovirus, including respiratory, secretion, and stool precautions.[94]

Adenoviruses causing respiratory disease may be isolated from sputum and conjunctival specimens and from throat or rectal swabs. Because the virus is stable at room temperature and in the presence of bile, proteolytic enzymes, and low pH, transport of viable virus to the laboratory is not usually a problem. Adenoviruses grow best in human epithelial cell lines or primary human embryonic kidney tissue and produce fairly characteristic, rounded cells that appear as grape-like clusters beginning at the periphery of the cell sheet. Growth is usually slow, with appearance of cytopathic effect no sooner than 3 to 5 days. Virus is released as cells die, and it is often necessary to freeze and thaw the initial culture and pass the lysate to fresh cells to recover virus from a specimen. Adenoviruses can be grouped by differential hemagglutination of rat, rhesus, and human erythrocytes and serotyped by hemagglutination inhibition or neutralization with specific antisera.

Recovery of an adenovirus from a stool specimen or a rectal swab does not prove its role in current disease, because virus shedding at this site may persist for months or years after an illness. Recovery from a throat swab or sputum is more suggestive, and recovery from a conjunctival swab probably indicates current acute infection. Demonstration of adenovirus antigens in exfoliated cells of respiratory or conjunctival origin by immunofluorescence is much quicker than virus isolation and is highly suggestive of current infection. Another, more sensitive use of immunofluorescence is early detection of adenovirus after amplification in tissue culture for a few days. If intranuclear inclusions are seen in biopsy material, the possibility of confusing adenovirus and herpesvirus inclusions should be recognized, and the diagnosis should be confirmed by virus isolation or immunofluorescence or both.[95] The distinctive appearance of adenoviruses on electron microscopy can also be used to identify them. Serodiagnosis essentially proves that an adenovirus infection has recently occurred, and it is more sensitive than virus isolation for detection of respiratory infections. Serodiagnosis can be accomplished by demonstrating a fourfold or greater increase in the antibody titer of convalescent compared with acute serum, using CF assays for antibodies to group antigen or hemagglutination inhibition or neutralization for type-specific antibodies. Enzyme-linked immunosorbent assay (ELISA) techniques are playing an increasingly important role in detection of adenovirus antigens and serodiagnosis.

There is no antiviral agent with demonstrated efficacy against adenoviral disease. The type of disease observed in volunteers after experimental infection with an adenovirus depends on the route of inoculation, with administration by aerosol reproducing the acute respiratory disease seen in military recruits, including atypical pneumonia.[96] Inoculation of the gastrointestinal tract with respiratory adenoviruses in an enteric-coated capsule produces no disease, but it nevertheless infects the intestines and provides effective immunization against subsequent respiratory disease with the serotypes included in the capsule.[97] Adenoviruses 4 and 7 grown in a human embryonic fibroblast cell line and administered in enteric-coated capsules have been used effectively and without complication for years for prevention of outbreaks of infection caused by these serotypes among military recruits,[98] although the viruses are not fully attenuated and remain capable of spread in the family setting.[99] Adenovirus 21 has also been administered in the same way as a vaccine, although decreased antigenicities of types 7 and 21 were observed when they were administered simultaneously with type 4.[100] Further development of adenovirus vaccines has been given a low priority, although a case can be made for continued work on them.[88] Another potential use of enteric infection with adenoviruses is to serve as a vehicle for vaccination against other agents using recombinant DNA technology.[101]

## MEASLES

Measles virus is a member of the *Paramyxoviridae* family, genus *Morbillivirus*.[102] Infection with this virus during childhood was formerly almost universal. A killed measles virus vaccine available in the mid-1960s was abandoned because of lack of durable immunity and the occurrence of severe, atypical measles (unusual, centripetal, petechial or vesicular rash and frequent pneumonia) if natural infection subsequently occurred. Measles has been eminently preventable since release of parenterally administered, live-attenuated vaccine in 1963. However, although the incidence is much lower than in the prevaccine era, cases continue to occur.[103] Major reasons are failure of vaccine delivery to young children belonging to medically underserved groups, imported cases, and vaccine failure in about 5% of recipients. As a consequence of the vaccine failures and the greatly diminished occurrence of natural measles among children, the infection periodically occurs in adolescents and young adults. The recent recommendation for routine administration of a second measles vaccination to older children should serve to reduce such outbreaks in the future.

The incubation period for natural measles virus illness is 10 to 14 days, during which a complex sequence of events unfolds.[104] Infection initially occurs in the respiratory tract. Virus spreads to and multiplies in regional lymphoid tissues, and then it spreads by means of a transient, primary viremia to the reticuloendothelial system (RES). Further replication in the RES then leads to a more prolonged, secondary viremia that seeds the skin and remaining organs. Initial symptoms, beginning a week or so after exposure, are fever, cough, rhinorrhea, and conjunctivitis. Koplik spots (ie, grayish spots surrounded by erythema on the buccal mucosa) appear at this time. A fine exanthem begins 2 to 4 days later on the skin of the head and neck and spreads to the trunk and upper and lower extremities over the next 2 to 3 days. Fever diminishes, and the rash begins to fade after a total illness of 5 to 10 days. Complications can include viral pneumonia, encephalitis, enteritis, secondary bacterial infection, reactivation of tuberculosis, and subacute sclerosing panencephalitis that becomes symptomatic 5 to 7 years after the initial infection of young children. Measles remains a major cause of morbidity and mortality among children worldwide.

If measles outbreaks occur in adolescents or young adults, the complication of pneumonia develops in 3% to 4%.[105] It is manifested by an interstitial infiltrate involving multiple lobes and coinciding with the skin rash. Nodular infiltrates and pleural effusions are more likely if the patient manifests an atypical, centripetal skin eruption, and the pulmonary nodules can persist for several months. Contraction of measles during pregnancy carries a higher risk of pneumonia (Fig. 40–2) and is often associated with abortion or preterm labor.[106] Secondary bacterial pneumonia occurs in about one third of the patients, often late in the course of the disease, as the rash is fading. Response to antimicrobial therapy is prompt, and deaths are rare.

The diagnosis of measles is usually made clinically without laboratory aid. The virus can be recovered from multiple sites, but this is usually reserved for unusual cases. If biopsy material is available, it typically reveals lymphoid hypertrophy and multinucleated giant cells with acidophilic inclusions in the cytoplasm and nuclei. A variety of serologic assays are available for documenting antibody responses to the infection, but the ELISA is most commonly employed.

No specific treatment exists for measles-related pneumo-

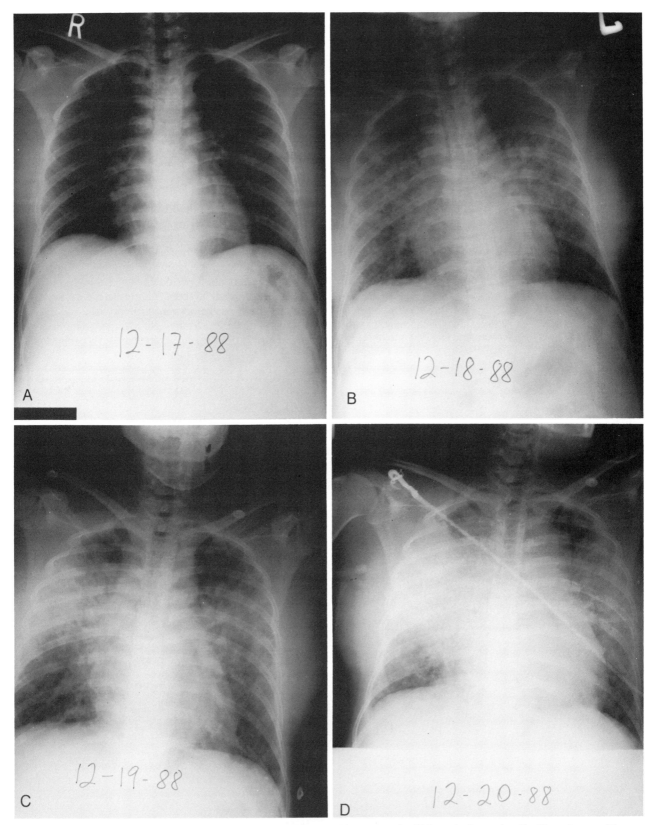

**Figure 40–2.** *A* through *D,* Progressive measles pneumonia in a 21-year-old woman in the 20th week of gestation. The illness began with coryza, conjunctivitis, and fever 1 week before admission, with the development of the morbilliform skin eruption, cough, and increasing dyspnea over the next few days. The course of progressive pneumonia and respiratory failure was not altered by therapeutic abortion or 5 days of therapy with aerosol ribavirin, and the patient died on the 15th hospital day.

nia. Prevention of the infection is best accomplished by routine childhood vaccination. If an unvaccinated person is exposed to measles, early administration of γ-globulin or of the live attenuated vaccine can prevent the natural illness. Trials in children have demonstrated the efficacy of orally administered vitamin A (200,000 IU on 2 consecutive days) for reducing morbidity and mortality from measles whether or not the child appears nutritionally deficient.[107]

## VARICELLA

The varicella-zoster virus (VZV) is a member of the *Herpesviridae* family.[108, 109] It causes two distinct illnesses, chickenpox as a primary infection in seronegative persons, and zoster (ie, shingles) by reactivation of latent virus in dorsal root ganglia of elderly or immunocompromised persons. Varicella pneumonia is primarily a complication of chickenpox (ie, primary infection). Chickenpox is typically a disease of childhood and is usually uncomplicated in normal children. However, infection with VZV in immunosuppressed patients poses a major threat for complications such as hemorrhagic skin lesions, pneumonia, hepatitis, and encephalitis, with mortality rates of about 10%;

approximately 100 deaths per year are attributed to acute varicella, mostly in such patients. Immunocompetent adults who missed VZV infection during childhood are also at a considerably greater risk than normal children for pneumonia (up to 16%) and death (about 3 per 10,000) if they develop chickenpox. Acute varicella infection during pregnancy can be associated with severe pneumonia,[110] and the fetus is at risk for various anomalies associated with congenital varicella or for severe neonatal varicella if the mother's infection occurs from 5 days before to 2 days after delivery. Adults raised in tropical climates are more likely to have missed VZV infection as a child than those raised in temperate climates;[111] most of the latter have serum antibody indicating prior VZV infection even if they are not aware of having had it.

VZV can be transmitted by contact or by aerosol. The latter route poses a particular risk for wide dissemination of the virus from patients with chickenpox in the hospital setting.[112] Acute varicella can occur throughout the year, but peak incidences occur in the spring in temperate climates. The incubation period for chickenpox is 10 to 21 days, during which a series of events analogous to that described for measles occurs. A prodrome of 1 to 2 days with fever, malaise, and myalgia may precede onset of the rash, or the two may begin simultaneously; some patients

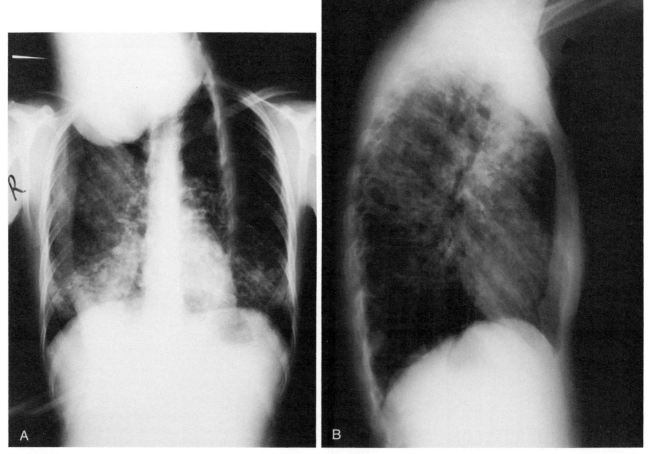

**Figure 40–3.** *A* and *B*, Varicella pneumonia in a 24-year-old woman exposed to three children with chickenpox. The typical vesicular eruption had begun 3 days before these roentgenograms and was associated with progressive cough and dyspnea. The patient's illness responded to therapy with intravenous acyclovir and she was discharged 1 week later.

with only a few scattered skin lesions have few systemic symptoms but remain infectious for others. Successive crops of skin lesions occur over a period of 2 to 4 days, and different sets of lesions may appear as maculopapules, vesicles, or scabs at the same time. The acute illness is generally finished by 5 days in uncomplicated cases, and it is followed by appearance on all skin lesions of crusts that eventually fall off and leave small scars.

Symptoms of varicella pneumonia in normal adults typically begin 1 to 6 days after the onset of the rash and may include cough, dyspnea, hemoptysis, and chest pain that can be pleuritic.[113] The physical findings of the chest examination may be relatively normal despite the appearance of a reticulonodular infiltrate with nodules about 0.5 cm in diameter throughout the lungs (Fig. 40–3). Pleural effusions and coalescence of the nodules to form larger ones may occur. Changes in the radiographic appearance of the lungs and the clinical course tend to correlate with changes in the skin lesions, which can become hemorrhagic in severe cases. Ventilatory support is sometimes necessary, and the deaths that occur are usually caused by respiratory insufficiency. Secondary bacterial pneumonias are uncommon. Calcified nodules[114] and prolonged defects in pulmonary function[115] can follow varicella pneumonia.

The diagnosis of chickenpox is usually made clinically, particularly in adults in whom confusion with impetigo, hand-foot-mouth disease, or disseminated herpes simplex lesions with atopic dermatitis or eczema is unlikely. The possibility of confusion with disseminated vaccinia lesions or smallpox is no longer applicable. Demonstration of multinucleated giant cells in a Tzanck smear from a vesicular lesion can occur with varicella or herpes simplex; differentiating these viruses requires culture or immunofluorescence staining. Serologic diagnosis of chickenpox can be done with CF tests, but serologic tests for susceptibility to VZV infection are best done with more sensitive immune adherence hemagglutination, fluorescence antibody to membrane antigen, or an ELISA assay.[116]

Treatment of varicella pneumonia with intravenous acyclovir reverses the process and speeds recovery.[117–120] Arguments can be made for routine, early administration of oral acyclovir to adults with varicella to prevent complications such as pneumonia from developing.[121] Prevention of the infection is best accomplished by isolation of infected persons. Susceptible persons exposed to varicella should be considered potentially infectious between 10 and 21 days after exposure, when the infection may become manifest. Varicella-zoster immune globulin given within 4 days of exposure can modify or prevent varicella in susceptible persons and, among adults, is indicated for those with any immunocompromising condition or pregnancy.[108] A live attenuated varicella vaccine has received extensive, successful trials in immunocompromised children, normal children, and adults.

## REFERENCES

1. Kendal A, Harmon MW: *Orthomyxoviridae*: The influenza viruses. *In* Lennette EH, Halonen P, Murphy FA (eds): Laboratory Diagnosis of Infectious Diseases: Principles and Practice. Viral, Rickettsial, and Chlamydial Diseases, vol 2. New York, Springer-Verlag, 1988:302–325.

2. Shaw MW, Arden NH, Maassab HF: New aspects of influenza viruses. Clin Microbiol Rev 5:74–92, 1992.

3. Webster RG, Bean WJ, Gorman OT, Chambers TM, Kawaoka Y: Evolution and ecology of influenza A viruses. Microbiol Rev 56:152–179, 1992.

4. Couch RB, Kasel JA, Six HR, Cate TR, Zahradnik JM: Immunological reactions and resistance to infection with influenza virus. *In* Stuart-Harris C, Potter CW (eds): The Molecular Virology and Epidemiology of Influenza. London, Academic Press, 1984:119–152.

5. Ada GL, Jones PD: The immune response to influenza infection. Curr Top Microbiol Immunol 128:1–54, 1986.

6. Kendal AP: Epidemiologic implications of changes in the influenza virus genome. Am J Med 82(suppl 6A):4–14, 1987.

7. Cate TR: Clinical manifestations and consequences of influenza. Am J Med 82 (suppl 6A):15–19, 1987.

8. Glezen WP, Couch RB: Interpandemic influenza in the Houston area, 1974–76. N Engl J Med 298:587–592, 1978.

9. Woodall J, Rowson KEK, McDonald JC: Age and Asian influenza, 1957. Br Med J 2:1316–1318, 1958.

10. Glezen WP, Six HR, Perrotta DM, Decker M, Joseph S: Epidemics and their causative viruses—Community experience. *In* Stuart-Harris C, Potter CW (eds): The Molecular Virology and Epidemiology of Influenza. London, Academic Press, 1984:17–38.

11. Glezen WP, Decker M, Joseph SW, Mercready RG Jr: Acute respiratory disease associated with influenza epidemics in Houston, 1981–1983. J Infect Dis 155:1119–1126, 1987.

12. Glezen WP: Serious morbidity and mortality associated with influenza epidemics. Epidemiol Rev 4:25–44, 1982.

13. Perrotta DM, Decker M, Glezen WP: Acute respiratory disease hospitalizations as a measure of impact of epidemic influenza. Am J Epidemiol 122:468–476, 1985.

14. Centers for Disease Control: Prevention and control of influenza. Recommendations of the Immunization Practices Advisory Committee (ACIP). MMWR 43:1–13, 1993.

15. Glezen WP, Payne AA, Snyder DN, Downs TD: Mortality and influenza. J Infect Dis 146:313–321, 1982.

16. Barker WH, Mullooly JP: Pneumonia and influenza deaths during epidemics. Arch Intern Med 142:85–89, 1982.

17. Murasko DM, Nelson BJ, Silver R, Matour D, Kaye D: Immunologic responses in an elderly population with a mean age of 85. Am J Med 81:612–618, 1986.

18. Stuart-Harris CH: Epidemiology of influenza in man. Br Med Bull 35:3–8, 1979.

19. Arden NH, Patriarca PA, Kendal AP: Experiences in the use and efficacy of inactivated influenza vaccine in nursing homes. *In* Kendal AP, Patriarca PA (eds): Options for the Control of Influenza. New York, Alan R. Liss, 1986:155–168.

20. Moser MR, Bender TR, Margolis HS, Noble GR, Kendal AP, Ritter DG: An outbreak of influenza aboard a commercial airliner. Am J Epidemiol 110:1–6, 1979.

21. Straub M, Mulder J: Epithelial lesions in the respiratory tract in human influenzal pneumonia. J Pathol Bacteriol 60:429–434, 1948.

22. Stinson SF, Ryan DP, Hertweck MS, et al: Epithelial and surfactant changes in influenzal pulmonary lesions. Arch Pathol Lab Med 100:147–153, 1976.

23. Nain M, Hinder F, Gong J-H, et al: Tumor necrosis factor-α production of influenza A virus-infected macrophages and potentiating effect of lipopolysaccharides. J Immunol 145:1921–1928, 1990.

24. Couch RB: The effects of influenza on host defenses. J Infect Dis 144:284–291, 1981.

25. Nickerson CL, Jakab GJ: Pulmonary antibacterial defenses during mild and severe influenza virus infection. Infect Immun 58:2809–2814, 1991.

26. Fainstein V, Musher DM, Cate TR: Bacterial adherence to pharyngeal epithelial cells during viral infection. J Infect Dis 141:172–176, 1980.

27. Betts RF, Douglas RG Jr: Influenza virus. *In* Mandell GL, Douglas RG Jr, Bennett JE (eds): Principles and Practice of Infectious Diseases, ed 3. New York, Churchill Livingstone, 1990:1306–1325.

28. Little JW, Hall WJ, Douglas RG Jr, Mudholkar GS, Speers DM, Patel K: Airway hyperreactivity and peripheral airway dysfunction in influenza A infection. Am Rev Respir Dis 118:295–303, 1978.

29. Johanson WG, Pierce AK, Sanford JP: Pulmonary function in uncomplicated influenza. Am Rev Respir Dis 100:141–146, 1969.

30. Homer GJ, Gray FD Jr: Effect of uncomplicated, presumptive influenza on diffusing capacity of the lung. Am Rev Respir Dis 108:866–869, 1973.

31. Little JW, Hall WJ, Douglas RG Jr, Hyde RW, Speers DM: Amantadine effect on peripheral airways abnormalities in influenza. Ann Intern Med 85:177–182, 1976.

32. Louria DB, Blumenfeld HL, Ellis JT, Kilbourne ED, Rogers DE: Studies on influenza in the pandemic of 1957–1958. II. Pulmonary complications of influenza. J Clin Invest 38:213–265, 1959.

33. Oswald NC, Shooter RA, Curwen MP: Pneumonia complicating Asian influenza. Br Med J 2:1305–1311, 1958.

34. Petersdorf RG, Fusco JJ, Harter DH, Albrink WS: Pulmonary infections complicating Asian influenza. Arch Intern Med 103:262–272, 1959.

35. Martin CM, Kunin CM, Gottlieb LS, Barnes MW, Liu C, Finland M: Asian influenza A in Boston. I. Observations in thirty-two influenza-associated fatal cases. Arch Intern Med 103:515–531, 1959.

36. Lindsay MI, Herrmann EC, Morrow GW, Brown AL Jr: Hong Kong influenza: Clinical, microbiologic, and pathologic features in 127 cases. JAMA 214:1825–1832, 1970.

37. Bisno AL, Griffin JP, Van Epps KA, Niell HB, Rytel MW: Pneumonia and Hong Kong influenza: A prospective study of the 1968–69 epidemic. Am J Med Sci 261:251–263, 1971.

38. Schwarzmann SW, Adler JL, Sullivan RJ, Marine WM: Bacterial pneumonia during the Hong Kong influenza epidemic of 1968–69. Arch Intern Med 127:1037–1041, 1971.

39. Lynn DJ, Wyman AC, Varma VM: Influenza A infection simulating pulmonary embolism. JAMA 238:1166–1168, 1977.

40. MacDonald KL, Osterholm MT, Hedberg CW, et al: Toxic shock syndrome: A newly recognized complication of influenza and influenza-like illness. JAMA 257:1053–1058, 1987.

41. Tashiro M, Ciborwski P, Klenk H-D, Pulverer G, Rott R: The role of *Staphylococcus* protease in the development of influenza pneumonia. Nature 325:536–537, 1987.

42. Knight V, Gilbert BE: Chemotherapy of respiratory viruses. Adv Intern Med 31:95–118, 1986.

43. Winterbauer RH, Ludwig WR, Hammar SP: Clinical course, management, and long-term sequelae of respiratory failure due to influenza viral pneumonia. Johns Hopkins Med J 141:148–155, 1977.

44. Warner JL, Todd SJ, Shalaby H, Murphy P, Wall LV: Comparison of Directogen Flu-A with viral isolation and direct immunofluorescence for rapid detection and identification of influenza A virus. J Clin Microbiol 29:479–482, 1991.

45. Millet VM, Dreisbach M, Bryson YJ: Double-blind controlled study of central nervous system side effects of amantadine, rimantadine and chlorpheniramine. Antimicrob Agents Chemother 21:1–4, 1982.

46. Wingfield WL, Pollack D, Grunert RR: Therapeutic efficacy of amantadine HCl and rimantadine HCl in naturally occurring influenza A2 respiratory illness in man. N Engl J Med 281:579–584, 1969.

47. Douglas RG Jr: Prophylaxis and treatment of influenza. N Engl J Med 322:443–450, 1990.

48. Belshe RB, Smith MH, Hall CB, Betts R, Hay AJ: Genetic basis of resistance to rimantadine emerging during rimantadine treatment of influenza virus infection. J Virol 62:1508–1512, 1988.

49. Belshe RB, Burk B, Newman F, Cerruti RL, Sim IS: Resistance of influenza A virus to amantadine and rimantadine: Results of one decade of surveillance. J Infect Dis 159:430–435, 1989.

50. Degelau J, Somani SK, Cooper SL, Guay DRP, Crossley KB: Amantadine-resistant influenza A in a nursing facility. Arch Intern Med 152:390–392, 1992.

51. Wilson SZ, Knight V, Wyde PR, Drake S, Couch RB: Amantadine and ribavirin treatment of influenza A and B infection in mice. Antimicrob Agents Chemother 17:642–648, 1980.

52. Aylward RB, Burdge DR: Ribavirin therapy of adult respiratory syncytial virus pneumonia. Arch Intern Med 151:2303–2304, 1991.

53. Davenport FM: Control of influenza. Med J Aust 1(suppl):33–38, 1973.

54. Barker WH, Mullooly JP: Effectiveness of inactivated influenza vaccine among non-institutionalized elderly persons. *In* Kendal AP, Patriarca PA (eds): Options for Control of Influenza. New York, Alan R. Liss, 1986:169–182.

55. Patriarca PA, Weber JA, Parker RA, et al: Efficacy of influenza vaccine in nursing homes: Reduction in illness and complications during an influenza A (H3N2) epidemic. JAMA 253:1136–1139, 1985.

56. Patriarca PA, Weber JA, Parker RA, et al: Risk factors for outbreaks of influenza in nursing homes: A case-control study. Am J Epidemiol 124:114–119, 1986.

57. Meiklejohn G, Hoffman R, Graves P: Effectiveness of influenza vaccine when given during an influenza A/H3N2 outbreak in a nursing home. J Am Geriatr Soc 37:407–410, 1989.

58. Foy HM, Cooney MK, McMahan R: A/Hong Kong immunity three years after vaccination. JAMA 226:758–761, 1973.

59. Budnick LD, Stricof RL, Ellis F: An outbreak of influenza A in a nursing home, 1982. N Y State J Med 84:235–238, 1984.

60. Hoskins TW, Davies JR, Smith AJ, Miller CL, Allchin A: Assessment of inactivated influenza A vaccine after three outbreaks of influenza A at Christ's Hospital. Lancet 1:33–35, 1979.

61. Oya A, Nerome K: Experiences with mass vaccination of young age groups with inactivated vaccines. *In* Kendal AP, Patriarca PA (eds): Options for Control of Influenza. New York, Alan R. Liss, 1986:183–192.

61a. Monto AS, Davenport FM, Napier JA, Francis T Jr: Modification of an outbreak of influenza in Tecumseh, Michigan by vaccination of school children. J Infect Dis 122:16–25, 1970.

62. Glezen WP: Guarding against influenzal pneumonia in 1991–1992. J Respir Dis 12:953–970, 1991.

63. Margolis KL, Lofgren RP, Korn JE: Organizational strategies to improve influenza vaccine delivery: A standing order in a general medical clinic. Arch Intern Med 148:2205–2207, 1988.

64. Fedson DS, Wajda A, Nicol JP, Roos LL: Disparity between influenza vaccination rates and risks for influenza-associated hospital discharge and death in Manitoba in 1982–1983. Ann Intern Med 116:550–555, 1992.

65. Horadam VW, Sharp JG, Smilack JD, et al: Pharmacokinetics of amantadine hydrochloride in subjects with normal and impaired renal function. Ann Intern Med 94:454–458, 1981.

66. Aoki FY, Stiver HG, Sitar DS, Boudreault A, Ogilvie RI: Prophylactic amantadine dose and plasma concentration affect relationships in healthy adults. Clin Pharmacol Ther 37:128–136, 1985.

67. Aoki FY, Sitar DS: Amantadine pharmacokinetics in healthy elderly men: Implications for influenza prevention. Clin Pharmacol Ther 37:137–144, 1985.

68. Bryson YJ, Monahan C, Pollack M, Shield WD: A prospective double-blind study of side effects associated with administration of amantadine for influenza A virus prophylaxis. J Infect Dis 141:543–547, 1980.

69. Dolin R, Reichman RC, Madore HP, Maynard R, Linton PN, Webber-Jones J: A controlled trial of amantadine and rimantadine in the prophylaxis of influenza infection. N Engl J Med 307:580–584, 1982.

70. Arden NH, Patriarca PA, Fasano MB, et al: The roles of vaccination and amantadine prophylaxis in controlling an outbreak of influenza A (H3N2) in a nursing home. Arch Intern Med 148:865–868, 1988.

71. Degelau J, Somani S, Cooper SL, Irvine PW: Occurrence of adverse effects and high amantadine concentrations with influenza prophylaxis in a nursing home. J Am Geriatr Soc 38:428–432, 1990.

72. Reuman PD, Bernstein DI, Keefer MC, Young EC, Sherwood JR, Schiff GM: Efficacy and safety of low dosage amantadine hydrochloride as prophylaxis for influenza A. Antiviral Res 11:27–40, 1989.

73. Paylor DK, Purdham PA: Influenza A prophylaxis with amantadine in a boarding school. Lancet 1:502–504, 1984.

74. Atkinson WL, Arden NH, Patriarca PA, Leslie N, Lui K-J, Gohd R: Amantadine prophylaxis during an institutional outbreak of type A (H1N1) influenza. Arch Intern Med 146:1751–1756, 1986.

75. Timberlake WH, Vance MA: Four-year treatment of patients with parkinsonism using amantadine alone or with levodopa. Ann Neurol 3:119–128, 1978.

76. Hoffman PC, Dixon RE: Control of influenza in the hospital. Ann Intern Med 87:725–728, 1977.

77. Wadell G: *Adenoviridae*: The adenoviruses. *In* Balows A, Hausler WJ Jr, Lennette EH (eds): Laboratory Diagnosis of Infectious Diseases, Principles and Practice. Viral, Rickettsial, and Chlamydial Diseases, vol 2. New York, Springer-Verlag, 1988:284–300.

78. Baum SG: Adenovirus. *In* Mandell GL, Douglas RG Jr, Bennett JE (eds): Principles and Practice of Infectious Diseases, ed 3. New York, Churchill Livingstone, 1990:1185–1191.

79. Rivadeneira ED, Henshaw EG: Adenoviruses and adeno-associated viruses. *In* Joklik WK, Willett HP, Amos DB, Wilfert CM (eds): Zinsser Microbiology, ed 20. Norwalk, CT, Appleton & Lange, 1992:968–974.

80. Hierholzer JC, Wigand R, Anderson LJ, Adrian T, Gold JWM: Adenoviruses from patients with AIDS: A plethora of serotypes and

a description of five new serotypes of subgenus D (types 43–47). J Infect Dis 158:804–813, 1988.

81. Rowe WP, Heubner RJ, Gilmore LK, Parrott RH, Ward TG: Isolation of a cytopathic agent from human adenoids undergoing spontaneous degeneration in tissue culture. Proc Soc Exp Biol Med 84:570–573, 1953.

82. Gooding LR, Elmore LW, Tollefson AE, Brady HA, Wold WSM: A 14,700 MW protein from the E3 region of adenovirus inhibits cytolysis by tumor necrosis factor. Cell 53:341–346, 1988.

83. Kalvakolanu DVR, Bandyopadhyay SK, Harter ML, Sen GC: Inhibition of interferon-inducible gene expression by adenovirus E1A proteins: Block in transcriptional complex formation. Proc Natl Acad Sci U.S.A. 88:7459–7463, 1991.

84. Routes JM, Cook JL: Adenovirus persistence in man. Defective E1A gene product targeting of infected cells from elimination by natural killer cells. J Immunol 142:4022–4026, 1989.

85. Andersson M, Pääbo S, Nilsson T, Peterson PA: Impaired intracellular transport of class I MHC antigens as a possible means for adenoviruses to evade immune surveillance. Cell 43:215–222, 1985.

86. Schultz I, Gundelfinger B, Rosenbaum M, Woolridge R, De Berry P: Comparison of clinical manifestations of respiratory illnesses due to Asian strain influenza, adenovirus, and unknown cause. J Lab Clin Med 55:497–509, 1960.

87. George RB, Ziskind MM, Rasch JR, Mogabgab WJ: *Mycoplasma* and adenovirus pneumonias: Comparison with other atypical pneumonias in a military population. Ann Intern Med 65:931–942, 1966.

88. Zahradnik JM: Adenovirus pneumonia. Semin Respir Infect 2:104–111, 1987.

89. Ellenbogen C, Graybill JR, Silva J Jr, Homme PJ: Bacterial pneumonia complicating adenoviral pneumonia: A comparison of respiratory tract bacterial culture sources and effectiveness of chemoprophylaxis against bacterial pneumonia. Am J Med 56:169–178, 1974.

90. Ferstenfeld JE, Schlueter DP, Rytel MW, Molloy RP: Recognition and treatment of adult respiratory distress syndrome secondary to viral interstitial pneumonia. Am J Med 58:709–718, 1975.

91. Aach R, Kissane J (eds): Clinicopathologic Conference: Adult respiratory distress syndrome. Am J Med 50:521–529, 1971.

92. Dudding BA, Wagner SC, Zeller JA, Gmelich JT, French GR, Top FH Jr: Fatal pneumonia associated with adenovirus type 7 in three military trainees. N Engl J Med 286:1289–1292, 1972.

93. Brummitt CF, Cherrington JM, Katzenstein DA, et al: Nosocomial adenovirus infections: Molecular epidemiology of an outbreak due to adenovirus 3a. J Infect Dis 158:423–432, 1988.

94. Valenti WM, Hruska JF, Menegus MA, Freeburn MJ: Nosocomial viral infections: III. Guidelines for prevention and control of exanthematous viruses, gastroenteritis viruses, picornaviruses, and uncommonly seen viruses. Infect Control 2:38–49, 1981.

95. Landry ML, Fong CKY, Neddermann K, Solomon L, Hsiung GD: Disseminated adenovirus infection in an immunocompromised host; pitfalls in diagnosis. Am J Med 83:555–559, 1987.

96. Couch RB, Cate TR, Fleet WF, Gerone PJ, Knight V: Aerosol-induced adenoviral illness resembling the naturally occurring illness in military recruits. Am Rev Respir Dis 93:529–535, 1966.

97. Couch RB, Chanock RM, Cate TR, Lang DJ, Knight V, Heubner RJ: Immunization with types 4 and 7 adenovirus by selective infection of the intestinal tract. Am Rev Respir Dis 88(suppl):394–403, 1963.

98. Top FH Jr: Control of adenovirus acute respiratory disease in U.S. Army trainees. Yale J Biol Med 48:185–195, 1975.

99. Mueller RE, Muldoon RL, Jackson GG: Communicability of enteric live adenovirus type 4 vaccine in families. J Infect Dis 119:60–66, 1969.

100. Takafuji ET, Gaydos JC, Allen RG, Top FH Jr: Simultaneous administration of live, enteric-coated adenovirus types 4, 7, and 21 vaccines: Safety and immunogenicity. J Infect Dis 140:48–53, 1979.

101. Gurwith MJ, Horwith GS, Impellizzeri CA, Davis AR, Lubeck MD, Hung PP: Current use and future directions of adenovirus vaccine. Semin Respir Infect 4:299–303, 1989.

102. Norrby E: *Paramyxoviridae*: Measles virus. *In* Balows A, Hausler WJ Jr, Lennette EH (eds): Laboratory Diagnosis of Infectious Diseases, Principles and Practice. Viral, Rickettsial, and Chlamydial Diseases, vol 2. New York, Springer-Verlag, 1988:525–539.

103. National Vaccine Advisory Committee: The measles epidemic; the problems, barriers and recommendations. JAMA 266:1547–1552, 1991.

104. Katz SL: Measles and subacute sclerosing panencephalitis. *In* Joklik WK, Willett HP, Amos DB, Wilfert CM (eds): Zinsser Microbiology (ed 20). Norwalk, CT, Appleton & Lange, 1992:1011–1015.

105. Gremillion DH, Crawford GE: Measles pneumonia in young adults; an analysis of 106 cases. Am J Med 71:539–542, 1981.

106. Atmar RL, Englund JA, Hammill H: Complications of measles during pregnancy. Clin Infect Dis 14:217–226, 1992.

107. Hussey GD, Klein M: A randomized, controlled trial of vitamin A in children with severe measles. N Engl J Med 323:160–164, 1990.

108. Straus SE, Ostrove JM, Inchauspé G, et al: Varicella-zoster infections; biology, natural history, treatment, and prevention. Ann Intern Med 108:221–237, 1988.

109. Whitley RJ: Varicella-zoster virus. *In* Mandell GL, Douglas RG Jr, Bennett JE (eds): Principles and Practice of Infectious Diseases, ed 3. New York, Churchill Livingstone, 1990:1153–1159.

110. Haake D, Kennedy C, Goetz MB: Pyelonephritis, rash, and progressive respiratory failure in a pregnant woman. Clin Infect Dis 14:599–607, 1992.

111. Gershon AA, Raker R, Steinberg S, Topf-Olstein B, Drusin LM: Antibody to varicella-zoster virus in parturient women and their offspring during the first year of life. Pediatrics 58:692–696, 1976.

112. Leclair JM, Zaia JA, Levin MJ, Congdon RG, Goldmann DA: Airborne transmission of chickenpox in a hospital. N Engl J Med 302:450–453, 1980.

113. Triebwasser JH, Harris RE, Bryant RE, Rhoades ER: Varicella pneumonia in adults; report of seven cases and a review of the literature. Medicine (Baltimore) 46:409–423, 1967.

114. Mackay JB, Cairney P: Pulmonary calcification following varicella. N Z Med J 59:453–457, 1960.

115. Stokes DC, Feldman S, Sanyal S, Mackert PW: Pulmonary function following varicella-zoster pneumonia in children with leukemia. Pediatr Pulmonol 3:236–241, 1987.

116. Forghani B, Schmidt NJ, Dennis J: Antibody assays for varicella-zoster virus; comparison of enzyme immunoassay with neutralization, immune adherence hemagglutination and complement fixation. J Clin Microbiol 8:545–552, 1978.

117. Eder SE, Apuzzio JJ, Weiss G: Varicella pneumonia during pregnancy; treatment of two cases with acyclovir. Am J Perinatol 5:16–18, 1988.

118. Boyd K, Walker E: Use of acyclovir to treat chickenpox in pregnancy. Br Med J 296:393–394, 1988.

119. Schlossberg D, Littman M: Varicella pneumonia. Arch Intern Med 148:1630–1632, 1988.

120. Haake DA, Zakowski PC, Haake DL, Bryson YJ: Early treatment with acyclovir for varicella pneumonia in otherwise healthy adults: Retrospective controlled study and review. Rev Infect Dis 12:788–798, 1990.

121. Feder HM Jr: Treatment of adult chickenpox with oral acyclovir. Arch Intern Med 150:2061–2065, 1990.

# PART

# IV

# Diagnostic Methods

# CHAPTER 41

# An Approach to Diagnostic Methods

GREGORY P. THOMPSON and GLENN D. ROBERTS

Treatment of respiratory infections depends on the results of laboratory investigations. Specific therapy targeted at an identified pathogenic organism is the preferred action, but empiric therapy based on nonspecific results is not an uncommon occurrence. In addition to the initial clues to the etiologic agent of a lower respiratory tract infection obtained from the history and physical examination, the microscopic examination of lower respiratory tract specimens can sometimes provide the most rapid laboratory evidence of the presence of a pathogenic organism. If the initial microscopic examination is not helpful, it may take days or weeks for culture or serologic results to become available. Even then, the results may be nonspecific. However, the newer molecular techniques may provide more rapid results with improved sensitivity and specificity than do the current methods. The improved methods employ the polymerase chain reaction (PCR) and DNA probes.

## SPECIMEN COLLECTION, HANDLING, AND SCREENING

Appropriate specimen collection and handling are essential to maximize the diagnostic utility of laboratory investigations. Sputum specimens contaminated with oropharyngeal flora or thoracentesis fluid sent for anaerobic culture in aerobic vials are examples of inappropriate collection. Clinically indicated expectorated sputum specimens should be obtained after appropriate instruction by medical or paramedical personnel and from patients who are conscious, cooperative, and do not have neuromuscular weakness that limits production of an effective cough. Some patients may require induction of sputum with aerosolized hypertonic (3% or 10%) salt solution. All specimens should be col-

lected in sterile, leakproof, screw-capped containers. The specimens should be placed in a watertight plastic bag and rapidly transported to the laboratory.

The initial examination of the sputum should be screening by Gram stain to assess the quality of the specimen. If 10 or more squamous epithelial cells per 100-power field are found, the specimen is unsatisfactory because of the high probability of oropharyngeal flora contamination.[1] Others have qualified a specimen as acceptable if there are fewer than 10 squamous epithelial cells and more than 25 leukocytes per high-power field.[2]

An unsatisfactory specimen should not be cultured for general bacterial growth. Oropharyngeal flora may also contaminate specimens aspirated through nasotracheal or endotracheal tubes or bronchoscopes. Transtracheal aspiration may have the lowest risk of oropharyngeal contamination, but it is rarely performed.[3]

Lower respiratory tract specimens obtained for culture for which there is less concern about contamination during collection (eg, mycobacteria) can undergo laboratory evaluation without the same quality screening that expectorated sputum specimens for general bacterial culture require. However, these specimens should be obtained and processed with good technique. Any lower respiratory tract specimen obtained for the recovery of mycobacteria should undergo the appropriate staining, microscopic, and culturing procedures. The role of screening expectorated sputum samples before examination for fungal organisms or *Pneumocystis carinii* is not well defined. The prerequisite for high-quality specimens, however, remains.

Pooled 24-hour sputum collections from patients with suspected mycobacterial or fungal infections are not recommended. Bacterial overgrowth in these specimens hinders interpretation. Instead, a series of three successive,

**489**

single, early morning specimens should be collected. If the patient's cough is nonproductive, induction of a productive cough with aerosolized hypertonic saline solution may be attempted. Early morning gastric aspirates may also be obtained for mycobacteria, preferably after collection of the morning sputum specimen.[4]

Respiratory specimens can also be obtained by more invasive methods, such as bronchoscopy with bronchial washings, protected catheter brush, or bronchoalveolar lavage; thoracentesis or closed pleural biopsy; transthoracic needle aspiration; and thoracoscopic or open lung biopsy. These procedures, especially bronchoalveolar lavage, are often required in immunocompromised patients. For each procedure, the specimen should be obtained in a sterile fashion and placed in a sterile container for rapid transport to the laboratory. The transport time can be shortened if the appropriate laboratory slips are completed before the specimen is obtained.

The laboratory evaluation of viral respiratory tract infections usually consists of examination of nasopharyngeal swabs or aspirated secretion specimens. Nasal swabs usually are adequate for the recovery of influenza viruses, but in hospitalized or confined populations, secretions are superior. Nasopharyngeal swabs usually are adequate for adenovirus recovery. Respiratory syncytial viruses and parainfluenza viruses usually require aspirated secretion specimens. Secretions or tissue specimens are preferred for cytomegalovirus and herpes simplex virus. Varicella-zoster virus pneumonia often requires tissue for a definitive diagnosis. All clinical specimens should be transported to the laboratory as quickly as possible.

Delays in the transportation of lower respiratory tract secretions so that they are left at room temperature for 2 to 5 hours result in decreased recovery rates of pneumococci, staphylococci, and gram-negative bacilli and an increased number of microorganisms indigenous to the upper respiratory tract.[5] If specimens for mycobacterial culture cannot be processed immediately or must be shipped to another facility, they should be treated with a solution of cetylpyridinium chloride and sodium chloride.[6] Specimens for fungal culture should be processed as quickly as possible after they are obtained, but most clinically significant, pathogenic fungi can tolerate 4 to 5 days of transport and storage.[7] Specimens for viral isolation in cell culture should be transported at 4° to 6°C using cold packs or wet ice, but they should not be frozen.[8]

Specimens shipped by mail or by other carriers to reference laboratories must be properly packaged to protect the shippers and the receiving laboratory personnel. Clinical specimens may be shipped in a sealed, watertight container that is placed in a sealed, watertight secondary container with absorbent, cushioning material between the two. The container must be properly labeled and should not contain more than 1000 mL of clinical specimen per primary container, 2000 mL per secondary container, or 4000 mL per shipping container.[9]

## MICROSCOPIC EXAMINATION OF CLINICAL SPECIMENS

The initial microscopic examination of a lower respiratory tract specimen can sometimes provide important information about the cause of a respiratory tract infection. An acceptable Gram-stained specimen should be examined under oil immersion ($\times$ 1000 magnification) to determine if a predominant bacterium is present. Organisms should be identified based on morphologic features or at least classified as gram-positive or negative.

The diagnostic importance of an initial Gram stain of lower respiratory tract specimens was discussed in several reports. A Gram stain of expectorated sputum or tracheal aspirate collected immediately after intubation of a group of critically ill patients was diagnostic for 23 of 31 patients.[10] Culture results later confirmed the same predominant organism in these 23 patients. In a prospective study from 1988 of 59 patients with bacterial pneumonia, a Gram stain of expectorated sputum specimens provided enough information to aid in the selection of appropriate monotherapy for 94% of the cases.[11] However, in 3 of 5 patients with *Haemophilus influenzae* pneumonia, the sputum Gram stain suggested an alternative pathogen. In community-acquired pneumonia, the Gram stain had an 86% correlation with sputum culture results.[12]

Although some previous studies have questioned the value of the sputum Gram stain, it can be a reliable, but not infallible, guide to the selection of initial antibiotic therapy in patients with community-acquired pneumonia.[13, 14] A good-quality sputum specimen obtained from a febrile patient with pulmonary infiltrates without a predominant organism may be a clue to an atypical infection or a noninfectious cause.

Gram stains of specimens obtained by bronchoscopy or by bronchoalveolar lavage (BAL) may be useful. Oropharyngeal contamination may occur with passage of the bronchoscope through the oral cavity. The protected brush and telescope catheter brush were developed to decrease the incidence of false-positive results caused by oropharyngeal contamination.

### Acid-Fast Smear

The microscopic examination for acid-fast bacteria (AFB) provides a rapid, inexpensive, and specific method to evaluate a suspected mycobacterial respiratory infection. Overall, the sensitivity has been between 22% and 43%.[15-18] The sensitivity is influenced by the concentration of mycobacteria, the presence of acquired immunodeficiency syndrome (AIDS),[19] and the staining method used.[20] Increasing the number of specimens examined from a single patient increases the overall sensitivity, and it is recommended that a sputum specimen for AFB examination be obtained on three consecutive mornings from patients with suspected mycobacterial disease. In a study of patients infected with the human immunodeficiency virus (HIV) in which a delayed diagnosis of tuberculosis (TB) was associated with increased mortality, a frequent reason for delay in diagnosis was that fewer than three sputum specimens were submitted for AFB examination.[21]

The auramine-rhodamine stain is reliable and more sensitive than the carbolfuchsin stain.[20, 22] The auramine-rhodamine stain has been reported to detect AFB in 18% of specimens that were negative by the carbolfuchsin method.[26] In general, the acid-fast stain is less sensitive than

Table 41–1. **Microscopic Morphologic Features of Fungi Seen in the Direct Examination of Body Fluids and Tissue**

| Morphologic Form | Organism | Diameter (μm) | Hyphae | Comments |
|---|---|---|---|---|
| Spherules | *Coccidioides immitis* | 20–80 | Possible | Spherules vary in size and may contain endospores; hyphae may be found in cavitary lesions |
| Yeasts | *Histoplasma capsulatum* | 2–5 | No | Small, oval budding cells; sometimes intracellular |
| | *Blastomyces dermatitidis* | 8–15 | No | Large cells with broad-based, usually singular buds |
| | *Cryptococcus neoformans* | 2–15 | Rare pseudohyphae | Various sizes with "pinched off" buds and capsule may be present |
| | *Sporothrix schenckii* | 3–5 | No | Rare in clinical specimens, small cells ranging from oval to cigar-shaped with single or multiple buds |
| Yeasts and/or hyphae | *Candida* spp. | 3–4 yeasts 5–10 pseudohyphae | Pseudohyphae and true hyphae | Single budding cells; pseudohyphae appear as links of sausage; true hyphae have parallel walls and are septate |
| Septate hyphae | *Aspergillus* spp. | 3–12 | Hyaline hyphae | Hyphae are septate and exhibit dichotomous 45° angle branching |
| | *Pseudallescheria boydii, Fusarium,* and numerous other fungi | 5–10 | Septate | Hyphae almost impossible to distinguish from other hyaline molds |
| Sparsely septate hyphae | Zygomycetes (*Rhizopus, Mucor, Absidia*) | 10–30 | Wide nonseptate hyphae | Hyphae large and ribbon-like; may branch at right angles |

culture. The specificity of the acid-fast smear examination is high, and the false-positive rate ranges from 10% to 20%.[16, 23–25]

Acid-fast smear examination of stool specimens may have a role in the diagnosis of mycobacterial disease in HIV-infected patients. AFB-positive smears of stool specimens may be found in approximately 40% of patients with concomitant HIV and TB infections.[21, 26] However, most of these patients also have positive acid-fast smears of sputum and rarely have clinical features of gastrointestinal TB. Positive acid-fast smears of stool from HIV-infected patients having TB probably represent organisms swallowed and may not be indicative of extrapulmonary TB.[27] *Mycobacterium avium-intracellulare* complex, however, can cause a symptomatic gastrointestinal tract infection without evidence of respiratory system involvement in HIV-infected patients.[28–30] In most cases, AFB may be seen in stool specimens. Acid-fast smears of stool are probably not indicated in patients not having HIV infection.

Acid-fast smears may be positive in 30% to 73% of bronchial washings from immunocompetent patients having pulmonary TB.[31] However, in one report, only 19% of patients with HIV infection and pulmonary TB had acid-fast organisms detected.[21] The roles of bronchoscopy and acid-fast smear examination therefore need to be better defined. Bronchoscopy may elicit episodes of vigorous coughing, and measures must be taken to prevent possible transmission of TB during the procedure.

## Examination of Specimens for Fungi

Prompt microscopic detection and identification of fungal elements in respiratory secretions can be achieved days or weeks before culture results are available. The findings may also prompt the clinical laboratory to provide specialized media and extended time for incubation to enhance recovery of the etiologic agent. Direct microscopic examination of respiratory secretions cannot differentiate whether an organism has colonized or infected the respiratory tract.

A variety of stains can aid the microscopic detection of fungal elements. A Gram stain can sometimes detect fungal elements. Of the common respiratory fungal pathogens, *Histoplasma capsulatum* is too small to be routinely detected and *Cryptococcus neoformans* may not stain well with the Gram stain. The potassium hydroxide (KOH) preparation can be performed rapidly, but the background debris can make interpretation difficult. The calcofluor white stain is better; it is rapid and produces bright fluorescence of the cell wall of the fungi. A fluorescence microscope is required. The methenamine silver stain is considered the best to detect fungal elements, but it requires a specialized, 1-hour procedure and is not usually performed in a clinical microbiology laboratory. Other stains are available for the detection of fungal elements, such as the periodic acid-Schiff (PAS), Wright, and Pananicolau stains; these are well described in other sources.[32]

Fungal elements have characteristic features that may allow prompt identification of the etiologic agent. These are presented in Table 41–1. The frequency of positive direct microscopic examinations of fungal respiratory tract infections is not well defined. This may be a result of the variety of clinical conditions with which they can present, infrequency of direct examination of respiratory secretions before the availability of culture results, and the small number of cases studied. In a review of 30 patients with blastomycosis, the cytologic stains (Papanicolaou) of sputum or bronchial washings were more often positive than the "microbiologic" stains (e.g., KOH, PAS) for first specimens and cumulative specimens.[33] This was true for 70% and 93% of cytologic stains, compared with 32% and 61% for microbiologic stains, respectively.[33] Similarly, the cytologic examination of respiratory secretions from patients with culture-proven pulmonary coccidioidomycosis was more sensitive than examination of KOH preparations (38.5% versus 15.4%).[34]

## Stains for *Pneumocystis carinii*

A variety of methods are available for the direct microscopic detection of *P. carinii* in bronchial washings, BAL fluid, or induced sputum. The Giemsa stain or a rapid modification of it is sometimes considered to be the primary stain for the detection of *P. carinii*. Stains that readily detect the cysts of *P. carinii* include methenamine silver, toluidine blue, and calcofluor white. Immunofluorescent stains using specific monoclonal antibodies to detect *P. carinii* are considered to be immunologic stains. Each of these stains has unique attributes that must be considered before use in the clinical laboratory.

Immunofluorescent stains are the most sensitive method for detecting *Pneumocystis* in respiratory tract secretions.[35] The direct microscopic examination of induced sputa with the Giemsa stain has been reported to be 56% sensitive and to have a negative predictive value of 39% when used in a population of patients suspected to have AIDS.[36] The methenamine silver stain combined with Papanicolaou stains of induced sputa has a sensitivity of 55%.[37] Immunofluorescent staining of induced sputa has a sensitivity of 90%, better than Giemsa or toluidine blue O stains.[35] Immunofluorescent staining of BAL fluid or tissue taken at lung biopsy has shown a sensitivity comparable to that of toluidine blue O staining.[38] Calcofluor white staining of BAL specimens has been shown to have a sensitivity and specificity of 95% and 100%, respectively, compared with toluidine blue O and Giemsa stains.[39]

With several stains available for detecting *P. carinii*, familiarity with the stain, cost, and ability to detect other pathogens are among the factors that determine which stain a laboratory may choose. The clinical utility of induced sputa for direct microscopic detection of *P. carinii* in patients not infected with HIV remains to be determined.

## CULTURES

Although sometimes of benefit, bacterial cultures of expectorated sputum often fail to provide definitive results. The interpretation of sputum cultures is hindered by oropharyngeal contamination, lack of sensitivity, and problems associated with the collection of a good-quality specimen in patients having pneumonia. The initial therapeutic decisions are usually made before the culture results are available, and for the acutely ill patient with pneumonia, culture results can only supplement the initial therapeutic choices.

Cultures of sputum or of the nasopharynx fail to recover pneumococci in 45% of patients with bacteremic pneumococcal pneumonia.[13] Poor correlation has also been reported between quantitative sputum cultures and transtracheal needle aspirate cultures.[40] The low sensitivity of sputum cultures in bacteremic community-acquired pneumonia has been documented; cultures of expectorated sputum or an endotracheal specimen collected at the time of intubation recovered the identical pathogen that was isolated in blood cultures in only 64% of bacteremic pneumonias.[10] Bacterial culture of BAL fluid can assist in the diagnosis of lower respiratory tract infections. It was reported in 1987 that 13 (87%) of 15 patients with clinically active pneumonia had BAL cultures that yielded more than $10^5$ colony-forming units per mL (CFU/mL) of BAL fluid.[41] The sensitivity for semiquantitative cultures of BAL fluid from immunocompetent patients suspected of having acute bacterial pneumonia was 89%.[42] The specificity reported for both studies was 100%. General bacterial cultures of BAL fluid from HIV-infected patients have had a high sensitivity (83%) in detecting bacterial pneumonias if the specimens were obtained before antibiotics were administered. The sensitivity fell to 23% if BAL was performed after antibiotic therapy was initiated.[43]

The protected catheter brush can be a useful technique to obtain specimens from patients with nosocomial pneumonia (especially those who are mechanically ventilated) or those with refractory community-acquired pneumonia. Specimens should be quantitatively cultured for aerobic and anaerobic bacteria. In general, the finding of more than $10^3$ CFU/mL differentiates positive from negative results; this threshold can accurately identify patients with and without pneumonia.[44, 45]

Of 45 mechanically ventilated patients with suspected nosocomial pneumonia and positive protected brush cultures, 34 had pneumonia, 7 had an uncertain diagnosis, and only 4 did not have pneumonia.[44] Of 72 patients with negative cultures, none had a definite pneumonia. There was a good correlation between negative protected brush catheter culture specimens and no histologic evidence of pneumonia from postmortem examination of patients who were mechanically ventilated.[45] Positive culture results correlated well with histologic proof of pneumonia.

Anaerobic and mixed aerobic-anaerobic bacteria are responsible for causing most pleural space infections.[46] Aerobic and anaerobic bacterial cultures of pleural fluid should be obtained from all patients with suspected parapneumonic effusion or empyema. The frequency with which the pleural fluid becomes infected depends in part on the etiologic agent. Approximately 35% of patients with anaerobic pneumonia have culture-positive pleural effusions,[46] but only 5% or fewer patients with pneumococcal pneumonia have culture-positive pleural effusion.[47]

Several measures are required to increase the sensitivity of cultures for the recovery of mycobacteria in respiratory tract specimens. These include reduction or elimination of contaminating bacterial flora, release of mycobacteria trapped in mucin, and concentration of the mycobacteria. An *N*-acetyl-L-cysteine (NALC) and sodium hydroxide (NaOH) method is used by many laboratories for the decontamination and liquefaction of specimens. The mycobacteria are then concentrated by centrifugation. After centrifugation, the specimen is ready for culture and should be inoculated onto selective and/or nonselective media and/or a BACTEC bottle. Culture plates should be incubated in an atmosphere of 5% to 10% carbon dioxide for 8 weeks.

Growth of mycobacteria can be detected with the BACTEC radiometric system or by visual inspection of culture plates. The BACTEC system can detect growth of *Mycobacterium tuberculosis* and mycobacteria other than *M. tuberculosis* approximately 10 days earlier than conventional media.[48] Identification can be made based on growth characteristics, morphology, biochemical tests, gas chromatographic analysis of cell wall lipids, and nucleic acid probes. High-performance liquid chromatography is also being used successfully as a means of identifying mycobacteria in growing cultures.

Nucleic acid probes (Gen-Probe, Inc., San Diego, CA) first became commercially available in 1987. Originally, these single-stranded DNA probes, which were complementary to the rRNA of the target organism, were labeled with iodine 125. Their ability to accurately identify *M. avium*, *M. intracellulare*, and *M. tuberculosis* complex was clearly demonstrated.[49–51] However, the radioactive label hindered widespread use because of costs and stability.

In 1991, nonisotopic nucleic acid probes for the culture identification of *M. tuberculosis* complex, *M. avium*, *intracellulare*, *M. kansasii*, and *M. gordonae* were introduced. These single-stranded DNA probes, complementary to the rRNA of the target organism, incorporate an acridinium ester label. If target organisms are present, the DNA probes bind to the complementary rRNA that is released during cell lysis. Chemiluminescence from the acridinium ester can be measured after a differential hydrolysis reaction. These probes have demonstrated good sensitivity and specificity for identifying mycobacteria grown in culture.[48] In addition, these probes are able to identify mycobacteria directly from BACTEC vials.[48] Nonisotopic DNA probes are continuing to have a rapidly expanding role in the clinical microbiology laboratory, but these probes have not been sensitive enough to detect mycobacteria in clinical specimens without culture.

Gas-liquid chromatography and high-performance liquid chromatography can identify mycobacterial species.[52, 53] Both will probably have a continued role in the identification of mycobacteria for which nonisotopic probes are not available.

The definitive method for the diagnosis of legionnaires disease is culture and identification of the etiologic agents. *Legionella* spp. have not been considered part of the normal flora of the respiratory tract. The primary medium for the culture of *Legionella* spp. is a buffered charcoal yeast extract agar with α-ketoglutarate (BCYEα). Semiselective media may also be used but should not be used alone. The sensitivity of cultures ranges from 50% to 80%, and the specificity is 100%.[54] After growth occurs on a culture medium, a modified Gram stain should be performed to visualize the characteristic pleomorphic gram-negative bacilli. If the organism demonstrates growth only with L-cysteine–containing media, it can be classified as the genus *Legionella*. Further species identification can then be made with direct fluorescent antibody testing or DNA probes.

Most fungal cultures require 1 to 2 mL of specimen to adequately inoculate three to four media. Liquefaction of respiratory secretions with a mucolytic agent (eg, NALC) before inoculation is optional. However, most fungi do not survive the NaOH treatment used to enhance recovery of mycobacteria from respiratory secretions. No one fungal medium is best for all clinically important fungi. A medium containing blood, one containing antibacterial agents, and one containing cycloheximide with or without antibacterial agents are recommended for the recovery of fungi from cultures of respiratory secretions. Another medium containing no antifungal or antibacterial agents and no blood is optional and should not be used. All specimens should be incubated for at least 4 weeks at 30°C. Fastidious fungi such as *H. capsulatum* and *Blastomyces dermatitidis* may sometimes require 6 weeks of incubation if the inoculum is small. All filamentous fungi should be handled in a certified, Class II laminar flow biological safety cabinet.

After fungal growth has been seen in the cultures, several methods are available for identification. Direct microscopic examination may provide enough evidence for complete identification of the isolated organism or at least narrow the differential list. An exoantigen technique can identify *Coccidioidomyces immitis*, *H. capsulatum*, *B. dermatitidis*, and *Paracoccidioidomyces brasiliensis*.[55] Nonisotopic, acridinium-labeled DNA probes are commercially available for rapid culture identification of *H. capsulatum*, *B. dermatitidis*, *C. neoformans*, and *C. immitis*. Preliminary studies indicate that these probes are sensitive and specific (both near 100%) and require only 1 hour for performance.[56]

In diagnostic virology, viruses isolated from the upper respiratory tract are usually assumed to be the cause of an associated pneumonia in an immunocompetent patient. A throat or nasopharyngeal swab or nasopharyngeal aspirate is usually adequate for the diagnosis of most viral pneumonias.[57] Sputum specimens, bronchial aspirates, and open lung biopsy specimens can also be used for viral isolation. Specimens should be collected as early as possible in the course of the illness, because viral shedding is greatest at that time.[57] The common cell culture types used for virus isolation include primary monkey kidney, human diploid cells, primary embryonic kidney, and continuous epithelial cells.[58] Five to 7 days are required to detect viral replication.

Historically, blood cultures were reported to be positive in 20% to 30% of patients early in the course of pneumococcal pneumonia.[59] More recently, blood cultures have been reported to be positive in 35% of patients with pneumonia who required admission to an intensive care unit.[10] Blood cultures should be obtained from any patient hospitalized with pneumonia.

If mycobacteremia is suspected, blood may be inoculated onto the appropriate mycobacterial culture media if the lysis-centrifugation system (Isolator) is used or with a radiometric system (BACTEC 13A). Twenty-six percent of HIV-positive patients with TB have blood cultures positive for *M. tuberculosis*.[60] Blood cultures are one of the preferred tests for AIDS patients with disseminated *M. avium-intracellulare* disease. Hawkins and colleagues reported that 98% of cases of autopsy-confirmed disseminated *M. avium-intracellulare* disease in AIDS patients had positive blood cultures.[61] Two blood cultures are usually adequate to make the diagnosis.[62]

Fungal pneumonia may represent disseminated fungal infection, and fungal blood cultures are an important consideration in systemically ill patients with pneumonia of undetermined cause. The lysis-centrifugation method (Isolator) provides the highest recovery rate and shortest recovery time of the accepted culturing methods used today.[63] *H. capsulatum* and *C. neoformans* are most commonly isolated from blood cultures.[63]

## IMMUNOFLUORESCENCE AND ELISA

Immunofluorescence and enzyme-linked immunosorbent assay (ELISA) techniques have made rapid viral diagnosis possible. Immunofluorescence is applicable to the diagnosis of infections caused by influenza, parainfluenza, respiratory syncytial virus, adenoviruses, measles, rubella, corona, and herpesviruses.[57] Nasopharyngeal aspirates are generally superior to nasopharyngeal swabs for detection by immunofluorescence. ELISA testing is available for the detection of parainfluenza, respiratory syncytial virus, herpes simplex, influenza A, and adenoviruses. Immunofluorescence and ELISA tests can detect viral antigens when the virus can no longer be recovered by culture methods.

Direct fluorescent antibody testing of respiratory tract secretions or tissue to detect *Legionella* has also been described.[64] These tests are specific, but the testing is hindered by the low number of organisms in the specimen.

## IMMUNODIAGNOSIS

The cause of pneumonia can often be difficult to determine. Direct microscopic examination and cultures of clinical specimens may be unrewarding. An alternative approach such as serologic testing is required. However, serologic tests (Table 41–2) usually provide a "retrospective" diagnosis.

### Legionella

Indirect fluorescent antibody (IFA) testing of serum for *Legionella* antibody should detect all classes of immunoglobulins, because the immune response to *Legionella* is variable.[65] The sensitivity of the standard IFA test is estimated to be 75% to 78% in patients with culture or epidemiologic proof of pneumonia caused by *Legionella pneumophila* serogroup 1.[66, 67] The specificity of the IFA test is estimated to be 96% to 99% for serogroup infections caused by *L. pneumophila*.[66, 68] A fourfold or greater rise in antibody titer up to 1:128 or higher between acute-phase (ie, 1 week after onset of symptoms) and convalescent-phase (ie, 3 to 6 weeks after onset) serum samples from a patient with a compatible illness is accepted for the diagnosis of legionnaires disease.[66] A single titer of 1:256 or greater establishes a presumptive diagnosis in patients having a compat-

ible illness.[69] An ELISA test has been developed for the serologic diagnosis of legionnaires disease, but it is not completely standardized.

### Mycoplasma

Because the complex growth requirements for *Mycoplasma pneumoniae* result in a culturing process that is technically difficult, lengthy, and often unrewarding, serologic testing has a significant role in diagnosis. Cold agglutinins, IgM antibodies that agglutinate human erythrocytes, have been used as a traditional serologic test for the diagnosis of *M. pneumoniae* infection. A titer of 1:128 or higher in a patient with pneumonia is highly suggestive of *M. pneumoniae* infection; lower titers are less specific. The titer may become elevated early in the second week of illness and provide an early, inexpensive clue to the diagnosis.

Complement fixation (CF) testing for antibodies to *M. pneumoniae* uses an extracted glycolipid antigen to detect specific IgG or IgM antibodies. Serum should be collected within the first week of illness (ie, acute phase) and after the third week of illness (ie, convalescent phase). The sera should be tested concurrently. A fourfold or greater increase in CF titer is acceptable for the diagnosis of *M. pneumoniae* pneumonia in a patient having a compatible clinical picture. Single titers of 1:32 or greater have been used to make a presumptive diagnosis.[65] CF titers, however, can remain elevated for long periods after infection, which makes it difficult to separate recent from past infection.[70] ELISA and microimmunofluorescence tests are under development and may play a significant role in the diagnosis of *M. pneumoniae* in the future.

### Fungal Infections

Serologic testing may aid in the diagnosis of fungal infections of the respiratory tract. These tests are most useful

**Table 41–2. Common Serologic Tests Useful for the Diagnosis of Respiratory Infections**

| Organism | Method* | Positive Result | Comment† |
|---|---|---|---|
| *Legionella* spp. | IFA | 4-fold increase to ≥1:128 | Acute to convalescent phase |
| | IFA | Single titer ≥1:256 | Presumptive diagnosis |
| *Mycoplasma pneumoniae* | Cold agglutinins | ≥1:128 | |
| | CF | 4-fold increase of titer | Acute to convalescent phase |
| | | Single titer ≥1:32 | Presumptive diagnosis |
| *Histoplasma capsulatum* | CF | ≥1:8 | |
| | CF | 4-fold increase or ≥1:32 | Likely cause of an acute illness‡ |
| | ID | H and M bands | Highly specific |
| | | M band | More sensitive, less specific than H and M bands |
| *Blastomyces dermatitidis* | CF | ≥1:8 or 1:16 | Suggestive of active infection‡ |
| | ID | | If positive, suggests active infection |
| *Coccidioides immitis* | CF | >1:16 | Suggests disseminated disease§ |
| *Aspergillus* spp. | ID | Positive precipitins | Seen with allergic bronchopulmonary aspergillosis and aspergilloma‖ |

*IFA, indirect fluorescent antibody; CF, complement fixation; ID, immunodiffusion.
†All examples assume a compatible clinical condition. Negative serology does not rule out a diagnosis.
‡Crossreactions between *H. capsulatum* and *B. dermatitidis* can occur.
§Titers as low as 1:2 or 1:4 may be seen in patients with active infection.
‖May be falsely negative in immunocompromised patients.

for the diagnosis of histoplasmosis, blastomycosis, coccidioidomycosis, cryptococcosis, and aspergillosis. Most tests detect specific antibodies to fungal antigens, and some detect specific fungal antigens found in body fluids of infected patients.

CF and immunodiffusion (ID) are often used in serologic testing for histoplasmosis. A histoplasmosis CF antibody titer of 1:8 or greater is considered positive.[71] A titer of 1:32 or greater or a fourfold rise in titers establishes histoplasmosis as the likely cause of an acute illness.[71] The CF test usually becomes positive within 21 to 28 days after primary exposure, and approximately 70% of patients develop elevated titers within 6 weeks. Of the two antigens used, yeast and mycelial forms, the former is the more sensitive. However, elevated CF titers may not be seen in patients with severe disseminated infection, and patients from endemic areas may have elevated titers in the absence of an active infection.

Precipitating antibodies to *H. capsulatum* can be detected as two precipitin bands (designated H and M bands) by ID testing. The H and M bands are highly specific for histoplasmosis, although they occur together in only approximately 10% of patients with pulmonary histoplasmosis.[71] Fifteen percent to 20% of patients with disseminated disease exhibit both H and M bands.[71] An M band occurs alone in approximately 50% of patients with active histoplasmosis and is the first antibody to appear.[71] Negative ID tests do not rule out active infection. The M band may persist after recovery, during chronic infection, or after recent skin testing. The ID test is most helpful when interpreted with CF test results.

Enzyme or radioimmunoassays for *H. capsulatum* antibodies or antigens have been reported.[72, 73] Although these tests may be more sensitive and serve as possible screening tests for histoplasmosis, further clinical testing is needed, and they are not widely used by clinical laboratories.

CF and ID testing have been used in the serologic evaluation of blastomycosis. CF titers greater than 1:8 or 1:16 suggest active infection.[71] Fewer than 25% of culture-proved cases of blastomycosis have positive CF titers.[71] Crossreactions occur in sera of patients with histoplasmosis, making interpretation difficult unless concurrent testing for histoplasma antibody is done. ID testing has questionable sensitivity reported in the literature and requires further clarification.[74]

In coccidioidomycosis, the mycelial form of antigen, coccidioidin, is the most useful for detecting humoral antibodies. Serum IgM-precipitating antibodies may be detected by tube precipitation, latex agglutination, or ID methods. In addition, serum IgG complement-fixing antibodies can be demonstrated. Serum IgM antibodies can be detected 1 to 3 weeks after the symptoms of a primary infection appear in 90% of cases.[71] Serum IgM antibodies usually disappear after 4 to 7 months. Serum IgG complement-fixing antibodies occur later and may persist for months to years. Fifty percent to 90% of patients with primary symptomatic infection have demonstrable IgG antibodies within 3 months after the onset of primary symptoms.[71] CF titers greater than 1:16 strongly suggest the presence of disseminated disease, and titers generally parallel the course of the disease.[71]

ID testing for detection of precipitating antibodies appears to be the most readily available and reliable of the tests used for serologic evaluation of patients having aspergillosis. Antigens of *Aspergillus fumigatus, Aspergillus flavus,* and *Aspergillus niger* are most commonly used. Precipitins are present in approximately 70% of patients with allergic bronchopulmonary aspergillosis and in more than 95% of patients with aspergilloma.[71] However, in immunocompromised patients, who are at the greatest risk of invasive aspergillosis, ID tests for the detection of antibodies to *Aspergillus* are often falsely negative.

The latex agglutination test for the detection of cryptococcal polysaccharide antigen is the test of choice for the serologic evaluation of patients having meningitis or disseminated cryptococcosis. The test is performed using cerebrospinal fluid or serum, and its use in the diagnosis of pulmonary infection is limited. Direct testing of respiratory tract secretions is under evaluation.

Serologic tests for the detection of *Candida* antigens or antibodies are not well validated and are not of use to the community clinical laboratory. Testing is not routinely available for the serologic diagnosis of pulmonary sporotrichosis, zygomycosis, or infection with *Pseudallescheria boydii.*

### Group A Streptococci and Other Pathogens

The agglutination test is based on a serologic reaction that requires the interaction of a specific antigen with an antibody. The clumping of particles by specific antibodies or antigens within controlled physical and chemical conditions results in agglutination. IgG and IgM are the two classes of immunoglobulins involved in agglutination. Commercially available agglutination kits are being used for the detection of microbial antigens in normally sterile body fluids. The difficulty with their use in testing of normally contaminated body fluids or of specimens that pass through the oropharynx is in differentiating colonization from active infection with an organism. Their use with the direct testing of respiratory tract secretions needs further clarification. However, the detection of group A streptococci from throat swabs should be considered significant, because the sensitivity of commercially available tests has been adjusted to discount low-level colonization.[75]

### MOLECULAR DIAGNOSTIC METHODS

The future for the rapid diagnosis of infection appears to rest on the development of molecular diagnostic methods. These are based on the detection in a clinical specimen of small amounts of nucleic acid specific for an etiologic agent. It is necessary to amplify the nucleic acid so that it can be detected by some indicator system. The PCR is a technique that provides amplification of targeted DNA. Recent advances in molecular biology have provided the specific DNA sequences of many microorganisms. After the DNA sequence of a microorganism is known, specific synthetic oligonucleotide primers can be made. The combination of the primers and the techniques of PCR provide amplification of a target DNA segment unique to the microorganism being studied. The amplified DNA is usually detected with gel electrophoresis or nucleic acid probes. The process of amplification and detection is usually accomplished in 48 hours or less.

Initial research with PCR focused on perfecting the technique on pure cultures of microorganisms, but reports regarding the application of this technique to the testing of clinical specimens have appeared. The primary benefit of PCR is in the detection of slowly growing organisms, such as mycobacteria or fungi, that are not always detected by direct microscopic examination of specimens and that require lengthy incubation and identification methods. Several reports indicate that PCR techniques can be used to rapidly detect mycobacteria in clinical specimens and differentiate the mycobacterial species.[76, 77] However, most specimens positive by PCR techniques were also positive on direct acid-fast stain examination. Further work is needed in perfecting the technique so that the results are positive for the specimens for which PCR would be most helpful: those negative by direct examination and positive by culture.

One report suggests that improvement in PCR detection of mycobacteria in smear-negative, culture-positive specimens is occurring.[78] In addition, the specificity of the PCR method for *Mycobacterium tuberculosis* has been found to be clinically useful.[79, 80] The AFB smear is unable to differentiate *M. tuberculosis* from nontuberculous organisms, but the PCR method can make that differentiation. The problems associated with molecular methods may include the clinical correlation of oversensitive results and the lack of distinction between viable and nonviable organisms in a clinical specimen. Even after molecular diagnostic methods become available, it will probably be a long time before clinical correlative studies substantiate the results generated by the laboratory. However, the future appears bright for the use of these diagnostic methods in all areas of microbiology, including virology, mycology, and bacteriology.

# REFERENCES

1. Murray PR, Washington JA II: Microscopic and bacteriologic analysis of expectorated sputum. Mayo Clin Proc 50:339, 1975.
2. Verghese A, Berk SL: Bacterial pneumonia in the elderly. Medicine (Baltimore) 62:271, 1983.
3. Bartlett JG, Rosenblatt JE, Finegold SM: Percutaneous transtracheal aspiration in the diagnosis of anaerobic pulmonary infection. Ann Intern Med 79:535, 1973.
4. Carr DT, Karlson AG, Stillwell GG: A comparison of cultures of induced sputum and gastric washings in the diagnosis of tuberculosis. Mayo Clin Proc 42:23, 1967.
5. Jefferson H, Dalton HP, Escobar MR, et al: Transportation delay and the microbiological quality of clinical specimens. Am J Clin Pathol 64:689, 1975.
6. Smithwick RW, Stratigos CB, David HL: Use of cetylpyridinium chloride and sodium chloride for the decontamination of sputum specimens that are transported to the laboratory for the isolation of *Mycobacterium tuberculosis*. J Clin Microbiol 1:411, 1975.
7. Hariri AR, Hempel HO, Kimberlin CL, et al: Effects of time lapse between sputum collection and culturing on isolation of clinically significant fungi. J Clin Microbiol 15:425, 1982.
8. Lennette DA: Preparation of specimens for virological examination. In Balows A, Hausler WJ Jr, Hermann KL, et al (eds): Manual of Clinical Microbiology. Washington, DC, American Society for Microbiology, 1990:818.
9. U.S. Postal Service: Mailability of etiologic agents. 37 CFR part III. Fed Regist 54:11970–11972, 1989.
10. Potgieter PD, Hammond JMJ: Etiology and diagnosis of pneumonia requiring ICU admission. Chest 101:199, 1992.
11. Gleckman R, deVita J, Hilbert D, et al: Sputum Gram stain assessment in community acquired bacteremia pneumonia. J Clin Microbiol 26:846, 1988.
12. Levy M, Drumer F, Brion N, et al: Community-acquired pneumonia: Importance of initial non-invasive bacteriologic and radiographic investigations. Chest 93:43, 1988.
13. Barrett-Connor E: The non-value of sputum culture in the diagnosis of pneumococcal pneumonia. Am Rev Respir Dis 103:845, 1971.
14. Geckler RW, Gremillion DH, McAllister CK, et al: Microscopic and bacteriological comparison of paired sputa and transtracheal aspirates. J Clin Microbiol 6:396, 1977.
15. Boyd JC, Marr JJ: Decreasing reliability of acid-fast smear techniques for detection of tuberculosis. Ann Intern Med 82:489, 1975.
16. Burdash NM, Manos JP, Ross D, et al: Evaluation of the acid-fast smear. J Clin Microbiol 4:190, 1976.
17. Murray PR, Elmore C, Krogstad CJ: The acid-fast stain: A specific and predictive test for mycobacterial disease. Ann Intern Med 92:512, 1980.
18. Marraro RV, Rodgers EM, Roberts TH: The acid-fast smear: Fact or fiction? J Am Med Technol 37:277, 1975.
19. Klein NC, Duncanson FP, Lenox TH, et al: Use of mycobacterial smears in the diagnosis of pulmonary tuberculosis in AIDS/ARC patients. Chest 95:1190, 1989.
20. Sommers HM, McClatchy JK, Monella JA: Laboratory diagnosis of the mycobacterioses. In Sommers HM, McClatchy JK (eds): Cumitech 16. Washington, DC, American Society for Microbiology, 1983:1.
21. Kramer F, Modilevsky T, Waliany AR, et al: Delayed diagnosis of tuberculosis in patients with human immunodeficiency virus infection. Am J Med 89:451, 1990.
22. Strumpf IJ, Tsang AY, Sayre JW: Reevaluation of sputum staining for the diagnosis of pulmonary tuberculosis. Am Rev Respir Dis 119:599, 1979.
23. Stottmeier KD: Acid-fast smears and tuberculosis. Ann Intern Med 83:429, 1975.
24. Fierer J, Merino R: Acid-fast smears and tuberculosis. Ann Intern Med 83:430, 1975.
25. Rickman TW, Moyer NP: Increased sensitivity of acid-fast smears. J Clin Microbiol 11:618, 1980.
26. Modilevsky T, Sattler FR, Barnes PF: Mycobacterial disease in patients with human immunodeficiency virus infection. Arch Intern Med 149:2201, 1989.
27. Barnes PF, Bloch AB, Davidson PT, et al: Tuberculosis in patients with human immunodeficiency virus infection. N Engl J Med 324:1644, 1991.
28. Gray JR, Rabeneck L: Atypical mycobacterial infection of the gastrointestinal tract in AIDS patients. Am J Gastroenterol 84:1521, 1989.
29. Roth RI, Owen RL, Keren DF, et al: Intestinal infection with *Mycobacterium avium* in acquired immune deficiency syndrome. Dig Dis Sci 30:497, 1985.
30. Klatt EC, Jensen DF, Meyer PR: Pathology of *Mycobacterium avium intracellulare* infection in acquired immunodeficiency syndrome. Hum Pathol 18:709, 1987.
31. So SY, Lam WK, Yu DYC: Rapid diagnosis of suspected pulmonary tuberculosis by fiber optic bronchoscopy. Tubercle 63:195, 1982.
32. Merz WG, Roberts GD: Detection and recovery of fungi from clinical specimens. In Balows A, Hausler WJ Jr, Hermann KL, et al (eds): Manual of Clinical Microbiology. Washington, DC, American Society for Microbiology, 1991:588.
33. Trumbull ML, Chesney TM: The cytologic diagnosis of pulmonary blastomycosis. JAMA 245:836, 1981.
34. Warlick MA, Quan SF, Sobonya RE: Rapid diagnosis of pulmonary coccidioidomycosis. Cytologic vs potassium hydroxide preparations. Arch Intern Med 143:723, 1983.
35. Kovacs JA, Ng VL, Masur H, et al: Diagnosis of *Pneumocystis carinii* pneumonia: Improved detection in sputum with use of monoclonal antibodies. N Engl J Med 318:589, 1988.
36. Bigby TD, Margolskee D, Curtis JL, et al: The usefulness of induced sputum in the diagnosis of *Pneumocystis carinii* pneumonia in patients with the acquired immunodeficiency syndrome. Am Rev Respir Dis 133:515, 1986.
37. Pitchenik AE, Ganjei P, Torres A, et al: Sputum examination for the diagnosis of *Pneumocystis carinii* pneumonia in the acquired immunodeficiency syndrome. Am Rev Respir Dis 133:226, 1986.
38. Gill VJ, Evans G, Stock F, et al: Detection of *Pneumocystis carinii* by fluorescent antibody stain using a combination of three monoclonal antibodies. J Clin Microbiol 25:1837, 1987.

39. Baselski VS, Robison MK, Pifer LW, et al: Rapid detection of *Pneumocystis carinii* in bronchoalveolar lavage samples by using cellufluor staining. J Clin Microbiol 28:393, 1990.

40. Hahn HH, Beaty HN: Transtracheal aspiration in the evaluation of patients with pneumonia. Ann Intern Med 72:183, 1970.

41. Thorpe JE, Baughman RP, Frame PT, et al: Bronchoalveolar lavage for diagnosing acute bacterial pneumonia. J Infect Dis 155:855, 1987.

42. Kahn FW, Jones JM: Diagnosing bacterial respiratory infection by bronchoalveolar lavage. J Infect Dis 155:862, 1987.

43. Magnenat JL, Nicod LP, Auckenthaler R, et al: Mode of presentation and diagnosis of bacterial pneumonia in human immunodeficiency virus-infected patients. Am Rev Respir Dis 144:917, 1991.

44. Fagon JY, Chastre J, Hance AJ, et al: Detection of nosocomial lung infection in ventilated patients. Use of a protected specimen brush and quantitative culture techniques in 147 patients. Am Rev Respir Dis 138:110, 1988.

45. Chastre J, Viau F, Brun P, et al: Prospective evaluation of the protected specimen brush for the diagnosis of pulmonary infections in ventilated patients. Am Rev Respir Dis 130:924, 1984.

46. Bartlett JG, Gorbach SL, Thadepalli H, et al: Bacteriology of empyema. Lancet 1:338, 1974.

47. Light RW, Girard WM, Jenkinson SG, et al: Parapneumonic effusions. Am J Med 69:507, 1980.

48. Roberts GD, Koneman EW, Kim YK: Mycobacteria. *In* Balows A, Hausler WJ Jr, Herrmann KL, et al (eds): Manual of Clinical Microbiology. Washington, DC, American Society for Microbiology, 1991:304.

49. Drake TA, Hindler JA, Berlin OGW, et al: Rapid identification of *Mycobacterium avium* complex in culture using DNA probes. J Clin Microbiol 25:1442, 1987.

50. Gonzalez R, Hanna BA: Evaluation of Gen-Probe DNA hybridization systems for the identification of *Mycobacterium tuberculosis* and *Mycobacterium avium-intracellulare*. Diagn Microbiol Infect Dis 8:69, 1987.

51. Musial CE, Tice LS, Stockman L, et al: Identification of mycobacteria from culture using the Gen-Probe rapid diagnostic system for *Mycobacterium avium* complex and *Mycobacterium tuberculosis* complex. J Clin Microbiol 26:2120, 1988.

52. Jiminez J, Larsson L: Heating cells in acid methanol for 30 minutes without freeze-drying provides adequate yields of fatty acids and alcohols for gas chromatographic characterization of mycobacteria. J Clin Microbiol 24:844, 1986.

53. Tisdall PA, DeYoung DR, Roberts GD, et al: Identification of clinical isolates of mycobacteria with gas-liquid chromatography: A 10-month follow-up study. J Clin Microbiol 16:400, 1982.

54. Rogers FC, Pasculle AW: *Legionella. In* Balows A, Hausler WJ Jr, Herrmann KL, et al (eds): Manual of Clinical Microbiology. Washington, DC, American Society for Microbiology, 1991:442.

55. Kaufman L, Standard PG: Specific and rapid identification of medically important fungi by exoantigen detection. Ann Rev Microbiol 41:209, 1987.

56. Stockman L, Clark KA, Hunt JM, Roberts GD: Evaluation of commercially available acridinium ester-labeled chemiluminescent DNA probes for culture identification of *Blastomyces dermatitidis, Coccidioides immitis, Cryptococcus neoformans,* and *Histoplasma capsulatum.* J Clin Microbiol 31:845, 1993.

57. Sullivan CJ, Jordan MC: Diagnosis of viral pneumonia. Semin Respir Infect 3:148, 1988.

58. Friedman HM, Forrer CB: Diagnosis of viral respiratory infections in the 1980s. Clin Lab Med 2:383, 1982.

59. Austrian R, Gold J: Pneumococcal bacteremia with especial reference to bacteremic pneumococcal pneumonia. Ann Intern Med 60:759, 1964.

60. Shafer RW, Goldberg R, Sierra M, et al: Frequency of *Mycobacterium tuberculosis* bacteremia in patients with tuberculosis in an area endemic for AIDS. Am Rev Respir Dis 140:1611, 1989.

61. Hawkins CC, Gold JWM, Whimbey E, et al: *Mycobacterium avium* complex infections in patients with the acquired immunodeficiency syndrome. Ann Intern Med 105:184, 1986.

62. Yagupsky P, Menegus MA: Cumulative positivity rates of multiple blood cultures for *Mycobacterium avium-intracellulare* and *Cryptococcus neoformans* in patients with the acquired immunodeficiency syndrome. Arch Pathol Lab Med 114:923, 1990.

63. Telenti A, Roberts GD: Fungal blood cultures. Eur J Clin Microbiol Infect Dis 8:825, 1989.

64. Cherry WB, Pittman B, Harris PP, et al: Detection of legionnaires disease bacteria by direct immunofluorescent staining. J Clin Microbiol 8:329, 1978.

65. Campbell JF, Spika JS: The serodiagnosis of nonpneumococcal bacterial pneumonia. Semin Respir Infect 3:123, 1976.

66. Edelstein PH, Meyer RD, Finegold SM: Laboratory diagnosis of legionnaires disease. Am Rev Respir Dis 121:317, 1980.

67. Wilkinson HW, Cruce DR, Broome CV: Validation of *Legionella pneumophilia* indirect immunofluorescent assay with epidemic sera. J Clin Microbiol 13:139, 1981.

68. Wilkinson HW, Reingold AL, Brake BJ, et al: Reactivity of serum from patients with suspected legionellosis against 29 antigens of Legionellaceae and *Legionella*-like organisms by indirect immunofluorescence assay. J Infect Dis 147:23, 1983.

69. Beaty HN, Miller AA, Broome CV, et al: Legionnaire's disease in Vermont, May to October 1977. JAMA 240:127, 1978.

70. Chamberlain P, Saeed AA: A study of the specific IgM antibody response in *Mycoplasma pneumoniae* infection in man. J Hyg 90:207, 1983.

71. Sarosi GA, Armstrong D, Davies, SF: Laboratory diagnosis of mycotic and specific fungal infections. Am Rev Respir Dis 132:1373, 1985.

72. George RB, Lambert RS, Bruce MJ, et al: Radioimmunoassay: A sensitive test for histoplasmosis and blastomycosis. Am Rev Respir Dis 124:407, 1981.

73. Wheat LJ, Kohler RB, Tewari RP: Diagnosis of disseminated histoplasmosis by detection of *Histoplasma capsulatum* antigen in serum and urine specimens. N Engl J Med 314:83, 1986.

74. Williams JE, Murphy R, Standard PG, et al: Serologic response in blastomycosis: Diagnosis value of double immunodiffusion assay. Am Rev Respir Dis 128:209, 1981.

75. Tinghitella TJ, Edberg SC: Agglutination tests and limulus assay for the diagnosis of infectious disease. *In* Balows A, Hausler WJ Jr, Hermann KL, et al (eds): Manual of Clinical Microbiology. Washington, DC, American Society for Microbiology, 1991:61.

76. Eisenach KD, Sifford MD, Cave MD, et al: Detection of *Mycobacterium tuberculosis* in sputum samples using a polymerase chain reaction. Am Rev Respir Dis 144:1160, 1991.

77. Brisson-Noel A, Gicquel B, Lecossier D, et al: Rapid diagnosis of tuberculosis by amplification of mycobacterial DNA in clinical samples. Lancet 2:1069, 1989.

78. Kolk AHJ, Schuitema ARJ, Juijper S, et al: Detection of *Mycobacterium tuberculosis* in clinical samples by using polymerase chain reaction and a nonradioactive detection system. J Clin Microbiol 30:2567, 1992.

79. Jonas V, Alden MJ, Curry JT, et al: Detection and identification of *Mycobacterium tuberculosis* directly from sputum sediments by amplification of rRNA. J Clin Microbiol 31:2410, 1993.

80. Wilson SM, McNerney R, Nye PM, et al: Progress toward a simplified polymerase chain reaction and its application to diagnosis of tuberculosis. J Clin Microbiol 31:776, 1993.

# Invasive Techniques for the Diagnosis of Lower Respiratory Tract Infections

ROBERT M. MIDDLETON, MICHAEL B. KIRKPATRICK,
and JOHN B. BASS, JR.

Whether it is community-acquired, nosocomial, or ventilator-associated, bacterial pneumonia usually is caused by the aspiration of oropharyngeal contents. The organisms that cause bacterial pneumonia are bacteria that first adhere to and colonize the oropharynx of the host. The spectrum of microbial pathogens is determined by the complex interaction between host defenses and the microenvironment. Variations in the clinical presentation warrant bacteriologic confirmation to direct antimicrobial therapy, particularly in the hospital setting or for immunocompromised hosts. A specific bacteriologic diagnosis can assist decision making, diminish the morbidity associated with broad-spectrum antimicrobial therapy, and improve the chance of survival.

Recovery of bacteria from blood or pleural fluid can establish the bacteriologic cause of the pneumonia, but positive cultures provide confirmation for only 15% to 25% of patients in most series.[1] Sputum is readily available from most patients. Some organisms found in sputum are always considered pathogenic (eg, *Mycobacterium tuberculosis*, *Mycoplasma pneumoniae*, some fungi, most viruses). However, most bacteria recovered from sputum can be pathogenic or oropharyngeal colonizers, and differentiation may be difficult in the clinical setting. In the classic 1971 Barrett-Connor report of 51 cases of bacteremic pneumococcal pneumonia, only 45% had recovery of the organism by sputum culture, and after isolation, the agent was not found on pure cultures for most patients.[2] Similar data are found for sputum cultures for bacteremic nosocomial pneumonia.[3] A negative endotracheal tube culture is highly predictive of the absence of lower airway infection in a patient not yet on antimicrobial therapy, but a positive culture remains difficult to interpret because of the presence of multiple colonizing species.[4, 5]

Because of the lack of sensitivity of cultures from "protected sites" and the potential contamination of sputum and endotracheal aspirates by colonizing organisms, a variety of methods have been proposed to access the lower airway and sample bacteria. This chapter reviews the techniques and their potential risks and benefits in the diagnosis of lower respiratory tract infection.

## OPEN LUNG BIOPSY

Although open lung biopsy (OLB) is considered the technique with the "highest likelihood of providing adequate tissue to achieve a specific microbiologic or histologic diagnosis," it is usually reserved for diagnosing immunocompromised patients rather than for the diagnosis of bacterial pneumonia.[6] The surgical technique remains largely unchanged from the 1949 description by Klasson and associates; however, the formal posterolateral thoracotomy approach occasionally is replaced by a modified small anterior thoracotomy incision.[7] In either case, general anesthesia is required, and a postoperative chest thoracostomy tube is usually placed. Complication rates are low, a mortality rate of 0.5% is quoted, and procedure-related complications include pneumothorax requiring thoracostomy tube drainage, bleeding, and problems related to anesthesia or the surgical technique.[7, 8]

Immediate specimen processing for bacterial culture (including anaerobes) and opportunistic pathogens is mandatory. A variety of rapid smears are available. The specimens should be divided so that appropriate preparation for histologic evaluation is performed. Reports of diagnostic accuracy vary widely.[6, 9–14] Negative results are obtained in the setting of nonspecific inflammatory changes, reminding us that the differential diagnosis of pulmonary infiltrates in the immunocompromised host includes noninfectious processes.

OLB results can be important in guiding patient management. For the most part, practitioners use OLB after less invasive means of diagnosis have been exhausted. The clinician may use OLB to exclude treatable diseases not apparent by other means, but OLB has not been found to significantly improve patient management or the patient's clinical course.[12, 15–18] OLB frequently offers more risk than benefit. Although OLB has been designated in many studies as the ''gold standard'' for the diagnosis of bacterial pneumonia, the physician must consider the fact that the specimen includes gas exchange units with distal airways. It is better to use quantitative culture methods for optimal interpretation of results.

## TRANSTHORACIC NEEDLE ASPIRATION

Direct acquisition of lower respiratory tract specimens through transthoracic needle aspiration (TTNA) was initially described in the late 1800s. It was not until the 1930s that Sappington and Favorite and Bullowa reported that the procedure was a safe and effective method for obtaining these specimens.[19, 20] Although used primarily for the cytologic evaluation of peripheral pulmonary nodules, some studies have focused on the use of TTNA in specific groups, such as pediatric patients,[21] immunocompromised hosts,[22, 23] and mechanically ventilated patients.[24] The technique has been described in many publications.[25, 26] In general, fluoroscopy is used to identify the parenchymal abnormality, although nonfluoroscopic TTNA has been evaluated. Needle selection varies from the ultra-thin 25-gauge needle to the 18- to 22-gauge spinal needle. Sterile technique is mandatory, and the chest should be appropriately cleaned and draped. Preparation of sterile, nonbacteriostatic transport media and slides at the site accelerates specimen processing. Sedation is commonly employed and is thought to decrease the likelihood of cough in this procedure. Oxygen administration is not routine, but it is advisable in patients with borderline arterial oxygenation. Topical 1% lidocaine is used for skin infiltration. Some researchers suggest the use of a small incision to facilitate entry of the aspiration needle into the chest. To prevent the risk of venous air embolism, a locking syringe is placed on the needle hub, and the unit is then passed through the rib interspace, over the rib in a line perpendicular to the chest wall. Readjustment of this position should be achieved by complete withdrawal and repositioning, not by angulation of the needle. After the needle is in position, suction may be applied to the syringe. A small amount of nonbacteriostatic saline may facilitate sample acquisition if none is obtained by dry suction. After the needle is withdrawn, repeated fluoroscopy is used to evaluate the possibility of pneumothorax. Aspirated material is transported immediately for appropriate cultures (eg, aerobic, anaerobic, mycobacterial, fungal) and stains (eg, Gram, acid-fast, methenamine silver, direct fluorescent antibody for *Legionella*). An erect expiratory chest roentgenogram is then obtained.

The major complications include pneumothorax, hemoptysis, venous air embolism, and hemorrhage. Patients with bullous lung disease and those who could not tolerate a pneumothorax, patients with bleeding diathesis, and uncooperative patients should not be subjected to the procedure. Until recently, positive pressure mechanical ventilation was also considered to be a contraindication, but Torres and colleagues reported that 41 mechanically ventilated patients underwent TTNA, with pneumothorax developing in only 7%.[24] Overall, a 20% to 30% risk of pneumothorax can be expected, with chest thoracostomy tube drainage required in approximately half of these cases.[25] Miller and Sahn report that the likelihood of pneumothorax is inversely proportional to $FEV_1$.[26] Hemoptysis, reported in 3% to 10% of cases, is usually transient, with onset immediately after the procedure, but cases of fatal hemorrhage have been described.[27] Pulmonary hemorrhage is usually of no clinical importance, appearing only as a transient chest roentgenogram abnormality. Air embolism is rare and is prevented by using a locking syringe-needle unit.

Diagnostic yield ranges from approximately 40% to 90%, depending on the series.[28–34] As in all bacteriologic techniques, prior administration of antimicrobial therapy significantly affects interpretation of the results. It appears that diagnostic yield for bacterial infection is represented by the lower end of the range described, and diagnostic yield for nonbacterial infection is represented by the upper end of the range. The reasons may include a lower sampling error in the setting of diffuse parenchymal disease or nodular and cavitary lesions and operator and processing factors. Moser and colleagues, in an animal model of pneumococcal pneumonia, reported that TTNA provided the highest sensitivity and specificity compared with other invasive techniques. TTNA was consistently associated with a 20% to 30% pneumothorax risk, and TTNA was the major cause of pneumothorax in their study.[28] The risk of pneumothorax continues to limit the usefulness of this technique in clinical practice despite its ease of performance and potential for diagnostic accuracy.

## TRANSTRACHEAL ASPIRATION

Observations that cultures of expectorated sputum did not reliably represent lower respiratory tract infections because of oropharyngeal contamination led to the description by Pecora and Brook, in 1959, of transtracheal aspiration (TTA).[35]

The technique is a modification of that used for transtracheal anesthesia. Although unnecessary in the obtunded patient, sedation is recommended in the awake patient. Atropine administration is also advised to prevent a vagal reaction. The patient is placed in the supine position with a pillow beneath the shoulders. The neck is extended, and the skin cleaned with antiseptic solution; a sterile drape is widely applied. Topical anesthesia is provided by a small cutaneous wheal of 1% lidocaine over the membranous trachea at the level of the cricoid cartilage in the midline. After the anatomy has been defined and topical anesthesia achieved, a 14-gauge needle is passed a few millimeters into the trachea and angled caudally. A small length of polyvinyl chloride tubing is placed through the needle to facilitate removal of the needle. Although the patient may be asked to suppress cough at this time, the urge to cough is usually overwhelming.

An aliquot of 3 mL of nonbacteriostatic saline is instilled from a syringe, locked to the tubing, into the trachea. Suction is applied as the patient coughs freely, and the specimen is collected in the syringe. After adequate specimen is obtained (ie, a few drops), the syringe and tubing are removed from the trachea. Light pressure with sterile gauze is applied to the puncture site, and a chest roentgenogram is obtained. Some physicians suggest that the initial secretions expectorated directly after the procedure is performed should also be collected, but this is not useful for bacteriologic evaluation. Periodic clinical evaluation of the patient for several hours after the procedure is advised.

The specimen is immediately delivered to the microbiology laboratory for processing. Semiquantitative or quantitative aerobic and anaerobic bacterial cultures and cultures for fungus, mycobacteria, and *Legionella* may be obtained. Acid-fast smears, fungal smears, and smears for opportunistic pathogens should be reviewed.

The potential complications related to TTA are many, but they are limited by appropriate patient selection.[36, 37] Bleeding and infection at the puncture site, onset or worsening of hypoxemia, subcutaneous emphysema, and vasovagal reaction may occur.[36, 37] Death, fortunately rare, has been reported. TTA is a potentially noxious procedure, occasionally requiring abortion before completion. In one evaluation, TTNA was preferred over TTA if another study was necessary.[30] This leads to the common belief that if a patient cannot give consent for this procedure, an alternative procedure should be performed. Absolute contraindications include bleeding diathesis, severe hypoxemia uncorrected with supplemental oxygen, and inability to cooperate during the procedure.

The diagnostic accuracy of TTA for nonbacterial pathogens is good. Recovery of organisms that are not part of the respiratory flora and are therefore pathogens (eg, mycobacteria, *Nocardia, Pneumocystis, Legionella*) has been reported.[25, 38]

The diagnosis of bacterial lower respiratory tract infection is based on two assumptions. First, it is assumed that the airways below the vocal cords are normally sterile and that bacteria recovered from this source represent lower respiratory tract pathogens rather than contaminants. Second, it is assumed that organisms recovered in central airways represent organisms that are causing infection in the gas exchange units.

The first assumption deals with the potential for false-positive results. Several studies have revealed that the airways below the vocal cords may be colonized with bacteria in a variety of settings.[36, 39–44] Patients with cultures positive for *Legionella* and patients recently treated for pneumococcal pneumonia have been found to have bacterial growth in TTA specimens. This suggests the potential for concurrent nonbacterial respiratory infection or recent bacterial illness to result in lower airway colonization. Patients with respiratory disease such as chronic bronchitis, bronchiectasis, or exacerbation of asthma or those who are at risk for aspiration of oropharyngeal secretions have been found to have bacterial growth by TTA even if acute lower respiratory tract infection was not suspected. Patients with bronchogenic carcinoma were found to have bacterial growth by TTA. Healthy volunteers were not observed to have bacterial growth by TTA.[45]

Because of the potential for contamination, even below the vocal cords, quantitative or semiquantitative bacteriology must be relied on. Using the quantitative growth cutoff of $10^5$ CFU/mL and semiquantitative growth of $3+$ as "significant," most subjects in the previously described clinical scenarios had growths of "insignificant" amounts. Patients with chronic respiratory disease, however, were likely to be colonized by potential pathogens in quantities of $10^4$ to $10^5$ CFU/mL or more. Although the assumption that the airways below the vocal cords are sterile is not correct in all cases, a quantitative growth cutoff point can be used to separate contaminants from pathogens in most cases.

The second assumption deals with the potential for false-negative culture results. Pecora reported animal data in which a small aliquot of *Serratia* suspension and direct sky blue dye was injected peripherally in the lungs of dogs and TTA was performed approximately 30 minutes afterward. The results of this experiment indicated that even a small number of organisms injected peripherally were detected proximally if bronchial communication existed.[46] In data comparing TTNA to TTA reported by Davidson and associates, agreement was found in 17 of 25 specimens; if sterile TTNA specimens were eliminated, agreement was observed in 17 of 20 specimens.[30] This suggests that false-negative TTA results are possible but uncommon. Although in the cited study no concurrent antimicrobial therapy was given, such therapy would have significantly affected results, increasing the false-negative rate.

The largest study of overall diagnostic accuracy of TTA for aerobic bacterial lower airway infection was published by Bartlett in 1977.[47] Of 488 patients who underwent TTA, 383 satisfied the clinical criteria for pneumonia, and 23 were bacteremic. Potential pathogens were isolated from 235, leaving 48 negative TTA specimens; of those, 44 had received antimicrobial therapy. In the 23 bacteremic patients, TTA culture was concordant in 100%.

For selected patients who are not receiving concurrent antimicrobial agents and in whom bacterial or nonbacterial lower respiratory tract infection is likely, TTA offers a potentially useful means of achieving an accurate bacteriologic diagnosis. TTA is noxious and potentially dangerous if not performed by experienced personnel. Strict criteria for patient selection should be adhered to. Quantitative bacteriology is advised because of the possibility of colonization by potential pathogens in the lower airways of most of the patients in whom this technique is considered useful.

## BRONCHOSCOPIC METHODS

The introduction of the flexible bronchoscope in the late 1960s enabled access to the lower airway with direct visualization. Flexible bronchoscopy is safe and effective for the diagnosis and management of many pulmonary diseases.[48] The technique, unlike that for TTA and TTNA, was readily used in mechanically ventilated patients without adverse consequences. A natural extension of the usefulness of bronchoscopy was the acquisition of lower airway secretions to confirm presumed infection.

Initial efforts to use the bronchoscope for the diagnosis of bacterial pneumonia included washing lobar and segmental airways with nonbacteriostatic saline and then suctioning the secretions into a collecting trap for processing. Significant contamination from oropharyngeal flora occurred with this method.[41, 43] Jordan and colleagues observed that quantitative bacterial growth from bronchial wash specimens in normal patients (ie, those not suspected of having lower respiratory tract infection) and in patients with chronic bronchitis was significant.[49] Bacterial growth up to $10^{4.5}$ CFU/mL in the former subject group and up to $10^{5.5}$ CFU/mL in the latter group was observed. Recovery of organisms by simple wash and suction was not useful in differentiating contamination from lower airway bacterial infection.

The potential causes of contamination are thought to include aspiration related to laryngeal anesthesia or induced by the passage of the bronchoscope through the larynx, contamination of the bronchoscope suction channel during passage through the nasopharynx and upper airway, and mobilization of the oropharyngeal flora to the lower airway by passage of the bronchoscope or by application of lidocaine for local anesthesia. For useful information to be gained through bronchoscopic technique, these potential sources of contamination had to be eliminated. Suction could not be applied while the airway was traversed, and topical anesthesia could not be applied through the bronchoscope. Quantitative culture methods were necessary to differentiate contaminating from potentially infecting organisms.

Neil Wimberley, while working with L. J. Faling and John Bartlett, described an instrument and technique for obtaining uncontaminated specimens from the lower airway.[50] The bronchoscopic protected specimen brush (BPSB; Microvasive/Microbiology Specimen Brush #1650, Microvasive, Melford, MA) is composed of an inner wire terminating in a 10-mm brush made of nylon bristles arranged in eight spiraling rows. The wire brush apparatus is housed in a telescoping dual-catheter system occluded by a small polyethylene glycol plug. In vitro data for aerobic and anaerobic organisms and gravimetric analysis have shown that the specimen brush accumulates a sample volume of approximately 0.01 to 0.001 mL.[50, 51]

The technique used is outlined in Table 42–1. Because the potential for cough is great, we emphasize adequate topical anesthesia. We use a regimen of 1% phenylephrine plus 10 mL of 2% lidocaine jelly in combination with inhaled lidocaine 4% to maximize patient comfort.[52] The protected brush system is passed through the suction channel into the area corresponding to the roentgenographic abnormality under direct visualization. The inner cannula is then advanced and the brush extended. After secretions are collected, the brush is retracted into the cannula and the system is removed from the bronchoscope. At this time, topical anesthesia through the bronchoscope may be used and additional specimens obtained as desired. Meticulous processing of the brush specimen is essential, and sterile technique should be used to prevent contamination by skin

**Table 42–1. Technique of Protected Specimen Brush Bronchoscopy**

1. Routine preoperative medication.
2. Preprocedure inhalation of nebulized 4% preservative-free lidocaine and 0.3 mL of metaproterenol.
3. The nostril chosen for bronchoscope passage is anesthetized topically and lubricated with 10 mL of 2% lidocaine jelly/viscous.
4. The bronchoscope is advanced into the lower airways.*
5. The protected specimen brush system may be inserted before passage of the bronchoscope or after the trachea has been entered.†
6. When lower airway purulence or the bronchial orifice corresponding to the abnormal segment on chest roentgenogram is visualized, the protected brush inner cannula is advanced, and the polyethylene glycol plug is jettisoned.

*It is imperative that suction not be applied through the bronchoscope channel and that the injection of anesthetic through the channel be avoided. This helps prevent contamination of the bronchoscope and lower airways with oropharyngeal bacterial flora.

†We prefer to place the PSB system in the bronchoscopic channel before passage into the nostril, because the cough reflex in the lower airways remains very active without topical anesthesia, and prior positioning decreases the time needed to obtain a specimen.

Data from Broughton WA, Bass JB, Kirkpatrick MB: The technique of protected brush catheter bronchoscopy. J Crit Illness 2:63–70, 1987.

or environmental flora.[53] The brush is advanced, and secretions are placed on a sterile microscope slide for Gram staining. The brush is then transected into 1 mL Ringer's lactate solution. After vortexing, the solution is serially diluted (100-fold) for aerobic and anaerobic quantitative culture. The final culture plates represent $10^{-1}$, $10^{-3}$, and $10^{-5}$ dilutions of the brush specimen contained in 1 mL of Ringer's lactate. Given the dilution factor inherent to the brush, it is thought that growth on the 1:1000 dilution plate represents $10^5$ to $10^6$ CFU/mL from the original specimen. This correlates with the quantity of organisms in patients with pneumonia (ie, $10^6$–$10^8$ CFU/mL).[54]

The first report of the clinical use of this technique accompanied the in vitro testing.[50] Eight healthy volunteers and 6 patients with clinical evidence of pneumonia underwent bronchoscopy with BPSB. Of the 8 volunteers, 7 showed no growth, and 1 subject had growth of *Haemophilus influenzae* ($10^{2.4}$ CFU/mL). Of the subjects thought to have pneumonia clinically, all demonstrated growth of potential pathogens in ($\geq 10^3$ CFU/mL). Two of the patients were bacteremic, and in both instances, the blood culture and BPSB specimen ($\geq 10^3$ CFU/mL) yielded the same organism. Two patients with lung abscess demonstrated anaerobic isolates in significant ($\geq 10^3$ CFU/mL) quantity.

Additional studies in the setting of community-acquired pneumonia confirmed the validity and clinical utility of this technique. In 1982, Wimberley and associates described 41 patients with evidence of pneumonia.[55] Ten of these patients were bacteremic. The BPSB specimen demonstrated significant growth of an organism identical to the blood culture isolate in all cases. Twelve patients with nonbacterial illness diagnosed by alternate means demonstrated no significant bacterial growth by BPSB. Of the remaining 24 patients, 19 demonstrated at least one organism in significant quantity. All patients responded to treatment directed at the BPSB isolate. In 7 patients who were receiving antimicrobial therapy, no significant growth was observed. In these 41 patients, no complications related to bronchoscopy or the BPSB procedure were observed.

Bass and colleagues described a series of 78 patients who

were believed to have community-acquired pneumonia.[56] Results supported previous data and included the fact that Gram staining of BPSB material was a good predictor of subsequent significant growth ($\geq 10^3$ CFU/mL) with 78% sensitivity, providing a valuable guide to early antimicrobial therapy.

Many clinical studies have used BPSB to diagnose community-acquired pneumonia.[57–60] All suffer from a lack of standardization for the diagnosis of pneumonia in nonbacteremic patients, and all support the need for strict adherence to protocol for optimal results. Results from BPSB cultures have been disappointing for patients who were receiving antimicrobial therapy, although some results in this setting have been helpful clinically.[61] For patients receiving antimicrobial therapy, no definitive information suggests what length of time is necessary after discontinuation of antibiotics to ensure helpful BPSB culture results.

Flexible bronchoscopy with BPSB cultures may be used in mechanically ventilated patients with little risk. An 8-Fr (2.6-mm) or larger endotracheal tube is required for bronchoscope passage, and the patient is placed on 100% $FIO_2$ during the procedure. No further modification of the BPSB protocol is required in the mechanically ventilated patient. Complications attributable to the BPSB procedure are limited to transient reversible hypoxemia and, rarely, pneumothorax.

Studies of the diagnostic accuracy of BPSB in the setting of ventilator-associated pneumonia (VAP) are complicated by the lack of a unified standard of diagnosis. The studies may use clinical parameters or response to therapy as an end point, leaving the microbiologic data open to question. Studies using a histologic standard for the diagnosis of VAP are few. Higuchi and coworkers, using a baboon model of adult respiratory distress syndrome, compared BPSB, TTA, blood culture, and TTNA.[62] A sensitivity of 70% was observed, and 100% concordance was found between the BPSB, TTNA, and blood culture. The researchers suggested that the low sensitivity could be related to sampling error in the setting of diffuse infiltrates, a finding subsequently observed by Baughman and associates in their report of BPSB culture results from roentgenographically involved and noninvolved areas.[63]

Chastre and colleagues compared BPSB culture directly with open lung biopsy (histology and quantitative tissue culture) in 26 mechanically ventilated, recently deceased patients.[64] Samples were obtained immediately after the patient's death as mechanical ventilation was continued. Findings showed that the BPSB quantitative growth of $10^3$ CFU/mL or greater had a sensitivity of 100% and specificity of 60% when compared with histologic evidence of pneumonia or tissue growth of $10^4$ CFU/g or greater. The BPSB culture had a positive predictive value of 70% and a negative predictive value of 100%. The concurrent administration of antimicrobial therapy significantly affected results of the BPSB culture. In contrast to Chastre's work, in which no false-negative cultures were observed, deCastro and colleagues published data in patients in whom pneumonia was confirmed by blood culture, pleural fluid culture, or autopsy.[65] Eight patients in the cohort were found to have false-negative results.

Many clinical studies of the use of BPSB in defining the cause of VAP have been reported.[66–71] The consensus among investigators is that BPSB is a sensitive and relatively noninvasive method for delineating the microbiology of VAP in the absence of prior antibiotic therapy. The BPSB Gram stain provides useful preliminary results for rational antimicrobial therapy pending culture results. Given the data available, it may be that most mechanically ventilated patients suspected of having VAP have an alternate cause of their clinical syndrome.[72]

## Use of the Protected Specimen Brush in Special Circumstances

Acute chest syndrome is defined as an acute febrile episode associated with dyspnea, cough, chest pain, and a new pulmonary infiltrate in adults who have sickle cell hemoglobinopathy. The differential diagnosis includes lower respiratory tract infection and in situ pulmonary thrombosis, which cannot be differentiated on clinical grounds alone. Kirkpatrick and coworkers reported the use of the BPSB in 19 patients who had acute chest syndrome.[73] In this study, only 21% of patients had significant bacterial growth suggesting lower respiratory tract infection. Clinicians could therefore focus on supportive therapy, possibly using exchange transfusion, but withhold unnecessary antimicrobial therapy.

Pang and colleagues, from Hong Kong, described a series of 23 patients with bronchiectasis.[74] BPSB and bronchoalveolar lavage (BAL) were performed. Most patients had significant bacterial isolates, some of which were resistant to the routine antimicrobial therapy given for typical pathogens. We have performed BPSB in 8 patients with bronchiectasis.[75] All patients had significant bacterial isolates, and all demonstrated clinical improvement after therapy was directed at the isolate. Only 1 patient had concurrent growth of the pathogen from sputum.

Few studies have focused on the use of BPSB in the immunocompromised host. However, patients with acquired immunodeficiency syndrome or other immunocompromising conditions are at increased risk of acquiring bacterial lower airway infection, and often these manifest roentgenographically as atypical presentations. Xaubet and associates reported combined use of BAL and BPSB in this setting and found that a specific diagnosis was achieved for 20% more patients than with BAL alone.[76] However, the false-positive rate approached 40%. The researchers thought that the potential benefits supporting the use of a combined approach included direction of specific antimicrobial therapy and cessation of other potentially toxic empiric therapy. The use of BPSB in neutropenic hosts requires more evaluation.[77]

The BPSB is a device that, under bronchoscopic visual guidance, is able to obtain a 0.01-mL to 0.001-mL specimen of airway secretions. If rigid technical standards for specimen acquisition and handling are adhered to, the bacterial growth from this specimen is thought to accurately represent lower airway flora. The bacterial growth that conforms to the clinically accepted guidelines represents the infecting pathogen or pathogens in the gas exchange units. The potential disadvantages include error because of concurrent antimicrobial therapy, small sample size with resultant sampling error in cases of diffuse infiltrates, and the need for reliable clinical microbiologic support.

## Bronchoalveolar Lavage

BAL is of proven benefit for the diagnosis of opportunistic pulmonary pathogens in immunocompromised patients.[78–83] BAL has gained increasing popularity as a research tool for the study of staging, natural history, and response to therapy of interstitial inflammatory diseases such as interstitial pulmonary fibrosis, sarcoidosis, and hypersensitivity pneumonitis.[82, 84–86] In these circumstances, bacterial contamination of the specimen is not of vital concern, but for the diagnosis of lower respiratory tract infection, BAL is subject to the same potential for contamination by oropharyngeal flora as described for bronchial wash specimens.

Unlike the widely used and accepted protocol for obtaining and processing BPSB specimens, there is no consensus for standardization of the BAL technique. A general description of our technique is provided in Table 42–2. Lavage fluid return from normal airways ranges from 50% to 60% of the instilled volume, but this volume is observed to drop significantly (10% to 40%) if parenchymal disease exists or the patient is ventilated mechanically. Lidocaine recovered in lavage fluid is well below the concentration associated with antimicrobial activity.[87, 88] Complications related directly to BAL are few and usually minor; they include postbronchoscopy fever, transient reversible fall in $PaO_2$, transient chest roentgenogram abnormality, and rare major complications such as exacerbation of respiratory failure, pneumothorax, and hemoptysis.[85–87] The method of specimen processing has been described in several studies, but there is wide variation in technique.[66, 83, 87, 89, 90] All agree that some portions of lavage fluid should be used for the cytologic evaluation of opportunistic pathogens, acid-fast staining and culture, fungal smear and culture, staining for *Legionella* with direct fluorescence antibody, and viral culture. However, the methodology has not been standardized for bacterial cultures. Because of the likelihood of specimen contamination, quantitative bacterial culture techniques are necessary for accurate interpretation of results. Kirkpatrick and Bass reported quantitative BAL cultures for 8 normal subjects with no evidence of lung disease.[89] Bacteria were

### Table 42–2. Technique of Bronchoscopic Bronchoalveolar Lavage for Bacteriologic Diagnosis of Pneumonia

1. After inhaling nebulized lidocaine (10 mL of preservative-free 4% lidocaine), the patient sniffs 10 mL of 2% lidocaine jelly/viscous to anesthetize the nostril to be traversed by the bronchoscope.*
2. If needed for airway anesthesia, preservative-free 1% lidocaine can be injected through the bronchoscope suction channel. Nothing is aspirated through this channel before the bronchoalveolar lavage (BAL) procedure.
3. The bronchoscope tip is gently wedged into the subsegmental bronchus leading to the area of roentgenographic abnormality.
4. Room-temperature normal saline (60 mL) is hand injected and then gently hand aspirated with a syringe. One or two additional 60-mL aliquots may be injected if needed to increase lavage fluid recovery.†
5. The bronchoscope is then withdrawn, and the specimen is divided for cytologic analysis, acid-fast smears and cultures, fungal smears and cultures, and quantitative aerobic and anaerobic bacterial cultures.

*Topical anesthesia may not be needed in intubated mechanically ventilated patients who are sedated.

†Although we recover approximately 20% to 30% of the injected volume in nonintubated patients, the BAL volume retrieved from intubated, mechanically ventilated patients usually is less.

recovered from 7 of the 8 persons, but in all cases, growth was less than $10^4$ CFU/mL. Growth was attributed to oropharyngeal contamination, because cultures from bronchoscopes cleaned by a strict decontamination protocol were sterile.

Kahn and Jones reported quantitative BAL cultures from 57 nonintubated patients who had clinically defined pneumonia and from 18 noninfected control subjects.[90] Among the 18 control patients, the quantitative growth results varied widely. After specimens were analyzed according to the proportion of squamous epithelial cells (SEC) identified on Giemsa-stained cytocentrifuged smears of BAL fluid, two groups emerged. Lavage fluids containing less than 1% SEC had no isolates recovered in quantities equal to or greater than $10^5$ CFU/mL; however, for specimens with greater than 1% SEC, indicative of contamination by oropharyngeal flora, growth was likely to be observed in quantities greater than $10^5$ CFU/mL. Of the 57 patients thought to have a lower airway infection, 18 were thought to have a bacterial illness (ie, 13 pneumonia and 5 bronchitis). All had growth equal to or greater than $10^5$ CFU/mL with 1% SEC or less. Seven patients had positive blood cultures, and in all 7, the identical pathogen was isolated in quantities of $10^5$ CFU/mL or greater. Differential cell count of BAL fluid offered no distinguishing characteristic in this group. These data provide support for a clinically useful cutoff point for differentiation of oropharyngeal contamination from lower airway infection if the clinical specimen is examined in this manner. However, the usefulness of SEC as markers of oropharyngeal contamination has been questioned by Irwin and colleagues, who noticed the difficulty of differentiating buccal SEC from squamous metaplasia of airway mucosal cells by light microscopy alone.[91]

Thorpe and coworkers used a semiquantitative culture method in evaluating 92 patients, 15 of whom were thought to have bacterial pneumonia and were not on antimicrobial therapy.[83] For these 15, the BAL cultures yielded bacterial growth of $10^4$ CFU/mL or greater, and 94% had growth of $10^5$ CFU/mL or greater. Gram staining was performed on ctyocentrifuged BAL fluid and was predictive of subsequent growth in 11 (73%) of 15 with no false-positive results. The differential cell count of BAL fluid revealed a predominance of polymorphonuclear leukocytes in groups with active or resolving bacterial infection, offering no distinction between the two groups.

Henriquez and colleagues reported the use of BAL in patients with anaerobic lung abscess and compared BAL to TTA in 4 patients.[92] Anaerobic growth was observed in low concentration in 1 of 26 control subjects. In patients with lung abscesses, a mixture of aerobic and anaerobic isolates was observed. Sixteen anaerobic isolates were recovered by TTA, and 12 of these were also recovered by BAL. A ''high correlation'' between Gram stains of BAL fluid and subsequent culture results was observed by the researchers.

Several studies have reported quantitative bacteriology of BAL for mechanically ventilated patients and have compared BAL with BPSB. Johanson and colleagues used an animal model to provide a histologic definition for pneumonia.[93] Lobes with histologically more severe pneumonia were associated with higher bacterial growth concentration, and most were polymicrobial. A bacterial index (ie, sum of log growth concentration of each species) of BAL specimens was closely related to the bacterial index of lung tissue culture and to the histologic severity of pneumonia. This association was maintained whether the specimen was obtained from the same lobe or from a lobe different from that studied histologically. BAL recovered 74% of all pathogenic species isolated by culture of lung tissue, compared with 41% recovered by BPSB.

Chastre and associates reported the use of BAL in patients with VAP defined clinically and histologically, and achieved different results.[66] Five patients with confirmed bacterial pneumonia had eight organisms isolated in quantities equal to or greater than $10^3$ CFU/mL by BPSB. Among these, only four were observed in quantities of $10^5$ CFU/mL or greater by BAL (five in $\geqslant 10^4$ CFU/mL). All 5 patients with confirmed bacterial pneumonia had intracellular organisms in at least 25% of the polymorphonuclear leukocytes observed on Gram stain of cytocentrifuged BAL fluid. The organisms were morphologically similar to those grown in high concentration on BPSB for eight of the nine organisms, but they were grown in quantities equal to or greater than $10^4$ CFU/mL from BAL in only six of the nine, suggesting the potential for a complementary role between BAL and BPSB. The differential cell counts of BAL fluid offered no additional useful information. The proposed usefulness of BAL fluid analysis for intracellular organisms was confirmed by Chastre and coworkers. In a report of 61 patients, intracellular organisms were found in at least 7% of examined alveolar cells in 12 of 15 patients with pneumonia but in only 2 of 47 patients without pneumonia.[94]

Guerra and colleagues reported their experience with BAL semiquantitative cultures in mechanically ventilated patients.[95] These patients were divided into two groups without knowledge of their BAL culture results. Group 1 consisted of patients with clinically defined lower respiratory tract infection; group 2 consisted of patients proven by autopsy or clinical criteria not to have lower respiratory tract infection. Of the latter group (24 patients), none demonstrated bacterial growth of $10^4$ CFU/mL or greater. Most patients in this study had received antimicrobial therapy before the sample acquisition.

Torres and coworkers compared the effectiveness of BAL and BPSB in 34 mechanically ventilated patients who were suspected of having bacterial pneumonia.[96] All patients had received recent antimicrobial therapy. The diagnostic values of BAL and BPSB were observed to be similar, with culture agreement in approximately 89% of cases, and the results of Gram staining always agreed if significant ($\geqslant 10^3$ CFU/mL) culture results were observed. Organisms found in blood culture were always found in BAL and BPSB specimens.

Meduri and colleagues described the effectiveness of a new BAL technique—protected BAL (PBAL).[97] The technique incorporates a transbronchoscopic balloon-tipped catheter, used to avoid exposing the instilled and aspirated BAL solution to contaminants present in the suction channel of the bronchoscope. The aspiration and suction channel of the apparatus is protected by a thin polyethylene diaphragm that is easily expelled by flushing 2 mL of sterile saline through the channel. A large-channel bronchoscope is required for the procedure, which may limit its usefulness in some setting. Of 13 patients with a diagnosis of pneumonia defined by histology, blood culture, or clinical response to narrow-spectrum antimicrobial therapy, the PBAL culture yielded significant growth in 12. Using a cutoff of $10^4$ CFU/mL to diagnose pneumonia, PBAL culture had a 92% sensitivity and a 97% specificity. Prior antimicrobial therapy appeared to have less adverse effect on PBAL results than on BPSB culture results. Gram stain of cytospin PBAL specimen was positive with morphologically similar organisms in 92% of cases. Intracellular organisms were observed in 8 patients.

BAL offers a safe and effective means for the diagnosis of pulmonary infections. Quantitative bacterial cultures of BAL fluid have the potential to separate contaminant from pathogen and may prove useful in the diagnosis of lower respiratory tract bacterial infection. Cytocentrifuged Giemsa smears may offer a means by which the degree of oropharyngeal contamination may be assessed (%SEC). The Gram stain and cytocentrifuged preparation for the observation of intracellular organisms are rapidly available, are complementary, may suggest subsequent growth, and may guide the initial decisions about antimicrobial therapy. Differential cell counts offer limited useful information about lower respiratory tract infections. The new PBAL technique may offer a valuable alternate diagnostic method for lower respiratory tract infections in intubated and nonintubated patients. Direct comparisons with BPSB are necessary to determine its clinical utility.

## ACKNOWLEDGMENTS

The opinions in this manuscript are those of the authors and do not necessarily represent the opinions of the United States Air Force.

## REFERENCES

1. Austrian R, Gold J: Pneumococcal bacteremia with especial reference to bacteremic pneumococcal pneumonia. Ann Intern Med 60:759–777, 1964.
2. Barrett-Conner E: The non-value of sputum cultures in the diagnosis of pneumococcal pneumonia. Am Rev Respir Dis 103:845–848, 1971.
3. Bryan CS, Reynolds KL: Bacteremic nosocomial pneumonia. Am Rev Respir Dis 129:668–671, 1984.
4. Middleton RM, Kirkpatrick MB: Comparison of four methods to assess airway bacteriology in the intubated mechanically ventilated patient. Am Rev Respir Dis 143:A107, 1991.
5. El-Ebiary M, Torres A, Gonzales J, et al: Diagnosis of ventilator-associated pneumonia: Diagnostic value of quantitative cultures of endotracheal aspirates. Am Rev Respir Dis 143:A108, 1991.
6. Tobin MJ: Diagnosis of pneumonia: Techniques and problems. Clin Chest Med 8:513–527, 1987.
7. Klassen KP, Ahiyan AJ, Curtis GM: Biopsy of diffuse pulmonary lesions. Arch Surg 59:694–704, 1949.
8. Ray JF, Lawton BR, Myers WO: Open pulmonary biopsy: Nineteen year experience with 416 consecutive operations. Chest 69:43–47, 1976.
9. Robin ED, Burke CM: Lung biopsy in immunosuppressed patients. Chest 89:276–278, 1986.
10. McKenna RJ, Mountain CF, McMurtrey MJ: Open lung biopsy in immunocompromised patients. Chest 91:639–640, 1987.
11. Stulbarg MS: Open lung biopsy in the acquired immunodeficiency syndrome (AIDS). Chest 91:639–640, 1987.
12. Suffredini AF, Ognibene FP, Lack EE, et al: Nonspecific interstitial pneumonitis a common cause of pulmonary disease in the acquired immunodeficiency syndrome. Ann Intern Med 107:7–13, 1987.
13. Hiatt JR, Gong M, Mulder DG, et al: The value of open lung biopsy in the immunosuppressed patient. Surgery 92:785–791, 1982.
14. McCabe RE, Brooks RG, Mark JB, et al: Open lung biopsy in patients with acute leukemia. Am J Med 78:609–616, 1985.

15. Rosenow EC, Wilson WR, Cockerelli FR: Pulmonary disease in the immunocompromised host. Mayo Clin Proc 60:473–487, 1985.
16. Wardman AJ, Cook NJ: Pulmonary infiltrates in adult acute leukemia, empirical treatment or lung biopsy. Thorax 39:647–650, 1984.
17. Pennington JE, Feldman NT: Pulmonary infiltrates and fever in patients with hematologic malignancy. Am J Med 62:501–507, 1977.
18. Puksa S, Hutchenson MA, Hyland RM: Usefulness of transbronchial biopsy in immunosuppressed patients with pulmonary infiltrates. Thorax 36:146–150, 1983.
19. Suppington SW, Favorite GO: Lung puncture in lobar pneumonia. Am J Med Sci 191:225–234, 1936.
20. Bullowa JGM: The reliability of sputum typing and its relation to serum therapy. JAMA 105:1512–1513, 1935.
21. Berger R, Aragno L: The value and safety of percutaneous lung aspiration for children with serious pulmonary infections. Pediatr Pulmonol 1:309–313, 1985.
22. Castellino RA, Blank N: Etiologic diagnosis of focal pulmonary infection in immunocompromised patients by fluoroscopically guided percutaneous needle aspiration. Radiology 132:563–567, 1979.
23. Wallace JM, Batra P, Gong H Jr, et al: Percutaneous needle lung aspiration for diagnosing pneumonitis in the patient with AIDS. Am Rev Respir Dis 131:389–392, 1985.
24. Torres A, Jimenez P, de la Bellacasa JP, et al: Diagnostic value of non-fluoroscopic percutaneous lung needle aspiration in patients with pneumonia. Chest 98:839–844, 1990.
25. Bartlett JG: Invasive diagnostic techniques in pulmonary infection in respiratory infections. In Pennington JE (ed): Respiratory Infections Diagnosis and Management, ed 2. New York, Raven Press, 1988:69–96.
26. Miller KS, Sahn SA: The technique of transthoracic needle aspiration. J Crit Illness 3:101–107, 1988.
27. Pearce JG, Putt NL: Fatal pulmonary hemorrhage after percutaneous aspiration lung biopsy. Am Rev Respir Dis 110:346–349, 1974.
28. Moser KM, Maurer J, Jassy L, et al: Sensitivity, specificity and risk and diagnostic procedures in a canine model of *Streptococcus pneumoniae* pneumonia. Am Rev Respir Dis 125:436–442, 1982.
29. Bandt PD, Blank N, Castellino RA: Needle diagnosis of pneumonitis: Value in high risk patients. JAMA 220:1578–1580, 1972.
30. Davidson M, Tempest B, Palmer DL: Bacteriologic diagnosis of acute pneumonia: Comparison of sputum, transtracheal aspirates and lung aspirates. JAMA 235:158–163, 1976.
31. Palmer DL, Davidson M, Lusk R: Needle aspiration of the lung in complex pneumonias. Chest 78:16–21, 1980.
32. Berger R, Arraongo L: Etiologic diagnosis of bacterial nosocomial pneumonia in seriously ill patients. Crit Care Med 13:833–836, 1985.
33. Berger R: Letter to the editor. Chest 100:591–592, 1991.
34. Sagel SS, Ferguson TB, Forrest JV, et al: Percutaneous transthoracic aspiration needle biopsy. Ann Thorac Surg 26:399–405, 1978.
35. Pecora DV, Brook R: A method of securing uncontaminated tracheal sections for bacterial examination. J Thorac Surg 37:653–654, 1959.
36. Kulinske RW, Parker RH, Brandt D, et al: Diagnostic usefulness and safety of transtracheal aspiration. N Engl J Med 276:604–608, 1967.
37. Pratter MR, Irvin RS: Transtracheal aspiration, guidelines for safety. Chest 76:518–520, 1979.
38. Thadepalli M, Rhambhatla K, Miden A: Transtracheal aspiration in the diagnosis of sputum smear-negative tuberculosis. JAMA 238:1037–1040, 1977.
39. Berman SZ, Mathisen DA, Stevenson DD, et al: Transtracheal aspiration studies in asthmatic patients in relapse with "infective" asthma and in subjects without respiratory disease. J Allergy Clin Immunol 56:206–214, 1975.
40. Bjerkestrand G, Digranes A, Schreiner A: Bacteriologic findings in transtracheal aspirates from patients with chronic bronchitis and bronchiectasis: A preliminary report. Scand J Respir Dis 56:201–207, 1975.
41. Fossieck BE, Parker RH, Cohen MN, et al: Fiberoptic bronchoscopy and culture of bacteria from the lower respiratory tree. Chest 73:5–9, 1977.
42. Lober D, Swenson RM: Bacteriology of aspiration pneumonia. Ann Intern Med 81:329–331, 1974.
43. Okinaka AJ, Dineen P: Bacterial colony counts in bronchial washings. Ann Surg 167:47–50, 1968.
44. Benner EJ, Muzinger JP, Chan R: Superinfections of the lung: An evaluation by serial transtracheal aspiration. West J Med 121:173–178, 1974.
45. Hoeprich DD: Etiologic diagnosis of lower respiratory tract infections. Calif Med 112:1–8, 1970.
46. Pecora DV: How well does transtracheal aspiration reflect pulmonary infection? [Letter] Chest 66:220, 1974.
47. Bartlett JG: Diagnostic accuracy of transtracheal aspiration. Bacteriologic studies. Am Rev Respir Dis 115:777–782, 1977.
48. Fulkerson WJ: Fiberoptic bronchoscopy. N Engl J Med 311:511–515, 1984.
49. Jordan GW, Wong GA, Koeprich PD: Bacteriology of the lower respiratory tract as determined by fiberoptic bronchoscopy and transtracheal aspiration. J Infect Dis 134:428–435, 1976.
50. Wimberley N, Faling LJ, Bartlett JG: A fiberoptic bronchoscopy technique to obtain uncontaminated lower airway secretions for bacterial culture. Am Rev Respir Dis 119:337–343, 1979.
51. Middleton RM, Seibert A, Sawyer L, et al: An in vitro comparison of two microbiology specimen brushes. Am Rev Respir Dis 141:277A, 1990.
52. Middleton RM, Shah A, Kirkpatrick MB: Topical nasal anesthesia for flexible bronchoscopy: A comparison of four methods in normal subjects and in patients undergoing transnasal bronchoscopy. Chest 99:1093–1096, 1991.
53. Broughton WA, Bass JB, Kirkpatrick MB: The technique of protected brush catheter bronchoscopy. J Crit Illness 2:63–70, 1987.
54. Bartlett JG, Finegold SM: Bacteriology of expectorated sputum with quantitative culture and wash technique compared to transtracheal aspirates. Am Rev Respir Dis 117:1010–1027, 1978.
55. Wimberley N, Bass JB, Boyd BW, et al: Use of a bronchoscopic protected catheter brush for the diagnosis of pulmonary infections. Chest 81:556–562, 1982.
56. Bass JB, Hawkins EL, Bonner JR, et al: Use of a bronchoscopic protected catheter technique in the clinical evaluation of a new antibiotic. Diagn Microbiol Infect Dis 1:95–106, 1983.
57. Glanville AR, Marlin GE, Hartnett BJS, et al: The use of fiberoptic bronchoscopy with sterile catheter in the diagnosis of pneumonia. Aust N Z J Med 15:309, 1985.
58. Lorch DG Jr, John JF Jr, Tomlinson JR, et al: Protected transbronchial needle aspiration and protected specimen brush in the diagnosis of pneumonia. Am Rev Respir Dis 136:565–569, 1987.
59. Ortqvist AKE, Kalin M, Lejdeborn L, et al: Diagnostic fiberoptic bronchoscopy and protected brush culture in patients with community-acquired pneumonia. Chest 97:576–582, 1990.
60. Pollock HM, Hawkins EL, Bonner JR, et al: Diagnosis of bacterial pulmonary infections with quantitative protected catheter cultures obtained during bronchoscopy. J Clin Microbiol 17:255–259, 1983.
61. Broughton WA, Kirkpatrick MB: Acute necrotizing pneumonia caused by *Enterobacter cloacae*. South Med J 81:1061–1062, 1988.
62. Higuchi JH, Coalson JJ, Johanson WG Jr: Bacteriologic diagnosis of nosocomial pneumonia in primates. Usefulness of the protected specimen brush. Am Rev Respir Dis 125:53–57, 1982.
63. Baughman RP, Thorpe JE, Staneck J, et al: Use of protected specimen brush in patients with endotracheal or tracheostomy tubes. Chest 91:733–736, 1987.
64. Chastre J, Viau F, Brun P, et al: Prospective evaluation of the protected specimen brush for the diagnosis of pulmonary infections in ventilated patients. Am Rev Respir Dis 130:928–929, 1984.
65. DeCastro Fr, Violan JS, Capuz BL, et al: Reliability of the bronchoscopic protected catheter brush in the diagnosis of pneumonia in mechanically ventilated patients. Crit Care Med 19:171, 1991.
66. Chastre J, Fagon JY, Soler P, et al: Diagnosis of nosocomial pneumonia in intubated patients undergoing ventilation: Comparison of the usefulness of bronchoalveolar lavage and the protected specimen brush. Am J Med 85:499, 1988.
67. Fagon JY, Chastre J, Hance AJ, et al: Detection of nosocomial lung infection in ventilated patients. Use of a protected specimen brush and quantitative culture techniques in 147 patients. Am Rev Respir Dis 138:110–116, 1988.
68. Fagon JY, Chastre J, Domart Y, et al: Nosocomial pneumonia in patients receiving continuous mechanical ventilation. Prospective analysis of 52 episodes with use of a protected specimen brush and quantitative culture techniques. Am Rev Respir Dis 139:877–884, 1989.
69. Martos JA, Ferrer M, Torres A, et al: Specificity of quantitative cultures of protected specimen brush and bronchoalveolar lavage in mechanically ventilated patients. Am Rev Respir Dis 141:A276, 1990.
70. Villers D, Derriennic M, Raffi F, et al: Reliability of the bronchoscopic protected catheter brush in intubated and ventilated patients. Chest 88:527, 1985.
71. Meduri GU: Ventilator associated pneumonia in patients with respiratory failure. A diagnostic approach. Chest 97:1208–1219, 1990.

72. Mauldin GL, Meduri GU, Wonderink RG, et al: Causes of fever and pulmonary infiltrates in mechanically ventilated patients. Am Rev Respir Dis 143:109A, 1991.

73. Kirkpatrick MB, Haynes J, Bass JB: Results of bronchoscopically obtained lower airway cultures from adult sickle cell disease patients with the acute chest syndrome. Am J Med 90:206–210, 1991.

74. Pang JA, Cheng A, Chan HS, et al: The bacteriology of bronchiectasis in Hong Kong investigated by protected catheter brush and bronchoalveolar lavage. Am Rev Respir Dis 139:14–17, 1989.

75. Middleton RM, Segarra J, Kirkpatrick MB, et al: Role of bronchoscopy in the diagnosis and management of adult patients with bronchiectasis. Clin Res 39:814A, 1991.

76. Xaubet A, Torres A, Marco F, et al: Pulmonary infiltrates in immunocompromised patients. Diagnostic value of telescoping plugged catheter and bronchoalveolar lavage. Chest 95:130–135, 1989.

77. Brunet F, Armaganidis A, Vaxelarie JF, et al: Evaluation of the Wimberley-Bartlett catheter-brush (WBCB) in the diagnosis of pneumonia in neutropenic patients. Am Rev Respir Dis 141:A278, 1990.

78. Baughman RP, Dohn MN, Loudon RG, et al: Bronchoscopy with bronchoalveolar lavage in tuberculosis and fungal infections. Chest 99:92–97, 1991.

79. Cordonnier C, Bernaudin JF, Fleury J, et al: Diagnostic yield of bronchoalveolar lavage in pneumonitis occurring after allogeneic bone marrow transplantation. Am Rev Respir Dis 132:1118–1123, 1985.

80. Glatt AE, Chirgwin K: *Pneumocystis carinii* pneumonia in human immunodeficiency virus-infected patients. Arch Intern Med 150:271–279, 1990.

81. Luce JM, Clement MJ: Pulmonary diagnostic evaluation in patients suspected of having an HIV-related disease. Semin Respir Infect 4:93–101, 1989.

82. Reynolds HY: Bronchoalveolar lavage. Am Rev Respir Dis 135:250–263, 1987.

83. Thorpe JE, Baughman RP, Frame PT, Wessler TA, Staneck JL: Bronchoalveolar lavage for diagnosing acute bacterial pneumonia. J Infect Dis 155:855–861, 1987.

84. Crystal RG, Reynolds HY, Kalica AR: Bronchoalveolar lavage: The report of an international conference. Chest 90:122–131, 1986.

85. Helmers RA, Hunninghake GW: Bronchoalveolar lavage in the non-immunocompromised patient. Chest 96:1184–1190, 1989.

86. Anonymous: Clinical guidelines and indications for bronchoalveolar lavage (BAL): Report of the European Society of Pneumology Task Group on BAL. Eur Respir J 3:937–976, 1990.

87. Rankin JA: Role of bronchoalveolar lavage in the diagnosis of pneumonia. Chest 95:187S–190S, 1989.

88. Wimberley N, Willey S, Sullivan N, et al: Antibacterial properties of lidocaine. Chest 76:37–40, 1979.

89. Kirkpatrick MB, Bass JB Jr: Quantitative bacterial cultures of bronchoalveolar lavage fluids and protected brush catheter specimens from normal subjects. Am Rev Respir Dis 139:546–548, 1989.

90. Kahn FW, Jones JM: Diagnosing bacterial respiratory infection by bronchoalveolar lavage. J Infect Dis 155:862–869, 1987.

91. Irwin RS, Demers RR, Pratter MR, Erickson AD, Farrugia R, Teplitz C: Evaluation of methylene blue and squamous epithelial cells as oropharyngeal markers: A means of identifying oropharyngeal contamination during transtracheal aspiration. J Infect Dis 141:165–171, 1980.

92. Henriquez AH, Mendoza J, Gonzalez PC: Quantitative culture of bronchoalveolar lavage from patients with anaerobic lung abscesses. J Infect Dis 164:414–417, 1991.

93. Johanson WG, Seidenfeld JJ, Gomez P, et al: Bacteriologic diagnosis of nosocomial pneumonia following prolonged mechanical ventilation. Am Rev Respir Dis 137:259–264, 1988.

94. Chastre J, Fagon JY, Soler P, et al: Quantification of lavage cells containing intracellular bacteria: A useful adjunct in the evaluation of patients suspected of having nosocomial pneumonia. Am Rev Respir Dis 137:360, 1988.

95. Guerra LF, Baughman RP: Use of bronchoalveolar lavage to diagnose bacterial pneumonia in mechanically ventilated patients. Crit Care Med 18:169–173, 1990.

96. Torres A, de la Bellacasa JP, Xaubet A, et al: Diagnostic value of quantitative cultures of bronchoalveolar lavage and telescoping plugged catheters in mechanically ventilated patients with bacterial pneumonia. Am Rev Respir Dis 140:306–310, 1989.

97. Meduri GU, Beals DM, Maijab AG, et al: Protected bronchoalveolar lavage: A new bronchoscopic technique to retrieve uncontaminated distal airway secretions. Am Rev Respir Dis 143:855–864, 1991.

# Therapy

# Antimicrobials for the Treatment of Respiratory Infection

STEVEN W. SONNESYN and DALE N. GERDING

Pneumonia, lung abscess, empyema, sinusitis, and bronchitis are commonly encountered infections in all fields of medicine. A basic understanding of the antimicrobial agents available to treat these infections is an essential component of respiratory infection treatment. This chapter emphasizes the oral and parenteral antibacterial, antifungal, and antiviral agents available to treat respiratory infections. The spectrum of activity, pharmacokinetics, toxicity, and limitations of individual agents are reviewed. Whenever possible, pharmacokinetic data are summarized in tabular or graphic form. Particular attention is focused on a comparison of antimicrobials within a given class. The discussion addresses antimicrobials from a respiratory standpoint, but specific applications are described in other chapters.

## ANTIBACTERIAL AGENTS

### Penicillins

The penicillins remain an important class of antibiotics in the treatment of respiratory infections. They provide the broadest spectrum of activity of any class of antibiotics. They are best divided into four categories: penicillinase-sensitive or natural penicillins, penicillinase-resistant or antistaphylococcal penicillins, extended-spectrum semisynthetic or antipseudomonal penicillins, and β-lactamase inhibitors.

The first ''antistaphylococcal'' penicillin was penicillin G. Widespread use of this drug led to 80% of the clinical isolates of *Staphylococcus aureus* being resistant by 1960. Today, 85% to 95% of isolates of *S. aureus* are resistant to penicillin G and other natural penicillins. Nonetheless, this class of penicillins remains useful in treating many respiratory infections. They remain the most active agents in vitro against streptococci, and penicillin G remains the drug of choice in treating pneumococcal pneumonia in the United States. Its streptococcal activity includes coverage against *Streptococcus pyogenes, Streptococcus viridans,* and group B and group G streptococci. There have been alarming reports of pneumococcal resistance, but these have been rare. Penicillin G also provides activity against most oropharyngeal anaerobes such as peptostreptococci, fusobacteria, and actinomyctes, although β-lactamase–mediated resistance among oral *Bacteroides* spp. has increased. *Pasteurella multocida, Listeria monocytogenes,* and *Neisseria meningitidis* are also susceptible to penicillin G. Few aerobic gram-negative bacillary organisms are sensitive to penicillin G, and other agents are preferred.

In contrast to penicillin G, penicillin V is acid stable, resulting in better oral absorption and providing peak serum levels of 3 μg/mL after a 500-mg dose. Penicillin V has a spectrum of activity similar to that of penicillin G. Its use should be limited to mild cases of pneumococcal pneumonia, continued therapy of lung abscess after initial parenteral therapy, and bronchitis, sinusitis, and pharyngitis if streptococci are the documented pathogens. As with penicillin G, most gram-negative bacillary organisms, *Bacteroides fragilis,* and β-lactamase–producing strains of *S. aureus* and *Haemophilus influenzae* should be expected to be resistant to penicillin V. Penicillin V is even less active than penicillin G against *H. influenzae, Neisseria,* and enteric gram-negative bacteria.

Ampicillin is a natural penicillin available in parenteral and oral forms. It is slightly less active than penicillin G in vitro against pneumococci and most other streptococci. However, it is much more active against enterococci and gram-negative organisms. Its spectrum includes many strains of *Escherichia coli, Proteus mirabilis, Salmonella, Shigella, L. monocytogenes,* and *H. influenzae.* Most strains of *Klebsiella, Enterobacter,* and *Serratia* and all strains of *Pseudomonas* are resistant. Patients with known pneumococcal pneumonia should be treated with penicillin G or penicillin V, based on better in vitro activity, lower cost, and less toxicity. The emergence of ampicillin-resistant strains of *H. influenzae* (30% in many hospitals) is a concern in the treatment of sinusitis, bronchitis, and pneumonia. If *H. influenzae* is a possibility, the empiric use of a second- or third-generation cephalosporin, ampicillin-sulbactam, ticarcillin-clavulanate, amoxicillin-clavulanate, a fluoroquinolone, newer macrolides or azalides, or trimethoprim-sulfamethoxazole is preferred over ampicillin. Oral ampicillin is only 50% absorbed and rarely provides peak serum levels greater than 3 $\mu$g/mL. Amoxicillin has a bacterial spectrum similar to that of ampicillin and is more completely absorbed, providing peak serum levels 2 to 2.5 times higher than ampicillin, although gastrointestinal side effects are less common. Amoxicillin has been at least as effective as ampicillin in the treatment of otitis media, sinusitis, and bronchitis.

The first penicillinase-resistant penicillin, methicillin, became available in 1960. These newer agents are most useful for treating penicillinase-producing strains of *S. aureus.* Although clinically they are adequate in streptococcal infections, their in vitro activity against streptococci is less than that of penicillin G. Methicillin-resistant *S. aureus* (MRSA) has become an increasingly prevalent problem. The incidence of MRSA varies geographically and by institution but constitutes 5% to 30% of the pathogens in some centers. MRSA seems to be most common in university teaching facilities and in nursing homes. Resistance of penicillinase-resistant penicillins to $\beta$-lactamases is conveyed by steric hindrance caused by the addition of an acyl side chain, which prevents opening of the $\beta$-lactam ring. Changes in the penicillin-binding proteins in isolates of MRSA alter their affinity to methicillin, producing resistance.

Methicillin is little used clinically because of a higher risk of interstitial nephritis compared with nafcillin or oxacillin. The latter agents provide similar activity to methicillin with a few minor exceptions. Penicillinase-resistant penicillins are ineffective against all gram-negative bacteria. Between 30% and 50% of the *Staphylococcus epidermidis* isolates are resistant. For the 10% of *S. aureus* isolates that remain sensitive to penicillin G, it remains the drug of choice, based on lower inhibitory concentrations, lower cost, and lower toxicity compared with oxacillin or nafcillin. Nafcillin is slightly more stable than oxacillin against penicillinase. Both of these agents are approximately four times more active against *S. aureus* than methicillin, with nafcillin the most active. The minimum inhibitory concentration (MIC) of *S. aureus* for these agents is slightly lower for penicillin-sensitive than for penicillin-resistant isolates

(0.1–0.4 $\mu$g/mL versus 0.1–0.8 $\mu$g/mL). Synergism, as demonstrated by lower inhibitory and bactericidal concentrations and increased killing rates, has been shown with rifampin and aminoglycosides for oxacillin and nafcillin. Nafcillin provides slightly better in vitro activity against pneumococci and hemolytic streptococci than oxacillin. The activity is adequate against most anaerobic gram-positive bacilli, peptostreptococci, and clostridial species. Enterococci and all gram-negative bacilli are resistant.

Nafcillin and oxacillin are not reliably absorbed after oral administration, and serum levels are unpredictable. Oral antistaphylococcal penicillins available in the United States include dicloxacillin and cloxacillin. Dicloxacillin is the preferred agent, based on peak serum levels which are 1.5 to 2 times higher than those provided by cloxacillin. A dose of 500 mg orally provides a peak of 7 to 9 $\mu$g/mL. Dicloxacillin use is limited by gastrointestinal side effects, especially at high doses (>2 g/d).

The extended-spectrum penicillins were developed to broaden penicillin coverage to include gram-negative organisms, particularly *Pseudomonas aeruginosa.* The first such penicillin was carbenicillin. Its spectrum is similar to that of ampicillin except that it provides increased in vitro activity against *P. aeruginosa,* indole-positive *Proteus,* and *Enterobacter. Klebsiella* and *Serratia* are resistant. The inhibitory concentration of carbenicillin for most gram-negatives is 10 to 25 $\mu$g/mL, but it is 25 to 100 $\mu$g/mL for *P. aeruginosa;* hence the need to use this agent at very high dosages (18–24 g/d).

Ticarcillin has a spectrum similar to that of carbenicillin except that it is two to four times more active against *P. aeruginosa.* It is also relatively inactive against *Klebsiella* and *Serratia.* Mezlocillin, piperacillin, and azlocillin are parenteral extended-spectrum penicillins that are even more active than carbenicillin and ticarcillin against *P. aeruginosa.* They also provide much better activity against anaerobes, *Enterobacter, Serratia, Citrobacter, E. coli,* and *Klebsiella* than carbenicillin or ticarcillin. Mezlocillin is equal to ticarcillin in antipseudomonal activity and two to four times more active than carbenicillin. Piperacillin and azlocillin are two to four times more active than mezlocillin or ticarcillin against *P. aeruginosa.*[1,2,3] The in vitro activity of these extended-spectrum penicillins against *E. coli* and *Klebsiella* is inferior to that provided by a third-generation cephalosporin. Mezlocillin is the most active antipseudomonal penicillin in vitro against enterococcus and is slightly more active against anaerobes. Ticarcillin and piperacillin provide the best activity against *Acinetobacter.* Piperacillin and mezlocillin provide slightly better in vitro coverage against *H. influenzae* and *Neisseria.* Aminoglycosides are synergistic with extended-spectrum penicillins against *P. aeruginosa,* and combination treatment has been shown to reduce the development of resistance to the antipseudomonal penicillins by *P. aeruginosa.*

The extended-spectrum penicillins provide good in vitro activity against streptococci and penicillin-sensitive staphylococci. None of these agents is active against $\beta$-lactamase–positive *H. influenzae* and *S. aureus* or against MRSA. They are also susceptible to inactivation by $\beta$-lactamases produced by other gram-positive and gram-negative organisms.

$\beta$-Lactamases constitute the primary mode of resistance used by bacteria to combat penicillin and cephalosporin therapy. A detailed discussion of the mechanism of these β-lactamases is beyond the scope of this chapter. β-Lactamases produced by *S. aureus* are produced by plasmids and are inducible. Those produced by gram-negative organisms and anaerobes may be produced chromosomally or by plasmids. β-Lactamase inhibitors were developed to improve the antibacterial spectrum of penicillins by circumventing resistance problems caused by penicillinase-producing organisms. Certain β-lactam agents such as sulbactam and clavulanic acid were found to inhibit certain β-lactamases of gram-positive and gram-negative organisms. Clavulanic acid itself does not provide any significant antibacterial effect at clinically achievable concentrations. It acts as a ''suicide inhibitor'' by forming an intermediate complex with the β-lactamase before destroying the enzyme and allowing the companion β-lactam agents (eg, ticarcillin, amoxicillin) to inhibit or kill the organism.

The combination of ticarcillin and clavulanic acid (Timentin) enhances the gram-positive, gram-negative, and anaerobic activity of ticarcillin alone. The activity against *P. aeruginosa*, however, is not improved because this β-lactamase is not inhibited by clavulanic acid. The amoxicillin-clavulanic acid combination (Augmentin) provides extended coverage against anaerobes, *H. influenzae, E. coli, Klebsiella, Moraxella catarrhalis,* and *S. aureus*. This combination makes amoxicillin potentially more efficacious in patients with otitis media, sinusitis, bronchitis, and pneumonia if β-lactamase–producing *H. influenzae* is a pathogen. It also provides possible increased efficacy in chronic sinusitis if anaerobes play a role.

Sulbactam, a β-lactamase inhibitor, has been combined with ampicillin to provide a parenteral combination (Unasyn). Like clavulanic acid, sulbactam has little intrinsic antimicrobial activity. In combination with ampicillin, it acts to improve the in vitro activity of ampicillin against *S.*

*aureus, H. influenzae, E. coli, Klebsiella,* and anaerobic bacteria.

The pharmacokinetic characteristics of all the penicillins are summarized in Table 43–1.[4] Certain penicillins require dose reduction in patients with renal insufficiency, as displayed in Table 43–2.[4] Adverse effects associated with penicillins are found in Table 43–3.[4]

## Cephalosporins

The cephalosporins constitute a large and often confusing category of antibiotics that provide broad antibacterial activity against a wide array of respiratory pathogens. In moving from first to third generations, gram-positive activity decreases, gram-negative activity increases, β-lactamase stability increases, central nervous system (CNS) penetration increases, and cost increases. Cephalosporins resemble penicillins in that they contain a β-lactam ring. They differ in that a six-member dihydrothiazine ring replaces the five-member thiazolidine ring found in penicillins. Minor structural changes are associated with changes in pharmacokinetics and in activity.[5]

The first-generation cephalosporins provide excellent activity against most streptococci and *S. aureus* (including penicillin-resistant *S. aureus*). They do not provide adequate activity against enterococci, penicillin-resistant *Streptococcus pneumoniae*, MRSA, or methicillin-resistant *S. epidermidis*. Their gram-negative spectrum is limited to some isolates of *E. coli, P. mirabilis,* and *Klebsiella pneumoniae*.[6] Cefazolin and cephalothin are almost identical in their in vitro activity except that cefazolin is less active against *S. aureus* and more active against gram-negative organisms.[7] Cephalothin is used infrequently because of its short half-life; however, it is considered by some authorities to be the

Table 43–1. **Pharmacokinetic Properties of Penicillins**

| Antibiotic | Oral Absorption (%) | Food Decreases Absorption | Protein Binding (%) | % Dose Metabolized | Serum Level* Total Drug (μg/mL) | Serum Level* Free Drug (μg/mL) | Serum T$_{1/2}$ (h)† Normal (C$_{cr}$ > 90 mL/min) | Serum T$_{1/2}$ (h)† Renal Failure (C$_{cr}$ < 10 mL/min) | Liver Impairment Increases (T$_{1/2}$) | Na$^+$ Content (mEq/g)‡ |
|---|---|---|---|---|---|---|---|---|---|---|
| Penicillin G | 20 | Yes | 55 | 20 | 2 | 0.9 | 0.5 | 10 | + | 2.7 |
| Penicillin V | 60 | No | 80 | 55 | 4 | 0.8 | 1 | 4 | | 3.1 |
| Methicillin | 0 | | 35 | 10 | | | 0.5 | 4 | | 3.1 |
| Oxacillin | 30 | Yes | 93 | 45 | 6 | 0.4 | 0.5 | 1 | | |
| Cloxacillin | 50 | Yes | 94 | 20 | 10 | 0.6 | 0.5 | 1 | + + | |
| Dicloxacillin | 50 | Yes | 97 | 10 | 15 | 0.45 | 0.5 | 1.5 | + + | |
| Nafcillin | Erratic | Yes | 87 | 62 | | | 0.5 | 1.5 | + + + | |
| Ampicillin§ | 40 | Yes | 17 | 10 | 3.5 | 2.9 | 1 | 8 | + + | 3.4 |
| Amoxicillin | 75 | No | 17 | 10 | 7.5 | 6.2 | 1 | 8 | + | |
| Carbenicillin | 0 | | 50 | <10 | | | 1.1 | 15 | + +, 18–20 h | 4.7 |
| Indanyl carbenicillin | 30 | No | 50 | <10 | 15 | 7.5 | 1.1 | 15 | + +, 18–20 h | |
| Ticarcillin | 0 | | 50 | 15 | | | 1.2 | 15 | + +, 18–20 h | 4.7 |
| Mezlocillin | 0 | | 25 | <10 | | | | 1.1 | 4 | + + |
| Piperacillin | 0 | | 16 | 0 | | | 1.3 | 4 | + + | 1.8 |
| Azlocillin | 0 | | 30 | <10 | | | 0.8 | 4 | + + | 2.2 |

*After 500-mg oral dose taken while fasting; data not shown if drug is not absorbed orally.
†Values have been rounded off to approximate values for half-life (T$_{1/2}$).
‡Na$^+$ content based on intravenous preparations.
§Proampicillins (eg, bacampicillin, pivampicillin) are absorbed twice as well as ampicillin, and food does not decrease absorption, but other properties are those of the parent ampicillin. Bacampicillin gives a serum level of 9 μg/mL after 500 mg.
Adapted from Mandell GL, Douglas RG Jr, Bennett JE (eds): Principles and Practice of Infectious Diseases, ed 3. Churchill Livingstone, New York, 1990:236–237.

Table 43–2. **Antibiotic Dosage Change in Renal Disease and After Dialysis**

| Agent | Dosage Change in Renal Failure* | | |
|---|---|---|---|
| | *Creatinine Clearance (30–50 mL/min)* | *Creatinine Clearance (<10 mL/min)* | **Dosage After Hemodialysis** |
| Penicillin G | NC† | $1.6 \times 10^6$ U/6 h | Yes ($1.6 \times 10^6$ U) |
| Penicillin V | NC | 250 mg/6 h | Yes (250 mg) |
| Methicillin | 1–2 g/8 h | 1–2 g/12 h | Yes (1–2 g) |
| Oxacillin | NC | NC | NC |
| Cloxacillin | NC | NC | NC |
| Dicloxacillin | NC | NC | NC |
| Nafcillin | NC | NC | NC |
| Ampicillin | NC | 0.5–1 g/8 h | Yes (500 mg) |
| Amoxicillin | NC | 500 mg/12 h | Yes (250 mg) |
| Carbenicillin‡ | 3 g/4 h | 2 g/8 h | Yes (2 g) |
| Ticarcillin‡ | 2 g/4 h | 2 g/12 h | Yes (2 g) |
| Indanyl carbenicillin | NC | Avoid | |
| Azlocillin | NC | 3 g/8–12 h | Yes (2 g) |
| Mezlocillin | NC | 3 g/8–12 h | Yes (2 g) |
| Piperacillin | NC | 3 g/8–12 h | Yes (2 g) |

*Refers to maximum dose used.

†NC, no change.

‡Only carbenicillin and ticarcillin need adjustment of dosage after peritoneal dialysis.

Adapted from Mandell GL, Douglas RG Jr, Bennett JE (eds): Principles and Practice of Infectious Diseases, ed 3. Churchill Livingstone, New York, 1990:236–237.

cephalosporin of choice against serious *S. aureus* infections.

Cefazolin has become the most used first-generation agent based on its longer half-life (1.7 versus 0.7 hours for cephalothin), superior tissue levels, slower renal clearance, and higher serum levels per gram. Cefazolin is slightly more sensitive to β-lactamases produced by *S. aureus.* Cephalothin has been implicated as a cause of dose-dependent acute renal failure when used in combination with aminoglycosides.[8]

Oral first-generation cephalosporins include cephradine, cephalexin, and cefadroxil. The spectra of activity of these agents are similar to those of first-generation parenteral agents, but they are slightly less active on a weight basis than parenteral agents. Cefadroxil has the advantage of a longer half-life (1.5 versus 1.0 hours), which allows twice-daily dosing.

The second-generation cephalosporins provide increased activity against *H. influenzae* and other aerobic gram-negative bacilli, improved anaerobic activity (eg, cefoxitin, cefotetan), and decreased gram-positive activity. Parenteral agents include cefuroxime, cefamandole, cefoxitin, cefotetan, ceforanide, cefmetazole, and cefonicid. None of these agents is active against *Pseudomonas* spp. Their activity compared with first-generation cephalosporins is much improved against *E. coli, Klebsiella,* and indole-negative *Proteus.* Cefuroxime provides the best coverage against *S. aureus* and also is active against *H. influenzae* and some strains of *Enterobacter, Serratia,* indole-positive *Proteus, N. meningitidis,* and anaerobes.[9] It is a useful agent for treating community-acquired pneumonia in bronchitics or nursing home residents if causes of atypical pneumonia (eg, *Mycoplasma pneumoniae, Chlamydia pneumoniae, Legi-*

*onella pneumophila)* are unlikely and *H. influenzae* is likely. Cefamandole has similar activity to cefuroxime, but it is less stable against gram-negative β-lactamases. Cefonicid has less staphylococcal activity, a very long half-life (4.5 hours), and high protein binding (98%), and it is otherwise similar to cefuroxime and cefamandole. Cefotetan is the most active of these agents against gram-negative aerobic bacilli.

Cefoxitin and cefotetan are less active than cefuroxime against gram-positive cocci, *Enterobacter,* and *H. influenzae.* They are much more active against anaerobes, particularly *B. fragilis.*[10] Although limited data exist, these agents may be useful in treating mixed aerobic-anaerobic infections such as aspiration pneumonia or lung abscess.[11, 12]

Second-generation oral agents include cefaclor, cefuroxime axetil, and cefprozil. The spectrum of cefuroxime axetil is the same as that of parenteral cefuroxime, and it is more active than cefaclor against *H. influenzae.* The oral form of cefuroxime has the advantage of twice-daily dosing. Cefprozil has good activity against gram-positive cocci and is comparable to cefuroxime axetil against gram-negative bacilli.

Table 43–3. **Adverse Reactions to Penicillins and Cephalosporins**

| Type of Reaction | Frequency (%) | Occurs Most Frequently With* |
|---|---|---|
| Allergic | | |
| IgE antibody | 0.004–0.4 | Penicillin G |
| Anaphylaxis | | |
| Early urticaria (<72 h) | | |
| Cytotoxic antibody | Rare | Penicillin G |
| Hemolytic anemia | | |
| Ag-Ab complex disease | Rare | Penicillin G |
| Serum sickness | | |
| Delayed hypersensitivity | 4–8 | Ampicillin |
| Contact dermatitis | | |
| Idiopathic | 4–8 | Ampicillin |
| Rash | | |
| Fever | | |
| Late-onset urticaria | | |
| Gastrointestinal | 2–5 | |
| Diarrhea | 2–5 | Ampicillin |
| Enterocolitis | <1 | Ampicillin |
| Hematologic | | |
| Hemolytic anemia | Rare | Penicillin G |
| Neutropenia | 1–4 | Penicillin G Oxacillin Piperacillin |
| Platelet dysfunction | 3 | Carbenicillin |
| Hepatic | | |
| Elevated SGOT level | 1–4 | Oxacillin Nafcillin Carbenicillin |
| Electrolyte disturbance | | |
| Sodium overload | Variable | Carbenicillin |
| Hypokalemia | Variable | Carbenicillin |
| Hyperkalemia (acute) | Rare | Penicillin G |
| Neurologic | | |
| Seizures | Rare | Penicillin G |
| Bizarre sensations | | Procaine Penicillin |
| Renal | | |
| Interstitial nephritis | 1–2 | Methicillin |
| Hemorrhagic cystitis | Rare | Methicillin |

*All the reactions can occur with any of the penicillins.

From Mandell GL, Douglas RG Jr, Bennett JE (eds): Principles and Practice of Infectious Diseases, ed 3. Churchill Livingstone, New York, 1990:236–237.

Table 43–4. **Pharmacokinetics of Selected Cephalosporins and Related β-Lactams**

| Cephalosporins | Administration | Half-life (h) | Protein Binding (%) | CNS Penetration | Excretion* | Dose Reduction in Renal Failure |
|---|---|---|---|---|---|---|
| Cefaclor | PO | 0.7 | 25 | − | R | Minimal |
| Cefadroxil | PO | 1.3 | 20 | − | R | Minimal |
| Cefamandole | IV, IM | 0.7 | 70 | ± | R,H | Minimal |
| Cefazolin | IV, IM | 2.0 | 86 | − | R | Moderate |
| Cefixime | PO | 3.0 | 65–69 | − | R,H | Minimal |
| Cefonicid | IV, IM | 4.5 | 98 | − | R | Major |
| Cefoperazone | IV, IM | 2.0 | 90 | − | R,H | Minimal |
| Cefotaxime | IV, IM | 1.2 | 40 | + | R,H | Minimal |
| Cefotetan | IV, IM | 3.2 | 90 | ± | R | Moderate |
| Cefoxitin | IV, IM | 0.8 | 73 | ± | R,H | Minimal |
| Cefprozil | PO | 1.3 | 42 | − | R,H | Minimal |
| Ceftazidime | IV, IM | 1.9 | 10 | + | R | Major |
| Ceftizoxime | IV, IM | 1.7 | 30 | + | R | Major |
| Ceftriaxone | IV, IM | 6.5 | 95 | + | R,H | Minimal |
| Cefuroxime | IV, IM, PO† | 1.3 | 50 | + | R | Major |
| Cephalexin | PO | 0.8 | 15 | − | R | Minimal |
| Cephalothin | IV, IM | 0.5 | 65 | − | R,H | Minimal |
| Cephradine | IV, IM, PO | 0.7 | 10 | − | R | Minimal |
| Imipenem | IV | 1.0 | 20 | ± | R | Major |
| Aztreonam | IV, IM | 1.7 | 40 | ± | R,H | Major |

*R, renal; H, hepatic.
†Cefuroxime axetil PO.

The third-generation cephalosporins may be divided into two groups: those with good antipseudomonal activity and those with poor antipseudomonal activity. The latter include cefotaxime, ceftizoxime, and ceftriaxone. Cefotaxime has the longest clinical experience and was the first of these agents released. These agents have similar spectra of activity, with a few exceptions. All of them are unreliable against *P. aeruginosa* and should not be used if *P. aeruginosa* is a likely pathogen. These agents have good grampositive activity, but better agents are available for documented gram-positive infections. Because of their β-lactamase stability, these agents are highly active against a broad range of gram-negative organisms. Most strains of Enterobacteriaceae are inhibited. *E. coli* and *Klebsiella* are highly susceptible, but strains of *Escherichia cloacae, Serratia marcescens,* and *Acinetobacter* show variable susceptibility. Their anaerobic activity is moderate and, with the exception of ceftizoxime, is inferior to cefoxitin and cefotetan against *B. fragilis.*

The main advantage of ceftriaxone is its extended half-life, allowing for once- or twice-daily administration. It can also be given intramuscularly, but this requires a large volume and is quite painful. In renal insufficiency, ceftizoxime requires a greater reduction in dosage than do cefotaxime or ceftriaxone.

Ceftazidime and cefoperazone are the most active antipseudomonal cephalosporins. Ceftazidime remains the most potent cephalosporin agent available for *P. aeruginosa*; it inhibits 90% of strains at 8 μg/mL or less.[13, 14] Its activity against other gram-negative bacilli approximates that of other third-generation cephalosporins. It has moderate activity against gram-positive cocci and anaerobes.[15, 16] Cefoperozone is slightly less active against gram-negative bacilli (except *P. aeruginosa*) than other third-generation cephalosporins,[17] but it is more active against *P. aeruginosa* than all other cephalosporins except ceftazidime. Cefoperozone penetrates the CNS poorly. It is hepatically excreted, making dose adjustment in renal insufficiency unnecessary.

Cefixime is the only available oral third-generation cephalosporin. It is inactive against *P. aeruginosa,* anaerobes, and *S. aureus.* It has very good activity against most other gram-negative bacilli and good activity against *S. pneumoniae.* A long half-life (3–4 hours) allows once- or twice-daily dosing.[18] Clinical experience with cefixime is limited. The pharmacokinetics and side effects of the cephalosporins (which are similar to those of penicillins) are detailed in Tables 43–3 and 43–4.

## Imipenem

Imipenem, a synthetic analog of thienamycin, is a carbapenem, similar in structure to conventional (penicillin and cephalosporin) β-lactam antibiotics. Its early development was complicated by problems with chemical instability and extensive metabolism by dehydropeptidase. Cilastatin, an inhibitor of dehydropeptidase, was developed as a companion agent with imipenem to circumvent this metabolism problem. Cilastatin has a pharmacokinetic profile similar to that of imipenem.

Like other β-lactam antibiotics, imipenem acts by binding to penicillin-binding proteins (PBPs), causing spherical cells that are easily lysed. Imipenem penetrates bacterial cell walls well because of its small size and zwitterion structure. It hydroxyethyl side chain possesses a unique *trans*-configuration that conveys stability against β-lactamases. Imipenem exhibits little cross-resistance between penicillin and cephalosporin-resistant isolates. Although most β-lactams confer a postantibiotic effect (PAE, a continued inhibition of bacterial growth after antibiotic levels have declined to a level below an organism's inhibitory concentration) against gram-positive organisms only, imipenem also exerts a significant PAE against many gram-negative organisms.[19]

The in vitro spectrum of imipenem exceeds that of any other single agent. It provides bactericidal activity with little inoculum effect. The concentration needed to inhibit bacteria approximates the concentration needed to kill them.[20] Imipenem is active against all gram-positive organisms except *Enterococcus faecium,* some strains of *S. epidermidis,* MRSA, and *Corynebacterium* JK. Against streptococci and *S. aureus,* its in vitro activity approaches that of penicillin G. As with penicillin, there is a large discrepancy between inhibition and killing of enterococci, and it is not bactericidal for these organisms. Imipenem should not be used as monotherapy for serious enterococcal infection and should only be considered in the treatment of infections caused by *E. faecalis.* Synergy with aminoglycosides (particularly gentamicin) has been documented in vitro, but not to the degree seen with penicillin.[21]

Among gram-negative organisms, its in vitro activity is independent of that for other β-lactams and aminoglycosides. *Xanthomonas maltophilia* and *Pseudomonas cepacia* are resistant. *Proteus, Providencia,* and *Morganella* are the least sensitive. *Enterobacter, Serratia,* and *Citrobacter* are also not as susceptible as most gram-negative organisms (MICs of 1–4 μg/mL). The susceptibility level for *P. aeruginosa* is usually 4 μg/mL or less.[19] Imipenem is more active against *P. aeruginosa* than aztreonam or ticarcillin and is sometimes synergistic with tobramycin (30% of isolates tested in one study).[22] Antagonism with other β-lactams has been seen against *P. aeruginosa,* and these combinations should be avoided. In cystic fibrosis patients with *P. aeruginosa* respiratory infections, resistance has emerged on therapy.[23] In the treatment of *P. aeruginosa* pneumonia in patients without cystic fibrosis, a high rate of failure has been noted.[24–26] After therapy with imipenem, the rate of *P. aeruginosa* resistance was 17% in one study.[27] For these reasons, imipenem probably should not be used alone in patients with serious *P. aeruginosa* infections, especially in the respiratory tract. Imipenem seems to be highly active against cephalosporin-resistant *Acinetobacter, Nocardia asteroides, L. monocytogenes* (discrepancy exists between inhibition and killing), *H. influenzae,* and *N. meningitidis.*[28] It has poor activity against *Flavobacterium, Chlamydia trachomatis, Mycobacterium fortuitum,* and *M. pneumoniae.*

The pharmacokinetic properties of imipenem are displayed in Table 43–4. Although imipenem does not seem to accumulate in cases of renal insufficiency, cilastatin does accumulate, requiring dose adjustment if this combination is used. It is marketed for use with cilastatin as a fixed-ratio combination (Primaxin). It is available in intravenous form only.

Adverse side effects are similar to those of other β-lactams. Rare effects include nausea, vomiting, diarrhea, phlebitis at the site of intravenous administration, fever, rash, and seizures. Seizures occur in 0.3% to 1% of patients and are most frequent in the elderly, in patients with renal insufficiency, in chronic alcoholics, and in patients with a history of head trauma, seizures, or cerebrovascular insults.[29] There is a risk of inducing β-lactamase production in gram-negative organisms if imipenem is used in combination with other β-lactams, and this practice is inadvisable.[30]

### Aztreonam

Aztreonam is a synthetic monobactam (a β-lactam with only the β-lactam ring) that is effective in treating gram-

negative pneumonia, particularly nosocomial pneumonia. Aztreonam acts by binding penicillin-binding protein 3 of susceptible Enterobacteriaceae, *P. aeruginosa,* and other aerobic gram-negative rods. This action produces elongated or filamentous forms that undergo cell lysis. Aztreonam does not bind the PBPs of gram-positive or anaerobic organisms. It is not hydrolyzed by most plasmid- or chromosome-mediated gram-negative β-lactamases. Aztreonam is inactivated by β-lactamases produced by many strains of *Klebsiella oxytoca,* by *P. cepacia,* and by plasmid-derived enzymes that inactivate cefotaxime.[31] The development of resistance during therapy is not common.[32]

The antimicrobial spectrum of aztreonam is quite narrow and is limited to gram-negative organisms. It is inactive against gram-positive cocci and anaerobes. Most Enterobacteriaceae are inhibited at drug concentrations of 0.5 μg/mL. It is active against most strains of *E. coli, Klebsiella, S. marcescens, Proteus, H. influenzae, N. meningitidis, Salmonella, M. catarrhalis, Morganella morganii,* and *Enterobacter agglomerans.* Aztreonam is slightly less active in vitro against *P. aeruginosa* than are ceftazidime and imipenem.[21, 33] The bactericidal concentration for sensitive strains of *P. aeruginosa* usually exceeds the MIC by 4 to 16 times.[33] In one study, synergy in vitro with aminoglycosides was found for 30% to 60% of isolates of *P. aeruginosa* and aminoglycoside-resistant gram-negative rods.[34] Aztreonam has not been shown to be synergistic in vitro with other β-lactams.[34]

Aztreonam is only moderately active against *E. cloacae, Enterobacter aerogenes,* and *Citrobacter freundii.* Enterobacter species resistant to cefotaxime are usually resistant to aztreonam. Aztreonam is often active against aminoglycoside-resistant strains of *Enterobacter, Serratia,* and *Klebsiella.*[21] Many strains of *Acinetobacter* and most *X. maltophilia* and *P. cepacia* are resistant to aztreonam.

Aztreonam is poorly absorbed orally and is available in a parenteral formulation only. It is excreted unchanged by glomerular filtration and tubular secretion. Dose adjustment is required in renal failure. It penetrates tissues similarly to other β-lactams, including pulmonary secretions. The pharmacokinetic details are summarized in Table 43–4.

Adverse side effects are rare and usually benign. The most common side effects include nausea, vomiting, diarrhea, rash, and a slight elevation in transaminase levels. Only 2.1% of patients treated with aztreonam developed toxicity requiring cessation of therapy.[33] Coagulation problems have not been reported, in contrast to some β-lactams. Because minimal cross-immunogenicity has occurred in patients with penicillin or cephalosporin allergies, aztreonam may be used safely in patients who are allergic to penicillins and cephalosporins.[32]

### Quinolones

The exact role of the new fluoroquinolones in respiratory infections has not been established. They are most appropriate for clinical situations in which gram-negative organisms are implicated, such as nosocomial pneumonia or pneumonia in the elderly, in nursing home residents, and in patients with cystic fibrosis, alcoholism, or chronic obstructive pulmonary disease. Their utility in treating community-

Table 43–5. **Pharmacokinetic Properties of Fluoroquinolones**

| Property | Ciprofloxacin | Ofloxacin | Pefloxacin | Enoxacin | Lomefloxacin |
|---|---|---|---|---|---|
| Oral dose (mg) | 500 | 400 | 400 | 600 | 400 |
| Peak levels ($\mu$g/mL) | 2.5 | 5.5 | 4.0 | 4.0 | 2.8 |
| Absorption (%) | 75–85 | 70–80 | 80–95 | 80–90 | 95 |
| Protein binding (%) | 20–40 | 10–20 | 20–30 | 30–40 | 10 |
| Urinary recovery (%) | 30 | 90 | 5 | 60 | 65 |
| Half-life (h) | | | | | |
| $C_{cr}$* normal | 4 | 7 | 8–12 | 6 | 8 |
| $C_{cr}$* <10 mL/min/1.75 m$^2$ | 10 | 30 | 12–15 | 9.4 | 45 |

*$C_{cr}$, creatinine clearance.
Adapted from Walker RC, Wright AJ: The fluoroquinolones. Mayo Clin Proc 66:1249, 1991.

acquired pneumonia or aspiration pneumonia has been questioned because of their marginal activity in vitro against *S. pneumoniae* and poor activity against anaerobes. Ciprofloxacin, ofloxacin, and lomefloxacin have been approved in the United States for use in lower respiratory infections. Norfloxacin is poorly absorbed and is useful only for urinary tract and gastrointestinal infections. Other agents likely to become available in the United States include enoxacin, pefloxacin, and sparfloxacin.

All the newer fluoroquinolones provide excellent in vitro activity against common gram-negative respiratory pathogens including *H. influenzae, Klebsiella, S. marcescens, M. catarrhalis, P. aeruginosa, Neisseria, Enterobacter, Proteus, Acinetobacter,* and *Citrobacter.*[35] *P. cepacia* and *X. maltophilia* are resistant, with an MIC greater than or equal to 3 $\mu$g/mL.[35] Ciprofloxacin is the most active quinolone against gram-negative organisms, including *P. aeruginosa*; it is two to eight times more active than ofloxacin. Against *P. aeruginosa,* the $MIC_{90}$ for ciprofloxacin is less than 1 $\mu$g/mL. Ofloxacin has slightly better in vitro activity against *S. aureus* than other quinolones. Most strains of *S. aureus* are sensitive to ciprofloxacin (MIC < 1 $\mu$g/mL), including many strains of MRSA; however, resistance has developed readily in MRSA.[35] Against *S. pneumoniae,* enterococci, and other streptococci, ciprofloxacin activity is intermediate at best (MIC 1–2 $\mu$g/mL). Anaerobic cocci are intermediately susceptible or are resistant, and most gram-negative anaerobic bacilli are resistant to ciprofloxacin.[35] *Actinomyces* and *Nocardia* are also not susceptible at concentrations below 2 $\mu$g/mL.

The quinolones have moderate to good activity against *L. monocytogenes, M. pneumoniae, Mycobacterium tuberculosis, M. fortuitum, C. trachomatis, C. pneumoniae, Legionella, Brucella,* and *P. multocida.*[35] Clinical efficacy in infections caused by many of these pathogens has yet to be demonstrated.

Clinical studies of ciprofloxacin and ofloxacin in pneumococcal pneumonia have demonstrated high clinical cure rates despite only moderate in vitro susceptibility. This observation may be related to relatively high tissue penetration, which is discussed later in this chapter. In these studies, a high MIC did not necessarily predict therapeutic failure. In one series, 95% of patients with pneumococcal respiratory infections from multiple centers were cured clinically.[36] In another study, 9 of 26 patients improved, and 21 of 48 isolates persisted after therapy.[37] There have also been reports of pneumococcal bacteremia and meningitis while patients were receiving ciprofloxacin for pneumococcal pneumonia.[38, 39] In the treatment of upper respiratory infec-

tions (for which there is no approved indication), complications on ciprofloxacin have been anecdotally reported, including *S. pneumoniae* meningitis and pneumonia and group A streptococcal epidural piriform abscess.[40] Delayed clinical response and failure to eradicate pneumococcus from sputum have been reported.[41] In the treatment of lower respiratory tract infections, doses of ciprofloxacin lower than 750 mg twice daily probably should not be used. A 500-mg oral dose achieves a maximum serum level of only 2.5 $\mu$g/mL, which is inadequate against many *S. pneumoniae.*

Fluoroquinolones are concentrated intracellularly in most tissues, including bronchial mucosa, which may enhance their effectiveness against pathogens with intermediate susceptibility. They are also concentrated in neutrophils and macrophages, which may provide efficacy in the treatment of intracellular pathogens such as *Legionella, Mycoplasma, Chlamydia,* and *Mycobacteria.* Tissue penetration by quinolones is favored by their zwitterion structure, their small molecular size, and their low degree of protein binding. Tissue concentration often exceeds serum levels. The activity of quinolones is reduced by an acidic pH, divalent cations, a large bacterial inoculum, and urine (lowers pH and contains $Mg^{2+}$).[35]

The pharmacokinetics of fluoroquinolones are detailed in Table 43–5.[42] Pharmacokinetic advantages of all the quinolones include high oral bioavailability, low protein binding, and an extended half-life (3–10 hours) allowing once- or twice-daily dosing. Many of the fluoroquinolones can be administered in intravenous or oral forms. Toxicity with the quinolones is minimal. Most commonly, nausea, abdominal discomfort, and dizziness have been reported. Patients given theophylline[43] (Table 43–6) and warfarin (Coumadin) require close monitoring because the metabolism of these

Table 43–6. **Interaction Between Fluoroquinolones and Theophylline**

| Fluoroquinolone | Plasma Theophylline Concentration (% Increase) | Total Body Clearance (% Decrease) |
|---|---|---|
| Ciprofloxacin | 23 | 30 |
| Enoxacin | 111 | 64 |
| Ofloxacin | No change | No change |
| Pefloxacin | 20 | 29 |
| Nalidixic acid | No change | No change |
| Lomefloxacin | No change | No change |

Data from Wijnands WJA, Vree TB: Interaction between the fluoroquinolones and the bronchodilator theophylline. J Antimicrob Chemother 22(suppl C):109, 1988.

drugs is reduced by some fluoroquinolones. Cations in antacids, sucralfate, multivitamins with zinc, and iron preparations bind the quinolones and prevent gastrointestinal absorption. Because of possible detrimental effects on cartilage development, fluoroquinolones are contraindicated in children, adolescents, and pregnant or lactating women.

## Aminoglycosides

The aminoglycosides remain important agents in the treatment of serious gram-negative pulmonary infections. The parenteral agents available in the United States include gentamicin, tobramycin, amikacin, netilmicin, kanamycin, and streptomycin. Kanamycin and streptomycin are much less active in vitro against Enterobacteriaceae and *P. aeruginosa* than other aminoglycosides and are little used clinically to treat gram-negative pneumonia. Streptomycin and kanamycin are of clinical use primarily in the treatment of mycobacterial infections.

The various mechanisms by which bacteria develop resistance to aminoglycosides warrant brief discussion. Three mechanisms have been identified: production of inactivating enzymes (the most common mechanism), alteration of the ribosomal site of attachment, and cellular transport system inhibition. Aminoglycoside-inactivating enzymes are a much more common problem with tobramycin and gentamicin than with amikacin or netilmicin. Amikacin possesses structural advantages that make it the least susceptible to enzymatic inactivation. It is, therefore, active against many strains resistant to gentamicin and tobramycin.[44] Major geographic and interhospital variations exist with respect to bacterial susceptibility to the aminoglycosides and should be considered when selecting among these agents.

The antimicrobial spectra of activity of gentamicin, tobramycin, and netilmicin are similar. Against gram-negative organisms, despite some in vitro variation, there are no clinical data to favor one aminoglycoside over another, if both are active in vitro. Gentamicin is somewhat more active against *S. marcescens* than is tobramycin. Tobramycin has greater activity against some strains of *Acinetobacter calcoaceticus* and has slightly more intrinsic activity against *P. aeruginosa*.[45] Netilmicin is relatively resistant to aminoglycoside-inactivating enzymes and is occasionally active against some strains of *Enterobacteriaceae* (particularly *E. coli, Klebsiella, Enterobacter,* and *Citrobacter*) that are resistant to tobramycin and gentamicin.[46] However, netilmicin has significantly less intrinsic activity against *P. aeruginosa.* In general, aminoglycosides are highly active against almost all aerobic and facultative gram-negative rods. They also are active in vitro against *S. aureus* and coagulase-negative staphylococci, and against enterococci they demonstrate synergistic activity if combined with certain β-lactam antibiotics or vancomycin.

Amikacin is the most potent aminoglycoside in vitro, as measured by the percentage of strains susceptible to the drug. The fact that it is unaffected by most aminoglycoside-inactivating enzymes has been a significant advantage in treating many gram-negative infections caused by gentamicin- and tobramycin-resistant organisms. Although concern over the development of resistance has often led to restrictions of amikacin use, there has been very little amikacin resistance despite high-level amikacin use in some hospitals.[47]

Significant pharmacokinetic differences exist among the aminoglycosides. None of them is absorbed orally. The half-life is approximately 2 hours for all the aminoglycosides, although significant patient-to-patient variation occurs.[48] The usual loading and maintenance doses may produce inadequate therapeutic levels in a significant percentage of patients. Several studies have shown that following the usual dosing nomograms for gentamicin and tobramycin led to peak serum concentrations that failed to exceed the level of susceptibility of the infecting organism in 17% to 33% of cases.[49, 50] Clinical efficacy has been correlated with a gentamicin peak of 4 to 8 μg/mL. In gram-negative sepsis, a favorable clinical response was obtained in 84% of patients if peak levels were in this range, compared with only 23% if levels were subtherapeutic.[52] Amikacin may demonstrate less variation in drug levels and possesses a higher ratio of peak serum concentration to MIC; it therefore has a greater therapeutic ratio. Minor variations in serum amikacin concentration have little effect.[51] Additional pharmacokinetic data are displayed in Table 43-7. In general, concentrations in pulmonary secretions are 20% to 40% of serum concentrations. This topic is discussed in detail later in this chapter.

The toxicity of aminoglycosides primarily affects the kidney and eighth cranial nerve. Tobramycin, amikacin, and netilmicin are less nephrotoxic than gentamicin. Netilmicin has been shown to be the least ototoxic in humans.[53] Ototoxicity has been associated with gentamicin or tobramycin peaks greater than 12 μg/mL and with amikacin peaks greater than 35 μg/mL. Nephrotoxicity has been associated with gentamicin or tobramycin troughs greater than 2 μg/mL and amikacin troughs greater than 10 μg/mL; it is essential to monitor levels. Trough levels often begin to rise as an early sign of nephrotoxicity, before any

Table 43-7. **Pharmacokinetic Data for the Aminoglycosides**

| Agent | Usual Dose* | Desirable Range of Serum Concentration (μg/mL) | | Apparent Volume of Distribution (L/kg) | Serum Half-life (h) | | Renal Clearance (mL/min/1.73 m²) |
| | | Peak | Trough | | NRF† | Anephric | |
|---|---|---|---|---|---|---|---|
| Gentamicin | 5 mg/kg/d, divide q 8 h | 8–10 | <2 | 0.25 | 2 | 55 | 50–90 |
| Tobramycin | 5 mg/kg/d, divide q 8 h | 8–10 | <2 | 0.22 | 2 | 70 | 50–90 |
| Amikacin | 15 mg/kg/d, divide q 12 h | 25–30 | <10 | 0.28 | 2–3 | 80 | 75–100 |
| Netilmicin | 6.5 mg/kg/d, divide q 8 h | 10–14 | <4 | 0.26 | 2 | 60 | 70–85 |

*Intravenous route preferred for adults.
†NRF, normal renal function in adults.
Adapted from Ristuccia AM: Aminoglycosides. *In* Ristuccia AM, Cunha BA (eds): Antimicrobial Therapy. New York, Raven Press, 1984:305.

elevation in creatinine.[44, 54] Excretion of aminoglycosides occurs exclusively through glomerular filtration, although other factors are important in determining blood levels. Age, fever, obesity, and the presence of semisynthetic penicillins that may inactivate aminoglycosides play a role in determining drug levels.

## Macrolides and Azalides

Erythromycin has long been the mainstay of the macrolide class of antibiotics, and it has been joined by the newer agents, clarithromycin and roxithromycin, and the related azalide compound, azithromycin. Erythromycin continues to be an important antibiotic for use in treating infections in the respiratory tract, although it is no longer considered to be a broad-spectrum antibiotic. It has developed new uses against more recently identified causes of atypical pneumonia, including *M. pneumoniae, L. pneumophila, C. trachomatis,* and *C. pneumoniae* (TWAR).

Erythromycin binds the 50S ribosome to inhibit the translocation step of protein synthesis. In doing so, it may interfere with the action of clindamycin and chloramphenicol by competitive binding at the ribosome.[55] The antibacterial action of erythromycin may be bacteriostatic or bactericidal, depending on the drug concentration, inoculum size, the organism, its sensitivity, and the growth phase.[56] Resistance by gram-negative organisms seems to be related to an inability of erythromycin to penetrate these bacteria. Resistance by gram-positive organisms is usually plasmid-mediated, although chromosomal mutations also occur.

Erythromycin lacks activity against Enterobacteriaceae, gram-negative anaerobes, and *P. aeruginosa.* Its activity against *H. influenzae* is only moderate.[57] If *H. influenzae* is a concern, as it often is in sinusitis, bronchitis, and pneumonia, other agents are preferred. Against gram-positive bacteria, erythromycin continues to have excellent activity against *S. pneumoniae,* group A streptococci and *S. aureus.* There have been rare reports of erythromycin-resistant pneumococci, including several strains with an MIC of 2000 μg/mL.[56, 58] Resistance to *S. aureus* has also been observed to occur on therapy.[56] Use in *S. aureus* infections should be limited to mild or moderate infections. The spectrum of erythromycin also includes activity against *N. meningitidis, Bordetella pertussis, L. monocytogenes, Corynebacterium diphtheriae,* and *N. asteroides.* The activity against *N. asteroides* is inadequate for treatment with erythromycin alone, and erythromycin should be combined with ampicillin.[59] Erythromycin is considered the drug of choice for *M. pneumoniae* pneumonia, resulting in a reduction in the duration of symptoms and fever. Although the rate of radiographic resolution is improved, erythromycin does not enhance bacterial eradication.[60, 61] Erythromycin has been shown to be 50 times more active in vitro than tetracycline against *M. pneumoniae.*[64] Erythromycin is also the drug of choice against *L. pneumophila* pneumonia and *C. trachomatis* pneumonia in children and is an alternate choice for *C. pneumoniae* pneumonia.

Erythromycin is available in several parenteral and oral preparations (Table 43–8).[56] Bioavailability is limited in oral formulations by acid lability. At doses of 500 mg using any of the oral preparations, serum levels of erythromycin

**Table 43–8. Peak Serum Levels of Erythromycin in Adults**

| Preparation | Dose (mg) | Route | Time After Dose (h) | Peak Levels (range, μg/mL) |
|---|---|---|---|---|
| Base | 250 | PO | 4 | 0.3–0.7 |
| | 500 | PO | 4 | 0.3–1.9 |
| | 500 | Rectal | 1 | 0.9 |
| Stearate | 250 | PO | 2–3 | 0.2–0.8 |
| | 500 | PO | 3 | 0.4–1.8 |
| Estolate | 250 | PO | 2–4 | 1.4–1.7* |
| | 500 | PO | 3.5–4 | 4.2* (1.1)† |
| Ethylsuccinate | 250 | PO | 0.5 | 0.45 |
| | 500 | PO | 0.5–2.5 | 1.5* (0.6)† |
| | 1000 | PO | 1 | 5.7 |
| Lactobionate | 500 | IV | 1 | 9.9 |
| | 1000 | IV | 0.5 | 15.5 |
| Gluceptate | 300 | IV | 2 | 2.6 |
| | 1000 | IV | 1 | 9.9 |

*Total drug (ester plus base).
†Free base.
From Chow AW: Erythromycin. *In* Ristuccia AM, Cunha BA (eds): Antimicrobial Therapy. New York, Raven Press, 1984:214.

base are limited to 0.3 to 1.9 μg/mL.[56] However, serum levels do not seem to correlate with clinical efficacy. There does not seem to be any significant advantage of one oral preparation over another. The only active form is erythromycin base, into which the various forms are converted. Parenteral administration allows much higher serum levels, 8 to 15 μg/mL, which may be important in treating serious infections.[56]

Erythromycin penetrates most tissues well, with the exception of the CNS. Alveolar macrophages and neutrophils also concentrate the drug, providing intracellular concentrations 9 to 23 times and 10 to 13 times greater than those found extracellularly, respectively.[63] This may explain the high degree of efficacy against intracellular pathogens observed for erythromycin despite its inhibitory (rather than bactericidal) activity against many organisms.

Adverse reactions to erythromycin are common. The most common side effects are gastrointestinal: nausea, vomiting, diarrhea, and epigastric discomfort. Phlebitis is common with parenteral use. Rash, fever, and eosinophilia occur rarely. The most serious toxic effect is reversible cholestatic hepatitis, which occurs rarely. The estolate form has most often been implicated (93% of cases),[56] but the ethylsuccinate form has also been implicated. Most cases caused by the estolate form have occurred in patients older than 12 years of age. Reversible sensorineural hearing loss has been observed rarely, usually in association with high-dose intravenous therapy in patients with renal failure. Erythromycin also interferes with the hepatic metabolism (through the cytochrome P-450 enzyme system) of certain medications, which can lead to toxic levels of digoxin, theophylline, carbamazepine, warfarin, and cyclosporine.[55]

Clarithromycin is a new macrolide antibiotic, recently approved in the United States, which has demonstrated efficacy against a broad range of respiratory pathogens. Clarithromycin and its active 14-hydroxy metabolite are similar to erythromycin, but they have certain pharmacokinetic advantages, greater activity against many respiratory pathogens, and lower toxicity. In clinical trials, clarithromycin has demonstrated efficacy equivalent to standard antibiotics in the treatment of acute maxillary sinusitis, acute exacerbations of chronic bronchitis, and community-acquired pneumonia.[64–66]

Clarithromycin demonstrates the same antibacterial spectrum as erythromycin. Its activity ranges from equal to four times more active against *S. pneumoniae, S. pyogenes, M. catarrhalis, M. pneumoniae, L. pneumophila,* and *Chlamydia* species.[67] Its activity against *H. influenzae* in vitro is approximately half that of erythromycin. However, when its activity is combined with that of its 14-hydroxy metabolite, its in vitro activity against *H. influenzae* exceeds that of erythromycin or cefaclor.[65, 68] The activity of clarithromycin in humans may be underestimated by in vitro results or animal models (ie, they do not produce the 14-hydroxy metabolite) if the activity of its active metabolite is not accounted for. Clarithromycin also has activity against nontuberculous mycobacteria, including *Mycobacterium avium-intracellulare* complex. Clinical efficacy in *M. avium-intracellulare* infection in patients with acquired immunodeficiency syndrome (AIDS) has been favorable in early trials.

Clarithromycin possesses pharmacokinetic advantages over erythromycin. These include greater acid stability, greater bioavailability (55%), and a long half-life, allowing less frequent dosing (ie, 5 hours for clarithromycin and 7 hours for its active metabolite). Clarithromycin also achieves higher tissue levels and has a postantibiotic effect (PAE) that is three times longer than that of erythromycin. Clarithromycin serum levels are considerably higher than those of erythromycin, and tissue levels are much higher than serum levels.[69] High concentrations are achieved in neutrophils and macrophages, enhancing efficacy against intracellular pathogens. Dose adjustment is necessary in renal insufficiency. In hepatic insufficiency, less of the 14-hydroxy metabolite is produced.[70]

Clarithromycin is well tolerated. Gastrointestinal complaints are milder than with erythromycin but include nausea, diarrhea, and abdominal pain. Clarithromycin seems to have a lower propensity to interact with drugs that undergo hepatic metabolism, particularly theophylline.[71]

Azithromycin is a new azalide antibiotic, approved for use in the United States, which should become a useful oral agent in the treatment of respiratory infections. Azithromycin possesses certain pharmacokinetic advantages over erythromycin and has greater in vitro activity against gram-negative organisms.

Azithromycin demonstrates a similar activity profile against gram-positive cocci to that seen with erythromycin. It is four times more active in vitro against *H. influenzae* and two times more active against *M. catarrhalis* and *L. pneumophila.*[72, 73] It is also significantly more active against most Enterobacteriaceae and has mycobacterial activity, including activity against *M. avium-intracellulare* complex. Against *Fusobacterium necrophorum,* azithromycin is 10 times more active than erythromycin, but against other anaerobes, its relative activity is equivalent. It also provides equivalent activity against *Chlamydia* species.[72] In an animal model, azithromycin was shown to be bactericidal by virtue of its high and sustained tissue levels.[74] This contrasts with the usually bacteriostatic action of erythromycin. However, in one study of acute exacerbations of chronic bronchitis, azithromycin failed to eradicate *H. influenzae* and was associated with significant clinical failure.[75] This study used an initial dose of 500 mg followed by 250 mg

once daily; however, this lower dosage was still associated with a relatively high sputum level (mean 3.66 μg/mL). Subsequent studies have used a dosage of 500 mg daily.

Azithromycin has greater acid stability, a longer half-life, and higher tissue but lower serum concentrations if compared with erythromycin.[76, 77] Azithromycin achieves intracellular concentrations in polymorphonuclear leukocytes and macrophages that are more than 10 times higher than those for erythromycin. Tissue concentrations generally exceed serum concentration by 10 to 100 times, and tissue levels tend to persist for days after serum levels decline. These advantages allow once-daily dosing and potentially briefer duration of therapy (5 days) than with previous agents. Azithromycin is well tolerated, with mild gastrointestinal side effects being most common. Asymptomatic elevation of liver function tests has also been reported. Because of the low serum levels, patients with suspected bacteremia should not be treated with azithromycin.

## Tetracyclines

The tetracyclines are useful agents in the treatment of bronchopulmonary infections. Although some gram-negative organisms have developed resistance, tetracyclines remain broad-spectrum agents with unique efficacy in certain infections. Their widespread use in livestock feeds has exacerbated problems with resistance among gram-negative organisms. Intracellularly, these agents bind the 30S ribosome and prevent access of aminoacyl transfer RNA to messenger RNA. An energy-dependent active transport system must pump tetracycline through the inner cytoplasmic membrane. Minocycline and doxycycline are more lipophilic and pass directly through the lipid bilayer. Resistance develops slowly, in a stepwise fashion; it is primarily plasmid-mediated and usually involves inhibition of the active transport system. The antibacterial action of the tetracyclines is primarily bacteriostatic.

The antimicrobial spectra of all the tetracyclines are similar. The lipophilic analogs, minocycline and doxycycline, are somewhat more active than other agents. If an organism is resistant to one tetracycline analog, it is resistant to all tetracyclines. Many gram-negative aerobic bacilli are resistant to tetracyclines. The tetracyclines are active against aerobic gram-positive cocci, but better agents are available. Pneumococcal resistance is not uncommon and has been reported in up to 14% of clinical isolates.[78, 79] Better agents also exist for the treatment of most anaerobic infections.

Tetracycline compounds have clinical efficacy in several respiratory infections. They are considered the drugs of choice in *C. pneumoniae* (TWAR) pneumonia and psittacosis. They are useful alternative agents in the treatment of infections caused by *M. pneumoniae, L. pneumophila, Actinomyces,* and *P. multocida.* Minocycline has been useful in the prophylaxis of meningococcal pharyngeal carriers if rifampin is contraindicated. Tetracycline and doxycycline are often used in the treatment of acute exacerbations of chronic bronchitis.

The tetracyclines have numerous pharmacokinetic differences that require discussion. Absorption is impaired by dairy products, divalent cations such as those found in antacids, iron preparations, and decreased gastric acidity.

Doxycycline and minocycline have the highest oral absorption, 90% to 100%. They also have extended half-lives (18–24 hours), allowing less frequent dosing. The half-lives of the tetracycline analogues are determined by the rate of renal excretion. Doxycycline does not accumulate in cases of renal insufficiency, and it alone is safe for use in patients with this diagnosis. It is primarily excreted as an inactive conjugate in the feces. Minocycline undergoes enterohepatic circulation but still accumulates in renal insufficiency. Minocycline and doxycycline are available in intravenous forms. Intramuscular injection causes excessive pain and should not be used. A more detailed pharmacokinetic description of the various tetracyclines is provided in Table 43–9.[79]

The most common side effects that occur with tetracycline analogs are nausea, vomiting, epigastric distress, sun sensitivity, hypersensitivity reactions, and in children younger than 8 years of age, discoloration of teeth and depression of skeletal growth. Superinfections are common and include oral and vaginal candidiasis, diarrhea, and pseudomembranous colitis caused by *Clostridium difficile*. Hepatotoxicity, particularly in pregnancy, anaphylaxis, and periorbital edema occur rarely. Increased azotemia occurs in patients with renal insufficiency.

## Clindamycin

Clindamycin continues to be an important agent in the treatment of respiratory infections. It is highly effective in the treatment of aspiration pneumonia, lung abscess, empyema, and pneumococcal or staphylococcal pneumonia.[80] In clinical use, it has replaced lincomycin because of its superior absorption, serum concentration, and activity. There are limited data suggesting that clindamycin may be superior to penicillin in the treatment of anaerobic pulmonary infections.[81, 82] There is some evidence that 15% to 25% of anaerobic lung infections may involve β-lactamase–producing strains of *Bacteroides* that may be resistant to penicillin. The clinical utility of clindamycin seems to be increasing.

Clindamycin inhibits protein synthesis by binding the 50S ribosomal subunit. It is primarily bacteriostatic, but against certain organisms it may be bactericidal. Its mechanism is similar to that of erythromycin and chloramphenicol; these agents should not be used in combination. Resistance to clindamycin develops slowly, in a stepwise fashion, usually by chromosomal or plasmid mutations.[80] Resistance of *S. aureus* has occurred on therapy.[83]

The antibacterial spectrum of clindamycin is limited to gram-positive and anaerobic organisms. All aerobic gram-negative organisms are resistant (slight activity is seen with *H. influenzae*). Activity against streptococcal species (enterococci are resistant) is similar to that of erythromycin. Against *S. aureus,* its activity is four times greater than that of erythromycin, with an MIC of 0.1 μg/mL.[84] MRSA strains are generally resistant. Most anaerobic cocci are sensitive to clindamycin, but 10% are resistant. Oropharyngeal anaerobes, including most *Bacteroides* species, are sensitive. In documented *B. fragilis* infections, metronidazole is preferred because of increasing resistance to clindamycin. *B. fragilis* resistance to clindamycin varies significantly between institutions, ranging from 1% to 20%. A recent study of *B. fragilis* from multiple centers revealed that 6% of isolates were resistant.[85] Clindamycin also has activity against many clostridial species, *N. asteroides,* and *Actinomyces israelii*. Its activity against *M. pneumoniae* is minimal and too little to be useful clinically. *L. pneumophila* and *N. meningitidis* are resistant.

Clindamycin is available in parenteral and oral formulations. The oral formulations are characterized by high bioavailability (90%) and good serum levels.[80, 86] The drug is metabolized by the liver and excreted in the bile and urine. Dose adjustment is necessary in both renal and liver failure. As with the macrolides, the drug is concentrated by neutrophils, by alveolar macrophages, and probably within abscesses.[80, 86]

The most important toxic effect related to clindamycin is *C. difficile* diarrhea or pseudomembranous colitis. This complication occurs much less commonly than originally reported: in 0.01% to 10% of treated patients.[82, 87] It is probably at least as common with ampicillin and cephalosporins. It occurs with intravenous and oral use but is more common with oral clindamycin. Diarrhea unrelated to *C. difficile* occurs commonly (up to 20% of patients). Other side effects include rash, a metallic taste (for intravenous form), transient transaminase elevations, neutropenia, and thrombocytopenia.

**Table 43–9. Pharmacologic Characteristics of the Tetracyclines**

| Characteristic | Tetracycline | Oxytetracycline | DMTC* | Minocycline | Doxycycline |
|---|---|---|---|---|---|
| Dose (mg) | 250 | 250 | 150–300 | 50–100 | 50–100 |
| (daily dose) | (1–2 g) | (1–2 g) | (300–1200 mg) | (100–200 mg) | (100–200 mg) |
| Interval (h) | 6 | 6 | 6–12 | 12 | 12–24 |
| Route | PO | PO | PO | PO, IV | PO, IV |
| Percent absorbed | 77–80 | 58 | 66 | 95 | 93 |
| Peak serum levels (μg/mL) | 2–4 | 2 | 1.3 | 2–4 | 2–4 |
| Protein binding (%) | 55–65 | 25–35 | 75 | 80–95 | 80–95 |
| Lipid solubility† | 0.09 | 0.007 | | 30 | 0.48 |
| Half-life, $T_{1/2}$ (h) | 8.5 | 9–10 | 15 | 12–16 | 12–18 |
| Renal failure, $T_{1/2}$ (h) | 33–79 | 48–66 | | 30 | 15–36 |
| Renal clearance (mL/min) | 70–90 | 90–100 | 30–40 | 5–15 | 15–25 |
| Renal excretion, eliminated in urine following IV administration (%) | 60 | 70 | 40 | 10 | 35 |

*Demethylchlortetracycline.
†Chloroform water partition coefficient at pH 7.4.
Adapted from Jonas M, Comer JB, Cunha BA: Tetracyclines. *In* Ristuccia AM, Cunha BA (eds): Antimicrobial Therapy. New York, Raven Press, 1984:226.

## Metronidazole

Metronidazole is rarely used in respiratory infections. It may be occasionally useful in the treatment of anaerobic lung abscess, aspiration pneumonia, or empyema. Clinical studies have been characterized by a high failure rate, perhaps related to the mixed aerobic-anaerobic nature of many of these infections.[88] Its mechanism of action involves the reduction of its nitro group within bacteria that possess nitro reductase. This reaction produces short-lived, highly cytotoxic intermediates that disrupt bacterial DNA. Resistance develops rarely through decreased uptake of the drug by bacteria or by decreased nitro reduction.

Metronidazole is potently bactericidal against most obligate anaerobes. Against *Fusobacterium, Bacteroides* species (including *B. fragilis*), and *Clostridium perfringens,* metronidazole is characterized by nearly uniform sensitivity. There have been a few reports of resistant organisms.[89] Against microaerophilic organisms, its activity is variable. *Actinomyces* and *Propionibacterium acnes* are generally resistant. Approximately 15% of peptostreptococci are resistant. Metronidazole has no activity against aerobic or facultatively aerobic bacteria, perhaps explaining clinical failures in mixed aerobic-anaerobic pulmonary infections.

Metronidazole is metabolized by the liver to produce an acid and a hydroxy metabolite that possess 5% and 65% of the activity of the parent compound, respectively. Dose adjustment is necessary in liver failure. Metronidazole penetrates most tissues well, including the CNS and abscesses. It is available parenterally and orally. Pharmacokinetic advantages include a high degree of oral bioavailability, a long half-life (6.1–7.1 hours), and low protein binding.[89]

Adverse effects are most commonly gastrointestinal and occur in 5% to 10% of patients. They include nausea, vomiting, a metallic taste, anorexia, and diarrhea. Neurologic toxicity is rare but includes seizures, confusion, vertigo, headache, ataxia, and a usually reversible, dose-related, peripheral neuropathy.[89]

## Vancomycin

The role of vancomycin in the treatment of gram-positive infections has increased dramatically. Shortly after vancomycin became available in 1958, it was relegated to second-line therapy for staphylococcal and streptococcal infections by the less toxic methicillin, lincomycin, and cephalosporins. The widespread occurrence of infections caused by MRSA and resistant *S. epidermidis* has provided new demands for the antibiotic. More purified preparations have reduced toxicity.

Vancomycin acts at an earlier stage of cell wall synthesis than do β-lactams, and competition for binding sites and β-lactam cross-resistance are not a problem. Vancomycin complexes with a D-alanyl-D-alanine precursor to inhibit the synthesis and assembly of cell wall peptidoglycan polymers. It also injures protoplasts by altering the permeability of their cytoplasmic membranes and inhibiting RNA synthesis. Its action is bactericidal, and the killing concentration for most organisms approximates the MIC.

Vancomycin's spectrum of activity is limited to gram-positive organisms. It has no significant activity against gram-negative organisms. Against *S. aureus* and *S. epidermidis,* most strains are inhibited by less than 1 to 5 μg/mL. Against MRSA, all strains are susceptible, but some have shown tolerance (minimum bactericidal concentration ≥ 8 times the MIC).[90, 91] Strains that exhibit tolerance may require treatment with a synergistic combination of vancomycin and an aminoglycoside (eg, gentamicin exhibits the best in vitro activity against gram-positive cocci) or rifampin.[92] Against enterococci, vancomycin is bacteriostatic, with an $MIC_{90}$ less than or equal to 6 μg/mL. However, strains have been reported with an MIC greater than or equal to 2000 μg/mL.[93] Most enterococci are not killed at serum concentrations less than 100 μg/mL. Other aerobic streptococci are uniformly susceptible. Anaerobic or microaerophilic streptococci, *Actinomyces,* lactobacilli, *L. monocytogenes,* clostridial species, and *Corynebacterium* including JK diphtheroids are generally susceptible to vancomycin.

The pharmacokinetics of vancomycin have been reviewed previously.[94, 95] Advantages include a long half-life (6–8 hours), but extensive accumulation in renal insufficiency occurs, and in these patients a marked reduction in dosage is required. Vancomycin penetrates cerebrospinal fluid (CSF) and the CNS only in the presence of inflammation, and in these patients it produces CSF levels 5% to 19% of serum levels.[93] To ensure bactericidal activity against most staphylococci and streptococci, a dose of 15 mg/kg intravenously every 12 hours is recommended in patients with normal renal function. Vancomycin is available in an intravenous but not in an intramuscular form, and it is not absorbed if administered orally.

The most common adverse side effect is the "red man" syndrome, which consists of pruritis, erythema, flushing, and tingling of the torso, neck, and face, angioedema, and occasionally hypotension or cardiac arrest. This effect seems to be the result of a nonimmunologic release of histamine from basophils and mast cells. It is associated with a rapid infusion of vancomycin and is prevented by slow infusion and antihistamines. Other toxicities occur much less frequently since a more purified preparation became available.

Ototoxicity occurs rarely at concentrations below 30 μg/mL and is usually seen with levels exceeding 80 to 100 μg/mL. If high-tone hearing loss results, it may be reversible with cessation of therapy. More typically, deterioration in auditory nerve function progresses. Nephrotoxicity with vancomycin alone is rare. The otic and renal toxicities of vancomycin and the aminoglycosides are additive. Other side effects include fever, chills, phlebitis, and a dose- and time-dependent neutropenia.[93]

## Sulfonamides and Trimethoprim

The sulfonamides and trimethoprim-sulfamethoxazole (TMP-SMX) remain important agents in treating respiratory infections. TMP-SMX is active against *H. influenzae* and *S. pneumoniae* and has good clinical efficacy in the treatment of otitis media, sinusitis, bronchitis, and pneumonia. TMP-SMX is particularly useful in infections caused by ampicillin-resistant *H. influenzae.* This combination of agents is the treatment of choice in pneumonia caused by *Pneumo-*

*cystis carinii,* and sulfonamides alone or TMP-SMX are the agents of choice for *N. asteroides.*

The sulfonamides act by competitively inhibiting the bacterial enzyme responsible for the incorporation of *p*-aminobenzoate into dihydropteroic acid, the immediate precursor of folic acid. Trimethoprim competitively inhibits the activity of bacterial dihydrofolate reductase. The usefulness of sulfamethoxazole alone has been diminished by the widespread acquisition of resistance, particularly by many staphylococci, Enterobacteriaceae, *N. meningitidis,* and *P. aeruginosa.* Resistance is usually the result of hyperproduction of paraminobenzoic acid or by the synthesis of a different form of dihydropteroate synthetase that is not susceptible to inhibition by sulfonamide.

TMP-SMX provides synergistic bactericidal activity against many gram-positive and gram-negative organisms. The sulfonamides and TMP-SMX are inactive against anaerobes and have poor activity against *P. aeruginosa, M. pneumoniae,* and *M. tuberculosis.* The combination of TMP-SMX provides activity against a wide array of other pathogenic bacteria. In the respiratory tract this includes activity against *S. aureus, S. pneumoniae, H. influenzae, C. trachomatis, M. catarrhalis, N. asteroides, P. carinii, Pseudomonas pseudomallei, L. monocytogenes, Brucella* species, *Legionella micdadei, Toxoplasma gondii, Mycobacterium kansasii,* and *Mycobacterium scrofulaceum.*

TMP-SMX is available in oral and intravenous forms. An intramuscular form is rarely used because of pain at the injection site. Trimethoprim and the various sulfonamides are well absorbed alone or in combination. A serum ratio (TMP:SMX) of 1:20 provides optimal synergy against most susceptible bacteria.[96] This ratio is achieved by using a fixed oral or intravenous combination of 1:5 (TMP:SMX): 80 mg TMP and 400 mg SMX in single-strength tablets or 5-mL intravenous vials, or 160 mg TMP and 800 mg SMX in double-strength tablets. In tissues, this optimal synergistic ratio is often not preserved, because trimethoprim penetrates tissues to a greater degree. The plasma half-lives of trimethoprim and sulfamethoxazole are approximately 11 and 9 hours, respectively. In renal insufficiency, the dosage should be reduced and the serum sulfonamide level should be monitored whenever the creatinine clearance falls below 30 mL/min.[97]

Adverse effects of TMP-SMX are usually the result of sulfamethoxazole rather than trimethoprim. Common side effects include nausea, vomiting, diarrhea, and hypersensitivity reactions (eg, rash). Less common reactions include fever, headache, and jaundice. Serious adverse reactions are rare but include anaphylaxis, thrombocytopenia, leukopenia, hemolytic anemia, renal insufficiency, erythema nodosum, and erythema multiforme (including Stevens-Johnson syndrome). Side effects occur in as many as 65% of AIDS patients, particularly rashes, cytopenias, and hepatotoxicity.[98–100] The use of sulfonamides should be avoided in pregnancy, in infants younger than 2 years of age because of the risk of kernicterus, and in patients taking methotrexate. TMP-SMX may potentiate the effects of warfarin, tolbutamide, and chlorpropamide.

## ANTIFUNGAL AGENTS

### Amphotericin B

Amphotericin B remains the most reliable antifungal agent available in the treatment of systemic fungal infec-

tions. Despite significant toxicity and the development of newer antifungal agents (imidazoles), amphotericin B remains the standard in the treatment of most deep-seated mycotic infections. Its mechanism of action is thought to include binding of sterol components in the fungal cell membrane, causing altered membrane permeability leading to cytoplasmic leakage, and fungal cell damage secondary to auto-oxidation.[101, 102] Its action can be fungistatic or fungicidal, depending on its concentration. Resistance develops through loss of ergosterol from fungal cell membranes. Until recently, resistance was thought to be limited to *Pseudallescheria boydii* and a few uncommon pathogens. Tolerance has now been described for *Candida parapsilosis,*[103] and resistant strains of *Coccidioides immitis, Candida* species, and *Mucor* have been reported.

Amphotericin remains active against *Candida albicans* and other *Candida* species, *Histoplasma capsulatum, Blastomyces dermatitidis, C. immitis, Cryptococcus neoformans, Aspergillus fumigatus* and other *Aspergillus* species, *Sporothrix schenckii,* and *Mucor* species.[104] In vitro sensitivity does not necessarily predict clinical efficacy. As clinical experience with the newer imidazoles increases, the indications for amphotericin B may decrease.

The pharmacokinetics of amphotericin B are poorly understood. Little is known of the proper dose, dosing schedule, or treatment duration for various infections. The drug does not penetrate body fluids well and does not penetrate the CSF well even in cases of inflammation. No more than 40% of a dose can be accounted for in the serum or extracellular fluid. Apparently, a large portion of the drug is bound tightly to tissues and plasma proteins and is released very slowly. Autopsy studies have revealed fungicidal tissue concentrations in the presence of persistent infection.[105] The half-life is approximately 24 hours, but the terminal half-life is almost 15 days. Blood levels are unaffected by hepatic or renal insufficiency. Administration recommendations are covered adequately elsewhere.

Amphotericin B causes a multitude of side effects, the most serious being nephrotoxicity. Although the renal toxicity is poorly understood, it seems to be the result of proximal and distal tubular damage. The role of renal vasoconstriction remains unclear. Virtually all patients develop some degree of azotemia. Other renal effects include hyposthenuria, renal tubular acidosis, hypokalemia, hypomagnesemia, nephrocalcinosis, pyuria, and cast formation. Azotemia usually reaches a plateau and rarely leads to end-stage renal failure. Other common reactions include fever, chills, rigors, anorexia, nausea, vomiting, headache, phlebitis at the site of intravenous administration, and a normochromic normocytic anemia. Tolerance to the febrile reaction, chills, and rigors occurs over time, and these symptoms may be ameliorated with hydrocortisone, meperidine, or acetaminophen. Rare side effects include thrombocytopenia, leukopenia, rash, anaphylaxis, burning paresthesias, and hepatic dysfunction.

### Flucytosine

Flucytosine is a synthesized fluorinated pyrimidine related to 5-fluorouracil that is rarely used in respiratory infections. It interferes with pyrimidine metabolism to inhibit RNA and protein synthesis. Flucytosine is never adequate

Table 43–10. **Pharmacokinetics of Triazole Agents**

| Drug | Bioavailability (%) | Protein Binding (%) | CNS Penetration (% of Serum) | $T_{1/2}$ (h) | Excretion |
|---|---|---|---|---|---|
| Ketoconazole | 75 | 99 | <10 | 8 | Inactive form in urine or bile |
| Fluconazole | >90 | 11 | 60–80 | 22–30 | 80% unchanged in urine |
| Itraconazole | 79 | 95 | <10 | 17 | Inactive form in urine or bile |

empiric treatment alone, because some fungi are inherently resistant (eg, 5–10% of *C. neoformans,* up to 50% of *C. albicans* serotype B) and resistance develops frequently on therapy.[105]

The antifungal spectrum of flucytosine is narrow, with activity against *Candida* species, *C. neoformans,* some agents of chromomycosis, and *Aspergillus.* Standardized methods are available for testing fungal susceptibility to flucytosine which correlate with clinical efficacy. Its activity in vitro, in combination with amphotericin B, is at least additive against *Candida* species and *Cryptococcus.* Sporadic reports suggest some added benefit against *Aspergillus.*[106, 107] The only clinical trial which has demonstrated greater efficacy and lower toxicity for flucytosine plus amphotericin, compared with amphotericin alone, was in cryptococcal meningitis.

Flucytosine is available in oral formulation only, although it may be obtained in intravenous form through the manufacturer under special circumstances. The drug is 90% absorbed and provides blood levels of 50 to 100 µg/mL if administered in standard doses to patients with normal renal function. Flucytosine is converted to 5-fluorouracil in the gastrointestinal tract, and at flucytosine levels exceeding 100 µg/mL, a therapeutic 5-fluorouracil level results (1 µg/mL).[103] Regular measurement of drug levels is recommended, especially during concomitant amphotericin B administration, because the renal toxicity of amphotericin B leads to accumulation of flucytosine, which can result in bone marrow suppression. Flucytosine penetrates CSF well, producing levels that are 65% to 90% of serum levels. It is excreted unchanged in the urine by glomerular filtration, with a half-life of 3 to 6 hours.

The most important toxicity with flucytosine is myelosuppression, which may include anemia, leukopenia, or thrombocytopenia and is associated with peak serum levels greater than 100 µg/mL. Diarrhea, nausea, and vomiting are common. Elevated liver function tests are less common.

## Ketoconazole

Ketoconazole was the first oral imidazole to be made available, and it has a broad spectrum of activity against many respiratory fungal pathogens. Its role in antifungal therapy will probably diminish after clinical trials with fluconazole and itraconazole are completed. It acts like other imidazoles by blocking the synthesis of ergosterol, causing a defective fungal cell membrane.

Ketoconazole provides good in vitro activity against many *Candida* species, *B. dermatitidis, H. capsulatum, Paracoccidioides brasiliensis, C. immitis,* and *C. neoformans.* Its in vitro activity is inadequate against many isolates of *Candida tropicalis, Candida glabrata, Sporothrix* species, and *P. boydii.* It is inactive against *Aspergillus* and

*Mucor.*[108] Its in vivo activity against most fungi is fungistatic.

Ketoconazole is available in oral formulation only. Several of its pharmacokinetic features are less favorable compared with the newer imidazoles (Table 43–10). In contrast to fluconazole, CSF penetration is very poor.[105] Ketoconazole is inadequate treatment for any meningeal fungal disease. Gastric acidity is necessary for absorption; antacids and $H_2$-blockers are contraindicated during treatment with ketoconazole.

Ketoconazole is associated with significantly more side effects than itraconazole or fluconazole. Nausea, vomiting, and anorexia occur commonly and are dose dependent.[108, 109] Abdominal pain (which often resolves on therapy or if the drug is taken with food) and pruritus occur in 1% to 2% of patients. Hepatotoxicity, rarely severe, with elevated transaminases and alkaline phosphatase, occurs in 1% to 5%. Ketoconazole causes a dose-dependent suppression of testosterone and adrenocorticotropic hormone-stimulated cortisol response. This effect is manifested by impotence, gynecomastia, oligospermia, decreased libido, menstrual abnormalities, and rarely, symptomatic adrenal insufficiency.[110]

## Miconazole

Miconazole is a synthetic imidazole with broad activity against virtually all pathogenic fungi except *Aspergillus* and *Phycomycetes.* Clinical studies with miconazole have been limited, and comparison trials with amphotericin B have not been done. In the respiratory tract, its sole indication is in the treatment of pseudoallescheriaisis, for which it is considered the drug of choice. Intravenous treatment has been complicated by a multitude of side effects. These include local phlebitis, rash, pruritus, nausea, fevers, chills, anemia, thrombocytosis, hyponatremia, and hyperlipidemia. Less common side effects include drowsiness, headache, blurred vision, diarrhea, and anxiety. Tachycardia, cardiac arrhythmias, anaphylaxis, and cardiac arrest have occurred rarely and are thought to be related to the use of too concentrated preparations or too rapid infusion of the drug.[105]

## Fluconazole

The precise role of fluconazole in the management of fungal pulmonary infections is not yet defined. It may prove useful in patients with pulmonary candidiasis, cryptococcosis, blastomycosis, histoplasmosis, or coccidioidomycosis. Early data suggest that fluconazole has little role in pulmonary aspergillosis. Fluconazole seems to have significant promise in the treatment of *C. neoformans* and *C. immitis* meningitis. It has currently been approved for use in serious *Candida* infections, particularly oropharyngeal and esophageal candidiasis, and cryptococcal meningitis. Like other azole derivatives, fluconazole exerts it effect through the inhibition of fungal cytochrome P450 enzymes. These enzymes are necessary for the demethylation of 14-alpha-methylsterols to form ergosterol. Unlike ketoconazole, fluconazole has a minimal effect on mammalian enzymes and should not be implicated in toxicity related to steroid hormone production.

In vitro susceptibility testing for antifungal agents has never had a well-defined clinical role, because results have not correlated well with clinical efficacy. In vivo models are often preferred to assess efficacy of antifungal agents. For fluconazole, the in vitro MIC for an organism is generally much higher than might be anticipated from a clinically effective antifungal.[111–114] Fluconazole was shown to be 16 times less active in vitro against *C. albicans* than ketoconazole, even though it was 24 times more effective in an in vitro model using the same organism.[115] A similar discrepancy for fluconazole between in vitro activity and clinical efficacy was shown to exist for *H. capsulatum*.[112, 113] In vitro tests for fluconazole are poorly standardized, and results vary according to medium composition, pH, and size of the starting inoculum.[116] Studies in animal models have shown improved survival of animals challenged with a lethal inoculum of *Candida, Cryptococcus, Aspergillus, Blastomyces, Coccidioides,* or *Histoplasma.*[117]

Fluconazole possesses several unique pharmacokinetic properties. These include water solubility, excellent sputum and CSF penetration (with and without inflammation), a prolonged half-life (30 hours), and low protein binding (11%).[118, 119] In contrast to itraconazole and ketoconazole, fluconazole is metabolically stable and is renally excreted, with more than 80% of the administered dose recovered from the urine unchanged. Dose reduction is required in renal insufficiency. Fluconazole is available in oral and intravenous preparations. It is well absorbed orally, with bioavailability exceeding 90%.[120] In contrast to ketoconazole, absorption is not diminished in patients taking antacids or H$_2$-blockers.

Fluconazole is well tolerated. The most common side effects are nausea, vomiting, abdominal pain, diarrhea, and headache. In contrast to ketoconazole, fluconazole does not seem to affect testicular and adrenal steroid production. Hepatoxicity, occasionally severe but usually consisting of transient mild transaminase elevation, has been reported. Exfoliative skin reactions have been seen rarely. Patients on phenytoin, cyclosporin, oral hypoglycemics, and oral anticoagulants should be monitored closely, because the metabolism of these drugs may be reduced by fluconazole.

## Itraconazole

Itraconazole is a new triazole antifungal agent with broad-spectrum antifungal activity. Compared with ketoconazole, it is more potent, has a broader spectrum of activity in vitro and in vivo, and is less toxic.[121–123] The primary advantage of itraconazole over fluconazole is its greater activity against aspergillus. Its role in the treatment of respiratory fungal infections has yet to be defined. Like other antifungal azoles, it acts by binding fungal cyto-chrome P450 enzymes to inhibit ergosterol synthesis. Unlike ketoconazole, itraconazole has no significant effect on mammalian cytochrome P450 and no significant effect on testicular and adrenal hormone production.

Itraconazole has demonstrated good in vitro activity against a broad range of yeasts, molds, and dimorphic fungi, including dermatophytes (eg, microsporum, trichophyton, and epidermophyton species), yeasts (eg, *Candida* and *C. neoformans*), dimorphic fungi (eg, *H. capsulatum, P. brasiliensis, B. dermatitidis,* and *S. schenckii*) and *A. fumigatus.* Itraconazole seems to be 5 to 100 times more active than ketoconazole, and, unlike ketoconazole, it is active against *Aspergillus* species, *S. schenckii,* and meningeal cryptococcosis. In vitro results vary with the culture medium, inoculum size, and conditions of incubation. Clinical responses have been reported with aspergillosis, coccidioidomycosis, sporotrichosis, blastomycosis, and histoplasmosis.[124–127]

Itraconazole's oral absorption is variable but is improved with meals and reduced by decreased gastric acidity. It is widely distributed in tissue, and tissue concentrations may exceed plasma concentrations 10-fold. Penetration into CSF is poor. Itraconazole is highly protein bound (95%), is lipophilic, and undergoes extensive hepatic metabolism before being excreted in inactive form in the urine and bile. No dose adjustment is required in renal insufficiency. Insufficient data exist concerning dose adjustment in hepatic insufficiency. The elimination half-life ranges from 20 hours after a single dose to 30 hours after 2 to 4 weeks of therapy. Itraconazole is available in oral form only.

Itraconazole is well tolerated. Mild gastrointestinal side effects predominate. No effect on androgen or cortisol metabolism was demonstrated at doses up to 400 mg/d.[128] At a high dose (600 mg/d), 1 of 8 patients developed evidence of adrenal insufficiency.[124] Other reported side effects include mild, reversible liver function test abnormalities, dizziness, headache, pruritus, edema, hypertension, and hypokalemia.[129] Rifampin may lower serum levels, and cyclosporine levels may be increased by itraconazole.[123]

## ANTIVIRALS

### Acyclovir

There are only a few clinical uses for acyclovir in respiratory tract infections. Its main indications include herpes simplex tracheobronchitis, herpes simplex pneumonitis, and varicella pneumonia. It is an acyclic guanosine nucleoside analog that inhibits DNA synthesis through a complex mechanism. Acyclovir initially is phosphorylated by viral thymidine kinase. It then inhibits viral DNA polymerase and competes with guanosine triphosphate as a substrate for this enzyme. In vitro resistance is mediated by changes in thymidine kinase or DNA polymerase.[130] In vivo resistance is usually the result of thymidine kinase-deficient isolates and is usually seen in immunocompromised patients who have received multiple courses of therapy. Resistant isolates of herpes simplex have been an increasing problem in AIDS patients.

Acyclovir provides good in vitro activity against most isolates of herpes simplex virus (HSV) types I and II and varicella-zoster virus (VZV).[131] It is much less active against Epstein-Barr virus (EBV) and cytomegalovirus (CMV). Clinical trials have failed to establish any clear benefit from the use of acyclovir in the treatment of CMV pneumonitis.[132, 133] Acyclovir is less active in vitro against HSV type I than HSV type II. In one trial, acyclovir was shown to be superior to vidarabine in the treatment of severe VZV infections in immunocompromised patients.[134]

Acyclovir is available in oral and intravenous formulations. The pharmacokinetic features include low oral bioavailability (15–20%), a half-life of 2 to 3 hours with normal renal function, and good CSF levels (50% of serum levels). Acyclovir is excreted renally, with 80% excreted unchanged. Dose adjustment is necessary in cases of renal insufficiency.

The most important adverse effects of acyclovir are a reversible nephrotoxicity and neurotoxicity. Nephrotoxicity seems to be limited to patients undergoing intravenous therapy. Acyclovir crystallizes in the renal tubules. Risk factors include high doses, rapid infusion, preexisting renal insufficiency, and dehydration.[131] CNS effects include lightheadedness, delirium, tremors, lethargy, seizures, and confusion. Other side effects include nausea, vomiting, and rash.

## Vidarabine

Vidarabine has little or no role in the treatment of viral respiratory infections. It has largely been replaced in clinical use by acyclovir, which has a lower toxicity profile and superior clinical efficacy. The spectrum of activity of vidabarine in vitro includes HSV types I and II, VZV, EBV, vaccinia and variola viruses, rhabdo viruses, and some RNA tumor viruses. Its activity against CMV is variable. Toxicity is primarily gastrointestinal and neurologic. It is not recommended as a first-line therapeutic agent in the respiratory tract.

## Ganciclovir

The role of ganciclovir, an acyclic nucleoside analog of guanine, in the treatment of CMV pneumonitis has yet to be defined. Clinical efficacy has been demonstrated only in CMV retinitis and CMV colitis. CMV retinitis in immunocompromised patients remains the only approved indication for ganciclovir. Ganciclovir acts by competitively inhibiting DNA polymerase by preventing the binding of deoxyguanosine triphosphate to DNA polymerase. Ganciclovir-resistant strains of CMV have been reported rarely[135–137] and are largely related to mutations in viral DNA polymerase genes. In resistant isolates, cross-resistance to other antivirals is common. Ganciclovir-resistant strains of CMV may become more prevalent as ganciclovir use increases.

Ganciclovir has in vitro activity against all herpesviruses and is particularly active against CMV. In vitro inhibitory concentrations are much lower than those of acyclovir against CMV and slightly lower against HSV.[138, 139] Activity against VZV is similar to that of acyclovir. Acyclovir remains the drug of choice for herpes simplex and varicella infection of the respiratory tract, based on lower toxicity and comparable in vitro activity. Despite good in vitro

activity against CMV, successful therapy for CMV pneumonitis is rare. CMV pneumonia has a particularly ominous prognosis in bone marrow transplant patients. In one study of 10 bone marrow allograft recipients with biopsy-proven CMV pneumonia treated with ganciclovir, CMV was eliminated from respiratory secretions after a median of 8 days of therapy; however, only 1 of 10 patients survived the pneumonia.[139] The results in other series have been slightly better. In one study, 5 of 11 patients improved, but only 3 of 11 patients survived for more than 100 days after transplant.[140] In another series, 8 of 21 patients survived past 90 days, but they were concomitantly treated with CMV immunoglobulin.[141] In this study 2 additional patients responded to ganciclovir; 1 patient relapsed after 60 days with fatal CMV pneumonia, and the other died of disseminated aspergillosis. Another study showed improved survival in patients treated with a combination of ganciclovir and CMV immunoglobulin; 13 of 25 patients survived the initial episode of CMV pneumonitis.[142] Solid organ transplant patients with CMV pneumonia fare somewhat better, with survival as high as 60%.[140, 143] Generally, survival seems to be improved in patients treated early and before intubation.

Ganciclovir is available in intravenous form only. In patients with normal renal function, its half-life is 3 to 4 hours. Compared with acyclovir, it has a narrow therapeutic range. It is excreted unmetabolized by the kidney and must be dose-adjusted for a creatinine clearance less than 50 mL/min. It achieves lung tissue levels that are 99% of serum levels. Ganciclovir triphosphate persists in CMV-infected cells for several days after the drug has been removed from cell culture supernatants.[144]

The most limiting side effects of ganciclovir are neutropenia (40% of patients) and thrombocytopenia (20%), which are usually reversible. These effects are dose-related and are particularly common in AIDS patients on zidovudine. Granulocyte-macrophage colony-stimulating factor may prove helpful in alleviating problems with neutropenia. Other adverse effects include nausea, vomiting, anorexia, elevated liver function tests, anemia, rash, confusion, eosinophilia, obstructive uropathy, and in animal models, inhibition of spermatogenesis.

## Foscarnet

Foscarnet is an inorganic pyrophosphate analog that has an undefined role in the treatment of certain viral respiratory infections. It acts to inhibit herpesvirus DNA polymerases and retroviral reverse transcriptases. Clinically, it has shown efficacy in the treatment of CMV retinitis in AIDS patients unresponsive to ganciclovir or in certain HSV infections resistant to acyclovir. In the respiratory tract, it may prove to have efficacy in CMV pneumonitis, HSV tracheobronchitis, and HSV pneumonitis. Resistance to foscarnet has not been a problem with CMV in clinical isolates or in vitro. Resistant mutants of HSV have been readily produced in vitro and are related to changes in viral DNA polymerase.[145]

Foscarnet has in vitro activity against most herpesviruses, including CMV, and human immunodeficiency virus (HIV). It has been useful in severe HSV infections resistant to acyclovir.[146] Foscarnet may prove to have some efficacy in CMV pneumonitis. CMV excretion is decreased in patients receiving foscarnet for CMV pneumonitis; however, viral replication resumes as early as 3 days after cessation of therapy.[143] In CMV pneumonia, experience with foscarnet is greatest in bone marrow and renal transplant patients. Survival has been reported in 2 marrow transplant patients treated with foscarnet in one study; however, no survivors were reported in a series of 14 marrow transplant patients who received foscarnet for CMV pneumonia.[143] Many of these patients were treated late and had other complications that may have contributed to their deaths. There have been reports of renal and liver transplant patients surviving CMV pneumonia after treatment with foscarnet.[143]

Foscarnet is available in intravenous form only. Intermittent infusion has been shown to be adequate and to minimize nephrotoxicity, but the optimal dosing regimen has not been defined. It is excreted unmetabolized in the urine by glomerular filtration and tubular secretion, with a half-life of 3 to 6 hours. Approximately 20% is deposited in bones, which may account for some of its effect on serum calcium and phosphorous.

An advantage of foscarnet over ganciclovir is that it does not suppress the granulocyte count. Nephrotoxicity secondary to acute tubular necrosis is the most limiting side effect. A twofold to threefold rise in serum creatinine occurs in up to 45% of patients.[145] Nausea and vomiting occur in 20% to 30%. Anemia occurs in 20% to 50%. Hypercalcemia and hyperphosphatemia have been reported in as many as 66% of patients.[145] Other side effects include malaise, hypocalcemia, phlebitis, elevated transaminases, headache, seizure, tremor, irritability, hallucinations, and penile ulceration. Concomitant therapy with pentamidine is contraindicated because of additive nephrotoxicity.

## Amantadine and Rimantadine

Amantadine and rimantadine are antiviral agents with proven efficacy against influenza A infections. Only amantadine has gained approval for use in the United States, although rimantadine may be better tolerated. Rimantadine, an analog of amantadine, offers several advantages over amantadine, including a longer half-life, lower CNS toxicity, greater activity against influenza A, and higher secretion concentrations. These agents are similar with respect to mechanism, spectrum of activity, and clinical indications. Although their precise mechanisms remain unclear, they seem to act by preventing viral uncoating after the virus enters the cell. Resistance occurs in a small percentage of treated patients.[147, 148] Resistance is readily achieved in vitro by the serial passage of virus through media containing amantadine or rimantadine. Isolates developing resistance to one agent develop cross-resistance to the other.

Amantadine and rimantadine have clinical efficacy only against influenza A. Neither agent has activity against influenza B. Although high concentrations have some inhibitory effect against influenza C, rubella-causing togavirus, Sendai virus, paramyxovirus, and arenavirus, these concentrations are too high to be clinically useful. Rimantadine is 3 to 4 times more active against influenza A than is amantadine. In young patients, these agents have been shown to reduce

fever and symptoms of influenza A by 50% if treatment is begun within 48 hours of the onset of illness.[149, 150] These patients have more rapid resolution of pulmonary function abnormalities and reduced viral shedding, and college students have returned to class more rapidly.[149, 150] In the elderly, studies demonstrate more rapid defervescence among treated patients but no significant effect on other symptoms.[151, 152] In one rimantadine study, elderly patients in the highest risk group did have significant improvement in symptoms.[151] In the prevention of influenza A, most studies have demonstrated a 50% to 70% reduced incidence of clinical cases.[153] Candidates for amantadine prophylaxis include high-risk contacts of index cases, those who are vaccinated after an outbreak of influenza and before the 2-week period necessary to form antibody elapses,[154] young children, elderly persons, those with underlying pulmonary or cardiac problems, nursing home populations, unvaccinated adults older than 65 years of age, adults with immunodeficiencies, and unvaccinated at-risk adults such as medical personnel.

Amantadine and rimantadine are available only in oral form. Serum levels are higher with amantadine, but rimantadine achieves higher concentrations in secretions.[151] The half-life of rimantadine exceeds that of amantadine (30 hours versus 15 hours).[153] Amantadine is excreted unmetabolized in the urine by glomerular filtration and tubular secretion. Dosage must be reduced in renal insufficiency. In the elderly, a 50% reduction is recommended. Rimantadine is excreted as a hydroxylated metabolite in the urine.

Clinical use of amantadine has gained slow acceptance in the medical community, partly because of its side effects. Side effects are dose related, and approximately 10% of patients have adverse effects at 200 mg/d. The most important side effect is neurotoxicity, including insomnia, difficulty concentrating, anxiety, lightheadedness, depression, confusion, lethargy, and seizures. In the elderly, confusion can lead to falls. The gastrointestinal effects are more common with rimantadine and include nausea, vomiting, and anorexia, which occurred in 10% of elderly patients in one study.[151]

## Interferons

The interferons continue to have an undefined role in the treatment and prophylaxis of viral respiratory infections. They are cytokines produced by leukocytes and fibroblasts in response to viral infection or other stimuli. They have no virucidal activity but inhibit viral protein synthesis through a complex mechanism. They also act as immunomodulators, with effects on T-cell–mediated cytotoxicity, natural killer cell activity, antibody synthesis, and macrophage function.[155]

Interferons-$\alpha$, -$\beta$ and -$\gamma$ have in vitro activity against a broad range of respiratory viruses (except adenovirus), including DNA and RNA viruses. In the respiratory tract, intranasal interferon-$\alpha$ has demonstrated efficacy in preventing colds if given prophylactically to family members of an index case. Several studies have demonstrated an approximately 80% reduction in rhinovirus-related colds and a 40% reduction in colds in general if the drug is given within 48 hours of symptoms in the index case.[156, 157] Long-term daily prophylaxis has been associated with prohibitive toxicity.[158] Intranasal interferon-α2 has been ineffective therapeutically in established rhinovirus colds.[159] Evidence suggesting some efficacy of intranasal interferon against experimentally induced influenza A and coronaviruses was not confirmed in further studies.[160, 161]

Interferons are available in intravenous, intramuscular, subcutaneous, and topical forms. Little is understood of their pharmacokinetics, metabolism, or optimal dosing schedules.

Parenteral interferon is associated with dose-dependent fever and bone marrow suppression. Toxicity also includes gastrointestinal complaints, weight loss, parasthesias, fatigue, and confusion. A flu-like illness consisting of fever, headache, malaise, chills, and lymphopenia may occur 2 to 4 hours after a dose. Intranasal therapy is associated with sore throat, hoarseness, nasal burning, increased nasal secretions, mucosal friability, bleeding, and ulcerations. A major problem in the further development of interferons for use in the respiratory tract is balancing clinical efficacy against toxicity.

## PHARMACOKINETICS OF ANTIMICROBIALS IN RESPIRATORY INFECTION SITES

Antimicrobial levels vary considerably at different sites in the respiratory tract. The concentration of an antimicrobial at a specific site is dependent on many factors, including serum concentration, lipid solubility, protein binding to serum and tissue site proteins, ionization state, active and passive transport mechanisms, extravascular site geometry (ie, surface area to volume ratio), and the degree of inflammation.[162] A serum level that exceeds the MIC or MBC of an organism does not necessarily assure an inhibitory or bactericidal concentration at the site of infection. Tables 43–11 through 43–15 contain representative data for antibiotic concentrations in sputum and bronchial secretions, in lung tissue, in infected and noninfected pleural fluid, in sinus secretions, and within cells.[163] Data not previously available for ofloxacin, azithromycin, and clarithromycin have been included.[67, 71, 75, 77, 163–165] These tables demonstrate that site antibiotic concentration is usually a small fraction of that obtained in the serum. The details of tissue penetration are beyond the scope of this discussion, but some of the pertinent clinical points are addressed.

After systemic administration, antimicrobials are bound to serum proteins, particularly albumin, or remain free. Only free antibiotic is available for tissue penetration or to exert an antimicrobial effect. In general, dosing regimens that produce high free serum concentrations favor tissue penetration because of the high concentration gradient from serum to interstitial fluid in the tissue. Aminoglycosides kill organisms rapidly, possess a prolonged PAE against aerobic or facultative gram-negative rods, and are associated with increased toxicity with elevated trough levels. For these agents, the serum level after intermittent dosing can be allowed to drop below the lethal level for the bacteria without a loss of efficacy. By contrast, most β-lactams kill slowly, are characterized by a lag time to onset of killing, and do not exhibit a PAE against gram-negative bacilli. For

β-lactam antibiotics, it is more important to maintain serum concentrations above the MIC of treated organisms.

Antibiotics that are highly protein bound have lower free drug levels and diffuse into interstitial fluids more slowly. With low serum protein binding, higher free drug levels are available for diffusion into tissues, resulting in more rapid tissue levels. The ultimate drug concentration achieved at an extravascular site is dependent on the protein content of the extravascular fluid; highly bound drugs achieve higher concentrations in fluids with high protein content. In general, serum protein binding plays a minor role in extravascular tissue fluid concentrations except when more than 90% of an antibiotic is bound to serum proteins. The importance of protein binding with respect to clinical outcome is minimal, and an effect is seen only if the free drug levels are below the concentration needed to inhibit or kill the organisms. There is evidence that agents that are highly protein bound, such as cefonicid (98% protein bound), are impaired in their ability to cure S. aureus endocarditis because the free drug level fails to exceed the MIC of S. aureus.[166]

In the lung, there are two important barriers to tissue penetration by antibiotics: the blood-bronchus barrier (between bronchial capillary and bronchial wall) and the blood-alveolar barrier (between alveolar capillary and alveolus). Lipid-soluble antimicrobials such as chloramphenicol, doxycycline, minocycline, erythromycin, clarithromycin, azithromycin, and clindamycin penetrate tissues more readily than lipid insoluble antibiotics such as the β-lactams and aminoglycosides. Aminoglycosides penetrate cell membranes slowly but become bound intracellularly to lysosomes and mitochondria, which allows accumulation leading to nephrotoxicity and ototoxicity.[167] After an antibiotic crosses a membrane, it can bind to extracellular and cellular proteins. Drugs that are highly bound to serum proteins also bind to extracellular proteins, resulting in high concentrations, particularly if the extravascular albumin concentrations is high. β-lactams are bound primarily to extracellular serum proteins, and quinolones are primarily bound intracellularly.[167]

The degree of local inflammation exerts important influence on the ability of an antibiotic to penetrate biological membranes. Antibiotic dependence on inflammation for extravascular tissue penetration is inversely related to lipid solubility. Inflammation-independent antibiotics are generally highly lipid soluble and include chloramphenicol, the macrolides, clindamycin, the tetracyclines, the quinolones, and TMP-SMX. Inflammation-dependent antibiotics include the penicillins, cephalosporins, aminoglycosides, carbapenems, and monobactams. These latter agents are relatively lipid-insoluble.[168] As an infectious process improves, the tissue concentration of an inflammation-dependent antibiotic may decline. In clinical practice, the inflammation dependence of an antibiotic is rarely a consideration in choosing an antibiotic.

Disease may change the character of any of the major factors influencing tissue penetration to cause an increase or decrease in membrane permeability. The complexities of tissue penetration make it evident that the precise concentration of an antibiotic at an infected tissue site is not highly predictable. Most clinical studies of tissue penetration do not simulate the conditions in infected or damaged tissues. It is assumed that extravascular site concentration is corre-

Table 43–11. **Antimicrobial Concentrations in Sputum and Bronchial Secretions***

| Antimicrobial | Administration Method | Dose (g) | No. of Patients | Serum Concentration Mean (Range) | Site Concentration Mean (Range) | Time Site Specimen Obtained (h) | Ratio of Site/ Serum (%) | Notes |
|---|---|---|---|---|---|---|---|---|
| Aminoglycosides | | | | | | | | |
| Amikacin | IM | 7.5 mg/kg (M) | 6 | 20.7 ($\pm$2.7 SD) | 4.4 ($\pm$.75 SD) | 4 | 21 | I,B |
| Gentamicin | IM | 2.8 mg/kg (S) | 4 | 3.0 | 0.3 | 2.0 | 10 | I,B |
| Netilmicin | IV | 7.5 mg/kg (S) | 10 | 3.3 ($\pm$0.3 SD) | 0.6 ($\pm$0.1 SD) | 1–8 | 18 | I,B |
| Tobramycin | IV | 2–3.5 mg/kg (S) | 7 | 3.6 (1.9–6.0) | 0.7 (0.2–2.2) | 2–8 | 20 | I,B,P |
| Cephalosporins and related β-lactams | | | | | | | | |
| Cefazolin | IV | 1.0 (S) | 9 | 100 ($\pm$30 SD) | 2.3 ($\pm$0.5 SD) | 0–2 | 2 | I,SP |
| Cephradine | PO | 1.0 (S) | 8 | 7.8 | 1.3 | 2–3.3 | 20 | I,B |
| Cefuroxime | IM | 0.75 (M) | 4 | 17.3 (14–25) | 2.4 (1.4–4.8) | 1.0 | 14 | I,B |
| Cefoxitin | IV | 2.0 (S) | 36 | 13.9 | 1.6 | 1.0 | 11 | I,B |
| Cefotaxime | IV | 2.0 (S) | 10 | 26.7 (24.5–29) | 2.6 (2.0–3.2) | 2 | 10 | I,B |
| Ceftizoxime | IV | 2.0 (S) | 8 | 109 ($\pm$45 SD) | 4.3 ($\pm$4.3 SD) | 2.6 | 4 | I,SP |
| Ceftriaxone | IV | 2.0 (S) | 22 | 43 (22–80) | 1.9 (0–6.5) | 3 | 2 | I,B |
| Ceftazidime | IV | 2.0 (S) | 8 | 32 ($\pm$6.1 SD) | 5.6 ($\pm$4.1 SD) | 2 | 18 | I,B |
| Aztreonam | IV | 2.0 (S) | 9 | 39 (12–69) | 4.2 (0.04–14.1) | 2 | 21 | I,B |
| Imipenem | IV | 1.0 (S) | 8 | 10.5 ($\pm$6.9 SD) | 2.1 ($\pm$1.0 SD) | 2 | 20 | U,B |
| Penicillins | | | | | | | | |
| Amoxicillin | PO | 0.5 (M) | 22 | 11.0 (<2->16) | 0.5 (<0.12->1) | 2–3 | 5 | I,SP,P |
| Ampicillin | PO | 1.0 (M) | 20 | 5.5 (3.5–9.8) | 0.25 (0–0.5) | 0–24 | 5 | I,SP |
| Carbenicillin | IV | 5.0 (S) | 12 | 463 ($\pm$89 SD) | 3.4 ($\pm$0.4 SD) | 0–2 | 1 | I,SP |
| Piperacillin | IV | 2.0 (M) | 18 | 101 | 3.6 | 2 | 4 | I,B |
| Ticarcillin | IV | 5.0 (S) | 11 | 469 ($\pm$65 SD) | 4.1 ($\pm$1.0 SD) | 0–2 | 1 | I,SP |
| Quinolones | | | | | | | | |
| Ciprofloxacin | PO | 0.50 (M) | 34 | 3.8 (2.0–7.5) | 1.0 | 2 | 26 | I,SP,AUC |
| Enoxacin | PO | 0.6 (S) | 15 | 3.2 | 3.1 | 3 | 95 | I,E |
| Ofloxacin | PO | 0.2 (M) | 15 | 3.9 (2.3–8.2) | 4.5 (1.3–15) | 2 | 115 | I |
| Pefloxacin | PO | 0.4 (S) | 30 | 5.1 | 4.6 | Peak | 89 | I,E,AUC |
| Tetracyclines | | | | | | | | |
| Doxycycline | PO | 0.1 (S) | 10 | 2.3 (1.1–4.4) | 0.4 (0.4–0.6) | 2–3 | 17 | I,SP |
| Minocycline | PO | 0.1 (S) | 11 | 4.5 (2.7–8.7) | 1.1 (0.4–2.6) | 2–3 | 24 | I,SP |
| Tetracycline | PO | 0.25 (S) | 12 | 4.0 (1.2–10) | 1.2 (0.3–2.3) | 4–5 | 30 | I,SP |
| Others | | | | | | | | |
| Clindamycin | PO | 0.3 (S) | 24 | 2.7 | 1.6 (0.3–4.8) | 2–4 | 60 | B |
| Erythromycin | PO | 1.0 (M) | 8 | 4.4 ($\pm$1.6 SD) | 1.1 ($\pm$0.5 SD) | 2 | 25 | I,B |
| Azithromycin[75] | PO | 0.25 (M) | 21 | 0.63 ($\pm$0.52) | 3.66 ($\pm$2.4) | 2–24 | 580 | I,SP |
| Clarithromycin[163] | PO | 0.25 (M) | 12 | 2.67 ($\pm$0.6) | 4.22 ($\pm$1.51) | NA | 158 | I,SP |
| 14-OH clarithromycin[163] | PO | 0.25 (M) | 12 | 1.23 ($\pm$0.21) | 1.89 ($\pm$0.63) | NA | 153 | I,SP |
| Trimethoprim | PO | 0.16 (M) | 10 | 2.6 | 4.51 | 3–7 | 173 | I,SP |
| Sulfamethoxazole | PO | 0.8 (M) | 6 | 58 | 12.4 | 3–7 | 20 | I,SP |

*AUC, area under the serum and sputum curve used to calculate penetration; B, bronchial secretions; E, extrapolated from graphs; I, infected; M, multiple dose; NA, not available; P, pneumonia; S, single dose; SP, sputum; U, uninfected.

Adapted from Gerding DN, Peterson LR, Hughes CE, et al: Extravascular antimicrobial distribution and the respective blood concentrations in humans. *In* Lorian V (ed): Antibiotics in Laboratory Medicine, ed 3. Baltimore, Williams & Wilkins, 1991:900–903.

lated with clinical efficacy, but this has been difficult to prove conclusively because serum levels usually parallel tissue levels. The advent of the new azalide antimicrobial, azithromycin, which has low serum and high tissue (cellular) levels, should permit better evaluation of the clinical importance of tissue levels.

Neutrophil and alveolar macrophage antimicrobial levels may be important in the treatment of respiratory infections caused by intracellular pathogens such as *L. pneumophila*, *C. pneumoniae*, *M. pneumoniae*, *M. tuberculosis*, *P. multocida*, *L. monocytogenes*, *Salmonella*, and *H. influenzae*. The antimicrobial concentrations within neutrophils and alveolar macrophages are displayed in Table 43–15.[162] Lipid-insoluble antibiotics, such as the penicillins, cephalosporins, aminoglycosides, and imipenem, penetrate neutrophils poorly. Alveolar macrophage levels for most β-lactams and

aminoglycosides are only 10% of serum levels.[169] Certain antibiotics, such as clindamycin, the tetracyclines, the quinolones, the macrolides, and chloramphenicol, are concentrated within alveolar macrophages to attain levels that exceed those found in serum or lung tissue.

It has been difficult to correlate intracellular antibiotic concentrations with killing or clinical efficacy.[170] Some antibiotics are active in vitro against intracellular pathogens but are clinically ineffective because of poor cellular penetration. Other agents seem to penetrate phagocytic cells adequately but are inactive intracellularly despite good in vitro activity. For instance, certain penicillins and cephalosporins exhibit in vitro activity against *L. pneumophila* but have never demonstrated clinical efficacy in legionellosis. This lack of efficacy may reflect poor penetration into phagocytes. It is likely that the clinical efficacy of erythro-

Table 43–12. **Antimicrobial Concentrations in Lung Tissue***

| Antimicrobial | Administration Method | Dose (g) | No. of Patients | Serum Concentration Mean (Range) | Site Concentration Mean (Range) | Time Site Specimen Obtained (h) | Ratio of Site/ Serum (%) | Notes |
|---|---|---|---|---|---|---|---|---|
| Aminoglycosides | | | | | | | | |
|   Amikacin | IM | 0.5 (S) | 10 | 20.7 ($\pm$1.5 SE) | 8.3 ($\pm$1.0 SE) | 0.8–1.5 | 40 | SR |
| Cephalosporins and related $\beta$-lactams | | | | | | | | |
|   Cefadroxil | PO | 1.0 (S) | 22 | 11.5 ($\pm$1.3 SD) | 7.4 ($\pm$0.7 SD) | 2–4 | 64 | SR |
|   Cefamandole | IV | 2.0 (S) | 6 | 23.1 ($\pm$9.4 SD) | 18.1 ($\pm$9.7 SD) | 1–2 | 78 | SR |
|   Cefoxitin | IV | 1.0 (S) | 11 | 23.7 (14–42) | 10.0 (7–12) | 2 | 46 | SR,C |
|   Cefoperozone | IV | 2.0 (S) | 10 | 97 (44–149) | 45 (21–68) | 2 | 46 | SR,C |
|   Ceftriaxone | IV | 2.0 (S) | 13 | 127 ($\pm$17.6 SD) | 57.4 ($\pm$13.3 SD) | 1–2 | 45 | SR |
|   Imipenem | IV | 1.0 (S) | 10 | 20 ($\pm$4) | 12 ($\pm$9) | 1.0 | 60 | SR,E |
| Penicillins | | | | | | | | |
|   Amoxicillin | PO | 0.5 (M) | 10 | 3.3 (2.0–7.1) | 3.1 (0.6–5.8) | 3 | 94 | SR |
|   Oxacillin | IM | 0.5 (S) | 9 | 11.9 (6.6–16.2) | 2.4 (0.5–4.4) | 1 | 20 | SR |
|   Piperacillin | IV | 2.0 (M) | 6 | 85.2 (54–108) | 25.4 (5.7–57) | 0.5–0.75 | 30 | T |
| Quinolones | | | | | | | | |
|   Ciprofloxacin | PO | 0.75 (S) | 10 | 2.0 | 4.9 ($\pm$1.7 SD) | 3.4 | 275 | T |
|   Ofloxacin[164] | PO | 0.2 (S) | 10 | 0.85 $\pm$ 0.23 | 2.17 $\pm$ 0.5 | 3–8 | 255 | SR |
|   Ofloxacin[165] | PO | 0.6 (S) | 11 | 8.7 $\pm$ 4.2 | 17.7 $\pm$ 9.2 | 0.9–3.5 | 203 | SR,C |
| Tetracyclines | | | | | | | | |
|   Tetracycline $PO_4$ | PO | 0.5 (M) | 6 | 3.9 (1.9–7.6) | 2.1 (0–3.6) | >3 | 54 | SR,C |
| Macrolides | | | | | | | | |
|   Erythromycin | | | | | | | | |
|     Stearate | PO | 0.5 (M) | 14 | 3.1 | 4.7 (3.3–6.4) | 3–4 | 152 | SR |
|   Clarithromycin[71] | PO | 0.5 (M) | 53 | 2.51 $\pm$ 0.87 | 17.47 $\pm$ 3.29 | 4 | 696 | SR |
| Trimethoprim | PO | 0.2 (M) | 31 | 2.7 (0.7–11) | 10.9 (2–34) | 11–15 | 403 | SR |

*SR, surgical resection; C, lung tissue corrected for hemoglobin concentration; E, data extrapolated from graphs; T, transbronchial biopsy; S, single dose; M, multiple dose.
Adapted from Gerding DN, Peterson LR, Hughes CE, et al: Extravascular antimicrobial distribution and the respective blood concentrations in humans. *In* Lorian V (ed): Antibiotics in Laboratory Medicine, ed 3. Baltimore, Williams & Wilkins, 1991:880.

Table 43–13. **Antimicrobial Concentrations in Pleural Fluid***

| Antimicrobial | Administration Method | Dose (g) | No. of Patients | Serum Concentration Mean (Range) | Site Concentration Mean (Range) | Time Site Specimen Obtained (h) | Ratio of Site/ Serum (%) | Notes |
|---|---|---|---|---|---|---|---|---|
| Aminoglycosides | | | | | | | | |
|   Amikacin | IV | 7.5 mg/kg (S) | 10 | 27.6 ($\pm$2.0) | 11.0 ($\pm$3.1) | 0–1 | 40 | U,T,PD |
|   Gentamicin | IV | 1.5 mg/kg (S) | 5 | 5.1 ($\pm$0.4) | 2.9 ($\pm$0.3) | 0.5–1 | 57 | U,T,PD |
|   Netilmicin | IV | 6.0 mg/kg (S) | 5 | 18.2 ($\pm$6.3) | 7.2 ($\pm$2.8) | 3–4 | 40 | U,PD |
| Cephalosporins and related $\beta$-lactams | | | | | | | | |
|   Cefazolin | IV | 1.0 (S) | 6 | 63.1 ($\pm$6.7) | 9 ($\pm$2) | 3 | 14 | U |
|   Cefadroxil | PO | 0.5 (S) | 7 | 2.15 | 2.46 | 8 | 114 | U |
|   Cefuroxime | IV | 1.0 (S) | 6 | 24 (14–40) | 7.3 (5.6–9.1) | 1.5–4.5 | 30 | U |
|   Cefoxitin | IV | 2.0 (S) | 6 | 11.8 (4–18) | 3.6 (1–6.4) | 1–5 | 31 | U |
|   Cefotaxime | IV | 1.0 (S) | 6 | 28 | 7.2 ($\pm$3.1 D) | 3.0 | 26 | U |
|   Ceftizoxime | IV | 1.0 (S) | 5 | 24.1 ($\pm$4.4 SD) | 7.8 ($\pm$2.2 SD) | 2–3 | 32 | U |
|   Ceftriaxone | IV | 1.0 (S) | 5 | 39.4 (34–50) | 7.9 (7.0–8.7) | 4 | 20 | I,U |
|   Ceftazidime | IV | 2.0 (S) | 5 | 80 ($\pm$10) | 17 ($\pm$3) | 1 | 21 | U,E |
|   Aztreonam | IV | 2.0 (S) | 3 | 64 ($\pm$12 SE) | 51 ($\pm$31 SE) | 1–3 | 79 | |
| Penicillins | | | | | | | | |
|   Amoxicillin | PO | 0.75 (S) | 9 | 4.5 | 1.6 | 5.3 | 36 | U,T |
|   Ampicillin | PO | 1.0 (S) | 6 | 21.4 ($\pm$3.7) | 10.5 ($\pm$1.5) | 3 | 49 | U |
|   Penicillin | PO | 1–2 $\times$ 10[6] U (M) | 5 | 20.4 (11–25) | 13.6 (3–26) | 1–3 | 67 | U |
|   Ticarcillin | IV | 5.0 (S) | 5 | 63 (56–70) | 9 (6–11) | 3 | 14 | U,PD |
|   Mezlocillin | IV | 10 (S) | 6 | 778 ($\pm$270) | 100 ($\pm$38) | 1 | 13 | U,T,PD |
| Quinolones | | | | | | | | |
|   Ciprofloxacin | IV | 1.5 mg/kg (S) | 5 | 0.55 ($\pm$0.11) | 0.52 ($\pm$0.19) | 1 | 95 | |
| Others | | | | | | | | |
|   Doxycycline | IV | 0.3 (S) | 16 | 5.0 ($\pm$0.4) | 1.8 ($\pm$0.2) | 10 | 36 | |
|   Clindamycin | PO | 0.15 (M) | 3 | 10.1 | 9.3 (1.3–22) | 1–2 | 92 | U |
|   Vancomycin | IV | 0.5 (S) | 12 | 7.3 (2.9–10) | 3.0 (0–8.1) | 1.2–4.5 | 41 | U |

*I, infected; U, uninfected; T, tube drainage; PD, peak serum and peak pleural fluid data; E, values extrapolated from graphs; S, single dose; M, multiple dose.
Adapted from Gerding DN, Peterson LR, Hughes CE, et al: Extravascular antimicrobial distribution and the respective blood concentrations in humans. *In* Lorian V (ed): Antibiotics in Laboratory Medicine, ed 3. Baltimore, Williams & Wilkins, 1991:880.

Table 43–14. **Antimicrobial Concentrations in Sinus Secretions\***

| Antimicrobial | Administration Method | Dose (g) | No. of Patients | Serum Concentration Mean (Range) | Site Concentration Mean (Range) | Time Site Specimen Obtained (h) | Ratio of Site/ Serum (%) | Notes |
|---|---|---|---|---|---|---|---|---|
| Ampicillin | PO | 0.5 (M) | 4 | 3.8 (1.8–8.0) | 0.125 (0–0.3) | 2–3 | 3 | AS |
| Cephalexin | PO | 0.5 or 15 mg/kg | 9 | 8.8 (1.9–19) | 1.1 (<0.1–4.0) | 2.0 | 10 | |
| Erythromycin stearate | PO | 0.5 (M) | 10 | 2.2 (0.3–5.0) | 1.3 (0.3–2.5) | 4.7 | 59 | AS |
| Tetracycline HCl | PO | 0.25 (M) | 21 | 2.4 (0.9–6.0) | 1.9 (0.5–3.6) | 2.1 | 79 | P |
| Doxycycline | PO | 0.1 (M) | 24 | 3.5 (1.2–6.0) | 2.0 (0.5–7.5) | 2–7 | 57 | |
| Sulfadiazine | PO | 0.5 (M) | 10 | 42 (24–66) | 6.6 (2.3–15) | 2–4 | 20 | AS |
| Trimethoprim | PO | 0.16 (M) | 10 | 3.0 (2.1–5.6) | 3.9 (1.1–10.8) | 2–4 | 133 | AS |

\*AS, acute sinusitis; M, multiple doses; P, purulent; S, single dose.

Adapted from Gerding DN, Peterson LR, Hughes CE, et al: Extravascular antimicrobial distribution and the respective blood concentrations in humans. *In* Lorian V (ed): Antibiotics in Laboratory Medicine, ed 3. Baltimore, Williams & Wilkins, 1991:880.

mycin in the treatment of legionellosis is dependent on its intracellular activity against *L. pneumophila,* because the organism resists killing when ingested by macrophages.[63]

Although extravascular antibiotic concentrations exceeding the MIC for an organism should correlate with clinical efficacy, other factors such as the host immune response, antibiotic inactivation, inoculum effect, and other pharmacokinetic considerations are also important. The actual measurement of local antibiotic concentration is difficult, especially if tissue homogenates are used, because this does not permit intracellular or extracellular localization of the antimicrobial.[171]

The ratio of local antibiotic concentrations to organism MIC has been used as an indicator of the likelihood a given antibiotic will have clinical efficacy at a given site of infection. It is expressed as the amount of antibiotic available at the site relative to the amount necessary to inhibit or kill the organism. It is customary to express this ratio as the local antibiotic concentration divided by the $MIC_{90}$. It is calculated value, and only large differences in the ratio are likely to be significant. An antibiotic that is characterized by a high ratio against a given organism is likely to be more efficacious than an antibiotic with a lower ratio. The

$S/MIC_{90}$ ratios of selected antibiotics, calculated using sputum concentrations for typical and for atypical bacterial causes of pneumonia (*M. pneumoniae, C. pneumoniae,* and *L. pneumophila*), are provided in Tables 43–16 and 43–17, respectively.[67, 75, 162, 163, 172–177] The occasional failure of ciprofloxacin to effectively treat pneumonia caused by *S. pneumoniae* is supported by $S/MIC_{90}$ ratios that are less than 1.0. The utility of the quinolones in the treatment of gram-negative infections is apparent from the $S/MIC_{90}$, which exceeds 10 for most gram-negative organisms. Similarly, the difficulty in treating infections caused by *P. aeruginosa* is emphasized by the fact that there are only a few antibiotics with an $S/MIC_{90}$ that exceeds 1. Unfortunately, there are no clinical data to support the use of these ratios in predicting clinical efficacy as yet.

## PHARMACOKINETIC ANTIMICROBIAL CONSIDERATIONS IN TREATING RESPIRATORY INFECTIONS

### Sputum and Bronchial Secretions

The clinical importance of antimicrobial penetration into sputum and bronchial secretions remains controversial.

Table 43–15. **Antimicrobial Concentrations Within Cells\***

| Antimicrobial | Cell Type | No. of Samples | Extracellular Concentration (μg/mL) | Time of Incubation (h) | Cellular Concentration (μg/mL) | C/E Ratio (%) | Notes |
|---|---|---|---|---|---|---|---|
| Ampicillin | PMN | 4 | 50 | 0.5 | 13 | 26 ± 3 SE | SO |
| Cefotaxime | PMN | 6 | R | 2 | R | 34 ± 8 SD | SO |
| Imipenem | PMN | 6 | R | 2 | R | 33 ± 14 SD | SO |
| Enoxacin | PMN | | 10 | 1 | 40 | 400 | CW |
| Ciprofloxacin | PMN | 3 | 10 | 0.5 | 46 | 460 ± 10 SD | |
| Ciprofloxacin | AM | 6 | 10 | 0.5 | 81 | 810 ± 110 SD | |
| Azithromycin | PMN | 12 | 4 | 0.66 | 1192 | 29,800 ± 9,700 | SO |
| Azithromycin | AM | 3 | 4 | 0.66 | 2672 | 66,800 ± 19,800 SD | SO |
| Clarithromycin | PMN | 3 | 2 | 0.5 | 18 | 920 ± 200 SE | SO |
| Clindamycin | PMN | 22 | 10 | 1–3 | 95.3 | 953 ± 42 SE | SO |
| Erythromycin | PMN | 19 | 10 | 0.5 | 80 | 800 ± 100 SD | CW |
| Erythromycin (nonsmoker) | AM | 2 | R | 2 | R | 1770 ± 640 SE | SO |
| Rifampin | AM | 10 | R | 1–2 | R | 522–978 | SO |
| Sulfonamides | RBC | 40 | 10–30 | | 10–30 | 80–200 | CW |
| Tetracycline | AM | 6 | R | 1–2 | R | 241–449 | SO |
| Trimethoprim | PMN | 13–16 | R | 0.02–1 | R | 430–902 | SO |

\*C/E, cellular to extracellular concentration ratio as a percent; SO, centrifugation through silicone oil; R, radiolabeled drug only; CW, centrifugation and washing; PMN, polymorphonuclear leukocytes; AM, alveolar macrophage; RBC, red blood cell.

Adapted from Gerding DN, Peterson LR, Hughes CE, et al: Extravascular antimicrobial distribution and the respective blood concentrations in humans. *In* Lorian V (ed): Antibiotics in Laboratory Medicine, ed 3. Baltimore, Williams & Wilkins, 1991:880.

**Table 43–16. The Minimum Inhibitory Concentration of 90% (MIC$_{90}$) of Common Respiratory Pathogens for Selected Antimicrobials and the Ratio of Sputum Concentration of the Antimicrobials to MIC$_{90}$ (S/M$_{90}$)**

| Antimicrobial | Haemophilus influenzae S/M$_{90}$* | MIC$_{90}$ | Streptococcus pneumoniae S/M$_{90}$ | MIC$_{90}$ | Moraxella catarrhalis S/M$_{90}$ | MIC$_{90}$ | Escherichia coli S/M$_{90}$ | MIC$_{90}$ | Klebsiella pneumoniae S/M$_{90}$ | MIC$_{90}$ | Pseudomonas aeruginosa S/M$_{90}$ | MIC$_{90}$ | Staphylococcus aureus† S/M$_{90}$ | MIC$_{90}$ |
|---|---|---|---|---|---|---|---|---|---|---|---|---|---|---|
| Amikacin | 0.8 | ~5.5 | <0.09 | >50 | | | 0.7–1.5 | 3–5 | 0.9–1.1 | 4–5 | 0.3–1.7 | 2.6–16 | 2.2 | ~2 |
| Gentamicin | 0.25 | ~1.2 | <0.012 | >25 | 1.2 | 0.25 | 0.025–0.12 | 2.5–12 | 0.1–0.15 | 2–3 | 0.04–0.1 | 3–>8 | 0.4–1 | 0.3–0.7 |
| Netilmicin | 0.3–1.2 | 0.5–2 | <0.02 | >32 | | | 0.4 | 1.6 | 0.3 | 2 | 0.02–0.12 | 5–25 | 0.75–3 | 0.2–0.8 |
| Tobramycin | 0.47 | 1.5 | <0.33 | >128 | | | 0.175–0.23 | ~3–4 | 0.23–0.44 | 1.6–~3 | 0.12–0.44 | 1.6–6 | 1.2–1.75 | 0.4–0.6 |
| Aztreonam | **42** | 0.1 | | | | | **21** | 0.2 | 5.25 | 0.8 | 0.17 | 25 | <0.33 | >128 |
| Cefazolin | 0.23 | 10 | 7.7 | ~0.3 | 0.29–2.3 | 1.0–8 | 0.23–0.46 | 5.0–10 | 0.4 | 6.0 | <0.02 | >100 | 2.3 | 1.0 |
| Cephradine | <0.03–0.06 | 20–>50 | >1.3 | <1.0 | | | 0.1 | 12–<25 | 0.1 | 12–<25 | <0.003 | >400 | 0.4 | 3.2 |
| Cefotaxime | **26–87** | 0.03–0.1 | 6.5 | 0.4 | 2.6–5.2 | 0.5–1 | **10.4–52** | 0.05–0.25 | **6.5–10.4** | 0.25–0.4 | <0.08 | >32 | 0.8–1.3 | 2.0–3.1 |
| Cefoxitin | 0.2–0.3 | 6.0–8 | >0.5 | <3 | **12.8** | 0.125 | 0.2 | 8.0 | <0.13–0.32 | 5.0–<12 | 0.016 | >100 | 0.32–0.53 | 3.0–5 |
| Ceftazidime | **56** | 0.1 | **22.5** | 0.25 | **22–>93** | <0.06–0.25 | **11** | 0.5 | **11** | 0.5 | 1.4 | 4 | 0.35 | 16 |
| Ceftizoxime | **430** | 0.01 | **43** | 0.1 | 1.9–7.6 | 0.25–1.0 | **33–107** | 0.1 | **12–86** | 0.05–0.25 | <0.13 | >32 | 1.4 | 3.0 |
| Ceftriaxone | **19** | 0.1 | 7.6 | 0.25 | | | **19** | 0.1 | **19** | 0.1 | <0.06 | >32 | 0.3–0.5 | 4.0–6.3 |
| Cefuroxime | 1.2–3 | 0.8–2.0 | **12** | 0.2 | 1.2–2.4 | 1.0–2 | 0.43–0.6 | 4.0–6 | 0.1–0.6 | 4.0–25 | <0.024 | >100 | 1.2–3 | 0.8–2.0 |
| Imipenem | **21** | 0.1 | **210** | 0.01 | | | 5.25 | 0.4 | 5.25 | 0.4 | 0.17 | 12.5 | **21** | 0.1 |
| Carbenicillin | 2.3–3.4 | 1.0–1.5 | **13.6** | 0.25 | | | <0.03 | >128 | <0.01 | 256 | <0.06 | >64 | <0.5 | >6.25 |
| Piperacillin | 1.2–3.6 | 1–3 | **120** | <0.03 | **29** | 0.125 | <0.04 | >100 | <0.06 | 64–>100 | 0.3 | 12 | 1.4–4.5 | 0.8–2.5 |
| Ticarcillin | 5.1 | 0.8 | **64** | 0.08 | 0.5 | 8.0 | <0.04 | 100 | <0.02 | ~200 | <0.04–0.14 | 30–100 | 0.33 | 12.5 |
| Ticarcillin-clavulanate‡,§ | **8–16** | 0.25–0.5 | | | | | 0.06–0.2 | 16–64 | 0.03–0.1 | 32–128 | 0.001 | 512 | 0.1–2 | 2–32 |
| Amoxicillin | 0.8–2 | 0.2–0.6 | **25** | 0.02 | 8 | 0.5 | <0.005 | >100 | <0.005 | >100 | <0.005 | >100 | 0.5–0.6 | 0.8–1.0 |
| Amoxicillin-clavulanate‡,§ | | | | | 8 | 0.06[17] | 0.02 | 16 | 0.01 | 32[23] | | | | |
| Ampicillin | 0.25 | 1.0 | 4.2 | 0.06 | 0.125–8 | 0.03–2 | <0.002 | >100 | <0.004 | >50–>400 | <0.007 | >128 | 0.625 | 0.4 |
| Ampicillin-sulbactam‡,§ | 0.125 | 2 | | | 0.3–0.1 | 0.25–0.8 | 0.016 | 16 | 0.03 | 8[22] | | | 0.06 | 4 |
| Ciprofloxacin | **67** | 0.015 | 1.0 | 1 | **67** | 0.015 | **33** | 0.03 | 8 | 0.125 | 2 | 0.5 | 2 | 0.5 |
| Enoxacin | **25** | 0.125 | 0.2 | 16 | | | 6 | 0.5 | 6 | 0.5 | 0.8 | 4 | 1.5 | 2 |
| Ofloxacin | **67** | 0.03 | 1 | 2 | | | **16** | 0.125 | 8 | 0.25 | | | 4 | 0.5 |
| Pefloxacin | **77** | 0.06 | >1 | 8 | | | **37** | 0.125 | 9.2 | 0.5 | 1.15 | 4 | 9.2 | 0.5 |
| Doxycycline | 0.13 | 3.1 | 0.17 | <0.4 | | | <0.016 | >25 | <0.016 | >25 | <0.016 | >25 | <0.016 | >25 |
| Minocycline | | | | | | | <0.04 | >25 | | | <0.04 | >25 | 0.37 | 3 |
| Tetracycline | 0.2–2.4 | 0.5–6 | 0.17 | 7 | 2.4–8.0 | 0.125–0.5 | <0.05 | >25 | <0.05 | >25 | 0.024 | 50 | 0.05–12 | 0.1–>25 |
| Clindamycin | 0.13–0.32 | 5–12.5 | **27** | 0.06 | 0.32–1.6 | 1.0–5 | 0.19 | >6.2 | 0.03 | >50 | <0.004 | >400 | **16–27** | 0.06–0.1 |
| Erythromycin | 0.2–2.75 | 0.4–6 | **11** | 0.1 | 4.4–8.8 | 0.125–0.25 | | | <0.04 | >25 | <0.01 | >100 | 2.2–2.8 | 0.4–0.5 |
| Azithromycin | 4.7[75] | 0.78[174] | **73.2**[75] | 0.05[174] | **122**[75] | 0.03[174] | 0.92[75] | 4[174] | 0.23[75] | 16[174] | 0.06[75] | 64[174] | 2.35[75] | 1.56[174] |
| Clarithromycin | 0.53[163] | 8.0[67] | **281**[163] | 0.015[175] | **16.9**[163] | 0.25[175] | | | | | | | 0.03–140.7[163] | 0.03–>128[177] |
| Sulfamethoxazole | **4.1–12.4** | 1.0–3 | 0.39 | 32 | **<1–450** | 4 | | | | | <0.01–1.24 | 10–>1000 | <0.124 | >100 |
| Trimethoprim‖ | **0.36–45** | 0.1–12.5 | **1–1100** | 0.004–5 | <1–>5 | 0.01–>5 | **1–30** | 0.15–5 | | | 0.004–0.15 | 30–>1000 | **2.9–11** | 0.4–1.6 |

*S/M 90 ratios of >10 indicate that the sputum concentration of the antimicrobial is at least 10 times as high as the amount of drug needed to inhibit 90% of the strains of that species. These ratios of >10 are shown in boldface in the table.

†Includes only methicillin-sensitive strains.

‡Site concentration of β-lactam used to approximate site concentration of drug combination.

§MIC$_{90}$s are expressed as the β-lactam concentration.

‖MIC$_{90}$ of trimethoprim (TMP) in combination with sulfamethoxazole is generally much lower than TMP alone with a resultant higher S/M$_{90}$ ratio.

Adapted from Hitt JA, Gerding DN: Sputum antibiotic levels and clinical outcome in bronchitis. Semin Respir Infect 6:122, 1991.

**Table 43–17. The Minimum Inhibitory Concentration of 90% (MIC$_{90}$) of Common Respiratory Pathogens for Selected Antimicrobials and the Ratio of Sputum Concentration of the Antimicrobials to MIC$_{90}$ (S/M$_{90}$)**

| Drug | *Mycoplasma pneumoniae* | | *Chlamydia pneumoniae* (TWAR) | | *Legionella pneumophila* | |
|------|---------|---------|---------|---------|---------|---------|
| | S/M$_{90}$* | MIC$_{90}$ | S/M$_{90}$ | MIC$_{90}$ | S/M$_{90}$ | MIC$_{90}$ |
| Ciprofloxacin | 0.125 | 8.0 | 1.0 | 1.0[173] | **33** | 0.03 |
| Tetracycline | 1.2 | 1.0 | 9.6 | 0.125[173] | 0.3 | 4 |
| Erythromycin | **18** | 0.06 | **18**[173] | 0.06[173] | 2.2 | 0.5 |
| Azithromycin | **3660**[75] | 0.001[175] | **29**[75] | 0.125[173] | **>29**[75] | <0.125[175] |
| Clarithromycin | **136**[163] | 0.03[176] | **281**[163] | 0.015[173] | **>34**[163] | <0.125[175] |

*S/M$_{90}$ ratios of >10 indicate that the sputum concentration of the antimicrobial is at least 10 times as high as the amount of drug needed to inhibit 90% of the strains of that species. These ratios of >10 are shown in boldface in the table.

Unless otherwise indicated, data from Gerding DN, Peterson LR, Hughes CE, et al: Extravascular antimicrobial distribution and the respective blood concentrations in humans. *In* Lorian V (ed): Antibiotics in Laboratory Medicine, ed 3. Baltimore, Williams & Wilkins, 1991:880.

Most studies have failed to show any correlation between antimicrobial concentration in sputum and therapeutic outcome. Sputum levels should not be used to predict drug levels in other parts of the respiratory tract, and they do not correlate well with serum levels. Sputum antimicrobial concentrations seem to correlate only with the eradication of colonizing organisms from sputum and not with their elimination from bronchial fluid, lung tissue, or pleural fluid.[168] Bronchial fluid levels seem to be important only in the treatment of patients who have chronic bronchitis or cystic fibrosis.

Antibiotic concentrations in sputum and bronchial secretions are depicted in Table 43–11.[162] Bronchial secretions were obtained by bronchoscopy in patients with chronic bronchitis, cystic fibrosis, or pneumonia, and sputum secretions were coughed specimens. Ciprofloxacin and trimethoprim achieved levels that exceeded serum levels. For most β-lactam antibiotics, sputum penetration is poor.[168] In general, quinolones, TMP-SMX, minocycline, and rifampin have the best penetration into sputum. The quinolones, TMP-SMX, the tetracyclines, clindamycin, and erythromycin have the best bronchial fluid penetration.[168] Aminoglycosides penetrate bronchial fluid poorly.[178] In fact, aminoglycosides achieve sputum levels that are below the MIC for many gram-negative organisms, particularly *P. aeruginosa*. Quinolones achieve high levels in sputum, which may explain their efficacy in the treatment of many patients with pneumococcal pneumonia despite marginal activity in vitro against *S. pneumoniae*.

### Lung Tissue

Most antibiotics penetrate lung tissues well. Much of the data concerning antibiotic levels in lung tissue is obtained from surgical resection of lung tumors or at autopsy and may not adequately represent conditions in infected patients. Lung tissue levels usually represent a mean concentration of all lung tissue and fluids and correlate best with bronchial fluid concentrations. Lung tissue concentrations are possibly the most important site concentration in the treatment of pneumonia.

The concentration of specific antimicrobials in lung tissue is displayed in Table 43–12.[162] The data indicate that ciprofloxacin, trimethoprim, and erythromycin penetrate lung tissue well and achieve concentrations that exceed serum concentrations. Doxycycline and minocycline are not listed, but in other studies they also achieved high concentrations.[179] The β-lactam agents also penetrated lung tissue well and achieved significantly higher concentrations than those attained in sputum or bronchial secretions. Amikacin achieved levels that exceeded the MIC for most gram-negative organisms. There is as yet little definitive evidence to support a correlation between lung tissue antibiotic concentration and clinical efficacy in treating pneumonia.

### Pleural Fluid

The data available on antimicrobial penetration into pleural empyemas are sparse. As Table 43–13 demonstrates, most antimicrobials penetrate uninfected pleural fluid reasonably well. Antimicrobials that demonstrate excellent pleural penetration include aztreonam, ciprofloxacin, and clindamycin. The penetration of penicillin into empyema fluid approximates that found with parapneumonic effusions.[180, 181] Similarly, cefotaxime achieved comparable levels in infected and noninfected pleural fluid.[181] Thys[182] showed that aminoglycoside levels are low in empyema fluid compared with uninfected pleural fluid. Undetectable levels were observed with gentamicin and netilmicin in empyemas.[182] Gentamicin has been shown to be inactivated in the presence of purulent exudate and at an acidic pH, conditions which are likely in empyema fluid.[181, 183] It remains unclear how antimicrobial penetration into empyema fluid relates to clinical efficacy, particularly in view of the well-demonstrated need for mechanical drainage and antimicrobial treatment in managing empyemas.

### Sinusitis

There are few data available concerning antibiotic penetration into infected sinus mucosa and sinus secretions. There is also controversy about which site (ie, sinus mucosa or sinus secretions) is primarily infected. Lundberg postulated that acute maxillary sinusitis is an infection of retained sinus secretions that produces an inflammatory response of the sinus mucosa.[184, 185]

The data in Table 43–14 demonstrate that ampicillin achieves only marginally adequate levels in sinus secretions. Erythromycin, tetracyclines, and trimethoprim achieve much better penetration. Tissue penetration in sinusitis may be adversely affected by the degree of purulence.[162] β-Lactam agents are known to penetrate purulent secretions poorly, but clinical studies with regard to efficacy have not demonstrated any significant difference between β-lactams and other alternatives in the treatment of sinusitis.[184] Ampicillin and amoxicillin have proven efficacy in some studies despite the presence of β-lactamase–producing organisms.[184, 186]

## REFERENCES

1. Coppen L, Kastersky J: Comparative study of antipseudomonas activity of azlocillin, mezlocillin, and ticarcillin. Antimicrob Agents Chemother 15:396, 1979.
2. White GW, Malow JB, Zimelis VM, et al: Comparative in vitro activity of azlocillin, ampicillin, mezlocillin, piperacillin, and ticarcillin, alone and in combination with an aminoglycoside. Antimicrob Agents Chemother 15:540, 1979.
3. Parry MF, Pancoast SJ: Antipseudomonal penicillins. In Ristuccia AM, Cunha BA (eds): Antimicrobial Therapy. New York, Raven Press, 1984:197.
4. Mandell GL, Douglas RG Jr, Bennett JE (eds): Principles and Practice of Infectious Diseases, ed 3. New York, Churchill Livingstone, 1990:236–237.
5. New HC: Relation of structural properties of beta-lactam antibiotics to antibacterial activity. Am J Med 79(suppl 2A):2, 1985.
6. Donowitz GR, Mandell GL: Beta-lactam antibiotics. N Engl J Med 318:490, 1988.
7. Phair JP, Carleton J, Tan JS: Comparison of cefazolin, a new cephalosporin antibiotic, with cephalothin. Antimicrob Agents Chemother 2:329, 1972.
8. Pickering MJ, Spooner GR, Quesada ADE, et al: Declining renal function associated with administration of cephalothin. South Med J 63:426, 1970.
9. Neu HC, Fu KP: Cefuroxime, a beta-lactamase–resistant cephalosporin with a broad spectrum of gram-positive and -negative activity. Antimicrob Agents Chemother 15:273, 1978.
10. Goldberg DM: The cephalosporins. Med Clin North Am 71:1113, 1987.
11. McCloskey RV: Results of a clinical trial of cefoxitin, a new cephamycin antibiotic. Antimicrob Agents Chemother 12:636, 1977.
12. Kirby BD, Busch DF, Citron DM, et al: Cefoxitin for treatment of infections due to anaerobic bacteria. Rev Infect Dis 1:113, 1979.
13. Bodey GP, Fainstein V, Hinkle AM: Comparative in vitro study of new cephalosporins. Antimicrob Agents Chemother 20:226, 1981.
14. Chattopadhyay B, Hall I, Curnow SR: Ceftazidime (GR 20263), a new cephalosporin derivative with excellent activity against *Pseudomonas* and Enterobacteriaceae. J Antimicrob Chemother 8:491, 1981.
15. Neu HC, Labthavikul P: Antimicrobial activity and β-lactamase stability of ceftazidime, an aminothiazolyl cephalosporin potentially active against *Pseudomonas aeruginosa*. Antimicrob Agents Chemother 21:11, 1982.
16. Gentry LO: Antimicrobial activity, pharmacokinetics, therapeutic indications and adverse reactions of ceftazidime. Pharmacotherapy 5:254, 1985.
17. Neu HC: The new beta-lactamase–stable cephalosporins. Ann Intern Med 97:408, 1982.
18. Neu HC: In vitro activity of a new broad spectrum beta-lactamase–stable oral cephalosporin, cefixime. Pediatr Infect Dis 6:958, 1987.
19. Lipman B, Neu HC: Imipenem: a new carbipenem antibiotic. Med Clin North Am 72:567, 1988.
20. Wise R, Andrews JM, Patel N: *N*-Formimidoyl-thienamycin, a novel beta-lactam: An in vitro comparison with other beta-lactam antibiotics. J Antimicrob Chemother 7:521, 1981.
21. Sobel JD: Imipenem and aztreonam. Infect Dis Clin North Am 3:613, 1989.
22. Zar FA, Kany RJ Jr: In vitro studies of investigational beta-lactams as possible therapy for *Pseudomonas aeruginosa* endocarditis. Antimicrob Agents Chemother 27:1, 1985.
23. Krilov LR, Blumer JL, Stern RC, et al: Imipenem/cilastatin in acute pulmonary exacerbations of cystic fibrosis. Rev Infect Dis 7(suppl 3):482, 1985.
24. Salata RA, Gebhart RC, Palmer DL, et al: Pneumonia treated with imipenem/cilastatin. Am J Med 78:104, 1985.
25. Nielsen DM, Katz JR, AhLoy RD, et al: Imipenem/cilastatin therapy for serious bacterial infections. Rev Infect Dis 7:S506, 1985.
26. Acar JF: Therapy for lower respiratory tract infections with imipenem/cilastatin: A review of worldwide experience. Rev Infect Dis 7:S513, 1985.
27. Calandra GB, Ricci FM, Wang C, et al: The efficacy results and safety profile of imipenem/cilastatin from the clinical research trials. J Clin Pharmacol 28:120, 1988.
28. Kropp H, Gerckens L, Sundelof JG, et al: Antibacterial activity of imipenem: The first thienamycin antibiotic. Rev Infect Dis 7(suppl 3):389, 1985.
29. Barza M: Imipenem: First of a new class of beta-lactam antibiotics. Ann Intern Med 103:552, 1985.
30. Norrby SR: Imipenem/cilastatin. In Peterson PK, Verhoef J (eds): The Antimicrobial Agents Annual 3. Amsterdam, Elsevier Science Publishers, 1988:151.
31. Mandell GL, Douglas RG Jr, Bennett JE (eds): Principles and Practice of Infectious Diseases, ed 3. New York, Churchill Livingstone, 1990:259.
32. Williams JD: Aztreonam. In Peterson PK, Verhoef J (eds): The Antimicrobial Agents Annual 3. Amsterdam, Elsevier Science Publishers, 1988:51.
33. Neu HC: Aztreonam: The first monobactam. Med Clin North Am 72:555, 1988.
34. Donowitz GR, Mandell GL: Beta-lactam antibiotics. N Engl J Med 318:490, 1988.
35. Wolfson JS, Hooper DC: The fluoroquinolones: Structures, mechanisms of action and resistance, and spectra of activity in vitro. Antimicrob Agents Chemother 28:581, 1985.
36. Khan FA: Ciprofloxacin for respiratory tract infections. In Sanders WE, Sanders CC (eds): Fluoroquinolones in the Treatment of Infectious Diseases. Glenview, Physicians and Scientists Publishing, 1990:87.
37. Davies BI, Maesen FPV, Baur C: Ciprofloxacin in the treatment of acute exacerbations of chronic bronchitis. Eur J Clin Microbiol 5:226, 1986.
38. Righter J: Pneumococcal meningitis during intravenous ciprofloxacin therapy. Am J Med 88:548, 1990.
39. Cooper B, Lawlor M: Pneumococcal bacteremia during ciprofloxacin therapy for pneumococcal pneumonia. Am J Med 87:475, 1989.
40. Lee BL, Kimbrough RC, Jones SR, et al: Infectious complications with respiratory pathogens despite ciprofloxacin therapy. [Letter] N Engl J Med 325:520, 1991.
41. Thys JP: Quinolones in the treatment of bronchopulmonary infections. Rev Infect Dis 10(suppl 1):212, 1988.
42. Walker RC, Wright AJ: The fluoroquinolones. Mayo Clin Proc 66:1249, 1991.
43. Wijnands WJA, Vree TB: Interaction between the fluoroquinolones and the bronchodilator theophylline. J Antimicrob Chemother 22(suppl C):109, 1988.
44. Ristuccia AM: Aminoglycosides. In Ristuccia AM, Cunha BA (eds): Antimicrobial Therapy. New York, Raven Press, 1984:305.
45. Sanders CC, Sanders WE Jr, Goering RV: In vitro studies with Sch 21420 and Sch 22591: Activity in comparison with six other aminoglycosides and synergy with penicillin against enterococci. Antimicrob Agents Chemother 14:178, 1978.
46. Kabins SA, Nathan C, Cohen S: In vitro comparison of netilmicin, a semisynthetic derivative of sisomicin and four other aminoglycoside antibiotics. Antimicrob Agents Chemother 10:139, 1976.
47. Gerding DN, Larson TA, Hughes RA, et al: Aminoglycoside resistance and aminoglycoside usage: Ten years of experience in one hospital. Antimicrob Agents Chemother 35:1284, 1991.
48. Walker JM, Wise R: The pharmacokinetics of amikacin and gentamicin in volunteers: A comparison of individual differences. J Antimicrob Chemother 5:95, 1979.
49. Riff JJ, Jackson GG: Pharmacology of gentamicin in man. J Infect Dis 124:S98, 1971.
50. Reymann MT, Bradac JA, Cobbs JA, et al: Correlations of aminoglycoside dosages with serum concentrations during therapy of serious gram-negative bacillary disease. Antimicrob Agents Chemother 16:353, 1979.
51. Baltch AL, Hammer M, Smith RP, et al: *Pseudomonas aeruginosa* bacteremia. J Lab Clin Med 94:201, 1979.
52. Noone P, Parson TM, Paltison JR, et al: Experience in monitoring

gentamicin therapy during treatment of serious gram-negative sepsis. Br Med J 1:477, 1974.

53. Kahlmeter G, Dahlager JI: Aminoglycoside toxicity: A review of clinical studies published between 1975 and 1982. J Antimicrob Chemother 13(suppl A):9, 1984.

54. Dahlgren JG, Anderson ET, Hewitt WL: Gentamicin blood levels: A guide to nephrotoxicity. Antimicrob Agents Chemother 8:58, 1975.

55. Brittain DC: Erythromycin. Med Clin North Am 71:1147, 1987.

56. Chow AW: Erythromycin. *In* Ristuccia AM, Cunha BA (eds): Antimicrobial Therapy. New York, Raven Press, 1984:209.

57. Fernandes PB, Hardy D, Bailer R, et al: Susceptibility testing of macrolide antibiotics against *Hemophilus influenza* and correlation of in vitro results with in vivo efficacy in a mouse septicemia model. Antimicrob Agents Chemother 31:1243, 1987.

58. Dixon JM, Lipinski AE: Pneumococci resistant to erythromycin. Can Med Assoc J 119:1044, 1978.

59. Finland M, Bach MC, Garner C, et al: Synergistic action of ampicillin against *Nocardia asteroides*: Effect of time of incubation. Antimicrob Agents Chemother 5:344, 1974.

60. Rasch JR, Mogabgab WJ: Therapeutic effect of erythromycin on *Mycoplasma pneumoniae* pneumonia. Antimicrob Agents Chemother 5:693, 1965.

61. Smith CB, Fiedewald WT, Cjanock RM: Shedding of *Mycoplasma pneumoniae* after tetracycline and erythromycin therapy. N Engl J Med 276:1172, 1967.

62. Jao RL, Finland M: Susceptibility of *Mycoplasma pneumoniae* to 21 antibiotics in vitro. Am J Med Sci 253:639, 1967.

63. Hand WL, Corwin RW, Steinberg TH, et al: Uptake of antibiotics by human alveolar macrophages. Am Rev Respir Dis 129:933, 1984.

64. Karma P, Pukander J, Penttilia M, et al: The comparative efficacy and safety of clarithromycin and amoxycillin in the treatment of outpatients with acute maxillary sinusitis. J Antimicrob Chemother 27(suppl A):83, 1991.

65. Bachand RT, Jr: Comparative study of clarithromycin and ampicillin in the treatment of patients with acute bacterial exacerbations of chronic bronchitis. J Antimicrob Chemother 27(suppl A):91, 1991.

66. Anderson G, Esmonde TS, Coles S, et al: A comparative safety and efficacy study of clarithromycin and erythromycin stearate in community-acquired pneumonia. J Antimicrob Chemother 27(suppl A):117, 1991.

67. Vallée E, Azoulay-Dupuis E, Swanson R, et al: Individual and combined activities of clarithromycin and its 14-hydroxy metabolite in a murine model of *Haemophilus influenzae* infection. J Antimicrob Chemother 27(suppl A):31, 1991.

68. Hardy DJ, Swanson RA, Rode RN, et al: Enhancement of the in vitro and in vivo activities of clarithromycin against *Haemophilus influenzae* by 14-hydroxy-clarithromycin, its major metabolite in humans. Antimicrob Agents Chemother 34:1407, 1990.

69. Fraschini F, Scaglione F, Pintucci G, et al: The diffusion of clarithromycin and roxithromycin into nasal mucosa, tonsil and lung in humans. J Antimicrob Chemother 27(suppl A):61, 1991.

70. Neu HC: The development of macrolides: Clarithromycin in perspective. J Antimicrob Chemother 27(suppl A):1, 1991.

71. Aldons PM: A comparison of clarithromycin with ampicillin in the treatment of outpatients with acute bacterial exacerbation of chronic bronchitis. J Antimicrob Chemother 27(supp A):101, 1991.

72. Retsema J, Girard A, Schelkly W, et al: Spectrum and mode of action of azithromycin (CP-62,993) a new 15-membered-ring macrolide with improved potency against gram-negative organisms. Antimicrob Agents Chemother 31:1939, 1987.

73. Maskell JP, Sefton AM, Williams JD: Comparative in vitro activity of azithromycin and erythromycin against gram-positive cocci, *Haemophilus influenzae*, and anaerobes. J Antimicrob Chemother 27(suppl A):19, 1990.

74. Retsema JA, Girard AE, Girard D, et al: Relationship of high tissue concentrations of azithromycin to bactericidal activity and efficacy in vivo. J Antimicrob Chemother 27(suppl A):83, 1990.

75. Davies BI, Maesen FPV, Gubbelmans R: Azithromycin (CP-62,993) in acute exacerbations of chronic bronchitis: An open clinical, microbiological and pharmacokinetic study. J Antimicrob Chemother 23:743, 1989.

76. Girard AE, Girard D, English AR, et al: Pharmacokinetic and in vivo studies with azithromycin (CP-62,993), a new macrolide with an extended half-life and excellent tissue distribution. Antimicrob Agents Chemother 31:1948, 1987.

77. Foulds G, Shepard RM, Johnson RB: The pharmacokinetics of azith-

romycin in human serum and tissues. J Antimicrob Chemother 25(suppl A):73, 1990.

78. Gopalakrishna KV, Lerner PI: Tetracycline-resistant pneumococci: Increasing incidence and cross resistance to newer tetracyclines. Am Rev Respir Dis 108:1007, 1973.

79. Jonas M, Comer JB, Cunha BA: Tetracyclines. *In* Ristuccia AM, Cunha BA (eds): Antimicrobial Therapy. New York, Raven Press, 1984:226.

80. Dhawan VK, Thadepalli H: Clindamycin: A review of fifteen years of experience. Rev Infect Dis 4:1133, 1982.

81. Levison ME, Mangura CT, Lorber B, et al: Clindamycin compared with penicillin for treatment of anaerobic lung abscess. Ann Intern Med 98:466, 1983.

82. Bartlett JG: Anti-anaerobic antibacterial agents. Lancet 2:478, 1982.

83. Watanakunakorn C: Clindamycin therapy of *Staphylococcus aureus* endocarditis. Clinical relapse and development of resistance to clindamycin, lincomycin, and erythromycin. Am J Med 60:419, 1976.

84. Sutter VL: In vitro susceptibility of anaerobes: Comparison of clindamycin and other antimicrobial agents. J Infect Dis 135(suppl):S7, 1977.

85. Cuchural GJ, Tally FP, Jacobus NV, et al: Comparative activities of newer β-lactam agents against members of the *Bacteroides fragilis* group. Antimicrob Agents Chemother 34:479, 1990.

86. Klainer AS: Clindamycin. Med Clin North Am 71:1169, 1987.

87. Tedesco FJ: Clindamycin and colitis: A review. J Infect Dis 135(suppl):S95, 1977.

88. Tally FP: The treatment of anaerobic infections with metronidazole. Antimicrob Agents Chemother 7:672, 1975.

89. Gerding DN: Metronidazole. *In* Peterson PK, Verhoef J (eds): The Antimicrobial Agents Annual 3. Amsterdam, Elsevier Science Publishers, 1988:138.

90. Watanakunakorn C: Treatment of infections due to methicillin-resistant *Staphylococcus aureus*. Ann Intern Med 97:376, 1982.

91. Sabath L, Wheeler N, Laverdiere M, et al: A new type of penicillin resistance in *Staphylococcus aureus*. Lancet 1:443, 1977.

92. Watanakunakorn C, Tisone J: Synergism between vancomycin and gentamicin or tobramycin for methicillin-susceptible and methicillin-resistant *Staphylococcus aureus* strains. Antimicrob Agents Chemother 22:903, 1982.

93. Ingerman MJ, Santoro J: Vancomycin: A new old agent. Infect Dis Clin North Am 3:641, 1989.

94. Cheung RPF, DiPiro JT: Vancomycin: An update. Pharmacotherapy 6:153, 1986.

95. Matzke GR, Zhanel GG, Guay DRP: Clinical pharmacokinetics of vancomycin. Clin Pharmacokinet 11:257, 1986.

96. Cockerill FR III, Edson RS: Trimethroprim-sulfamethoxazole. Mayo Clin Proc 66:1260, 1991.

97. Craig WA, Kunin CM: Trimethoprim-sulfamethoxazole: Pharmacodynamic effects of urinary pH and impaired renal function. Ann Intern Med 78:491, 1973.

98. Cockerill FR III, Edson RS: Trimethoprim-sulfamethoxazole. Mayo Clin Proc 66:1260, 1991.

99. Wofsy CB: Use of trimethoprim-sulfamethoxazole in the treatment of *Pneumocytis carinii* pneumonitis in patients with acquired immunodeficiency syndrome. Rev Infect Dis 9(suppl 2):S184, 1987.

100. Lawson DH, Paice BJ: Adverse reactions to trimethoprim-sulfamethoxazole. Rev Infect Dis 4:429, 1982.

101. Brajtburg J, Elberg S, Schwartz D, et al: Involvement of oxidative damage in erythrocyte lysis induced by amphotericin B. Antimicrob Agents Chemother 27:172, 1985.

102. Sokol-Anderson ML, Brajtburg J, Medoff G: Amphotericin B-induced oxidative damage and killing of *Candida albicans*. J Infect Dis 154:76, 1986.

103. Graybill JR: Therapeutic agents. Infect Dis Clin North Am 2:805, 1988.

104. Christinasen KJ, Bernard EM, Gold JWM, et al: Distribution and activity of amphotericin B in humans. J Infect Dis 152:1037, 1985.

105. Bodey GP: Topical and systemic antifungal agents. Med Clin North Am 72:637, 1988.

106. Polak A: Synergism of polyene antibiotics with 5-fluorocytosine. Chemotherapy 24:2, 1978.

107. Medoff G, Comfort M, Kobayashi GS: Synergistic action of amphotericin B and 5-fluorocytosine against yeast-like organisms. Proc Soc Exp Biol Med 138:571, 1971.

108. Dismukes WE, Stamm AM, Graybill JR, et al: Treatment of systemic mycoses with ketoconazole: Emphasis on toxicity and clinical response in 52 patients. Ann Intern Med 98:13, 1983.

109. Sugar AM, Alsip SG, Galgiani JN, et al: Pharmacology and toxicity of high-dose ketoconazole. Antimicrob Agents Chemother 31:1874, 1987.

110. Pont A, Graybill JR, Craven PC, et al: High-dose ketoconazole therapy and adrenal and testicular function in humans. Arch Intern Med 144:2150, 1984.

111. Rogers TE, Galgiani JN: Activity of fluconazole (UK 49,858) and ketoconazole against *Candida albicans* in vitro and in vivo. Antimicrob Agents Chemother 30:418, 1986.

112. Kobayashi GS, Travis S, Menoff G: Comparison of the in vitro and in vivo activity of the bis-triazole derivative UK 49,858 with that of amphotericin B against *Histoplasma capsulatum.* Antimicrob Agents Chemother 29:660, 1986.

113. Graybill JR, Palou E, Ahrens J: Treatment of murine histoplasmosis with UK 49,858 (fluconazole). Am Rev Respir Dis 134:768, 1986.

114. Odds FC, Cheesman SL, Abbott AB: Antifungal effects of fluconazole (UK 49858), a new triazole antifungal in vitro. J Antimicrob Chemother 18:473, 1986.

115. Saag MS, Dismukes WE: Azole antifungal agents: Emphasis on new triazoles. Antimicrob Agents Chemother 32:1, 1988.

116. Galgiani JN: Susceptibility of *Candida albicans* and other yeasts to fluconazole: Relation between in vitro and in vivo studies. Rev Infect Dis 12:S272, 1990.

117. Grant SM, Chissold SP: Fluconazole: A review of its pharmacodynamic and pharmacokinetic properties, and therapeutic potential in superficial and systemic mycoses. Drugs 39:877, 1990.

118. Perfect JR, Durack DT: Penetration of imidazoles and triazoles into cerebrospinal fluid of rabbits. J Antimicrob Chemother 16:81, 1985.

119. Arndt CA, Walsh TJ, McCully CL, et al: Fluconazole penetration into cerebrospinal fluid: Implications for treating fungal infections of the central nervous system. J Infect Dis 157:178, 1988.

120. Brammer KW, Farrow PR, Faulkner JK: Pharmacokinetics and tissue penetration of fluconazole in humans. Rev Infect Dis 12(suppl 3):S318, 1990.

121. Van Cutsem J, Van Gerven F, Janssen PAJ: Activity of orally, topically, and parentally administered itraconazole in the treatment of superficial and deep mycoses: Animal models. Rev Infect Dis 9(suppl 1):515, 1987.

122. Espinel-Ingroff A, Shadomy S, Gebhard RJ: In vitro studies with R51,211 (itraconazole). Antimicrob Agents Chemother 26:5, 1984.

123. Grant SM, Clissold SP: Itraconazole: A review of its pharmacokinetic properties, and therapeutic use in superficial and systemic mycoses. Drugs 37:310, 1989.

124. Sharkey PK, Rinaldi MG, Dunn JF, et al: High-dose itraconazole in the treatment of severe mycoses. Antimicrob Agents Chemother 35:707, 1991.

125. Cauwenbergh GP, DeDoncker D, Stoops A, et al: Itraconazole in the treatment of human mycoses: Review of three years of clinical experience. Rev Infect Dis 9(suppl 1):S146, 1987.

126. Ganer A, Arathoon E, Stevens DA: Initial experience in therapy for progressive mycoses with itraconazole, the first clinically studied triazole. Rev Infect Dis 9(suppl 1):S77, 1987.

127. DeBeule K, DeDoncker P, Cauwenbergh G, et al: The treatment of aspergillosis and aspergilloma with itraconazole, clinical results of an open international study. (1982–1987). Mycoses 31:476, 1988.

128. Phillips P, Graybill JR, Fetchick R, et al: Adrenal responses to corticotropin during therapy with itraconazole. Antimicrob Agents Chemother 31:647, 1987.

129. Tucker RM, Haq Y, Denning DW: Adverse events associated with itraconazole in 189 patients on chronic therapy. J Antimicrob Chemother 26:561, 1990.

130. Collins P: Viral sensitivity following the introduction of acyclovir. Am J Med 85(suppl 2A):129, 1988.

131. Dorsky DI, Crumpacker CS: Drugs five years later: Acyclovir. Ann Intern Med 107:859, 1987.

132. Wade JC, Hintz M, McGuffin RW, et al: Treatment of cytomegalovirus pneumonia with high-dose acyclovir. Am J Med 73(suppl 1A):249, 1982.

133. Balfour HH, Bean B, Mitchell CD, et al: Acyclovir in immunocompromised patients with cytomegalovirus disease: A controlled trial at one institution. Am J Med 73(suppl 1A):241, 1982.

134. Shepp DH, Dandliker PS, Meyer JD: Treatment of varicella-zoster virus infection in severely immunocompromised patients: A randomized comparison of acyclovir and vidarabine. N Engl J Med 314:208, 1986.

135. Erice A, Chou S, Biron KK, et al: Progressive disease due to ganci-

136. Cole NL, Balfour HH: In vitro susceptibility of cytomegalovirus isolates from immunocompromised patients to acyclovir and ganciclovir. Diagn Microbiol Infect Dis 6:255, 1987.

137. Shepp DH, Dandliker PS, de Miranda P, et al: Activity of 9-[(2-hydroxy-1-(hydroxymethyl) ethoxy) methyl] guanine in the treatment of cytomegalovirus pneumonia. Ann Intern Med 103:368, 1985.

138. Smee DF, Martin JC, Verheyden JPH, et al: Antiherpes virus activity of the acyclic nucleoside 9-(1,3-dihydroxy-2-propoxymethyl) guanine. Antimicrob Agents Chemother 23:676, 1983.

139. Faulds D, Heel RC: Ganciclovir: A review of its antiviral activity, pharmacokinetic properties and therapeutic efficacy in cytomegalovirus infections. Drugs 39:597, 1990.

140. Erice A, Jordan MC, Chace BA, et al: Ganciclovir treatment of cytomegalovirus disease in transplant recipients and other immunocompromised hosts. JAMA 257:3082, 1987.

141. Crumpacker C, Marlowe S, Zhang JL, et al: Treatment of cytomegalovirus pneumonia. Rev Infect Dis 10(suppl 3):S538, 1988.

142. Reed EC, Bowden RA, Dandliker PS, et al: Treatment of cytomegalovirus pneumonia with ganciclovir and intravenous cytomegalovirus immunoglobulin in patients with bone marrow transplants. Ann Intern Med 109:783, 1988.

143. Reed EC: Treatment of cytomegalovirus pneumonia in transplant patients. Transplant Proc 23(suppl 1):8, 1991.

144. Balfour HH Jr: Management of cytomegalovirus disease with antiviral drugs. Rev Infect Dis 12(suppl 7):S849, 1990.

145. Chrisp P, Clissold SP: Foscarnet: A review of its antiviral activity, pharmacokinetic properties, and therapeutic use in immunocompromised patients with cytomegalovirus retinitis. Drugs 41:104, 1991.

146. Chatis PA, Miller CH, Schrager LE, et al: Successful treatment with foscarnet of an acyclovir-resistant mucocutaneous infection with herpes simplex virus in a patient with acquired immunodeficiency syndrome. N Engl J Med 320:297, 1989.

147. Heider H, Adamczyk B, Presber HW, et al: Occurrence of amantadine- and rimantadine-resistant influenza A virus strains during the 1980 epidemic. Acta Virol (Praha) 25:395, 1981.

148. Belshe RB, Burk B, Neurman P, et al: Resistance of influenza A to amantadine and rimantadine: Results of one decade of surveillance. J Infect Dis 159:430, 1989.

149. Van Voris LP, Betts RF, Hayden FG, et al: Successful treatment of naturally occurring influenza A/USSR/77 H1N1. JAMA 245:1128, 1981.

150. Little JW, Hall WJ, Douglas RG, et al: Amantadine effect on peripheral airways abnormalities in influenza. Ann Intern Med 85:177, 1976.

151. Betts RF: Antiviral agents in respiratory infections. Semin Respir Infect 6:1, 1991.

152. Betts RF, Treanor JJ, Graman PS, et al: Antiviral agents to prevent or treat influenza in the elderly. J Respir Dis 8:556, 1987.

153. Bryson YJ: Antiviral agents. Clin Chest Med 7:453, 1986.

154. Gundelfinger BF, Stilla WT, Bell JA: Effectiveness of influenza vaccines during an epidemic of Asian influenza A. N Engl J Med 259:1005, 1958.

155. Haratshorn KL, Hirsch MS: Interferons. *In* Peterson PK, Verhoef J (eds): The Antimicrobic Agents Annual 2. Amsterdam, Elsevier Science Publishers, 1986:339.

156. Douglas RM, Moore BW, Miles HB, et al: Prophylactic efficacy of intranasal alpha-2-interferon against rhinovirus infections in the family setting. N Engl J Med 314:65, 1986.

157. Hayden FG, Albrecht JK, Kaiser DL, et al: Prevention of natural colds by contact prophylaxis with intranasal alpha-2-interferon. N Engl J Med 314:71, 1986.

158. Douglas RM, Albrecht JK, Miles HB, et al: Intranasal interferon-$\alpha_2$ prophylaxis of natural respiratory virus infection. J Infect Dis 151:731, 1985.

159. Hayden FG, Kaiser DL, Albrecht JK: Intranasal recombinant alpha-2b interferon treatment of naturally occurring common colds. Antimicrob Agents Chemother 32:224, 1988.

160. Phillpotts RJ, Higgins PG, Willman JS, et al: Intranasal lymphoblastoid interferon prophylaxis against rhinovirus and influenza virus in volunteers. J Interferon Res 4:535, 1984.

161. Higgins PG, Phillpotts RJ, Scott GM, et al: Intranasal interferon as protection against experimental respiratory corona virus infection in volunteers. Antimicrob Agents Chemother 24:713, 1983.

clovir-resistant cytomegalovirus in immunocompromised patients. N Engl J Med 320:289, 1989.

162. Gerding DN, Peterson LR, Hughes CE, et al: Extravascular antimicrobial distribution and the respective blood concentrations in humans. *In* Lorian V (ed): Antibiotics in Laboratory Medicine, ed 3. Baltimore, Williams & Wilkins, 1991:880.

163. Fraschini F: Distribution of clarithromycin and its metabolite in the therapeutically relevant respiratory spaces. [Abstract] International Conference on Chemotherapy, Berlin, 1991.

164. Serour F, Dan M, Gorea A, et al: Penetration of ofloxacin into human lung tissue after a single oral dose of 200 milligrams. Antimicrob Agents Chemother 35:380, 1991.

165. Wijnands WJA, Vree TB, Baars AM, et al: The penetration of ofloxacin into lung tissue. J Antimicrob Chemother 23(suppl C):85, 1988.

166. Drusano GL: Minireview: Role of pharmacokinetics in the outcome of infections. Antimicrob Agents Chemother 32:289, 1988.

167. Nix DE, Goodwin SD, Peloquin CA, et al: Antibiotic tissue penetration and its relevance: Impact of tissue penetration on infection response. Antimicrob Agents Chemother 35:1953, 1991.

168. Cunha BA: Antibiotic pharmacokinetic considerations in pulmonary infections. Semin Respir Infect 6:168, 1991.

169. Murdoch MB, Peterson LR: Antimicrobial penetration into polymorphonuclear leukocytes and alveolar macrophages. Semin Respir Infect 6:112, 1991.

170. Klempner MS: Antibiotic penetration into phagocytes. A determination of therapeutic efficacy? Drug Ther 12:44, 1982.

171. Nix DE, Goodwin SD, Peloquin CA, et al: Minireviews: Antibiotic tissue penetration and its relevance: Models of tissue penetration and their meaning. Antimicrob Agents Chemother 35:1947, 1991.

172. Hitt JA, Gerding DN: Sputum antibiotic levels and clinical outcome in bronchitis. Semin Respir Infect 6:122, 1991.

173. Chirgwin K, Roblin PM, Hammerschlag MR: In vitro susceptibilities of *Chlamydia pneumoniae (Chlamydia* sp. strain TWAR). Antimicrob Agents Chemother 33:1634, 1989.

174. Retsema J, Girard A, Schelkly W, et al: Spectrum and mode of action of azithromycin (CP-62,993), a new 15-membered-ring macrolide with improved potency against gram-negative organisms. Antimicrob Agents Chemother 31:1939, 1987.

175. Ball AP: Therapeutic considerations for the management of respiratory tract infections. Infect Med 8(suppl A):7, 1991.

176. Cassell GH: *Mycoplasma pneumoniae.* Infect Med 8(suppl A):23, 1991.

177. Hardy DJ, Guay DRP, Jones RN: Clarithromycin, a unique macrolide: A pharmacokinetic, microbiological, and clinical overview. Diagn Microbiol Infect Dis 15:39, 1992.

178. Klastersky J, Thys JP, Mombelli G: Comparative studies of intermittent and continous administration of aminoglycosides in the treatment of bronchoplumonary infections due to gram-negative bacteria. Rev Infect Dis 3:74, 1981.

179. Thadepalli H: Lower respiratory tract. *In* Ristuccia AM, Cunha BA (eds): Antimicrobial Therapy. New York, Raven Press, 1984:439.

180. Taryle DA, Good JT, Morgan EJ, et al: Antibiotic concentrations in human parapneumonic effusion. J Antimicrob Chemother 7:171, 1981.

181. Hughes CE, VanScoy RE; Antibiotic therapy of pleural empyema. Semin Respir Infect 6:94, 1991.

182. Thys JP, Vanderhoeft P, Herchuelz A, et al: Penetration of aminoglycosides in uninfected pleural exudates and in pleural empyemas. Chest 93:530, 1988.

183. Vandaux P, Waldvogel FA: Gentamicin inactivation in purulent exudates: Role of cell lysis. J Infect Dis 142:586, 1980.

184. Bamberger DM: Antimicrobial treatment of sinusitis. Semin Respir Infect 6:77, 1991.

185. Lundberg C: General discussion. Scand J Infect Dis Suppl 44:71, 1985.

186. Wald ER, Reilly JS, Casselbrant M, et al: Treatment of acute maxillary sinusitis in childhood: A comparative study of amoxicillin and cefaclor. J Pediatr 104:297, 1984.

# CHAPTER 44

# Inhaled Antibiotics

JONATHAN S. ILOWITE

Topical therapy for infectious lung disease is an appealing concept. Delivering therapy directly to the site of infection can achieve high levels of antibiotic while minimizing systemic effects and avoiding the poor penetration of antibiotics given systemically. Agents that are metabolized quickly by the oral or intravenous routes may have a longer duration of action if inhaled directly into the lung.

Several factors must be taken into account in delivering a dose of medication by aerosol to the lung. Nebulizers vary widely in efficiency, and much of the medication is wasted in the tubing or exhaled into the environment. Particle size, lung function, and the patient's breathing pattern affect the efficiency of aerosol delivery and the distribution within the lung. After delivery, the pharmacokinetics of the antibiotic and the local concentrations achieved in the lung are of paramount importance. Few studies have attempted to control for all these factors, which may account for the widely varying results reported. This chapter analyzes the role of aerosol therapy in cystic fibrosis (CF), nosocomial pneumonia, and *Pneumocystis carinii* pneumonia (PCP).

## TREATMENT OF INFECTION IN CYSTIC FIBROSIS

CF is a disease characterized by progressive destruction of the airways and parenchyma associated with bacterial infection by a variety of organisms. The most prevalent organism, and the one most often associated with worsening lung function and exacerbations of disease, is *Pseudomonas aeruginosa*. Several studies have examined the value of inhaled aminoglycosides in this setting. In 1971, Boxerbaum and associates[1] reported on their experience treating a group of CF patients with aerosolized gentamicin. Subjective symptoms (ie, cough and sputum production) were not improved as a whole, but a subset of outpatients appeared to benefit from the treatment.

In 1974, Hoff and colleagues[2] examined the addition of aerosolized tobramycin to systemic therapy for CF patients hospitalized with acute exacerbations. The bacteriologic response was improved in the group receiving systemic and aerosol therapy. Friis[3] found that the addition of aerosol tobramycin was of no clinical benefit in a similar study. Stephens and coworkers[4] also looked at the addition of inhaled tobramycin therapy for children with CF hospitalized with exacerbations of their disease. They found a higher percentage of patients in the treatment group had *P. aeruginosa* eradicated from their sputum, but this produced no clinical benefit.

In 1981, a well-designed, randomized, crossover trial evaluated a combination of aerosolized gentamicin and carbenicillin in CF patients.[5] Seventeen patients were treated with carbenicillin (1 g) and gentamicin (80 mg), both given twice daily by nebulizer. Improvements in pulmonary function were observed in the treated group. Fewer hospitalizations were required while patients were receiving the treatment. In a similar study, Wall and associates[6] treated 11 CF patients chronically infected by *P. aeruginosa* with tobramycin (80 mg) and ticarcillin (1 g), both given by aerosol twice daily. Hospital admissions decreased from 31 before treatment to 5 patients during the same period after treatment.

Kun and associates[7] compared the inhalation of 20 mg of nebulized gentamicin twice daily with placebo in 29 children and adolescents with CF over a 2-year period. Less deterioration in lung function was seen in the treated group, but there were no differences in antibiotic usage, days in hospital, or clinical symptoms between the two groups.

Stead and coworkers[8] used a randomized crossover study to compare nebulized ceftazidime with a combination of nebulized gentamicin and carbenicillin in 13 CF patients chronically infected with *P. aeruginosa*. They were unable to show any difference in efficacy between the two antibiotic regimens, but both regimens were effective in increasing body weight, improving pulmonary function, and reducing hospitalizations compared with an untreated control group.

Although these early studies were encouraging, many questions remained unanswered. What dosage of antibiotic was effective? What type of breathing pattern should be used? What dosage could be delivered to the lungs, and what was the regional distribution of that dosage? What sputum levels could be obtained? In a carefully designed study, investigators examined the dose and regional distribution of gentamicin (80 mg) given by a commercially available nebulizer.[9] They determined that a mean of 7.7% of the original amount placed in the nebulizer was deposited in the patient's lungs. The peak sputum levels of gentamicin were determined by immuoenzymatic assay and were an order of magnitude higher than levels achieved after systemic administration (mean, 377 $\mu$g/mL), but serum levels were undetectably low. Peak sputum levels were related to the dose deposited and the regional distribution of the aerosol. The regional distribution closely followed the patient's pulmonary function: the worse the $FEV_1$, the more centrally the aerosol was deposited. The dose deposited was a function of the patient's minute ventilation; it fell with very low or very high levels of minute ventilation.

Attention has been focused on the delivery systems available for the aerosolization of antibiotics. Newman and associates, in a series of articles,[10–12] delineated the aspects of the delivery system that affect particle size and efficiency of delivery. They found that the more powerful models of home compressors produce smaller, more respirable particles. Commercially available nebulizers vary widely in the particle size produced and in efficiency, and the nebulizer must be chosen carefully to achieve the desired effect. In one study, the peripheral distribution of aerosol was dramatically increased by choosing a nebulizer that produced a smaller particle size.

These principles of aerosol therapy have been used to advantage in other clinical studies. Steinkamp and colleagues[13] investigated the long-term efficacy and safety of aminoglycoside aerosol therapy in CF patients chronically colonized with *P. aeruginosa*. Fourteen patients received aerosol therapy for a mean of 20 months in an open, unblinded study. Patients were given 80 mg of tobramycin through a jet nebulizer designed to produce particles of a respirable size and distribution. A significant increase in their weight and clinical scores was seen. Hospital admissions decreased from 2 to 1.3 per patient during the year after the study, compared with the year before the beginning of the study. Oxygenation, pulmonary function, and the need for intravenous therapy significantly improved during the study. No serious side effects were seen. Resistance occurred in 5 patients but was not associated with clinical deterioration.

Smith and coworkers[14] examined the long-term toxicity of aerosol tobramycin administered for 3 months to patients with CF. Pulmonary function, body temperature, eighth cranial nerve function, serum creatinine, blood urea nitrogen, urinary creatinine clearance, and *P. aeruginosa* density were measured before, during, and 6 weeks after discontinuation of treatment. No detectable ototoxicity or nephrotoxicity were seen. Sputum concentration of *P. aeruginosa* decreased from $10^7$ colony-forming units (CFU) per gram

of sputum to $10^4$ CFU/g. A reduced cough frequency and weight gain were observed during the treatment period. Organisms resistant to tobramycin were isolated in 73% of all sputum samples during treatment; however, 1 year later, all sputum isolates of *P. aeruginosa* were susceptible to tobramycin.

A multicenter, randomized double-blind, placebo-controlled crossover study examined the efficacy and safety of short-term administration of aerosol tobramycin to CF patients colonized with *P. aeruginosa*.[14a] Seventy-one patients were randomly allocated to receive 600 mg of tobramycin in 30 mL of normal saline three times daily or placebo. The nebulizer used was the Devilbiss 99 ultrasonic nebulizer, which was chosen based on its suitable particle size and relative efficiency. Patients were stratified into categories of mild or severe disease based on their forced vital capacity (FVC). Those with an FVC less than 70% of the predicted value were considered to have severe disease, and those with an FVC greater than 70% of the predicted value to have mild disease. Pulmonary function data and density of *P. aeruginosa* (CFU per gram of sputum) were measured. Only the first 28 days (noncrossover) of the trial had been analyzed. Patients had a 2-log reduction in median *P. aeruginosa* density in sputum and a significant improvement in pulmonary function. These improvements were significant for patients with mild or severe lung disease, and no significant side effects of the treatment were reported.

Aerosolized antibiotics have a role in the management of patients with CF who are chronically infected with *P. aeruginosa*. Studies have shown a reduction in the quantity of *P. aeruginosa* in the airways, an improvement in pulmonary function, and improvements in clinical scores. However, many questions remain to be answered. The dosage used in these clinical studies varied widely, from 30 mg twice daily of gentamicin in Kun's study to 600 mg three times daily in Ramsey's study. The optimal dosage, particle size, regional distribution, and breathing pattern during therapy require further study. Although Ramsey's study established efficacy in mild and severe disease, it is unclear whether there are subsets of patients who do not respond well to this therapy. We also need to know whether resistant organisms will become a problem as the therapy becomes more widely established and longer follow-up is analyzed. The most effective agents or combinations are yet to be identified.

## ANTIBIOTICS FOR PNEUMONIA

### Prevention of Nosocomial Pneumonia

Pneumonia is a serious problem in the hospital, and the nosocomial infection is most likely to lead to the death of patients.[15] Persons treated with mechanical ventilators in the intensive care unit have a particularly high rate of nosocomial pneumonia, with an estimated incidence of 1% per day of mechanical ventilation.[16] The mortality rate among those infected may be as high as 50%.[17, 18]

Several factors may explain this high rate of nosocomial pneumonia, particularly in the intensive care unit. Some investigators cite the failure of traditional measures of infection control in the intensive care unit.[19] Unrecognized environmental reservoirs may be present, and spread from asymptomatically colonized patients may also occur. Patients are frequently admitted to the hospital with gram-negative colonization, and nosocomial infection is frequently the result of the patient's endogenous organisms, making traditional infection control methods ineffective. The lack of adherence to traditional policies regarding hand washing, intravenous tube changes, and similar measures during periods of crisis are common problems in intensive care units.

Investigators have searched for alternative therapies aimed at preventing nosocomial pneumonia in the intensive care unit, particularly in patients treated with mechanical ventilation. Aerosol therapy offers the potential advantage of high local concentrations of antibiotic delivered to the site of potential infection with low systemic concentrations of antibiotic and less toxicity.

Klastersky and associates examined the utility of endotracheally administered gentamicin for the prevention of infections of the respiratory tract in patients with tracheostomies.[20] Endotracheal gentamicin was administered in a double-blinded, placebo-controlled study to 85 patients in a neurosurgery intensive care unit, and biweekly cultures were obtained. The rate of pneumonia was significantly decreased, from 24% in the control group to 9% in the treated group. However, the overall mortality rate was unchanged, and strains resistant to gentamicin were detected.

In 1975, Klastersky and coworkers[21] compared endotracheal gentamicin with the combination of endotracheal polymyxin B and kanamycin in similar groups of patients. Both groups had reduced rates of gram-negative colonization and pneumonia compared with historic controls; however, the combination regimen seemed to prevent the emergence of resistant organisms.

A series of studies by Feingold and associates led to the abandonment of endotracheal therapy. In the first study,[22] 58 high-risk patients in an intensive care unit were randomized to receive aerosolized polymyxin B or placebo. Seventeen of 25 patients in the control group became colonized with gram-negative bacilli, compared with 7 of 33 polymyxin-treated patients. No patient in the treated group became colonized with *P. aeruginosa*.

A second study[23] enrolled all 744 patients admitted to the intensive care unit in a prospective fashion, comparing aerosol polymyxin to placebo in alternating 2-month cycles over a 22-month period. The incidence of colonization with *P. aeruginosa* was significantly reduced during the treatment cycles (1.6% versus 9.7%, $P < .01$). Similarly, the incidence of pneumonia caused by *P. aeruginosa* was significantly reduced during the treatment cycles. Three patients developed *P. aeruginosa* pneumonia during the treatment phase, and 17 patients did so during the control cycles ($P < .01$). However, the overall mortality rates were comparable in the two groups (12.2% versus 12.0%, not significant).

In the third study,[24] aerosolized polymyxin B was administered to the upper airways of all 292 patients admitted to an intensive care unit over a 7 month period. Only 1 patient acquired pneumonia as a result of *P. aeruginosa* during the study. However, pneumonias caused by organisms resistant to polymyxin B were seen in 10 patients. Seven of these pneumonias were caused by unusual organisms not normally seen as pathogens. The mortality rate for pneumonias

caused by these resistant organisms was exceedingly high (64%) and led the researchers to conclude that "continuous use of polymyxin B aerosol appears to be a dangerous form of therapy."

Aerosolized antibiotics given as prophylaxis have not been effective in altering mortality rates among intensive care unit patients. The studies did show a reduction in oropharyngeal colonization and nosocomial pneumonia rates, results that are similar to those obtained with selective digestive decontamination. The results are not surprising in view of the methods used. Klastersky administered endotracheal antibiotics by injecting them through a plastic catheter. Feingold sprayed the solution into the oropharynx and through the endotracheal tube using a hand atomizer. Neither of these methods produced an aerosol that was likely to penetrate down the tracheobronchial tree. These studies were actually early studies in oropharyngeal and endotracheal tube decontamination, and in no study have dosage, regional distribution, pharmacokinetics, and other aspects of aerosol delivery been studied in a careful manner. Perhaps by delivery of aerosol to the lower respiratory tract, bypassing the oropharynx, prophylaxis of nosocomial pneumonia could be achieved without altering the normal flora of the oropharynx and without the emergence of resistant organisms. This deserves properly designed studies.

## Treatment of Pneumonia

Several studies have examined the use of aerosolized or endotracheally administered antibiotics for the treatment of respiratory infections. These studies have yielded conflicting results and have been plagued by methodologic difficulties. In many studies, lack of a precise end point other than clinical success or failure makes objective interpretation difficult. Most of the studies have not been blinded or placebo controlled and with the success of intravenous antibiotics, it is difficult to show an incremental benefit from inhaled agents.

Much of the research on treatment of pneumonia in intubated patients has been spurred by the hypothesis that an efficacious antibacterial agent must exceed the minimum inhibitory concentration (MIC) of the pathogen. The penetration of antibacterial agents, particularly aminoglycosides, to the lung parenchyma when delivered by the intravenous route may be poor. Levels may be much greater when delivered by aerosol route. For example, Odio and associates[25] measured serum and sputum gentamicin levels after administration to tracheostomized patients by intravenous or by bolus injection down the tracheal tube. After intravenous administration, sputum levels averaged less than 2.0 $\mu$g/mL, lower than the MIC for many pathogens and lower than the serum levels of greater than 6 $\mu$g/mL. When the same dose was delivered endotracheally, sputum levels were greater than 400 $\mu$g/mL, and serum levels were less than 1 $\mu$g/mL. However, these data must be interpreted with caution. Binding of gentamicin to sputum mucins may interfere with its bioavailability and with the assay for its measurement. Sputum levels of antibiotic may not accurately reflect tissue levels, and the extent of parenchymal injury may affect the accumulation of antibiotic in the injured tissue over time (ie, levels resulting from intravenous therapy may continually increase after multiple doses). Nevertheless, the extremely high sputum levels of antibiotic achievable by the aerosol route have led to several trials of this form of therapy.

Pines and associates[26] reported the treatment of purulent bronchial infections with gentamicin administered as an aerosol or intramuscularly. No additional benefit was seen in the group receiving aerosol therapy in combination with intramuscular therapy, compared with the group receiving intramuscular therapy alone. The same researchers[27] later reported that the addition of aerosolized gentamicin to the combination of intramuscular gentamicin and carbenicillin produced no advantage.

Sisomicin, an aminoglycoside, has been examined by several investigators. Klastersky and associates[28] investigated the endotracheal administration of sisomicin in conjunction with systemic sisomicin and carbenicillin in patients with bronchopneumonia. The group receiving endotracheal therapy with sisomicin had a better clinical response rate and a lower mortality rate than the control group. Sculler and associates[29] also evaluated the addition of endotracheal sisomicin to a combination of systemic mezlocillin and sisomicin. No difference was observed after adding the topical antibiotic.

Stockley and coworkers[30] administered aerosolized amoxicillin to patients with chronic, purulent bronchial secretions who had not responded to oral amoxicillin. Despite the emergence of resistant organisms during therapy, clinical improvement and a reduction of sputum purulence and volume were seen during therapy.

Brown and associates[31] performed a double-blind, randomized study comparing administration of 40 mg of tobramycin every 8 hours by endotracheal tube with placebo in patients with gram-negative pneumonia. Patients also received intravenous therapy with tobramycin and cefazolin or pipercillin. Eighty-one patients were enrolled in the study, but only 41 were assessable. *P. aeruginosa* accounted for 41% of the isolates, other gram-negative organism for 15%, and a mixture of organisms for 32%. The causitive organism was eradicated from the sputum in a greater percentage of patients receiving the aerosolized therapy. However, no difference in clinical outcome was seen.

Brown's study was the only randomized, blinded study performed that showed a bacteriologic response without any clinical benefit. Additional basic research needs to be done to determine the dosage, regional distribution, and pharmacokinetics before further clinical studies can be accomplished. New technologies to achieve a more uniform distribution may prove valuable for treating this subset of patients. Animal studies have shown that aerosolizing an agent with the addition of surfactant provides a more uniform distribution of the agent; it may enable the antibiotic to penetrate into areas of atelectasis or pneumonia. However, no conclusive evidence exists for the use of aerosolized or endotracheally administered antibiotics for the treatment of bacterial pneumonia.

## Treatment of *Pneumocystis carinii* Pneumonia

PCP is a common opportunistic infection in patients with acquired immunodeficiency syndrome (AIDS). Despite ef-

fective therapy, it is thought to be a direct cause of mortality in 24% of patients.[32] Standard therapy is frequently associated with significant side effects, requiring a change of therapy for 40% of patients, and patients may become intolerant to intravenous trimethoprim-sulfamethoxazole and intravenous pentamidine.[33] Attention has focused on aerosol therapy to provide an effective means of combatting the protozoal infection while avoiding toxic side effects.

Debs and associates[34] examined the tissue distribution of pentamidine after the intravenous or aerosolized route in rodents. Aerosol delivery produced substantially higher levels of pentamidine in the lungs than delivery by the intravenous route, with negligible blood or extrapulmonary drug levels. Surprisingly little metabolism or clearance of pentamidine from the lung occurred in the first 48 hours, making the agent ideal for aerosol administration. The group also examined the administration of aerosolized pentamidine in rodents with PCP. The drug was delivered in free form and encased in liposomes. Both treatments were effective in eradicating PCP, although they were less effective if the infection was severe.

Initial human studies were concerned with the development of a suitable delivery system. Montgomery and associates[35] designed a nebulizer (RespirGard II, Marquest Inc., Englewood, CO) that produced particles of appropriate size to deposit in the alveoli (approximately 1 μm). One-way valves and filters were designed to trap exhaled aerosol to minimize environmental contamination. Pilot studies using human volunteers showed that high levels of pentamidine could be delivered to the lung with little systemic absorption.[35] Using 300 mg of pentamidine in 6 mL of distilled water, levels in the alveoli, as reflected by concentrations in the bronchoalveolar lavage sediment, were $705 \pm 242$ ng/mL. When the same dose was given by intravenous route, the level in the sediment was $9.34 \pm 1.74$ ng/mL. The side effects were minor, with cough and bronchospasm occurring in a small percentage of patients.

Initial human studies were promising. Conte and coworkers[36] administered reduced-dose intravenous pentamidine (3 mg/kg of body weight per day) or aerosolized pentamidine (4 mg/kg of body weight per day) to patients with mild to moderate PCP. The rates of initial response to therapy and major toxicity were 89% and 22%, respectively, in the group that received intravenous pentamidine and 90% and 20%, respectively, in the group that received aerosolized pentamidine. Three patients who received aerosolized pentamidine relapsed within 3 months, but none of the patients who received systemic therapy relapsed.

Montgomery and coworkers[37] examined the utility of aerosolized pentamidine in an open trial of 15 patients with PCP. Severely ill patients, defined as having a PaO$_2$ of less than 50 mm Hg on room air, were excluded. Treatment consisted of inhalation of pentamidine aerosol daily for 21 days, with 600 mg of pentamidine solution delivered by the RespirGard II nebulizer. Thirteen of 15 patients had subjective and objective improvement during treatment with aerosolized pentamidine, with a marked reduction in dyspnea, respiratory rate, and fever. Eleven of 13 had improvement in arterial oxygenation and vital capacity. No adverse systemic reactions occurred in any patient during therapy, and serum pentamidine levels were less than 10 ng/mL in 12 of 14 patients. Minor complaints of coughing occurred in 12 patients, although no changes in spirometry were observed.

Miller and associates[38] used nebulized pentamidine to treat 30 patients infected with PCP in an open, unblinded study. Patients with severe hypoxemia were excluded. Pentamidine, in two dose regimens, was delivered by a standard jet nebulizer (Acorn, System 22), with a median aerodynamic diameter of 2.6 μ. Only 3 of the 14 patients responded clinically to this regimen, although the higher dose (8 mg/kg versus 4 mg/kg pentamidine) was slightly better. An additional 16 patients received 8 mg/kg of pentamidine through the RespirGard II nebulizer, and treatment was successful in 13 of these patients.

A randomized trial comparing intravenous with inhaled pentamidine for treatment of PCP in AIDS was completed by Conte and coworkers.[39] Forty-five patients were randomized to receive aerosolized pentamidine or intravenous pentamidine (3 mg/kg intravenously daily for 2–3 weeks). Pentamidine isothionate (600 mg) was delivered by Respirgard II nebulizer. The rate of initial response to therapy was similar in the two groups. However, early recrudescence of symptoms occurred in 35% of the patients receiving aerosol therapy and in none of the systemically treated patients. Relapse occurred in 24% of patients receiving aerosolized pentamidine and in none of the systemically treated group, despite greater levels of pentamidine achieved in the bronchoalveolar lavage with aerosol therapy. The overall conclusion of this randomized study suggests that intravenous therapy is more effective than aerosolized pentamidine for treatment of mild to moderate PCP.

Aerosolized pentamidine has been investigated in other settings. Montgomery and coworkers[33] used aerosolized pentamidine in 10 patients with AIDS and PCP who had previous or concurrent severe adverse reactions to standard therapy. All patients showed clinical improvement. The researchers concluded that aerosolized pentamidine was safe and effective in this group of patients. Golden and associates (personal communication) are studying the utility of aerosolized pentamidine as completion therapy for a shortened course of systemic therapy.

Aerosolized pentamidine cannot be recommended for routine use in the treatment of PCP. Although the initial pilot studies were encouraging, a randomized study showed conclusively the relative advantage of systemic therapy. Perhaps the dose delivered to the lung in the study of aerosolized therapy was inadequate. The RespirGard II is an inefficient nebulizer, with approximately 5% of the dose depositing in the patient's lungs.[40] Perhaps by increasing the dose or by switching to a more efficient nebulizer, the efficacy of aerosol therapy could be increased. One study compared the efficiency, particle size, and regional distribution of four commercially available nebulizers for patients with AIDS.[40] This study showed that the nebulizers studied varied fivefold in efficiency and produced widely different regional distributions in the lungs. It would also be worthwhile to examine the reason for failure in the study by Conte and coworkers.[39] Reports have suggested that aerosol delivery by standard means is inefficient at delivering medication to the apex of the lung.[41] If the failures in Conte's study were caused by poor apical delivery, perhaps altering the patient's breathing pattern and body position could improve apical delivery of drug and clinical efficacy.[42]

Aerosol therapy for lung infection is still in its developmental stages. Additional research is needed to determine the delivery systems, pharmacokinetics, and other factors necessary to enhance the dosage delivered and regional distribution of these agents.

# REFERENCES

1. Boxerbaum B, Pittman S, Doershuck CF, et al: Use of gentamicin in children with cystic fibrosis. J Infect Dis 124(suppl):293–295, 1971.
2. Hoff GE, Schiotz PO, Paulsen J: Tobramycin treatment of *Pseudomonas aeruginosa* infections in cystic fibrosis. Scand J Infect Dis 6:333–337, 1974.
3. Friis B: Chemotherapy of chronic infections with mucoid *Pseudomonas aeruginosa* in lower airways of patients with cystic fibrosis. Scand J Infect Dis 11:211–217, 1979.
4. Stephens D, Garey N, Isles A, et al: Efficacy of inhaled tobramycin in the treatment of pulmonary exacerbations in children with cystic fibrosis. Pediatr Infect Dis 2:209–211, 1983.
5. Hodson ME, Penketh AR, Batten JC: Aerosol carbenicillin and gentamicin treatment of *Pseudomonas aeruginosa* infection in patients with cystic fibrosis. Lancet 2:1137–1139, 1981.
6. Wall MA, Terry AB, Eisenberg J, et al: Inhaled antibiotics in cystic fibrosis. Lancet 1:1325, 1983.
7. Kun P, Landau LI, Phelan PD: Nebulized gentamicin in children and adolescents with cystic fibrosis. Aust Paediatr J 20:43–45, 1984.
8. Stead RJ, Hodson ME, Batten JC: Inhaled ceftazidime compared with gentamicin and carbenicillin in older patients with cystic fibrosis infected with *Pseudomonas aeruginosa*. Br J Dis Chest 81:272–278, 1987.
9. Ilowite JS, Gorvoy JD, Smaldone GC: Quantitative deposition of aerosolized gentamicin in cystic fibrosis. Am Rev Respir Dis 136:1445–1449, 1987.
10. Newman SP, Pellow PG, Clarke SW: Choice of nebulisers and compressors for delivery of carbenicillin aerosol. Eur J Respir Dis 69:160–168, 1986.
11. Newman SP, Pellow PG, Clay MM, et al: Evaluation of jet nebulisers for use with gentamicin solution. Thorax 40:671–676, 1985.
12. Newman SP, Woodman G, Clarke SW: Deposition of carbenicillin aerosols in cystic fibrosis: Effects of nebuliser system and breathing pattern. Thorax 43:318–322, 1988.
13. Steinkamp G, Tummler B, Gappa M, et al: Long-term tobramycin aerosol therapy in cystic fibrosis. Pediatr Pulmonol 6:91–98, 1989.
14. Smith AL, Ramsey BW, Hedges DL, et al: Safety of aerosol tobramycin administration for 3 months to patients with cystic fibrosis. Pediatr Pulmonol 7:265–271, 1989.
14a. Ramsey BW, Darkin HL, Eisenberg JD, et al: Efficacy of aerosolized tobramycin in patients with cystic fibrosis. N Engl J Med 328:1740–1746, 1993.
15. Gross PA, Neu HC, Aswapikee P, et al: Deaths from nosocomial infection: Experience in a university hospital and a community hospital. Am J Med 68:219–223, 1980.
16. Haley RW, Hooton TM, Culver DH, et al: Nosocomial infections in U.S. hospitals, 1975–1976: Estimated frequency by selected characteristics of patients. Am J Med 70:947–959, 1981.
17. Celis R, Torres A, Gatell JM, et al: Nosocomial pneuminia: A multivariate analysis of risk and prognosis. Chest 93:318–324, 1988.
18. Stevens RM, Teres D, Skillman JJ, et al: Pneumonia in an intensive care unit: A thirty month experience. Arch Intern Med 134:106–111, 1974.
19. Flaherty JP, Weinstein RA: Infection control and pneumonia prophylaxis strategies in the intensive care unit. Semin Respir Infect 5:191–203, 1990.
20. Klastersky J, Huysmans E, Weerts D, et al: Endotracheally administered gentamicin for the prevention of infections of the respiratory tract in patients with tracheostomy: A double-blind study. Chest 65:650–664, 1974.
21. Klastersky J, Hensgens C, Noterman J, et al: Endotracheal antibiotics for the prevention of tracheobronchial infections in tracheostomized unconscious patients. A comparative study of gentamicin and aminosidin-polymyxin B combination. Chest 68:302–306, 1975.
22. Greenfield S, Teres D, Bushnell LS, et al: Prevention of gram-negative bacillary pneumonia using aerosol polymyxin as prophylaxis. I. Effect on colonization pattern of the upper respiratory tract of seriously ill patients. J Clin Invest 52:2935–2940, 1973.

23. Klick JM, DuMoulin GC, Hedley-Whyte J, et al: Prevention of gram-negative bacillary pneumonia using polymyxin aerosol as prophylaxis. II. Effect on the incidence of pneumonia in seriously ill patients. J Clin Invest 55:514–519, 1975.

24. Feeley TW, DuMoulin GC, Hedley-White J, et al: Aerosol polymyxin and pneumonia in seriously ill patients. N Engl J Med 293:471–475, 1975.

25. Odio W, Vanlaer E, Klastersky J: Concentrations of gentamicin in bronchial secretions after intramuscular and endotracheal administration. J Clin Pharmacol 15:518–524, 1975.

26. Pines A, Raafat H, Plucinsky K: Gentamicin and colistin in chronic purulent bronchial infections. Br Med J 2:543–545, 1967.

27. Pines A, Raafat H, Siddigui GM, et al: Treatment of severe *Pseudomonas* infections of the bronchi. Br Med J 1:663–665, 1970.

28. Klastersky J, Meunier-Carpentier F, Kahan C: Endotracheally administered antibiotics for gram-negative pneumonia. Chest 75:586–591, 1979.

29. Sculler J, Coppens I, Klastersky J: Effectiveness of mezlocillin and endotracheally administered sisomicin with or without parenteral sisomicin in the treatment of gram-negative bronchopneumonia. J Antimicrob Chemother 9:63–68, 1982.

30. Stockley RA, Hill SI, Burnett D: Nebulized amoxicillin in chronic purulent bronchiectasis. Clin Ther 7:593–598, 1985.

31. Brown RB, Kruse JA, Counts GW, et al: Double blind study of endotracheal tobramycin in the treatment of gram-negative bacterial pneumonia. Antimicrob Agents Chemother 34:269–272, 1990.

32. Devita VT, Broder S, Fauci AS, et al: Developmental therapeutics and the acquired immunodeficiency syndrome. Ann Intern Med 106:568–581, 1987.

33. Montgomery AB, Debs RJ, Luce JM, et al: Aerosolized pentamidine as second line therapy in patients with AIDS and *Pneumocystis carinii* pneumonia. Chest 95:747–750, 1989.

34. Debs R, Straubinger R, Brunette E: Selective enhancement of pentamidine uptake in the lung by aerosolization and delivery in liposomes. Am Rev Respir Dis 135:731–737, 1987.

35. Montgomery A, Debs R, Luce J: Selective delivery of pentamidine to the lung by aerosol. Am Rev Respir Dis 137:477–478, 1987.

36. Conte JE, Hollander H, Golden JA: Inhaled or reduced-dose intravenous pentamidine for *Pneumocystis carinii* pneumonia. Ann Intern Med 107:495–498, 1987.

37. Montgomery A, Debs R, Luce J: Aerosolized pentamidine as sole therapy for *Pneumocystis carinii* pneumonia in patients with acquired immunodeficiency syndrome. Lancet 2:480–483, 1987.

38. Miller RF, Godfrey FP, Semple SJ: Nebulised pentamidine as treatment for *Pneumocystis carinii* pneumonia in the acquired immunodeficiency syndrome. Thorax 44:565–569, 1989.

39. Conte JEJ, Chernoff D, Feigal DWJ, et al: Intravenous or inhaled pentamidine for treating *Pneumocystis carinii* pneumonia in AIDS. A randomized trial. Chest 98:386–388, 1990.

40. Ilowite JS, Baskin MI, Sheetz MS, et al: Delivered dose and regional distribution of aerosolized pentamidine using different delivery systems. Chest 99:1139–1144, 1991.

41. Abd A, Nierman D, Ilowite J, et al: Bilateral upper lobe *Pneumocystis carinii* pneumonia in a patient receiving inhaled pentamidine prophylaxis. Chest 94:329–331, 1988.

42. Baskin MI, Abd AG, Ilowite JS: Regional deposition of aerosolized pentamidine. Effects of body position and breathing pattern. Ann Intern Med 150:2167–2168, 1990.

# CHAPTER 45

# Adjunctive Measures in the Treatment of Respiratory Infections

MARK J. ROSEN and ROBERT J. GLENNON

Innate host defenses and specific antimicrobial therapy are the most important factors in the outcome of respiratory infections. However, these infections may be complicated by other problems that require therapeutic interventions. Tracheobronchial secretions may accumulate because of increased production of purulent material as a consequence of infection and because of impaired clearance by inadequate mucociliary function and cough. Retained secretions may lead to hypoxemia because of inadequate ventilation of local areas of the lung. If secretions completely occlude an airway, atelectasis of a segment, lobe, or entire lung may occur. Excessive secretions can produce a clinical spectrum that ranges from mild hypoxemia to respiratory failure necessitating endotracheal intubation and mechanical ventilation.

Adjunctive measures in the treatment of respiratory infections focus on assisting the patient in clearing secretions and correcting hypoxemia. Chest physiotherapy, suctioning, fiberoptic bronchoscopy, and the administration of bronchodilators, mucolytics, and hydration are often employed for patients with pneumonia. The rationale for these measures is often based on empiric impressions and tradition rather than on scientific proof. Besides increasing the costs of medical care, these therapies may be harmful in some situations. In 1979, the National Heart, Lung, and Blood Institute of the National Institutes of Health convened a conference on the Scientific Basis of In-Hospital Respiratory Therapy. The conference attempted to summarize the state of knowledge about these treatments and recommended avenues of investigation to answer questions about which modalities are useful in specific disease states.[1] Most of the questions remain unanswered. The variability in physiotherapy techniques among centers, disparate populations under study, and the lack of widely available methods to assess tracheobronchial clearance are impediments to valid controlled studies of these therapies.

## CHEST PHYSIOTHERAPY

Orders and suggestions for ''vigorous chest PT'' or ''aggressive pulmonary toilet'' often appear on patients' hospital charts. The aim of chest physiotherapy is to assist the patient in removing sputum from the large airways. The process is like ''getting ketchup out of a bottle: turn it upside down, thump it on the back several times, and a splash of the desired material usually appears.''[2] Methods used to achieve this goal include postural drainage, chest percussion, chest wall vibration, and forced expiration techniques.[3–5] These maneuvers are intended to augment the patient's own cough and mucociliary clearance mechanisms. Although the removal of excessive secretions is desirable to reduce the work of breathing and improve gas exchange in some patients,[6, 7] the efficacy of chest physical therapy in facilitating the resolution of respiratory infections is unproved.

Chest physiotherapy appears to be most useful in chronic conditions in which there is a large amount of sputum production, as in bronchiectasis, cystic fibrosis, and some cases of chronic bronchitis,[8–12] although it may offer no advantages to persons who have effective cough and mucociliary mechanisms. In acute exacerbations of chronic bronchitis, data on the efficacy of physiotherapy generally show little benefit.[13, 14]

Chest physiotherapy can have deleterious effects. Postural drainage in a head-down position increases the work of breathing by forcing the diaphragm to contract against gravity, which may provoke respiratory distress in a compromised patient. Chest percussion may be uncomfortable, and it has led to bronchospasm in patients with chronic bronchitis and cystic fibrosis.[5, 15]

Hypoxemia can also occur during chest percussion and postural drainage. Connors and associates investigated the effect of these modalities used together in 22 hospitalized patients with acute, nonsurgical pulmonary disorders.[16] Ten patients produced little or no sputum, and their mean $PaO_2$ fell by 16.8 mm Hg after percussion and postural drainage and by another 5.3 mm Hg 30 minutes later. There was no significant change in $PaO_2$ in 12 patients who produced moderate or large amounts of mucopurulent secretions.

Because the aim of chest physiotherapy is to clear secretions from the central airways, it is unlikely to be effective in most cases of pneumonia, in which the site of infection is predominantly the distal airways and alveoli. In a randomized, prospective clinical trial, Graham and Bradley found that patients with pneumonia who were treated with postural drainage, percussion, vibration, and intermittent positive-pressure breathing had no improvement in the duration of fever, rate of radiographic resolution, length of hospital stay, or mortality compared with controls.[17] In another prospective, randomized trial, 171 patients with pneumonia received postural drainage with percussion and vibration or advice on expectoration, deep breathing, and exercise to prevent thrombosis; the latter was considered a placebo-control group.[18] Patients with underlying pulmonary diseases such as chronic bronchitis and asthma were excluded. There were no differences in the length of hospital stay, improvement in spirometry, or the rate of radiographic resolution. Younger patients, smokers, and patients with predominantly interstitial infiltrates who received physiotherapy had a longer duration of fever.

Although conclusive data are lacking, chest physiotherapy appears to be most effective in selected patients with excessive sputum who are unable to expectorate effectively. The routine use of postural drainage, percussion, and vibration should be abandoned for patients with pneumonia who do not fulfill these criteria.

## SUCTIONING

Tracheal suctioning can remove excessive secretions from a patient who does not cough effectively. Secretions are removed directly, and the introduction of a suction catheter into the trachea can provoke vigorous coughing, even in a patient who has a depressed mental status. Endotracheal suctioning is part of the routine care of patients with endotracheal tubes, partly because the presence of the tube usually precludes effective coughing. Nasotracheal suctioning may be performed in patients without endotracheal tubes, but the passage of the suction catheter into the trachea is difficult to achieve, and it is uncomfortable for the patient. It is indicated only rarely, because obtunded or comatose patients are usually intubated.

Several complications may occur as a result of endotracheal suctioning, including tissue trauma, laryngospasm, and bronchospasm.[19] Hypoxemia is a common occurrence because of alterations in ventilation induced by the catheter and temporary discontinuation of mechanical ventilation and because gas is suctioned from the airway.[20] Supplemental oxygen should be administered to patients before suctioning. The introduction of a catheter into the lower airway may deposit pathogenic bacteria and set the stage for infection, although the magnitude of this risk remains undefined. Adherence to proper techniques in suctioning patients appears important to prevent pneumonia, especially in intubated patients.

## FIBEROPTIC BRONCHOSCOPY

The role of fiberoptic bronchoscopy in the diagnosis of respiratory infections has been discussed. In patients with respiratory infections, bronchoscopy may be used as a therapeutic measure, usually to remove secretions that obstruct an airway and lead to atelectasis.[21–26] Bronchoscopy has also been used to facilitate the drainage of lung abscess and to remove foreign bodies.[21, 25]

Bronchoscopy permits direct visualization of the tracheobronchial tree and aspiration of visible secretions. However, the bronchoscope can visualize only the proximal airways. The procedure must be performed by experienced personnel, entails cost and discomfort, and may be difficult to perform repeatedly in the same patient. Potential complications include respiratory depression from premedications, respiratory compromise due to airway narrowing in the presence of the bronchoscope, and cardiac arrhythmias.[27–29] Various degrees of hypoxemia usually occur during bronchoscopy and for several hours afterward.[30–32] The use of bronchial lavage for diagnostic purposes or to facilitate removal of secretions may cause transient hypoxemia.

Several studies support the efficacy of fiberoptic bronchoscopy in the management of retained secretions and atelectasis, usually in critically ill, intubated patients.[22, 23] However, convincing evidence attesting to superior results compared with more conservative treatment is lacking. In a prospective randomized study, 31 subjects with acute lobar atelectasis had immediate fiberoptic bronchoscopy, followed by respiratory therapy every 4 hours for 48 hours, or received respiratory therapy alone.[26] The respiratory therapy regimen included deep breathing (or hyperinflation with an anesthesia bag in intubated patients), coughing or endotracheal suctioning, inhalation of bronchodilator aerosols, and chest percussion with postural drainage. Bronchoscopy did not add significantly to the respiratory therapy regimen in resolution of the atelectasis. Of the patients in both groups in whom 24 hours of respiratory therapy was not effective, most had a visible air bronchogram on frontal chest radiograph, signifying that the central airways were not obstructed. In these cases, lobar atelectasis can be explained by pneumonitis or extensive microatelectasis, conditions where bronchoscopy and respiratory therapy are ineffective. Bronchoscopy should be used for clearance of secretions and atelectasis only if there is no response to more conservative measures, and if no air bronchogram is visible on chest radiograph.

In some cases, patients with pneumonia should undergo bronchoscopic inspection of the major airways if an intraluminal obstruction caused by a neoplasm or foreign body is suspected. Patients with cavitary lung lesions may have fiberoptic bronchoscopy to differentiate a carcinoma from lung abscess. In a retrospective review of 52 patients undergoing bronchoscopy in the evaluation of cavitary lung lesions with an air-fluid level, 19 (36.5%) had associated carcinomas.[33] Patients who had fevers exceeding 101°F, leukocyte counts exceeding 14,000/mm[3], predisposing factors for aspiration, systemic symptoms, or extensive infiltrates seen on the chest radiographs were more likely to have a lung abscess without associated malignancies, and bronchoscopy added little to their evaluations.

## BLAND AEROSOLS, MUCOLYTICS, EXPECTORANTS, AND BRONCHODILATORS

In addition to antibiotics, several agents are commonly used in treating respiratory infections. Bland aerosols, bronchodilators, mucolytics, and expectorants are often ordered in an attempt to enhance clearance of secretions and improve respiratory function.

Bland aerosols are mists of water or saline solutions that are sometimes employed to add water to desiccated, inflamed upper airway mucosa or to facilitate expectoration. If expectoration does increase, it is probably the result of stimulation of cough. Most of the particles constituting mists are deposited above the vocal cords, and deposition of liquid on the airways probably does not significantly alter the properties of sputum. A review of the literature by Wanner and Rao led to the conclusion that these treatments offer no benefit to patients with asthma, chronic bronchitis, or respiratory infections.[34]

In theory, mucolytic agents like *N*-acetylcysteine may facilitate the expectoration of excessive thick tracheobronchial secretions in patients with airway disease. In vitro studies of mucolytic agents show that they reduce sputum viscosity, but the clinical importance of altering sputum characteristics is unknown. Because many of these agents have irritant and bronchoconstricting effects, especially in patients with airway disease,[35] the use of mucolytics, detergents, or enzymes is not recommended in the treatment of most lung infections.

Expectorants may be employed with the goal of facilitating mucous clearance, but objective data demonstrating efficacy are scarce, even in patients with stable chronic bronchitis. A double-blind, placebo-controlled trial of iodinated glycerol in stable patients with stable chronic bronchitis demonstrated that, compared with placebo, treatment with 60 mg four times daily improved cough symptoms, chest discomfort, ease in bringing up sputum, and overall patient well-being.[36] Although there was no difference between groups in the overall incidence of acute exacerbations, the mean duration of exacerbations was 6.3 days in the iodinated glycerol group and 10.2 days in the placebo-control group. The efficacy of starting treatment with this or any other expectorant agent as adjunctive treatment for an acute respiratory infection is unsubstantiated.

Bronchodilating aerosols are useful in some patients with chronic pulmonary disease, particularly asthma and cystic fibrosis. They are effective in relieving airway obstruction caused by smooth muscle contraction. Because bronchospasm may inhibit clearance of foreign material from airways through cough, bronchodilators may improve the mobilization of secretions produced by lung infection. However, most patients with pneumonia do not have significant airway obstruction caused by bronchospasm, and bronchodilating drugs are of little benefit to them.

Bronchodilators may improve the clearance of secretions by mechanisms other than smooth muscle relaxation. Although the precise mechanisms are unknown, theophylline and sympathomimetic agents enhance mucociliary transport by alteration of the physical characteristics of sputum or by increasing airway ciliary beat frequency.[37] Although these effects may improve the transport of purulent material from the small airways, benefits are theoretical, and the efficacy of bronchodilators for this purpose in patients with pneumonia is unproven.

## HYDRATION

Patients with bronchitis and pneumonia are often urged to drink large volumes of water, and hospitalized patients may be given intravenous fluids, on the premise that hydration thins the sputum and makes it easier to expectorate. However, the benefits of fluid intake are unproven in the management of acute respiratory infections or even in chronic bronchitis. Shim and coworkers tested three regimens in 12 patients with chronic bronchitis and daily sputum production: drinking 1 glass of any fluid except alcohol every waking hour after supper and upon waking the next morning; drinking no fluid after supper or the next morning; and drinking fluid ad libitum. There was no difference in sputum volume or elasticity, respiratory symptoms, or ease of expectoration.[38] There is no justification for vigorous hydration of euvolemic patients to facilitate sputum expectoration.

## OXYGEN

All lower respiratory tract infections impose some ventilation-perfusion mismatch or shunt, which may be clinically important if hypoxemia ensues. In 1921, Meakins underscored the importance of oxygen therapy in lobar pneumonia, stating, "It is most important—perhaps the most important—factor in the treatment of pneumonia, apart from the specific cure of infection that the patient should be prevented from developing an anoxemia. . . ."[39] In 1979, Snider and Renaldo reviewed the indications for oxygen therapy and modes of administration as part of the Conference on the Scientific Basis of In-Hospital Respiratory Therapy and proposed a definition of "treatable hypoxemia" as a value of $PaO_2$ less than 60 mm Hg.[40] At this level, the hemoglobin saturation is 90%, and large increments in $PaO_2$ are necessary to achieve a minimal increase in arterial oxygen content. However, many patients with pneumonia have abrupt changes in gas exchange, and supplemental oxygen may be appropriate despite a $PaO_2$ higher than 60 mm Hg in a patient who is deemed unstable.

Oxygen may be administered by a variety of devices. A

nasal cannula has the advantages of greatest comfort and convenience of use. However, the precise $F_{IO_2}$ the patient is receiving depends on the $O_2$ flow rate and on the respiratory frequency and depth. It also cannot deliver high concentrations of oxygen. Nasal cannulas are most appropriate for patients with mild hypoxemia or chronic hypercapnia who have stable breathing patterns, in whom relatively low concentrations of supplemental oxygen are appropriate.

Venturi masks deliver a more precise $F_{IO_2}$ up to 0.40, and they should be used if titration of inhaled oxygen is important, usually in patients with chronic hypercapnia in whom excessive oxygen administration may increase the $PaCO_2$.[41] Standard oxygen masks deliver higher $O_2$ concentrations, and nonrebreathing reservoir masks can deliver $F_{IO_2}$ up to 0.90.

A simple maneuver that may improve gas exchange in patients with pneumonia makes use of the effects of gravity on pulmonary blood flow. At normal lung volumes, there is a gradient of hydrostatic and pleural pressure that results in increased ventilation and perfusion of dependent areas. By positioning a patient with an asymmetric lung disease with the less-involved lung in a dependent position, blood flow is directed preferentially to the better-ventilated lung, improving ventilation-perfusion matching and increasing the $PaO_2$.[42] Gravitational maneuvers may be a useful temporizing measure for patients with hypoxemia refractory to supplemental oxygen delivered by mask.

A patient who requires high concentrations of oxygen to maintain the $PaO_2$ at or above 60 mm Hg usually has a severe shunt and may require airway pressure therapy in the form of continuous positive airway pressure therapy by mask or positive end-expiratory pressure delivered by an endotracheal tube.

Oxygen should be used as a drug with specific indications and doses. The aim of therapy is the correction of hypoxemia, and the $F_{IO_2}$ should be titrated to provide the patient with an adequate $PaO_2$. The prolonged administration of excessive oxygen causes decreased mucociliary clearance, tracheobronchial inflammation, and alveolar damage.[43] Although the precise $F_{IO_2}$ and duration of use that can be deemed ''safe'' is unknown, there is a consensus that an $F_{IO_2}$ of more than 0.50 to 0.60 should not be maintained longer than 48 hours.[40]

## REFERENCES

1. National Heart, Lung, and Blood Institute of the National Institutes of Health: Proceedings of the Conference on the Scientific Basis of Respiratory Therapy. Am Rev Respir Dis 122(Suppl):1–161, 1979.
2. Murray JF: The ketchup-bottle method. N Engl J Med 300:1155, 1979.
3. Campbell AH, O'Connell JM, Wilson F: The effect of chest physiotherapy upon the $FEV_1$ in chronic bronchitis. Med J Aust 1:33–35, 1975.
4. Rochester DF, Goldberg SK: Techniques of respiratory physical therapy. Am Rev Respir Dis 122:133–146, 1979.
5. Sutton PP: Chest physiotherapy: Time for a reappraisal. Br J Dis Chest 82:127–137, 1988.
6. Mackenzie CF, Shin B, Hadi F, et al: Changes in total lung/thorax compliance following chest physiotherapy. Anesth Analg (Cleve) 59:207, 1980.
7. Mackenzie CF, Shin B, McAslan TC: Chest physiotherapy: The effect on arterial oxygenation. Anesth Analg (Cleve) 57:28, 1978.
8. Lorin MI, Denning CR: Evaluation of postural drainage by measurement of sputum volume and consistency. Am J Phys Med 50:215, 1971.
9. Cochrane GM, Webber BA, Clarke SW: Effects of sputum on pulmonary function. Br Med J 2:1181, 1977.
10. Bateman JRM, Newman SP, Daund KM, et al: Regional lung clearance of excessive bronchial secretions during chest physiotherapy in patients with stable chronic airways obstruction. Lancet 1:294, 1979.
11. Bateman JRM, Newman SP, Daunt KM, et al: Is cough as effective as chest physiotherapy in the removal of excessive tracheobronchial secretions? Thorax 36:683, 1981.
12. Mazzoco MC, Owens GR, Kirilloff LH, et al: Chest percussion and postural drainage in patients with bronchiectasis. Chest 88:360, 1985.
13. Anthonisen P, Riis P, Sogaard-Andersen T: The value of lung physiotherapy in the treatment of acute exacerbations in chronic bronchitis. Acta Med Scand 175:715, 1964.
14. Newton DAG, Stephenson A: Effect of physiotherapy on pulmonary function. Lancet 1:228, 1978.
15. Feldman J, Traver GA, Taussig LM: Maximal expiratory flows after postural drainage. Am Rev Respir Dis 119:239–245, 1979.
16. Connors AF, Hammon WE, Martin RJ, Rogers RM: Chest physical therapy: The immediate effect of oxygenation on acutely ill patients. Chest 78:559, 1980.
17. Graham WBCB, Bradley DA: Efficacy of chest physiotherapy and intermittent positive-pressure breathing in the resolution of pneumonia. N Engl J Med 299:624, 1978.
18. Britton S, Bejstedt M, Vedin L: Chest physiotherapy in primary pneumonia. Br Med J 290:1703, 1975.
19. Demers RR: Complications of endotracheal suctioning procedures. Respir Care 27:453, 1982.
20. Boutros AR. Arterial blood oxygenation during and after endotracheal suctioning in the apneic patient. Anesthesiology 32:114, 1970.
21. Wanner A, Landa JF, Nieman RE, et al: Bedside bronchofiberoscopy for atelectasis and lung abscess. JAMA 224:1281, 1973.
22. Lindholm CE, Ollman B, Snyder J, et al: Flexible fiberoptic bronchoscopy in critical care medicine: Diagnosis, therapy and complications. Crit Care Med 2:250, 1974.
23. Mahajan VK, Catron PW, Huber GL: The value of fiberoptic bronchoscopy in the management of pulmonary collapse. Chest 73:817, 1978.
24. Barrett CR: Flexible fiberoptic bronchoscopy in the critically ill patient: Methodology and indications. Chest 73:746, 1978.
25. Dreisin RB, Albert RK, Talley PA, et al: Flexible fiberoptic bronchoscopy in the teaching hospital: Yield and complications. Chest 74:144, 1978.
26. Marini JJ, Pierson DJ, Hudson LD: Acute lobar atelectasis: A prospective comparison of fiberoptic bronchoscopy and respiratory therapy. Am Rev Respir Dis 119:971, 1979.
27. Credle WF, Smiddy JF, Elliot RC: Complications of fiberoptic bronchoscopy. Am Rev Respir Dis 109:67, 1974.
28. Suratt PM, Smiddy JF, Gruber B: Deaths and complications associated with fiberoptic bronchoscopy. Chest 69:747, 1976.
29. Pereira W, Kovnat DM, Snider GL: A prospective cooperative study of complications following flexible fiberoptic bronchoscopy. Chest 73:813, 1978.
30. Albertini RE, Harrell JH, Kurihara N, et al: Arterial hypoxemia induced by fiberoptic bronchoscopy. JAMA 230:1666, 1974.
31. Pierson DJ, Iseman MD, Sutton FD, et al: Arterial blood gas changes in fiberoptic bronchoscopy during mechanical ventilation. Chest 66:495, 1974.
32. Shrader DL, Lakshminarayan S: The effect of fiberoptic bronchoscopy on cardiac rhythm. Chest 73:821, 1978.
33. Sosenko A, Glassroth J: Fiberoptic bronchoscopy in the evaluation of lung abscesses. Chest 87:489, 1985.
34. Wanner A, Rao A: Clinical indications for and effects of bland, mucolytic and antimicrobial aerosols. Am Rev Respir Dis 122(suppl):79, 1980.
35. Rao S, Wilson DB, Brooks RC, et al: Acute effects of nebulization of N-acetylcysteine on pulmonary mechanics and gas exchange. Am Rev Respir Dis 102:17, 1970.
36. Petty TL: The National Mucolytic Study: Results of a randomized, double-blind, placebo-controlled study of iodinated glycerol in chronic obstructive bronchitis. Chest 97:75, 1990.
37. Wanner A: Alteration of tracheal mucociliary transport in airway disease. Effect of pharmacologic agents. Chest 80(suppl):867, 1981.
38. Shim C, King M, Williams MH: Lack of effect of hydration on sputum production in chronic bronchitis. Chest 92:679–682, 1987.

39. Meakins J: Observations on the gases in human arterial blood in certain pathological pulmonary conditions and their treatment with oxygen. J Pathol Bacteriol 24:70, 1921.

40. Snider GL, Rinaldo JE: Oxygen therapy in medical patients hospitalized outside the intensive care unit. Am Rev Respir Dis 122(suppl):29–36, 1980.

41. Cohen JL, Demers RR, Saklad M: Air-entrainment oxygen masks: A performance evaluation. Respir Care 22:277, 1977.

42. Kvetan V, Carlon GC, Howland WS: Acute pulmonary failure in asymmetric lung disease: Approach to management. Crit Care Med 10:114, 1982.

43. Jackson RM: Molecular, pharmacologic and clinical aspects of oxygen-induced lung injury. Clin Chest Med 11:73, 1990.

44. Fanburg BL: Oxygen toxicity: Why can't a human be more like a turtle? Intensive Care Med 3:134, 1988.

# New Therapeutic Strategies for Sepsis and Pneumonia

STEVE NELSON and WARREN R. SUMMER

Respiratory tract infections are major causes of excessive morbidity and mortality in hospitalized patients.[1, 2] Patients with systemic sepsis have an especially high risk of acquiring these respiratory infections, which suggests that their antibacterial defenses are uniquely compromised.[3, 4] In this review, we examine these sepsis-induced alterations in pulmonary host defense mechanisms, and new strategies are discussed in the context of systemic- and lung-related therapeutic targets.

The poor prognosis of patients who develop nosocomial pneumonia strongly suggests that host factors may be more important determinants of outcome than current treatment modalities. Surgery, trauma, underlying systemic infection, and chronic illnesses have been shown to alter the indices of immune function.[5] Aspirated bacterial challenges that enter the lower respiratory tract rarely cause pneumonia in healthy persons, because the pulmonary defense mechanisms are remarkably effective under normal circumstances in maintaining the sterility of the distal airways.[6] The antibacterial defenses of the lung include the resident alveolar macrophages (AM) and the polymorphonuclear leukocytes (PMN) that are mobilized from the bloodstream into the alveoli in response to bacterial stimuli.

Evidence indicates that the underlying condition of the host is the primary determinant of response to therapy and survival of patients with pneumonia.[5] When pneumonia develops, some element of the normal defense apparatus has failed or is inadequate. Extrapulmonary infections are commonly associated with the subsequent development of nosocomial pneumonia. Sepsis is the most common clinical antecedent of the adult respiratory distress syndrome (ARDS) and is a major risk factor for the subsequent development of pneumonia.[7-9] As many as 45% of patients with ARDS have sepsis as the primary predisposing factor. Moreover,

pneumonia, the most common secondary infection in these patients, is associated with the poorest survival rate of all secondary infections (<10%).[10] In one report, the mortality rate of ARDS patients with nosocomial infection was not affected by appropriate antibiotic administration,[10] indicating that endogenous host defense factors are critical determinants of susceptibility to infection and survival. Alternatively, the host defense system may be one of multiple failing organs in a patient with poor physiologic reserve, or standard approaches in antibiotic therapy may be inadequate.

Although the role of sepsis in the pathogenesis of acute lung injury is a focus of numerous investigations, the effects of systemic sepsis on pulmonary antibacterial defenses are poorly defined. Bacterial pneumonia, rather than respiratory failure, appears to be a primary cause of death of these patients. Measures focused on reducing the exposure of the host to potential pathogens (eg, selective decontamination) and optimizing antimicrobial delivery have been reviewed.[11, 12] Two other potential therapeutic approaches are prevention of the sequence of systemic events induced by sepsis that lead to lung immunosuppression and immune restoration of the lung.

## EXTRAPULMONARY SEPSIS

The limitations of currently available therapy for sepsis are evidenced by the high, relatively fixed mortality rates associated with this disease despite improvements in antibiotic therapy and critical care technology. If the various steps in the pathogenesis of sepsis are considered, beginning with tissue invasion by the offending pathogen and culminating in the pathophysiologic sequelae associated with the septic shock syndrome, it is clear that conventional therapy addresses only the initial and final stages of this process (Fig. 46–1). Current therapy includes antibiotics directed against the bacteria and supportive measures that attempt to compensate for failing organs. Standard approaches fail to target key intermediate steps, which probably play a critical role in the evolution of this disease process. Newer strategies are directed at the intermediate stages of this disease and entail the selective attenuation of host responses to the invading pathogen or its products (Fig. 46–2).

## Lipopolysaccharide Neutralization

Lipopolysaccharide (LPS), or endotoxin, is an integral component of the outer membrane of gram-negative bacteria. LPS plays a pivotal role in the pathophysiology of sepsis and its sequelae.[13] The pathogenic function of LPS makes it a prime target for new therapies that aim to neutralize the toxic properties of LPS, remove LPS from potential in vivo sites of action, inactivate functional LPS molecules, or prevent LPS interaction with receptors on susceptible host cells.

### Antibiotics

Antibiotics, the mainstay of current therapy, can have a dramatic influence on circulating endotoxin levels. It has been suggested that under certain circumstances shock might be precipitated in susceptible hosts by bacterial cell lysis and the sudden release of endotoxin from the gram-negative bacteria exposed to antibiotics.[14, 15] In vitro studies have demonstrated that endotoxin is released when bacteria are exposed to antibiotics.[16–18] Direct evidence that antibiotic therapy can promote endotoxin release in vivo has been provided by studies in rabbits infected with *Escherichia coli.*[19] Rokke and colleagues demonstrated that endotoxin is liberated during antibiotic therapy in a porcine sepsis model and that this increase is associated with cardiac dysfunction.[20] In patients undergoing antibiotic therapy for sepsis, endotoxin release can be induced after antibiotic administration and leads to hypotension and an increased level of plasma lactate.[21]

An antimicrobial agent that minimizes the release of endotoxin is desirable. In general, the use of antibiotics acting

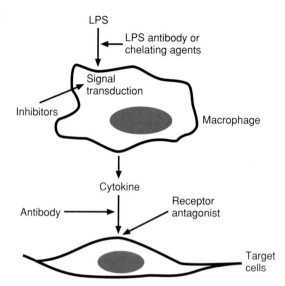

**Figure 46–2.** Possible sites for therapeutic intervention during sepsis. LPS, lipopolysaccharide.

on the bacterial cell wall (eg, β-lactam agents) tends to be associated with greater endotoxin release than the use of those whose action leaves the cell wall intact.[19] Such considerations in the selection of antibiotic therapy must be balanced by the fact that bacteriostatic drugs may not be as efficient as bactericidal agents in decreasing the number of viable bacteria. There are also differences even between the various β-lactam antibiotics that may be related to the binding and inhibition of penicillin-binding proteins.[22] These differences in binding have been proposed as a possible mechanism for an in vitro study showing that *E. coli* organisms incubated in the presence of various β-lactams exhibit significant differences in the release of tumor necrosis factor from mononuclear cells stimulated by filtrates of these antibiotic-killed bacteria.[23] It has also been suggested that a lower initial dose of antibiotics should be administered to patients with presumed sepsis or that antibiotic treatment should be delayed until the patient has been resuscitated and hemodynamically stabilized. Alternatively, pretreatment of the patient with an antibody to LPS or a chelating agent (eg, polymyxin B) before antibiotic administration may be an effective strategy.

### Antibodies to Endotoxin

Historically, immunization (active and passive) has proven effective against several bacterial infections, but this approach has been limited to antitoxic immunity or type-specific immunity to a limited number of serologic types. However, the many species and serotypes responsible for gram-negative sepsis render type-specific or passive immunization impractical for the prevention or treatment of these infections.

The virtually identical composition of the core or lipid A regions of LPS from gram-negative bacteria suggests that shared or common epitopes may be exposed on the bacterial surfaces and that an antibody to these common antigens may enhance resistance. Animal and human investigations support this hypothesis. Ziegler demonstrated that human antiserum to the core glycolipid of the rough mutant *E. coli*

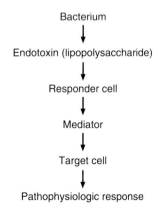

**Figure 46–1.** Pathophysiologic sequence of events during sepsis.

Bacterium
↓
Endotoxin (lipopolysaccharide)
↓
Responder cell
↓
Mediator
↓
Target cell
↓
Pathophysiologic response

J5 strain reduced the mortality rate in patients with gram-negative bacteremia from 39% to 22% ($P = .011$); in patients with shock, the mortality rate was reduced by the J5 antiserum from 77% to 44% ($P = .003$).[24] Prophylactic intravenous administration of standard immune globulin or core-lipopolysaccharide immune globulin in adults at high risk of abdominal sepsis failed to alter the rates of systemic infection, septic shock, and mortality.[25] There are substantial problems involved in the isolation and purification of commercially useful amounts of antibody suitable for human use. To circumvent these difficulties, murine and human monoclonal antibodies have been developed.

Two monoclonal antibodies—a murine IgM monoclonal antibody (E5; XOMA, Berkeley, CA) and a human IgM monoclonal antibody (Centoxin, HA-1A; Centocor, Malvern, PA) reactive with the lipid A portion of LPS—have undergone clinical trials. In the HA-1A trial, the mortality rate for patients with gram-negative bacteremia was reduced from 49% in the placebo group to 30% in the HA-1A group ($P = .014$).[26] For patients with gram-negative bacteremia and shock, the mortality rate was reduced by HA-1A from 57% to 33% ($P = .017$). In the E5 clinical trial, the mortality rate was reduced only for those with gram-negative infections in the absence of shock (ie, 23% mortality rate in the placebo group and 12% in the E5 group, $P < .05$).[27]

The mechanism of clinical protection afforded by these antibodies is unclear, although it is widely assumed to involve direct endotoxin neutralization. A placebo-controlled study of 82 patients with gram-negative sepsis by Wortel and coworkers reported that treatment with HA-1A reduced the mortality rate primarily for patients with endotoxemia (ie, 73% to 31%, $P < .01$).[28] However, comparable reductions in circulating endotoxin were observed in the HA-1A and placebo groups. Serum tumor necrosis factor-$\alpha$ (TNF) levels were lower in the HA-1A treated patients. These data suggest that HA-1A may interfere with endotoxin-induced activation of the cytokine cascade rather than enhancing endotoxin clearance. Complete delineation of the clinical efficacy of monoclonal antibodies to lipid A in the treatment of gram-negative sepsis requires careful analysis and scrutiny of the results of these clinical trials and will probably entail additional clinical studies. This is particularly important in light of a study of sepsis in a canine model in which HA-1A did not alter levels of endotoxemia and actually decreased survival.[28a]

### Bactericidal Permeability-Increasing Protein

The bactericidal permeability-increasing protein (BPI) of neutrophils is a potent cytotoxin, specific for gram-negative bacteria, that also inhibits endotoxin activity by binding to the lipid A region of LPS.[29, 30] It is a 57-kd membrane-associated protein isolated from the granules of PMN. It binds to the surface of susceptible gram-negative bacteria, alters membrane permeability, and causes cell death. BPI prevents neutrophil activation by LPS in vitro and inhibits LPS-induced TNF production in whole blood.[31] Together with its potent antibacterial properties, these findings suggest that BPI may be able to down-regulate responses to LPS by halting the proliferation of bacteria producing LPS and by binding directly with LPS.[32] The availability of

cloned protein will greatly facilitate future studies of the efficacy of BPI in animal models of gram-negative infection and sepsis.

### Polymyxin B

Polymyxin B is a cell-wall active antibiotic that avidly binds to LPS. Polymyxin B attenuates many of the functional and toxic activities of LPS, including its ability to induce TNF and interleukin-1 (IL-1) secretion by macrophages, to prime PMN for release of oxygen radicals, and to cause death in various animal models.[33–35] Polymyxin B has also been shown to protect animals from various LPS-induced physiologic derangements and death related to *Haemophilus influenzae* and *E. coli* septicemia.[36, 37] A major limitation of polymyxin B as an antibiotic is its toxicity. However, many of its anti-LPS properties are operational at concentrations that are subinhibitory in terms of antibiotic activity and relatively nontoxic. The clinical strategy for using low-dose polymyxin B in combination with other antibiotics should be explored.

### Lipid A Analogs

Lipid X is a monosaccharide biosynthetic precursor of lipid A, the major toxic moiety of endotoxin.[38] The structural similarities of lipid A and lipid X, combined with the substantially lower toxicity of lipid X, suggest that lipid X may serve as a competitive inhibitor (ie, receptor antagonist) of lipid A and of native LPS.[39, 39a] Lipid X has protected animals against LPS-induced lethality and blocked LPS-induced secretion of TNF by macrophages,[40, 41] although one study could not demonstrate a survival benefit in an animal model of sepsis utilizing live *E. coli*.[39a] However, data suggest that lipid X probably acts on postreceptor signal transduction or secretory systems.[42]

Monophosphoryl (MPL) lipid A is another nontoxic derivative of lipid A. MPL is as much as 1000 times less toxic in animals than LPS.[43] MPL lipid A has significantly reduced mortality rates for animals given lethal challenges of *E. coli*.[44] If the toxicity of endotoxin is mediated solely by the production of TNF by the macrophage, it would be expected that, in contrast to LPS or lipid A, the low toxicity of MPL is a result of its inability to induce high levels of TNF in vivo. However, both MPL and LPS induce high levels of TNF, but only LPS induces shock and death.[45] These findings suggest that factors other than TNF are required for the lethal consequences of endotoxin.

## Cytokine Antagonism

### Tumor Necrosis Factor

Cytokines are potent polypeptide humoral and paracrine mediators that modulate the host defense response to invasive disorders. TNF is one of these proinflammatory mediators derived from mononuclear phagocytes that elicits myriad responses in the host. TNF is detected in the circulation of approximately one third of critically ill patients.[46] Waage and colleagues reported higher serum TNF activity in patients who subsequently died from meningococcal meningitis than in those who survived.[47] Other investigators found that high circulating levels of TNF appear to correlate with the severity of illness, but this has not been uniformly observed.[48-53] Moreover, Calandra and coworkers found the severity of the underlying disease, patient age, documented bacteremia, urine output, and arterial pH to be more significant predictors of patient outcome than serum TNF levels.[49]

To speculate that higher TNF levels are causally related to the detrimental consequences of infections is tempting, but this conclusion cannot be firmly drawn from elevated TNF levels alone. Several studies of patients and animals demonstrated that the high TNF levels were not by themselves sufficient to produce the full complement of adverse symptoms seen during overwhelming infections. Feuerstein and associates found TNF levels reached their highest when sublethal doses of LPS were administered.[54] Toxic and nontoxic forms of the lipid A component of LPS produce similar increases in TNF levels.[45] Several investigators have increased serum TNF concentrations to levels typically seen in patients by administering purified recombinant human TNF itself or by injecting low doses of bacterial endotoxins under controlled conditions.[55-58] In these experiments, flu-like symptoms such as fever, chills, nausea, headache, tachycardia, increases in stress hormones, and hypermetabolism were observed, but a severe life-threatening disease state did not develop. Collectively, these findings suggest that other factors, such as the duration of the TNF response, the presence of synergistic mediators, or the site of infection (eg, systemic, localized) may be critical factors necessary to evoke a role for TNF as a cause of mortality resulting from sepsis.

In most instances, increases in serum TNF after experimental administration of bacteria or endotoxin are transient.[51, 55, 59, 60] Moreover, septic patients do not consistently exhibit a detectable increase in systemic TNF. However, Leroux-Roels and Oftner reported low but persistently detectable serum levels in 23 patients with sepsis.[50] The significance of this sustained elevation is unknown, but experiments indicate that continuous exposure of animals to TNF can have more severe consequences than episodic exposure to this cytokine.[61-63]

The consequences of passive immunization with antibodies directed against TNF offer the best means for determining the role TNF plays during severe infections. Pretreatment of animals with these antibodies protects them from lethal doses of bacterial LPS and certain kinds of bacterial and parasitic insults. Beutler and colleagues first demonstrated that passive immunization with anti-TNF serum rendered mice less sensitive to E. coli LPS.[64] Other laboratories, including our own, have substantiated this finding.[59, 65, 66] Such data provide compelling evidence that TNF elicited by endotoxin administration participates in the lethal consequences of sepsis. The detrimental role of TNF has been extended to lethal bacteremia by studies in baboons. Tracey and coworkers found that neutralizing monoclonal anti-TNF F(ab')$_2$ prevented death from a lethal intravenous challenge of live E. coli if administered 2 hours before the bacterial challenge.[67] An anti-TNF antibody used by Hinshaw and associates was similarly effective when administered to baboons up to 30 minutes after initiating a 2-hour infusion of bacteria.[68] However, the murine monoclonal

anti-TNF antibody did not improve overall survival in patients with sepsis.[68a]

The relevance of these findings cannot be extended to all types of bacterial infections. A study conducted in our laboratory indicates that an intravenous injection of heat-killed E. coli produces a TNF response and percent lethality similar to an equivalent dose of live bacteria.[66] This implies that when large doses of bacteria are administered intravenously, their lethal effects do not depend on their viability or proliferation, but instead they are related to their inherent heat-stable chemical composition (eg, LPS and other virulence factors). Bacteremia produced by the rapid intravenous administration of microorganisms may more closely mimic LPS toxicity than a septic state in which bacterial proliferation is occurring and the infection is substantially compartmentalized.

Lethality from severe infections is not uniformly prevented by using antibodies against TNF. A lack of efficacy with anti-TNF antibodies has been reported in animals subjected to bacterial peritonitis. Evans and associates were unable to prevent mortality from cecal ligation and puncture by pretreating mice with a monoclonal antibody directed against murine TNF.[65] Their results are not particularly surprising, because TNF was not detected in the serum or the peritoneal cavity of the mice subjected to this insult. We have also attempted to reduce the mortality induced by bacterial peritonitis in an E. coli fecal inoculum model without success.[66] In this case, low levels of TNF, which are completely neutralized by pretreatment with a goat anti-TNF immunoglobulin G, were detected in serum and the peritoneal cavity. Despite demonstrating that more than sufficient antibody was administered, mortality from gram-negative bacterial peritonitis was not abrogated in this model.

These results suggest that TNF is not an essential component in the cascade of events resulting in death during bacterial peritonitis. However, secreted TNF could produce adverse effects within a microenvironment before being neutralized. Moreover, a cell-associated form of TNF that may be relatively inaccessible to administered anti-TNF has been identified.[69] This cell membrane-associated protein is biologically active and serves as the precursor to the secreted form.[70] Keogh and colleagues found such a protein in the liver of rats 3 days after being subjected to thermal injury combined with topical application of Pseudomonas aeruginosa.[71] In an earlier experiment, these investigators were able to detect TNF in the circulation in only 18% of similarly treated animals.[72]

Anti-TNF therapy fails to protect animals against all forms of infections, and in some cases, using these antibodies may exacerbate the condition. Mice infected with Listeria monocytogenes are adversely affected if pretreated with anti-TNF antibodies. Havell found spleen TNF levels to be increased between 1 to 3 days after intravenous inoculation with a sublethal dose of Listeria.[73] Treatment of infected mice on the first day with a monospecific anti-TNF immunoglobin resulted in an exponential growth of Listeria in the liver and spleen and death within 3 days.[73, 74] The antibody converted a nonlethal infection into a lethal infection by neutralizing tissue expression of TNF. A similar negative effect of antiserum against TNF was reported by Nakane and colleagues.[75]

Cross and coworkers conducted interesting experiments

in C3H/HeJ mice.[76] This murine strain is resistant to endotoxin-induced shock and death because of the inability of its macrophages to produce TNF in direct response to LPS. However, these investigators found C3H/HeJ mice to be 100-fold more sensitive to *E. coli*-induced lethality. Pretreatment of C3H/HeJ mice with a combination of recombinant murine TNF and IL-1 protected mice from intraperitoneal bacterial challenge. To further define the role of TNF in mediating pulmonary antibacterial defenses, we similarly challenged C3H/HeJ mice and control animals (C3H/HeN) with intrapulmonary *Klebsiella pneumoniae*. The C3H/HeJ animals were unable to generate an inflammatory response, and the bacteria proliferated within their lungs (Fig. 46–3), in contrast to the findings for control animals.

Local TNF synthesis is thought to play a vital role in eliminating bacillus Calmette-Guérin (BCG) infections in the liver and *P. aeruginosa* instilled into the lungs. Kindler and associates found that the development of bactericidal granulomas within the liver after a systemic infection with *Mycobacterium bovis* (ie, BCG strain) coincided with TNF expression.[77] Treatment with anti-TNF 1 to 2 weeks after initiating the infection suppressed the development of granulomas and resulted in subsequent elimination of these bacteria. In studies completed in our laboratory, treatment of rats with anti-TNF IgG before an aerosol inhalation challenge with *P. aeruginosa* suppressed PMN recruitment into the alveolar compartment by approximately eightfold and significantly suppressed intrapulmonary bactericidal activity against this pathogen.[78] These data indicate that TNF can play an important role in mediating normal host defenses designed to eliminate pathogens from the internal environment.

### Interleukin-1

IL-1 is another cytokine that shares many similarities with TNF and acts synergistically with TNF in various model systems to enhance tissue damage and death.[79, 80]

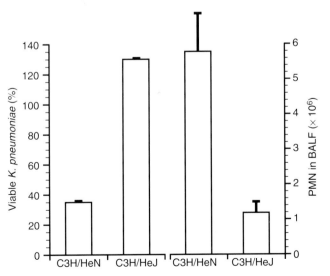

**Figure 46–3.** The percentage of *Klebsiella pneumoniae* organisms remaining viable in the lung and the number of polymorphonuclear leukocytes (PMN) recovered in bronchoalveolar lavage fluid (BALF) in C3H/HeJ and C3H/HeN (control) mice 4 hours after a bacterial challenge.

Several lines of evidence implicate IL-1 in the development of sepsis. Serum IL-1 levels are frequently elevated in patients with sepsis, and administration of low doses of IL-1 induces many of the signs and symptoms of sepsis.[81–83] IL-1 occurs in two forms: IL-1α and IL-1β. IL-1β is usually elevated in sepsis.[84] The actions of both forms are regulated at the receptor level; the receptor for IL-1α and IL-1β is a plasma membrane glycoprotein with broad distribution.[85–87] At least one IL-1 receptor antagonist (IL-1ra) occurs naturally and was originally discovered in the urine of patients with monocytic leukemia.[88] IL-1ra is a 26-kd protein produced by monocytes.[89] Recombinant technology has produced a nonglycosylated form of IL-1ra that blocks the action of IL-1 and seems to have no detectable agonist activity.[90] When given immediately before and several times after injection of endotoxin in rabbits, IL-1ra increased survival from 20% to 90%.[91] When injected before a continuous infusion of live *E. coli*, IL-1ra improved survival and hemodynamics and reduced the severity of lactic acidemia in baboons.[92] Studies of the safety and efficacy of IL-1ra in patients with sepsis are under way. However, it is possible that IL-1 (like TNF) may produce more benefit than harm in septic patients.

### Pharmacologic Interventions

Numerous pharmacologic agents including glucocorticoids, nonsteroidal antiinflammatory agents, pentoxifylline, oxygen radical scavengers, and inhibitors of nitric oxide have been shown to attenuate LPS- and cytokine-induced toxicity in various model systems.[93–100] However, the therapeutic efficacy of these agents in patients with sepsis awaits proof in controlled clinical trials. Although no pharmacologic treatment of sepsis has been as extensively studied as glucocorticoids with overwhelming supportive preclinical data, no benefit could be found in controlled clinical trials.[101, 102] This may reflect the fact that clinicians cannot recognize the imminent septic state, identify these high-risk patients, and administer an agent in time to prevent the adverse sequelae of sepsis. The more we learn, the more we realize how extraordinarily complex the host defense system is. The complexity of this system makes it unlikely that any one agent can be effective for most patients. Information is needed about how best to titrate these agents in an individual patient. The host defense response normally functions to restore homeostasis after an infectious insult, and it is reasonable to assume that any agent we administer that interferes with its operation must be carefully titrated to avoid destruction of the body's own defense mechanisms.

### PNEUMONIA

The lung is particularly prone to developing infection in a patient with underlying sepsis. Nosocomial pneumonia is one of the most common secondary infections in these patients, and it is frequently fatal. A better understanding of how extrapulmonary sepsis predisposes to pneumonia is beginning to emerge from ongoing basic and clinical studies, and strategies may soon develop that prevent this lethal complication.

The AM is positioned as the central cell in responding to an infectious challenge in the lung, and invading microbes would flourish without this essential first line of host defense. The migration of PMN into the alveoli provides critical auxiliary phagocytic defenses.[6, 103] Expression of the antimicrobial function of the PMN depends on the ability of these cells to leave the systemic circulation and enter infected sites. PMN movement into the alveoli is an orderly reaction initiated from the alveolar side.[104] Potential mediators for this inflammatory response include complement and AM-derived chemotactic factors (eg, bioactive lipids, cytokines).[105]

We have been actively investigating the role of cytokines in the normal pulmonary inflammatory response to an invading pathogen. We initially determined the effects of LPS on TNF activity and the pulmonary inflammatory response in rats challenged intravenously or intratracheally with LPS.[60] In the unchallenged lung, bronchoalveolar lavage (BAL) fluid contains no measurable TNF, and the cell population is 99% AM. After acute stimulation with intratracheal LPS, TNF rapidly increases and is followed by the development of a marked inflammatory response. These temporal observations are compatible with a potential role of TNF as a factor in recruiting PMN into the lung in response to an infectious challenge. In vivo and in vitro data also support this finding.[78, 106–108]

After intravenous LPS, the serum TNF level peaks in 90 minutes, and by 3 hours, it returns to near-nondetectable levels. Similar findings have been reported by other investigators.[55–57] Histopathologic analysis of these lungs shows that intravenous LPS causes a marked sequestration of PMN within the pulmonary vasculature with no increase in PMN within the air spaces of the lung. Other studies have shown that intravenous LPS or recombinant TNF administration causes similar histologic findings.[109–111] These experiments showed that LPS-induced TNF release was confined to the LPS-challenged compartment. When LPS was administered intravenously, TNF was not detected in BAL fluid, and intratracheal LPS resulted in high BAL fluid TNF without spillover into the vascular compartment.

These data demonstrate that the normal host synthesizes and releases TNF within the lung in response to a local LPS challenge. We and others have shown a similar response in normal animals challenged locally within the lung with gram-negative or gram-positive bacteria.[112–114] Under these conditions, TNF functions as an immune response augmentor of lung host defense. These data are supported by other studies showing that endogenous and exogenous TNF promotes lung host defense against *Staphylococcus aureus, Legionella pneumophila,* and *Pneumocystis carinii.*[115–117] We have found that pharmacologic agents such as glucocorticoids and alcohol, which are widely recognized risk factors for the development of pneumonia, markedly suppress the intrapulmonary TNF response and lung antibacterial defenses.[112, 118] In preliminary experiments, we have shown that systemic administration of an anti-TNF antibody impairs PMN recruitment and lung bactericidal activity against an intrapulmonary challenge with *P. aeruginosa.*[78]

We previously showed in animals that *E. coli* peritonitis or systemic LPS markedly impaired lung host defense.[119–121]

This impairment was characterized by a failure of PMN to enter the infected lung, which led to proliferation of the pathogen (Fig. 46–4). The mechanisms compromising lung antibacterial defenses during extrapulmonary sepsis may involve a systemic-induced suppression of intrapulmonary signals and responses.

We next investigated the hypothesis that systemic sepsis leads to a down-regulation of AM production of TNF in response to a secondary infectious challenge. In these experiments, rats were divided into three groups and subjected to a 5-day pretreatment protocol.[122] On days 1 through 4, saline and acute LPS groups of rats received an intravenous injection of saline. Rats in the chronic LPS group were intravenously injected with LPS on days 1 through 4. On day 5, rats in the saline group received saline, and rats in the other two groups received LPS. Two hours after either saline or LPS injection, rats in all three groups were then challenged by aerosol inhalation with *P. aeruginosa.*

In response to acute systemic LPS, serum TNF peaked after about 90 minutes. However, with successive days of chronic LPS injection, the serum TNF response decreased. By the fifth consecutive day, the rats lacked a detectable TNF response, signifying the development of LPS-tolerance.

Saline-control rats challenged with aerosolized *P. aeruginosa* expressed high levels of TNF in the BAL fluid. In contrast, rats injected with LPS 2 hours before this bacterial challenge showed a marked reduction in the BAL fluid TNF response. Rats rendered LPS-tolerant by 5 daily injections of LPS exhibited a normal lung TNF response to the pulmonary bacterial challenge. This indicates that when rats are chronically injected intravenously with LPS, AM are not exposed to sufficient LPS to render them incapable of responding to subsequent intrapulmonary challenges. The diminished BAL fluid TNF response to a subsequent bacterial challenge in rats pretreated with a single injection of LPS was not caused by a direct effect of LPS itself on the AM. This was supported by our finding that macrophages removed from the lung of rats subjected to acute or chronic exposure to LPS and subsequently stimulated in vitro with

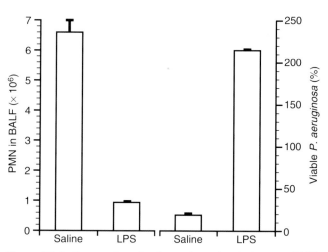

**Figure 46–4.** The number of polymorphonuclear leukocytes (PMN) recovered in bronchoalveolar lavage fluid (BALF) and the percentage of *Pseudomonas aeruginosa* organisms remaining viable in the lung in saline and lipopolysaccharide (LPS)-treated rats 4 hours after an aerosolized *P. aeruginosa* challenge.

LPS responded normally with respect to TNF expression. Removing AM from the lung after the acute LPS challenge restored responsiveness. This may indicate that a soluble factor is produced in response to acute systemic LPS challenge (eg, endogenous glucocorticoids, prostaglandin $E_2$) that suppresses the response of the AM to a subsequent in vivo stimulus. However, this suppression is not retained after removal of the macrophage from its endogenous environment.

In vivo, the development of a BAL fluid TNF response to an aerosol *P. aeruginosa* challenge was associated with the subsequent recruitment of PMN and effective pulmonary bactericidal activity. Rats pretreated with a single LPS injection showed a diminished pulmonary TNF response, recruited substantially fewer PMN into the alveolar compartment, and had an impaired ability to kill aerosolized bacteria. In the last case, net bacterial proliferation occurred, indicating a complete failure of lung host defense. However, chronic exposure to intravenous LPS resulted in normal numbers of PMN recruited into the lung and resulted in a return to normal bactericidal activity within the lung.

These preclinical data, which show that mononuclear phagocyte cytokine production is down-regulated after sepsis, have been supported by recent clinical investigations. In a study of AM recovered by BAL from septic and control patients, the AM from nonseptic patients produced significantly more TNF than AM from septic patients stimulated with LPS.[123] The peripheral blood mononuclear cells from patients with severe sepsis produced significantly less IL-1 in culture than normal controls, and in vitro stimulation of their cells did not induce IL-1 secretion.[124] An inability to produce IL-1 was associated with a poor prognosis.

These phenomena of down-regulation may, under most conditions, protect the host. It would not be advantageous to nonspecifically or continually activate the inflammatory cascade, which may inadvertently injure the host. This mechanism may localize the inflammatory responses at a specific site or within a selected compartment. However, this protective mechanism may then render the host vulnerable to a subsequent infection at an adjacent or distant site (eg, lung).

It is possible that early, effective blockade of the sequence of events that leads to fulminant sepsis by application of the previously discussed approaches may prevent the acquired immunodeficient state of the lung in these patients. Some of these therapies may increase lung susceptibility to infection by further suppressing the remaining vestiges of the lung host defense system.

In patients who have survived their initial septic episodes, immune restoration may be possible through the exogenous administration of cytokines. We and others have shown that cytokines can up-regulate the antibacterial defenses of the lung. As with mononuclear phagocytes elsewhere in the body, many biologic processes that are associated with host defense functions of AM can be augmented by interferon-γ (IFN).[125] IFN, although unable by itself to induce TNF synthesis, enhances LPS-induced TNF.[126] Because systemic administration of IFN may not deliver sufficient quantities of IFN into the lower respiratory tract and because the AM is the target cell, a more effective approach to augment selectively the host defense capabilities of this

cell may be to deliver IFN directly into the lower respiratory tract by aerosol or intratracheal administration.[125]

To determine the effects of exogenous IFN on pulmonary antibacterial defenses, we pretreated rats with $10^5$ U of recombinant murine IFN or saline intratracheally 24 hours before an aerosol challenge with *P. aeruginosa* (Fig. 46–5).[127] We found that local delivery of IFN significantly augmented the alveolar TNF response of rats to *P. aeruginosa*. PMN recruitment and lung bactericidal activity in response to this pathogen were enhanced. Pretreatment of these animals with anti-TNF antibody attenuated the IFN-induced enhancement of lung host defense. Similar beneficial results using IFN have been shown in animal models of *L. pneumophila* and *P. carinii* pneumonia.[128, 129]

Colony-stimulating factors are growth factors responsible for the proliferation and maturation of bone marrow stem cells to fully differentiated granulocytes and monocytes.[130] Granulocyte colony-stimulating factor (G-CSF) is a neutrophil-specific growth factor that stimulates the growth and differentiation of myeloid progenitor cells.[131] In addition to its effect on granulopoiesis, G-CSF primes mature cells for enhanced functional activity in response to physiologic stimuli, including adhesion, chemotaxis, phagocytosis, and oxidative metabolism.[132–137] Data show that human AM produce G-CSF when stimulated in vitro by LPS and that AM lavaged from the lungs of patients with pneumonia spontaneously release G-CSF in culture.[138] The serum levels of G-CSF are elevated in patients during the acute phase of a respiratory tract infection.[139] Such findings suggest an important function for G-CSF during pneumonia.

These data imply that exogenous G-CSF could assist in the recovery of the host from local or systemic infections by enhancing the activity of preexisting leukocytes or by increasing the number of these cells. The availability of large quantities of molecularly homogeneous and biologically active human G-CSF by recombinant DNA technology has made it possible to explore the efficacy of G-CSF in the treatment of pneumonia in the nonneutropenic host.

Even in persons with no other detectable underlying disease, splenectomy carries an increased risk of life-threatening pneumococcal infection.[140] In a splenectomized mouse

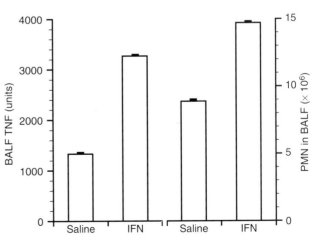

**Figure 46–5.** Bronchoalveolar lavage fluid (BALF) tumor necrosis factor (TNF) response and the number of polymorphonuclear leukocytes (PMN) recovered in BALF in saline and interferon-γ (IFN)-pretreated rats 4 hours after a *Pseudomonas aeruginosa* challenge.

model, G-CSF administered from 24 hours before bacterial challenge to 3 days after the challenge improved the survival of animals exposed to an aerosol of *Streptococcus pneumoniae*.[141] Splenectomized G-CSF treated mice had a 70% rate of survival compared with a 20% rate of survival in saline-treated controls. The circulating PMN counts were greatest for the G-CSF treated splenectomized mice compared with all other groups, presumably because of the absence of splenic sequestration. G-CSF also decreased the recovery of viable *S. pneumoniae* organisms from the lung and tracheobronchial lymph nodes in splenectomized and sham-operated mice compared with saline-treated controls.

Numerous clinical studies have reported evidence that alcohol abusers are at increased risk for severe pneumonia that is often fatal despite current antibiotic therapy.[142, 143] In human and animal studies, the most consistent immunologic defect induced by ethanol is an impairment in neutrophil delivery to a site of infection.[144, 145] We have previously shown that alcohol, like systemic LPS, markedly inhibits lung TNF production.[118] In a study of the effect of G-CSF on ethanol-treated rats with experimentally induced pneumonia, we pretreated rats with G-CSF or vehicle for 2 days and then administered intraperitoneal ethanol or saline, followed by an intratracheal challenge with *K. pneumoniae*.[146] Four hours after the intratracheal challenge, G-CSF was found to augment the recruitment of neutrophils into the lungs of control rats and significantly attenuated the adverse effects of ethanol on neutrophil entry into the infected lung. G-CSF therapy also enhanced the antibacterial defenses of the lung in normal and alchohol-treated rats. The survival of rats was markedly enhanced by G-CSF. Twelve of 12 intoxicated rats died within 72 hours of inoculation, but only 1 of 12 rats pretreated with G-CSF succumbed. Histologically, the lungs of the surviving rats sacrificed 2 weeks later showed complete resolution of their pneumonia.

In a clinically relevant experiment, G-CSF was administered to normal rats after a pulmonary *P. aeruginosa* infection. G-CSF or vehicle was administered subcutaneously 6 hours after the animals had received a lethal intratracheal inoculation of *P. aeruginosa* and then twice daily for the following 2 days. The survival of the infected animals was markedly enhanced by G-CSF (Fig. 46–6). All animals that received vehicle died within 48 hours, but 14 of 14 G-CSF treated animals survived. Similar beneficial results using G-CSF have been shown in lethal models of burn wound

infection, intramuscular infection, neonatal sepsis, and intraabdominal sepsis.[147–151] To date, G-CSF has not been found to enhance endotoxic-induced lung injury[151a, 151b] and, interestingly, in one animal model G-CSF attenuated LPS-induced acute lung injury.[152] Perhaps G-CSF-induced increases in BPI diminished LPS toxicity or G-CSF altered endothelial-PMN interactions.

## CONCLUSION

The care and management of the septic patient represents a formidable challenge to the physician. As long as the basic underlying host defense defects in these patients remain elusive, the clinician's approach will remain reactive and empiric. The development of a multimodal approach, including components of immune modulation and immune restoration, is needed to improve the multiple aberrations in the host defense system induced by sepsis. Although the thrust of experimental approaches to the treatment of patients with sepsis are focused on the selective down-regulation of the immune response, emerging data suggest that these patients are already immunosuppressed, and these interventions may predispose susceptible patients to the development of nosocomial pneumonia. However, the host defense system functions in a delicate balance, and efforts to stimulate the immune system nonselectively may prove to be as deleterious to these patients as the negative effects of their immunocompromised state.

## REFERENCES

1. Toews GB: Southwestern internal medicine conference: Nosocomial pneumonia. Am J Med Sci 291:355–366, 1986.
2. Niederman MS, Craven DE, Fein AM, et al: Pneumonia in the critically ill hospitalized patient. Chest 97:170–181, 1990.
3. Clowes GHA Jr, Zuschneid W, Turner M, et al: Observations on the pathogenesis of the pneumonitis associated with severe infections in other parts of the body. Ann Surg 167:630–650, 1968.
4. Richardson JD, Fry DE, Van Ardsall L, et al: Delayed pulmonary clearance of gram-negative bacteria: The role of intraperitoneal sepsis. J Surg Res 26:499–503, 1979.
5. Nelson S, Chidiac C, Summer WR: New strategies for preventing nosocomial pneumonia. J Crit Illness 3:12–24, 1988.
6. Green GM, Jakab GJ, Low RB, et al: Defense mechanisms of the respiratory membrane. Am Rev Respir Dis 115:479–514, 1977.
7. Ashbaugh DG, Bigelow DB, Petty TL, et al: Acute respiratory distress in adults. Lancet 2:319–323, 1967.
8. Fowler AA, Hamman RF, Good JT: Adult respiratory distress syndrome: Risk with common predispositions. Ann Intern Med 98:593–597, 1983.
9. Neiderman MS, Fein AM: Sepsis syndrome, the adult respiratory distress syndrome and nosocomial pneumonia: A common clinical sequence. Clin Chest Med 11:633–656, 1990.
10. Seidenfeld JJ, Pohl DF, Bell RC, et al: Incidence, site, and outcome of infections in patients with the adult respiratory distress syndrome. Am Rev Respir Dis 134:12–16, 1986.
11. Vandenbroucke-Grauls CM, Vandenbroucke JP: Effect of selective decontamination of the digestive tract on respiratory tract infections and mortality in the intensive care unit. Lancet 338:859–862, 1991.
12. Burlew BP, Noel P, Nelson S: Local antibiotic therapy in bronchopulmonary infections. Crit Care Rep 2:136–144, 1991.
13. Young LS, Proctor RA, Beutler B, et al: University of California/Davis interdepartmental conference on gram-negative septicemia. Rev Infect Dis 13:666–687, 1991.
14. Hopkin BDA: Too-rapid destruction of gram-negative organisms. Lancet 2:603–604, 1977.

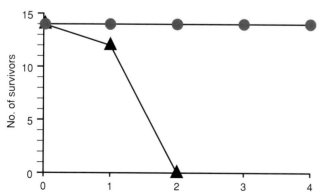

**Figure 46–6.** Survival of animals treated with granulocyte colony-stimulating factor (●) or 5% dextrose (▲) after an intratracheal challenge with *Pseudomonas aeruginosa*.

15. Hopkin BDA: A nasty shock from antibiotics. Lancet 2:594, 1985.
16. Cohen J, McConnell JS: Release of endotoxin from bacteria exposed to ciprofloxin and its prevention with polymyxin B. Eur J Clin Microbiol 5:13–17, 1986.
17. Cohen J, McConnell JS: Antibiotic induced endotoxin release. Lancet 2:1069–1070, 1985.
18. McConnell JS, Cohen J: Release of endotoxin from *Escherichia coli* by quinolones. J Antimicrob Chemother 18:765–773, 1986.
19. Shenep JL, Barton RP, Morgan KA: Role of antibiotic class in the rate of liberation of endotoxin during the therapy for experimental gram-negative bacterial sepsis. J Infect Dis 151:1012–1018, 1985.
20. Rokke O, Revhaug A, Osterud B, et al: Increased plasma levels of endotoxin and corresponding changes in circulatory performance in a porcine sepsis model: The effect of antibiotic administration. Prog Clin Biol Res 272:247–262, 1988.
21. Dofferhoff ASM, Nijland JH, deVries-Hospers HG, et al: Effects of different types and combinations of antimicrobial agents on endotoxin release from gram-negative bacteria: An in-vitro and in-vivo study. Scand J Infect Dis 23:745–754, 1991.
22. Neu HC: Relation of structural properties of beta-lactam antibiotics to antibacterial activity. Am J Med 79(suppl 2A):2–13, 1985.
23. Simon DM, Koenig G, Trenholme GM: Differences in release of tumor necrosis factor from THP-1 cells stimulated by filtrates of antibiotic-killed *Escherichia coli*. J Infect Dis 164:800–802, 1991.
24. Ziegler EJ, McCutchan A, Fierer J, et al: Treatment of gram negative bacteremia and shock with human antiserim to a mutant *Escherichia coli*. N Engl J Med 307:1225–1230, 1982.
25. The Intravenous Immunoglobulin Collaborative Study Group: Prophylactic intravenous administration of standard immune globulin as compared with core-lipopolysaccharide immune globulin in patients at high risk of postsurgical infection. N Engl J Med 327:234–240, 1992.
26. Ziegler EJ, Fisher CJ, Sprung CL, et al: Treatment of gram-negative bacteremia and septic shock with HA-1A human monoclonal antibody against endotoxin. N Engl J Med 324:429–436, 1991.
27. Greenman RL, Schein RMH, Martin MA, et al: A controlled clinical trial of E5 murine monoclonal IgM antibody to endotoxin in the treatment of gram-negative sepsis. JAMA 266:1097–1102, 1991.
28. Wortel CH, Sprung C, van Deventer SJH, et al: Anti endotoxin treatment with HA 1A: Possible mechanism of beneficial effects in patients with gram-negative septicemia. *In* Abstracts of the International Congress for Infectious Diseases. Montreal, Canadian Infectious Diseases Society and International Society for Infectious Disease, 1990.
28a. Quezado ZMN, Natanson C, Alling DW, et al: A controlled trial of HA-1A in a canine model of gram-negative septic shock. JAMA 269:2221–2227, 1993.
29. Schumann RR, Leong SR, Flaggs GW, et al: Structure and function of lipopolysaccharide binding protein. Science 249:1429–1431, 1990.
30. Tobias PS, Mathison JC, Ulevitch RJ: A family of lipopolysaccharide binding proteins involved in responses to gram-negative sepsis. J Biol Chem 263:13479–13481, 1988.
31. Ooi CE, Weiss J, Doerfler ME, et al: Endotoxin-neutralizing properties of the 25 kd N-terminal fragment and a newly isolated 30 kd C-terminal fragment of the 55–60 kd bactericidal/permeability-increasing protein of human neutrophils. J Exp Med 174:649–655, 1991.
32. Weiss J, Elsbach P, Olsson I, et al: Purification and characterization of a potent bactericidal and membrane active protein from the granules of human polymorphonuclear leukocytes. J Biol Chem 253:2664–2672, 1978.
33. Stokes DC, Shenep JL, Fishman M, et al: Polymyxin B prevents lipopolysaccharide induced release of tumor necrosis factor α from alveolar macrophages. J Infect Dis 160:52–57, 1989.
34. Danner RL, Joiner KA, Rubin M, et al: Purification, toxicity, and antiendotoxin activity of polymyxin B nonapeptide. Antimicrob Agents Chemother 33:1428–1434, 1989.
35. Craig WA, Turner JH, Kunin CM: Prevention of the generalized Shwartzman reaction and endotoxin lethality by polymyxin B localized in tissues. Infect Immun 10:287–292, 1974.
36. Walterspiel JW, Kaplan SL, Mason EO Jr: Protective effect of subinhibitory polymyxin B alone and in combination with ampicillin for overwhelming *Haemophilus influenzae* type B infection in the infant rat: Evidence for in vivo and in vitro release of free endotoxin after ampicillin treatment. Pediatr Res 20:237–241, 1986.
37. Flynn PM, Shenep JL, Stokes DC, et al: Polymyxin B moderates acidosis and hypotension in established, experimental gram-negative septicemia. J Infect Dis 56:706–712, 1987.
38. Takayama K, Qureshi N, Mascagni P, et al: Fatty acyl derivatives of glucosamine-1-phosphate in *Escherichia coli* and their relation to lipid A. J Biol Chem 258:7379–7385, 1983.
39. Raetz CRH: The enzymatic synthesis of lipid A: Molecular structure and biologic function of monosaccharide precursors. Rev Infect Dis 6:463–471, 1984.
39a. Danner RL, Eichacker PQ, Doerfler ME, et al: Therapeutic trial of lipid X in a canine model of septic shock. J Infect Dis 167:378–384, 1993.
40. Proctor RA, Will JA, Burhop KE, et al: Protection of mice against lethal endotoxemia by a lipid A precursor. Infect Immun 52:905–907, 1986.
41. Danner RL, Joiner KA, Parrillo JE: Inhibition of endotoxin induced priming of human neutrophils by lipid X and 3 aza-lipid X. J Clin Invest 80:605–612, 1987.
42. Hampton RY, Golenbock DT, Raetz CRH: Lipid A binding sites in membranes of macrophage tumor cells. J Biol Chem 263:14802–14807, 1988.
43. Takayama K, Qureshi N, Ribi E, et al: Separation and characterization of toxic and nontoxic forms of lipid A's. Rev Infect Dis 6:439–443, 1984.
44. Chase JJ, Kubey W, Dulek MH, et al: Effect of monophosphoryl lipid A on host resistance to bacterial infection. Infect Immun 53:711–712, 1986.
45. Keiner PA, Marek F, Rodgers G, et al: Induction of tumor necrosis factor, IFN-γ, and acute lethality in mice by toxic and non-toxic forms of lipid A. J Immunol 141:870–874, 1988.
46. Waage A, Espevik T, Lamvik J: Detection of tumor necrosis factor-like cytotoxicity in serum from patients with septicaemia, but not from untreated cancer patients. Scand J Immunol 24:739–743, 1986.
47. Waage A, Halstensen A, Espevik T: Association between tumor necrosis factor in serum and fatal outcome in patients with meningococcal disease. Lancet 1:355–357, 1987.
48. Cannon JG, Tompkins RG, Gelfand JA, et al: Circulating interleukin-1 and tumor necrosis factor in septic shock and experimental endotoxin fever. J Infect Dis 161:79–84, 1990.
49. Calandra T, Baumgartner J-D, Grau GE, et al: Prognostic values of tumor necrosis factor/cachectin, interleukin-1, interferon-alpha, and interferon-gamma in the serum of patients with septic shock. J Infect Dis 161:982–987, 1990.
50. Leroux-Roels G, Oftner F: Tumor necrosis factor in sepsis. JAMA 263:1494–1495, 1990.
51. Marks JD, Marks CB, Luce JM, et al: Plasma tumor necrosis factor in patients with septic shock: Mortality rate, incidence of adult respiratory distress syndrome, and effects of methylprednisolone administration. Am Rev Respir Dis 141:94–97, 1990.
52. Damas P, Reuter A, Gysen P, et al: Tumor necrosis factor and interleukin-1 serum levels during severe sepsis in humans. Crit Care Med 17:975–978, 1989.
53. DeGroote MA, Martin MA, Densen P, et al: Plasma tumor necrosis factor levels in patients with presumed sepsis. Results in those treated with antilipid A antibody vs placebo. JAMA 262:249–251, 1989.
54. Feuerstein G, Hallenbeck JM, Vanatta B, et al: Effect of gram-negative endotoxin on levels of serum corticosterone, TNF-alpha, circulating blood cells, and survival of rats. Circ Shock 30:265–278, 1990.
55. Michie HR, Manogue KR, Spriggs DR, et al: Detection of circulating tumor necrosis factor after endotoxin administration. N Engl J Med 318:1481–1486, 1988.
56. Michie HR, Spriggs DR, Manogue KR, et al: Tumor necrosis factor and endotoxin induce similar metabolic responses in human beings. Surgery 104:280–286, 1988.
57. Hesse DG, Tracey KJ, Fong Y, et al: Cytokine appearance in human endotoxemia and primate bacteremia. Surg Gynecol Obstet 166:147–153, 1988.
58. Fong Y, Marano MA, Moldawer LL, et al: The acute splanchnic and peripheral tissue metabolic response to endotoxin in humans. J Clin Invest 85:1896–1904, 1990.
59. Mathison JC, Wolfson E, Ulevitch RJ: Participation of tumor necrosis factor in the mediation of gram negative bacterial lipopolysaccharide-induced injury in rabbits. J Clin Invest 81:1925–1937, 1988.
60. Nelson S, Bagby GJ, Bainton BG, et al: Compartmentalization of

intraalveolar and systemic lipopolysaccharide-induced tumor necrosis factor and the pulmonary inflammatory response. J Infect Dis 159:189–194, 1989.

61. Darling G, Fraker DL, Jensen JC, et al: Cachectic effects of recombinant human tumor necrosis factor in rats. Cancer Res 50:4008–4013, 1990.

62. Michie HR, Sherman ML, Spriggs DR, et al: Chronic TNF infusion causes anorexia but not accelerated nitrogen loss. Ann Surg 209:19–24, 1989.

63. Mullen BJ, Harris RBS, Patton JS, et al: Recombinant tumor necrosis factor-α chronically administered in rats: Lack of cachectic effect. Proc Soc Exp Biol Med 193:318–325, 1990.

64. Beutler B, Milsark IW, Cerami AC: Passive immunization against cachectin/tumor necrosis factor protects mice from lethal effect of endotoxin. Science 229:869–871, 1985.

65. Evans GF, Snyder YM, Butler LD, et al: Differential expression of interleukin-1 and tumor necrosis factor in murine septic shock models. Circ Shock 29:279–290, 1989.

66. Bagby GJ, Plessala KJ, Wilson LA, et al: Divergent efficacy of anti-TNF α antibody in intravascular and peritonitis models of sepsis. J Infect Dis 163:83–88, 1991.

67. Tracey KJ, Fong Y, Hesse DG, et al: Anti-cachectin/TNF monoclonal antibodies prevent septic shock during lethal bacteraemia. Nature 330:662–664, 1987.

68. Hinshaw L, Tekamp-Olson P, Chang ACK, et al: Survival of primates in LD 100 septic shock following therapy with antibody to tumor necrosis factor (TNF α). Circ Shock 30:279–292, 1990.

68a. Fisher CJ Jr, Opal SM, Dhainaut J-F, et al: Influence of an anti-tumor necrosis factor monoclonal antibody on cytokine levels in patients with sepsis. Crit Care Med 21:318–327, 1993.

69. Chensue SW, Remick DG, Shmyr-Forsch C, et al: Immunohistochemical demonstration of cytoplasmic and membrane-associated tumor necrosis factor in murine macrophages. Am J Pathol 133:564–572, 1988.

70. Kriegler M, Perez C, DeFay K, et al: A novel form of TNF/cachectin is a cell surface cytotoxic transmembrane protein: ramifications for the complex physiology of TNF. Cell 53:45–53, 1988.

71. Keogh C, Fong Y, Marano MA, et al: Identification of a novel tumor necrosis factor α/cachectin from the livers of burned and infected rats. Arch Surg 125:79–85, 1990.

72. Marano MA, Moldawer LL, Fong Y, et al: Cachectin/TNF production in experimental burns and *Pseudomonas* infection. Arch Surg 123:1383–1388, 1988.

73. Havell EA: Evidence that tumor necrosis factor has an important role in antibacterial resistance. J Immunol 143:2894–2899, 1989.

74. Havell EA: Production of tumor necrosis factor during murine listeriosis. J Immunol 139:4225–4231, 1987.

75. Nakane A, Minagawa T, Kato K: Endogenous tumor necrosis factor (cachectin) is essential to host resistance against *Listeria monocytogenes* infection. Infect Immun 56:2563–2569, 1988.

76. Cross AS, Sadoff JC, Kelly N, et al: Pretreatment with recombinant murine tumor necrosis factor α/cachectin and murine interleukin 1 α protects mice from lethal bacterial infection. J Exp Med 169:2021–2027, 1989.

77. Kindler V, Sappino A-P, Grau GE, et al: The inducing role of tumor necrosis factor in the development of bactericidal granulomas during BCG infection. Cell 56:731–740, 1989.

78. Nelson S, Bagby G, Summer W: Anti-tumor necrosis factor-alpha antibody suppresses pulmonary antibacterial defenses. Am Rev Respir Dis 143S:393, 1991.

79. Dinarello CA, Cannon JG, Wolff SM, et al: Tumor necrosis factor (cachectin) is an endogenous pyrogen and induces production of interleukin 1. J Exp Med 163:1433–1450, 1986.

80. Okusawa S, Gelfand JA, Ikejima T, et al: Interleukin 1 induces a shock-like state in rabbits. Synergism with tumor necrosis factor and the effect of cyclooxygenase inhibition. J Clin Invest 81:1162–1172, 1988.

81. Casey L, Balk R, Bone R: Cytokines in patients with the sepsis syndrome. [Abstract] Program and abstracts of the Second International Congress on the Immune Consequences of Trauma, Shock, and Sepsis: Mechanisms and Therapeutic Approaches, Munich, Germany, March 6–9, 1991.

82. Zuckerman SH, Shelhaas J, Butler LD: Differential regulation of lipopolysaccharide-induced interleukin-1 and tumor necrosis factor synthesis: Effects of endogenous glucocorticoids and the role of the pituitary-adrenal axis. Eur J Immunol 19:301–305, 1989.

83. Evans GF, Snyder YM, Butler LD, et al: Differential expression of interleukin-1 and tumor necrosis factor in murine septic shock models. Circ Shock 29:279–290, 1989.

84. Dinarello CA, Cannon JG, Wolff SM: New concepts on the pathogenesis of fever. Rev Infect Dis 10:168–190, 1988.

85. Dower SK, Kronheim SR, March CJ, et al: Detection and characterization of high-affinity plasma membrane receptors of human interleukin-1. J Exp Med 162:501–515, 1985.

86. Dower SK, Kronheim SR, Hopp TP, et al: The cell surface receptors for interleukin-1 alpha and interleukin-1 beta are identical. Nature 324:266–268, 1986.

87. Bird TA, Saklatvala J: Identification of a common class of high affinity receptors for both types of porcine interleukin-1 on connective tissue cells. Nature 324:263–266, 1986.

88. Balavoine JF, deRochemonteix B, Williamson K, et al: Prostaglandin E₂ and collagenase production by fibroblasts and synovial cells is regulated by urine-derived human interleukin-1 and inhibitor(s). J Clin Invest 78:1120–1124, 1986.

89. Mazzei GJ, Seckinger PL, Dayer JM, et al: Purification and characterization of a 26-kDa competitive inhibitor of interleukin-1. Eur J Immunol 20:683–689, 1990.

90. Hannum CH, Wilcox CJ, Arend WP, et al: Interleukin-1 receptor antagonist activity of a human interleukin-1 inhibitor. Nature 343:336–340, 1990.

91. Ohlsson K, Bjork P, Bergenfeldt M, et al: An interleukin-1 receptor antagonist (IL-1ra) blocks effect of IL-1 beta in the rabbit, rat and mouse and reduces the mortality in endotoxin shock. [Abstract] Program and abstracts of the Second International Congress on the Immune Consequences of Trauma, Shock, and Sepsis: Mechanisms and Therapeutic Approaches, Munich, Germany, March 6–9, 1991.

92. Fischer E, Marano MA, vanZee KJ, et al: IL-1 receptor blockade attenuates the hemodynamic and metabolic consequences of lethal *E. coli* septic shock. [Abstract] Program and abstracts of the Second International Congress on the Immune Consequences of Trauma, Shock, and Sepsis: Mechanisms and Therapeutic Approaches, Munich, Germany, March 6–9, 1991.

93. Sheagren JN: Glucocorticoid therapy in the management of severe sepsis. *In* Sande MA, Root RK (eds): Septic Shock. New York, Churchill Livingstone, 1985:201–218.

94. Fletcher JR, Herman CM, Ramwell PW: Improved survival in endotoxemia with aspirin and indomethacin pretreatment. Surg Forum 27:11–12, 1976.

95. Jacobs ER, Soulsby ME, Bone RC, et al: Ibuprofen in canine endotoxin shock. J Clin Invest 70:536–541, 1982.

96. Strieter RM, Remick DG, Ward PA, et al: Cellular and molecular regulation of tumor necrosis factor-alpha production by pentoxifylline. Biochem Biophys Res Commun 155:1230–1236, 1988.

97. Nakamura C, Nelson S, Lippton H, et al: Contrasting effects of misoprostol on systemic and intrapulmonary lipopolysaccharide-induced tumor necrosis factor-alpha. Life Sci 50:1869–1872, 1992.

98. Zabel P, Schonharting MM, Wolter DT, et al: Oxpentifylline in endotoxaemia. Lancet 2:1474–1477, 1989.

99. Kunimoto F, Morita T, Ogawa R, et al: Inhibition of lipid peroxidation improves survival rate of endotoxemic rats. Circ Shock 21:15–22, 1987.

100. Kilbourn RG, Jubran A, Gross SS, et al: Reversal of endotoxin-mediated shock by NG-methyl-L-arginine, an inhibitor of nitric oxide synthesis. Biochem Biophys Res Commun 172:1132–1138, 1990.

101. Sprung CL, Caralis PV, Marcial EH, et al: The effects of high-dose corticosteroids in patients with septic shock: A prospective, controlled study. N Engl J Med 311:1137–1143, 1984.

102. The Veterans Administration Systemic Sepsis Cooperative Study Group: Effect of high-dose glucocorticoid therapy on mortality in patients with clinical signs of systemic sepsis. N Engl J Med 317:659–665, 1987.

103. Toews GB: Determinants of bacterial clearance from the lower respiratory tract. Semin Respir Infect 1:68–78, 1986.

104. Nelson RD, Herron MJ: Chemotaxis and motility of lung phagocytes. Semin Respir Infect 1:79–88, 1986.

105. Nathan CF: Secretory products of macrophages. J Clin Invest 79:319–326, 1987.

106. Ming WJ, Bersani L, Mantovani A: Tumor necrosis factor is chemotactic for monocytes and polymorphonuclear leukocytes. J Immunol 138:1469–1474, 1987.

107. Furie MB, McHugh DD: Migration of neutrophils across endothelial monolayers is stimulated by treatment of the monolayers with inter-

leukin-1 or tumor necrosis factor-α. J Immunol 143:3309–3317, 1989.

108. Salyer JL, Bohnsack JF, Knape WA, et al: Mechanisms of tumor necrosis factor-α alteration of PMN adhesion and migration. Am J Pathol 136:831–841, 1990.

109. Worthen GS, Haslett C, Rees AJ, et al: Neutrophil-medicated pulmonary vascular injury. Synergistic effect of trace amounts of lipopolysaccharide and neutrophil stimuli on vascular permeability and neutrophil sequestration in the lung. Am Rev Respir Dis 136:19–28, 1987.

110. Haslett C, Worthen GS, Giclas PC, et al: The pulmonary vascular sequestration of neutrophils in endotoxemia is initiated by an effect of endotoxin on the neutrophil in the rabbit. Am Rev Respir Dis 136:9–18, 1987.

111. Lilly CM, Sandhu JS, Ishizaka A, et al: Pentoxifylline prevents tumor necrosis factor-induced lung injury. Am Rev Respir Dis 139:1361–1368, 1989.

112. Bainton BG, Nelson S, Chidiac C, et al: Anti-inflammatory agents in sepsis and acute lung injury. Effects of methylprednisolone and ibuprofen on TNF and pulmonary host defenses. Crit Care Rep 1:201–207, 1990.

113. Nelson S, Bagby GJ, Summer WR: Alcohol-induced suppression of tumor necrosis factor—A potential risk factor for secondary infection in the acquired immunodeficiency syndrome. *In* Seminara D, Watson R, Pawlowski A (eds): Alcohol, Immunosuppression and AIDS. New York, Alan R Liss, 1990:211–220.

114. Blanchard DK, Djeu JY, Klein TW, et al: Induction of tumor necrosis factor by *Legionella pneumophila*. Infect Immun 55:433–437, 1987.

115. Nelson S, Noel P, Bokulic R, et al: Murine recombinant tumor necrosis factor enhances host defenses against *Staphylococcus aureus*. [Abstract] Am Rev Respir Dis 139:A357, 1989.

116. Blanchard DK, Djeu JY, Klein TW, et al: Protective effects of tumor necrosis factor in experimental *Legionella pneumophila* infections of mice via activation of PMN function. J Leukoc Biol 43:429–435, 1988.

117. Krishnan VL, Meager A, Mitchell DM, et al: Alveolar macrophages in AIDS patients: Increased spontaneous tumor necrosis factor-alpha production in *Pneumocystis carinii* pneumonia. Clin Exp Immunol 80:156–160, 1990.

118. Nelson S, Bagby GJ, Bainton BG, et al: The effects of acute and chronic alcoholism on tumor necrosis factor and the inflammatory response. J Infect Dis 160:422–429, 1989.

119. White J, Nelson S, Jakab G, et al: Methylprednisolone impairs the bactericidal activity of alveolar macrophages. J Surg Res 39:46–52, 1985.

120. Harris SE, Nelson S, Astry CL, et al: Endotoxin-induced suppression of pulmonary antibacterial defenses against *Staphylococcus aureus*. Am Rev Respir Dis 138:1439–1443, 1988.

121. Nelson S, Chidiac C, Bagby G, et al: Endotoxin-induced suppression of lung host defenses. J Med 21:85–103, 1990.

122. Nelson S, Summer WR, Bagby GJ, Kluger M, Powanda M, Oppenheim J: LPS-induced inhibition of lung TNF and host defenses. *In* Dinarello CA, et al (eds): The Physiological and Pathological Effects of Cytokines. New York, Wiley-Liss, 1990:141–146.

123. Simpson SQ, Modi HN, Balk RA, et al: Reduced alveolar macrophage production of tumor necrosis factor during sepsis in mice and men. Crit Care Med 19:1060–1066, 1991.

124. Luger A, Graf H, Schwarz HP, et al: Decreased serum interleukin-1 activity and monocyte interleukin-1 production in patients with fatal sepsis. Crit Care Med 14:458–461, 1986.

125. Jaffe HA, Buhl R, Mastrangeli A, et al: Organ specific cytokine therapy. J Clin Invest 88:297–302, 1991.

126. Luedke C, Cerami A: Interferon-γ overcomes glucocorticoid suppression of cachectin/tumor necrosis factor biosynthesis by murine macrophages. J Clin Invest 86:1234–1240, 1990.

127. Nelson S, Nakamura C, Shellito J, et al: Intratracheal gamma-interferon enhances pulmonary host defenses against *Pseudomonas aeruginosa*. Am Rev Respir Dis 145S:337, 1992.

128. Skerrett SJ, Martin TR: Intratracheal interferon gamma augments pulmonary clearance of *Legionella pneumophila* in immunosuppressed rats. Am Rev Respir Dis 145:A12, 1992.

129. Beck JM, Liggitt HD, Brunette EN, et al: Reduction in intensity of *Pneumocystis carinii* pneumonia in mice by aerosol administration of gamma interferon. Infect Immun 59:3859–3862, 1991.

130. Weisbart RH, Gasson JC, Golde DW: Colony-stimulating factors and host defense. Ann Intern Med 110:297–303, 1989.

131. Souza LM, Boone TC, Gabrilove J, et al: Recombinant human granulocyte colony-stimulating factor: Effects on normal and leukemic myeloid cells. Science 232:61–65, 1986.

132. Lindemann A, Herrmann F, Oster W, et al: Hematologic effects of recombinant human granulocyte colony-stimulating factor in patients with malignancy. Blood 74:2644–2651, 1989.

133. Cohen AM, Hines DK, Korach ES, et al: In vivo activation of neutrophil function in hamsters by recombinant human granulocyte colony-stimulating factor. Infect Immun 56:2861–2865, 1988.

134. Sartorelli KH, Silver GM, Gamelli RL: The effect of granulocyte colony-stimulating factor (G-CSF) upon burn-induced defective neutrophil chemotaxis. J Trauma 31:523–530, 1991.

135. Platzer E, Oez S, Welte K, et al: Human pluripotent hematopoietic colony stimulating factor: activities on human and murine cells. Immunobiology 172:185–193, 1986.

136. Weisbart RH, Kacena A, Schuh A, et al: GM-CSF induces human neutrophil IgA-mediated phagocytosis by an IgA Fc receptor activation mechanism. Nature 332:647–648, 1988.

137. Roilides E, Walsh TJ, Pizzo PA, et al: Granulocyte colony-stimulating factor enhances the phagocytic and bactericidal activity of normal and defective human neutrophils. J Infect Dis 163:579–583, 1991.

138. Tazi A, Nioche S, Chastre J, et al: Spontaneous release of granulocyte colony-stimulating factor (G-CSF) by alveolar macrophages in the course of bacterial pneumonia and sarcoidosis: Endotoxin-dependent and exotoxin-independent G-CSF release by cells recovered by bronchoalveolar lavage. Am J Respir Cell Mol Biol 4:140–147, 1991.

139. Kawakami M, Tsutsumi H, Kumakawa T, et al: Levels of serum granulocyte colony-stimulating factor in patients with infections. Blood 76:1962–1964, 1990.

140. Gopal V, Bisno AL: Fulminant pneumococcal infection in ''normal'' asplenic hosts. Arch Intern Med 137:1526–1530, 1977.

141. Hebert JC, O'Reilly M, Gamelli RL: Protective effect of recombinant human granulocyte colony-stimulating factor against pneumococcal infections in splenectomized mice. Arch Surg 125:1075–1078, 1990.

142. Kolb D, Gunderson EKE: Alcohol-related morbidity among older career navy men. Drug Alcohol Depend 9:181–189, 1982.

143. Capps JA, Coleman GH: Influence of alcohol on prognosis of pneumonia in Cook County Hospital. JAMA 80:750–752, 1923.

144. MacGregor RR, Safford M, Shalit M: Effect of ethanol on functions required for the delivery of neutrophils to sites of inflammation. J Infect Dis 157:682–689, 1988.

145. MacGregor RR, Gluckman SG: Effect of acute alcohol intoxication on granulocyte mobilization and kinetics. Blood 52:551–559, 1979.

146. Nelson S, Summer W, Bagby G, et al: Granulocyte colony-stimulating factor enhances pulmonary host defenses in normal and ethanol-treated rats. J Infect Dis 164:901–906, 1991.

147. Mooney DP, Gamelli RL, O'Reilly M, et al: Recombinant human granulocyte colony-stimulating factor and *Pseudomonas* burn wound sepsis. Arch Surg 123:1353–1357, 1988.

148. Silver GM, Gamelli RL, O'Reilly M: The beneficial effect of granulocyte colony-stimulating factor (G-CSF) in combination with gentamicin on survival after *Pseudomonas* burn wound infection. Surgery 106:452–456, 1989.

149. Yasuda H, Ajiki Y, Shimozato T, et al: Therapeutic efficacy of granulocyte colony-stimulating factor alone and in combination with antibiotics against *Pseudomonas aeruginosa* infections in mice. Infect Immun 58:2502–2509, 1990.

150. Cairo MS, Mauss D, Kommareddy S, et al: Prophylactic or simultaneous administration of recombinant human granulocyte colony-stimulating factor in the treatment of group B streptococcal sepsis in neonatal rats. Pediatr Res 27:612–616, 1990.

151. O'Reilly M, Silver GM, Greenhalgh D, et al: Treatment of intra-abdominal injection with granulocyte colony-stimulating factor. J Trauma 33:679–682, 1992.

151a. Koizumi T, Kubo K, Shinozak S, Koyama S, Kobayashi T, Sekigudri M: Granulocyte colony-stimulating factor does not exacerbate endotoxin-induced lung injury in sheep. Am Rev Respir Dis 148:132–137, 1993.

151b. Fink MP, O'Sullivan BP, Menconi MJ, et al: Effect of granulocyte colony-stimulating factor on systemic and pulmonary responses to endotoxin in pigs. J Trauma 34:571–578, 1993.

152. Kanazawa M, Ishizaka A, Hasegawa N, et al: Granulocyte colony-stimulating factor does not enhance endotoxin-induced acute lung injury in guinea pigs. Am Rev Respir Dis 145:1030–1035, 1992.

PART

VI

Prevention

# Infection Control Methods

JANIS WIENER and ROBERT A. WEINSTEIN

The Study on the Efficacy of Nosocomial Infection Control (SENIC Project), a large, complex study conducted between 1974 and 1983 by the Centers for Disease Control (CDC) and published in 1985, demonstrated a 27% reduction in postoperative pneumonia and a 13% reduction in pneumonia in medical patients after the establishment of infection control programs that included organized surveillance and control activities and a trained infection control physician and one infection control nurse per 250 hospital beds.[1] The overall infection rates were reduced by 32% in hospitals with these programs. Among hospitals without effective programs, the overall infection rate increased by 18%. This chapter reviews hygienic and environmental infection control practices that may contribute to the control of nosocomial pneumonia.

## HAND WASHING

Although hand washing is considered to be one of the few infection control practices with demonstrated efficacy (Table 47–1), there are few prospective trials evaluating a connection between hand washing and prevention of pulmonary infection.[2] The introduction of routine practice of

Table 47–1. **When to Use Hand Washing and Barrier Precautions**

| Precaution | Indication |
|---|---|
| Hand washing | Between patient contacts, even if gloves are worn |
| Gloving | When contact with body fluids is likely and as part of antibiotic resistance precautions |
| Gowning | Routine use not indicated; use if soiling or splashing by body fluids is anticipated |
| Masking | Routine use not indicated; limit use to strict and respiratory isolation and if splashing by body fluids is anticipated |

hand washing, antisepsis, and environmental hygiene by Semmelweis, Holmes, and Lister resulted in such dramatic decreases in morbidity and mortality from infectious processes that the idea of a randomized trial in which such activities would be withheld seems unethical. However, studies of puerperal fever and of transmission of staphylococcal disease to neonates have shown that hand washing decreases colonization and infection rates.[3] For example, in a neonatal nursery, there was a 43% transmission rate when nurses routinely handled a baby colonized with *Staphylococcus aureus* and then handled another baby without washing their hands. Antiseptic hand washing between infant contacts reduced this rate to 14%.[4]

Studies have shown that persistent hand carriage of pathogens is also a problem. An investigation of the hand flora of 103 hospital personnel showed that one or more of 22 different species of gram-negative bacteria were carried persistently on the hands of 21% of the workers.[5] Persons who washed their hands less than eight times per day were significantly more likely to carry the same species of gram-negative bacteria throughout the day; 21% of 541 nosocomial infections over a 7-month period were caused by species found on the hands of personnel. In another report, an outbreak of *Acinetobacter* pneumonia was traced to the chronically colonized hands of a respiratory therapist with dermatitis.[6]

A few trials have focused on efficacy of hand washing in intensive care units (ICUs).[7–9] A 1977 study identified the skin of patients and hands of nurses as reservoirs of certain strains of *Klebsiella* endemic to a British ICU.[7] The introduction of antiseptic hand washing practices into the ICU was associated with a significant reduction in the number of patients colonized or infected with *Klebsiella* spp. when sequential groups were compared. Two hospital-based trials of the effect of hand washing on ICU infection rates showed that after an antiseptic agent was used for hand washing, infection rates were almost half those seen after a nonantiseptic agent was used.[8, 9] Similar results were found after the same two products were compared in a crossover design trial, although the reduced infection rate was only seen in the medical ICU and not in the cardiac or surgical ICUs.

Despite the evidence linking hand washing and reduction of infection rates, compliance with hand washing guidelines is poor.[10] In one medical ICU study, health care workers washed their hands after only 41% of patient contacts.[11] Physicians were among the worst offenders, washing their hands after only 28% of contacts. The reasons cited for poor compliance included busy schedules, irritating soaps, inadequate numbers of sinks, inconvenient location of sinks, belief that gloves provide adequate protection, forgetfulness, and skepticism about the efficacy of hand washing in reducing infection rates.[10]

Attempts to improve hand-washing practices by changing washing agents, using private rooms with more convenient sinks, providing automated sinks, or offering education and feedback have had limited success.[10] Changing to an emollient hand-washing agent made no difference in hand-washing frequency, but providing feedback on a regular basis improved the rate of hand washing significantly, from 63% to 92%.[12] Conversion of a six-bed open ICU with only two hand-washing sinks to a new facility with 14 enclosed isolation rooms, each with an individual sink, did not increase hand-washing frequency and had no effect on overall colonization and infection rates.[13] A trial of automated sinks in which the dispensing of soap and water was controlled by electronic sensors showed that this approach resulted in better quality but less frequent hand washing by hospital personnel.[14] These studies suggest that unless totally new technologies are developed or attitudes can be improved, conventional physical plant or minor technologic upgrades are unlikely to improve hand-washing frequency.

### Recommendations

The absolute indications for and the ideal frequency of hand washing are not known because of the lack of well-controlled studies. The CDC guidelines published in 1985 make several recommendations.[15] In the absence of a true emergency, hospital workers should always wash their hands before performing invasive procedures; before taking care of immunocompromised patients and newborn infants; before and after touching wounds; after contact with mucous membranes, blood, body fluids, secretions, or excretions; after touching contaminated inanimate sources such as suction devices; after caring for a patient infected or colonized with multidrug-resistant organisms or other organisms of clinical and epidemiologic significance; and between contacts with different patients.

### Technique

The surfaces of lathered hands should be rubbed together for at least 10 seconds, followed by thorough rinsing under a stream of water. Plain soap should be used; bar soap is often avoided for asthetic reasons. Before caring for patients in high-risk units or for immunocompromised pa-

tients and newborns, antimicrobial hand-washing products are often used, although further study is necessary to confirm the efficacy of this practice.

## BARRIER PRECAUTIONS

### Gloves

The absolute indications for gloves, gowns, and other barrier precautions (see Table 47–1) as means of preventing nosocomial infection and pneumonia are unknown, but there is agreement that nonsterile examination gloves should be worn if hands are likely to become contaminated with potentially infectious material such as blood, body fluids, secretions, or excretions. Sterile gloves should be worn for performing invasive procedures, for suctioning intubated patients, or for touching open wounds.[15] Evidence suggests that, if applied aggressively, barrier precautions are effective in preventing the spread of multiple-antibiotic–resistant Enterobacteriaceae and methicillin-resistant S. aureus (MRSA).[16–18] The institution of barrier precautions resulted in a sustained 87% reduction in resistant Enterobacteriaceae in one center and controlled an ICU outbreak of MRSA in another.[17, 18]

### Glove Reuse

Several reports, particularly in the dental literature, have been interpreted as supporting the reuse of examination gloves.[19] However, a microbiologic study evaluating the effectiveness of three different types of cleaning agents for decontaminating gloved hands that had been inoculated with nosocomial pathogens showed that bacteria adhere to gloves and are not easily washed off, even in the best of hand-washing circumstances.[20] Moreover, after glove removal, up to 50% of hands were contaminated. Based on such findings, gloves should be changed between patients, and hands should be washed after removing gloves.

### Gowns

A prospective, controlled study showed a 50% reduction in the infection rate in a pediatric ICU after the use of nonsterile gloves and disposable nonwoven polypropylene gowns.[21] Although the incidence of pneumonia was similar in the glove-and-gown group and the standard-care group, there were almost four times as many cases of tracheobronchitis in the standard-care group. Extrapolation of these findings to the adult ICU may not be justified because of the much higher rate of viral infections in the pediatric setting. Data from a recent longitudinal pediatric intervention study conducted over three respiratory syncytial virus (RSV) seasons showed that gloves and gowns substantially reduced transmission of RSV.[22] The adjusted relative risk of nosocomial RSV transmission was almost three times greater during the first half of the study, when gloves and gowns were worn during only 38.5% of contacts, than during the second half, when compliance increased to 81%. However, because gloves and gowns were used together in both of these studies, the relative benefit of each of these barrier precautions is unknown.

Several studies specifically addressing the use of gowns have been carried out in neonatal and pediatric ICUs, in the newborn nursery, and with immunocompromised cancer patients.[23–26] Because none of these studies has shown a significant reduction in infection rates, the routine use of gowns cannot be recommended except in situations in which soiling or splashing of body fluids is expected.

## Masks

The use of masks usually does not play a role in preventing nosocomial pneumonia. For example, a study comparing the effect of masking and gowning on the rate of nosocomial RSV infections in infants and staff during two sequential periods showed a 32% rate during the intervention period and a 41% rate during the control period.[27]

An area of increasing importance, and one in which the use of masks is controversial, is the control of MRSA infections. Although several studies have shown that routine isolation in a private room without barrier precautions has not been effective in containing the spread of MRSA, the role of masks in particular has not been well studied.[28] CDC guidelines recommend masks for those coming close to the patient colonized or infected with MRSA and the use of gowns, gloves, and a single room.[29] The British Hospital Infection Society and Society for Antimicrobial Chemotherapy recommend that masks be worn only during procedures that may generate staphylococcal aerosols (eg, sputum suction, chest physiotherapy, procedures on patients with exfoliative skin conditions).[30] Because there have been no controlled trials to establish the efficacy of control measures used in MRSA outbreaks, the role of masks remains unknown. We do not advocate their routine use as a means of reducing pneumonia rates.

## RESPIRATORY THERAPY AND VENTILATOR EQUIPMENT

A discussion of the role of respiratory therapy equipment (Table 47–2) as a predisposing factor for nosocomial pneumonia requires differentiating nebulization from humidification, two markedly different principles used to increase the humidity of gases delivered to the tracheobronchial

Table 47–2. **Suggestions for Care of Respiratory Therapy Equipment**

| Equipment | Care and Handling |
| --- | --- |
| In-line medication nebulizers | Disinfect after each treatment |
| Humidifiers | Handle condensate as if it were a contaminated body fluid; consider use of systems that reduce or eliminate condensate; sterilize between patient uses |
| Ventilator tubing | Change and disinfect circuit at ≥ 48-h intervals |
| Other (eg, spirometers, oxygen analyzers) | Disinfect between patient uses |

tree.[31] Humidifiers are devices that saturate gas with water vapor but do not aerosolize droplet water. Nebulizers saturate the gas with water vapor and disperse an aerosol of droplet particles less than 4 μm in diameter.

The potential hazards of respiratory therapy equipment have been reviewed by Craven and associates,[32] and the areas amenable to intervention are summarized in the following sections.

## Nebulizers

In the 1960s, there were many reports of nosocomial pneumonia attributed to nebulization equipment.[33, 34] For example, a study of autopsy material from the Parkland Memorial Hospital showed that a 10-fold increase in the rate of necrotizing gram-negative pneumonia from 1952 through 1963 coincided with an increase in the use of inhalation therapy.[33] Disinfection of nebulization equipment with 25% acetic acid reduced the rates of gram-negative necrotizing pneumonia to levels that had been observed before the institution of reservoir nebulizers.

There has also been concern about the potential for cross-contamination from nebulization equipment. A canine model of *Pseudomonas aeruginosa* pneumonia indicated that bacteria could be recovered as far as 15 feet from an animal connected to a mechanical ventilator with a nebulizer.[35] Particles from a nebulizer can travel as far as 32 feet from the exhalation valve of a pressure ventilator.[36] Using such data, some investigators have recommended that filtering devices be placed on exhalation valves, but it is unknown whether such environmental contamination poses a true risk of cross-infection.

## In-Line Medication Nebulizers

Several outbreaks of nosocomial pneumonia have been attributed to contaminated medications used with the nebulizers.[37, 38] In-line medication nebulizers, which are inserted into the inspiratory tubing of the ventilator to administer bronchodilators, pose a greater risk of nosocomial pneumonia than wall nebulizers. In an outbreak of *Serratia* pneumonia, opened bottles of aerosol medications used for nebulization treatments were found to be contaminated with *Serratia marcescens*.[37] After all of the opened bottles were discarded and replaced with smaller bottles that were discarded every 8 hours, the outbreak ended.

Even without such common-source contamination, medication nebulizers may produce bacterial aerosols. A study of in-line nebulizers showed that during the first 24 hours after a circuit change, high levels of contamination ($>10^3$ organisms/mL) were present in 68% of 19 nebulizer reservoirs, and bacterial aerosols were produced by 71% of 14 nebulizers.[39] Nebulizer contamination apparently came from contaminated condensate that was refluxed from the ventilator circuit. When nebulizers were cleaned after each treatment, the contamination rate was reduced to 20%. Although no correlation between endemic nebulizer contamination and the development of sporadic nosocomial pneumonia has been shown, some investigators recommend that in-line nebulizers be disinfected after each treatment rather than every 24 hours, as recommended by the CDC.[39]

## Humidifiers

An alternate, more commonly used device for warming and moistening inspiratory phase gas is the humidifier. The tubing condensate that forms because of humidifier use easily becomes contaminated with the patient's own flora or exogenous pathogens and is a risk factor for ventilator-associated pneumonia even though ventilators with cascade humidifiers do not generate aerosols. Craven and coworkers have shown that there are high levels of humidifier-related tubing contamination within 2 hours of a circuit change.[40] Water condensation occurs at a mean rate of 30 mL per hour, and within 24 hours, 80% of condensate samples are contaminated, at a median level of $2 \times 10^5$ organisms/mL. The microbiology of the condensate usually correlates with that of the patient's sputum, suggesting that the patient's oropharyngeal flora is the source of circuit colonization.

Common activities, such as turning a patient, may wash the contaminated condensate directly into the patient's respiratory tract. Care should be taken to avoid such accidental instillation of contaminated fluid, and the circuit condensate should be frequently emptied away from the humidifier without allowing drainage back into the reservoir. Because heavily contaminated condensate can serve as a source for cross-infection, health care workers should treat the condensate as contaminated waste.

Because maintaining a sterile ventilator circuit for even 24 hours has proved to be an elusive goal, "the solution to the problem of contaminated condensate is not more frequent circuit changes but rather an improved circuit that will provide adequate humidification without contamination."[40] Several methods that have been developed to reduce collection of condensation and subsequent colonization include heated, nondisposable ventilator tubing; in-line devices with one-way valves to empty condensate from tubing; and heat-moisture exchangers that recycle exhaled heat and moisture and eliminate the need for a humidifier.[32] These methods, however, have been expensive, ineffective, or impractical, and there remains a need for moisture- and bacteria-free humidification systems.

## Ventilator Tubing

The guidelines for the frequency of ventilator circuit changes have evolved. In 1982, the CDC recommended changes every 24 hours.[41] In the same year, Craven and colleagues reported that levels of bacteria in inspiratory phase gas and ventilator tubing were not significantly different between circuit changes every 24 hours and those every 48 hours and that there were cost savings with 48-hour changes.[42] By 1984, a survey showed that 58% of hospitals were changing circuits every 48 hours.[43] In 1986, Craven reported that a policy of 24-hour rather than 48-hour circuit changes was an independent risk factor for nosocomial pneumonia in mechanically ventilated patients.[44] It has been suggested that no circuit changes are necessary. A prospective study from France showed no

difference in the incidence of ventilator-associated pneumonia if 48-hour circuit changes were compared with no changes in patients requiring prolonged (>48 hours) mechanical ventilation.[45]

## Spirometers and Oxygen Analyzers

Devices put in a patient's ventilator circuit may become contaminated and should not be shared between patients without adequate disinfection. For example, an increase in *Acinetobacter* respiratory infections was traced to contaminated spirometers that were transferred between patients.[46] An outbreak of *Pseudomonas maltophilia* sputum colonization in two ICUs was caused by a contaminated spirometer and oxygen analyzer T piece that had been shared among patients and between the units.[47]

## Resuscitation Bags

There have been several reports published on bedside resuscitation bags as a source of bacterial contamination.[48, 49] These bags are used by nursing and respiratory therapy personnel during suctioning of intubated patients or for urgent ventilation. One study showed that the practice of maintaining a resuscitation bag with a constant flow of oxygen to the bag's reservoir, as is routinely done, produces a bacterial aerosol in 25% to 30% of bags.[49] Some investigators have suggested discontinuing oxygen flow if the bag is not in use. Because the role of these aerosols is of questionable significance in contributing to nosocomial infection, such recommendations must be considered optional. Because positive cultures were obtained from 75% of the bag valve connectors within 24 hours of use, periodic replacement of the bag for an individual patient would need to be done on such a frequent basis as to be impractical in many ICUs. However, the transfer of bags between patients may serve as a source of cross-infection and should be avoided.

## Disinfection and Sterilization of Respiratory Therapy and Ventilator Equipment

Proper cleaning and reprocessing procedures for reusable components are necessary to prevent pneumonia related to use of respiratory therapy equipment. The most reliable approach is to sterilize devices with steam under pressure or with ethylene oxide. If this is not possible, high-level disinfection with an agent such as glutaraldehyde should be used. In some settings, pasteurization has been used for parts of circuits (eg, tubing) that do not directly contact patients. Additional information is available in a comprehensive text of sterilization and disinfection procedures.[50]

## ENDOTRACHEAL SUCTIONING

### Indications

Endotracheal suctioning is a routine and crucial aspect of ICU care for the mechanically ventilated patient. Besides

Table 47–3. **Continuous Lateral Rotation Therapy**

| Investigation | Patient Population | Pneumonia* | | | Mortality* | | |
|---|---|---|---|---|---|---|---|
| | | *Cases* | *Controls* | *P Value* | *Cases* | *Controls* | *P Value* |
| Gentilello[56] | Head injury or traction | 5/27 (18.5) | 13/38 (34.2) | NS | 7/27 (25.9) | 5/38 (13.2) | NS |
| Fink[57] | Blunt chest trauma | 7/51 (13.7) | 19/48 (39.6) | 0.006 | 10/51 (19.6) | 8/48 (16.7) | NS |
| Kelley[58] | Acute stroke | 5/18 (28) | 13/25 (52) | N/A | 6/18 (33.3) | 5/25 (20) | NS |
| Sumner[59] | Intensive care unit | 4/43 (9.3) | 7/43 (16.2) | NS | 10/41 (24.4) | 11/42 (26.2) | NS |

*Number of patients with indicated outcome/number of patients studied (%); NS, nonsignificant; N/A, not available.

the complications of arterial oxygen desaturation, cardiac arrhythmias, and cardiorespiratory instability associated with open suctioning technique, there is concern about suction material as a source of cross-infection and the potential for introducing pathogens into the lower respiratory tract during suctioning.

The CDC has issued guidelines for appropriate suction technique.[41] These include such commonsense measures as maintenance of "no-touch" technique, use of sterile gloves on both hands, use of a sterile catheter for suctioning, and use of sterile fluid when flushing the catheter. Suction collection tubing and suction canisters should be changed between patients. Nondisposable suction canisters should be thoroughly washed and then disinfected or sterilized before reuse. Disposable collection systems may be used for patients with known infectious secretions. There have also been recommendations that favor the use of high-efficiency bacterial filters in suction collection systems to minimize the aerosolization of microorganisms. However, we agree with the most recent CDC guidelines that the use of these filters can be limited to portable suction devices, because the use of filters with wall suction units has not been proven necessary for infection control.

### Closed Systems

A closed system has been introduced for suctioning intubated patients.[51] The major theoretical advantage of a closed system is lessened arterial desaturation, because mechanical ventilation of the patient can continue during the suctioning procedure. Other possible benefits include reduction in cross-colonization and lower costs. The potential disadvantages include growth of microorganisms on and in the catheter and on the diaphragm through which the catheter passes and cross-infection if the system is not handled appropriately.

Data from a microbiologic study of 30 patients showed that cultures of the surfaces of closed-system catheters after 24 hours of use have the same number of microorganisms as cultures from the surface of open-system catheters after a single use.[52] Baseline and serial sputum cultures showed that no new bacterial species were introduced into the respiratory secretions. Nevertheless, because cultures of the catheter luminal surface and the diaphragm were not performed, this study may have underestimated the degree of contamination. Further study of these parts of the closed system is necessary.

The only study to look prospectively at the closed catheter in a clinical setting found no difference in the incidence of nosocomial pneumonia between patients suctioned with

the closed system and those suctioned with the open system, although bacterial colonization of the respiratory tract was unexpectedly higher (67% versus 39%, $P<.02$) in the closed system group.[53] We have seen repeated miniclusters of cross-infection associated with disconnection of the closed-system and suction-tubing junction and with failure of personnel to wear gloves when using the closed system because of its sealed appearance.

## CONTINUOUS LATERAL ROTATIONAL THERAPY

Continuous lateral rotational therapy (CLRT) is an intervention that attempts to overcome the immobility that may predispose ICU patients to nosocomial pneumonia (Table 47–3). In the recumbent position and during sleep and sedation, there is a decrease in tidal volume, pulmonary blood flow, and mucociliary transport. These changes may lead to atelectasis and pneumonia.[54] In 1967, the first form of rotational therapy for critically ill patients was devised, based on the hypothesis that frequent automatic turning would promote mobilization of secretions.[55] Rotational therapy theoretically counters the effects of gravity on blood flow and ventilation.

There have been four published prospective, randomized trials evaluating the effect of CLRT on risk of nosocomial pneumonia.[56–59] Each study used a different type of patient population, but in each study, patients were randomized to a routine hospital bed with routine patient turning or to a study bed that provided 10 to 16 hours of slow rotation in the longitudinal axis from 40° to 62° in each direction. Two of the four studies showed a significant decrease in pulmonary complications.[56, 57] Gentilello and associates studied 65 critically ill patients immobilized because of head injury or traction and found that the total incidence of atelectasis and pneumonia was significantly greater in the control patients (66% versus 33% $P < .01$).[56] Considered separately, pneumonia and atelectasis rates were both lower in the CLRT patients, but the differences were not significant. In a study of 106 patients with blunt chest trauma, lower respiratory tract infection (ie, tracheobronchitis or pneumonia) occurred in 58% of control patients, compared with 26% of study patients ($P = .001$).[57] A study of 53 acute stroke patients found a trend toward a decreased rate of pneumonia in the CLRT-treated group, but the trend was not statistically significant.[58] However, the risk of infection at all sites was 2.9 times greater ($P = .02$) among control patients. The one study to evaluate a heterogeneous group of 86 medical ICU patients did not show any difference in pneumonia incidence between the CLRT patients and conventionally treated patients (9% versus 16%, not significant).[59]

The mortality rate was not improved in any of the CLRT studies. One study showed a trend toward increased mortality among acute stroke patients treated with CLRT; 33% of patients using the study bed died, compared with 20% of patients using the standard hospital bed.[58] This finding raises concern about the potential deleterious effect of CLRT on intracranial pressure, because all of the patients who died of transtentorial herniation had received CLRT. Other potential complications of CLRT include arrhythmias, hemodynamic instability, and dislodgement of intravascular catheters. The absolute contraindications to CLRT include unstable spinal cord injuries and traction of arm abductors; the relative contraindications include a rise in intracranial pressure, hemodynamic instability, cardiac arrhythmias, and marked patient agitation.[54]

The study of large numbers of patients is necessary to determine which groups may benefit from CLRT. It appears that trauma patients may benefit more than the general medical ICU patients. The minimum duration of time that CLRT should be used and the minimum degree of rotation also require further study. Cost effectiveness must be evaluated; two studies that included crude cost analyses showed no difference in costs between CLRT and conventionally treated patients.[57, 60]

## BRONCHOSCOPE CARE

Several outbreaks have highlighted the problems of pulmonary infections and pseudoinfections caused by inadequately cleaned fiberoptic bronchoscopes.[61–64] An outbreak of *S. marcescens* pulmonary infection associated with a contaminated fiberoptic bronchoscope ended after institution of a povidone-iodine sterilization procedure.[61] In 1983, transmission of tuberculosis by fiberoptic bronchoscope occurred despite povidone-iodine use.[62] Povidone-iodine was not reliably tuberculocidal, but glutaraldehyde was effective, and the routine use of glutaraldehyde was recommended. Recurrent episodes of mycobacterial contamination of bronchoscopy specimens and a case of pulmonary infection were caused by incomplete disinfection of the bronchoscope suction valves despite a standard protocol that used glutaraldehyde.[63] After the institution of routine autoclaving of heavily contaminated suction valves, no additional episodes of mycobacterial contamination occurred. The CDC has reported an automatic bronchoscope-reprocessing machine as the source of *Mycobacterium chelonae* contamination of bronchoscopy specimens.[64] The extent of contamination of bronchoscopes by use of such machines needs to be determined.

## OTHER ENVIRONMENTAL SOURCES AND RESERVOIRS OF INFECTION

In a nationwide survey of hospital infection control programs in 1976 and 1977, 74% of respondents reported performing routine microbiologic surveillance of the hospital environment despite the conclusion of the American Hospital Association in 1974 that "routine environmental microbiologic sampling programs done with no specific epidemiologic goal in mind are unnecessary and economically unjustifiable."[65, 66] Most infection control authorities agreed with the statement, but supportive scientific data were lacking at that time.

Maki and colleagues compared environmental cultures of air, surfaces, and fomites from the old (1924) University of Wisconsin hospital with those from the University's new (1979) hospital.[67] The new hospital was twice as large as the old hospital and was equipped with a modern ventilation system and "excellent isolation facilities." Despite the fact that 17% of environmental cultures from the old hospital were positive for pathogenic bacteria and fungi compared with 4.5% of cultures from the new hospital before occupancy (P<.001), the incidence of nosocomial infections, including pneumonia, was identical in both hospitals.

Another study monitored bacteria from air, staff, and patients in a medical ICU.[68] Hand-washing samples revealed potentially pathogenic bacteria from 30.8% of physicians and 16.6% of nurses. Air cultures yielded pathogens in 15% of sampling periods. Surveillance of patients showed that 17% were colonized with gram-negative bacteria, *S. aureus* or *Candida* species. The spectra of bacteria recovered from patients and air were generally different, but strains recovered from patients and the hands of health care workers were identical in most cases.

A 1984 study of cultures from ICU sink drains found that all of the sink drains harbored multiple strains of *P. aeruginosa* and that 56% of isolates had high-level resistance to gentamicin and tobramycin.[69] None of the strains of *P. aeruginosa* acquired by patients in that unit during the 6-week survey showed this pattern of resistance. Although sink drains may be reservoirs for large numbers of resistant bacteria, they are rarely the source of organisms that colonize patients.

Based on studies such as these, most bacteria causing endemic nosocomial infection derive predominantly from the hands of medical personnel or from the patient's endogenous flora and rarely from the environment. In the absence of a specific infection problem epidemiologically linked to the environment, routine microbiologic surveillance of the inanimate hospital environment cannot be recommended. However, there is a role for routine environmental surveillance and control measures, as described later, directed at nosocomial infections caused by *Legionella* and by filamentous fungi. This is particularly true in hospitals with large numbers of immunosuppressed patients, because they are particularly at risk for acquiring these infections.

## NOSOCOMIAL *LEGIONELLA* PNEUMONIA

Shortly after the Philadelphia outbreak of legionnaires disease in 1976, it became clear that *Legionella* was an important cause of endemic and epidemic nosocomial pneumonia. In some areas, *Legionella* infections are responsible for at least 10% of cases of nosocomial pneumonia.[70, 70a] Evidence suggests that water distribution systems, specifically hot water supplies, are the major source for most reported nosocomial cases. Nosocomial infection also has been linked to humidifiers, nebulizers, endotracheal intubation, and aspiration of contaminated water. An epidemiologic link between showerhead aerosols and acquisition of disease has never been shown in prospective studies, although retrospective analyses have suggested showers as a possible source.[71] In the setting of documented nosocomial *Legionella* infection, most authorities agree that cultures of hot water and of faucets and showerheads should be obtained. If cultures are positive for *Legionella* and typing of clinical and environmental isolates correlate, eradication measures should be instituted (Table 47–4).[71, 72]

If no nosocomial disease is documented in a hospital, the approach to prevention and the environment is more controversial. It has been argued that because *Legionella pneu-*

*mophila* is ubiquitous, merely documenting its presence in a hospital water supply does not necessitate eradication, and routine culturing of water is not needed unless cases of *Legionella* infection have been documented. However, Yu and colleagues have presented evidence that an apparent absence of cases often represents underdiagnosis. In a prospective study of three hospitals without recognized endemic nosocomial *Legionella,* the one hospital with a water supply shown to be contaminated with *Legionella* also was found to have clinical cases of *Legionella* infection after serologic testing, direct fluorescent antibody analysis, and sputum cultures on selective media were performed.[73]

**Table 47–4. Epidemiology and Control of Nosocomial Pneumonias Requiring Additional Environmental, Engineering, or Isolation Procedures**

| Factors Influencing Control | *Legionella*[70–80] | *Aspergillus*[81–91] | *Mycobacterium tuberculosis*[92–97] |
|---|---|---|---|
| Source | Environment (eg, water) | Environment (eg, spore-laden dust) | Patients with active pulmonary infection |
| At-risk population | Primarily immunocompromised patients | Immunocompromised patients | Primarily immunocompromised patients and hospital personnel |
| Epidemiology | Sporadic and epidemic cases related to contaminated potable water including water used for respiratory therapy | Endemic cases due to inhalation of low-level environmental spore load by immunosuppressed patients; epidemics related to release of spores during construction or to heavy environmental spore load | Sporadic person-to-person airborne infection and epidemics related to failure to recognize and isolate patients with active pulmonary disease |
| **Environmental Controls** | | | |
| Air handling | Unknown | Examine and clean air-handling systems on regular schedule and when infection problems are detected; prevent bird access to air intakes; involve infection control personnel in planning construction and when repairing air-handling systems | Isolate patient with active tuberculosis in private room with door closed; at least six air changes per hour and negative pressure |
| Air filtration | Unknown | HEPA filters should be used in areas housing immunocompromised patients and at hospital construction sites | Consider HEPA filters in areas with high incidence of tuberculosis (although no clinical experience) |
| Ultraviolet light | Only practical if it can be focused on water supply to specific high-risk units | Unknown | Used with some success in shelters and in some hospitals as wall-mounted and overhead fixtures |
| Construction precautions | Involve infection control when installing new water heaters and piping | Remove immunosuppressed patients from construction sites; place plastic barriers between patient areas and renovation sites; vacuum and damp-dust horizontal surfaces and false ceiling tiles (consider copper 8-quinolinolate application to air ducts and false ceiling tiles before construction) | Involve infection control when construction or other activities may involve air-handling systems or alter air flow or ventilation |
| Other environmental control measures | Water treatment with one or more of the following: thermal eradication, chlorination, instantaneous steam heating, ultraviolet light, or copper/silver electrodes | Unknown | Unknown |
| Barrier precautions | Not applicable | See construction-related precautions | Infected patients should wear surgical masks when leaving room for diagnostic tests; personnel and visitors should wear particulate respirators or HEPA-filter masks in patient's room; particulate respirators or HEPA-filter masks should be worn by personnel during bronchoscopy, sputum induction, and aerosolized pentamidine therapy for patients with known or suspected active tuberculosis |

Based on these findings, Yu and colleagues recommend that all hospital hot water tanks and selected distal sites (eg, ICUs, transplant wards) be cultured three times in 1 year. If no waterborne *Legionella* is isolated, clinical and continued environmental surveillance is not necessary. If *Legionella* is isolated, they recommend that clinicians should routinely culture for *Legionella* in all cases of nosocomial pneumonia. Others have suggested that such an approach be limited to high-risk patients (ie, organ transplant patients, patients receiving steroids or immunosuppressive drugs, those with chronic obstructive pulmonary disease or aspiration pneumonia).[74] If clinical cases of *Legionella* are identified, eradication measures should be considered.

## Eradication Measures

Disinfection methods have been summarized by Yu and colleagues and include thermal eradication, chlorination, instantaneous steam heating, and ultraviolet (UV) light or metal ionization treatment.[71, 72]

Thermal eradication should be considered if immediate implementation is needed.[75] The basic method requires that hot water tank temperatures be elevated above 70°C, followed by flushing of all faucets and showerheads with hot water. All water tanks should be shut down, drained, descaled with high-pressure steam, and then chlorinated to 100 ppm for 12 to 14 hours. The chlorinated water should be drained, and the tanks should be flushed with water to remove residual chlorine. All distal water sites should be flushed with water that exceeds a temperature of 60°C for 2 to 3 days. If cultures of distal sites show no *Legionella* on the fourth day, the procedure is complete; if *Legionella* are isolated on day 4, the protocol is repeated on days 9 and 10.

The major disadvantages of this approach are that large numbers of personnel are needed, there is a potential for scalding, and recontamination will gradually occur. Recontamination can be prevented by maintaining hot water tank temperatures at 60°C. With this additional measure, the heat and flush method may be needed only every 2 to 3 years, although steps (eg, signs at all water faucets) must be taken to reduce the risk of scalding patients and employees.

A chlorinator may be inserted into the water system and can be successful in controlling *Legionella* in institutional water distribution systems.[76, 77] The chlorinator continuously injects metered volumes of chlorinated salts to achieve the desired free chlorine residual level (2–6 ppm). Pipe corrosion will occur, although silicate coating of water pipes has reduced this problem.

Instantaneous steam-heating systems flash heat water to a temperature greater than 88°C and then blend hot water with cold water to achieve the desired temperature. These systems are most effective if installed as original heating systems in new buildings. In older systems, this approach is less efficacious because reseeding of *Legionella* into the system can occur. This system should not be relied on initially as the sole disinfection system if it is installed into a building with known water contamination; thermal eradication followed by hyperchlorination for several months should be done first.

UV light has proven effective if disinfection can be lo-

calized within the hospital. Installation of UV light into the pipes providing water to an eight-room renal transplant unit reduced the number of water samples positive for *Legionella micdadei* from 26 of 95 to 0 of 71.[78] UV sterilization provides no residual protection, and areas distal to the sterilizer must be disinfected after installation and start-up.

A commercial system using copper-silver electrodes that generate ions when an electrical current is applied has been shown to kill *Legionella* in vitro.[79] Installation in hospitals with *Legionella* problems has produced mixed results.[79a] One report suggests using this approach with UV light supplementation.[80]

## ASPERGILLOSIS

During the past 20 years, nosocomial aspergillosis has emerged as an important cause of morbidity and mortality in immunosuppressed patients. Most of our understanding of the epidemiology and prevention of this infection derives from more than 25 published reports of nosocomial aspergillosis outbreaks.[85] Patients acquire nosocomial aspergillosis through the inhalation of airborne spores. Contaminated, inadequate, or malfunctioning ventilation systems and hospital construction are the principal nosocomial sources of *Aspergillus* spores. Because these spores can be cultured from various reservoirs within the hospital, epidemiologic analysis and culture surveys for environmental sources are important for determining appropriate control measures (see Table 47–4).

Nonfiltered, nonventilated air was suggested as a source of *Aspergillus* in two reports.[82, 83] Rose reported that moving from an older hospital without filtered air to a new hospital with prefiltered, nonrecirculating air was associated with a decline in invasive aspergillosis from 11 cases over 5 years to no cases in the next 5 years.[82] In another report, a fivefold decrease in aspergillosis and zygomycosis cases was observed after patients were moved from an older hospital with no central ventilation to a new hospital with central, filtered ventilation.[83]

Contaminated or malfunctioning ventilation systems have frequently been implicated as a source of nosocomial aspergillosis.[81] *Aspergillus* has been shown to colonize air intake ducts, filters, and ventilation exhaust ducts.[84–86] A cluster of pulmonary aspergillosis in 4 renal transplant patients was associated with *Aspergillus*-containing pigeon excreta at the air intake ports of the transplantation unit.[84] The problem was resolved by making the system inaccessible to pigeons. Another outbreak investigation showed that *Aspergillus fumigatus* was present in dust and fibers within air intake ducts.[85] However, after the ducts were cleaned and the rooms were painted, subsequent cases of nosocomial aspergillosis occurred. The source of the continuing problem was contaminated air intake filters that had not been changed during the initial investigation. A malfunctioning exhaust fan on a renal transplant unit caused a reversal of air flow that blew *Aspergillus* conidia from a contaminated bird screen in the exhaust duct into the rooms of 3 renal transplant patients who subsequently developed nosocomial pulmonary aspergillosis.[86]

These outbreaks of nosocomial aspergillosis emphasize the need for the routine inspection of air handling equipment and filters for high-risk patient care areas. Birds should be prevented from having access to hospital air intake ducts, and there should be additional examination and cleaning of ventilator systems if infection problems are noted. Moreover, all hospital engineering repairs on air supply and exhaust systems must be coordinated with infection control personnel.

Even with all of these measures, ventilation systems may be inadequate. It is recommended that high-risk-patient areas (eg, bone marrow transplant units) be ventilated with high-efficiency particulate air (HEPA) filters.[81] HEPA filters remove at least 99.97% of particles larger than 0.3 μm and have been shown to be effective in cleansing the air of *Aspergillus* spores, which are 1.5 to 6 μm in diameter. At the University of Minnesota, the installation of in-room, wall-mounted HEPA filters reduced the frequency of *Aspergillus* infection in bone marrow transplant recipients from 15% to 8%.[87] The subsequent addition of HEPA filtration to the air in corridors outside of the bone marrow transplant patient rooms reduced the incidence of infection to 4%; air sampling showed a concomitant reduction in *Aspergillus* count from 2.0 colony-forming units (CFU)/mm³ to 0.17 CFU/m³. A study at the University of Florida bone marrow transplant unit used whole-wall HEPA filtration units with horizontal laminar air flow.[88] No cases of *Aspergillus* infection occurred among 39 bone marrow transplant recipients cared for in this environment, compared with 14 cases of nosocomial *Aspergillus* infection among 74 bone marrow transplant patients who were housed elsewhere in that hospital. Air counts of *Aspergillus* decreased from 0.16 to 0.4 CFU/m³ to only 0.009 CFU/m³ after installation of the whole-wall HEPA filters.

Construction and renovation outside and inside the hospital are an important source of airborne *Aspergillus* conidia. A retrospective autopsy review revealed that the occurrence of 10 cases of invasive aspergillosis correlated with contamination of air conditioners caused by road construction outside the hospital.[89] Similar problems have occurred during excavation and demolition near medical centers. A cluster of aspergillosis cases on a renal transplant ward revealed that renovation of the ward one floor above it had caused *Aspergillus*-laden dust to filter through holes in ceiling acoustical tiles.[90] It was recommended that immunosuppressed patients be removed from renovation sites during construction and renovation. Impermeable plastic barriers should be placed between patient areas and renovation sites, and horizontal surfaces and false ceiling tiles should be vacuumed and damp dusted.

A study that examined the efficacy of measures used to control an outbreak of renovation-associated pulmonary aspergillosis found a decrease, from 11 cases over 24 months during construction to 1 case over 18 months after the initiation of control measures, despite ongoing construction.[91] Control measures included the construction of airtight plastic and drywall barriers around the construction sites, use of negative-pressure ventilation in the work area, installation of portable HEPA filters in rooms housing immunocompromised patients, and the use of copper 8-quinolinolate for area decontamination in the airway plenums and the air handling systems.

Copper 8-quinolinolate was chosen as the antifungal agent for decontamination because it is easily applied in aerosolized form, dries to a nontoxic powder and has been proven safe near food. It was mixed at a 1:9 concentration and applied above the false ceilings and to air ducts. Patients were allowed to reoccupy the area within 36 hours. The major risk involved with the use of the chemical is upper airway irritation, but this can be avoided by the use of proper protective masks and evacuation of areas undergoing decontamination.

## PREVENTION OF NOSOCOMIAL TRANSMISSION OF TUBERCULOSIS

Reports of several outbreaks of tuberculosis (TB) in health care settings, including outbreaks of multidrug-resistant strains, prompted the CDC to publish updated guidelines for the prevention of nosocomial transmission of TB.[92, 92a] Much of the increased concern is related to the occurrence of TB among persons infected with the human immunodeficiency virus (HIV), who are at increased risk for new infection and for reactivation of latent TB.[92b]

The prevention of nosocomial transmission requires a well-organized, multifaceted approach that includes identifying and treating infected patients, maintaining appropriate isolation, ensuring adequate ventilation, providing supplemental measures as needed, attending to special circumstances, decontaminating equipment appropriately, and maintaining ongoing surveillance (see Table 47–4).

### Identification and Treatment of Patients With Tuberculosis

High-risk patients should be screened with a 5-TU Mantoux tuberculin skin test. Skin responses of 5 mm or greater in patients with acquired immunodeficiency syndrome or 10 to 15 mm or greater in immunocompetent patients, are considered positive. If there is a positive skin test, active disease should be sought, and prophylactic or therapeutic treatment should be initiated as indicated.[93]

### Isolation Precautions for Patients With Active Tuberculosis

Isolation precautions include the use of a private room with proper ventilation and a minimum of six air changes per hour, including at least two outside air changes per hour. In health care facilities, isolation precautions should be instituted for those patients considered to be infectious. In general, a patient with suspected or confirmed active pulmonary TB should be considered infectious if cough is present or cough-inducing procedures are performed, or if sputum smear is known to contain acid-fast bacilli (AFB) and the patient is not on chemotherapy, has received chemotherapy for less than 2 weeks, or is having a poor clinical or microbiologic response to chemotherapy.

A person with pulmonary TB on adequate chemotherapy for at least 2 weeks who has had clinical and bacteriologic response to therapy (ie, reduction in cough, resolution of fever, decreased quantity of AFB on smear) is probably not infectious. However, if drug resistance is suspected or confirmed, isolation precautions should be continued until the smear is negative for AFB. Most TB experts agree that noninfectiousness in pulmonary TB can be established by finding sputum free of AFB on 3 consecutive days for a patient on effective chemotherapy.

Patients with extrapulmonary TB usually are not infectious, except for those with nonpulmonary disease located in the upper respiratory tract or oral cavity (eg, laryngeal TB) and those with open lesions in which the concentration of organisms is high and aerosol production is likely.[94]

## Ventilation

Proper ventilation requires that the concentration of contaminants be diluted by introducing noncontaminated air into the room and that air be exhausted directly and completely to the outside. Air mixing must be adequate; ideally, air supply outlets located at ceiling level and exhaust inlets located near the floor provide downward air movement through the breathing zone to the floor area for exhaust. The patient's room should be under negative pressure so that air flows into the contaminated area from adjacent noncontaminated areas. Maintaining the direction of air flow and pressure differentials may be difficult because of open doors; movements of patient and staff; temperature changes; lint-clogged vents, ducts, and filters; inadequately maintained exhaust motors; adjustments made to the ventilation system elsewhere in the building; and automatic shutdown of outside air introduction during cold weather. Doors should remain closed, and the close fit of all doors and other closures between pressurized areas should be maintained.

## Supplemental Environmental and Other Measures

HEPA filters remove at least 99.97% of particles greater than 0.3 μm in diameter and have been effective in clearing the air of *Aspergillus* spores.[87] Their use in removing *Mycobacterium tuberculosis* bacilli has not been studied, but bacteria-containing droplet nuclei, which are 1 to 5 μm in diameter, are about the same size as *Aspergillus* spores. HEPA filters may be employed in general use areas such as emergency rooms where air recirculation is an alternative to using large volumes of outside air for ventilation, but we suggest that HEPA filters should not be used to recirculate air from TB isolation rooms back into the general circulation. If HEPA filters are used, proper installation, testing, and regular maintenance are critical.

The use of germicidal UV lamps (100–290 nm) to sterilize the air and prevent TB transmission is controversial. The theoretical and experimental basis for their effectiveness and several reports of their clinical utility have prompted recommendations for their use if TB transmission is high.[95] UV air disinfection has been used with success in shelters for the homeless.[96, 97] Stead has reported the control of an outbreak of TB in a shelter using wall-mounted UV light in rooms and in corridors.[96] In another shelter, skin test conversions among staff fell from 16 of 83 over a 14-month period to 0 of 83 over 10 months after the installation of overhead UV fixtures.[97] At Milwaukee County Hos-

pital, wall-mounted UV lights in each patient room and in the corridors dramatically decreased tuberculin conversions among staff from several per year to none during 10 years.[96]

The main concerns about UV lamps are safety (ie, short-term overexposure can cause keratoconjunctivitis and skin erythema) and the need for proper installation and maintenance to ensure that the wavelengths are maintained at the needed level. Routine cleaning is unnecessary if tubes are replaced yearly. UV lamps are less effective in areas with relative humidity greater than 70%. Even if UV units are installed in ducts, air should not be recirculated from a TB isolation room back into the general circulation.

Standard surgical masks may not be effective in preventing inhalation of droplet nuclei. "Particulate respirators" and HEPA-filter masks are cone-shaped, surgical-style face masks that were originally developed for industrial use and provide a better facial fit and better filtration capability; however, their efficacy in protecting susceptible persons from TB has not been demonstrated. Their use should be considered if appropriate ventilation is not available, in TB isolation rooms, or if bursts of droplet nuclei are likely to be generated (eg, during bronchoscopy). If particulate respirator or HEPA mask use is instituted, wearers should be trained in their use.

## Special Circumstances

Sputum induction in patients with suspected TB should be performed in a room or booth equipped with negative pressure. Ideally, air should be exhausted to the outside. Adequate time should be allowed between patients to remove infectious particles.

Before initiating *Pneumocystis* prophylaxis with aerosolized pentamidine, HIV-infected patients should be screened for TB, using history, tuberculin skin test, and chest radiograph. Before each subsequent treatment, evaluation for development of symptoms of TB should be performed. If active TB is suspected or diagnosed, antituberculosis treatment should be started, and aerosolized pentamidine should only be administered in a negative-pressure room or booth. Personnel in attendance may wear particulate respirators or HEPA-filter masks if patients receiving aerosol pentamidine have pulmonary TB.

Bronchoscopy should be performed in rooms with adequate ventilation, good distribution of air flow, and air exhausted to the outside in accordance with federal, state, and local regulations. Negative-pressure rooms are preferred; if bronchoscopy must be performed in positive-pressure areas, attempts to rule out infectious TB beforehand should be made. UV lamps, HEPA filters, and local exhaust ventilation near the patient's head may be considered.

Ventilation in ICUs should provide at least six total air changes per hour, including at least two outside air changes. HEPA filters and UV lamps should be considered in ICUs if there is high risk of TB transmission or if air is recirculated. Any ICU patient with suspected or proven active TB should be placed in a private room with isolation precautions.

Emergency room waiting areas should have 10 air changes per hour. In facilities serving populations with a high incidence of TB, the use of UV lamps and HEPA filters should be considered.

Autopsy rooms should have 12 air changes per hour and should be equipped with negative pressure. Room air should be exhausted directly to the outside of the building. Particulate respirators or HEPA-filter masks may be worn by those performing aerosol-producing procedures, such as sawing and irrigating.

## Tuberculosis Decontamination

Devices that are directly introduced into the bloodstream or other sterile sites should be sterilized. Items that may come in contact with mucous membranes (eg, bronchoscopes) should be sterilized or cleaned with high-level disinfectants.[62] Autoclaving of heavily contaminated equipment may be necessary.[63] Noncritical items need only be cleaned with detergent, because these items touch only intact skin and do not transmit TB infection. Extraordinary attempts to disinfect or sterilize environmental surfaces to remove tubercle bacilli are not indicated, because inhalation of the bacilli usually is required for infection to occur.

## Surveillance

Surveillance for TB among health care workers should be maintained with annual tuberculin skin testing. Health care workers who are frequently exposed to patients with TB or who are involved with potentially high-risk procedures, such as bronchoscopy or sputum induction of patients with suspected TB, should be tested every 6 months. Conversion rates should be calculated by area to determine if unrecognized high rates of transmission exist. Rates should be no higher than those in the surrounding community. Prophylactic treatment should be initiated as indicated.

## CONCLUSION

This review of hygienic and environmental infection control practices has focused on a basic soap, water, and common sense approach to preventing nosocomial pneumonias. Unfortunately, many proposed interventions have not received sufficient evaluation to warrant strong endorsement. Ongoing, prospective surveillance of nosocomial pneumonia rates, epidemiologic investigation if rates are high or increasing and regular review of control-related costs will help each hospital determine when its preventive measures need to be reassessed.

## REFERENCES

1. Haley RW, Culver DH, White JW, et al: The efficacy of infection surveillance and control programs in preventing nosocomial infections in US hospitals. Am J Epidemiol 121:159–167, 1985.
2. Larson E: A causal link between handwashing and risk of infection? Examination of the evidence. Infect Control Hosp Epidemiol 9:28–36, 1988.
3. Beck WC: Handwashing, Semmelweis, and chlorine. Infect Control Hosp Epidemiol 9:366–367, 1988.
4. Mortimer EA, Wolinsky E, Gonzaga AJ, et al: Role of airborne transmission in staphylococcal infections. Br Med J 1:319–322, 1966.
5. Larson EL: Persistent carriage of gram-negative bacteria on hands. Am J Infect Control 9:112–119, 1981.
6. Buxton FE, Anderson RL, Werdegar J, et al: Nosocomial respiratory tract infection and colonization with *Acinetobacter calcoaceticus*. Epidemiologic characteristics. Am J Med 65:507–513, 1978.
7. Casewell M, Phillips I: Hands as route of transmission for *Klebsiella* species. Br Med J 2:1315–1317, 1977.
8. Maki D, Hecht J: Antiseptic-containing handwashing agents reduce nosocomial infections—a prospective study. [Abstract] Presented at the 22nd Interscience Conference on Antimicrobial Agents and Chemotherapy, Miami Beach, FL, 1982.
9. Massanari RM, Hierholzer WJ: A crossover comparison of antiseptic soaps on nosocomial infection rates in intensive care units. [Abstract] Am J Infect Control 12:247–248, 1984.
10. Simmons B, Bryant J, Neiman K, et al: The role of handwashing in prevention of endemic intensive care unit infections. Infect Control Hosp Epidemiol 11:589–594, 1990.
11. Albert RK, Condie F: Hand-washing patterns in medical intensive care units. N Engl J Med 304:1465–1466, 1981.
12. Mayer JA, Dubbert PM, Miller M, et al: Increasing handwashing in an intensive care unit. Infect Control 7:259–262, 1986.
13. Preston MA, Larson E, Stamm WE: The effect of private isolation rooms on patient care practices, colonization and infection in an intensive care unit. Am J Med 70:641–645, 1981.
14. Larson E, McGeer A, Quraishi ZA, et al: Effect of an automated sink on handwashing practices and attitudes in high-risk units. Infect Control Hosp Epidemiol 12:422–428, 1991.
15. Garner JS, Favero MS: CDC guideline for handwashing and hospital environmental control. Infect Control 7:231–243, 1986.
16. Weinstein RA, Kabins SA: Strategies for prevention and control of multiple drug-resistant nosocomial infection. Am J Med 70:449–454, 1981.
17. Guiguet M, Rekacewicz C, Leclercq B, et al: Effectiveness of simple measures to control an outbreak of nosocomial methicillin-resistant *Staphylococcus aureus* infections in an intensive care unit. Infect Control Hosp Epidemiol 11:23–26, 1990.
18. Weinstein RA, Nathan C, Gruensfelder R, et al: Endemic aminoglycoside resistance in gram negative bacilli: Epidemiology and mechanisms. J Infect Dis 141:338–345, 1980.
19. Gobetti JP, Cerminara U, Shipman C: Hand asepsis: The efficacy of different soaps in the removal of bacteria from sterile gloved hands. J Am Dent Assoc 113:291–292, 1986.
20. Doebbeling BN, Pfaller MA, Houston AK, et al: Removal of nosocomial pathogens from the contaminated glove. Implications for glove reuse and handwashing. Ann Intern Med 109:394–398, 1988.
21. Klein BS, Perloff WH, Maki DG: Reduction of nosocomial infection during pediatric intensive care by protective isolation. N Engl J Med 320:1714–1721, 1989.
22. Leclair JM, Freeman J, Sullivan BF, et al: Prevention of nosocomial respiratory syncytial virus infections through compliance with glove and gown isolation precautions. N Engl J Med 317:329–334, 1987.
23. Haque KN, Chagla AH: Do gowns prevent infection in neonatal intensive care units? J Hosp Infect 14:159–162, 1989.
24. Donowitz LG: Failure of the overgown to prevent nosocomial infection in a pediatric intensive care unit. Pediatrics 77:35–38, 1986.
25. Cloney DL, Donowitz LG: Overgown use for infection control in nurseries and neonatal intensive care units. Am J Dis Child 140:680–683, 1986.
26. Nauseef WM, Maki DG: A study of the value of simple protective isolation in patients with granulocytopenia. N Engl J Med 304:448–453, 1981.
27. Hall CB, Douglas RG: Nosocomial respiratory syncytial viral infections. Am J Dis Child 135:512–515, 1981.
28. Brumfitt W, Hamilton-Miller J: Methicillin-resistant *Staphylococcus aureus*. N Engl J Med 320:1188–1196, 1989.
29. Garner JS, Simmons BP: Guideline for isolation precautions in hospitals. Infect Control 4:245–325, 1983.
30. Duckworth G: Report of a combined working party of the Hospital Infection Society and British Society for Antimicrobial Chemotherapy. Revised guidelines for the control of epidemic methicillin-resistant *Staphylococcus aureus*. J Hosp Infect 16:351–377, 1990.
31. Bennett JV, Brachman PS: Hospital Infections, ed 3. Boston, Little, Brown, 1992.
32. Craven DE, Steger KA: Nosocomial pneumonia in the intubated pa-

tient: New concepts on pathogenesis and prevention. Infect Dis Clin North Am 3:843–866, 1989.

33. Pierce AK, Sanford JP, Thomas GD, et al: Long-term evaluation of decontamination of inhalation-therapy equipment and the occurrence of necrotizing pneumonia. N Engl J Med 282:528–531, 1970.

34. Reinarz JA, Pierce AK, Mays BB, et al: The potential role of inhalation therapy equipment in nosocomial pulmonary infection J Clin Invest 44:831–839, 1965.

35. Christopher KL, Saravolatz LD, Bush TL, et al: The potential role of respiratory therapy equipment in cross infection. Am Rev Respir Dis 128:271–275, 1983.

36. Dyer ED, Peterson DE: How far do bacteria travel from the exhalation of IPPB equipment? Anesth Analg 51:516, 1972.

37. Sanders CV, Luby JP, Johanson WG, et al: *Serratia marcescens* infections from inhalation therapy medications: Nosocomial outbreak. Ann Intern Med 73:15–21, 1970.

38. Ringrose R, McKown B, Felton FG, et al: A hospital outbreak of *Serratia marcescens* associated with ultrasonic nebulizers. Ann Intern Med 69:719–729, 1968.

39. Craven DE, Lichtenberg DA, Goularte TA, et al: Contaminated medication nebulizers in mechanical ventilator circuits. Am J Med 77:834–838, 1984.

40. Craven DE, Goularte TA, Make BJ: Contaminated condensate in mechanical ventilator circuits. A risk factor for nosocomial pneumonia? Am Rev Respir Dis 129:625–628, 1984.

41. Simmons BP, Wong ES: Guideline for prevention of nosocomial pneumonia. Infect Control 3:327–333, 1982.

42. Craven DE, Connolly MG, Lichtenberg DA, et al: Contamination of mechanical ventilators with tubing changes every 24 or 48 hours. N Engl J Med 306:1505–1509, 1982.

43. Goularte TA, Craven DE: Results of a survey of infection control practices for respiratory therapy equipment. Infect Control 7:327–330, 1986.

44. Craven DE, Kunches LM, Kilinsky V, et al: Risk factors for pneumonia and fatality in patients receiving continuous mechanical ventilation. Am Rev Respir Dis 133:792–796, 1986.

45. Dreyfuss D, Djedaini K, Weber P, et al: Prospective study of nosocomial pneumonia and of patient and circuit colonization during mechanical ventilation with circuit changes every 48 hours versus no change. Am Rev Respir Dis 143:738–743, 1991.

46. Irwin RS, Demers RR, Pratter MR, et al: An outbreak of *Acinetobacter* infection associated with the use of a ventilator spirometer. Respir Care 25:232–237, 1980.

47. Carroll AR, Goularte TA, McGinley KN, et al: An outbreak of *Pseudomonas maltophilia* in intensive care units traced to contaminated respiratory therapy equipment. Presented at the 12th Annual Conference of the Association of Practitioners in Infection Control, Las Vegas, NV, 1985.

48. Weber DJ, Rutala WA, Wilson MB: Manual ventilation bags (MVB) as a source for bacterial colonization of intubated patients. [Abstract] Presented at the 28th Interscience Conference on Antimicrobial Agents and Chemotherapy, Los Angeles, CA, 1988.

49. Thompson AC, Wilder BJ, Powner DJ: Bedside resuscitation bag: A source of bacterial contamination. Infect Control 6:231–232, 1985.

50. Block SS: Disinfection, Sterilization, and Preservation, ed 4. Philadelphia, Lea & Febiger, 1991.

51. Mayhall CG: The Trach Care closed tracheal suction system: A new medical device to permit tracheal suctioning without interruption of ventilatory assistance. Infect Control Hosp Epidemiol 9:125–126, 1988.

52. Ritz R, Scott LR, Coyle MB, et al: Contamination of a multiple-use suction catheter in a closed-circuit system compared to contamination of a disposable, single-use suction catheter. Respir Care 31:1086–1091, 1986.

53. Deppe SA, Kelly JW, Thoi LL, et al: Incidence of colonization, nosocomial pneumonia and mortality in critically ill patient using a Trach Care closed-suction system versus an open-suction system: Prospective, randomized study. Crit Care Med 18:1389–1393, 1990.

54. Sahn SA: Continuous lateral rotational therapy and nosocomial pneumonia. Chest 99:1263–1267, 1991.

55. Keane FX: Roto-rest. Br Med J 3:731–733, 1967.

56. Gentilello L, Thompson DA, Tonnesen AS, et al: Effect of a rotating bed on the incidence of pulmonary complications in critically ill patients. Crit Care Med 16:783–786, 1988.

57. Fink MP, Helsmoortel CM, Stein KL, et al: The efficacy of an oscillating bed in the prevention of lower respiratory tract infection in critically ill victims of blunt trauma. Chest 97:132–137, 1990.

58. Kelley RE, Vibulsresth S, Bell L, et al: Evaluation of kinetic therapy in the prevention of complications of prolonged bed rest secondary to stroke. Stroke 18:638–642, 1987.

59. Sumner WR, Curry P, Haponik EF, et al: Continuous mechanical turning of intensive care unit patients shortens length of stay in some diagnostic related groups. J Crit Care 4:45–53, 1989.

60. Kelley RE, Bell LK, Mason RL: Cost analysis of kinetic therapy in the prevention of complications of stroke. South Med J 83:433–434, 1990.

61. Webb SF, Vall-Spinosa A: Outbreak of *Serratia marcescens* associated with the flexible fiberbronchoscope. Chest 68:703–708, 1975.

62. Nelson KE, Larson PA, Schraufnagel DE, et al: Transmission of tuberculosis by flexible fiberbronchoscopes. Am Rev Respir Dis 127:97–100, 1983.

63. Wheeler PW, Lancaster D, Kaiser AB: Bronchopulmonary cross-colonization and infection related to mycobacterial contamination of suction valves of bronchoscopes. J Infect Dis 159:954–958, 1989.

64. Nosocomial infection and pseudoinfection from contaminated endoscopes and bronchoscopes—Wisconsin and Missouri. MMWR 40:675–678, 1991.

65. Mallison GF, Haley RW: Microbiologic sampling of the inanimate environment in US hospitals, 1976–1977. Am J Med 70:941–946, 1981.

66. American Hospital Association: Statement on microbiologic sampling in the hospital. Hospitals 48:125–126, 1974.

67. Maki DG, Alvarado CJ, Hassemer CA, et al: Relation of the inanimate hospital environment to endemic nosocomial infection. N Engl J Med 307:1562–1566, 1982.

68. Bauer TM, Ofner E, Just HM, et al: An epidemiological study assessing the relative importance of airborne and direct contact transmission of microorganisms in a medical intensive care unit. J Hosp Infect 15:301–309, 1990.

69. Levin MH, Olson B, Nathan C, et al: *Pseudomonas* in the sinks in an intensive care unit: Relation to patients. J Clin Pathol 37:424–427, 1984.

70. Ching WTW, Meyer RD: *Legionella* infections. Infect Dis Clin North Am 1:595–614, 1987.

70a. Edelstein PH: Legionnaires' disease. Clin Infect Dis 16:741–749, 1993.

71. Nguyen MH, Stout JE, Yu VL: Legionellosis. Infect Dis Clin North Am 5:561–584, 1991.

72. Muraca PW, Yu VL, Goetz A: Disinfection of water distribution systems for *Legionella:* A review of application procedures and methodologies. Infect Control Hosp Epidemiol 11:79–88, 1990.

73. Yu VL, Beam TR, Lumish RM, et al: Routine culturing for *Legionella* in the hospital environment may be a good idea: A three-hospital prospective study. Am J Med Sci 30:97–99, 1987.

74. Marrie TJ: The presence of nosocomial legionellosis can be monitored in an institution by targeting surveillance in immunocompromised and intensive care unit patients with pneumonia. Am J Infect Control 19:79–85, 1991.

75. Best M, Yu VL, Stout J, et al: Legionellaceae in the hospital water supply. Lancet 2:307–310, 1983.

76. Helms CM, Massanari M, Wenzel RP, et al: Legionnaires' disease associated with a hospital water system. JAMA 259:2423–2427, 1988.

77. Snyder MB, Siwicki M, Wireman J, et al: Reduction in *Legionella pneumophila* through heat flushing followed by continuous supplemental chlorination of hospital hot water. J Infect Dis 162:127–132, 1990.

78. Farr BM, Gratz JC, Tartaglino JC, et al: Evaluation of ultraviolet light for disinfection of hospital water contaminated with *Legionella*. Lancet 2:669–672, 1988.

79. Landeen KL, Yahya M, Gerba CP: Efficacy of copper and silver ions reduced levels of free chlorine in inactivation of *Legionella pneumophilia*. Appl Environ Microbiol 55:3045–3050, 1989.

79a. Colville A, Crowley J, Dearden D, Slack RCB, Lee JV: Outbreak of Legionnaires' disease at University Hospital Nottingham. Epidemiology, microbiology, and control. Epidemiol Infect 110:105–116, 1993.

80. Baker RL, Stevens J, Fish L, et al: Nosocomial legionnaires disease controlled by UV light and low level Ag/Cu ions. Abstracts of the 3rd International Conference on Nosocomial Infections, Atlanta, GA, 1990.

81. Walsh TJ, Dixon DM: Nosocomial aspergillosis: Environmental microbiology. Hospital epidemiology. Diagnosis and treatment. Eur J Epidemiol 5:131–142, 1989.

82. Rose HD: Mechanical control of hospital ventilation and *Aspergillus* infections. Am Rev Respir Dis 105:306–307, 1972.

83. Rosen PR, Sternberg SS: Decreased frequency of aspergillosis and mucormycosis. N Engl J Med 295:1319–1320, 1976.

84. Burton JR, Zachary JB, Bessin R, et al: Aspergillosis in four renal transplant patients. Diagnosis and effective treatment with amphotericin B. Ann Intern Med 77:383–388, 1972.

85. Petheram IS, Seal RME: *Aspergillus* prosthetic valve endocarditis. Thorax 31:380–390, 1976.

86. Kyriakides GK, Zimmerman HH, Hall WH, et al: Immunologic monitoring in renal transplant patients. Am J Surg 131:246–252, 1976.

87. Rhame FS, Streifel AJ, Kersey JH, et al: Extrinsic risk factors for pneumonia in the patient at high risk of infection. Am J Med 76(suppl 5A):42–52, 1984.

88. Sherertz RJ, Belani A, Kramer BS, et al: Impact of air filtration on nosocomial *Aspergillus* infections. Unique risk of bone marrow transplant recipients. Am J Med 83:709–717, 1987.

89. Lentino JR, Rosenkranz MA, Michaels JA, et al: A retrospective review of airborne disease secondary to road construction and contaminated air conditioners. Am J Epidemiol 116:430–437, 1992.

90. Arnow PM, Andersen RL, Mainous PD, et al: Pulmonary aspergillosis during hospital renovation. Am Rev Respir Dis 118:49–53, 1978.

91. Opal SM, Asp AA, Cannady PB, et al: Efficacy of infection control measures during a nosocomial outbreak of disseminated aspergillosis associated with hospital construction. J Infect Dis 153:634–637, 1986.

92. Centers for Disease Control: Guidelines for preventing the transmission of tuberculosis in health care settings with special focus on HIV-related issues. MMWR 39(RR-17), 1990.

92a. Centers for Disease Control and Prevention: Guidelines for Preventing the Transmission of Tuberculosis in Health-Care Facilities, ed 2 (in press, Federal Register).

92b. Small PM, Shafer RW, Hopewell PC, et al: Exogenous reinfection with multidrug-resistant *Mycobacterium tuberculosis* in patients with advanced HIV infection. N Engl J Med 328:1137–1144, 1993.

93. Centers for Disease Control: Screening for tuberculosis and tuberculous infection in high risk populations and the use of preventive therapy for tuberculosis infection in the United States: Recommendations of the Advisory Committee for Elimination of Tuberculosis. MMWR 39(RR-8), 1990.

94. Hutton MD, Stead WW, Cauthen GM: Nosocomial transmission of tuberculosis associated with a draining tuberculous abscess. J Infect Dis 161:286–295, 1990.

95. Riley RL, Nardell EA: Clearing the air. The theory and application of ultraviolet air disinfection. Am Rev Respir Dis 139:1286–1294, 1989.

96. Stead WW: Clearing the air: The theory and application of ultraviolet air disinfection. [Letter] Am Rev Respir Dis 140:1832, 1990.

97. Nardell E, McInnis B, Riley R, et al: Ultraviolet light air disinfection to reduce tuberculosis transmission in a shelter for the homeless: Rationale, installation and preliminary results. [Abstract] Am Rev Respir Dis 137:257, 1988.

# CHAPTER 48

# Prevention of Respiratory Tract Infections in Intensive Care by Selective Decontamination of the Digestive Tract

CHRISTIAAN P. STOUTENBEEK, HENDRIK K.F. VAN SAENE, and ALEXANDRO LIBERATI

Respiratory tract infections include laryngitis, tracheitis, bronchitis, bronchopneumonia, and pneumonia, the whole spectrum of upper and lower tract infections (Fig. 48–1). Bronchopneumonia, the most common severe infection in mechanically ventilated patients, has traditionally received the most attention from clinicians.

## COLONIZATION AND INFECTION

The clinical dilemma is to differentiate infection from mere colonization. Conventional antibiotic policies rely on this distinction to avoid unnecessary antibiotic therapy and to minimize the emergence of antimicrobial resistance. If systemic antibiotics are administered too early (ie, before infection occurs), the acquisition of resistant strains with subsequent superinfection is promoted; if antibiotic therapy is delayed until an infection is well established, it often comes too late. In a study by Fagon and colleagues,[1] the mortality rate for pneumonia proven to be caused by gram-negative organisms was 69% and for pseudomonal pneumonia as high as 87%, despite adequate antibiotic treatment.

The most difficult problem is to differentiate tracheobronchitis from colonization. Although these infections are frequently overlooked in the setting of the intensive care unit (ICU), they constitute true illness, with specific histo-pathologic changes and with their own morbidity. The recommendation that these infections do not require antimicrobial therapy[2] is not based on sound clinical data.

## DIAGNOSIS OF BRONCHOPNEUMONIA

The diagnosis of bacterial pneumonia is based on classic clinical and bacteriologic criteria, including fever, leukocytosis, purulent tracheobronchial secretions, the appearance of new and persistent infiltrates on chest radiograph, more than 25 leukocytes and less than 5 squamous epithelial cells per low-power field in the Gram stained specimen of the tracheal aspirate, and the isolation of potentially pathogenic microorganisms (PPM) from tracheal aspirate. In intensive care, these criteria are not specific: many patients have fever, leukocytosis, and radiographic abnormalities from other causes; purulent sputum may be present with bronchitis; and the presence of PPM in tracheal aspirate may represent colonization.

To obtain uncontaminated specimens of secretions from terminal bronchioli, the protected specimen brush (PSB) and bronchoalveolar lavage (BAL), which are described in detail elsewhere in this book, have been developed.[3–5] Although these techniques may be valuable research tools, they are of limited value in daily clinical practice.

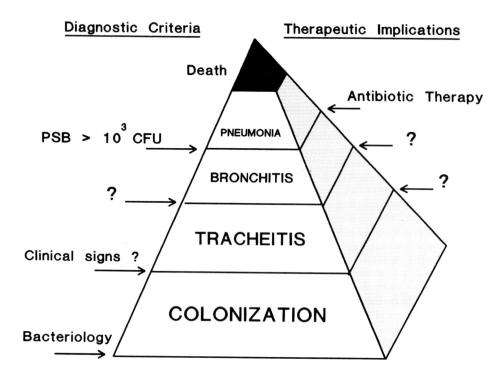

**Figure 48–1.** Pyramid representing the diagnostic criteria and therapeutic implications of the different stages of bacterial invasion of the respiratory tract. Conventional (ie, restrictive) antibiotic policies rely on the distinction between colonization and infection to avoid unnecessary antibiotic therapy. Protected specimen brush and bronchoalveolar lavage are valuable tools for diagnosing pneumonia. However, differentiation of colonization from tracheitis or bronchitis remains difficult, because the clinical signs are nonspecific. The dilemma of when to commence antibiotic therapy has not been solved.

## TERMINOLOGY OF PNEUMONIA

The terminology used for different types of pneumonia is confusing. Several commonly used classifications are based on time of onset: community-acquired or hospital-acquired; primary or ICU-acquired; early-onset or late-onset pneumonia (Fig. 48–2).

### Community-Acquired and Hospital-Acquired Pneumonias

Infections occurring within the first 48 hours after admission to the hospital are by definition community-acquired infections, i.e., those that were incubating at the time of admission. All infections occurring later are hospital-acquired or nosocomial infections (Fig. 48–2A). This distinction has no implications for prevention.

### Primary and Intensive Care Unit-Acquired Pneumonias

Infections occurring within the first 48 hours after admission to the ICU are defined as primary, because they were present or incubating on admission. Primary infections are identical to community-acquired infections if hospital admission coincides with ICU admission (see Fig. 48–2A). However, because ICU admission is often more than 48 hours after hospital admission, most primary infections in the ICU are nosocomial (Fig. 48–2B).

### Early-Onset and Late-Onset Pneumonias

Langer and coworkers[6] found that 40% to 50% of all acquired pneumonia episodes in the ICU develop within the

first 4 days of mechanical ventilation; these are early-onset pneumonias (see Fig. 48–2A). In a study of mechanically ventilated trauma patients not receiving any antibiotic prophylaxis, 55% to 75% of patients developed pneumonia within the first 4 days, depending on the Injury Severity Score.[7] Preventive measures should aim at these early-onset pneumonias.

### Pathogenesis of Pneumonia

A more useful classification of pneumonia in the ICU is based on the pathogenesis of disease.

#### Endogenous Infections

The most common route of lower respiratory tract infections is aspiration (or microaspiration) of saliva containing high concentrations of oropharyngeal PPM. This is the endogenous pathway. The presence of a cuffed endotracheal tube in mechanically ventilated patients is no safeguard against aspiration.[8]

Gastric colonization by gram-negative bacilli (GNB) has received much attention as a potential source of pneumonia pathogens.[9] High concentrations of GNB ($\geq 10^8$ organisms/mL) may be found in the stomach of mechanically ventilated patients at a gastric pH above 4, but at a low pH, no GNB are found.[10] Patients with a gastric pH of 3.5 or greater have a higher pneumonia rate than patients with a low gastric pH, but in only 30% of cases are the same GNB that were found in the stomach later recovered from the respiratory tract.[10, 11]

The role of the stomach in the pathogenesis of respiratory tract infections should not be overestimated. In most studies on the role of gastric colonization, no oropharyngeal cultures were taken. In one study in which gastric and oropharyngeal cultures were taken simultaneously, the oropharynx

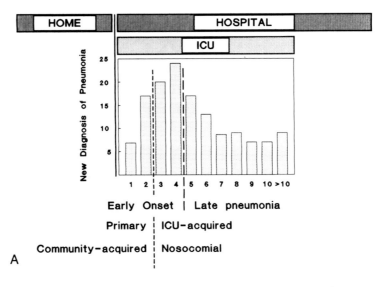

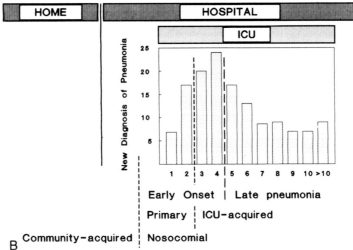

**Figure 48–2.** *A,* The common classification of pneumonia is based on the time of onset. Nosocomial infections are by definition infections arising more than 48 hours after hospital admission. Infections diagnosed within the first 2 days are community-acquired infections that were incubating or existed on admission. *B,* Community-acquired pneumonia usually is caused by *Streptococcus pneumoniae, Haemophilus influenzae,* or *Staphylococcus aureus,* and nosocomial pneumonia usually is caused by aerobic gram-negative bacteria. In mechanically ventilated patients who are not infected at the time of admission, 40% to 50% of all respiratory tract infections are diagnosed within the first 4 days (ie, early-onset pneumonia). All infections acquired in the intensive care unit (ICU) are nosocomial. Primary infections in the ICU may be community acquired, when a patient is admitted from home directly to the ICU (see *A*), or nosocomial, when the patient has been hospitalized before ICU admission. *C,* For infection prevention, the most useful classification is primary endogenous, secondary endogenous, and exogenous infections. The time of onset does not determine whether an infection is ICU acquired; the causative pathogen defines this. If a patient was carrying the pathogen on admission, it is defined as a primary endogenous infection, and if the pathogen is acquired from the hospital, the infection is exogenous or secondary endogenous. In an exogenous infection, there is no preceding stage of oropharyngeal carriage, but in a secondary endogenous infection, the acquired pathogen first multiplies in the oropharynx and gastrointestinal tract.

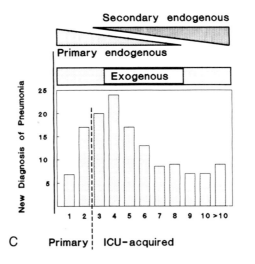

was the major source of respiratory pathogens.[12] However, the stomach may serve as an ''amplifier'' for oropharyngeal pathogens.

For infection prevention, it is useful to subdivide endogenous infections into primary endogenous infections and secondary endogenous infections.[13]

### Primary Endogenous Infections

Primary endogenous infections are caused by organisms that the patient is carrying at the time of admission to the hospital or ICU.

In a previously healthy person suffering multiple trauma

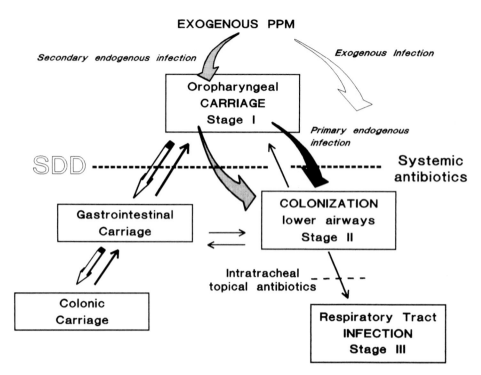

**Figure 48–3.** Oropharyngeal carriage is the first step in the development of an endogenous respiratory tract infection. The second stage is colonization of the respiratory tract, and the third stage is infection. The oropharynx is the most important reservoir of PPM causing respiratory tract infections. The patient may be carrying potentially pathogenic microorganisms (PPM) (ie, primary endogenous) or acquire exogenous PPM from the environment (ie, secondary endogenous). Acquisition of exogenous PPM occurs primarily in the oropharynx. The stomach is rarely the primary source of respiratory tract infections, but it may amplify the number of PPM carried by the patient. In exogenous infections, the multiplication of PPM must occur outside the patient to attain sufficient numbers to overcome the pulmonary defense mechanisms. Selective decontamination of the digestive tract aims to prevent colonization and infection of the respiratory tract by preventing secondary oropharyngeal and gastrointestinal carriage.

and admitted to the ICU for mechanical ventilation, most primary endogenous infections are caused by community PPM (eg, *Streptococcus pneumoniae, Staphylococcus aureus, Haemophilus influenzae, Moraxella catarrhalis, Escherichia coli*). However, in a patient with underlying diseases, such as diabetes or chronic obstructive pulmonary disease, a primary endogenous infection may be caused by GNB. A primary endogenous infection may be community acquired or hospital acquired (see Fig. 48–2C).

In the intensive care setting, primary endogenous infections develop mostly within the first 4 days. Most primary endogenous infections are early-onset infections, but not all early-onset infections are primary endogenous infections.

### Secondary Endogenous Infections

Secondary endogenous infections are mostly caused by GNB acquired after admission. The site of acquisition usually is the oropharynx or gut, where the organisms can proliferate (carriage) and then be aspirated into the respiratory tract (ie, colonization), leading to infection.

Secondary endogenous infections are always nosocomial, but nosocomial infections may be primary endogenous, secondary endogenous, or even exogenous infections (see Fig. 48–2C).

### Exogenous Infections

Another route of infection, the exogenous pathway, is the direct instillation or nebulization of PPM into the lung from an animate or inanimate source in the environment of the patient. For example, *Pseudomonas* pneumonia can be acquired in this manner through the use of a contaminated nebulizer. The numbers of microorganisms introduced must be sufficient to overcome the pulmonary defenses.

The term exogenous does not refer to the origin of the pathogens but to the site where multiplication occurs. Se-

condary endogenous infections and exogenous infections are caused by pathogens that are by definition "exogenous" to the patient; they are not found in the patient's oropharyngeal or gut flora. In a secondary endogenous infection, the causative agents multiply in the oropharynx or in the gut of the patient, but in an exogenous infection, multiplication occurs outside the patient, omitting the first stage of carriage.

Many of these infections are called cross-infections. A cross-infection is caused by PPM acquired from another patient through transmission on the hands of hospital personnel. Cross-infections may represent true exogenous infections (ie, the organisms were transmitted directly into the trachea) or secondary endogenous infections (ie, they were first transmitted to the oropharynx).

### Three Stages of Infection

In the development of an endogenous respiratory tract infection, three stages can be differentiated (Fig. 48–3). Each of these stages is the result of a breakdown of one of the three major lines of defense against infection:

Stage 1: Carriage of PPM in the oropharynx and gastrointestinal tract
Stage 2: Colonization of the lower respiratory tract
Stage 3: Infection of the respiratory tract

Carriage must be differentiated from colonization.[14] Carriage is defined as the presence of PPM among the indigenous flora on the skin and on the mucosal surfaces of the oropharynx (eg, nose), stomach, gut, and vagina. In practice, carriage defines a state in which the same strain is isolated from at least two consecutive surveillance samples (eg, saliva, gastric fluid, feces, throat swab, rectal swab), in any concentration over a period of at least 1 week.

Colonization refers to the presence of PPM on the mucosa of internal organs that are normally sterile (eg, lower airways, bladder, wounds), without clinical signs of infection. In practice, colonization can be defined as the repeated isolation of the same strain from successive samples of the relevant fluid (lower airway secretion, urine, wound fluid), in a concentration of less than 100,000 colony-forming units (CFU) per 1 mL of sampled fluid.

Bacterial or mycologic infection is a microbiologically proven clinical diagnosis. Apart from the clinical signs of infection, the diagnostic sample obtained from the internal organ generally yields at least 100,000 CFU per 1 mL of sample, or in the case of blood, the sample is positive.

In the conventional approach to infection prevention, the first two stages are considered to be harmless to the patient, and no attempts are made to interfere with the development of an infection. In many ICUs, surveillance cultures of the oropharynx and gastrointestinal tract are not even taken. Only after an infection has been fully established is antibiotic therapy started.

Alternative approaches have included the topical application of antibiotics to tracheal, oropharyngeal, and gastrointestinal mucosal sites to interfere with the development of infection in an early stage.

## INTRATRACHEAL APPLICATION OF TOPICAL ANTIBIOTICS

Feeley and colleagues studied polymyxin aerosolization,[15] and their data have been widely cited as proof that topical antibiotics are a dangerous form of prevention that leads to the emergence of antimicrobial resistance. In their study, 292 patients were treated with polymyxin aerosol during a 7-month period, and 11 patients (4%) acquired pneumonia, of whom 7 (64%) died. Because 10 of 11 pneumonias were caused by "polymyxin-resistant" microorganisms, which caused a higher mortality rate (64%) than in the period before polymyxin aerosol was used (48%), this form of prevention was abandoned.[15]

This decision does not seem justified by the data, which showed a consistently lower pneumonia rate during the periods of polymyxin nebulization (4% versus 11%). The absolute numbers of deaths from pneumonia must have actually decreased during polymyxin prophylaxis (48% of 11% = 5.3% versus 64% of 4% = 2.5%). In this study, true emergence of polymyxin-resistant strains was not observed. The observed secondary colonization with, for example, *Proteus*, *Morganella*, and *Serratia* spp., enterococci, and *Pseudomonas maltophilia* reflected the selection of strains that were naturally insensitive to polymyxin. Although the percentage of insensitive strains was high because of the elimination of the sensitive ones, these studies do not present any evidence for an increase in the absolute number of patients colonized by insensitive strains.[16]

Other studies on the intratracheal application of antibiotics used topical gentamicin and found a significant reduction in bacterial colonization of the tracheal tree and in the pneumonia rate.[17, 18] However, because of absorption of gentamicin, significant systemic gentamicin levels were found, and gentamicin resistance developed.[17] In a placebo-controlled, double-blind, multi-center study of intratracheal gentamicin application, a reduction in the pneumonia rate could not be demonstrated, although the colonization rate was significantly lower.[19] However, aerosolization with polymyxin E or other topical agents may be a valuable adjunctive therapy if exogenous bacterial colonization of the trachea develops.

## SELECTIVE DECONTAMINATION OF THE DIGESTIVE TRACT

Another approach to the prevention of respiratory tract infections is the selective decontamination of the oropharynx and gastrointestinal tract to intervene in the pathogenesis in the first stage of infection.

Selective decontamination of the digestive tract (SDD) is the abolition of oropharyngeal and gastrointestinal (GI) carriage of PPM by means of bactericidal salivary and fecal concentrations of topically applied, nonabsorbable antimicrobials that preserve the indigenous flora as much as possible.

### Rationale

The rationale for SDD is based on two observations. First, most infections are preceded by carriage of PPM in the oropharynx and GI tract. Second, most infections are caused by only 14 species, which make up less than 0.001% of the total body flora. The rest of the indigenous flora has a low pathogenic potential and is beneficial to the host.

### Potentially Pathogenic Microorganisms

An important concept is the difference in pathogenic potential among microorganisms, which can be expressed as the ratio of the number of infected patients divided by the number of symptom-free carriers (ie, the intrinsic pathogenicity index).[20] If the intrinsic pathogenicity index is close to 1, it indicates high-level pathogens (eg, *Salmonella* species). PPM are microorganisms with an index between 0.1 and 0.3. The indigenous throat, gut, and skin flora show a low intrinsic pathogenicity, with index values between 0.01 and 0.03, and are not regarded as PPM.

PPM can be subdivided into community and hospital microorganisms. Community PPM (eg, *S. pneumoniae*, *H. influenzae*, *M. catarrhalis*, *E. coli*, *S. aureus*, *Candida* species) are commonly carried by healthy persons. Hospital PPM (eg, *Klebsiella*, *Proteus*, *Morganella*, *Enterobacter*, *Citrobacter*, *Serratia*, *Acinetobacter*, *Pseudomonas*) are rarely carried by healthy persons.

### Indigenous Flora

The normal indigenous flora consists of anaerobic and aerobic microorganisms. A healthy person carries high concentrations of anaerobes such as *Veillonella* ($10^8$ CFU/mL of saliva) and *Bacteroides* spp. ($10^{12}$ CFU/g of feces). Among the aerobes, enterococci and viridans streptococci (now called $\alpha$-hemolytic streptococci) predominate at $10^6$ to $10^8$ CFU per gram of feces and per milliliter of saliva, respectively. On the skin, coagulase-negative staphylococci (eg, *S. epidermidis*) are the most common microorganisms, found at approximately $10^5$ CFU/cm$^2$. Anaerobes are represented by *Propionibacterium acnes* at $10^3$ CFU/cm$^2$. Normal vaginal flora consists mainly of anaerobes at a concentration of $10^8$ CFU/mL and aerobes at a concentration of $10^7$ CFU/mL of vaginal fluid.

## Carriage Defense

The normal flora is a stable ecosystem. Exogenous microorganisms ingested with food and beverages have little chance of survival in the body, and after a transient presence in throat, stomach, and gut, they are cleared by the defense mechanisms of the oropharynx and the GI tract. Carriage defense comprises the following seven factors, which operate in the oropharynx and gut to eliminate exogenous microorganisms from mucosal surfaces.

### Integrity of Anatomy and Physiology

The integrity of anatomy and physiology is crucial to the optimal functioning of the other clearing mechanisms.[21] The mucosal cell receptors are thought to be covered with a fibronectin layer that prevents enterobacterial and pseudomonal adherence and subsequent carriage.[22]

### Gastric pH

Gastric acidity contributes to the carriage defense of the alimentary canal by killing any incoming oropharyngeal flora. The low pH ($<2$) of the gastric juice is bactericidal for GNB but has little effect on yeasts or gram-positive cocci.[23, 24]

### Mechanical Clearance

Motility is the most important factor contributing to the mechanical removal of microorganisms.[25, 26] Chewing, deglutition, gastric emptying, and peristalsis promote the clearance of microorganisms present in the daily food intake.[27]

### Mucosal Cell Renewal

The alimentary canal is the most metabolically active cell mass in the body, repopulating its entire mucosal surface every 2 to 3 days under normal circumstances. Microorganisms adhering to the mucosal surfaces are removed by this high cell turnover.[28]

### Secretions

Secretions, including saliva, gastric and pancreatic juice, bile, and mucus, form an integral part of the carriage defense; the continuously renewed mucous layer prevents GNB from adhering to the mucosal lining.[29] Moreover, antibacterial products, including lysozyme, peroxidase, and other enzymes, are present in secretions.[30]

### Secretory Immunoglobulin A

The mechanism by which secretory immunoglobulin A contributes to the carriage defense is thought to be the coating of enterobacteria and pseudomonads to prevent bacterial adherence.[31, 32]

### Indigenous Flora

The indigenous flora covering the oropharyngeal and intestinal surfaces is thought to control exogenous GNB through competition for food and production of bacterial toxins and volatile fatty acids (ie, bacterial interference).[33, 34] This concept of bacterial interference has been called colonization resistance.[35, 36]

## Impaired Carriage Defense

The carriage defense is the first to fail during illness, and substantial GNB carriage is found in specific patient populations suffering from different underlying diseases. One third of diabetics and alcoholics[37] and more than half of patients with chronic obstructive pulmonary disease[38] or head and neck cancer[39] have been shown to carry GNB. Among neutropenic and severely ill trauma patients undergoing prolonged ventilation, the incidence of abnormal carriage is 60% to 90%.[40, 41]

During illness, the adherence of GNB to mucosal cells is greatly increased, because the loss of fibronectin from the surface of mucosal cells leads to the exposure of more receptors.[42, 43] Stasis in the GI tract due to paralytic ileus or mechanical obstruction leads to overgrowth of aerobic GNB.[44] In critically ill patients, gastric exocrine failure is common,[45] leading to a gastric pH of more than 4, even without the use of H$_2$-blockers or antacids. Gastroduodenal dysfunction with bile reflux is associated with increased bacterial colonization of the lower airways.[45a] Starvation and lack of enteral feeding may impair the mucosal cell turnover and lead to mucosal atrophy.[46] In this setting, the indigenous flora appears to become easily replaced by GNB.[47]

### Surgery, Intensive Care, and Anesthetic Procedures

The endotracheal tube, the nasogastric tube, sedative and narcotic drugs, and dopamine contribute to impairment of the carriage defense.[48] The presence of a nasogastric tube impairs the function of the gastroesophageal sphincter, leading to migration of gastric flora into the esophagus and oropharynx.[49] Salivary excretion may be reduced by atropine-like drugs.

### Antacids, H$_2$-Antagonists, Pirenzepine, and Sucralfate

Antacids and H$_2$-antagonists promote bacterial overgrowth in the stomach by increasing the pH to greater than 4. This may lead to high concentrations of throat flora, including viridans streptococci and *Neisseria* species, in the stomachs of healthy persons[50] and to gastric carriage of enterobacteria and *Pseudomonas* species in the critically ill patient.[10]

### Antimicrobial Agents

Administration of intravenous broad-spectrum β-lactam antibiotics, which are excreted into the oropharynx and the GI canal in saliva, bile, and mucus, may eradicate the indigenous flora and the sensitive community PPM. As a consequence, resistant GNB, *S. aureus*, and *Candida* spp. are selected, and overgrowth in the oropharynx and GI tract occurs. Volunteer studies have shown that antibiotics that are active against the indigenous anaerobic flora (eg, broad-spectrum penicillins) impair the carriage defense most.[51, 52] However, the contribution of antibiotics to the impairment of carriage defense is difficult to assess in patients.[53]

### Nutrition

Early enteral feeding is considered to be advantageous to prevent mucosal atrophy. However, continuous nasogastric feeding for longer than 24 hours promotes abnormal gastric carriage by maintaining an alkaline pH.[54, 55] An intermittent feeding regimen, 16 hours of feeding followed by an 8-hour fast, has been suggested to restore gastric pH during the fasting phase and prevent subsequent overgrowth in the stomach.[56]

## Abnormal Carrier State

In the critically ill patient, the impairment in carriage defense leads to high concentrations of bacilli, mostly GNB, in the saliva, stomach, and gut ($\geq 10^9$ CFU/mL or g).[57–59] These patients often carry high concentrations of *S. aureus* and *Candida* spp.

Critically ill patients are continuously contaminated by small amounts of PPM transmitted from other patients on the hands of personnel to the oropharynx. Oropharyngeal carriage readily develops because of the impaired local defenses described earlier. PPM carried in the oropharynx are subsequently found in the rest of the GI tract. Abnormal oropharyngeal carriage of gram-negative bacilli has been shown to persist for more than 2 weeks after hospital discharge.[59a]

## SELECTIVE DIGESTIVE TRACT DECONTAMINATION REGIMEN

### Topical Antibiotics

SDD aims at the abolition of oropharyngeal and GI carriage of PPM by the use of topical, nonabsorbable antimicrobials. Oropharyngeal and GI carriage, particularly of *Pseudomonas* and *Acinetobacter* spp., can only be treated with **topical** application of antibiotics, because extremely high levels of antibiotics are attained in throat, stomach, and gut, sufficient to eradicate even highly resistant PPM. With systemic antimicrobials, the salivary and fecal antimicrobial concentrations are generally lower than the minimum bactericidal concentrations (MBCs) required to kill most PPM at these sites.

The criteria for topical antibiotics to be used for selective decontamination are that they be nonabsorbable, bactericidal, synergistic, and not subject to inactivation by fecal compounds.

Nonabsorbable antimicrobials are used to maintain constantly high antimicrobial titers inside the lumen of the oropharynx and gut. The use of nonabsorbable agents avoids the systemic presence of antibiotics, which could be harmful and is unwarranted, particularly during prolonged use.

Eradication of carriage is thought to be more effective using a combination of bactericidal antimicrobials. Decontamination depends solely on the lethal activity of the topical antibiotics. Unlike carriage in the respiratory tract, gut carriage is generally not associated with high salivary or fecal leukocyte concentrations to assist or augment the bactericidal activity of the topical antibiotics.

Synergistic combinations of antimicrobials lower the effective MBCs of the components, which is possibly important in reducing the emergence of resistance. Glycoproteins in saliva, fecal compounds such as fiber, and bacterial proteins do bind antimicrobials in the alimentary canal. Although this interaction is likely to be reversible, the salivary and fecal inactivation of decontaminating agents vary substantially for different antimicrobials.[60, 61] Moreover, there seems to be a correlation between in vitro inactivation data and the in vivo results of abolition of carriage.

Another crucial factor is the **contact time** between antimicrobial drugs and PPM carried in oropharynx or gut. The contact time should allow killing. Earlier work in neutropenic patients showed a higher failure rate for oropharyngeal decontamination than gut decontamination. Apparently, the transit time in the oropharynx is substantially shorter than the transit time of stomach and gut. Aerosols and suspensions were partially effective, but the administration of a paste or tablet was associated with a high degree of eradication of oropharyngeal microorganisms. Gut decontamination is a lesser problem from the point of view of contact time because of stasis in stomach and gut, particularly in the critically ill ICU patient.

## Polymyxin-Tobramycin-Amphotericin Regimen

The original SDD regimen comprises polymyxin and tobramycin, which covers enterobacteria, *Pseudomonas* spp., *Acinetobacter*, and *S. aureus*.[41] The indigenous flora is not within their spectra. Polymyxin is active against all aerobic gram-negative PPM except *Proteus*, *Morganella*, and *Serratia* species. Tobramycin was added because of its activity against the latter three species and *S. aureus*. This combination fulfills the criteria of being nonabsorbable, bactericidal, synergistic, and minimally inactivated. In addition, this mixture was attractive because of its mode of bacterial action: both antimicrobials rapidly kill microorganisms, even in rest phase. Emergence of resistance to polymyxin has rarely been seen, and polymyxin is thought to protect tobramycin from being destroyed by inactivating enzymes. Amphotericin B was added to the regimen to control yeasts, completing the PTA regimen.

## Oral Decontamination

In unconscious, ventilated ICU patients, a sticky paste (Orabase) containing 2% each of polymyxin B or E, tobramycin, and amphotericin B is applied to the mucous membranes of the oropharynx four times daily. The composition of the paste base is of paramount importance: it sticks to the mucosa for several hours and releases the antibiotics gradually.

Before each application of the paste, the mouth is carefully cleaned and rinsed with a sterile saline solution. The teeth are brushed with normal toothpaste and a clean (disposable) toothbrush. A small amount of the Orabase paste (0.5–1 g) is applied to the buccal mucosa and the back of the tongue with a cotton swab or a gloved finger. The awake patient may be asked to distribute the paste in the mouth with the tongue. A thin film of the antibiotic paste is sufficient for decontamination. Awake patients may find the taste and the stickiness of the paste unpleasant. Careful application and frequent oral hygiene generally suffice to overcome these complaints.

A lozenge containing polymyxin B or E (2 mg) and tobramycin (1.8 mg) proved to be effective in ambulatory patients with head and neck cancer to eradicate abnormal carriage, and it was well tolerated.[62]

## Gastrointestinal Decontamination

The same combination of nonabsorbable antimicrobials is given through the nasogastric tube to abolish GI carriage. A 10-mL suspension containing 100 mg of polymyxin E, 80 mg of tobramycin, and 500 mg of amphotericin B is administered four times daily. The nasogastric tube is clamped, and gastric suctioning is discontinued for 1 hour. The aim of GI decontamination is to eradicate swallowed oral PPM and colonic PPM that have migrated into the intestines and stomach.

Oropharyngeal and gastric PPM usually can be eliminated by SDD within 48 hours. Eradication of PPM from the bowel or rectal cavity is achieved only after intestinal motility has been restored, which may take as long as 7 to 10 days in the critically ill patient. Measures to improve GI motility (eg, early enteral nutrition, avoiding the use of narcotic drugs) may accelerate decontamination.

SDD is primarily a preventive technique. In a patient with abnormal carriage of PPM in the bowel, it may take some time before these PPM are eliminated, but in a patient with normal bowel flora, pathologic carriage can almost completely be prevented.

## Duration of Therapy

SDD should be continued throughout the ICU stay until the carriage defense has recovered and the risk of infection diminishes. In practice, SDD can be discontinued after a patient is extubated and is able to eat and drink.

## Systemic Antibiotic Prophylaxis

In mechanically ventilated patients, SDD is often combined with a short course of intravenous antibiotics (1–4 days), for two reasons. First, the drugs eliminate oropharyngeal carriage of pneumococci and other hemolytic streptococci, which are insensitive to the PTA regimen. Second, they prevent primary endogenous infections.

To be effective for prophylaxis, systemic antibiotics should have an adequate spectrum, a good penetration into bronchial secretions, and a broad therapeutic range, and they should not affect the indigenous flora.

To prevent primary endogenous pneumonia in a patient having normal flora, the spectra of systemic antibiotics should include community PPM (eg, S. aureus, S. pneumoniae, H. influenzae); first- or second-generation cephalosporin would suffice. However, in a patient carrying hospital PPM, a cephalosporin with a broader spectrum should be used (ie, a third-generation cephalosporin).[13]

## Cefotaxime

In most studies, cefotaxime has been used for prophylaxis. Cefotaxime covers both community and hospital PPM, with the notable exception of Acinetobacter and Pseudomonas spp., and has an acceptable minimum inhibitory concentration for S. aureus. Cefotaxime penetrates well into bronchial secretions, has a relatively broad therapeutic range, and requires no dose adjustment for impaired renal function. Allergic reactions are rare, and cefotaxime is considered to be one of the few antibiotics that have minimal effects on the indigenous flora. However, some evidence suggests that cefotaxime does decrease the colonization resistance,[63] albeit less than broad-spectrum penicillins or ceftriaxone.

Other third-generation cephalosporins or monobactams (eg, ceftazidime, aztreonam), which could be used as alternatives to cefotaxime, have an extended gram-negative spectrum including Pseudomonas and Acinetobacter spp. but at the expense of S. aureus activity. The fluoroquinolones (eg, ciprofloxacin) fulfill all the criteria for systemic antibiotic prophylaxis but have a gap in the spectrum for hemolytic streptococci and pneumococci.

Broad-spectrum penicillins seriously affect the indigenous flora and should not be used for prophylaxis.

Mandelli and associates[64] studied the effect of narrow-spectrum antibiotic prophylaxis using penicillin G or cefoxitin in mechanically ventilated patients. Penicillin G was not effective; cefoxitin decreased the early-onset pneumonia rate but at the expense of more late-onset infections.

Although cefotaxime alone may be effective in preventing primary endogenous infections, it should be combined with SDD to prevent emergence of resistance and possible superinfections.

## Microbiologic Monitoring

The technique of SDD requires intensive microbiologic surveillance, and the regimen should be adjusted if necessary. Surveillance samples of the oropharynx (eg, throat swab) and GI tract (eg, gastric fluid, fecal sample, rectal swab) are obtained on admission and afterward at least twice weekly. Oral and throat swabs are processed semiquantitatively by the four-quadrant method combined with an enrichment broth.[20] Omission of the enrichment step may result in underestimation of the carriage rate. Semiquantitative estimation of microbial concentrations is made by grading growth density on a scale of $1+$ to $5+$.

Surveillance samples of gastric fluid and feces can be quantitatively and qualitatively cultured. One milliliter or 1g of specimen is suspended in 9 mL of brain-heart infusion broth, and serial tenfold dilutions are made.

Although implementation of SDD increases the number of cultures, the actual workload may decrease, because most surveillance and diagnostic samples are negative, and the time-consuming steps of pure culturing, identification, and sensitivity determination are reduced.

Reports on GNB may be available after 24 hours, but community flora may require 48 hours. It is of benefit to provide an overview chart of each patient showing patterns of carriage, colonization, and infection. This is more useful than a disjointed series of laboratory reports (Fig. 48–4).

Surveillance samples during SDD are necessary for three reasons: to control the effect of the topically applied antibiotics; to differentiate primary and secondary endogenous from exogenous infections; and to evaluate the carriage of resistant strains in an "early" stage.

Diagnostic samples of lower airways, bladder, wounds, and blood should be sent only if indicated clinically. Quantitative microbiology should be applied to all samples to maximize the relevance of interpretation of cultures.

## RESULTS OF CLINICAL TRIALS

Since the introduction of SDD in 1984, the reports of 29 trials have been published.[65–92] These studies varied greatly with respect to the basic elements of study design, such as patient selection, randomization, the SDD regimen, the use of other measures influencing the main endpoint, the microbiologic methods, and the definitions of infection (Table 48–1).

## Differences in Study Design

The randomized, controlled trial with concurrent control groups in a single ICU is not the ideal study design for SDD studies, because the use of SDD treatment in only half of the patients changes the ecology of the ICU profoundly. Because the oropharynxes and GI tracts of patients are the prime reservoir of PPM in the ICU, selective decontamination of some patients reduces the risk of contamination for the nontreated patients. The full benefit of SDD can only be achieved after all major reservoirs have been eliminated. A randomized, controlled trial with SDD in a single ICU may therefore mask the true treatment differences.

In SDD, the effect of the topical antibiotics should be monitored frequently by surveillance cultures of the throat and rectum. In a blinded, placebo-controlled SDD study, the investigator must be blinded to the results of the surveillance cultures, preventing him from adjusting the topical antibiotics in case decontamination is incomplete. The risk of ineffective decontamination in a blinded trial therefore may be considerable. This is particularly a problem in hospitals where methicillin-resistant *S. aureus* (MRSA) is endemic, because the PTA regimen has little effect on MRSA. To avoid these problems, many studies have relied on consecutive controls. The disadvantage of a consecutive study, the variation of infection rate with time, is largely avoided by a crossover design in two ICUs.[69, 73]

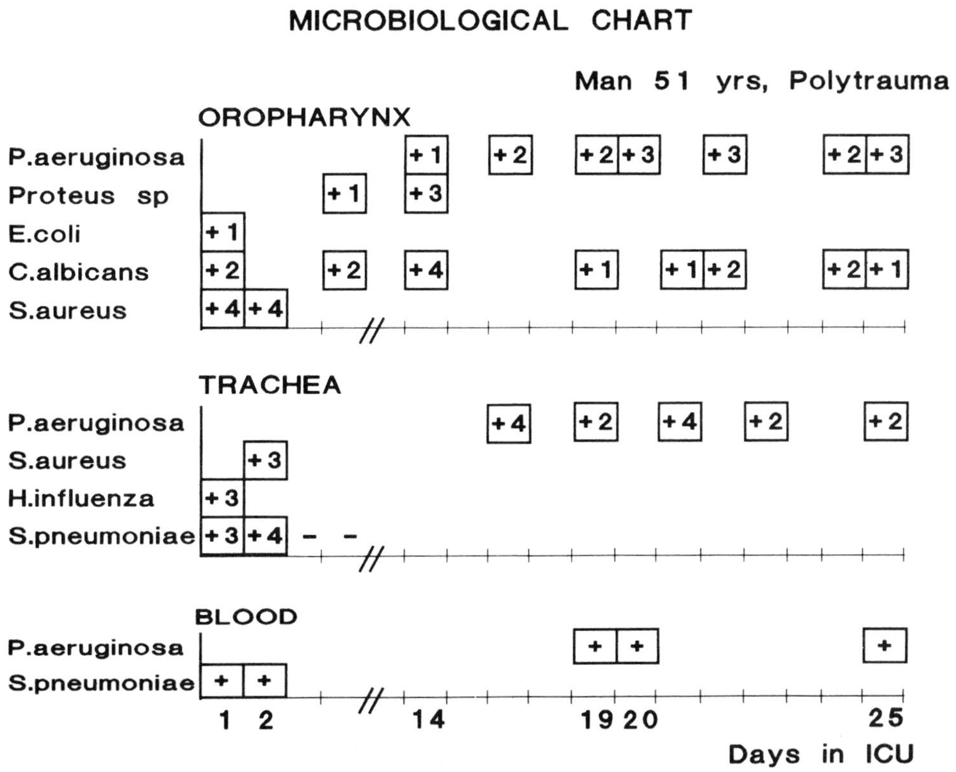

**MICROBIOLOGICAL CHART**

**Man 51 yrs, Polytrauma**

**Figure 48–4.** Microbiologic chart of a patient admitted to the intensive care unit after blunt chest trauma and splenectomy for a splenic rupture. The patient did not receive antibiotic prophylaxis. Each positive culture is represented by the name of the microorganism on the Y axis and a box with the semiquantitative concentration. The chart demonstrates the timely sequence of events (ie, carriage, colonization, infection), which enables the clinician to diagnose endogenous and exogenous infections and to take the appropriate measures.

**Table 48–1. Differences in Study Design in Clinical Trials of Selective Decontamination of the Digestive Tract**

**Study Design**
Observational cohort study
Treatment versus historic control group
Prospective consecutive treatment and control groups
Alternating treatment and control groups
Alternating treatment with crossover in two ICUs
Concurrent control groups
Double-blind, placebo-controlled study or blinded detection of end point

**Patient Selection Issues**
Primarily infected patients included
Medical or surgical patients
Homogeneous patient selection
Curable underlying disease
Intubated and mechanically ventilated patients
Prolonged mechanical ventilation
Prolonged intensive care unit stay

**Study Maneuvers**
Combination of topical antibiotics
Oral decontamination
Intestinal decontamination
Oral decontamination and intestinal decontamination
Systemic antibiotic prophylaxis
Microbiologic monitoring of decontamination effect

**Comaneuvers**
Stress ulcer prophylaxis with H$_2$-blockers or antacids
Sucralfate
Intermittent gastric feeding
Tracheotomy versus orotracheal intubation
Early mobilization
Minimal sedation
Protective isolation
Other specific infection control measures

**Outcome Events**
Carriage, colonization and infection rates
Respiratory tract infections
Pneumonia rate (definitions?)
Primary infections versus secondary infections
Mortality
Morbidity
Emergence of resistance
Control of outbreaks
Cost effectiveness
Intention-to-treat analysis

## Differences in Patient Population

Most studies included high-risk ICU patients requiring prolonged mechanical ventilation, but in one study,[66] all ICU patients were included, regardless of duration of stay or mechanical ventilation.

Only a few studies used a homogenous, noninfected patient population (eg, trauma patients).[41, 75, 81] Most other studies included heterogeneous patient populations, in mixed medical-surgical ICUs, with many different diagnostic groups, different prognoses, and different infection risks. Most centers did not stratify for age or underlying disease. A high proportion of patients enrolled in these trials had incubating or established infection on admission, such as respiratory tract infections, septicemia, or peritonitis. Only the rate of acquired infections and the effect of acquired infections on morbidity and mortality could be determined. In two studies, the effects of preoperative SDD in liver transplantation[75] and of esophageal resection[81] were investigated. These major differences in patient selection may explain the wide variation in overall infection rates (18%–81%) among the studies.

## Differences in Therapeutic Regimens

The topical antimicrobials used in several trials differ essentially from the original PTA regimen. Gentamicin and nystatin have been used because of the unavailability of oral tobramycin and amphotericin B in the United States.[75] Tobramycin was replaced by neomycin and netilmicin in other studies.[78, 86] Pugin and colleagues added vancomycin to the regimen to control MRSA.[86] Two Dutch groups administered the absorbable norfloxacin instead of tobramycin.[79, 85] Cerra and associates[88] used a high dose of norfloxacin (2000 mg/day) and nystatin. Not all investigators have applied the SDD technique in full (ie, both oral and gastrointestinal) decontamination. Rinsing of the oropharynx with povidone-iodine was used in two French studies.[69, 78] However, because no oropharyngeal cultures were taken in these studies, there is no evidence that this method is effective. In other studies, the antibiotics were instilled in the oropharynx instead of using the antibiotic paste.[76, 86] In another trial,[82] the antibiotic oral paste (Orabase) was applied to the oropharynx without concomitant gastrointestinal decontamination.

Many of the failures in these studies can be explained by the topical antibiotic regimen used, such as the failure to eradicate *Pseudomonas* species using norfloxacin or neomycin monotherapy.[78, 88]

## Differences in Systemic Antibiotic Prophylaxis

The systemic administration of a broad-spectrum antibiotic to cover primary endogenous colonization and infection has not been an integral part of the SDD regimen in all trials. However, in these trials, most patients received antibiotic therapy for primary infections existing on admission.[86, 90] In patients not receiving the systemic prophylaxis, primary endogenous infections with pneumococci, *H. influenzae*, and *S. aureus* were found.[86, 90]

## Differences in Microbiologic Methods

In some studies, no surveillance cultures of the oropharynx or the GI tract were taken to confirm the efficacy of the topical antibiotic regimen used.[69, 78, 90] No conclusions can be drawn about whether infections resulted because SDD was not applied properly, whether the SDD regimen used was not effective, or whether the infections were exogenous rather than endogenous.

## Differences in Comaneuvers

Several studies[93, 94] have shown that patients treated with H$_2$-blockers or antacids have a higher pneumonia rate than patients treated with sucralfate, which has no influence on gastric pH. This suggests that sucralfate may offset the increased pneumonia rate resulting from H$_2$-blockers or antacids. Although this may have a significant influence on the infection rates in the different studies, it is unlikely that sucralfate is an effective method for infection prevention. First, exocrine failure of the stomach is common in critically ill patients,[45] and 50% to 75% of patients not receiving any antacids or $H_2$-blockers have a gastric pH greater than 4.[93, 95] This implies that, in most patients, the gastric barrier cannot be effective, even when using sucralfate. Second, sucralfate has no appreciable effect on colonization of the oropharynx, whereas the oropharynx is the most important source of pulmonary infections. In one study, more than 30% of patients were colonized by gram-negative PPM, *S. aureus,* or yeasts in the oropharynx and trachea.[93] Third, GI decontamination with topical antibiotics without oropharyngeal decontamination did not reduce the pneumonia rate,[96] but oropharyngeal decontamination without gastric decontamination was effective.[82, 97]

There is no placebo-controlled, blinded trial proving that sucralfate is effective as stress ulcer prophylaxis in critically ill patients or that it reduces pneumonia rate. In one study, it was shown that critically ill patients with tetanus who were treated without any stress ulcer prophylaxis had a significantly lower pneumonia rate than patients treated with ranitidine, although there was no difference in the incidence of stress bleeding.[98]

Sucralfate does not seem to be an effective alternative to SDD. Flaherty compared sucralfate with SDD combined with $H_2$-blockers in postoperative cardiac surgical patients and found that, even with $H_2$-blockers, SDD was superior to sucralfate in preventing carriage of bacteria in the oral cavity and stomach and in reducing respiratory tract infections and other infections.

The potential interaction between ulcer prophylaxis medication and topical antibiotics should be kept in mind. Quinolones can be inactivated by antacids. In vitro studies showed that sucralfate inactivates tobramycin (unpublished observations). In a multicenter study of SDD, 40% of the patients received sucralfate.[90] Ineffective decontamination due to the inactivation of tobramycin may have influenced the clinical outcome of this study.

## RESULTS OF SELECTIVE DECONTAMINATION OF THE DIGESTIVE TRACT

### Effect of Selective Decontamination of the Digestive Tract on Colonization Rate

SDD reduced the colonization rate of the respiratory tract in all studies. However, oropharyngeal secretions containing topical antimicrobials may leak around the cuff of the endotracheal tube into the trachea.[76, 99] It has been suggested that the usual microbiologic criteria used to assess respiratory tract infections may be unreliable in this setting.[100] A French study showed that half of the tracheal aspirates of 15 patients contained more than 1 mg of tobramycin per liter.[99] However, detectable antimicrobial titers in the distal bronchial secretions were found in only 4 of 10 patients from whom bronchial secretions were obtained. Despite the presence of measurable tobramycin levels, *Pseudomonas* and *S. aureus* could be isolated from the tracheal aspirates of some patients.

## Effect of Selective Decontamination of the Digestive Tract on Primary Respiratory Tract Infections

Large differences exist in the definitions for the major endpoints, especially for the definition of primary infections. Most SDD studies defined primary infections as infections diagnosed within 48 hours after admission to the ICU and secondary or ICU-acquired infections as arising after 48 hours.[66, 68, 77] By this definition, primary infections include infections that are established or incubating on admission and the true early-onset infections that did not yet exist on admission to the ICU. Only the latter are preventable by systemic antibiotic prophylaxis.

An accurate assessment of the value of systemic antibiotic prophylaxis can be made only in a population of noninfected patients (eg, trauma patients), in whom all primary infections are theoretically preventable. In patients who are already hospitalized, it is impossible to differentiate existing or incubating infections from early-onset infections.

In one study of noninfected trauma patients receiving no antibiotic prophylaxis, the rate of primary endogenous respiratory tract infections was 44%.[96] These primary endogenous infections included all the primary infections (<48 hours) and part of the secondary infections (days 3 and 4; after day 4, most infections were secondary endogenous infections). The sole application of intestinal SDD did not reduce the pulmonary infection rate. The combined topical antimicrobial prophylaxis in the oropharynx and gut significantly reduced the rate of secondary infection of the respiratory tract with GNB but not the incidence of primary endogenous infections. The addition of a systemic broad-spectrum agent significantly reduced the incidence of primary endogenous respiratory tract infections (Fig. 48–5).[96] These findings were confirmed by other studies in which the systemic antibiotic prophylaxis was omitted.[86, 90] In those studies, SDD significantly reduced the ICU-acquired, gram-negative pneumonia rate but had no effect on the primary endogenous infection rate (by susceptible community PPM).

It is to be expected that a systemic antibiotic prophylaxis, without SDD, would reduce primary endogenous infections and reduce the overall infection rate, but at the expense of more secondary endogenous infections with resistant strains. This may be the explanation for the findings of Hammond and coworkers, who observed that the infection rate in the group receiving prophylaxis with cefotaxime did not have community-acquired infections but developed aerobic gram-negative nosocomial infections with *Acinetobacter* and *Pseudomonas* spp.[92]

## Effect of Selective Decontamination Digestive Tract on Secondary Respiratory Tract Infections

Large differences exist in the criteria used among studies to assess the main end point (ie, secondary or acquired respiratory tract infections). In most studies, microbiologically proven respiratory tract infections were the end point or exclusively clinical criteria were used to diagnose pneu-

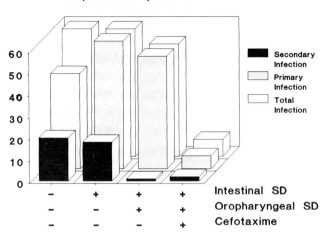

**PRIMARY and SECONDARY RTI**
**in multiple trauma patients**

**Figure 48–5.** Respiratory tract infections in multiple trauma patients requiring prolonged mechanical ventilation. Four consecutive groups were studied. The first group did not receive any antibiotic prophylaxis. The overall infection rate was 59%. Primary endogenous infections occurred in 44% and secondary endogenous infections in 18%. In the second group, which was treated with gastrointestinal decontamination, no reduction of the infection rate was found. Adding oropharyngeal decontamination successfully prevented secondary infections. Because the primary infection rate was not reduced, the overall infection rate did not change. In the last group, primary endogenous infections were effectively prevented by the addition of systemic antibiotic prophylaxis, but the secondary infections were prevented by selective decontamination of the digestive tract. (Data from Stoutenbeek CP, van Saene HKF, Miranda DR, et al: The effect of oropharyngeal decontamination using topical nonabsorbable antibiotics on the incidence of nosocomial respiratory tract infections in multiple trauma patients. J Trauma 27:357, 1987.)

monia;[66, 83, 86] in few studies, strict criteria were used to diagnose pneumonia by PSB and BAL.[69, 90]

A metanalysis of 22 randomized trials that were performed between January, 1984 and June, 1992 included 4142 patients. Analysis of the effect of SDD on respiratory tract infections was based on 3836 patients and 826 events (260 treated patients and 566 controls) and suggests a 64% reduction in the relative odds of developing a pulmonary infection (odds ratio [OR] = 0.37, 95% confidence interval [CI] of 0.31–0.43) when patients treated with SDD were compared with untreated controls.[100a] This effect was consistent in all subgroups, regardless of whether the diagnosis of pneumonia was made by protected catheter or whether the study was blinded.

The effect of SDD on infection rates should also be analyzed according to pathogenesis, using the classifications of exogenous, primary endogenous, and secondary endogenous infections. Only secondary endogenous infections, occurring during SDD, are true SDD failures; primary endogenous infections should be considered failures of the systemic antibiotic prophylaxis, and exogenous infections are failures of hygiene and asepsis. In a study by Hammond and colleagues,[92] the SDD-treated group developed gram-negative infections, although the oropharynx and GI-tract were effectively decontaminated. The most likely explanation is that these infections must have been exogenous.

### Effect of Selective Decontamination of the Digestive Tract on Mortality

In the first metanalysis of 6 published randomized and 6 historical controlled trials on SDD, it was concluded that

"despite a clear preventive effect on the occurrence of respiratory tract infections, the evidence is at best consistent with a very limited effect of SDD on survival in ICU patients."[101] The paper was, however, heavily criticized[102] because of the methodology adopted and the large numbers of trials not considered in the analysis.

Another quantitative metanalysis of data from randomized controlled trials (RCTs) was initiated under the auspices of the Paris Consensus Conference. The exercise was initiated with the following aims: (1) to assess the overall effects of SDD on mortality using all unconfounded available information; and (2) to quantify the plausible magnitude of the effects of the treatment on infection and the strength of the association between infection and mortality.

To perform an unconfounded analysis based on "intention-to-treat," only randomized trials were considered, and additional information on the number and outcomes of patients excluded after randomization in each study was sought. Twenty-two randomized controlled trials performed between January, 1984 and June, 1992 (totaling approximately 4142 patients) have been traced. Only 3 studies had results with an individually statistically significant reduction in mortality; the remaining 19, although showing most of the time a favorable trend, were inconclusive. The claimed heterogeneity of the patient populations included in these trials was clearly confirmed by the large variation in the mortality of the control groups (median = 30%, range = 18–52%).

To pool data from individual trials, a crude mortality rate was computed. Once the observed proportions of deaths were obtained, the OR (ie, the ratio of the odds of dying in the treated group to the odds of dying in the control group) was calculated for each trial. An OR of less than 1 indicated a beneficial treatment effect. The overall analysis, based on 4142 patients and 1160 deaths (553 among treated patients and 607 among controls), suggests a 10% non–statistically significant reduction in the odds of death (OR = 0.90; 95% CI of 0.79–1.04).

Results of a subgroup analysis of trials (in 2450 patients), in which topical antibiotics were combined with a short course of a systemic antibiotic, showed a significant reduction (20%) in the odds of death (OR = 0.80; CI of 0.67–0.97).[103]

Thus, the results of the metanalysis suggest that a modest reduction in mortality due to SDD may exist.

The key issue is whether the apparent discrepancy between the relatively small effect of SDD on overall mortality and the striking effect of the treatment in reducing infections comes as a disappointing negative result or whether its proper interpretation calls for a departure from the traditional "clinical perspective" and for a move toward discussion of issues related to biologic plausibility and epidemiologic or public health relevance.

A realistic appraisal of the benefit of SDD can be obtained only if proper expectations are set. Because not all deaths in patients with pneumonia are due to pneumonia, prevention of lung infection will not necessarily reduce mortality. For example, in a matched cohort study, mortality was found to be attributable to pneumonia in only one third of the crude mortality.[104] In another study of trauma patients, nosocomial pneumonia did not increase mortality.[7] The important conclusion to be drawn from the SDD trials is that ICU patients die with infection rather than of infection; the major cause of mortality is the underlying disease. This is consistent with the finding that SDD reduces mortality in subgroups of patients with primarily curable underlying disease (eg, trauma patients, postoperative cardiac surgical patients).[41, 66, 73, 79]

The most important conclusion from metanalysis is that future trials should be performed in homogeneous, well-defined populations at risk for the development of infection and that the patients should be stratified according to age and the severity of disease. This population should have a good prognosis if infectious complications are avoided (eg, trauma and burn patients, patients undergoing organ transplantation or high-risk surgery).

## Cost Effectiveness of Selective Decontamination of the Digestive Tract

The costs for the topical antibiotics vary from country to country. In some countries, polymyxin B and E and tobramycin can be purchased in bulk at relatively low prices. The suspension and the paste are prepared by the local hospital pharmacy. In Holland, the charge for the SDD antibiotics, including the Orabase paste, is $25 per patient per day.

The costs of surveillance cultures in decontaminated patients are much lower than those of diagnostic cultures in nondecontaminated patients, because in decontaminated patients, the number of PPM to be subcultured and identified usually is low.

None of the studies on SDD has evaluated the cost effectiveness of the SDD regimen. In some studies evaluating the amount of systemic antibiotics prescribed for acquired infections, a striking reduction[66, 90] in the drugs for SDD-treated patients has been found. However, the total amount of systemic antibiotics used did not differ because of the high percentage of patients (65%) being treated with systemic antibiotics for infections present on admission.[90]

A cost-effectiveness analysis should include all the costs of resources consumed by the individual patients that are linked to medical decisions.[100] The costs should be related to the number of survivors (eg, calculating the mean costs per survivor).

## Effect of Selective Decontamination of the Digestive Tract on the Emergence of Resistance

Evaluation of antimicrobial resistance in an ICU is complex. Calculating percentages of resistant strains may give a false impression of an increase in resistance. For example, if the total number of *Pseudomonas* isolates has been reduced by SDD, the few resistant strains might represent a substantial proportion of the total number of isolates, even if there is a decrease in absolute numbers. Analysis of resistance data should not include isolates with an identical sensitivity pattern taken from the same site of the same patient at different times (ie, copy strains). A clinically relevant analysis of resistance concerns patient-related phenomena such as carriage, colonization, and infection by resistant PPM.[105]

The oropharynx, stomach, and gut are the body sites where resistance in vivo develops. The usual systemic antimicrobials, such as β-lactams, aminoglycosides, and fluoroquinolones, are excreted in low concentrations into the oropharynx, stomach, and gut in saliva, bile, and mucus. Eradication of sensitive PPM is followed by selection and overgrowth of resistant GNB. In a successfully decontaminated patient, the emergence of resistance is highly unlikely because of the absence of PPMs, including the resistant mutants.

Resistance during SDD has been the end point of 16 studies,[106] only a few of which were conducted over a prolonged period.[107] Superinfections by resistant gram-negative PPM occurring as a consequence of carriage of resistant PPM have not been reported. Clinical resistance studies over prolonged periods are needed.

## Selective Decontamination of the Digestive Tract to Control Outbreaks With Multiresistant Potentially Pathogenic Microorganisms

After superinfections, outbreaks of multiresistant GNB and MRSA infections may be the second clinical consequence of resistance. The ICU is an enclosed environment in which PPM transmission by the hands of personnel readily occurs.[108, 109] The critically ill patient carries high concentrations of PPM, often multiresistant strains, and continuously excretes PPM during hospitalization. Transmission from one carrier to another patient is highly likely, even if the nurses and doctors do not neglect to wash their hands after every contact.[110]

Two reports have appeared about the control by SDD of an outbreak of multiresistant *Klebsiella* infections in ICUs.[78, 111] The underlying mechanism is thought to be a significant reduction of carriage, reducing transmission and leading to control of the outbreak. Hand-washing procedures may be more effective in units in which SDD is implemented.

## Effect of Selective Decontamination of the Digestive Tract on Gram-Positive Cocci

The isolation of enterococci, coagulase-negative staphylococci, and anaerobes (which rarely cause infections) during SDD should not be regarded as selection of resistance, because it is the consequence of the intentional choice of "selective" antimicrobials not active against low-level pathogens. None of the randomized, controlled SDD trials has shown an increase in the infection rate by these microorganisms during SDD.

In some SDD studies, selection of MRSA occurred.[90, 99] In ICUs in which MRSA is endemic, the SDD regimen should be adjusted to include an effective antibiotic against MRSA,[86] and other precautions should be taken.

## FUTURE DIRECTIONS: PREOPERATIVE SELECTIVE DECONTAMINATION OF THE DIGESTIVE TRACT

In most SDD studies in ICUs, nosocomial infections were already incubating or present in 50% to 70% of patients on admission. Although SDD is effective in preventing further infectious complications during intensive therapy, most of the damage is already done. Theoretically, some of these primary infections are preventable by earlier application of SDD in high-risk patients.

Future lines of research should focus on the application of SDD for prevention of perioperative infections in high-risk patients or patients undergoing high-risk surgery[81] (eg, transplantation, esophagus resection, head and neck surgery, colon resections). Topical antimicrobial prophylaxis may be commenced a few days before the operation to render the patient free of PPM on the day of operation. A single shot of a systemic agent at the induction of anesthesia may be sufficient to cover the indigenous flora. The major end points of these studies should be infection rate and cost effectiveness.

# REFERENCES

1. Fagon JY, Chastre J, Domart Y, et al: Nosocomial pneumonia in patients receiving continuous mechanical ventilation. Prospective analysis of 52 episodes with use of protected specimen brush and quantitative culture techniques. Am Rev Respir Dis 139:877, 1989.
2. Fagon JY, Chastre J, Hance AJ, et al: Detection of nosocomial lung infection in ventilated patients. Use of protected specimen brush and quantitative culture techniques in 147 patients. Am Rev Respir Dis 138:110, 1988.
3. Torres A, Gonzalez J, Ferrer M: Evaluation of the available invasive and non-invasive techniques for diagnosing nosocomial pneumonias in mechanically ventilated patients. Intensive Care Med 17:439, 1991.
4. Meduri GV, Beals DH, Maijub AG, et al: Protected bronchoalveolar lavage. Am Rev Respir Dis 143:855, 1991.
5. Chastre J, Viau F, Brun P, et al: Prospective evaluation of the protected specimen brush for the diagnosis of pulmonary infections in ventilated patients. Am Rev Respir Dis 130:924, 1984.
6. Langer M, Cigada M, Mandelli M, et al: Early onset pneumonia: A multicenter study in intensive care units. Intensive Care Med 13:342, 1987.
7. Rodriguez JL, Gibbons KJ, Bitzer LG, et al: Pneumonia: Incidence, risk factors, and outcome in injured patients. J Trauma 31:907, 1991.
8. Seegobin RD, van Hasselt GL: Aspiration beyond endotracheal cuffs. Can Anaesth Soc J 33:273, 1986.
9. Heyland D, Mandell LA: Gastric colonization by gram-negative bacilli and nosocomial pneumonia in the intensive care unit patient. Evidence for causation. Chest 101:187, 1992.
10. Daschner F, Reuschenbach K, Pfisterer J, et al: Der Einfluss von Stressulcus prophylaxe auf die Häufigkeit einer Beatmungspneumonie. Anaesthesist 36:9, 1987.
11. Cook DJ, Laine LA, Guyatt GH, et al: Nosocomial pneumonia and the role of gastric pH. A meta-analysis. Chest 100:7, 1991.
12. Reusser P, Zimmerli W, Scheidegger D, et al: Role of gastric colonization in nosocomial infection and endotoxaemia: A prospective study in neurosurgical patients on mechanical ventilation. J Infect Dis 160:414, 1989.
13. Stoutenbeek CP: The role of systemic antibiotic prophylaxis in infection prevention in intensive care by SDD. Infection 17:418, 1989.
14. Murray AE, Mostafa SM, van Saene HKF: Essentials in clinical microbiology. In Stoutenbeek CP, van Saene HKF (eds): Infection and the Anaesthetist. Bailliere's Clinical Anaesthesiology, vol 5. London, Bailliere Tindall, 1991:1.
15. Feeley TW, du Moulin GC, Hedley-Whyte J, et al: Aerosol polymyxin and pneumonia in seriously ill patients. N Engl J Med 293:471, 1975.
16. Klick JM, du Moulin GC, Hedley-Whyte J, et al: Prevention of gram-negative bacillary pneumonia using polymyxin aerosol as prophylaxis. II. Effect on the incidence of pneumonia in seriously ill patients. J Clin Invest 55:514, 1975.
17. Klastersky J, Huysmans E, Weert D, et al: Endotracheally administered gentamicin for the prevention of infections of the respiratory tract in patients with tracheostomy: A double-blind study. Chest 65:650, 1974.
18. Vogel F, Werner H, Exner M, et al: Prophylaxe und Therapie von

Atemwegsinfektionen bei beatmeten Patienten durch intratracheal Aminoglycosidegabe. Dtsch Med Wochenschr 106:899, 1981.
19. Lode H, Höffken G, Kemmerich B, et al: Systemic and endotracheal antibiotic prophylaxis of nosocomial pneumonia in ICU. Intensive Care Med 18:S24, 1992.
20. Leonard EM, van Saene HKF, Stoutenbeek CP, et al: An intrinsic pathogenicity index for microorganisms causing infection in a neonatal surgical unit. Microb Ecol Health Dis 3:151, 1990.
21. MacFarlane TW: Defense mechanisms of the mouth. In Lavelle CLB (ed): Applied Physiology of the Mouth. Bristol, John Wright & Sons, 1975:180.
22. Woods JDE, Straus DC, Johanson WG, et al: Role of fibronectin in the prevention of adherence of Pseudomonas aeruginosa to buccal cells. J Infect Dis 143:784, 1981.
23. Gray JDA, Shiner M: Influence of gastric pH on gastric and jejunal flora. Gut 8:574, 1967.
24. Gorbach SL, Plaut AG, Nahas L, et al: Studies of intestinal microflora. II. Microorganisms of the small intestine and their relations to oral and faecal flora. Gastroenterology 53:856, 1967.
25. Bloomfield AL: The fate of bacteria introduced into the upper air passages. Bull Johns Hopkins Hosp 30:317, 1919.
26. Dack GM, Petran E: Bacterial activity in different levels of the intestine. J Infect Dis 54:204, 1934.
27. Aitkenhead AR: Anaesthesia and the gastrointestinal system. Eur J Anaesthesiol 5:73, 1988.
28. Bradley JL: The relation of cellular elements of saliva to caries. Oral Surg Oral Med Oral Pathol 1:423, 1948.
29. Bloomfield AL: The dissemination of bacteria in the upper air passages. I. The circulation of foreign particles in the mouth. Am Rev Tuberc 5:903, 1922.
30. Cross CE, Halliwell B, Allen A: Antioxidant protection: A function of tracheobronchial and gastrointestinal mucus. Lancet 2:1328, 1984.
31. Van Saene HKF, van der Waaij D: A novel technique for detecting IgA coated potentially pathogenic microorganisms in the human intestine. J Immunol Methods 30:87, 1979.
32. Williams RC, Gibbons RJ: Inhibition of bacterial adherence by secretory immunoglobulin A: A mechanism of antigen disposal. Science 177:697, 1972.
33. Sprunt K, Redman W: Evidence suggesting importance of role of interbacterial inhibition in maintaining balance of normal flora. Ann Intern Med 68:579, 1968.
34. Wells CL, Maddaus MA, Jechorek RP, et al: Role of intestinal anaerobic bacteria in colonisation resistance. Eur J Clin Microbiol Infect Dis 7:107, 1988.
35. Van der Waaij D: Colonisation resistance of the digestive tract: Clinical consequences and implications. J Antimicrob Chemother 10:263, 1982.
36. Raibaud P, Ducluzeau R, Tancrede C: L'effect de barrière dans le tube digestif: Moyen de défense de l'hôte contre les bactéries exogenes. Med Mal Infect 7:130, 1977.
37. Mackowiak PA, Martin RM, Jones SR, et al: Pharyngeal colonisation by gram-negative bacilli in aspiration prone persons. Arch Intern Med 138:1224, 1978.
38. Valenti WM, Trudell RG, Bentley DW: Factors predisposing to oropharyngeal colonization with gram-negative bacilli in the aged. N Engl J Med 298:1108, 1978.
39. Spijkervet FKL, van Saene HKF, Panders AK, et al: Colonization index of the oral cavity: A novel technique for monitoring colonization defense. Microb Ecol Health Dis 2:145, 1989.
40. Wahlin YB, Holm AK: Changes in the oral microflora in patients with acute leukemia and related disorders during the period of induction therapy. Oral Surg Oral Med Oral Pathol 65:411, 1988.
41. Stoutenbeek CP, van Saene HKF, Miranda DR, et al: The effect of selective decontamination of the digestive tract on colonisation and infection in multiple trauma patients. Intensive Care Med 10:185, 1984.
42. Donaldson SC, Azizi SQ, Dal Nogare AR: Characteristics of aerobic gram-negative bacteria colonizing critically ill patients. Am Rev Respir Dis 144:202, 1991.
43. Dal Nogare AR, Toews GB, Pierce AK: Increased salivary elastase precedes gram-negative bacillary colonization in postoperative patients. Am Rev Respir Dis 135:671, 1987.
44. Sjöstedt S, Kager L, Heimdahl A, et al: Microbial colonization of tumors in relation to the upper gastrointestinal tract in patients with gastric carcinoma. Ann Surg 207:341, 1988.
45. Stannard VA, Hutchinson A, Morris DL, et al: Gastric exocrine

''failure'' in critically ill patients: Incidence and associated features. Br Med J 296:155, 1988.

45a. Inglis TJJ, Sherrat MJ, Sproat LJ, Gibson JS, Hawkey PM: Gastro-duodenal dysfunction and bacterial colonisation of the ventilated lung. Lancet 341:911–913, 1993.

46. Wilmore DW, Smith RJ, O'Dwyer ST, et al: The gut: A central organ after surgical stress. Surgery 104:917, 1988.

47. Van der Waaij D: Selective decontamination of the digestive tract: General principles. Eur J Cancer Clin Oncol 24:51, 1988.

48. Thülig B, van Saene HKF: Impact of anaesthetic procedures on the oropharyngeal and gastrointestinal defense against carriage. *In* Stoutenbeek CP and van Saene HKF (eds): Infection and the Anaesthetist. Bailliere's Clinical Anaesthesiology, vol 5. London, Bailliere Tindall, 1991:27.

49. Wynne JW, Modell JH: Respiratory aspiration of stomach contents. Ann Intern Med 87:466, 1977.

50. Snepar R, Poporad GA, Romano JM, et al: Effect of cimetidine and antacid on gastric microbial flora. Infect Immun 36:518, 1982.

51. Van Saene HKF, Willems FTC, Davies RJ: The abnormal carrier state and superinfection following antibiotic treatment of respiratory tract infection in general practice: A clinical, controlled trial. Eur Respir Rev 2:193, 1992.

52. Van Saene HKF, Stoutenbeek CP, Geitz JN, et al: Effect of amoxycillin on colonisation resistance in human volunteers. Microb Ecol Health Dis 1:169, 1988.

53. Van Saene HKF, Percival A: Bowel microorganisms—a target for selective antimicrobial control. J Hosp Infect 19(suppl C):19, 1991.

54. Pingleton SK, Hinthorn DR, Liu CH: Enteral nutrition in patients receiving mechanical ventilation. Multiple sources of tracheal colonization include the stomach. Am J Med 80:827, 1986.

55. Jacobs S, Chang RWS, Lee B, et al: Continuous enteral feeding: A major cause of pneumonia among ventilated intensive care unit patients. JPEN J Parenter Enter Nutr 14:353, 1990.

56. Lee B, Chang RWS, Jacobs S: Intermittent nasogastric feeding: A simple and effective method to reduce pneumonia among ventilated ICU patients. Clin Intensive Care 1:100, 1990.

57. Sprunt K: Practical use of surveillance for prevention of nosocomial infection. Semin Perinatol 9:47, 1985.

58. Sprunt K, Leidy G, Redman W: Abnormal colonization of neonates in an intensive care unit: Means of identifying neonates at risk of infection. Pediatr Res 12:998, 1978.

59. Van Saene HKF, Stoutenbeek CP, Torres A: The abnormal oropharyngeal carrier state: Symptom or disease? Respir Med 86:183, 1992.

59a. Ketai LH, Rypka G: The course of nosocomial oropharyngeal colonization in patients recovering from acute respiratory failure. Chest 103:1837–1841, 1993.

60. Van Saene JJM, van Saene HKF, Stoutenbeek CP, et al: Influence of faeces on the activity of antimicrobial agents used for decontamination of the alimentary canal. Scand J Infect Dis 17:295, 1985.

61. Edlund C, Lindqvist L, Nord CE: Norfloxacin binds to human fecal material. Antimicrob Agents Chemother 32:1869, 1988.

62. Spijkervet FKL, van Saene HKF, van Saene JJM, et al: Effect of selective elimination of the oral flora on mucositis in irradiated head and neck cancer patients. J Surg Oncol 46:167, 1991.

63. Vollaard EJ, Clasener HAL, Janssen JHM, et al: Influence of cefotaxime on microbial colonization resistance in healthy volunteers. J Antimicrob Chemother 26:117, 1990.

64. Mandelli M, Mosconi P, Langer M, et al: Prevention of pneumonia in an intensive care unit: A randomized multicenter clinical trial. Crit Care Med 17:501, 1989.

65. Korinek AM, Laisne MJ, Nicolas MH, et al: Selective decontamination of the digestive tract in neurosurgical intensive care unit patients: A double blind randomised study. Crit Care Med (in press).

66. Ledingham MCA I, Alcock SR, Eastaway AT, et al: Triple regimen of selective decontamination of the digestive tract, systemic cefotaxime, and microbiological surveillance for prevention of acquired infection in intensive care. Lancet 1:785, 1988.

67. Schardey M, Meyer G, Kern M, et al: Die nosokomiale Lungeninfektion: Präventive Massnahmen beim chirurgischen Intensivpatienten. Intensivmed Notfall Med 26:242, 1989.

68. Konrad F, Schwalbe B, Heeg K, et al: Kolonisations—Pneumoniefrequenz und Resistenzentwicklung bei langseitbeatmeten Intensivpatienten unter selektiver Dekontamination des Verdauungstraktes. Anaesthesist 38:99, 1989.

69. Godard J, Guillaume C, Reverdy ME, et al: Intestinal decontamination in a polyvalent ICU. A double-blind study. Intensive Care Med 16:307, 1990.

70. McClelland P, Murray AE, Williams PS, et al: Reducing sepsis in severe combined acute renal and respiratory failure by selective decontamination of the digestive tract. Crit Care Med 18:935, 1990.

71. Nardi G, Valentinis U, Bartaletti R, et al: Efficacia della sola decontaminazione selettiva, sensa profilassi antibiotica sistemica, nella prevensione delle infezioni polmonari in terapia intensiva. Minerva Anestesiol 56:19, 1990.

72. Sydow M, Burchardi H, Crozier TA, et al: Einfluss der selektiven Dekontamination auf nosokomiale Infektionen, Erregerspektrum und Antibiotikaresistenz bei langzeitbeatmeten Intensivpatienten. Anaesth Intensivther Notfallmed 25:416, 1990.

73. Hartenauer U, Thulig B, Diemer W, et al: Effect of selective flora suppression on colonisation, infection, and mortality in critically ill patients: A one-year, prospective consecutive study. Crit Care Med 19:463, 1991.

74. Mackie DP, van Hertum WAJ, Schumburg T, et al: Prevention of infection in burns: Preliminary experience with selective decontamination of the digestive tract in patients with extensive injuries. J Trauma 32:570, 1992.

75. Wiesner RH, Krom RAF, Hermans P: Selective bowel decontamination to decrease gram-negative aerobic bacterial and *Candida* colonization and prevent infection after orthotopic liver transplantation. Transplantation 45:570, 1988.

76. Unertl K, Ruckdeschel G, Selbmann HK, et al: Prevention of colonisation and respiratory infections in long-term ventilated patients by local antimicrobial prophylaxis. Intensive Care Med 13:106, 1987.

77. Kerver AJH, Rommes JH, Mevissen-verhage EAE, et al: Prevention of colonisation and infection in critically ill patients. A prospective randomised study. Crit Care Med 16:1087, 1988.

78. Brun-Buisson C, Legrand P, Rauss A, et al: Intestinal decontamination for control of nosocomial multiresistant gram-negative bacilli. Ann Intern Med 110:873, 1989.

79. Ulrich C, Harinck-de Weerd JE, Bakker NC, et al: Selective decontamination of the digestive tract with norfloxacin in the prevention of ICU-acquired infections: A prospective randomised study. Intensive Care Med 15:424, 1989.

80. Hunefeld G: Klinische Studie zur selektiven Darmdekolonisation bei 204 langzeitbeatmeten abdominal- und unfallchirurgischen Intensivpatienten. Anaesthesiol Reanimat 3:131, 1989.

81. Tetteroo GWM, Wagenvoort JHT, Castelein A, et al: Selective decontamination to reduce gram-negative colonisation and infections after oesophageal resection. Lancet 335:704, 1990.

82. Rodriguez-Roldan JM, Altuna-Cuesta A, Lopez A, et al: Prevention of nosocomial lung infection in ventilated patients: Use of an antimicrobial pharyngeal nonabsorbable paste. Crit Care Med 18:1239, 1990.

83. Blair P, Rowlands BJ, Lowry K, et al: Selective decontamination of the digestive tract: A stratified, randomised, prospective study in a mixed intensive care unit. Surgery 110:303, 1991.

84. Gaussorgues PL, Salord F, Sirodot M, et al: Efficacité de la décontamination digestive sur la survenue des bactériémies nosocomiales chez les patients sous ventilation mécanique et reçevant des beta-mimétiques. Rean Soins Intens Med Urg 7:169, 1991.

85. Aerdts SJA, van Dalen R, Clasener HAL, et al: Antibiotic prophylaxis of respiratory tract infection in mechanically ventilated patients. A prospective, blinded, randomised trial of the effect of a novel regimen. Chest 100:783, 1991.

86. Pugin J, Auckenthaler R, Lew DP, et al: Oropharyngeal decontamination decreases incidence of ventilator-associated pneumonia. JAMA 265:2704, 1991.

87. Zobel G, Kuttnig M, Grubbauer HM, et al: Reduction of colonisation and infection rate during pediatric intensive care by selective decontamination of the digestive tract. Crit Care Med 19:1242, 1991.

88. Cerra FB, Maddaus MA, Dunn DL, et al: Selective gut decontamination reduces nosocomial infections and length of stay but not mortality or organ failure in surgical intensive care unit patients. Arch Surg 127:163, 1992.

89. Palomar M, Barcenilla F, Alvarez F, et al: Prevencion de la neumonia nosocomial: Descontaminacion digestiva selectiva y sulcralfato. Med Intensiva 16:81, 1992.

90. Gastinne H, Wolff M, Delatour F, et al: A controlled trial in intensive care units of selective decontamination of the digestive tract with nonabsorbable antibiotics. N Engl J Med 326:594, 1992.

91. Fox MA, Peterson S, Fabri BM, et al: Selective decontamination of the digestive tract in cardiac surgical patients. Crit Care Med 19:1486, 1991.

92. Hammond JMJ, Potgieter PD, Saunders GL, et al: Double-blind study of selective decontamination of the digestive tract in intensive care. Lancet 340:5, 1992.

93. Driks MR, Craven DE, Celli BR, et al: Nosocomial pneumonia in intubated patients given sucralfate as compared with antacids or histamine type 2 blockers. The role of gastric colonization. N Engl J Med 217:1376, 1987.

94. Tryba M: Risk of acute stress bleeding and nosocomial pneumonia in ventilated intensive care patients; sucralfate versus antacids. Am J Med 83(suppl 3B):117, 1987.

95. Flaherty J, Nathan C, Kabins SA, et al: Pilot trial of selective decontamination for prevention of bacterial infection in intensive care unit. J Infect Dis 162:1393, 1990.

96. Stoutenbeek CP, van Saene HKF, Miranda DR, et al: The effect of oropharyngeal decontamination using topical nonabsorbable antibiotics on the incidence of nosocomial respiratory tract infections in multiple trauma patients. J Trauma 27:357, 1987.

97. Martinez-Pellús AE, Ruiz J, Garcia J, et al: Role of selective digestive decontamination (SDD) in the prevention of nosocomial pneumonia (NP): Is gastric decontamination necessary? Intensive Care Med 18:218, 1992.

98. Apte NM, Karnad DR, Medhekar TP, et al: Gastric colonization and pneumonia in intubated critically ill patients receiving stress ulcer prophylaxis. A randomized controlled trial. Crit Care Med 20:590, 1992.

99. Gastinne H, Wolff M, Lachartre G, et al: Antibiotic levels in bronchial tree and in serum during SDD. Intensive Care Med 17:215, 1991.

100. Consensus Conference on selective digestive decontamination in intensive care unit patients. Intensive Care Med 18:182, 1992.

101. VandenBroucke-Grauls CMJE, VandenBroucke JP: Effect of selective decontamination of the digestive tract on respiratory tract infections and mortality in the intensive care units. Lancet 338:859, 1991.

102. Brazzi L, Liberati A, Torres V, et al: Letter to the editor. Lancet 338:1389, 1991.

103. Selective Decontamination of the Digestive Tract Trialists' Collaborative Group: Meta-analysis of randomised controlled trials of selective decontamination of the digestive tract. Br Med J 307:525, 1993.

104. Leu HS, Kaiser DL, Mori M, et al: Hospital-acquired pneumonia: Attributable mortality and morbidity. Am J Epidemiol 129:1258, 1989.

105. van Saene HKF, Stoutenbeek CP, Zandstra DF: Eleven important definitions. Reanimat Urgences 1:485, 1992.

106. van Saene HKF, Stoutenbeek CP, Hart CA: Selective decontamination of the digestive tract (SDD) in intensive care patients: A critical evaluation of the clinical, bacteriological, and epidemiological benefits. J Hosp Infect 18:261, 1991.

107. Stoutenbeek CP, van Saene HKF, Zandstra DF: Effect of oral nonabsorbable antibiotics on the emergence of resistance ICU patients. J Antimicrob Chemother 19:513, 1987.

108. Larson EL: Persistent carriage of gram-negative bacteria on hands. Am J Infect Control 9:112, 1981.

109. Burnie JP, Odds FC, Lee W, et al: Outbreak of systemic *Candida albicans* in intensive care unit caused by cross-infection. Br Med J 290:746, 1985.

110. Nystrom B: Optimal design/personnel for control of intensive care unit infection. Infect Control 4:388, 1983.

111. Taylor ME, Oppenheim BA: Selective decontamination of the gastrointestinal tract as an infection control measure. J Hosp Infect 17:271, 1991.

# Prevention of Pneumococcal and Influenza Infections

MICHAEL S. SIMBERKOFF and MARIAM ESAT

## PNEUMOCOCCAL INFECTIONS AND PNEUMOCOCCAL VACCINE

Pneumococcal infections are an important cause of morbidity and mortality. *Streptococcus pneumoniae* is the pathogen most commonly isolated from adults with pneumonia.[1] Although the precise incidence of this infection is unknown, it has been estimated that 150,000 to 570,000 cases of pneumococcal pneumonia occur annually in the United States and that these are associated with a 5% case-fatality rate despite treatment with appropriate antibiotics.[2] Patients with bacteremia or meningitis have a substantially worse prognosis.

A variety of illnesses have been associated with increased incidence or severe manifestations of pneumococcal infections. These include anatomic or functional asplenia,[3-5] sickle cell anemia,[6, 7] Hodgkin disease,[8, 9] multiple myeloma,[10, 11] alcoholism,[12, 13] renal failure,[14, 15] and nephrotic syndrome.[16] Immunosuppressed patients[17] and those with nosocomial infections[18] may also experience more severe infections. An increased incidence and severity of pneumococcal infections has been documented among patients with acquired immunodeficiency syndrome (AIDS) and human immunodeficiency virus (HIV) infection.[19-22] Redd and colleagues reviewed microbiologic and clinical records at 10 hospitals in San Francisco and identified 294 city residents with pneumococcal bacteremia who were 20 to 55 years of age.[22] AIDS was documented in 15% of these patients before or soon after the pneumococcal bacteremia, and an additional 11% had less advanced HIV infection. The incidence of pneumococcal bacteremia among patients with AIDS in this San Francisco study was estimated to be 9.4 per 1000 years of patient follow-up. This is similar to the incidence of pneumococcal bacteremia

among patients with AIDS reported in New York City[19] and is far higher than the estimated annual incidence of 1 to 2 per 1000 patients in the general population.[2]

Penicillin is the treatment of choice for pneumococcal infections in nonallergic patients. Most pneumococcal strains are exquisitely sensitive to penicillin. However, reports from sites in the United States and abroad have documented a small number of isolates that are resistant or relatively resistant to this antibiotic.[23-25]

Pneumococcal vaccines have been advocated as a means to limit the morbidity and mortality of *S. pneumoniae* infection in high-risk populations. The initial work on pneumococcal vaccine was conducted in the early part of this century by Sir Almroth Wright.[26, 27] He conducted a series of six mass inoculation experiments among native South African miners who were at high risk for pneumococcal pneumonia. The vaccines for these trials were prepared by heat-killing whole pneumococcal isolates grown in broth media supplemented with blood and glucose. Despite the fact that these vaccines contained a limited sample of the *S. pneumoniae* serotypes prevalent among the miners, reduced incidences of pneumonia and mortality were observed among the inoculated miners. At the conclusion of his report, Sir Almroth made two comments that are still relevant:

1. The advantage derivable from a prophylactic inoculation will be limited by the patient's power of immunizing response . . . . 2. The advantage derivable from prophylactic inoculation will depend upon the degree to which the population . . . has already run the gauntlet of the particular microbic infection. . . .[28]

Pneumococcal capsules are composed of complex polysaccharide antigens that are important for virulence. In contrast to the influenza virus antigens, discussed later, these antigens have remained remarkably constant over the years. Antisera were used for treatment of pneumococcal infections in the preantibiotic era, and they currently are used for serotyping isolates. Among the 83 pneumococcal serotypes recognized by serologic reactions with their capsular polysaccharides are 19 serogroups consisting of two to four antigenically related serotypes. The test most often performed to serogroup or serotype pneumococcal isolates is the Neufeld quellung reaction, in which microscopic swelling of the bacterial capsule is detected in the presence of specific antiserum and methylene blue. The factor sera required to differentiate the serotypes in related serogroups are not readily available, and this has confused some of the available data.

Purified pneumococcal capsular polysaccharides (PCP) elicit an antibody response in inoculated volunteers and have been used as vaccines.[29, 30] Abundant evidence supports the safety of PCP vaccines for previously unimmunized persons and their immunogenicity in normal subjects.[31] However, a limited number of randomized trials and observational studies have evaluated the efficacy of these vaccines. Some of the studies of adult patients are summarized here.

Several trials were conducted with PCP vaccines from 1930 through 1947 (Table 49–1). Ekwurzel and coworkers studied the efficacy of a bivalent vaccine among Civilian Conservation Corps personnel.[32] Eighty per cent of the subjects studied in this trial were younger than 25 years of age, and although some World War I veterans were included, fewer than 2% were older than 50 years of age. The study was not randomized, because pneumococcal vaccine was administered to volunteers. However, a decrease in the incidence of pneumonia was observed among vaccine recipients. This difference was more dramatic among volunteers from the West Coast (6 and 80 cases of pneumonia in inoculated and control subjects, respectively) than among New Englanders (15 and 36 cases, respectively) and among subjects younger than 20 years of age than among older persons.

Kaufman conducted a trial of a trivalent PCP vaccine among older adults hospitalized at Goldwater Memorial Hospital, a chronic care facility in New York City.[33] This study was not blind, and vaccine was initially administered to volunteers. Nevertheless, the incidence of pneumonia observed during follow-up was 44 and 12.2 per 1000 among control and immunized subjects, respectively. Most of the differences between vaccinated and control subjects were observed during the first 8-month period after vaccine

administration. Thereafter, the incidence of pneumonia in the two groups was similar. Protection against vaccine-serotype pneumococcal infection was observed. There were 33 cases of vaccine-type pneumonia among 5153 control patients and only 3 among the 5750 vaccinees. However, a 50% reduction in the incidence of nonvaccine-type pneumonia also occurred among the vaccine recipients, an effect not adequately explained.

MacLeod and associates conducted a trial at an Army Air Force Technical school at which an unusually high incidence (150 cases per 1000 subjects annually) of pneumococcal pneumonia had been observed during the preceding winter seasons.[34] Recruits were randomly assigned to receive a tetravalent vaccine or saline placebo. A striking reduction in the incidence of vaccine-serotype pneumococcal pneumonia was observed among the vaccine recipients. There were four episodes of vaccine-type pneumococcal pneumonia among the vaccinees, all within the first 2 weeks after vaccination, and there were 26 cases among the control subjects. No effect on nonvaccine-serotype infections was observed; there were 56 and 59 nonvaccine-type cases among immunized and control subjects, respectively. The carrier rate of vaccine-serotype pneumococcal strains was also reduced among the vaccine recipients. This may have modified the incidence of vaccine-type pneumonia among the nonimmunized cohort of this closed population, because it was far lower than expected from previous experience.

Hexavalent PCP vaccines were initially licensed for use in the United States at the same time that penicillin became widely available. Interest in immunoprophylaxis vanished during that period, the available vaccines were withdrawn from the market, and the license to produce them was revoked.[35] However, interest in PCP vaccines was rekindled by the studies of Austrian and Gold[36] and Mufson and colleagues,[37] which demonstrated the continued morbidity and mortality of bacteremic pneumococcal infection in the antibiotic era. A second series of efficacy trials was initiated.

Austrian studied the efficacy of a 6- and 13-valent PCP vaccine in three trials conducted among South African gold miners (Table 49–2).[38] Preliminary studies showed that the attack rate was 90 cases of pneumococcal pneumonia per 1000 person-years among men coming to work for the first time in these mines. Trials were designed in which subjects were randomly assigned to receive the PCP vaccine or a saline or meningococcal vaccine placebo. The incidences of vaccine-type pneumococcal pneumonia occurring 2 weeks or more after inoculation among vaccine and placebo recipients were 11.4 and 53.3 per thousand patient-years, and

Table 49–1. **Trials of Pneumococcal Vaccine in Adults, 1930 to 1947**

| Investigation | Vaccine | Study Population | Results | Comments |
|---|---|---|---|---|
| Wright et al[27] | Whole, heat-killed pneumococci | South African gold miners | Limited efficacy | No serotyping |
| Ekwurzel et al[32] | 2-Valent PCP* | Conservation corps | Efficacy | Most effective in youngest patients |
| Kaufman[33] | 3-Valent PCP | Elderly adults, chronic care patients | Efficacy | Greatest difference in first 8 months; unexplained effect on nonvaccine serotypes |
| MacLeod et al[34] | 4-Valent PCP | Military recruits | Efficacy | Reduced carrier rate and pneumonia incidence among controls and vaccinees |

*PCP, pneumococcal capsular polysaccharides.

Table 49–2. **Trials of Pneumococcal High-Valent Vaccine in Adults**

| Investigation | Vaccine | Study Population | Results | Comments |
|---|---|---|---|---|
| Austrian[38] | 6- and 13-Valent PCP* | South African gold miners | Effective against pneumonia and bacteremia | |
| Smit et al[39] | 6- and 12-Valent PCP | South African gold miners | Effective against pneumonia | Small increase in nonvaccine serotype pneumonia |
| Riley et al[40] | 14-Valent PCP | New Guinea highlanders | Effectively diminished mortality, bacteremia, and lung aspirates | No efficacy against sputum isolates |
| Austrian[42] | 12-Valent PCP | Dorothea Dix Hospital, NC | Serologic data suggested efficacy | |
| Austrian[42] | 12-Valent PCP | Kaiser-Permanente Med Center, CA | Serologic data suggested efficacy | |
| Simberkoff et al[44] | 14-Valent PCP | Veterans Administration, high-risk patients | No efficacy | Results based on sputum isolates; "failures" had poor serologic responses |

*PCP, pneumococcal capsular polysaccharides.

the incidences of vaccine-type bacteremia were 2.5 and 14.1 per thousand patient-years, respectively. Protection rates of 78.5% and 82.5% against pneumonia and bacteremia, respectively, were demonstrated.

Similar results were reported by Smit and associates, who conducted another study of South African gold miners using 6- and 12-valent vaccines.[39] These studies and those by Ekwurzel and colleagues[32] and MacLeod and coworkers,[34] cited earlier, provide unequivocal evidence of PCP vaccine efficacy in preventing pneumonia and its invasive complications in young, immunocompetent persons who are exposed to pneumococcal infections under unusual environmental or occupational circumstances.

Riley and coworkers conducted a randomized trial of a 14-valent PCP vaccine and placebo in Papua New Guinea.[40] The subjects were native subsistence farmers who experienced a high incidence of lower respiratory infections associated with significant mortality. Riley did not observe a significant difference in the incidence of pneumonia or of the vaccine-type pneumococcal isolates from sputum cultures from the two groups. However, there was a lower rate of vaccine-type pneumococcal isolation from cultures of blood and lung aspirates of the vaccinees. Mortality, particularly from pneumonia, was reduced among the vaccine recipients.

Three contemporary randomized, controlled field trials of polyvalent PCP vaccines have been conducted in the United States. The first was among inpatients at the Dorothea Dix Hospital in Raleigh, North Carolina, a hospital for the mentally ill. The second trial was among ambulatory patients who were 45 years of age or older at the Kaiser Permanente Health Plan in San Francisco, California. Details of these studies are scanty and not generally available.[41, 42] They showed no significant differences in the incidence of radiographically confirmed pneumonia between vaccine recipients and placebo recipients. In both studies, seroconversion (ie, a twofold or greater rise in antibody titer to a vaccine-type pneumococcus) occurred more commonly among controls than among vaccine recipients. This was interpreted as evidence of more frequent vaccine-type *S. pneumoniae* infection among the placebo recipients. However, prior immunization is known to affect serum antibody responses to PCP antigens.[43] Therefore, differences in serologic response between vaccine recipients and controls after infection has occurred may not be significant.

A randomized trial of the 14-valent PCP vaccine was conducted by the Veterans Administration (VA) Cooperative Studies Program.[44] The trial was designed to test the hypothesis that the PCP vaccine would reduce the incidence of vaccine-type infections (eg, bacteremia, pneumonia, bronchitis) in patients with one or more high-risk conditions: age greater than 55 years; chronic cardiac, pulmonary, renal, or hepatic disease; alcoholism; or diabetes mellitus. It was hypothesized that the vaccine would have no effect on the incidence of nonvaccine-type infections in these patients. To test these hypotheses, a double-blind clinical trial was planned to compare the incidence of pneumococcal infections in ambulatory patients randomly assigned to receive the 14-valent vaccine or saline placebo.

A total of 2295 high-risk patients entered this study; 1150 received placebo and 1145 vaccine. Two proven infections occurred among the vaccine recipients and one in a placebo recipient. One organism isolated from blood cultures was discarded by the clinical laboratory before it could be serotyped. The two other blood or other sterile body fluid isolates were vaccine serotypes. Nineteen episodes of probable pneumococcal pneumonia occurred in vaccine recipients, and 15 occurred in placebo recipients. Seven and 6 of these, respectively, were associated with vaccine-type isolates. There were 22 episodes of probable pneumococcal bronchitis in vaccinees and 12 in placebo recipients; 6 and 4 of these, respectively, were associated with vaccine-type isolates. Infections occurred most frequently among patients with chronic pulmonary, cardiac, or renal diseases, and rates increased with the number of chronic diseases.

There was no difference in the rates of pneumococcal pneumonia and bronchitis between vaccine and placebo recipients and no evidence of vaccine efficacy in this study. Most vaccine failures occurred among patients with inadequate serum antibody responses to PCP antigens of their infecting organisms. Chronic diseases rather than age enhanced the risk of pneumococcal infections. The study did not provide data to support or refute the hypothesis that pneumococcal vaccine is effective in preventing bacteremia, and it has been criticized on that basis.[45] However, it was recognized that a much larger sample size would be required to test prospectively the vaccine's efficacy against bacteremic infections, and such a study was not planned.

The continuing controversy concerning the efficacy of PCP vaccine and recommendations for its use has resulted in a search for alternative methods to assess vaccine efficacy. Clemens and Shapiro presented a thoughtful analysis of some of the alternatives to randomized trial.[46] These may be logistically more feasible than randomized prospective trials. However, they must be rigorously conducted and frequently repeated to ensure their scientific validity.

The Centers for Disease Control (CDC) has been serotyping blood and sterile body fluid *S. pneumoniae* isolates from patients who received the PCP vaccine and from patients in hospitals participating in a national pneumococcal surveillance study. In 1980, these data were published with a formula for calculating PCP vaccine efficacy.[47] The formula is based on the assumption that vaccinated patients are not protected against nor predisposed toward the development of nonvaccine serotype infections. Additional data[48] published later is summarized here.

In patients with bacteremic disease, the efficacy was estimated to be 64% (95% confidence limits, 47%–76%). The estimates of efficacy (95% confidence limits) for individual groups of patients were as follows: renal failure 19% (−407, 86%); alcoholism 31% (−225, 83%); heart disease 76% (−136, 98%); pulmonary disease 47% (−112, 86%); diabetes mellitus 90% (−49, 100%); Hodgkin disease ≤0% (−29, 330, 83%); multiple myeloma 6% (−600, 84%). Efficacy was not statistically demonstrated for these groups of patients. However, after patients with chronic cardiovascular disease, pulmonary disease, and diabetes were analyzed together, the efficacy was estimated to be 55% (95% confidence limits, 2%–82%).

The major problem with the serotype distribution method of vaccine efficacy estimation is that it is based on the unverified assumption that vaccination does not affect the occurrence of nonvaccine-type infections. Although some data support this assumption,[34] others do not.[32, 42] Selection biases may be introduced in ascertaining vaccination histories from patients or records retrospectively and in submitting specimens to the CDC for serotyping. An interesting case, such as an apparent ''vaccine failure,'' may be more carefully scrutinized or referred for serotyping than a more routine isolate. These biases may influence the quality of the data available for efficacy calculations.

The case-control method has also been used to assess PCP vaccine efficacy. For these studies, patients with systemic pneumococcal infections were matched with controls. A history of prior PCP vaccination was determined for each patient-control pair, and the odds ratio of vaccination for groups of patients and controls was calculated. Because pneumococcal disease is rare, it was assumed that the odds ratio approximated the relative risk of disease in the vaccinated and nonvaccinated populations. This allowed calculation of protective efficacy (ie, 1 − relative risk).

PCP vaccine efficacy was not demonstrated in a small study of 89 bacteremic pneumococcal infections followed at the Denver VA Medical Center.[49] The vaccination status of cases and controls was taken from the VA hospital records only. Control subjects were matched with cases on the basis of age, date of admission, and comorbid conditions. Twenty-nine per cent of the patients and 24% of control subjects had been vaccinated within the VA hospital. Vaccine-serotype pneumococcal bacteremia occurred as commonly among the vaccinees (18 [69%] of 26) as among the nonvaccinated subjects (43 [68%] of 63). Efficacy was not demonstrated for any of the risk groups analyzed.

PCP vaccine efficacy was demonstrated in a much larger study involving 11 hospitals in Connecticut, which was conducted from September 1984 to June 1990 and in which hospital, clinic, and private physician records were reviewed to determine vaccine exposure.[50] A total of 1054 case-control pairs were established. Thirteen per cent of the cases had received PCP vaccine, as had 20% of the control subjects. The calculated efficacy against strains represented in the 14- or 23-valent pneumococcal vaccines was 61% (95% confidence intervals, 47%–72%) among immunocompetent case-control pairs and 21% (95% confidence intervals, −55%–60%) among immunoincompetent case-control pairs.

It was hoped that analysis of serum antibody concentrations in ''vaccine failures'' might result in determination of the minimal protective titer. Such data could be compared with the antibody responses of groups of patients with various diseases to determine which groups might benefit from PCP vaccination. On the basis of limited data (ie, 11 isolates; 6 vaccine serotypes), Landesman and Schiffman concluded that antibody concentrations equal to or greater than 300 ng Ab N/mL might be presumed to be protective.[51] However, many more isolates and sera must be studied before any conclusions can be drawn.

Patients with HIV infection have been considered an important target for pneumococcal vaccine use. Patients with HIV infection and those with AIDS have an increased incidence of pneumococcal infections.[19–22] The data suggest that patients with AIDS make an impaired response to pneumococcal vaccine[19, 52] and that the response of patients with earlier HIV infection is variable.[53, 54] Treatment with zidovudine appears to improve the response to pneumococcal vaccine.[55]

Additional studies of the PCP vaccine are required. Patients who clearly benefit from the pneumococcal vaccine include persons with intact immunologic systems who are at increased risk of infection because of unusual occupational or environmental factors and those with anatomic or functional asplenia.[56, 57] However, the efficacy of pneumococcal vaccine has not been established for other groups, including those whose immunologic status or antibody responses are suboptimal. Patients with debilitating or multiple chronic illnesses and those with diseases that affect the immunologic system should be included in this group. Healthy elderly persons respond well to PCP vaccine antigens.[58] However, their risk for pneumococcal infection does not appear to be excessive.[44] Debilitated elderly patients may be at increased risk of pneumococcal infection and relatively impaired in their capacity to respond to the PCP vaccine.[59, 60]

Use of the PCP vaccine has been advocated for prophylaxis against respiratory and invasive infection. It is essential that efficacy studies be conducted in cases of uncomplicated pneumonia, and pending completion of these studies, recommendations about use of the PCP vaccine should remain cautious. The vaccine is not harmful, but it is not clear that it benefits most of the patients for whom its use has been advocated. Alternatives for the current pneumococcal vaccines or new strategies for their use must be considered to provide effective immunoprophylaxis for the entire population.

The Advisory Committee on Immunization Practices (ACIP) recommends PCP vaccine for the groups of patients listed in Table 49–3.[61] It may be reasonable to administer PCP vaccine to these patients early in the course of their chronic illnesses to improve their chances of satisfactory antibody responses, although this approach has not been proven to be effective.

Fedson observed that most patients who are hospitalized for pneumonia have histories of prior hospitalizations during which chronic illnesses were recognized.[62] He and others have recommended that patients with the high-risk conditions listed earlier should receive PCP vaccine during the hospitalization at which these conditions are first recognized,[62–64] and this recommendation is supported by the ACIP.[61]

The duration of a "protective" antibody response after administration of PCP vaccine is unknown. However, the ACIP has recommended that revaccination should be strongly considered after 6 years in those with the greatest risk of rapid antibody concentration decline, including patients with chronic renal failure, transplant recipients, and those at substantially increased risk of fatal pneumococcal infections, such as asplenic patients.[61]

## INFLUENZA, PREVENTION, AND THERAPY

### Influenza Vaccine

Influenza is an acute respiratory infection characterized by fever, myalgia, and cough that affects children and adults and occurs in epidemics or pandemics. In temperate zones, influenza epidemics tend to occur during fall and winter months. In the tropics, they may occur during hot weather. Influenza is caused by viruses of the family *Orthomyxoviridae* named *influenza* A and *influenza* B.[65] A third member of this family, *influenza* C, probably represents another genus but has not been classified.[65, 66] Although other viruses may cause symptoms that are similar to those of influenza, none occurs in epidemics that involve as much of the population and none is associated with the excess mortality that regularly accompanies influenza outbreaks.

**Table 49–3. Recommendations for Pneumococcal Vaccine Use**

Immunocompetent adults at increased risk of pneumococcal disease or its complications because of chronic disease
  Chronic cardiovascular diseases
  Chronic pulmonary diseases
  Diabetes mellitus
  Chronic alcoholism
  Cirrhosis
  Adults with cerebrospinal leaks
  Adults older than 65 years of age
Immunocompromised adults at increased risk of pneumococcal disease or its complications
  Splenic dysfunction or anatomic asplenia
  Hodkin disease, lymphoma, multiple myeloma
  Chronic renal failure, nephrotic syndrome
  Transplant recipients
Asymptomatic or symptomatic human immunodeficiency virus infection
Persons living in special environments or social settings with an identified increased risk of pneumococcal disease or its complications

Data from Centers for Disease Control: Update on adult immunization: Recommendations of the Immunization Practices Advisory Committee (ACIP). MMWR 40:1–94, 1991.

Isolates of *influenza* A and *influenza* B were originally obtained from patients during epidemics in 1933[67] and 1940,[68] respectively. The viruses are enveloped, spherical or filamentous particles that are 80 to 120 nm in diameter, and their genetic material is carried in segmented RNA. Two glycoproteins on the surface of the influenza virus induce antibodies that may be protective. These are the hemagglutinin antigen (HA) and the neuraminidase antigen (NA). Thirteen distinct hemagglutinins (H1–H13) and nine neuraminidases (N1–N9) have been identified in human, swine, equine, and avian influenza viruses.[65] However, only the H1N1, H2N2, and H3N2 combinations have been associated with human disease. Repeated infections in individual patients result from mutations or substitutions in the RNA segments coding for these viral surface antigens, leading to "antigenic drift" of the HA or NA, or from reassortment of RNA segments, which may occur when a host is simultaneously infected with two or more viruses, leading to "antigenic shift" or new viruses. The existence of neutralizing antibodies to prior epidemic strains in the population creates a selective pressure for continual antigenic change in the HA and NA of the virus.

Epidemics of influenza occur annually and may involve 5% to 40% of the population of a community.[65] Epidemics often begin in children and spread rapidly among school and family contacts throughout the community. Naturally acquired immunity to the infecting influenza strain limits the rapidity and extent of spread. For example, Miller and associates showed that prior exposure to the H3N2 Hong Kong influenza strain protected Air Force personnel against exposure to a similar strain 1 year later.[69] The naturally acquired immunity may persist for many years. Mulder and Masurel showed that elderly persons who had been exposed to the H2 influenza hemagglutinin during a pandemic in the winter of 1889 to 1890 had at least partial immunity, as judged by mouse protective antibody titer, when that hemagglutinin reappeared in the Asian influenza pandemic of 1957.[70]

Vaccines were first used to limit the morbidity and mortality of influenza infection soon after the first isolates of this virus were made.[71] However, attempts to eliminate this disease by vaccination have been hampered by difficulties in producing adequate quantities of a suitable vaccine in a timely manner, real and perceived reactions to the virus vaccine preparations, the transient immune response that is elicited by purified viral antigen vaccines, and the rapidity with which the virus changes its antigenic characteristics.

Preparation, distribution, and appropriate use of an adequate supply of vaccine requires coordinated scientific and technologic effort. It is made more difficult by the antigenic changes in the influenza virus HA and NA, which occur rapidly and which require annual reformulation of the vaccine preparations. Selection of appropriate vaccine strains requires a worldwide surveillance system to monitor and characterize the antigens of influenza virus isolates in the early stages of their spread. After the virus is characterized, appropriate vaccine must be produced in quantity, vaccine preparations must be standardized and distributed, and targeted populations must be inoculated in a timely manner to limit the morbidity and mortality of the ensuing epidemic. In recent years, trivalent vaccine preparations have been recommended for use.[61, 65, 66] These contain antigens (two type A and one type B) from influenza virus strains that are predicted to circulate in the population during the following fall and winter seasons.

Whole influenza virus vaccines are prepared in the allantoic sacs of chick embryos. Industrial production of large quantities of influenza virus vaccine is accomplished by recombining patient isolate strains bearing the appropriate hemagglutinin and neuraminidase antigens with strains of virus that have been adapted for rapid growth in chick embryos. The virus is harvested and rendered noninfective by treatment with formalin. It is then purified from contaminating egg proteins and endotoxins by gradient centrifugation and chromatography. Further purification of viral antigens by treatment with organic solvents or detergents results in split or subunit vaccines.

Influenza vaccine preparations are standardized by their hemagglutinin content. A radial diffusion assay has replaced the chick cell agglutination assay used to standardize the vaccine HA potency; the former is more reproducible, less time consuming, and better correlated to clinical immune response in patients than the latter method.[72]

Reactions to influenza vaccines are common. These may be local or systemic. Local reactions occur at the vaccination site 12 to 24 hours after inoculation and consist of erythema, edema, pain, tenderness, and itching. Local symptoms occur more commonly in adults than in children.[73]

Systemic reactions to influenza vaccines include myalgia, arthralgia, fever, headache, and malaise. Although transient, these symptoms are similar to those that are commonly described in influenza infection, and patients may confuse these reactions with the disease. Systemic reactions, particularly fever, are more common in children than in adults.[73] Neurologic complications may also follow administration of influenza vaccine. Of these, Guillian-Barré syndrome is noteworthy. In 1976, 43 million Americans were given a monovalent swine influenza virus vaccine. After reports of a Guillian-Barré syndrome temporally associated with vaccine administration were received, the program was suspended. Subsequent investigation of approximately 1300 cases confirmed this association.[74]

The efficacy of influenza vaccines has been assessed in terms of the antibody titer they elicit and their ability to reduce morbidity and mortality (Table 49–4). Antibody responses to influenza vaccines are influenced by the type of vaccine preparation used, the vaccine potency, the route of vaccine administration, the age and prior influenza or vaccine history of the host, and underlying diseases in the vaccine recipient.

**Table 49–4. Factors That Affect the Efficacy of Influenza Vaccine**

Host factors
  Age and influenza or influenza-vaccine experience of host
  Immunologic status and chronic disease
Vaccine factors
  Type of vaccine
    Killed vaccines (eg, whole, split, subunit)
    Live vaccines (eg, attenuated, temperature sensitive, cold adapted)
  Potency and dose of vaccine
  Route of vaccine administration
Viral factors
  Unexpected appearance of mutant or recombinant strain
  Antigenic drift

Whole, inactivated influenza vaccines are more immunogenic than split virus vaccines of similar potency.[75, 76] However, the whole virus vaccines are far more likely to elicit adverse reactions, particularly in children, and the split virus or subunit vaccine is recommended for primary immunization of children. Other types of vaccines have been proposed and used in some experiments or models. These include live, attenuated influenza viruses,[77] temperature-sensitive mutants that cannot proliferate at the temperatures normally found in the lower respiratory tract,[78] and cold-adapted influenza viruses that proliferate best at 25°C.[79] The live viruses usually elicit an immune response that lasts for much longer than that observed after killed or split vaccine administration. However, use of live virus vaccines in clinical situations has been hampered by concerns about the possibility that these strains could revert to virulence.

The vaccine dose affects the antibody response. McLean and colleagues first showed a linear relation between the log dose of vaccine inoculated and the log titer of antibody resulting in the sera of inoculated swine.[80] Subsequent studies in humans have confirmed a similar relation.[72, 81]

The route of vaccine administration may affect the antibody responses. Brown and coworkers studied the antibody responses of healthy adults to intradermal and intramuscular doses of influenza A/New Jersey/76 (Hsw1N1) virus vaccine and found that the latter elicited a stronger antibody response than the former.[82] However, the dose of vaccine inoculated intradermally was only one fifth of that administered intramuscularly. Gwaltney and colleagues compared subcutaneous inoculation with nasal instillation of a killed monovalent Hong Kong (A$_2$/Aichi/2/68) influenza virus vaccine.[83] A comparable dose of vaccine (ie, 400 chick cell agglutination units) was administered by both routes. The subcutaneous inoculation resulted in a greater than 80% seroconversion in all adults studied, but only 16% and 20% of the youngest and oldest adults, respectively, who received nasal vaccine seroconverted.

The age and immunologic experience of the host affects antibody response to influenza vaccine. Children and young adults usually produce a poorer antibody response to vaccine than older adults.[84, 85] Elderly persons, especially those without chronic diseases, have excellent responses to the vaccine.[86]

The ACIP advises annual vaccination of persons who are considered to be at high risk for complications of influenza infection and others who are in close contact with them (Table 49–5).[61, 87] The latter category includes all health care workers. Most of these high-risk patients have excellent antibody responses to influenza vaccines. However, transplant recipients[88, 89] and some patients with malignant diseases on chemotherapy[90, 91] have poor antibody responses to the vaccine.

Patients with HIV infection have profound immunologic dysfunction. Data on their responses to influenza vaccine have suggested that response may worsen as the HIV infection progresses. Huang and colleagues showed a satisfactory antibody response to influenza vaccine in a relatively small group of HIV-seropositive men who were asymptomatic or had generalized lymphadenopathy.[92] Nelson and coworkers found a poor antibody response to a single dose of vaccine in patients at all stages of HIV infection,[93] and Miotti and colleagues reported an impaired antibody re-

Table 49–5. **Recommendations for Influenza Vaccine Use**

Groups at Increased Risk for Influenza-Related Complications
Persons older than 65 years of age
Residents of nursing homes or chronic care facilities
Adults and children with chronic cardiovascular or pulmonary diseases, including asthma
Adults and children with chronic metabolic diseases (eg, diabetes mellitus), renal dysfunction, hemoglobinopathies, or immunosuppression
Children and teenagers who receive long-term aspirin therapy
Groups Capable of Transmitting Influenza to High-Risk Patients
Physicians, nurses, and other health care personnel who have occupational contact with high-risk patients
Employees of nursing homes and chronic care facilities who have occupational contact with high-risk patients
Home care providers who have occupational contact with high-risk patients
Household members of high-risk patients

Data from Centers for Disease Control: Update on adult immunization: Recommendations of the Immunization Practices Advisory Committee (ACIP). MMWR 40:1–94, 1991.

sponse to one or two doses of influenza vaccine in patients with AIDS or AIDS-related complex but a near-normal response in asymptomatic HIV-seropositive patients.[94]

Studies to evaluate the efficacy of influenza vaccine have been hampered by the lack of precision in determining the cause of respiratory infections occurring in vaccine recipients and by the antigenic drift of the influenza virus itself. Nonetheless, several studies have provided convincing evidence of influenza vaccine efficacy. For example, Patriarca and associates studied nursing homes during an epidemic of *Influenza* A (H3N2) infection during the winter of 1982 to 1983.[95] Twenty-seven per cent of the nursing home residents were affected. Unvaccinated nursing home residents were more likely than vaccinees to become ill, to develop roentgenologic evidence of pneumonia, and to require hospitalization. This study was nonrandomized, and the data were reviewed retrospectively.

Hoskins and coworkers studied the attack rate of an epidemic influenza A strain at a boarding school among boys 11 to 19 years of age who had been randomly assigned to receive an influenza A or influenza B (placebo) vaccine.[96] The former provided substantial protection in this young population, and no infections were observed among vaccine recipients with antibody titers greater than 10 against the epidemic strain. Similarly, Stiver and colleagues studied the efficacy of "Hong Kong" vaccine in preventing "England" variant influenza A infection in U.S. Air Force recruits.[97] Laboratory-confirmed influenza attack rates were reduced from 46 per thousand placebo recipients to 18.4 per thousand vaccinees.

Keitel and coworkers conducted a randomized, prospective trial of influenza vaccine and placebo in employees of Texas Medical Center and surrounding industries in Houston, Texas, from 1983 to 1985.[98] A placebo group, a group who received one vaccination, and a group who received two or more vaccinations within 3 years were compared. Specimens from patients with influenza-like illness were cultured for influenza virus, and acute and convalescent sera were collected. Sera also were collected from all volunteers before and after vaccination and in the spring after the influenza season. Persons with influenza virus isolates and those who demonstrated fourfold rise in antibody titer

during acute illness or in the comparison between the post-vaccination and spring titers were considered to have been infected. By these criteria, vaccine recipients, compared with placebo recipients, were protected against influenza except against the influenza A (H1N1) in the first vaccine group and against influenza B in the multivaccine group.

## Amantadine and Rimantadine

Antiviral drugs may be used to treat or prevent influenza virus infections. Amantadine (1-adamantanamine hydrochloride), a symmetric tricyclic amine, and its structural analog, rimantadine ($\alpha$-methyl-1-adamantanemethylamine hydrochloride) are approximately as effective as influenza vaccine in preventing influenza A. Unfortunately, they are not active against influenza B, which is responsible for approximately 20% of all influenza epidemics and in a given year may be the only virus circulating. Amantadine is licensed in the United States for the prophylaxis and therapy of influenza A. Rimantadine is still experimental.

The two drugs have similar mechanisms of action and antiviral spectra but differ with respect to pharmacokinetics (Table 49–6). Replication of the influenza virus requires cleavage of hemagglutinin by proteolytic enzymes, followed by acidification to open the cleaved hemagglutinin and release viral RNA, which then gains access to the cytoplasm of infected cells. According to Belshe and Hay, amantadine and rimantadine block the acidification process.[99] Hay and colleagues reported that sensitivity to amantadine is primarily a property conferred by plasma membrane proteins, such as the M2 proteins, although the gene that codes for the hemagglutinin may influence sensitivity of certain strains.[100]

Table 49–6. **Comparison of Amantadine and Rimantadine**

| Characteristic | Amantadine | Rimantadine |
|---|---|---|
| Efficacy against influenza A | Similar | Similar |
| Prophylaxis and treatment of influenza A | Yes | Yes |
| Prophylaxis and treatment of influenza B | No | No |
| Prophylaxis or treatment of pulmonary complications | Unknown | Unknown |
| Licensed in United States | Yes | No |
| Mechanism of action | Similar | Similar |
| Oral absorption | Good | Good |
| Time to peak plasma levels | 2–4 h | 2–6 h |
| Excretion | Renal (unmetabolized) | Renal (90% metabolized) |
| Plasma half-life | 12–18 h (usual) | 24–36 h |
| Frequency of adverse effects | | |
| Gastrointestinal | Similar | Similar |
| Central nervous system | | |
| At 300 mg daily dose | Greater | Few |
| At comparable plasma concentrations | Similar | Similar |
| Usual adult prophylactic dose | 100 mg | 200 mg |
| Usual adult treatment dose | 100–200 mg | 300 mg |
| Aerosol therapy | Proven effective | Limited study |

Resistance occurs because of point mutations in the RNA coding for the M2 protein resulting in a single amino acid change. It may be that the M2 protein functions as an ion channel to facilitate virus acidification and that amantadine and rimantadine block this channel.

Resistance to amantadine and rimantadine is easily produced in the laboratory by serial passage of influenza virus strains through low concentrations of drugs, and the resulting isolates are cross-resistant, as shown by Oxford and Galbraith.[101] The administration of amantadine or rimantadine to birds with avian influenza yielded virulent, drug-resistant viruses that were able to compete with wild-type viruses, resulting in continued transmission of drug-resistant virus after cessation of amantadine or rimantadine use.[102]

A 10-year study of one community by Belshe and coworkers failed to detect naturally occurring drug-resistant influenza virus strains in untreated patients,[103] but such strains have been recovered after 6 or 7 days of illness in children on antiviral therapy[104] and in family members who are receiving postexposure prophylaxis. Hayden and colleagues showed that after rimantidine was used for the treatment and prophylaxis of influenza, transmission of resistant virus occurred within families, and clinical disease caused by rimantidine-resistant virus resulted.[105] Adults treated with amantadine shed smaller quantities of the influenza virus than children, and they shed the virus for shorter periods. This may be because the presence of antibodies in older patients results in more rapid clearance of the virus. The findings regarding resistance affect the recommendations for routine treatment in children and recommendations for postexposure prophylaxis in families.

In persons older than 65 years of age, the daily dosage of amantidine is 100 mg. Persons 10 to 64 years of age should be given 200 mg once daily or in divided doses. Children 1 to 9 years of age require larger doses (4.4 mg/kg/d) once daily or in divided doses, to a maximum of 150 mg/d. Dose adjustment is required for patients with impaired renal function. Amantadine is excreted unmetabolized in the urine. Its half-life is usually 12 to 18 hours but may vary greatly. In elderly patients, the half-life is twice as long, and it is even longer in patients with impaired renal function.

Disproportionate increases in plasma concentrations of amantadine as a function of dose may account for the high rates of neurotoxicity, including delirium, confusion, hallucinations, and seizures. Only a small amount of amantadine is removed by dialysis. Monitoring of plasma concentrations in patients with renal insufficiency is desirable but impractical.

Rimantadine is at least 90% metabolized.[106] Its half-life is 24 to 36 hours, twice as long as that of amantadine. Unlike amantadine, its pharmacokinetics are not appreciably altered in patients with chronic liver or renal disease.[107]

The most common adverse effects of amantadine are minor gastrointestinal and central nervous system symptoms, including nervousness, lightheadedness, insomnia, loss of appetite, and nausea. They are typically dose related and reversible after discontinuation of the drug. Rimantidine causes few central nervous system adverse effects but similar gastrointestinal complaints.

Acute overdose of amantadine results in anticholinergic activity, causing dry mouth, pupillary dilatation, urinary retention, toxic psychosis,[108] and serious neurotoxic reactions that may be transiently reversed by neostigmine. Antihistamine or anticholinergic agents used concomitantly may potentiate the central nervous system adverse effects. Long-term complications include livedo reticularis, peripheral edema, loss of vision, urinary retention, orthostatic hypotension, and occasionally, congestive heart failure.[109] One case of malignant ventricular arrhythmia after amantadine overdose has been described.[110]

For prophylaxis, amantadine should be taken as soon as possible after an outbreak is identified in a community. It should be taken daily for the duration of the outbreak (usually 4–6 weeks).

According to the recommendations of the ACIP,[111] amantadine prophylaxis may be used in several situations:

1. To control outbreaks of influenza A in institutions housing unvaccinated, high-risk persons. All residents of the institution should be given amantadine, whether or not they have received influenza vaccine the previous fall. It should also be offered to unvaccinated staff who provide care to the high-risk patients.
2. To reduce the spread of infection and to maintain care of unvaccinated, high-risk patients at home. Unvaccinated persons providing home care for high-risk patients (eg, visiting nurses, household members) should receive prophylaxis during an outbreak.
3. As an adjunct to late vaccination in high-risk persons. Even if influenza A is known to be in the community, vaccine may be given to high-risk persons. However, a protective antibody response takes 2 weeks to develop. Because amantadine does not interfere with antibody formation, it may be used during this period.
4. For patients with immunodeficiency. Amantadine may be used as a supplement to vaccination in high-risk patients who produce a poor antibody response to vaccine. Adults with AIDS may be expected to have some residual immunity to influenza from prior infections, but children with AIDS may have little or no immunity.
5. For high-risk persons in whom vaccination is contraindicated (eg, those with vaccine allergy or toxicity).

Although amantadine has been shown to reduce the severity and duration of influenza A, there have been no well-controlled studies to show its efficacy in the treatment or prevention of complications of influenza A, such as pneumonia. For treatment of influenza A illness, the drug should be given within 24 to 48 hours after the onset of illness and should be continued until 48 hours after signs and symptoms resolve.

Amantadine-treated students infected with influenza A returned to class sooner than placebo recipients.[112] A study by Younkin and colleagues comparing the efficacy of aspirin and amantadine treatment of disease caused by a naturally occurring H1N1 subtype showed a more rapid reduction in fever and fewer adverse effects in the aspirin-treated group but faster symptomatic improvement in the amantadine-treated group.[113] Intermittent amantadine aerosol therapy proved successful in the treatment of naturally occurring influenza A infection.[114]

Rimantadine, in daily dosages of 200 mg in adults and of 5 mg/kg/d in children, proved effective in preventing influenza A.[115] Because of rimantadine's slower absorption, low initial plasma levels, and long half-life, larger doses (400–600 mg in divided doses) in the first 24 hours of treatment may provide greater antiviral and clinical effects.[116] Aerosolized rimantadine has received limited study.[117]

In children with influenza A (H3N2) infection, rimantadine treatment for 5 days resulted in less fever, lower viral titers, and fewer symptoms during the first 2 days of treatment compared with acetaminophen administration, but rimantadine-treated children had more prolonged viral shedding.[118] The optimal dose and duration of therapy have not been established for children, and the problem of rapid emergence of drug-resistant virus may limit the therapeutic application of rimantadine in this age group.

Although amantadine and rimantadine are equally effective, rimantadine may be preferred in patients with renal impairment and patients older than 65 years of age because of lower risk of central nervous system toxicity due to undetected changes in renal function.

Several questions about the use of amantadine and rimantadine remain unanswered. We need to know more about the optimal dosage, frequency of administration, and efficacy of the drugs in the elderly, in children, and in patients with complications of influenza, such as viral or mixed viral and bacterial pneumonia. In these patients, the possibility of clinical synergy with other antiviral or with antibacterial drugs must be evaluated.[119] More studies are needed to define the effect of drug resistance on influenza virus infection.

The combination of antiviral drugs and vaccine needs to be studied more fully in children, in nursing home patients, and in debilitated patients in hospitals. The strategy of using vaccine before an epidemic and an antiviral drug at the time of an epidemic warrants further study. We need to find antiviral drugs active against influenza A and influenza B viruses.

# REFERENCES

1. Woodhead MA, MacFarlane JT, McCracken JS, et al: Prospective study of the aetiology and outcome of pneumonia in the community. Lancet 1:671–674, 1987.
2. Recommendations of the Immunization Practices Advisory Committee (ACIP): Update: Pneumococcal polysaccharide vaccine usage—United States. MMWR 33:273–281, 1984.
3. Erakklis AJ, Kevy SV, Diamond LK, et al: Hazard of overwhelming infection after splenectomy in childhood. N Engl J Med 176:1225–1229, 1967.
4. Gopal V, Bisno AL: Fulminant pneumococcal infections in "normal" asplenic hosts. Arch Intern Med 137:1526–1530, 1977.
5. Winkelstein JA: Splenectomy and infection. Arch Intern Med 137:1516–1517, 1977.
6. Barrett-Connor E: Bacterial infection and sickle cell anemia. Medicine (Baltimore) 50:97–112, 1971.
7. Falter ML, Robinson MG, Kim OS, et al: Splenic function and infection in sickle cell anemia. Acta Haematol 50:154–161, 1973.
8. Weitzman S, Aisenberg AC: Fulminant sepsis after the successful treatment of Hodgkin's disease. Am J Med 62:47–50, 1977.
9. Notter DT, Grossman PL, Rosenberg SA, Remington JS: Infections in patients with Hodgkin's disease: A clinical study of 300 consecutive adult patients. Rev Infect Dis 2:761–800, 1980.
10. Zinneman HH, Hall WH: Recurrent pneumonia in multiple myeloma and some observations on immunologic response. Ann Intern Med 41:1152–1163, 1954.
11. Glenchur H, Zinneman HH, Hall WH: A review of fifty-one cases

12. Mufson MA, Oley G, Hughey D: Pneumococcal disease in a medium-sized community in the United States. JAMA 248:1486–1489, 1982.
13. Burman LA, Norrby R, Trollfors B: Invasive pneumococcal infections: Incidence, predisposing factors and prognosis. Rev Infect Dis 7:133–142, 1985.
14. Montgomery JZ, Kalmanson GM, Guze LB: Renal failure and infection. Medicine (Baltimore) 47:1–32, 1968.
15. Keane WF, Shapiro FL, Raij L: Incidence and type of infections occurring in 445 chronic hemodialysis patients. Trans Am Soc Artif Intern Organs 23:41–47, 1977.
16. Pahmer M: Pneumococcus peritonitis in nephrotic and non-nephrotic children. J Pediatr 17:90–106, 1940.
17. Wisholtz SJ, Hartman BJ, Roberts RB: Effect of underlying disease and age on pneumococcal serotype distribution. Am J Med 75:199–205, 1983.
18. Mylotte JM, Beam TR: Comparison of community-acquired and nosocomial pneumococcal bacteremia. Am Rev Respir Dis 123:265–268, 1981.
19. Simberkoff MS, ElSadr W, Schiffman G, et al: *Streptococcus pneumoniae* infection in patients with acquired immune deficiency syndrome, with report of a pneumococcal vaccine failure. Am Rev Respir Dis 130:1174–1176, 1984.
20. Polsky B, Gold JWM, Whimbey E, et al: Bacterial pneumonia in patients with the acquired immunodeficiency syndrome. Ann Intern Med 104:38–41, 1985.
21. Witt DJ, Craven DE, McCabe WR: Bacterial infections in adult patients with the acquired immune deficiency syndrome (AIDS) and AIDS-related complex. Am J Med 82:900–906, 1987.
22. Redd SC, Rutherford GW, Sande MA, et al: The role of human immunodeficiency virus infection in pneumococcal bacteremia in San Francisco residents. J Infect Dis 162:1012–1017, 1990.
23. Ward J: Antibiotic-resistant *Streptococcus pneumoniae*: Clinical and epidemiological aspects. Rev Infect Dis 3:254–256, 1981.
24. Simberkoff MS, Lukaszewski M, Cross A, et al: Antibiotic-resistant isolates of *Streptococcus pneumoniae* from clinical specimens: A cluster of serotype 19A organisms in Brooklyn, New York. J Infect Dis 153:78–82, 1986.
25. Pallares R, Gudiol F, Linares J, et al: Risk factors and response to antibiotic therapy in adults with bacteremic pneumonia caused by penicillin-resistant pneumococci. N Engl J Med 317:18–22, 1987.
26. Wright AE, Morgan WP, Colebrook L, Dodgson RW: Prophylactic inoculation against pneumococcus infection and on the results which have been achieved by it. Lancet 1:1–10, 1914.
27. Wright AE, Morgan WP, Colebrook L, Dodgson RW: Prophylactic inoculation against pneumococcus infection and on the results which have been achieved by it. Lancet 1:87–95, 1914.
28. Wright AE, Morgan WP, Colebrook L, Dodgson RW: Prophylactic inoculation against *Pneumococcus* infection and on the results which have been achieved by it. Lancet 1:93, 1914.
29. Francis T, Tillet WS: Cutaneous reactions in pneumonia: The development of antibodies following the intradermal injection of type specific polysaccharide. J Exp Med 52:573–585, 1930.
30. Felton LD: Studies on the immunizing substances in pneumococci. VII. Response in human beings to antigenic pneumococcus polysaccharide type I and II. Public Health Rep 53:1855–1877, 1938.
31. Hilleman MR, Carlson AJ, McLean AA, et al: *Streptococcus pneumoniae* polysaccharide vaccine: Age and dose responses, safety, persistence of antibody, revaccination, and simultaneous administration of pneumococcal and influenza vaccines. Rev Infect Dis 3:S31–S42, 1981.
32. Ekwurzel GM, Simmons JS, Dublin LI, Felton LD: Studies on immunizing substances in pneumococci. VIII. Report on field tests to determine the prophylactic value of a pneumococcus antigen. Public Health Rep 53:1877–1893, 1938.
33. Kaufman P: Pneumonia in old age: Active immunization against pneumonia with pneumococcus polysaccharide: Results of a six year study. Arch Intern Med 79:518–531, 1947.
34. MacLeod CM, Hodges RG, Heidelberger M, Bernhard WG: Prevention of pneumococcal pneumonia by immunization with specific capsular polysaccharide. J Exp Med 82:445–465, 1945.
35. Austrian R: Random gleanings from a life with the pneumococcus. J Infect Dis 131:474–484, 1975.
36. Austrian R, Gold J: Pneumococcal bacteremia with especial refer-

ence to bacteremic pneumococcal pneumonia. Ann Intern Med 60:759–776, 1964.

37. Mufson MA, Kruss DM, Wasil RE, Metzger WI: Capsular types and outcome of bacteremic pneumococcal disease in the antibiotic era. Arch Intern Med 134:505–510, 1974.

38. Austrian R: Prevention of pneumococcal pneumonia by vaccination. Trans Assoc Am Physicians 89:184–194, 1976.

39. Smit P, Oberholzer D, Hayden-Smith S, et al: Protective efficacy of pneumococcal polysaccharide vaccines. JAMA 238:2613–2616, 1977.

40. Riley ID, Tarr PI, Andrews M, et al: Immunization with a polyvalent pneumococcal vaccine: Reduction of adult respiratory mortality in a New Guinea highlands community. Lancet 1:1338–1341, 1977.

41. Austrian R: Some observations on the pneumococcus and on the current status of pneumococcal disease and its prevention. Rev Infect Dis 3:S1–S17, 1981.

42. Austrian R: Surveillance of Pneumococcal Infection for Field Trials of Polyvalent Pneumococcal Vaccines. Springfield, VA, National Technical Information Service, 1980:1–84.

43. Heidelberger M, Dilapi MM, Siegel M, Walter AW: Persistence of antibodies in human subjects injected with pneumococcal polysaccharide. J Immunol 65:535–541, 1950.

44. Simberkoff MS, Cross AP Al-Ibrahim M, et al: Efficacy of pneumococcal vaccine in high-risk patients: Results of a Veterans Administration Cooperative Study. N Engl J Med 315:1318–1327, 1986.

45. Shapiro ED: Pneumococcal vaccine failure. N Engl J Med 317:1272–1273, 1987.

46. Clemens JD, Shapiro ED: Resolving the pneumococcal vaccine controversy: Are there alternatives to randomized clinical trials? Rev Infect Dis 6:589–600, 1984.

47. Broome CV, Facklam RR, Fraser DW: Pneumococcal disease after pneumococcal vaccination: An alternative method to estimate the efficacy of pneumococcal vaccine. N Engl J Med 303:549–552, 1980.

48. Bolan G, Broome CV, Facklam RR, et al: Pneumococcal vaccine efficacy in selected populations in the United States. Ann Intern Med 1:1–6, 1986.

49. Forrester HL, Jahnigen DW, LaForce FM: Inefficacy of pneumococcal vaccine in a high-risk population. Am J Med 83:425–430, 1987.

50. Shapiro ED, Berg AT, Austrian R, et al: The protective efficacy of polyvalent pneumococcal polysaccharide vaccine. N Engl J Med 325:1453–1460, 1991.

51. Landesman SH, Schiffman G: Assessment of the antibody response to pneumococcal vaccine in high-risk populations. Rev Infect Dis 3:S184–S196, 1981.

52. Amman AJ, Schiffman G, Abrams D, et al: B-cell immunodeficiency in acquired immune deficiency syndrome. JAMA 251:1447–1449, 1984.

53. Huang KL, Ruben FL, Rinaldo CR, et al: Antibody responses after influenza and pneumococcal immunization in HIV-infected homosexual men. JAMA 257:2047–2050, 1987.

54. Ballet JJ, Sulcebe G, Couderc LJ, et al: Impaired antipneumococcal antibody response in patients with AIDS-related persistent generalized lymphadenopathy. Clin Exp Immunol 68:479–487, 1987.

55. Glaser JB, Volpe S, Aguirre A, et al: Zidovudine improves response to pneumococcal vaccine among persons with AIDS and AIDS-related complex. J Infect Dis 164:761–764, 1991.

56. Amman AJ, Addiego J, Wara DW, et al: Polyvalent pneumococcal-polysaccharide immunization of patients with sickle-cell anemia and patients with splenectomy. N Engl J Med 297:897–900, 1977.

57. Giebink GS, Foker JE, Kim Y, Schiffman G: Serum antibody and opsonic response to vaccination with pneumococcal capsular polysaccharide in normal and splenectomized children. J Infect Dis 141:404–412, 1980.

58. Simberkoff MS, Cross AP, Schiffman G, et al: Further analysis of antibody responses to pneumococcal vaccine among patients enrolled in a trial of efficacy. Abstracts of the 27th Interscience Conference on Antimicrobial Agents and Chemotherapy, New York, NY, 1987.

59. Bentley DW: Pneumococcal vaccine in the institutionalized elderly: Review of past and recent studies. Rev Infect Dis 3:S61–S70, 1981.

60. Bentley DW, Ha K, Mamot K, et al: Pneumococcal vaccine in the institutionalized elderly: Design of a nonrandomized trial and preliminary results. Rev Infect Dis 3:S71–S81, 1987.

61. Centers for Disease Control: Update on adult immunization: Recommendations of the Immunization Practices Advisory Committee (ACIP). MMWR 40:1–94, 1991.

62. Fedson DS, Harward MP, Reid RA, Kaiser DL: Hospital-based pneumococcal immunization: Epidemiologic rationale from the Shenandoah study. JAMA 264:1117–1122, 1990.

63. Fedson DS, Chiarello LA: Previous hospital care and pneumococcal bacteremia: Importance for pneumococcal immunization. Arch Intern Med 143:885–889, 1983.

64. Magnussen CR, Valenti WM, Mushlin AI: Pneumococcal vaccine strategy: Feasibility of a vaccination program directed at hospitalized and ambulatory patients. Arch Intern Med 144:1755–1757, 1984.

65. Kilbourne ED: Influenza. New York, Plenum Medical Book Company, 1987.

66. Betts RF, Douglas RG: Influenza virus. In Mandell GL, Douglas RG, Bennett JE (eds): Principles and Practice of Infectious Diseases, ed 3. New York, Churchill Livingstone, 1990:1306–1325.

67. Smith W, Andrews CH, Laidlaw PP: A virus obtained from influenza patients. Lancet 2:66–68, 1933.

68. Francis T: A new type of virus from epidemic influenza. Science 92:405–408, 1940.

69. Miller DL, Reid D, Diamond JR, et al: Hong Kong influenza in the Royal Air Force 1968–70. J Hyg 71:535–547, 1973.

70. Mulder J, Masurel N: Pre-epidemic antibody against 1957 strain of Asiatic influenza. Lancet 2:810–814, 1958.

71. Chenowith A, Waltz AD, Stokes J: Active immunization with the viruses of human and swine influenza. Am J Dis Child 52:757–758, 1936.

72. Ennis FA, Mayner RE, Barry DW, et al: Correlation of laboratory studies with clinical responses to A/New Jersey influenza vaccines. J Infect Dis 136:S397–S405, 1977.

73. Barry DW, Mayner RE, Hochstein HD, et al: Comparative trial of influenza vaccines. II. Adverse reactions in children and adults. Am J Epidemiol 104:47–59, 1976.

74. Langmuir AD, Bregman DJ, Kurland LT, et al: An epidemiologic and clinical evaluation of Guillian-Barré syndrome reported in association with the administration of swine influenza vaccines. Am J Epidemiol 119:841–879, 1984.

75. Barry DW, Mayner RE, Staton E, et al: Comparative trial of influenza vaccines. I. Immunogenicity of whole virus and split product vaccines in man. Am J Epidemiol 104:34–46, 1976.

76. Hilleman MR: Serologic responses to split and whole swine influenza virus vaccines in light of the next influenza pandemic. J Infect Dis 136:S683–S685, 1977.

77. Beare AS, Schild GC, Craig JW: Trials in man with live recombinants made from A/PR/8/34(H0N1) and wild H3N2 influenza viruses. Lancet 2:729–738, 1975.

78. Mills J, Chanock RM: Temperature-sensitive mutants of influenza virus. I. Behavior in tissue culture and in experimental animals. J Infect Dis 123:145–157, 1971.

79. Maasab HR, Kendal AP, Abrams GD, et al: Evaluation of a cold-recombinant influenza virus in ferrets. J Infect Dis 146:780–790, 1982.

80. McLean IW, Beard D, Taylor AR, et al: The relation of antibody response in swine to dose of the swine influenza inactivated with formalin and with ultraviolet light. J Immunol 51:65–99, 1945.

81. Mostow SR, Schoenbaum SC, Dowdle WR, et al: Studies on inactivated influenza vaccines. II. Effect of increasing dosage on antibody response and adverse reactions in man. Am J Epidemiol 92:248–256, 1970.

82. Brown H, Kasel JA, Freeman DM, et al: The immunizing effect of Influenza A/New Jersey/76(Hsw1N1) virus vaccine administered intradermally and intramuscularly to adults. J Infect Dis 136:S466–471, 1977.

83. Gwaltney JM, Edmondson WP, Rothenberg R, White PW: A comparison of subcutaneous, nasal, and combined influenza vaccination. I. Antigenicity. Am J Epidemiol 93:472–479, 1971.

84. Betts RF, Douglas RG: Comparative study of reactogenicity and immunogenicity of Influenza A/New Jersey/8/76(Hsw1N1) virus vaccines in normal volunteers. J Infect Dis 136:S443–S449, 1977.

85. Gross PA: Reactogenicity and immunogenicity of bivalent influenza vaccine in one- and two-dose trials in children: A summary. J Infect Dis 136:S616–625, 1977.

86. Barker WH, Mullooly JP: Influenza vaccination of elderly persons. JAMA 244:2547–2549, 1980.

87. Centers for Disease Control: Prevention and control of influenza; Recommendations of the Immunization Practices Advisory Committee (ACIP). MMWR 40:1–15, 1991.

88. Pabico RC, Douglas RG, Betts RF, et al: Antibody response to

influenza vaccination in renal transplant patients: Correlation with allograft function. Ann Intern Med 85:431–436, 1976.

89. Versluis DJ, Beyer WEP, Masurel N, et al: Impairment of the immune response to influenza vaccination in renal transplant recipients by cyclosporine, but not azathioprine. Transplantation 42:376–379, 1986.

90. Ortbals DW, Liebhaber H, Presant CA, et al: Influenza immunization of adult patients with malignant diseases. Ann Intern Med 87:552–557, 1977.

91. Gross PA, Gould AL, Brown AE: Effect of cancer chemotherapy on the immune response to influenza virus vaccine: Review of published studies. Rev Infect Dis 7:613–618, 1985.

92. Huang KL, Ruben FL, Rinaldo CR, et al: Antibody responses after influenza and pneumococcal immunization in HIV-infected homosexual men. JAMA 257:2047–2050, 1987.

93. Nelson KE, Clements ML, Miotti P, et al: The influence of human immunodeficiency virus (HIV) infection on antibody responses to influenza vaccines. Ann Intern Med 109:383–388, 1988.

94. Miotti PG, Nelson KE, Dallabetta GA, et al: The influence of HIV infection on antibody responses to a two-dose regimen of influenza vaccine. JAMA 262:779–783, 1989.

95. Patriarca PA, Weber JA, Parker RA, et al: Efficacy of influenza vaccine in nursing homes: Reduction in illness and complications during an influenza A (H3N2) epidemic. JAMA 253:1136–1139, 1985.

96. Hoskins TW, Davies JR, Allchin A, et al: Controlled trial of inactivated influenza vaccine containing the A/Hong Kong strain during an outbreak of influenza due to the A/England/42/72 strain. Lancet 2:116–120, 1973.

97. Stiver HG, Graves P, Eickhoff TC, Meikeljohn G: Efficacy of ''Hong Kong'' vaccine in preventing ''England'' variant influenza A in 1972. N Engl J Med 289:1267–1271, 1973.

98. Keitel WA, Cate TR, Couch RB: Efficacy of sequential, annual vaccination with inactivated influenza virus vaccine. Am J Epidemiol 127:353–364, 1988.

99. Belshe RB, Hay AJ: Drug resistance and mechanisms of action on influenza A viruses. J Respir Dis 10(suppl):S52–S61, 1989.

100. Hay AJ, Zambon MC, Wolstenholme AJ, et al: Molecular basis of resistance of influenza A viruses to amantadine. J Antimicrob Chemother 18(suppl B):19–29, 1986.

101. Oxford JS, Galbraith A: Antiviral activity of amantadine: A review of laboratory and clinical data. Pharmacol Ther 11:181–262, 1980.

102. Beard CW, Brugh M, Webster RG: Emergence of amantadine-resistant H5N2 avian influenza virus during a simulated layer flock treatment program. Avian Dis 31:533–537, 1987.

103. Belshe RB, Burk B, Newman F, et al: Resistance of influenza A virus to amantadine and rimantadine: Results of one decade of surveillance. J Infect Dis 159:430–435, 1989.

104. Belshe RB, Smith MH, Hall CB, Beth R, Hay AJ: Genetic basis of

105. Hayden FG, Belshe RB, Clover RD, et al: Emergence and apparent transmission of rimantidine-resistant influenza A virus in families. N Engl J Med 321:1696–1702, 1989.

106. Hayden FG, Minocha A, Spyker DA, Hoffman HE: Comparative single-dose pharmacokinetics of amantadine hydrochloride and rimantadine hydrochloride in young and elderly adults. Antimicrob Agents Chemother 28:216–221, 1985.

107. Capparelli EV, Stevens RC, Chow MS, et al: Rimantidine pharmacokinetics in healthy subjects and patients with end-stage renal failure. Clin Pharmacol Ther 43:536–544, 1988.

108. Tominack TL, Hayden FG: Rimantidine hydrochloride and amantadine hydrochloride use in influenza A virus infection. Infect Dis Clin North Am 1:459–478, 1987.

109. Atkinson WL, Arden NH, Patriarca PA, et al: Amantadine prophylaxis during an institutional outbreak of type A(H1N1) influenza. Arch Intern Med 1751–1756, 1986.

110. Sartori M, Pratt CM, Young JB: Malignant cardiac arythmia as induced by amantadine poisoning. Am J Med 77:388–391, 1984.

111. Advisory Committee on Immunization Practices: Prevention and control of influenza. MMWR 37:361–373, 1988.

112. Van Voris LP, Betts RF, Hayden FG, et al: Successful treatment of naturally occurring influenza A/USSR/77 H1N1. JAMA 245:1128–1131, 1981.

113. Younkin SW, Beth RF, Roth FK, et al: Reduction in fever and symptoms in young adults with influenza A/Brazil/78 H1N1 infection after treatment with aspirin or amantadine. Antimicrob Agents Chemother 23:577–582, 1983.

114. Hayden FG, Hall WJ, Douglas RG: Therapeutic effects of aerosolized amantadine in naturally acquired infection due to influenza A virus. J Infect Dis 141:535–542, 1980.

115. Clover RD, Crawford SA, Abell TD, et al: Effectiveness of rimantadine prophylaxis of children within families. Am J Dis Child 140:706–709, 1986.

116. Hayden FG, Monto AS: Oral rimantadine hydrochloride therapy of influenza A virus H3N2 subtype infection in adults. Antimicrob Agents Chemother 29:339–241, 1986.

117. Hayden FG, Zylidnikov DM, Iljenkovi, et al: Comparative therapeutic effect of aerosolized and oral rimantadine hydrochloride in experimental human influenza A virus infection. Antiviral Res 2:147–153, 1982.

118. Belshe RB, Smith MH, Hall CB, et al: Genetic basis of resistance to rimantadine emerging during treatment of influenza virus infections. J Virol 62:1508–1512, 1988.

119. Hayden FG: Combinations of antiviral agents for treatment of influenza virus infections. J Antimicrob Chemother 18(suppl B):177–183, 1986.

# CHAPTER 50

# Preventive Interventions for Persons Infected With the Human Immunodeficiency Virus

PETER T. FRAME and MICHAEL N. DOHN

Pulmonary infections are a major problem in persons infected with the human immunodeficiency virus (HIV). As the immune-based pulmonary defenses become less effective, "opportunistic" infections caused by virulent and less virulent pathogens become more common. This chapter describes preventive strategies for the most common respiratory infections in HIV-infected patients: *Pneumocystis carinii* pneumonia (PCP), bacterial pneumonia, tuberculosis (TB), and viral influenza.

Pneumonia caused by *P. carinii* was the most common life-threatening infection for acquired immunodeficiency syndrome (AIDS) patients in the 1980s. Early data indicate that as many as 80% of patients with AIDS eventually develop PCP.[1] During the 1980s, *Pneumocystis* pneumonia was the most common cause of death in AIDS patients, and those who survived their first episode of PCP had a 40% to 60% chance of developing it again within the next year.[2] During the late 1980s, the use of prophylactic measures to prevent PCP became widespread in the United States. As a result, PCP has become less common as a first AIDS-defining infection, and early recognition and treatment have made PCP less common as the cause of death in AIDS patients. Nevertheless, because many HIV-infected persons are not receiving medical care for their HIV infection, primary PCP is still a common presentation of AIDS. PCP still affects most AIDS patients during their illness, and PCP still carries a mortality rate of 15% to 20%.[1, 3-7]

The incidence of bacterial infection in general and bacterial pneumonia specifically is high in adults infected with HIV. Although bacterial infections have long been recognized as significant problems in HIV-infected children, and have been included as an AIDS-defining illness in the pediatric population, the Centers for Disease Control and Prevention (CDC) has only recently added recurrent bacterial pneumonia to the criteria for the definition of AIDS in adults.[8] Bacterial pneumonias have occurred 10 to 100 times more commonly in AIDS patients than in the general population.[9-12] Deaths attributable to bacterial pneumonia in CDC surveillance records have increased by 176% among persons 25 to 44 years of age. This increase has been seen predominantly in cities with a high incidence of AIDS, and a retrospective review of reported pneumonia deaths from New York City indicates that 80% of the persons who died could be categorized as members of groups at increased risk for AIDS.[12] *Streptococcus pneumoniae* and *Haemophilus influenzae* are the most commonly reported bacterial causes of pneumonia in AIDS patients.[9-11, 13] Among patients with pneumococcal pneumonia, bacteremic disease is more common than in the general population, and unusual pneumococcal infections may also be more common.[9-14]

In HIV-infected patients, TB is a more virulent disease than in the general population, with a high incidence of extrapulmonary and disseminated disease and a rapid progression from infection to disease to death.[15-17] The gradual fall in the incidence of TB which the United States had enjoyed for the past few decades was reversed in the mid-1980s, with a new epidemic of TB occurring in large inner city populations. Even more disturbing was the rapid spread of multidrug-resistant strains of *Mycobacterium tuberculosis* in these populations. Coinfection with HIV facilitated the changes in *M. tuberculosis* epidemiology, and the combination of these two infections in some developing countries has been particularly deadly.[18]

It is unclear whether viral influenza is more common or more severe in HIV-infected patients compared with the general population. Studies of influenza outbreaks have not shown an increased incidence of influenza in HIV-infected patients.[19, 20] A study of 6 HIV-infected patients at San Francisco General Hospital during the influenza outbreak of 1988 to 1989 did not show a particularly severe influenza virus infection. Although the level of hypoxemia seemed higher than expected, no control groups were available for comparison.[21] However, an increased mortality rate for young adults during influenza outbreaks in areas with high incidence of AIDS suggested the possibility of increased mortality during influenza outbreaks.[12] Because most influenza-related mortality is caused by bacterial pneumonia, it is possible that the occurrence of influenza in HIV-infected patients may increase the likelihood of bacterial pneumonia or other respiratory infections that carry higher morbidity.

Other serious pulmonary infections occur in AIDS patients. Often these are part of a systemic process in which the pulmonary component is less life threatening than the systemic disease. Examples include histoplasmosis, coccidioidomycosis, disseminated *Mycobacterium avium* infections, and systemic cytomegalovirus infection. If the initial route of infection is through the lung, diagnosis may be made by examination of pulmonary secretions or biopsies, but respiratory failure is an uncommon complication of the systemic process. In these patients, chronic fever, weight loss, and pancytopenia are more frequent manifestations.

This chapter reviews several strategies for preventing pulmonary infection in HIV-infected patients: enhancing host defenses, using therapeutic agents to prevent or suppress infection, and preventing transmission of respiratory pathogens from other actively infected persons. Infection control in health care workers is essential to prevent morbidity and mortality among the workers and to prevent transmission of infection to their highly susceptible patients. Table 50–1 summarizes the strategies for preventing pulmonary infections in HIV-infected patients and their caregivers.

## ENHANCING HOST DEFENSES

### Smoking

Cessation of smoking should be a preventive measure emphasized to HIV-infected patients. If immune-based defenses of the lung become compromised by HIV, other pulmonary defense mechanisms, such as mucociliary clearance, become more important. HIV-infected smokers have a higher incidence of bacterial pneumonia than nonsmokers,[22] and two reports suggest that smoking increases the risk of PCP in patients with HIV infection.[23, 24] The difference between smokers and nonsmokers could not be attributed to differences in immune status as measured by peripheral blood CD4 count.

### Diagnosing and Treating Human Immunodeficiency Infection

HIV infection must be recognized before preventive measures can be applied. To do this, all health care providers must be able to assess HIV risk factors in their patients and be prepared to counsel and test patients for HIV infection or refer them to an appropriate counseling and testing site.[24a] Because HIV infection is present for approximately 10 years before the development of AIDS, patients must be questioned about present and past high-risk behaviors, such as injection drug use (including androgenic steroids), nonintravenous cocaine use, multiple sex partners, and the receipt of blood products before 1985. The CDC now recommends that all patients with newly diagnosed TB be offered HIV testing because of the common coexistence of these infections and the different management of TB in those coinfected with HIV. Patients with recurrent bacterial pneumonia or unusual manifestations of pneumonia also should be considered candidates for HIV testing. The essence of any preventive therapy is to institute

Table 50–1. **Specific Strategies to Prevent Pulmonary Infections in HIV-Infected Patients and Their Caregivers**

| Preventive Measure | Recipient | Pulmonary Infection | | | |
| | | *Viral Influenza* | *Bacterial Pneumonia* | Pneumocystis carinii *Infection* | *Tuberculosis* |
| --- | --- | --- | --- | --- | --- |
| Vaccination | Patient | Yearly | Pneumococcal vaccine* H. influenzae B*,† | No | No |
| | HCW‡ | Yearly | No | No | No |
| Prophylaxis | Patient | Amantadine§ | Selected cases‖ | Yes¶ | Yes |
| | HCW | Amantadine§ | No | No | Yes |
| In-hospital isolation | Patient | No# | No# | No# | Yes |
| Masks | HCW | No** | No** | No** | Yes |

*For patients beginning anti-HIV therapy (eg, zidovudine), a delay of 4 to 8 weeks after starting anti-HIV therapy may improve vaccination responses.
†With severe immune deficiency (CD4 ≤ 200), use unconjugated vaccine (PRP); with less severe immune depression, use conjugated vaccine (PRP-CRM).
‡HCW, health care worker.
§For unvaccinated patients or those unlikely to have responded to vaccine. Amantadine is used only if influenza A is known to be present in the community.
‖Penicillin V for patients with recurrent episodes of pneumococcal pneumonia is sometimes recommended.
¶Trimethoprim-sulfamethoxazole (one double-strength tablet daily) is the first-choice agent.
#Respiratory isolation is appropriate for patients with these infections until tuberculosis coinfection can be excluded.
**Masks should be worn in the presence of these patients until tuberculosis coinfection has been excluded.

it before clinical disease occurs, and to be effective, the ideal time to recognize HIV infection is in the *asymptomatic* patient.

The treatment of HIV infection with antiviral agents such as zidovudine (AZT), didanosine (DDI), and zalcitabine (DDC) enhances the function of the immune system and prevents or delays the onset of opportunistic infections, including pulmonary infections. This effect is seen in patients with evidence of suppressed immunity, regardless of whether they have already experienced an opportunistic infection.[25–27] The strategies of combining anti-HIV agents and alternating between them is beyond the scope of this discussion, but evidence is mounting that anti-HIV treatment with multiple drugs can further delay the onset of opportunistic infection beyond the effect of a single drug.[28, 29] Many new antiretroviral strategies are being investigated, and long-term control of HIV infection and subsequent maintenance of immune system function are realistic expectations for the future.

Although the proportion of total CD4+ lymphocytes that circulate in the peripheral blood is relatively small, quantifying the peripheral blood CD4 count has value in assessing the level of immune deficiency caused by HIV infection and has prognostic value regarding the occurrence of opportunistic infections.[30] Most HIV-infected patients who develop PCP have peripheral blood CD4 counts below 200 $CD4^+/mm^3$ (normal >500 cells/$mm^3$), and the risk of PCP increases as the CD4 count falls.[31] Preventive drug therapy for PCP is now instituted according to peripheral blood CD4 count, and preventive strategies for other opportunistic infections are being investigated according to the results of this test.

As recommended by a National Institute of Allergy and Infectious Disease Consensus Panel,[32] all physicians should become familiar with the procedures for recognizing and diagnosing HIV infection. Diagnosis in the asymptomatic patient is optimum so that treatments to prevent or delay the onset of AIDS can be instituted. Patients with HIV infection should have their immune function monitored by regular (3–6 months) examinations and assessment of peripheral blood CD4 count.[32] Patients with evidence of immune deficiency (CD4 count <500/$mm^3$ or the development of an opportunistic infection or neoplasm) caused by HIV infection should receive antiretroviral therapy, which can reduce their risk for opportunistic infections, including pulmonary infections.[33] AZT is the first drug of choice in 1993, with DDI and DDC used as alternative therapies for those who cannot tolerate AZT. Sequential use of these agents further extends the suppressive effect on HIV, and combination antiretroviral therapy is under investigation.

## Immunization

Some researchers have suggested that the use of vaccines may have a deleterious effect on the HIV-infected recipient. This theoretical concern is based on an in vitro experiment that demonstrated that stimulation of an HIV-infected T-cell culture with tetanus toxoid resulted in amplification of HIV replication.[33] However, studies of immunization in children and adults with several different vaccines have shown no serious or unusual events and no evidence that the vaccines stimulate progressive immune deficiency.[34–37]

### Influenza Virus Vaccine

Protection against influenza virus infection develops in as many as 80% of the normal members of the population who receive influenza vaccine of the same serotype as the epidemic strain. Immunity appears to be subtype specific, but a prior antigenic experience with a related strain may provide partial protection or allow for amelioration of disease. However, major genetic variation in the external proteins of the virus allows repeated infection with new viral strains. Long-term immunity to reinfection with the same strain of virus has been well documented. During outbreaks of influenza A (H1N1) in the 1970s, disease occurred only in persons who had not been living during previous outbreaks of this virus; older persons in the population were not affected.[38]

Although cell-mediated responses occur after influenza virus infection or influenza vaccine, antibody responses appear to be the primary protective immune responses, because variation in protection is closely linked with specificity and titers of immunoglobulin responses. Because humoral immune responses to glycoproteins are T-cell–mediated B-cell responses, adequate helper T-cell function is probably required for a response to a new influenza virus antigen. However, anamnestic humoral immune responses to previously recognized antigens may be T-cell independent.

The ability of HIV-infected patients to respond to influenza vaccine has been studied by several investigators. In an early study of volunteers in the multicenter AIDS Cohort Study in Pittsburgh, asymptomatic HIV-infected men usually responded to influenza vaccine with antibody titers that did not significantly differ from those of HIV-negative homosexual or heterosexual controls.[36] In another study, a diminished antibody response to the influenza A component of trivalent influenza vaccine was observed in HIV-infected hemophilia patients, particularly those with advanced AIDS-related complex (ARC) or AIDS. Immune responses to the influenza B component of the vaccine were similar to those of controls.[39]

After finding that HIV-infected subjects were less likely to develop protective levels (1:64 or greater) of hemagglutination inhibition antibodies after influenza vaccine, investigators at Johns Hopkins studied the antibody responses to a two-dose regimen of influenza vaccine, with the second dose 1 month after the first. The second dose of vaccine did not significantly increase the frequency or magnitude of influenza antibody responses in the HIV-positive subjects or in the HIV-negative controls. In these studies, a graded response was again observed; HIV-seropositive patients with no symptoms had better vaccine responses than those who had AIDS or ARC.[36–40]

As recommended by the CDC,[41] all HIV-infected persons should receive influenza vaccine annually. The earlier in the course of HIV infection influenza immunization begins, the more likely it is that the patient will develop protective antibody responses.

## Streptococcus pneumoniae Vaccine

Although the use of pneumococcal polysaccharide vaccine is recommended by the CDC for HIV-infected persons, evidence that this strategy prevents pneumococcal disease in this population is lacking. However, several lines of evidence suggest that the strategy is safe and may be at least partially effective.

The human immune response to polysaccharide antigens, such as pneumococcal vaccine, are T-cell–independent responses. However, B-cell dysfunction also occurs in HIV infection, and the response to pneumococcal polysaccharide vaccine may not always be adequate. Some studies have demonstrated that HIV-infected patients with a normal number of circulating CD4 cells have antibody responses to pneumococcal vaccine that do not differ from those of HIV-negative controls.[34, 35, 42–44] A study of HIV-infected patients by Rodriguez-Barradas and coworkers showed that the percentage of possible antipneumococcal antibody responses to polyvalent vaccine achieved was 75% in patients with more than 500 CD4 cells/mm³ and 74% in healthy controls. HIV-infected patients with fewer than 500 CD4 cells/mm³ had a response rate of only 24%. Subjects who responded to an antigen developed similar antibody titers against that antigen, regardless of the CD4 count. The investigators were careful to remove pneumococcal cell wall antigens, which are ubiquitous in the normal human population but not protective against pneumococcal infection.[42]

Helper T cells may facilitate the transition of B cells from IgM to IgG or IgA production. The proportion of these three antibody classes produced in response to vaccine stimulation may be expected to differ in HIV-infected patients. However, Janoff and coworkers have shown that antibody production, although lower in HIV-infected men than in normal controls, was proportional for each of the immunoglobulin classes. They found that all HIV-infected men responded to pneumococcal antigens, but the responses of subjects with AIDS were lower than those of HIV-infected men without AIDS. The researchers reexamined some subjects after 1 year and found that antibody levels in all three classes remained elevated above baseline values.[44]

HIV-infected patients with prior antibody to a specific pneumococcal serotype are able to develop an anamnestic response after exposure to the vaccine. In asymptomatic persons, these responses are sufficient to elevate antibody titers above 400 ng Ab N/mL, a level which is considered to be protective.[34]

Glaser and associates have shown that pneumococcal antibody responses among AIDS and ARC patients receiving AZT were higher than in a similar group of HIV-infected patients who were not receiving AZT. In this study, AIDS and ARC patients with a median CD4 count of 119 were administered 23-valent pneumococcal polysaccharide vaccine. Those who were not receiving AZT at the time of immunization had no response to any of 12 pneumococcal serotypes studied. The 24 AIDS/ARC patients who were receiving AZT had responses in antibody titer that were not significantly different from the responses of asymptomatic HIV-infected controls, who had a median CD4 count of 510. Although this study was not prospective, blinded, nor randomized, it does suggest that the improvement in cell-mediated immune response that has been demonstrated with AZT therapy also may apply to the antibody response to pneumococcal antigens.[43]

HIV-infected persons should receive 23-valent pneumococcal vaccine as soon as HIV infection is identified.[45] If immune deficiency exists (CD4 count <500 cells/mm³) and antiretroviral therapy will be started soon, a delay of 6 to 8 weeks after beginning anti-HIV therapy may improve the antibody response to pneumococcal vaccine. As in transplant recipients, a booster dose of pneumococcal vaccine after 6 years may be considered.[45] Consideration should be given to immunizing HIV-seronegative persons who are at increased risk for HIV infection and pneumonias, such as injection drug users. These persons would be able to mount anamnestic responses in the future, even if they became immunocompromised.

## Haemophilus influenzae Vaccine

Although the serotypes of H. influenzae infections in HIV-infected adult patients have not been well studied, at least some of the cases are reported as type B and may be prevented by the use of H. influenzae type B polysaccharide vaccine. An extensive study of antibody responses to H. influenzae type B vaccines was performed in HIV-infected men by Steinhoff and associates. They compared a T-cell–independent vaccine, prepared from the bacterial capsular polysaccharide polyribosylribitol phosphate (PRP), with a T-cell–dependent vaccine in which the PRP polysaccharide was conjugated with a protein derived from mutant diphtheria toxin (PRP-CRM). Both of these vaccines are licensed for use in the United States. The researchers found that the response to the unconjugated PRP (T-cell–independent) vaccine was similar in all of the subjects, regardless of their level of immune suppression. However, in normal control subjects and HIV-infected men without AIDS, the researchers reproduced the previously reported superior immunogenicity of the T-cell–dependent protein conjugated vaccine, PRP-CRM. The superiority of this vaccine was lost in HIV-infected patients with severe immunodeficiency (ie, patients with AIDS). Antibody levels induced by PRP-CRM usually were lower in HIV-infected patients with CD4 counts below 200/mm³. The investigators also demonstrated an anamnestic response with the conjugated vaccine in patients who had preexisting detectable antibody to the diphtheria toxoid carrier protein.[37]

The Immunization Practices Advisory Committee of the CDC suggests that immunization with H. influenzae type B vaccine in HIV-infected adults "might be considered."[46] The equivocation is in part due to the lack of knowledge about the prevalence of type B H. influenzae in this population. If immunization for H. influenzae type B is to be undertaken, the conjugated vaccine (PRP-CRM) would be the appropriate agent in HIV-positive patients who are not severely immunocompromised (eg, those with CD4 counts >200/mm³). For those with more severe immune deficiency (CD4 count <200/mm³), the unconjugated vaccine (PRP) would be a more appropriate choice.

## Tuberculosis Vaccine

Because bacille Calmette-Guérin (BCG) vaccine contains live attenuated Mycobacterium bovis, administration of

BCG should be avoided by HIV-infected patients, even if measures of immune function are normal. Some HIV-positive patients have had local suppurative adenopathy or disseminated "BCG-osis" after administration of BCG vaccine.[47–50] Some of these patients have developed disease from BCG months or years after the vaccination, suggesting that BCG infection can be reactivated if the immune system fails.[49–51]

In areas where TB is a major health problem, such as sub-Saharan Africa and Asia, the risk of TB may outweigh the risk of disease caused by BCG. In these situations, it may be prudent to continue with BCG vaccination programs even in asymptomatic patients with HIV infection.[47, 52]

## PREVENTIVE DRUG THERAPY

The term prophylactic therapy usually implies administration of a drug to prevent the acquisition of infection, but it is sometimes used to refer to treatment of a patient with subclinical infection in an attempt to prevent the infection from progressing to clinical disease. Penicillin given to prevent streptococcal infection falls into the first category, and isoniazid to prevent clinical TB falls into the second. In some cases, the relationship between host and pathogen is unknown, as with *P. carinii* prophylaxis. In this chapter, the terms preventive drug therapy and prophylaxis are used interchangeably.

### *Pneumocystis carinii* Prophylaxis

The mortality rate for all episodes of PCP in AIDS patients is about 10% to 20%, with a range of 5% to 95%. The highest rates have been reported for patients with respiratory failure and recurrent episodes. Advances in the diagnosis and management of PCP have improved the outcome of moderate to severe disease and recurrent disease, independently of the introduction of prophylactic treatment.[1, 5, 7, 53, 54]

Several studies have demonstrated the beneficial effect of PCP prophylaxis on slowing the progression of AIDS. Graham and colleagues reviewed 2512 cases of HIV-seropositive men in the U.S. Multicenter AIDS Cohort Study. The period of this study, 1986 to 1990, includes the years before and after the widespread introduction of prophylactic measures to prevent *Pneumocystis* pneumonia in the United States. Comparing the patients who received PCP prophylaxis with those who did not, the investigators demonstrated that the use of PCP prophylaxis significantly reduced the incidence of PCP in the cohort. The PCP reduction was most apparent in those who had reduced numbers of CD4 lymphocytes at the time of study entry. Overall, the relative risk of developing PCP for patients receiving prophylaxis was one quarter of the risk for comparable subjects who were not receiving PCP prophylaxis during the 24 months each subject was followed. The effect of PCP prophylaxis on reducing the incidence of PCP in this group was independent of the effect of AZT in reducing the overall incidence of AIDS.[3]

The efficacy of *P. carinii* prophylaxis was also demonstrated in Amsterdam by Bindels and coworkers. In a retrospective review of patients who survived their first episode of *Pneumocystis* pneumonia, the researchers were able to show an improved survival rate after the introduction of secondary *Pneumocystis* prophylaxis in 1985, several years before AZT became available. The improved survival was attributed to a reduced incidence of *Pneumocystis* pneumonia.[55]

In a study of AIDS patients receiving chemotherapy for Kaposi sarcoma, Fischl and colleagues showed that prophylaxis reduced the incidence of *Pneumocystis* pneumonia and prolonged survival. No antiviral agents were available for these patients, who were studied in 1984 and 1985.[56]

A large, multicenter study conducted by the AIDS Clinical Trials Group compared two forms of *Pneumocystis* prophylaxis in 310 patients who had survived their first episode of PCP and were also taking AZT. During the next 2 years, only 16% of subjects had recurrent episodes of PCP, in contrast to an expected relapse rate of 60%. Only 10% died of their second episodes of PCP. This and other studies show that *Pneumocystis* pneumonia is now an uncommon cause of death in AIDS patients receiving prophylaxis.[2, 4, 6]

In patients with HIV infection, there is a clear correlation between the level of immunosuppression and the incidence of PCP. The Public Health Service (PHS) has twice convened a task force to determine recommendations for PCP prophylaxis. The advice of the task force has been that PCP prophylaxis should be offered to patients after their peripheral blood CD4 count approaches 200 cells/mm$^3$.[57] The PHS task force also recommends *P. carinii* prophylaxis if patients with higher CD4 counts have thrush or unexplained fever, because these patients have a higher risk for the subsequent development of PCP.[25, 31] This strategy reaches most HIV-infected patients with increased risk of PCP, although 5% to 10% of AIDS patients who develop PCP have CD4 counts greater than 200/mm$^3$. Because some patients with HIV infection have rapidly deteriorating cellular immunity and CD4 counts, regular determinations of CD4 count are recommended to identify those who fall into the range for prophylaxis recommendations. An HIV-infected person with a CD4 count below 500 cells/mm$^3$ who is not receiving PCP prophylaxis should have CD4 counts measured every 3 months.[57]

### Trimethoprim-Sulfamethoxazole

In the mid-1970s, the combination of trimethoprim and sulfamethoxazole (Co-trimoxazole) was demonstrated to be effective for the treatment and prevention of *P. carinii* in children with lymphocytic leukemia.[58, 59] In AIDS patients, it has been demonstrated to be more effective than aerosolized pentamidine, and it may have the added benefit of preventing bacterial infections and cerebral toxoplasmosis in these patients.[4, 60, 61] The most common treatment-limiting adverse events are rash and fever. Although the incidence of these complications among non-HIV–infected patients is relatively low (3%–5%), it is quite high among those with HIV infection, requiring cessation of therapy in 25% to 30% of HIV-infected patients who receive the drug.[4, 56, 61] Interstitial nephritis, hemolytic anemia, thrombocytopenia, neutropenia, hepatitis, interstitial pneumonitis, and Stevens-Johnson syndrome have been reported with this drug combination. Most investigators think that the sulfamethoxazole component is more frequently the cause of these reactions, but allergic reactions and bone marrow suppression caused by trimethoprim have also been reported.

Dosage regimens of the trimethoprim-sulfamethoxazole combination have not been completely defined. In adults with HIV infection, the most commonly prescribed dose is one double-strength tablet (160 mg of trimethoprim plus 800 mg of sulfamethoxazole) daily. This dose has been shown to be almost 100% effective in several clinical trials, and it is the dose recommended by the PHS Task Force on *Pneumocystis* Prophylaxis.[57] A Dutch study showed that a single-strength tablet (80 mg of trimethoprim and 400 mg of sulfamethoxazole) was equally effective and had a lower rate of side effects.[61] Even lower doses of trimethoprim-sulfamethoxazole (one double-strength tablet three times each week) have been shown to be effective in uncontrolled studies, but these doses have not been subjected to randomized comparative trials.[62, 63]

## Pentamidine

Intravenous pentamidine was the first drug shown to be effective for the treatment of active PCP. Because of the toxicity of the drug and the requirement for parenteral administration, pentamidine was not widely used for prophylaxis in the pre-AIDS era. Later, the high frequency of intolerance to trimethoprim-sulfamethoxazole and the fact that *P. carinii* is primarily a pulmonary infection led to the use of inhaled aerosolized pentamidine for PCP prophylaxis. Early investigators studied dose, frequency of delivery, and type of nebulizer required to deliver the proper particle size for deposition of pentamidine in the alveoli.[64–66]

The largest studies have been done with the Respigard II nebulizer (Marquest, Englewood, CO) and the Fisoneb nebulizer (Fisons Corp., Rochester, NY). The Respigard II is disposable and requires a compressed air source to generate an aerosol with predominance of particles 0.5 to 2 μm in diameter. The patient inhales the generated aerosol for 15 to 30 minutes, during which time about 10% of the aerosolized pentamidine is deposited in the alveoli of the lungs. The Fisoneb apparatus is an ultrasonic nebulizer and requires a larger initial cash outlay, but it does not require a compressed air source and uses less pentamidine to deliver a similar dose to the lung. The two devices have not been directly compared, but they appear to be roughly equivalent in ability to prevent PCP.

Results of studies of aerosol deposition in various patient positions and with various breathing techniques have been inconsistent. One study demonstrated no differences in regional deposition of pentamidine in patients treated in the sitting position only.[67] Patients with abnormal lungs, such as those with emphysema or restrictive lung disease, may have incomplete distribution of the pentamidine.

The adverse effects of aerosolized pentamidine include cough and bronchospasm, which are usually effectively managed by pretreatment with an inhaled bronchodilator. Because pentamidine delivery is limited to the lung and very little drug is absorbed, systemic toxicity has not been a problem.

Complete studies for determining the range of effective doses of aerosolized pentamidine have not been done. How-

ever, the current recommended dosage of 300 mg of pentamidine administered with the Respigard II nebulizer every 4 weeks has been shown to be more effective than lower doses.[65] Whether higher doses or more frequent administration of aerosol would be more effective has not been completely studied, nor have other nebulizers been compared with the Respigard II.

Aerosolized pentamidine delivered by the Respigard II nebulizer at a dose of 300 mg every 4 weeks was prospectively compared with a regimen of one double-strength trimethoprim-sulfamethoxazole tablet per day in adult AIDS patients who had recovered from their first episode of PCP. Treatment at this stage is referred to as secondary prophylaxis; primary prophylaxis is the delivery of prophylactic treatment before an episode of PCP. Several important findings resulted from this large, multicenter study. The major finding was that aerosolized pentamidine delivered in this fashion was less effective than trimethoprim-sulfamethoxazole, with an estimated recurrence rate of 27.6% at 18 months, compared with 11.4% for those randomized to trimethoprim-sulfamethoxazole.[4] Almost all of the *Pneumocystis* pneumonia episodes in the patients randomized to trimethoprim-sulfamethoxazole occurred after they stopped taking the drug; most had been switched over to pentamidine because of trimethoprim-sulfamethoxazole intolerance.

In this study, aerosolized pentamidine was less toxic and better tolerated. Because the yearly incidence of recurrent *Pneumocystis* pneumonia in AIDS patients receiving AZT without prophylaxis is approximately 60%,[2] aerosolized pentamidine is clearly an effective means of *Pneumocystis* prophylaxis, although less effective than trimethoprim-sulfamethoxazole. It is also more expensive. Daily trimethoprim-sulfamethoxazole remains the first choice in therapy for *Pneumocystis* prevention. However, aerosolized pentamidine is an effective alternative choice and should be provided for patients with a high risk of developing PCP who cannot tolerate trimethoprim-sulfamethoxazole.[7, 57]

Parenteral pentamidine has been used as a prophylactic agent, usually given as one intramuscular or intravenous dose monthly. The side effects of systemic pentamidine, such as altered renal function and β-cell pancreatic toxicity, are of concern with long-term parenteral pentamidine.[68, 69] This regimen has not been studied in large comparative trials, and its relative efficacy and toxicity are unknown.

There have been reports that the administration of aerosolized pentamidine for prophylaxis can alter the pattern of subsequent PCP such that upper lobe disease is more prominent on chest radiograph. However, the severity of disease is not different in patients receiving aerosolized pentamidine prophylaxis.[70, 71] Although earlier studies reported that the diagnostic yield of bronchoalveolar lavage was reduced in patients receiving aerosolized pentamidine, later studies did not support this finding.[71, 72] Baughman and colleagues demonstrated by differential lavage that *P. carinii* has a predilection for the upper lobes regardless of whether the patient is receiving aerosol prophylaxis.[73]

## Dapsone-Containing Regimens

Dapsone, a sulfone, is active against *Pneumocystis* in animal models, and in combination with trimethoprim, it is an effective agent for the treatment of PCP.[73] Some unpublished reports and small series have suggested that dapsone is useful for the prevention of PCP, alone or in combination with pyrimethamine or trimethoprim.[74–77] The doses and dosing intervals in these studies varied widely. In a randomized, prospective comparison with aerosolized pentamidine, 100 mg dapsone administered twice weekly resulted in a PCP incidence of 18% during a median follow-up period of 18 months. This rate was similar to the 17% incidence in the pentamidine group, but this study was not statistically significant.[77] The PHS *Pneumocystis* Task Force made no recommendations for the use of dapsone for *Pneumocystis* prevention, because no comparative trials of sufficient size had then been reported. A large, multicenter trial comparing dapsone, trimethoprim-sulfamethoxazole, and aerosolized pentamidine for primary *Pneumocystis* prophylaxis has been in progress since 1989 (ie, ACTG 081), and results should become available in 1993.

The most common dapsone toxicity is hemolysis. This can be particularly severe in patients with glucose-6-phosphate dehydrogenase (G6PD) deficiency, and most studies evaluating its use have screened for and excluded subjects with G6PD deficiency. If future studies show reasonable efficacy of dapsone for *P. carinii* prophylaxis, the results will only be applicable to patients with normal G6PD levels, and screening for G6PD deficiency will be necessary before administration of dapsone for prophylaxis.

HIV-infected patients with a previous episode of PCP, a peripheral blood CD4 count less than 200 cells/mm$^3$, or the presence of thrush or unexplained fever should be prescribed trimethoprim-sulfamethoxazole (one double-strength tablet per day), indefinitely.[57] Patients who cannot tolerate trimethoprim-sulfamethoxazole should be prescribed aerosolized pentamidine (300 mg every 4 weeks using the Respigard II nebulizer or 60 mg every 2 weeks using the Fisoneb nebulizer). Proper instruction in the use of the nebulizer is important, and pretreatment with a rapid-onset inhaled bronchodilator, such as metaproterenol, may be required to prevent bronchospasm.[57, 65, 66]

All patients should be fully evaluated for TB before aerosolized pentamidine is given. Treatment should be administered in a negative-pressure, closed room with outside exhaust, or in a booth ventilated to the outside or with a high-efficiency filtered exhaust. Personnel entering the room should wear a tight-fitting face mask designed to filter particles 1 to 3 μm in diameter, which can prevent TB exposure and repeated inhalation of pentamidine.[78] Dapsone (100 mg twice weekly) may be an equivalent alternative to aerosolized pentamidine, but data are not yet available to make a complete comparison between the two.[77]

## Tuberculosis Prophylaxis

### Identification of Patients With Mycobacterium tuberculosis Infection

Patients with HIV infection are less likely to have a diagnostic reaction to intradermal 5 TU tuberculin purified protein derivative (PPD), and the likelihood of a false-negative result is increased in patients with more advanced HIV disease. A reaction of 5 mm of induration or more is considered by the CDC to be positive for patients coin-

fected with HIV.[78–80] Graham and coworkers have shown that induration of 2 mm or more may be the most appropriate definition of a positive PPD reaction in HIV-infected persons.[81] Because patients with immune deficiency have a reduced reactivity to PPD, a careful history of prior skin test reaction and TB exposure should also be obtained. If patients have had extended or intimate exposure to an active TB case and have a negative PPD associated with cutaneous anergy, they should be considered possibly infected and prescribed preventive therapy.[78, 82]

### Exclusion of Active Tuberculosis

A chest radiograph to exclude active TB should be obtained for all HIV-positive persons with reactive PPD and all skin test-negative persons with associated cutaneous anergy or laboratory evidence of immune deficiency (eg, peripheral blood CD4 count <500/mm$^3$). Those with exposure to known cases of active TB should be evaluated with a chest radiograph regardless of skin test or immune status. All HIV-positive persons with chest radiograph abnormalities attributed to other pulmonary diseases should also be evaluated for TB with acid-fast bacilli (AFB) smears and cultures of sputum or respiratory secretions, because simultaneous opportunistic infections are common in HIV-infected patients, and radiographic findings of TB may be atypical in this population.[83]

### Evaluation of the Risk of Developing Active Tuberculosis

The likelihood of developing active TB is considerably higher in persons coinfected with HIV and *M. tuberculosis.* For example, 38% of HIV-infected persons exposed in a San Francisco TB outbreak developed active TB within 4 months, but the expected rate for the normal population was 5% to 10% over 2 years.[15] Coinfection with HIV renders a person infected with *M. tuberculosis* 10 times more likely to develop active disease than persons with other immunocompromising conditions and 100 times more likely than a PPD-positive person with no other risk factors for TB progression.[17, 84, 85]

### Selection of a Preventive Drug Regimen

The efficacy of isoniazid for prevention of active TB has been well established. Most of the studies have been conducted in normal populations, but one study in Zambia showed that isoniazid prophylaxis for patients coinfected with HIV and *M. tuberculosis* was effective in reducing the rate of active disease by 87% compared with placebo.[82, 86] If the infecting strain of *M. tuberculosis* is known to be resistant to isoniazid but sensitive to rifampin, rifampin is recommended as preventive therapy, but an appropriate preventive therapy for multidrug-resistant TB has not been determined. In these cases, the susceptibility pattern of the organism with which the patient is presumed to be infected must be weighed against the side effects of the available drugs.[17] Even in an area with a high rate of multidrug-resistant TB, isoniazid prophylaxis is appropriate for patients with positive skin tests and unknown exposure histories, because isoniazid-sensitive TB is still common in these areas.[17, 87]

### Appropriate Follow-up

The recommended duration of isoniazid preventive therapy is 12 months in persons coinfected with HIV, rather than 6 months as now recommended for persons with no other risk factors for the development of active TB. During this period, it is extremely important to ensure compliance with the treatment regimen. If the patient is unlikely to be compliant (eg, the patient is homeless), directly observed prophylaxis should be considered.[88]

Before beginning preventive treatment for TB the presence of active disease should be excluded with appropriate clinical examinations and chest radiographs. All HIV-infected patients who have been infected with *M. tuberculosis* at any time should receive preventive therapy with isoniazid (300 mg daily for 1 year). A directly observed dose of 15 mg/kg of body weight twice weekly for 1 year is an alternative for potentially noncompliant patients.[78, 82, 88] Immunodeficient HIV-infected patients (anergic or CD4 count $<500/mm^3$) without evidence of *M. tuberculosis* infection but with significant history of exposure to active cases should also receive isoniazid for 1 year.[78]

Patients with significant exposure to isoniazid-resistant, rifampin-sensitive TB cases should receive rifampin (10 mg/kg/d; maximum, 600 mg) for 1 year, daily or twice weekly in a directly observed preventive therapy program.[17] HIV-infected patients who are possibly infected with multidrug–resistant *M. tuberculosis* should receive preventive therapy with specially designed multidrug regimens, depending on the likely susceptibility pattern of the infecting organism.[17] HIV-infected patients should be evaluated for active TB each time they have pulmonary disease, even if another etiologic agent is present.

### Influenza Virus A Prophylaxis

Two oral antiviral agents, amantadine and rimantadine, are effective in the prophylaxis and treatment of all strains of influenza A. Only amantadine has been licensed for use in the United States. Amantadine interferes with viral replication, and if given prophylactically, it can prevent 70% to 90% of influenza A infections. It is not active against influenza B. Amantadine can also ameliorate the symptoms of influenza A if it is started within 24 to 48 hours of the onset of disease. Amantadine does not interfere with antibody responses to influenza vaccine.[41, 89]

Patients taking amantadine have experienced several side effects, most of which are mild. Nausea, vomiting, or loss of appetite occurs in about 5% of patients. Central nervous systems side effects occur in about 7%; these consist of nervousness, lightheadedness, insomnia, and difficulty concentrating. These side effects diminish with continued use of the drug and, in one study, did not affect psychomotor or academic performance.[90] Amantadine is excreted unchanged by the kidneys and is not removed by hemodialysis. Patients with renal failure require dosage adjustments.[91]

Amantadine-resistant influenza A virus has been docu-

mented, usually after prolonged use of the drug. Resistant viruses can be transmitted and do cause disease.[92]

During a community outbreak of influenza A, amantadine (100 mg twice daily) should be given to HIV-infected patients who have not received influenza vaccine. The dosage can be reduced to 100 mg daily if side effects occur. Amantadine is not effective against influenza B. To prevent institution-centered outbreaks, amantadine should be offered to unvaccinated health care workers during an influenza A outbreak at the same time that the currently formulated vaccine is administered. The amantadine can be discontinued 2 to 3 weeks after the administration of vaccine.

Immunocompromised HIV-infected patients (those with ARC, AIDS, or moderate to severe depression of CD4 count) should be considered candidates for amantadine therapy during influenza A outbreaks, even if they have received influenza vaccine. Patients who develop influenza symptoms during an influenza outbreak should be treated with amantadine if it can be started within 48 hours of the onset of symptoms. Amantadine and rimantadine appear to be equally effective.[89]

### Pneumococcal Prophylaxis

The chronic administration of antibiotics for the prevention of pneumonia has not been generally recommended, because the incidence of untoward effects and drug resistance exceed the risk of pneumonia. In populations with an exceptional risk for a pneumococcal pneumonia, such as South African miners, prophylactic antibiotics sometimes have been recommended. The incidence of bacterial pneumonia in AIDS patients does not justify the widespread use of prophylactic antibiotics. However, in a large trial comparing trimethoprim-sulfamethoxazole with aerosolized pentamidine for *P. carinii* prophylaxis, the total incidence of bacterial infections was lower and the onset to first bacterial infection was delayed in those taking the systemic antibiotic. No details were given about the types of infection prevented or the pathogens involved.[4]

In AIDS patients with frequent recurrences of documented pneumococcal pneumonia, long-term antibiotic suppression with penicillin V may be considered. The selection of penicillin-resistant organisms and the risk of penicillin allergy must be considered.

## ISOLATION OF HIV-INFECTED PATIENTS WITH RESPIRATORY INFECTIONS

Many of the opportunistic infections associated with AIDS are characterized by low virulence, and they are often the result of reactivation of endogenous pathogens. Most of these pathogens are not considered transmissible from person to person and do not require isolation of patients infected with them. Examples of this group are cytomegalovirus, *Histoplasma, Candida albicans,* and *M. avium.* The risk of person-to-person spread of *P. carinii, H. influenzae,* and *S. pneumoniae* is low or unknown.

*M. tuberculosis,* is spread only by personal contact. Coinfection with HIV and *M. tuberculosis* is in large part responsible for the increasing incidence of TB in the United States. Respiratory precautions directed at *M. tuberculosis* would also be effective against other respiratory pathogens that might be transmitted, with possible exception of viral influenza. Isolation procedures for TB patients are outlined in Chapter 38; here we review special considerations for HIV-infected patients.

## Tuberculosis

TB is spread by droplet nuclei that are small enough to remain suspended in the air for long periods. The keys to protecting other patients or health care personnel are to reduce the generation of these particles, exhaust the air containing droplet nuclei, and prevent the breathing of air containing droplet nuclei.[93] Methods are the same for TB patients with and without HIV coinfection. The major difference for HIV-infected persons is in recognizing the patient who requires isolation procedures.

The drawbacks of relying on skin test reactivity to identify patients infected with *M. tuberculosis* have been previously discussed. Unlike TB patients from the general population, who often develop TB by reactivation of an old infection, many AIDS patients with TB are newly infected and have progressive primary disease rather than reactivation cavitary disease. A history of positive skin tests or remote TB exposure is less common for AIDS patients, but a recent TB exposure may be more common. HIV-TB coinfected persons are unusually susceptible to acquiring new exogenous TB infection. Although they already have TB, they are always at risk for newly acquired TB infection.[94] The clinical presentation of AIDS patients with TB may be atypical, with diffuse or lower lobe infiltrates without cavities. The absence of classic disease may lead to failure to recognize TB. HIV-infected patients with TB may also have other pulmonary pathogens, such as *P. carinii*, cytomegalovirus, or *Histoplasma*. The recognition of another pulmonary pathogen does not exclude the possibility of TB.

Evaluation for TB should be carried out for all AIDS patients admitted to the hospital with respiratory syndromes. AIDS patients with respiratory infections who are admitted to the hospital should be placed in negative-pressure private rooms with outside exhaust if TB cannot be satisfactorily excluded. Patients who have had previous negative evaluations for TB and have no history of TB exposure since that evaluation may not require TB isolation.[17, 19] Three sputum specimens, expectorated or induced, with negative AFB stain results permit removing a patient from respiratory isolation. A negative AFB smear of bronchial secretions obtained by bronchoscopy is sufficient to remove a patient from respiratory isolation. Patients with multidrug-resistant TB should be continued in respiratory isolation for the duration of their hospitalization.

## Pneumocystis carinii

The ability to reduce exposure of HIV-infected patients to *P. carinii* is limited because of poor understanding of the epidemiology of this infection. Because the organism cannot be consistently cultured, studies to identify the natural reservoir have not been done. It is clear that the organism is ubiquitous in the environment of young children, because most humans have developed antibody to the organism by the time they are 4 years of age.[95–97] *P. carinii* is found worldwide, as evidenced by serosurveys of persons from different continents. Smulian and associates have demonstrated that the organism is common around the world and that there may be strain differences in *P. carinii* isolated from different continents. Using Western blot analysis of multiple *P. carinii* antigens, the investigators showed that antigen recognition patterns differed in serum specimens collected from different continents. However, the prevalence of anti-*Pneumocystis* antibody approached 80% of all sera tested.[97]

*P. carinii* is acquired through the respiratory route. Although there may be some differences between human and animal *P. carinii*, animal studies have shown that uninfected immunosuppressed rat colonies can be infected by noncontact exposure to infected colonies, suggesting an airborne route of transmission.[98] These experiments did not demonstrate whether transmission was directly animal to animal or occurred through a secondary environmental stage, as occurs with dimorphic fungi.

The mechanism of development of PCP may be reactivation of dormant pulmonary infection acquired years earlier. Observations supporting this hypothesis include the fact that isolated immunosuppressed animals develop PCP; human cases have most often been sporadic; and patient-to-patient transmission has not been recognized in epidemiologic studies. On the other hand, the apparently ubiquitous nature of the organism, the failure to demonstrate an endogenous reservoir of the organism in autopsy lungs, and a few apparent outbreaks of *Pneumocystis* infection in humans suggest that reinfection may be the origin of many cases of PCP. The pathology of PCP shows an intraalveolar, extracellular infection, unlike the interstitial, intracellular pattern seen in most long-term pulmonary infections with dormant or inactive states. None of the reports sheds light on the distinction between an environmental or human reservoir as the source of *Pneumocystis*, making strategies to prevent exposure difficult to design.[99–102] Walzer[15] reviewed the limited evidence available for person-to-person spread and recommended isolation of immunocompromised patients with *P. carinii* infection from other immunocompromised patients on the basis of the case clustering which has been reported.[103]

Because PCP in AIDS patients often is accompanied by bacterial, fungal, or viral infection, respiratory isolation is prudent until transmissible agents, such as *M. tuberculosis*, can be ruled out. No isolation procedures are required to prevent PCP transmission to hospital personnel or other patients with normal immunity. The policies and procedures for administering aerosolized pentamidine, which are designed to prevent transmission of TB in the clinic, should be adequate for any potential transmission of *P. carinii*.

## Bacterial Pneumonia

Pneumococcal and *H. influenzae* pneumonias are endogenous infections of the airways. Pneumonia occurs in patients previously colonized by these agents, but colonization without disease is common in the general population. Colonization rates are higher in children than adults and more common in crowded conditions, such as military camps and institutional housing.[104, 105] However, epidemics caused by *S. pneumoniae* and *H. influenzae* pneumonia are rare. Colonization by *S. pneumoniae* is not prevented by the presence of type-specific antibody to the colonizing strain. There is no recommendation for isolation of patients with pneumococcal infection in the community or in the hospital.

### Viral Influenza

During influenza outbreaks in a community, virtually all persons are exposed during the 4 to 8 weeks that an epidemic lasts. Avoidance of exposure is difficult and would require reclusive avoidance of human contact for the duration of the influenza season (approximately 6 months). Influenza outbreaks in institutions such as hospitals have been well documented. Although these outbreaks can be devastating to hospitalized patients, monitoring for outbreaks and isolation of patients is neither practical nor likely to interrupt transmission, because persons infected with an influenza virus are most infectious before the onset of symptoms.[106]

## DISEASE PREVENTION AMONG HEALTH CARE STAFF

Health care workers have been vectors for the transmission of TB and viral influenza in hospital outbreaks among patients. Vigorous control programs for these infections in health care workers are appropriate to protect the workers and the patients.

### Tuberculosis

In addition to isolation procedures, an active program of surveillance for TB is appropriate to protect the health care workers and monitor for hospital outbreaks of TB. Because immunodeficient AIDS patients often do not respond to PPD testing, testing of the health care worker population is useful for monitoring TB activity in the HIV-infected patients they care for. A skin test program is also a measure of the adequacy of TB control policies and procedures. Investigations of several hospital outbreaks indicated serious deficiencies in TB control measures.[107, 108] HIV-infected patients with respiratory syndromes in whom TB has not been excluded should be promptly isolated in a room with proper air control.

The CDC and the National Institute for Occupational Safety and Health have proposed specific masking procedures for different levels of potential TB exposure. These recommendations are strict and expensive.[93, 109] Nevertheless, a tight-fitting particulate mask designed to filter particles of 1 to 2 μm in diameter should be worn at all times by personnel entering respiratory isolation rooms and during procedures likely to produce cough.[78]

Health care workers involved in the care of HIV-infected

patients should be given an intradermal tuberculin test at least every 6 months. In hospital units with a high incidence of TB cases, multidrug resistance, noncompliant patients, or inadequate air handling facilities, the frequency of testing should be increased to every 3 months.[17, 79] A reaction of 5 mm of induration in a health care worker previously known to be negative is considered a conversion.[78, 79] All skin test-positive persons should be examined by chest radiographs at the time of the initial positive test result. Routine follow-up radiographs are not indicated, but the possibility of reactivation TB must be considered if symptoms consistent with TB occur. Health care workers with positive skin tests and no evidence of active disease should be considered candidates for isoniazid prophylaxis according to the CDC guidelines.[78]

### Viral Influenza

Several outbreaks of influenza in health care settings have involved health care workers as vectors of disease. The CDC recommends that regular immunization of health care workers be undertaken to minimize this phenomenon.[41, 45] Health care workers are more likely to develop protective antibody than their HIV-infected patients, and this may protect patients from transmission in the health care setting. In one hospital-associated outbreak, an immunization program directed at the physician and nursing staff was credited with controlling the outbreak, although the contribution of the immunization program was hard to substantiate.[106]

Health care workers, regardless of the level of patient contact, should receive yearly influenza vaccine.[41] During an influenza A outbreak, nonimmunized personnel should be offered amantadine prophylaxis and vaccine. The amantadine can be stopped after 2 weeks, after which a vaccine response should be expected.

## ACKNOWLEDGMENT

The authors are grateful for the patience and skill of Angela Birch Smith, who prepared the manuscript.

## REFERENCES

1. Dohn MN, Baughman RP, Vigdorth EM, et al: Equal survival rates for first, second, and third episodes of *Pneumocystis carinii* pneumonia in patients with acquired immunodeficiency syndrome. Arch Intern Med 152:2465, 1992.
2. Fischl MA, Parker CB, Pettinelli C, et al: A randomized controlled trial of reduced daily dose of zidovudine in patients with the acquired immunodeficiency syndrome. N Engl J Med 323:1010, 1990.
3. Graham NMH, Zeger SL, Park LP, et al: Effect of zidovudine and *Pneumocystis carinii* prophylaxis on progression of HIV-1 infection to AIDS. Lancet 338:265, 1991.
4. Hardy WD, Feinberg J, Finkelstein DM, et al: A controlled trial of trimethoprim-sulfamethoxazole or aerosolized pentamidine for secondary prophylaxis of *Pneumocystis carinii* pneumonia in patients with the acquired immunodeficiency syndrome. N Engl J Med 327:1842, 1992.
5. Brenner M, Ognibene FP, Lack EE, et al: Prognostic factors and life expectancy of patients with acquired immunodeficiency syndrome and *Pneumocystis carinii* pneumonia. Am Rev Respir Dis 136:1199, 1987.

6. Yarchoan R, Venzon DJ, Pluda JM, et al: CD4 count and the risk for death in patients infected with HIV receiving antiretroviral therapy. Ann Intern Med 115:184, 1991.

7. Mazur H: Prevention and treatment of *Pneumocystis* pneumonia. N Engl J Med 327:1853, 1992.

8. Centers for Disease Control: 1993 Revised classification system for HIV infection and expanded surveillance case definition for AIDS among adolescents and adults. MMWR 41(RR-17):1–19, 1992.

9. Simberkoff MS, El Sadr W, Schiffman G, et al: *Streptococcus pneumoniae* infections and bacteremia in patients with acquired immune deficiency syndrome, with report of a pneumococcal vaccine failure. Am Rev Respir Dis 130:1174, 1984.

10. Polsky B, Gold JWM, Whimbey E, et al: Bacterial pneumonia in patients with the acquired immunodeficiency syndrome. Ann Intern Med 104:38, 1986.

11. Witt DJ, Craven DE, McCabe WR: Bacterial infections in adult patients with the acquired immune deficiency syndrome (AIDS) and AIDS-related complex. Am J Med 82:900, 1987.

12. Centers for Disease Control: Increase in pneumonia mortality among young adults and the HIV epidemic—New York City, United States. MMWR 37:593, 1988.

13. Redd SC, Rutherford GW III, Sandy MA, et al: The role of human immunodeficiency virus infection in pneumococcal bacteremia in San Francisco residents. J Infect Dis 162:1012, 1990.

14. Rodriguez-Barradas MC, Musher DM, Ha RJ, et al: Unusual manifestations of pneumococcal infection in human immunodeficiency virus infected individuals: The past revisited. Clin Infect Dis, 14:192, 1992.

15. Daley CL, Small PM, Schecter GF, et al: An outbreak of tuberculosis with accelerated progression among persons infected with the human immunodeficiency virus. An analysis using restriction length polymorphisms. N Engl J Med 326:231, 1992.

16. Centers for Disease Control: Tuberculosis outbreak among persons in a residential facility for HIV-infected persons—San Francisco. MMWR 40:649, 1991.

17. Centers for Disease Control: Management of persons exposed to multidrug-resistant tuberculosis. MMWR 41:61, 1992.

18. Murray JF: Tuberculosis and human immunodeficiency virus infection during the 1990's. Bull Int Union Tuberc Lung Dis 66:21, 1991.

19. Cohen JP, Macauley C: Susceptibility to influenza A in HIV-positive patients. JAMA 261:245, 1989.

20. Maldarelli F, McPhee J, Ellner P, et al: Influenza in HIV-exposed adults. Clin Res 36:800A, 1988.

21. Safrin S, Rush JD, Mills J: Influenza in patients with human immunodeficiency virus infection. Chest 98:33, 1990.

22. Hirschtick R, Glassroth J, Jordan M, et al: Bacterial pneumonia in patients infected with human immunodeficiency virus. Am Rev Respir Dis 147(suppl 4):1003, 1993.

23. Buskin SE, Hopkins SG, Farizo KM: Heavy smoking increases the risk of *Pneumocystis carinii* pneumonia (PCP). [Abstract WeC 1030] In Program and Abstracts of the Eighth International AIDS Conference, Amsterdam, The Netherlands, July 19–24, 1992.

24. Nieman R, Fleming J, Coker RJ, et al: Cigarette smoking by HIV infected individuals is associated with a more rapid progression to AIDS. In [Abstract PoC4407] Program and Abstracts of the Eighth International AIDS Conference, Amsterdam, The Netherlands, July 19–24, 1992.

24a. Centers for Disease Control: Recommendations for HIV testing services for inpatients and outpatients in acute-care hospital settings and technical guidance on HIV counseling. MMWR 42:1–17, 1993.

25. Fischl MA, Richman DD, Grieco MH, et al: The efficacy of azidothymidine (AZT) in the treatment of patients with AIDS-related complex. N Engl J Med 317:185, 1987.

26. Volberding PA, Lagakos SW, Koch MA, et al: Zidovudine in asymptomatic human immunodeficiency virus infection. N Engl J Med 322:941, 1990.

27. Fischl MA, Richman DD, Hausen N, et al: The safety and efficacy of zidovudine (AZT) in the treatment of subjects with mildly symptomatic known immunodeficiency virus type 1 (HIV) infection. Ann Intern Med 112:727, 1990.

28. Kahn JO, Lagakos SW, Richman DD, et al: A controlled trial comparing continued zidovudine with didanosine in human immunodeficiency virus infection. N Engl J Med 327:581, 1992.

29. Skowron G, Bozette SA, Lim L, et al: Alternating and intermittent regimens of zidovudine and dideoxyinosine in patients with AIDS or AIDS-related complex. Ann Intern Med 118:321, 1993.

30. Stein DS, Korvick JA, Vermund SH: CD4 lymphocyte cell enumeration for prediction of clinical course of human immunodeficiency virus disease: A review. J Infect Dis 165:352, 1992.

31. Phair J, Múnoz A, Detels R, et al: The risk of *Pneumocystis carinii* pneumonia among men infected with human immunodeficiency virus type 1. N Engl J Med 322:161, 1990.

32. National Institute of Allergy and Infectious Disease: Recommendations for zidovudine: Early intervention. JAMA 263:1606–1609, 1990.

33. Morgolick JB, Volkman DJ, Folks TM, et al: Amplification of HTLV-III/LAV infection by antigen-induced activation of T cells and direct suppression by virus of lymphocyte blastogenic responses. J Immunol 138:1719, 1987.

34. Klein RS, Selwyn PA, Maude D, et al: Response to pneumococcal vaccine among asymptomatic heterosexual partners of persons with AIDS and intravenous drug users infected with human immunodeficiency virus. J Infect Dis 160:826, 1989.

35. Huang K-L, Ruben FL, Rinaldo Jr CR, et al: Antibody responses after influenza and pneumococcal immunization in HIV-infected homosexual men. JAMA 257:2047, 1987.

36. Nelson KE, Clements ML, Miotti P, et al: The influence of human immunodeficiency virus (HIV) infection on antibody responses to influenza vaccines. Ann Intern Med 109:383, 1988.

37. Steinhoff MC, Auerbach BS, Nelson KE, et al: Antibody responses to *Haemophilus influenzae* type B vaccines in men with human immunodeficiency virus infection. N Engl J Med 325:1837, 1991.

38. Couch RB, Kasel JA: Immunity to influenza in man. Annu Rev Microbiol 37:529, 1983.

39. Ragni MV, Ruben FL, Winkelstein A, et al: Antibody response to immunization of patients with hemophilia with and without evidence of human immunodeficiency virus (human T-lymphotropic virus type III) infection. J Lab Clin Med 109:545, 1987.

40. Miotti PG, Nelson KE, Dallabetta GA, et al: The influence of HIV infection on antibody responses to a two-dose regimen of influenza vaccine. JAMA 262:779, 1989.

41. Centers for Disease Control: Prevention and control of influenza. Recommendations of the Immunization Practices Advisory Committee (ACIP). MMWR 42(RR-6):1–14, 1993.

42. Rodriguez-Barradas MC, Musher DM, Lahart C, et al: Antibody to capsular polysaccharides of *Streptococcus pneumoniae* after vaccination of human immunodeficiency virus-infected subjects with 23-valent pneumococcal vaccine. J Infect Dis 165:553, 1992.

43. Glaser JB, Volpe S, Aguirre A, et al: Zidovudine improves response to pneumococcal vaccine among persons with AIDS and AIDS-related Complex. J Infect Dis 64:761, 1991.

44. Janoff EN, Douglas Jr JM, Gabriel M, et al: Class-specific antibody response to pneumococcal polysaccharides in men infected with human immunodeficiency virus type 1. J Infect Dis 158:983, 1988.

45. Centers for Disease Control: Recommendations of the Immunization Practices Advisory Committee: Pneumococcal polysaccharide vaccines. MMWR 38:64, 1989.

46. Centers for Disease Control: Recommendations of the Advisory Committee on Immunization Practices (ACIP): Use of vaccines and immune globulins in persons with altered immunocompetence. MMWR 42(RR-4):1–18, 1993.

47. Quinn TC: Interaction of the human immunodeficiency virus and tuberculosis and the implications for BCG vaccination. Rev Infect Dis 2(suppl 2):S379, 1989.

48. Von Reyn CR, Clements CJ, Mann JM: Human immunodeficiency virus infection and routine childhood immunization. Lancet 2:669, 1987.

49. Anonymous: Disseminated *Mycobacterium bovis* infection from BCG vaccination of a patient with acquired immunodeficiency syndrome. MMWR 34:227, 1986.

50. Smith E, Thybo S, Bennedsen J: Infection with *Mycobacterium bovis* in a patient with AIDS. A late complication of BCG vaccination. Scand J Infect Dis 24:109, 1992.

51. Armbruster C, Junker W, Vetter N, et al: Disseminated bacille Calmette-Guérin infection in an AIDS patient 30 years after BCG vaccination. J Infect Dis 162:1216, 1990.

52. Tarantola D, Mann JM: Acquired immunodeficiency syndrome (AIDS) and expanded programmes on immunization. Special Programme on AIDS. Geneva, World Health Organization, 1987.

53. Bozette SA, Sattler FR, Chin J, et al: A controlled trial of early adjunctive treatment with corticosteroids for *Pneumocystis carinii* pneumonia in the acquired immunodeficiency syndrome. N Engl J Med 323:1451, 1990.

54. Montaner JSG, Lawson LM, Levitt N, et al: Corticosteroids prevent early deterioration in patients with moderately severe *Pneumocystis carinii* and the acquired immunodeficiency syndrome (AIDS). Ann Intern Med 113:14, 1990.

55. Bindels PJ, Poos RMJ, Jong JT, et al: Trends in mortality among AIDS patients in Amsterdam, 1982–1988. AIDS 5:853, 1991.

56. Fischl MA, Dickinson GM, La Voie L: Safety and efficacy of sulfamethoxazole and trimethoprim chemoprophylaxis for *Pneumocystis carinii* pneumonia in AIDS. JAMA 259:1185, 1988.

57. U.S. Public Health Service Task Force on Antipneumocystis Prophylaxis for Patients with Human Immunodeficiency Virus Infection: Recommendations for prophylaxis against *Pneumocystis carinii* pneumonia for adults and adolescents infected with human immunodeficiency virus. MMWR 41(RR-4):1–11, 1992.

58. Hughes WT, Kuhn S, Chaudhary S, et al: Successful chemoprophylaxis for *Pneumocystis carinii* pneumonia. N Engl J Med 297:1419, 1977.

59. Hughes WT, McNabb PC, Makres TD, et al: Efficacy of trimethoprim and sulfamethoxazole in the prevention and treatment of *Pneumocystis carinii* pneumonia. Antimicrob Agents Chemother 5:289, 1974.

60. Heald A, Flepp M, Chave J-P, et al: Treatment for cerebral toxoplasmosis protects against *Pneumocystis carinii* pneumonia in patients with AIDS. Ann Intern Med 115:760, 1991.

61. Schneider MME, Hoepelman AIM, Schattenkerk JKME, et al: A controlled trial of aerosolized pentamidine or trimethoprim-sulfamethoxazole as primary prophylaxis against *Pneumocystis carinii* pneumonia in patients with human immunodeficiency virus infection. N Engl J Med 327:1836, 1992.

62. Wormser GP, Horowitz HW, Duncanson FP et al: Low-dose intermittent trimethoprim-sulfamethoxazole for prevention of *Pneumocystis carinii* pneumonia in patients with human immunodeficiency virus infection. Arch Intern Med 151:688, 1991.

63. Ruskin J, LaRiviere M: Low-dose co-trimoxazole for prevention of *Pneumocystis carinii* pneumonia in human immunodeficiency virus disease. Lancet 337:468, 1991.

64. Golden JA, Chernoff D, Hallander H, et al: Prevention of *Pneumocystis carinii* pneumonia by inhaled pentamidine. Lancet 1:654, 1989.

65. Leoung GS, Feigal Jr, DW, Montgomery AB, et al: Aerosolized pentamidine prophylaxis following *Pneumocystis carinii* pneumonia in AIDS patients: The San Francisco Community Prophylaxis trial. N Engl J Med 323:769, 1990.

66. Montaner JSG, Lawson LM, Gervais A, et al: AIDS related *Pneumocystis carinii* pneumonia. Ann Intern Med 114:948, 1991.

67. O'Riordan T, Baughman R, Dohn M, et al: Lobar pentamidine levels and *Pneumocystis carinii* pneumonia following aerosolized pentamidine. Chest (in press).

68. Karaffa C, Rehm S, Calabrese L: Efficacy of monthly pentamidine infusions in preventing recurrent *Pneumocystis carinii* pneumonia (PCP) in the AIDS patient. [Abstract 690] Program and Abstracts of the 1986 International Conference on Antimicrobial Agents and Chemotherapy. 1986:224.

69. Sands M, Kron MA, Brown RB: Pentamidine: A review. Rev Infect Dis 7:625, 1985.

70. Jules-Elysee KM, Stover DE, Zaman MB, et al: Aerosolized pentamidine: Effect on diagnosis and presentation of *Pneumocystis carinii* pneumonia. Ann Intern Med 112:750, 1990.

71. Fahy JV, Chin DP, Schnapp LM, et al: Effect of aerosolized pentamidine prophylaxis on the clinical severity and diagnosis of *Pneumocystis carinii* pneumonia. Am Rev Respir Dis 146:844, 1992.

72. Baughman RB, Dohn MN, Shipley R, et al: Increased *Pneumocystis carinii* recovery from the upper lobes in *Pneumocystis* pneumonia: The effect of aerosol pentamidine prophylaxis. Chest 103:426, 1993.

73. Medina I, Mills J, Leoung G, et al: Oral therapy for *Pneumocystis carinii* pneumonia in the acquired immunodeficiency syndrome. N Engl J Med 323:776, 1990.

74. Lucas CR, Saudland AM, Mijch A, et al: Primary dapsone chemoprophylaxis for *Pneumocystis carinii* pneumonia in immunosuppressed patients infected with human immunodeficiency virus. Med J Aust 151:30, 1989.

75. Hughes WT, Kennedy W, Dugdale M, et al: Prevention of *Pneumocystis carinii* pneumonia in AIDS patients with weekly dapsone. Lancet 336:1066, 1990.

76. Kemper CA, Tucker RM, Lang DS, et al: Low dose dapsone prophylaxis of *Pneumocystis carinii* pneumonia in AIDS and AIDS-related complex. AIDS 4:1145, 1990.

77. Slavin MA, Hoy JF, Stewart K, et al: Oral dapsone versus nebulized pentamidine for *Pneumocystis carinii* pneumonia prophylaxis: An open randomized prospective trial to assess efficacy and haematological toxicity. AIDS 6:1169, 1992.

78. Centers for Disease Control: Guidelines for preventing the transmission of tuberculosis in health-care setting, with special focus on HIV-related issues. MMWR 39(RR-17):1–29, 1990.

79. American Thoracic Society, Centers for Disease Control: Diagnostic standards and classification of tuberculosis. Am Rev Respir Dis 142:725, 1990.

80. Centers for Disease Control: Purified protein derivative (PPP)-tuberculin anergy and HIV infection: Guidelines for anergy testing and management of anergic persons at risk of tuberculosis. MMWR 40:27, 1991.

81. Graham NMH, Nelson KE, Solomon L, et al: Prevalence of tuberculin positivity and skin test anergy in HIV-1-seropositive and -seronegative intravenous drug users. JAMA 267:369, 1992.

82. Centers for Disease Control: The use of preventive therapy for tuberculosis infection in the United States: recommendations of the Advisory Committee for Elimination of Tuberculosis. MMWR 39(RR-8):9–12, 1990.

83. Pitchenik AE, Robinson HA: The radiographic appearance of tuberculosis in patients with the acquired immune deficiency syndrome (AIDS) and pre-AIDS. Am Rev Respir Dis 131:393, 1985.

84. Rieder HL, Cauthen GM, Comstock GW, et al: Epidemiology of tuberculosis in the United States. Epidemiol Rev 11:79, 1989.

85. Selwyn PA, Hartel D, Lewis VA, et al: A prospective study of the risk of tuberculosis among intravenous drug users with human immunodeficiency virus infection. N Engl J Med 320:545, 1989.

86. Wadhawan D, Hira S, Mwansa N, et al: Preventive tuberculosis chemotherapy with isoniazid among persons infected with human immunodeficiency virus. [Abstract WB2261] Proceedings of the Seventh International Conference on AIDS, Florence, Italy, June 16–21, 1991.

87. American Thoracic Society, Centers for Disease Control: Treatment of tuberculosis and tuberculosis infection in adults and children. Am Rev Respir Dis 134:355, 1986.

88. Centers for Disease Control: Prevention and control of tuberculosis in U.S. communities with at-risk minority population and prevention and control of tuberculosis among homeless persons. MMWR 41(RR-5):1–23, 1992.

89. Mostow SR: Prevention, management, and control of influenza. Role of amantadine. Am J Med 82(suppl 6A):35, 1987.

90. Monto AS, Gunn RA, Bandyk MG, et al: Prevention of Russian influenza by amantadine. JAMA 241:1003, 1979.

91. Horadam VW, Sharp JG, Smilack JD, et al: Pharmacokinetics of amantadine hydrochloride in subjects with normal and impaired renal function. Ann Intern Med 94(part 1):454, 1981.

92. Belshe RB, Burk B, Newman F, et al: Resistance of influenza A virus to amantadine and rimantadine: Results of one decade of surveillance. J Infect Dis 159:430, 1989.

93. Iseman MD: A leap of faith: What can we do to curtail ultrainstitutional transmission of tuberculosis? Ann Intern Med 117:251, 1992.

94. Small PM, Shafer RW, Hopewell PC, et al: Exogenous infection with multidrug-resistant *Mycobacterium tuberculosis* in patients with advanced HIV infection. N Engl J Med 328:1137, 1993.

95. Pifer LL, Hughes WT, Stagno S, et al: *Pneumocystis carinii* infection: Evidence for high prevalence in normal and immunosuppressed children. Pediatrics 61:35, 1978.

96. Peglow SL, Smulian AG, Linke MJ, et al: Serologic responses to *Pneumocystis carinii* antigens in health and disease. J Infect Dis 161:298, 1990.

97. Smulian AG, Sullivan DW, Linke MJ, et al: Geographic variation in the humoral response to *Pneumocystis carinii*. J Infect Dis 167:123, 1993.

98. Walzer PD, Schnell V, Armstrong D, et al: Nude mouse: A new experimental model for *Pneumocystis carinii* infection. Science 197:177, 1977.

99. Jacobs JL, Libby DM, Winters RA, et al: A cluster of *Pneumocystis carinii* pneumonia in adults without predisposing illnesses. N Engl J Med 324:246, 1991.

100. Goesch TR, Götz G, Stellbrinck KH, et al: Possible transfer of *Pneumocystis carinii* between immunodeficient patients. Lancet 336:627, 1991.

101. Chave J, David S, Wauters J, et al: Transmission of *Pneumocystis carinii* from AIDS patients to other immunosuppressed patients: A

cluster of *Pneumocystis carinii* pneumonia in renal transplant recipients. AIDS 5:927, 1991.

102. Hover DR, Graham NMH, Bacellar H, et al: Epidemiologic patterns of upper respiratory illness and *Pneumocystis carinii* pneumonia in homosexual men. Am Rev Respir Dis 144:756, 1991.

103. Walzer PD: *Pneumocystis carinii*—New clinical spectrum? N Engl J Med 324:263, 1991.

104. Hendley JO, Sande MA, Stewart PM, et al: Spread of *Streptococcus pneumoniae* in families. I. Carriage rates and distribution of types. J Infect Dis 132:55, 1975.

105. Gwaltney Jr JM, Sande MA, Austrian A, et al: Spread of *Streptococcus pneumoniae* in families. II. Relation of transfer of *S. pneumoniae* to incidence of colds and serum antibody. J Infect Dis 132:62, 1975.

106. Pachucki CT, Pappas SA, Fuller GF, et al: Influenza A among hospital personnel and patients. Arch Intern Med 149:77, 1989.

107. Centers for Disease Control: Nosocomial transmission of multi-drug resistant tuberculosis to health care workers and HIV infected patients in an urban hospital—Florida. MMWR 39:718, 1990.

108. Centers for Disease Control: Nosocomial transmission of multi-drug resistant tuberculosis among HIV-infected persons—Florida and New York, 1988–1991. MMWR 40:585, 1991.

109. Centers for Disease Control, National Institute for Occupational Safety and Health: NIOSH Recommended guidelines for personal respiratory protection of workers in health-care facilities potentially exposed to tuberculosis. Atlanta, GA, September 14, 1992.

# CHAPTER 51

# Chronic Bronchitis: Role of Antibiotics

CARLOS M. ISADA and JAMES K. STOLLER

Since the early 1900s, physicians have postulated that the purulent exacerbations of chronic bronchitis were caused by infection. Although the flares of chronic bronchitis were associated with numerous microorganisms in the sputum, the bacteriologic analysis of chronic bronchitis remained incomplete. Because of the lack of effective therapy, there was a general sense of futility in managing this disease.[1] In 1953, May[2] reported a statistically significant correlation between exacerbations of bronchitis and recovery of *Haemophilus influenzae* and *Streptococcus pneumoniae* from the sputum. There followed a resurgence of interest in chronic bronchitis, motivated by factors such as an increasing incidence of the disease, a growing recognition of its economic impact, a stable or declining rate of other infections such as tuberculosis, and the introduction of effective antimicrobial agents.

Penicillin and oxytetracycline were among the first antibiotics to come into widespread use in the early 1950s. These new agents were embraced as revolutionary treatment options for chronic bronchitis. The initial reports of antibiotic efficacy were excellent. Pilot studies were carried out for other broad-spectrum agents, including sulfadiazine, chloramphenicol, and streptomycin, with promising results. Antimicrobial therapy soon became an accepted standard of practice in several situations: short-term treatment of acute bronchitic exacerbations, continuous daily prophylaxis against future exacerbations, and seasonal prophylaxis during the winter months. Some researchers even suggested that antibiotics might be useful in altering the natural history of chronic bronchitis.

Large-scale clinical trials were conducted in the 1950s and 1960s to examine the physiology of chronic bronchitis, the pathogenesis of acute exacerbations, the role of bacteria and viral agents, and the efficacy of specific antibiotics. The results of these larger studies were difficult to interpret and often conflicting. Critics at the time pointed out numerous flaws in the study designs. Nevertheless, there emerged a considerable body of literature supporting the importance of bacterial infection in chronic bronchitis.

Clinical testing of antimicrobial agents in chronic bronchitis has continued, and most classes of antibiotics have been formally studied: penicillins, tetracyclines, cephalosporins, aminoglycosides, macrolide antibiotics, rifamycins, and sulfonamides. The quinolones (eg, ciprofloxacin, ofloxacin, temafloxacin) and other newer agents (eg, azithromycin, clarithromycin, loracarbef) have been formally tested and are being advocated as effective monotherapy for bronchitic flares.

Despite numerous studies and years of clinical experience, the role of antibiotics in chronic bronchitis remains controversial. There appears to be little agreement on the indications for antibiotics, the optimal agent, the duration of treatment, and the efficacy of antibiotic intervention. Some physicians think that antibiotics should be administered in a traditional fashion for proven bacterial infection only. Other physicians argue that antibiotics should be prescribed liberally and, if necessary, empirically for exacerbations of chronic bronchitis. The reasons cited are an inability to differentiate bacterial from nonbacterial flares using current microbiologic techniques, difficulties in interpreting sputum cultures because of heavy bacterial colonization of the upper and lower respiratory tract, incomplete knowledge of viral and other nonbacterial precipitants, low cost and low toxicity of an empiric course of oral antibiotics, and almost continuous relapses in some patients. Patients are instructed to self-administer antibiotics at the first sign of a "chest cold." In most cases, this is done without knowledge of the sputum Gram stain result, culture find-

**621**

ings, or bacterial susceptibility pattern. This approach appears to be more popular than the withholding of therapy until cultures are obtained.

At the heart of this controversy are two clinical observations concerning bronchitic patients: they are prone to frequent and prolonged hospitalizations, and respiratory decompensation is the most commonly identified cause of death. From these observations, it has been inferred that rapid decompensation occurs commonly if antibiotics are withheld or delayed during acute flares.

In formulating a rational policy for antibiotics, it is important to revisit the basic data concerning the pathogenesis of bronchitic flares, the role of infection, and the microbiologic spectrum associated with chronic bronchitis. The clinical trials exploring the efficacy of antibiotic therapy are also reviewed in this chapter, with emphasis placed on the methodologic and interpretive difficulties inherent in these studies.

## TERMINOLOGY

One of the difficulties in interpreting the chronic bronchitis literature lies in the definitions of some basic terms. In 1986, the American Thoracic Society[3] defined chronic obstructive pulmonary disease (COPD) as a group of disorders characterized by abnormal tests of expiratory airflow that are unchanged over several months. The three diseases subsumed by this definition of COPD are emphysema, peripheral airways disease, and chronic bronchitis. Other disorders causing specific airflow obstruction, such as bronchiectasis, asthma, cystic fibrosis, and localized disease of the upper airways, are deliberately excluded. Earlier studies evaluating antibiotics in COPD or chronic bronchial disease loosely referred to chronic bronchitis alone, chronic bronchitis and emphysema, or in some cases, bronchiectasis and tuberculosis. The conclusions drawn from studies of COPD are not necessarily applicable to the other respiratory diseases characterized by chronic cough and sputum production.

Chronic bronchitis has been defined as excessive sputum production on a daily basis for 3 months each year for a minimum of 2 consecutive years. This clinical definition was popularized by the Medical Research Council of Great Britain and by the American Thoracic Society in the early 1960s. Before then, British and North American terminology differed significantly; for example, the term "chronic bronchitis" in Great Britain was equivalent to "emphysema" in North America.[4] Although there was an orderly transition to the new terminology, some large clinical studies adopted the new definition of chronic bronchitis only with certain modifications: unspecified duration of illness, chronic cough for a minimum of 1 year instead of 2,[5] additional criteria for absenteeism from work,[6] winter invalidism, and dyspnea on exertion.[7] These alterations in the consensus definition are common in the literature but pose only minor difficulties in interpretation compared with the many studies that fail to define chronic bronchitis.

The most significant problem in terminology is the lack of a rigorous definition for an acute exacerbation of bronchitis. This is particularly troublesome because the dependent (outcome) variable measured in antibiotic trials is the frequency or duration of acute exacerbations. Various criteria have been applied by investigators, including subjective worsening of dyspnea, an increase in the quantity or appearance of sputum (but not wheezing and dyspnea alone), symptoms of upper or lower respiratory tract infections, and the investigator's clinical impression (which is the most commonly used). Most studies rely on clinical criteria alone to define the acute exacerbation. Only a limited number of studies incorporate microbiologic data.

Much of the confusion results from the variability in objective findings during an uncomplicated exacerbation. Fever, rigors, and mental status changes are unusual, and their presence suggests a complicating pneumonitis or bacteremia. Auscultation of the chest usually reveals some combination of rhonchi, wheezes, or rales, which can be difficult to differentiate from baseline findings. Basic laboratory studies, including the leukocyte count, are unremarkable. The chest radiograph is typically normal or nondiagnostic. Sputum analysis with Gram stain and wet preparations is a promising means of objectively documenting inflammation, but its role is still controversial and the technique is underused. Clinicians and investigators have come to rely almost exclusively on patients' self-reports. This sometimes includes ambiguous symptoms such as changes in sputum color and subtle changes in the baseline level of dyspnea. In a subgroup of patients with severe chronic bronchitis, it may be almost impossible to determine whether an exacerbation is occurring.

This level of precision is inadequate for research purposes, particularly in the patient with moderate to severe bronchitis. A 1980 pilot study[8] attempted to define an exacerbation objectively using spirometry, erthrocyte sedimentation rate, and transtracheal aspiration. These and other parameters were measured in bronchitic patients at baseline and at the onset of worsening respiratory symptoms (eg, increased cough, mucopurulent expectoration, dyspnea). Significant differences were reported in the forced vital capacity, forced expiratory volume in 1 second ($FEV_1$), and sedimentation rate during clinical exacerbations in all patients, and these parameters returned to baseline levels after symptoms had resolved. This type of approach is impractical for the routine management of the bronchitic patient but is long overdue in clinical research.

Acute bacterial exacerbation is an even more ambiguous term in the literature. A precise definition is not likely to be forthcoming until the basic pathogenesis of a bacterial exacerbation is better understood. It seems clear, however, that subjective reports of dyspnea and cough are inadequate for differentiating bacterial from nonbacterial exacerbations. Antibiotic trials have avoided the challenge of defining this term by accepting all patients with respiratory exacerbations, regardless of the cause. This is a reflection of clinical practice, but such an approach inevitably captures many patients without true infection. A notable exception is the work by Chodosh and colleagues,[9, 10] in which a bacterial exacerbation is defined in terms of increased bacterial flora and increased bronchial inflammation; nonbacterial exacerbations are excluded using sputum cytology.

## THE ROLE OF INFECTION IN ACUTE EXACERBATIONS OF CHRONIC BRONCHITIS

Data from longitudinal studies of chronic bronchitis estimate that one to four exacerbations occur per patient each year. Most episodes are managed on an ambulatory basis, with only a small percentage requiring hospitalization. Nevertheless, these seemingly minor episodes are often disabling for the patient and are the major manifestation of infectious disease in this population. With more than 7.5 million Americans suffering from chronic bronchitis,[11] these flares constitute a major source of morbidity, medical expenditure, and absenteeism from the workplace.

Several pathologic mechanisms predispose the bronchitic patient to increased mucus production and bacterial infection. Data derived from animal studies, autopsy studies, and epidemiologic surveys suggest that these abnormalities are largely the result of prolonged exposure to cigarette smoke.[12, 13] Although tobacco use is the premier risk factor for the development of chronic bronchitis, other factors are involved. Some lifetime nonsmokers have developed chronic bronchitis, but other persons with more than 50 pack-years of tobacco use have remained disease free. Infection is probably not a significant factor in the early years of chronic bronchitis, but in the later stages, infection becomes increasingly common and may contribute to the underlying pathogenesis of the disease.

A significant finding in early chronic bronchitis is the hypertrophy of the submucosal glands in the walls of the large bronchi, a process that results in mucus hypersecretion. Copious amounts of a thick, tenacious material are secreted into the large airways. The glycoprotein and lipid composition of this mucus differs slightly from that of normal bronchial secretions and resists airway clearance. Clinically, the patient complains of a persistent daily cough productive of clear or white sputum, the ''smoker's morning cough,'' but may otherwise feel quite well. Little or no airways obstruction is present. Infection plays a minor role at this stage. Expectorated sputum is nonpurulent, and cultures are usually sterile.

As the disease progresses, hypersecretion of mucus begins to involve the small airways. Submucosal glands located in the medium-sized bronchi and bronchioles begin to enlarge in response to continued exposure to cigarette smoke. Another histologic finding, which usually parallels gland hypertrophy, is the proliferation of goblet cells in the respiratory epithelium. These secretory cells are normally found scattered infrequently through the epithelium of the large bronchi. In severe chronic bronchitis, goblet cells can account for almost all the respiratory epithelium and are found encroaching on the small airways. Mucociliary clearance is further impaired by this loss of the normal ciliated epithelium. Impaction of mucus in the lumen of the small airways, along with the structural changes associated with submucosal gland hypertrophy, leads to progressive obstruction of the peripheral airways. Although a chronic low-grade inflammation often exists, the sputum is not frankly purulent at this stage, and only a moderate number of polymorphonuclear leukocytes are present.

These morphologic features of chronic bronchitis probably represent a nonspecific response to a chronic irritant. Animal studies suggest that infection need not be present for these changes to take place; many of the histologic changes of human chronic bronchitis have been duplicated in animals exposed to cigarette smoke in the absence of infection. In murine and canine models, chronic inhalation of cigarette smoke has led to submucosal hypertrophy, increased secretory cell activity, and chronic lymphocytic in-

flammation.[12, 14, 15] Tobacco smoke has also been shown to directly inhibit mucociliary function, as shown by impaired particle transport in vitro, ciliostasis, decreased tracheal mucous velocity in animals, and reduced clearance of inhaled aerosols in humans.[16] In vitro studies have demonstrated subtle defects in the local host immune system, particularly in persons who continue to smoke. These include impaired neutrophil phagocytosis, impaired neutrophil bactericidal function, and decreased levels of sputum immunoglobulin A.[17, 18]

These mechanisms work in concert to impair clearance of inhaled bacteria. Studies have shown that the oropharynx (normally nonsterile) and the large bronchi (normally sterile) become colonized with the same aerobic bacteria.[19] Organisms of relatively low pathogenicity assume residence in the oropharynx initially and are then aspirated continuously into the large bronchi. If mucociliary clearance is impaired, these bacteria may persist in deeper bronchial epithelium, sometimes even after antibiotic therapy. This new tracheobronchial flora represents a classic state of bacterial colonization: organisms are replicating in or on host tissues, but tissue invasion does not take place, and the host immune response is minimal.

For reasons that remain unclear, this baseline state of colonization may periodically progress to active disease. Microscopically, there is evidence of bacterial proliferation and acute inflammation with polymorphonuclear leukocytes. Clinically, the patient complains of worsened cough, dyspnea, or sputum production (ie, acute bacterial exacerbation). Little is known about the precise host defense mechanisms or microbial virulence factors that lead to active infection in the patient with previously stable chronic bronchitis. Presumably, the same factors that permit bacterial colonization to occur also predispose to acute bacterial exacerbations, but this has been difficult to prove microbiologically.

This problem is best illustrated in the efforts to implicate *H. influenzae* as a specific cause of infectious flares. As reviewed by Murphy and Apicella,[20] four strategies have been adopted. The first strategy is to demonstrate an association between *H. influenzae* and purulent sputum or clinical exacerbations. This approach has met with only limited success; some studies demonstrated an association[2, 21, 22] and others did not.[23, 24] The second strategy is to demonstrate a rise in specific antibody titers before and after infections. Paired serologic studies are an established means of identifying an infecting organism. Prospective studies have examined paired antibody levels to *H. influenzae* with exacerbations. The results have been conflicting, with some studies showing significant antibody rises with exacerbations but others demonstrating no association. In part, this disparity has been explained by the use of a single surface antigen in the serologic assay, rather than heterogeneous *H. influenzae* antigens.[20] The third strategy is to demonstrate a similar respiratory illness caused by the same organism in normal patients. Acute febrile tracheobronchitis due to *H. influenzae* has been well described outside the chronic bronchitis population. Some researchers think this is indirect evidence that *H. influenzae* is capable of causing tracheobronchitis in the bronchitic patient. The fourth strategy is to determine the clinical response to specific antibiotic therapy directed against *H. influenzae,* an approach that is discussed later in this chapter.

The final step in the putative pathogenesis of bacterial exacerbations is only partially supported by microbiologic data. The literature is even more problematic for infections caused by *S. pneumoniae* and *Moraxella catarrhalis*. Nevertheless, clinicians usually attribute infectious exacerbations to one of these colonizing bacteria, although most agree that the role of infection is still uncertain.[18, 23, 25–28]

## NONBACTERIAL EXACERBATIONS OF CHRONIC BRONCHITIS

More than 50% of acute exacerbations of bronchitis may be caused by factors other than bacterial infection.[19, 23, 29–32] A sizable body of data confirms the importance of respiratory viruses and *Mycoplasma pneumoniae* infections in bronchitic flares. Sachs[28] reviewed the evidence relating viral infections to acute exacerbations. Results are divergent, with prevalence rates ranging from 4.4% to 63% because of differences in study design, viral culture techniques, and use of viral antibody studies. The most commonly isolated viruses are respiratory syncytial virus, influenza, parainfluenza, and coronavirus. Studies showed a clear trend for seasonal, especially winter, proclivity. The relatively long turnaround time required for viral identification precludes its routine use in clinical practice, but the frequency of isolation should not be overlooked. *M. pneumoniae* appears to be of lesser importance but may be a sporadic cause of exacerbations. The prevalence of *M. pneumoniae* as a cause of acute exacerbations is estimated at 1% to 10%.

Worsening respiratory symptoms can also be caused by noninfectious agents,[18] such as toxic inhalations (eg, recent cigarette use, exposures to pollutants or irritant gases); recent exposure to allergens; thickening in bronchial secretions (eg, poor humidification, winter months, medication noncompliance); congestive heart failure; and less commonly, pulmonary embolism. A differential diagnosis should be constructed in all cases, because the presenting signs and symptoms of nonbacterial precipitants are difficult to differentiate from true infection. As summarized in Table 51–1, some investigators think that these nonbacterial causes may be diagnosed accurately using the sputum Gram stain, sputum cellular analysis, and certain historic clues.[18, 24, 25, 33, 34] The presence of more than 5% eosinophils or swollen bronchial epithelial cells on cytologic examination of expectorated sputum suggests an allergic cause and has been used to exclude patients from some antibiotic trials.

## SPUTUM ANALYSIS IN ACUTE EXACERBATIONS OF CHRONIC BRONCHITIS

Although the usual presence of organisms in the trachea and bronchi of chronic bronchitics complicates the laboratory diagnosis of bacterial infection, analysis of expectorated sputum may still be a useful means of diagnosis.

The sputum Gram stain continues to be advocated as a means of demonstrating objectively an increase in bacterial flora and an increase in bronchial inflammation. Baigelman and colleagues[35] examined more than 1000 sputum Gram stains from patients with chronic bronchitis during stable states, acute bacterial exacerbations, acute allergic exacerbations, and recoveries from acute bacterial exacerbations. The mean number of microorganisms was determined for 20 oil-immersion fields during each of these phases. Fewer than two bacteria per oil-immersion field were found for stable-state samples. Calculating three standard deviations from the mean, the investigators found that 12 or more organisms resembling *H. influenzae*, 8 or more resembling *S. pneumoniae*, or 18 or more resembling *M. catarrhalis* per oil-immersion field clearly differentiated acute bacterial infection from stable bronchitis, allergic exacerbation, or recovery from bacterial infection. The researchers proposed that 99% of chronic bronchitis patients without clinical evidence of bacterial infection would fall below these thresholds. These findings suggest that an upper limit may be set for the numbers of microorganisms seen on a Gram stain of sputum from a bronchitic patient in the absence of bacterial infection. In this and other studies, gram-negative bacilli and fungi were infrequently observed on Gram stain. The presence of even small numbers of gram-negative bacilli may be significant.

The routine sputum culture plays a more limited role and can be misleading in some instances.[19, 23, 27, 28, 35] Studies examining sputum cultures before, during, and after bacterial exacerbations have correlated poorly with clinical parameters and Gram stain results. Gram-negative bacilli often have been recovered in sputum culture although they were absent on Gram stain, and clinical recovery has occurred without specific gram-negative antibiotic coverage. In one series,[18] more than 50% of sputum cultures remained

**Table 51–1. Differential Diagnosis for Acute Exacerbations of Chronic Bronchitis**

| Condition | Historic Clues | Gram Stain Results |
|---|---|---|
| Acute bacterial infection | Cough, increased sputum volume; purulent sputum, dyspnea; fever and chills if pneumonia | Numerous bacteria; numerous polymorphonuclear leukocytes |
| Acute viral infection | History of family member with recent viral illness; winter months | Few or no bacteria; many polymorphonuclear leukocytes |
| Allergy | Known history of allergies; recent allergen exposure; background of bronchospasm on spirometry | Few or no bacteria; possible sputum eosinophilia |
| Toxic inhalation | Recent increased cigarette use; exposure to pollutants; exposure to irritant gases at workplace | Few or no bacteria; possible increase in polymorphonuclear leukocytes (variable) |
| Change in bronchial secretions | Dry house, no humidification; winter months; medication noncompliance | Few or no bacteria; no polymorphonuclear leukocytes |
| Congestive heart failure | Dyspnea, wheezing, orthopnea; weight gain, edema; no change in sputum | Few or no bacteria; no polymorphonuclear leukocytes |
| Pulmonary embolism | Dyspnea, hemoptysis; pleuritic chest pain | Few or no bacteria; no polymorphonuclear leukocytes |

positive long after clinical recovery. However, culture of expectorated sputum may be useful in certain circumstances: identification of unknown bacteria seen on Gram stain, confirmation of gram-negative baccilli or staphylococci-like forms, and antimicrobial susceptibility testing if drug resistance is suspected. The role of quantitative and semiquantitative sputum cultures (in which the number of bacterial colony-forming units per milliliter is estimated) appears to be limited.

The presence of numerous polymorphonuclear leukocytes on sputum Gram stain indicates bronchial damage. Although consistent with a bacterial infection, this result also accompanies viral infections and some noninfectious conditions. A 24-hour sputum collection has been suggested as a more accurate indicator of bronchial inflammation than the traditional Gram stain.[9, 10, 33] With this technique, the concentration of cells in the sputum is determined by means of a hemocytometer, and the percentage of each cell type is calculated from a Papanicolaou-stained smear.

Bacterial colonization of the lower respiratory tract does not invalidate routine examination of the sputum, as claimed by some.[36] For patients with advanced bronchitis, sputum analysis should be performed when the patient is at a baseline state, and the Gram stain should be permanently saved for later comparison.

## MICROBIOLOGY OF CHRONIC BRONCHITIS

The bronchi of normal patients usually are sterile, but in some, the upper airways may be colonized with *H. influenzae* or *S. pneumoniae*. In patients with chronic bronchitis, pathogenic bacteria can be cultured from respiratory secretions in as many as 80%.[27] *H. influenzae*, *S. pneumoniae*, and *M. catarrhalis* are the bacterial species most commonly cultured from sputum in large airways, with at least one organism recovered in 30% to 50% of bronchitic patients. However, the literature is conflicting, and many reports are at variance with this belief.[25, 37] This is probably a result of differences in severity of bronchitis in the populations sampled and of frequent reliance on sputum cultures alone.

In an attempt to minimize upper airway contamination, some studies have adopted more invasive techniques for sampling the lower airways. In one well-designed trial,[19] 20 patients with chronic bronchitis underwent transtracheal aspiration during stable periods. Bacteria were recovered from the bronchial tree in only 50% of patients. The most common isolate was viridans streptococci (now called α-hemolytic streptococci). The investigators concluded that the tracheobronchial microflora in patients with chronic bronchitis is more diverse than previously appreciated and that viridans streptococci species, normally considered oral commensals, should instead be considered potential pathogens. The same group performed transtracheal aspirations on bronchitic patients during acute exacerbations.[37] In this well-designed pilot study, oropharyngeal contamination was ruled out by nebulizing 1% methylene blue in the pharynx and assaying for its presence spectrophotometrically in transtracheal specimens. No microorganisms were cultured in 22% of patients. A variety of bacteria were recovered in the remainder, including *Neisseria* species,

viridans streptococci, and *Haemophilus parainfluenzae*. The researchers concluded that *H. influenzae* and *S. pneumoniae* may not be the predominant organisms during exacerbations of bronchitis and that other pathogens should be considered.

Fagon and coworkers[38] used fiberoptic bronchoscopy with a protected specimen brush to obtain samples of the distal bronchial microflora in a homogeneous group of patients with chronic bronchitis. All 54 patients required mechanical ventilation for severe respiratory exacerbations of bronchitis despite clear chest radiographs on admission. In 50% of patients, cultures of protected brush specimens failed to yield any organisms, supporting the notion that bronchitic flares are frequently nonbacterial in origin. The most common isolate was *H. parainfluenzae* (25%), followed by *S. pneumoniae* (16%) and *H. influenzae* (14%). Several other organisms were recovered in 7% to 9% of cultures: *M. catarrhalis*, *Pseudomonas aeruginosa*, *Proteus mirabilis,* and *Staphylococcus aureus*. The investigators concluded that, in distal bronchial infection, the usual pathogens such as *H. influenzae* and *S. pneumoniae* may not be the sole or even predominant cause of bronchitic flares.

Although these studies suggest a fairly diverse tracheobronchial flora, *H. influenzae* continues to be the organism most intensively studied.[20, 39–42] Experimental evidence suggests that nontypable (nonencapsulated) *H. influenzae* is able to elaborate an IgA protease enzyme that inactivates a secretory IgA in the bronchi, allowing this organism to adhere to the epithelium. Studies using restriction endonuclease technology have further elucidated this phenomenon.[39, 41] Nontypable *H. influenzae* strains display morphologic changes during persistent infections in COPD. The major outer membrane proteins of *H. influenzae* appear to change over time. It has been proposed that host antibodies against outer membrane proteins may eventually select for reinfection with strains containing different major outer membrane proteins. In this way, *H. influenzae* further escapes immunologic defenses.

An increasing number of nontypable and typable strains of *H. influenzae* also express the enzyme β-lactamase, which cleaves the amide bond of ampicillin. The percentage of *H. influenzae* strains that elaborate this plasmid-mediated β-lactamase varies considerably from one laboratory to another, depending in part on the patient population served, and ranges from less than 5% to more than 20% in some hospitals. Other strains of *H. influenzae* exhibit altered penicillin-binding proteins, further contributing to ampicillin resistance. Recognition of these resistance mechanisms has prompted formal testing of newer classes of antibiotics and antibiotic combinations during acute exacerbations of chronic bronchitis.

## CLINICAL TRIALS OF ANTIBIOTICS

Data from available clinical trials examining the efficacy of antibiotics are reviewed separately for several clinical scenarios: patients with stable chronic bronchitis, patients with histories of numerous exacerbations, patients with acute exacerbations of mild to moderate severity, and patients who are hospitalized for severe exacerbations requiring parenteral antibiotics.

## Stable Chronic Bronchitis

The patient with early chronic bronchitis and only mild airway obstruction may produce sputum on a daily basis but may never suffer a purulent exacerbation. Few studies have examined the efficacy of antibiotics in this population. However, one large study from the Medical Research Council in Britain[43] deliberately selected patients with ''early'' chronic bronchitis to determine whether progression of chronic bronchitis could be delayed by the control of recurrent infection. Patients with ''mild disability'' were recruited, defined in terms of baseline symptoms (ie, no more than two chest illnesses in the preceding 3 years) and an $FEV_1$ exceeding 1.4 L. Winter prophylaxis was administered for a 5-year period using oxytetracycline at a dose of 2 g per day in a double-blind, placebo-controlled fashion. No benefit was found for the antibiotic group. Prophylaxis had no consistent effect on the number of exacerbations in patients who normally had few exacerbations. The average rate of decline of $FEV_1$ over 5 years was not influenced by antibiotics.

The natural history of untreated chronic bronchitis (without any antibiotic intervention) is unknown.[44] The often cited notion that antibiotics given early in chronic bronchitis can forestall progressive pulmonary deterioration remains unsupported by available evidence. Since the early 1950s, some researchers have considered it unethical to treat a patient with moderately severe bronchitis with a placebo over an extended period. Because few studies have examined the natural history of chronic bronchitis in the preantibiotic era, the true influence of long-term prophylactic antibiotics on the overall disease course may never be known.

## Numerous Exacerbations of Chronic Bronchitis

For patients who experience multiple, disabling exacerbations each year, prophylactic therapy is often considered. This has been a subject of controversy for more than 40 years. Although most of the large-scale, controlled studies were performed in the 1950s and 1960s, their impact continues. Early studies demonstrated a trend favoring the use of prophylactic antibiotics. In one of the earliest controlled trials, McVay and Sprunt recruited 30 patients with chronic bronchial disease.[1] Patients received either daily chlortetracycline (250 mg, orally twice daily) or placebo for 11 months. The incidence of respiratory infections in the group receiving antibiotics was 50% lower than among controls. However, there were several flaws in the study design: the patient population was heterogeneous, including subjects with bronchiectasis and emphysema; patients were not randomly assigned to placebo or control groups; and the investigators were not blinded in treating 4 of 30 patients.

Other contemporary trials have reported good results with continuous administration of tetracycline during the winter months.[45–48] In general, these studies are small and contain design flaws. A representative study performed by

Buchanan and associates[49] chose low-dose tetracycline (250 mg, orally twice daily) over oxytetracycline or chlortetracycline because of a more favorable side effect profile. A total of 51 patients with chronic bronchitis of unspecified severity were randomized to tetracycline or placebo for 12 months. The study was deliberately left unblinded because of concerns about ''staphylococcal gastroenterocolitis'' ascribed to tetracycline. In assessing outcomes, the investigators maintained that a clinical exacerbation was ''a sufficiently objective index of therapeutic effect'' and that bias was negligible. In this study, an acute flare of bronchitis was defined as ''a severe exacerbation of the bronchitic state requiring the patient to remain in bed for at least 5 days.'' The investigators reported a clear benefit for the group receiving antibiotics. The incidence of exacerbations was less in the group receiving tetracycline than for controls (ie, 0.33 exacerbations per patient per year versus 1.13 exacerbations in controls). The antibiotic-treated group demonstrated significant subjective improvement compared with the placebo-treated group, but this finding is suspect, because it is easily biased in an unblinded study. The mean serum level of tetracycline was reported as 1.35 μg/mL, a level that is now recognized as inadequate for treating pulmonary infections. The investigators concluded that continuous tetracycline prophylaxis was indicated in the long-term management of chronic bronchitis, and they further recommended using antibiotics during the winter months.

This strategy of winter prophylaxis was examined in a small but reasonably designed trial by Murdoch and co-workers.[50] At the time of the study, the researchers thought that acute exacerbations were caused by *H. influenzae* and *S. pneumoniae,* that antibiotic prophylaxis was clearly beneficial, and that the only issues to be settled were optimal drug dosage, proper patient selection, and emergence of tetracycline-resistant *S. aureus.* Patients with moderate to severe chronic bronchitis were randomized to tetracycline or placebo during the winter months over a 2-year period. There were fewer patients off work because of bronchitis in the antibiotic group than in the placebo group (13 and 27, respectively). Unfortunately, the patient withdrawal rates were quite high in both groups, up to 50% in the placebo-treated group.

Large-scale controlled studies conducted in the 1960s demonstrated less impressive benefit from continuous antibiotic therapy. Many of these studies were coordinated at a national level to increase patient enrollment and improve study design.

In an attempt to find a less expensive alternative to tetracycline prophylaxis, the British Tuberculosis Association[6] recruited 226 patients with moderate chronic bronchitis and randomized them to penicillin VK (312 mg, orally twice daily), tetracycline (250 mg, orally twice daily) or placebo. The investigators acknowledged that the dose of tetracycline was low, but they were encouraged by the findings of Buchanan and associates.[49] The average time off work as a result of bronchitis was greater in the control group (14.2 days) than in the group treated with penicillin VK (6.8 days) or the group treated with tetracycline (7.5 days). The favorable results found with the tetracycline-treated group have come into question, because most of the beneficial effects were reported from 3 of 16 participating centers, accounting for fewer than 15% of patients.[51] In contrast to previous studies, the number of exacerbations was the same in all groups. The researchers were also surprised by the equivalent efficacy of penicillin and tetracycline, because they expected penicillin VK to suppress *S. pneumoniae* and not *H. influenzae* and expected tetracycline to suppress *S. pneumoniae* and some *H. influenzae*. Bacteriologic examination of the sputum was thought to be impractical at the beginning of the study and was not performed. One year later (1961), the same group conducted a prospective study of 519 patients with chronic bronchitis to include more bacteriologic information, reassess the previous year's results, and include an alternative prophylactic regimen in which acute exacerbations were treated with a short course of antibiotics or placebo.[52] Patients were randomly allocated to one of four treatment regimens: (1) daily placebo with intermittent oral penicillin VK (624 mg, orally three times daily) for exacerbations, (2) daily tetracycline (250 mg, orally twice daily) with placebo for exacerbations, (3) daily penicillin (312 mg, orally twice daily) with placebo for exacerbations, or (4) daily placebo with tetracycline (500 mg, orally three times daily) for exacerbations. Overall, there was a modest benefit shown in the group receiving daily tetracycline (regimen 2) with respect to days missed from work (ie, 4 days missed in regimen 2 versus 8 days in all other groups). No reduction in exacerbation rate was found in those receiving maintenance tetracycline compared with those on tetracycline for exacerbations only.

The 1966 study of winter chemoprophylaxis by the Medical Research Council,[43] although intended for the early chronic bronchitis patient, included many patients with multiple exacerbations. Oxytetracycline prophylaxis was associated with a 16% reduction in days lost from work. However, this benefit was modest and statistically surprising; the 95% confidence interval included the possibility of a detrimental effect from the prophylaxis. No improvements in the number of exacerbations or the rate of decline of $FEV_1$ were found. A follow-up study in 1968 focusing on a small subgroup of these study patients yielded conflicting results. Fewer exacerbations occurred after chemoprophylaxis was extended an additional 2 years.

As reviewed by Tager and Speizer,[25] many smaller and less carefully designed studies conducted in the late 1960s showed conflicting results for chemoprophylaxis. In one of the few trials in which confidence intervals were provided,[53] chemoprophylaxis with a sulfonamide was thought to have decreased the percentage of patients with relapses (ie, 38% relapse rate with antibiotics versus 68% with placebo). However, the 95% confidence interval for relapses in patients on antibiotics was wide (3%–57%).

Johnston and coworkers[54] examined the efficacy of winter chemoprophylaxis over a 5-year period. Patients were randomly assigned to one of four groups: placebo during the winter for 5 consecutive years; tetracycline daily for the first two winters and then placebo for the next three; placebo for two winters and then tetracycline for 3 years; or daily tetracycline for five winters. The number of exacerbations was similar in all groups, and no benefit was found for prophylaxis. However, in analyzing specific patient subsets, the researchers found that patients who experienced frequent flares while on placebo appeared to benefit from prophylaxis. They concluded that antibiotics may have a limited role in these more "susceptible" patients (two or more exacerbations per winter), but this post hoc analysis has been criticized[25] for revising the initial study design.

Only a limited number of chemoprophylaxis trials were performed in the 1970s. The practice of prolonged low-dose antibiotic therapy was coming under criticism because of increasing reports of ampicillin-resistant *H. influenzae* and tetracycline-resistant pneumococci. Newer antibiotics were tested as prophylactic agents, including cephalexin versus placebo,[55] trimethoprim-sulfamethoxazole (320 mg/1600 mg each day) versus placebo,[56] co-trimoxazole versus amoxicillin (no placebo),[57] and cefadroxil versus doxycyline (no placebo). These studies are difficult to interpret because of the small numbers of patients in each treatment arm and differences in methodologies; no single antibiotic afforded a clear advantage.

In 1987, Finnish investigators reopened this issue.[58] Although this study recruited a small number of patients, the format was double blinded and controlled. Twenty-four chronic bronchitics with three or more exacerbations per season were randomized to trimethoprim (300 mg, orally each day) or placebo for 6 months. No benefit of antibiotic prophylaxis was shown.

On review of these conflicting studies, there is little evidence to support the prophylactic use of antibiotics, even for moderate to severe chronic bronchitis. The trials that demonstrate a benefit from prophylactic antibiotics contain serious methodologic flaws. For the problematic patient who relapses in a continuous fashion, some researchers have proposed individualizing therapy.[28] If exacerbations seem primarily seasonal, a trial of limited prophylaxis may be warranted (eg, October through March). If exacerbations occur throughout the year, prophylaxis is less appealing because of cost, drug toxicity, and selection of resistant bacteria. As logical as this approach appears, it should only be adopted with the understanding that it is not supported strongly by available literature (Table 51–2).

## Mild or Moderate Acute Exacerbations of Bronchitis

Studies in the 1960s yielded conflicting results about the efficacy of antibiotics for mild to moderate exacerbations. Table 51–3 summarizes the major placebo-controlled trials that clearly defined entry and response criteria. Of these earlier trials, four of six showed borderline benefits of antibiotic therapy, none of which was statistically significant. In 1957, Elmes and coworkers[59] randomized 88 patients to oxytetracycline or placebo. Therapy was started at patient discretion at the onset of a respiratory illness. No significant differences were found between the antibiotic and placebo groups. Berry and associates[60] studied oxytetracycline in acute exacerbations and found no difference for mild attacks but a trend toward earlier recovery for moderate attacks. In 1965, Elmes and associates[61] conducted a controlled trial of ampicillin in patients who required hospitalization. Several trends in favor of antibiotics were found, but no overall statistical advantage was observed. In 1967, Petersen and coworkers[51] randomized patients with acute exacerbations to chloramphenicol or placebo and included measurements of pulmonary function. No beneficial trends were found for any observed objective parameters (eg, pulmonary function tests, arterial blood gas analysis, leukocyte count).

Table 51–2. **Trials of Antibiotic Prophylaxis in Chronic Bronchitis**

| Investigation | No. of Patients | Antibiotic and Dose | Results and Comments |
|---|---|---|---|
| British Tuberculosis Association, 1960 | 226 | Tetracycline (250 mg, PO bid) vs penicillin VK (312 mg PO bid) vs placebo | Frequency of acute exacerbations comparable in all groups; number of days lost from work decreased for antibiotic group |
| British Tuberculosis Association, 1961 | 519 | Four regimens: A. Placebo maintenance, penicillin for exacerbations (312 mg PO bid) B. Tetracycline maintenance (250 mg bid), placebo for exacerbations C. Maintenance penicillin, placebo for exacerbations D. Maintenance placebo, tetracycline for exacerbations | Frequency of exacerbations decreased somewhat for regimens B, C, D; no difference between intermittent and continuous tetracycline (B and D are the same) |
| Medical Research Council, 1966 | 373 | Oxytetracycline (500 mg qd to 1 g bid) during winter months over 5 y vs placebo | Frequency of exacerbations not improved with antibiotics |
| Johnston et al, 1969 | 79 | Four regimens: A. Placebo for 5 winters B. Tetracycline (500 mg bid) × 2 winters, then placebo × 3 winters C. Placebo × 2 winters, then tetracycline × 3 winters D. Tetracycline × 5 winters | Frequency of exacerbations comparable for all groups; possible benefit reported for antibiotic in high-risk patient, ignored in original study design |
| Liipo et al, 1987 | 24 | Trimethoprim (300 mg PO qd) vs placebo | No benefit with antibiotic prophylaxis |

The two studies from this era that did show statistical benefit have been questioned. In a limited pilot study, Pines and associates[62] reported 30 patients who were judged moderately or severely ill, clearly a more symptomatic group than in other studies. Patients were randomized to receive a penicillin-streptomycin combination or placebo. The study was terminated early because of "disastrous results" in the placebo group, in which 9 of 15 patients deteriorated rapidly and 3 died. In the treatment group, only 3 of 15 had adverse outcomes. The statistical methods used to calculate significance in the study have been questioned.[25] A much larger study was performed by the same investigators,[63] randomizing 259 patients to tetracycline and chloramphenicol or placebo. Clinical parameters improved significantly in the treatment group, but these benefits appeared to be short-lived. By 7 days after therapy, the groups were comparable, and at 28 days, relapses were frequent in both groups.

Many studies were performed in the 1970s, with different study designs, lengths of therapy, measured variables, exclusion criteria for pneumonia, and criteria for successful outcome. As a group, these trials are difficult to interpret and are not readily applied to clinical practice.

Two trials readdressed the efficacy of antibiotics for acute exacerbations of chronic bronchitis. In 1982, Nicotra and colleagues[64] demonstrated no benefit for tetracycline in acute exacerbations. Patients were allocated to receive tetracycline (40 patients) or placebo (40 patients) for 1 week in the hospital. Patients with severe exacerbations (ie, temperature $>38.5°C$, leukocyte count $>12,000/mm^3$, pneumonia, recent failure of antibiotic therapy, or respiratory failure) were excluded. After 1 week of therapy, no differences were found in blood gases, sputum analysis, spirometry, or subjective status in the compared groups.

A similarly designed but larger trial was conducted by Anthonisen and associates.[65] Unlike the previous study, pa-

Table 51–3. **Trials of Antibiotics for Acute Exacerbations of Chronic Bronchitis**

| Investigation | No. of Patients | Antibiotic and Dose | Results and Comments |
|---|---|---|---|
| Elmes et al, 1957 | 88 | Oxytetracycline (250 mg PO qid) × 5 to 7 d vs placebo for days off work | No significant difference; insignificant trend favoring antibiotics |
| Berry et al, 1960 | 53 | Oxytetracycline (250 mg qid) × 5 d vs placebo | Mild attacks showed no difference; severe attacks revealed trend in favor of antibiotics |
| Elmes et al, 1965 | 56 | Ampicillin (1 g q 6 h) × 3 d, then 500 mg q 6 h × 4 d vs placebo | Trend in favor of antibiotic therapy, but no statistical advantage |
| Peterson et al, 1967 | 43 | Chloramphenicol vs placebo | Control group had more flares; no difference on any parameters |
| Pines et al, 1968 | 30 | Penicillin (3 million units IM bid) in combination with streptomycin (500 mg IM bid) × 14 d vs placebo | Pilot study terminated early due to deterioration in placebo group; statistical analysis questioned |
| Pines et al, 1972 | 259 | Tetracycline and chloramphenicol vs placebo | Significant improvement with antibiotics but numerous relapses at 7 days |
| Nicotra et al, 1982 | 40 | Tetracycline (500 mg qid) × 7 d vs placebo | No differences observed |
| Anthonisen et al, 1987 | 106 | Trimethoprim-sulfamethoxazole (160 mg/800 mg bid), amoxicillin (250 mg qid), or doxycycline (100 mg qd) vs placebo | Significant improvement with all antibiotics compared with placebo; increased peak flow at 21 days |

tients in this trial were healthy enough to be managed as outpatients. Exacerbations were defined as worsened dyspnea, sputum purulence, and increased sputum volume, measures that, although somewhat "soft" by the researchers' admission, were thought to reflect criteria applied in actual practice. Microbiologic confirmation of infection was not needed, and patients received trimethoprim-sulfamethoxazole (160 mg/800 mg, orally twice daily), doxycycline (200 mg, orally initially, followed by 100 mg, orally daily), amoxicillin (250 mg, orally four times daily), or placebo. Unlike the study by Nicotra and colleagues,[64] antibiotic recipients did experience demonstrable benefit. Symptoms resolved more rapidly, and the success rate was higher with antibiotics than with placebo. Almost twice as many patients in the placebo group deteriorated and required hospitalization. An accelerated improvement in peak expiratory flow was also documented in the treatment group, a finding lacking in previous studies.

The results of reasonably well-designed, placebo-controlled trials of the efficacy of antibiotics for acute exacerbations of chronic bronchitis have been conflicting. There appears to be a modest trend favoring the efficacy of antibiotics in this setting. Antibiotic toxicity in these trials has proven negligible, and the consequences of incorrectly withholding antibiotics, as documented by Pines and associates,[62] remain a valid clinical concern. In their view, the weight of available evidence favors the use of antibiotics during acute exacerbations of chronic bronchitis.

No single oral antibiotic has emerged as a clear favorite, but several appear effective. Studies claiming efficacy of a particular antibiotic in exacerbations of bronchitis abound in the literature but tend to be small, uncontrolled, or unblinded. Few studies directly compare multiple oral antibiotics at the same time; most studies limit the comparison to only two agents (usually a newer drug against an established "control" antibiotic). Methodologic differences among the numerous studies examining oral antibiotics in this setting make a metanalysis difficult.

In 1987, Chodosh[18] summarized the clinical trials that employed a double-blind crossover format. The outcomes examined included the percentage of treatment failures and the relative infection-free period associated with each antibiotic. According to this analysis, the leading oral antibiotics (in descending order of efficacy) are ampicillin, bacampicillin, amoxicillin, doxycycline, and minocycline. Trimethoprim-sulfamethoxazole was an effective alternative agent, with a clinical response rate over 80% but with a relatively short infection-free period. The investigator had doubts about cefaclor, cephalexin, and erythromycin because of a relatively high incidence of treatment failures in some of the studies reviewed. However, other investigators do not share this opinion, particularly about cefaclor.[67, 68]

Since Chodosh's study, newer broad-spectrum oral agents have come into common usage, in part because of concerns about increasing bacterial resistance to ampicillin and, to a lesser extent, concerns about tetracycline. The combination of amoxicillin-clavulanate tested favorably in bronchitic exacerbations caused by β-lactamase–producing strains of *H. influenzae* and *M. catarrhalis,* but frequent recurrences have been reported within 1 week of ending treatment.[66] Another widely prescribed antibiotic is cefaclor, a second-generation oral cephalosporin that also resists cleavage by β-lactamase. This agent shares the same broad antibacterial coverage as amoxicillin-clavulanate but also some of its drawbacks, including high cost, diarrhea, and antibiotic-associated colitis. The role of cefaclor as a first-line agent in treating moderate exacerbations is somewhat unclear; some researchers have discouraged its use,[18] but others have chosen cefaclor as the "control" antibiotic against which experimental antibiotics are compared.[67, 68]

In 1988, investigators compared cefaclor, amoxicillin, cephalexin, and enoxacin against doxycycline in four separate crossover arms.[69] In acute exacerbations, doxycycline appeared comparable to the other antibiotics except cefaclor, to which doxycycline was superior. Early rebound infections were similar for doxycycline, amoxicillin, and enoxacin in this study, but they were significantly more frequent for cephalexin and cefaclor. Doxycycline was found to have the longest infection-free period.

The fluoroquinolones may play a role in treating acute exacerbations of chronic bronchitis in selected cases. As a class, these agents demonstrate excellent penetration into repiratory secretions and bronchial mucosa, with tissue-plasma ratios of approximately 1:1 and 2:1, respectively. The spectrum of activity is broad, including β-lactamase–producing *H. influenzae* and *M. catarrhalis,* Enterobacteriaceae, *P. aeruginosa, M. pneumoniae,* and *Chlamydia pneumoniae.* There is also excellent penetration of the quinolones into phagocytic cells, a finding that may affect the treatment of intracellular organisms such as *M. pneumoniae.*

Doubts have been raised concerning the efficacy of certain quinolones in eliminating *S. pneumoniae,* one of the major pathogens implicated in bronchitic flares. The mean inhibitory concentration ($MIC_{90}$) of ciprofloxacin for *S. pneumoniae* is relatively high compared with the level achieved in the serum and bronchial secretions. For example, the $MIC_{90}$ of ciprofloxacin for *S. pneumoniae* is about 2 μg/mL, with levels of drug in respiratory tissues after oral administration also approximately 2 μg/mL (or less), a somewhat unfavorable ratio. The $MIC_{90}$ of ciprofloxacin for *M. catarrhalis* is about 0.03 μg/mL, and for *H. influenzae,* the breakpoint is even better at 0.01 μg/mL.[70]

Evidence demonstrates that other quinolones besides ciprofloxacin lack predictable bactericidal activity against *S. pneumoniae* in vitro; lomefloxacin and ofloxacin have only intermediate activity against *S. pneumoniae.* However, the clinical significance of these findings is not clear. As reviewed by Thys and colleagues,[71] there was an unexpectedly high clinical response to ciprofloxacin in several studies of acute exacerbations of chronic bronchitis, including among patients with *S. pneumoniae* infection. In randomized clinical trials comparing ciprofloxacin against ampicillin,[9, 72] amoxicillin,[73] amoxicillin-clavulanate,[74] or cefaclor[75] in treating exacerbations of bronchitis, clinical cure or improvement was found in 70% to 100% of patients receiving ciprofloxacin. In general, cure rates among patients receiving ciprofloxacin were similar to those for patients receiving the more established antibiotics.

Other quinolones have been tested in clinical trials involving treatment of moderate exacerbations of bronchitis. Lomefloxacin has the advantage of once-daily dosing, and it appears to be effective in treating acute exacerbations caused by *H. influenzae* and *M. catarrhalis.*[76] In vitro resistance of some *S. pneumoniae* to lomefloxacin has been documented, and this agent is contraindicated if gram-pos-

itive cocci predominate on the Gram stain of sputum. Ofloxacin appears to be useful against lower respiratory tract
infections, including some exacerbations of bronchitis.[77-79]
The $MIC_{90}$ of ofloxacin for *S. pneumoniae* is roughly the
same as for ciprofloxacin, approximately 2 µg/mL. Temafloxacin was originally introduced as a quinolone capable of
eradicating a higher percentage of *S. pneumoniae* isolates
than ciprofloxacin.[80, 81] This agent was withdrawn from the
commercial market (June 1992) because of serious adverse
reactions, including hepatic dysfunction, renal failure, severe hypoglycemia, and death.

The quinolones are most useful in acute exacerbations of
bronchitis caused by gram-negative bacilli, such as *P. aeruginosa,* but this constitutes a relatively small percentage of
bronchitic flares. *H. influenzae* and *M. catarrhalis* are
highly susceptible to the quinolones, but other equally effective and less expensive agents are available, such as
amoxicillin-clavulanate and trimethoprim-sulfamethoxazole. If gram-positive cocci are seen on a smear of expectorated sputum, the quinolones should not be used as first-
line agents. Similarly, if atypical bacteria are strongly suspected as the cause of a bronchitic flare (eg, *M. pneumoniae*
or *C. pneumoniae*), the quinolones should be reserved as
alternative agents to use after the macrolide antibiotics.

Preliminary studies suggest that clarithromycin, a macrolide antibiotic related to erythromycin, may be effective
in acute bacterial exacerbations. This new-generation macrolide contains a 6-methoxy group on its 14-membered
lactone ring, a modification that affords greater stability in
gastric acid and minimizes the gastrointestinal upset commonly seen with erythromycin. Clarithromycin has fourfold
greater in vitro activity against *S. pneumoniae* and other
gram-positive cocci than erythromycin. Other respiratory
pathogens usually susceptible to clarithromycin include *M.
catarrhalis, Legionella* species, *M. pneumoniae,* and *C.
pneumoniae.* In vitro studies suggest that the combination
of clarithromycin and its metabolite (14 hydroxy-clarithro-
mycin) is more active against *H. influenzae* than erythromycin or some oral cephalosporins.[82-84]

Another macrolide derivative, azithromycin, is notable
for its rapid penetration into a variety of tissues, particularly
lung parenchyma, and higher antibiotic concentrations are
achieved in infected tissues than in noninfected tissues or
serum.[85] Azithromycin exhibits greater in vitro activity
against *H. influenzae* than erythromycin or clarithromycin,
but it is two to four times less potent than clarithromycin
against *S. pneumoniae* and other gram-positive cocci. In a
randomized clinical trial comparing azithromycin with cefaclor for acute exacerbations of bronchitis, azithromycin
elicited excellent clinical and bacteriologic responses.[86] Cefaclor also performed well in this study (>90% clinical
cure or improvement) but required dosing every 8 hours
over a 10-day period; azithromycin is given every 24 hours
over a 5-day period.

Despite the concerns about bacterial resistance, the newer
broad-spectrum agents have not demonstrated clear-cut superiority over more established and less expensive agents.
Ampicillin is able to achieve clinical and bacteriologic cure
rates approaching 80% to 90% in mild exacerbations of
bronchitis, and newer agents have not consistently exceeded
those rates. It seems logical and practical to begin with
established agents such as ampicillin, amoxicillin, or trimethoprim-sulfamethoxazole if the Gram stain of expecto-

rated sputum shows a predominance of gram-positive cocci
(resembling *S. pneumoniae*) or gram-negative coccobacilli
(resembling *H. influenzae*). In communities in which β-
lactamase–producing *H. influenzae* organisms are prevalent,
amoxicillin-clavulanate may be appropriate as a first-line
agent. The same is true if gram-negative cocci (resembling
*M. catarrhalis*) are found in large numbers in the sputum
smear; if there is a high incidence of β-lactamase–producing *M. catarrhalis* infections in the area, ampicillin or
amoxicillin is not the optimal initial therapy. In the unusual
case in which the Gram stain reveals gram-negative bacilli,
empiric treatment with a quinolone is a reasonable option
if the patient is not acutely ill.

If a person with a mild to moderate exacerbation fails to
respond to the initial antibiotic chosen, reevaluation by a
physician is mandatory. Antibiotic therapy may fail for a
variety of reasons: the exacerbation is caused by a viral
infection; the exacerbation is not infectious in origin (eg,
cigarette smoking, allergen exposure, toxic inhalations); the
patient is not taking the antibiotic as prescribed because of
high cost, inconvenient dosing schedule, or toxicity; the
antibiotic chosen is inappropriate for the specific bacteria
involved; the route of administration is inappropriate for
the severity of the exacerbation; or, an underlying pneumonia exists.

Data are lacking to support the practice of ''rotating
antibiotics'' during an acute exacerbation (ie, empirically
changing from one class of oral antibiotic to another if a
patient is slow to respond). Empiric changes are likely to
be useful only in a limited number of situations. This practice is time-consuming and can cause dangerous delays in
recognizing the patient who has become seriously ill. It is
far more important for the clinician to promptly reexamine
such patients, reassess the level of disease severity, obtain
additional microbiologic data as needed, and determine the
precise cause of the antibiotic failure. In all cases, it is vital
to exclude the possibility of an evolving pneumonia, which
would require hospitalization and parenteral antibiotic therapy.

## Severe Acute Exacerbations of Chronic Bronchitis

Parenteral antibiotics usually are administered to the
bronchitic patient in respiratory distress. The parenteral
route may also be considered if an infectious exacerbation
has not improved on oral antibiotics, if pneumonia exists,
if the patient is receiving corticosteroids or other immunosuppressive agents, if gram-negative bacilli are prevalent on
the Gram stain, or if oral antibiotics are poorly tolerated.

Few systematic trials have been conducted in these situations, because physicians are unlikely to withhold antibiotics from a seriously ill patient. Most studies in this setting
have been performed without placebo controls, and their
design is a two-arm comparison study (eg, cefazolin versus
ceftazidime) or a single-arm observational study (eg, imipenem alone).

Some authorities consider ampicillin the preferred parenteral agent, but this has not been proven rigorously. Several other antibiotics have been reasonably successful in
clinical trials: ceftazidime, the combination of cefazolin and

tobramycin, cefoperazone, cefotaxime, imipenem, and the combination of ampicillin and sulbactam.[87–91] Among these newer agents, none has emerged as clearly superior. However, some antibiotics performed poorly in formal testing: moxalactam (new or recurrent infection occurred in 40% of patients within 7 days of completing therapy[92]), mezlocillin (14 of 36 patients became infected with β-lactamase–producing bacteria[93]), ceftriaxone (12 of 36 patients developed reinfections with *M. catarrhalis*[94]), and aztreonam (13 of 36 patients developed serious pneumococcal infections during therapy[95]).

Objective criteria for assessing or grading the severity of an exacerbation are lacking in these trials, and it is difficult to judge the seriousness of a patient's illness, an important factor when cross-study drug comparisons are being made. There are also no conventional indications for using parenteral antibiotics in many of these studies. In some trials, it appears that even mildly ill patients are being treated with a parenteral study drug in situations in which an oral agent may suffice. The presence or absence of pneumonia is not addressed in most analyses.

Guidelines for the antibiotic management of the acutely ill patient are limited by the available data. The prompt administration of antibiotics is indicated, but the specific agent, route, and duration remain undefined. The usual microbial flora of bronchitic patients should be covered, for which parenteral ampicillin appears reasonable. If high-level bacterial resistance is suspected, expanded-spectrum agents such as ampicillin-sulbactam, cefotaxime, or imipenem may be warranted alone or in combination. Moxalactam, mezlocillin, ceftriaxone, and aztreonam should probably be avoided as monotherapy. If an underlying pneumonia is diagnosed, the differential diagnosis must be widened, and it becomes impossible to recommend a single antibiotic of choice. If a bronchitic patient is receiving high-dose steroids, the possibility of opportunistic pathogens must be entertained, as outlined by Wiest and coworkers.[96]

## CONCLUSIONS

The available literature suggests that antibiotics are indicated in the chronic bronchitic with a mild to moderate acute exacerbation and in the chronic bronchitic with a severe exacerbation. There is little evidence to support the prophylactic use of antibiotics in managing chronic bronchitis. The antimicrobial agent chosen should be active against organisms such as *H. influenzae, S. pneumoniae,* and possibly *M. catarrhalis*. The clinician should bear in mind the wide spectrum of pathogens that may be involved, including gram-negative bacilli. The newer antimicrobial agents have theoretical advantages over the traditional ampicillin and tetracycline, but they have not been proven clearly superior in clinical trials. Nonbacterial causes for an acute exacerbation may be present in more than 50% of cases, and an aggressive search for historic clues should be undertaken. The Gram stain of expectorated sputum is still useful in confirming the diagnosis of a bacterial exacerbation and selecting appropriate antimicrobial therapy; this simple technique is probably underused. The clinician and the researcher can benefit from a more objective approach.

## REFERENCES

1. McVay LV, Sprunt DH: Antibiotic prophylaxis in chronic respiratory diseases. Arch Intern Med 92:833–846, 1953.
2. May JR: The bacteriology of chronic bronchitis. Lancet 2:534–537, 1953.
3. American Thoracic Society: Standards for the diagnosis and care of patients with COPD and asthma. Am Rev Respir Dis 136:225–228, 1987.
4. Ciba Guest Symposium Report: Terminology, definitions, and classification of chronic pulmonary emphysema and related conditions. Thorax 14:286–299, 1959.
5. Cherniak NS, Vosti KL, Dowling HF, et al: Long-term treatment of bronchiectasis and chronic bronchitis. Arch Intern Med 103:345–353, 1959.
6. Francis RS, Spicer CC: Chemotherapy in chronic bronchitis: Influence of daily penicillin and tetracycline on exacerbations and their cost. A report to the research committee of the British Tuberculosis Association by their Chronic Bronchitis subcommittee. Br Med J 1:297–303, 1960.
7. Murdoch JM, Leckie WJH, Downie J, et al: An evaluation of continuous antibiotic therapy in chronic bronchitis. Br Med J 2:1277–1285, 1959.
8. Irwin RS, Corrao WM, Erickson AD, et al: A true exacerbation of chronic obstructive bronchitis can be objectively defined. [Abstract] Am Rev Respir Dis 121:151, 1980.
9. Chodosh S, Tuck J, Stottmeier KD, et al: Comparison of ciprofloxacin with ampicillin in acute exacerbations of chronic bronchitis. Am J Med 87(suppl 5A):107S–112S, 1989.
10. Chodosh S, Eichel B, Ellis C, et al: Trimethoprim-sulfamethoxazole compared with ampicillin in acute infectious exacerbations of chronic bronchitis: A double-blind, crossover study. J Infect Dis 128 (suppl):S710–S718, 1978.
11. Higgins M: Epidemiology of COPD: State of the art. Chest 85(suppl 6):35, 1984.
12. Reid LM: Chronic obstructive pulmonary disease. *In* Fishman AP (ed): Pulmonary Diseases and Disorders. New York, McGraw-Hill, 1988:1247–1272.
13. Tager IB, Speizer FE: Risk estimates for chronic bronchitis in smokers: A study of male-female differences. Am Rev Respir Dis 113:619–625, 1976.
14. Chakrin LW, Saunders LZ: Experimental chronic bronchitis: Pathology in the dog. Lab Invest 30:145–154, 1974.
15. Seltzer J, Scanlon PD, Drazen JM, et al: Morphologic correlation of physiologic changes caused by $SO_2$-induced bronchitis in dogs. Am Rev Respir Dis 129:790–797, 1984.
16. Warner A: Clinical aspects of mucociliary transport. Am Rev Respir Dis 116:73–115, 1977.
17. Green GM, Jakab GJ, Low RB, Davis GS: Defense mechanisms of the respiratory membrane. Am Rev Respir Dis 115:479–513, 1977.
18. Chodosh S: Acute bacterial exacerbations in bronchitis and asthma. Am J Med 82(suppl 4A):154–163, 1987.
19. Irwin RS, Erickson AD, Pratter MR, et al: Prediction of tracheobronchial colonization in current cigarette smokers with chronic bronchitis. J Infect Dis 145:234–241, 1982.
20. Murphy TF, Apicella MA: Nontypable *Haemophilus influenzae:* A review of clinical aspects, surface antigens, and the human response to infection. Rev Infect Dis 9:1–15, 1987.
21. May JR: Antibiotics in chronic bronchitis. Lancet 2:899–902, 1953.
22. Elmes PC, Knox K, Fletcher CM: Sputum in chronic bronchitis: Effects of antibiotics. Lancet 2:903–906, 1953.
23. Gump DW, Phillips CA, Forsyth BR, et al: Role of infection in chronic bronchitis. Am Rev Respir Dis 113:465–474, 1976.
24. McHardy VU, Inglis JM, Calder MA, et al: A study of infective and other factors in exacerbations of chronic bronchitis. Br J Dis Chest 74:228–238, 1980.
25. Tager I, Speizer FE: Role of infection in chronic bronchitis. N Engl J Med 292:563–571, 1975.
26. Bates JH: The role of infection during exacerbations of chronic bronchitis. Ann Intern Med 97:130–131, 1982.
27. Reynolds HY: Chronic bronchitis and acute infectious exacerbations. *In* Mandel GL, Douglas RG, Bennett JE (eds): Principles and Practice of Infectious Diseases, ed 3. New York, Churchill Livingstone, 1989:531–535.
28. Sachs FL: Chronic bronchitis. *In* Pennington JE (ed): Respiratory

Infections: Diagnosis and Management. New York, Raven Press, 1989:142–158.

29. Lambert HP, Stern H: Infective factors in exacerbations of bronchitis and asthma. Br Med J 3:323–327, 1972.

30. Eadie MB, Scott EJ, Grist NR: Virological studies in chronic bronchitis. Br Med J 2:671–673, 1966.

31. Smith CB, Golden C, Klauber MR, et al: Interactions between viruses and bacteria in patients with chronic bronchitis. J Infect Dis 134:552–561, 1976.

32. Smith CB, Golden C, Kanner RE, et al: Association of viral and *Mycoplasma pneumoniae* infections with acute repiratory illness in patients with COPD. Am Rev Respir Dis 121:225–232, 1980.

33. Medici TC, Chodosh S: Sputum cell dynamics in bacterial exacerbations of chronic bronchial disease. Arch Intern Med 129:597–603, 1972.

34. Chodosh S: Examination of sputum cells. N Engl J Med 282:854–857, 1970.

35. Baigelman W, Chodosh S, Pizzuto D, et al: Quantitative sputum Gram stains in chronic bronchial disease. Lung 156:265–270, 1979.

36. Paterson IC, Petrie GR, Crompton GK, et al: Chronic bronchitis: Is bacteriological examination of the sputum necessary? Br Med J 2:537–538, 1978.

37. Irwin RS, Corrao WM, Erickson AD, et al: Characterization by transtracheal aspiration of the tracheobronchial microflora during acute exacerbations of chronic obstructive bronchitis. [Abstract] Am Rev Respir Dis 121:150–151, 1980.

38. Fagon JY, Chastre J, Trouillet JL, et al: Characterization of distal bronchial microflora during acute exacerbations of chronic bronchitis. Am Rev Respir Dis 142:1004–1008, 1990.

39. Groenveld K, van Alphen L, Eijk PP, et al: Change in outer membrane proteins of nontypable *Haemophilus influenzae* in patients with COPD. J Infect Dis 158:360–365, 1988.

40. Turk DC: The pathogenicity of *Haemophilus influenzae*. J Med Microbiol 18:1–16, 1984.

41. Loeb MR, Smith DH: Outer membrane protein composition in disease isolates of *Haemophilus influenzae:* Pathogenic and epidemiological implications. Infect Immun 30:709–717, 1980.

42. Clancy R, Cripps A, Murree-Allen K, et al: Oral immunization with killed *Haemophilus influenzae* for protection against acute bronchitis in chronic obstructive lung disease. Lancet 2:1395–1397, 1985.

43. Fletcher CM, Ball JD, Carstairs LW, et al: Value of chemoprophylaxis and chemotherapy in early chronic bronchitis: A report to the Medical Research Council by their Working Party on trials of chemotherapy in early chronic bronchitis. Br Med J 1:1317–1322, 1966.

44. Lepper MH, Dowling HF, Jackson GG, et al: Natural history of placebo-treated patients with chronic bronchial disease observed for 7 years. Antimicrob Agents Chemother 4:692–698, 1964.

45. Helm WH, May JR, Livingstone JL: Long-term oxytetracycline (Terramycin) therapy in advanced chronic respiratory infections. Lancet 1:775–777, 1956.

46. Edwards G, Fear EC: Adult chronic bronchitis—continuous antibiotic therapy. Br Med J 2:1010–1014, 1958.

47. Moyes EN, Kalinowski SZ: Prophylactic chemotherapy in chronic bronchitis. Tubercle 40:112–116, 1959.

48. May JR, Oswald NC: Prophylactic antibiotic therapy in adult chronic bronchitis. Lancet 2:814–819, 1956.

49. Buchanan J, Buchanan WW, Melrose AG, et al: Long-term prophylactic administration of tetracycline to chronic bronchitics. Lancet 1:719–722, 1958.

50. Murdoch JM, Leckie WJH, Downie J: An evaluation of continuous antibiotic therapy in chronic bronchitis. Br Med J 2:1277–1285, 1959.

51. Petersen ES, Esmann V, Honcke P, et al: A controlled study of the effects of treatment on chronic bronchitis. Acta Med Scand 182:293–305, 1967.

52. Francis RS, May JR, Spicer CC: Chemotherapy of bronchitis: Influence of penicillin and tetracycline administered daily, or intermittently, for exacerbations. Br Med J 2:979–985, 1961.

53. Pines A: Controlled trials of a sulphonamide given weekly to prevent exacerbations of chronic bronchitis. Br Med J 3:202–204, 1967.

54. Johnston RN, McNeill RS, Smith DH, et al: Five-year winter chemoprophylaxis for chronic bronchitis. Br Med J 4:265–269, 1969.

55. Pines A: Cephalexin in the prevention of purulent exacerbations of chronic bronchitis. Br J Clin Pract 26:209–210, 1972.

56. Pines A: Trimethoprim-sulfamethoxazole in the treatment and prevention of purulent exacerbations of chronic bronchitis. J Infect Dis 128(suppl):S706–709, 1973.

57. Cooper J, Inman JS, Currie WJC: Prophylactic treatment of chronic bronchitis comparing co-trimoxazole and amoxycillin. Br J Clin Pract 29:307–310, 1975.

58. Liipo K, Pelliniemi TT, Lehto H: Trimethoprim prophylaxis in acute exacerbations of COPD. Acta Med Scand 221:455–459, 1987.

59. Elmes PC, Fletcher CM, Dutton AAC: Prophylactic use of oxytetracycline for exacerbations of chronic bronchitis. Br Med J 2:1272–1275, 1957.

60. Berry DG, Fry J, Hindley CP, et al: Exacerbations of chronic bronchitis treated with oxytetracycline. Lancet 1:137–139, 1960.

61. Elmes PC, Langlands JHM, Wallace WFM, et al: Value of ampicillin in the hospital treatment of exacerbations of chronic bronchitis. Br Med J 2:904–908, 1965.

62. Pines A, Raafat H, Plucinski K, et al: Antibiotic regimens in severe and acute purulent exacerbations of chronic bronchitis. Br Med J 2:735–738, 1968.

63. Pines A, Raafat H, Greenfield JSB, et al: Antibiotic regimens in moderately ill patients with purulent exacerbations of chronic bronchitis. Br Med J 66:107–115, 1972.

64. Nicotra MB, Rivera M, Awe RJ: Antibiotic therapy of acute exacerbations of chronic bronchitis. Ann Intern Med 97:18–21, 1982.

65. Anthonisen NR, Manfreda J, Warren CP, et al: Antibiotic therapy in exacerbations of chronic obstructive pulmonary disease. Ann Intern Med 106:196–204, 1987.

66. Maesen FPV, Davies BI, Baur C: Amoxycillin/clavulanate in acute purulent exacerbations of chronic bronchitis. J Antimicrob Chemother 19:373–383, 1967.

67. Hurst DJ: A comparison of cefaclor and tetracycline in the treatment of bacterial bronchitis. Clin Ther 6:163–169, 1982.

68. Smialowicz CR: Clinical and bacteriological evaluation of cefaclor and tetracycline in acute episodes of bacterial bronchitis. Clin Ther 5:113–119, 1982.

69. Chodosh S, Tuck J, Pizzuto D: Comparative trials of doxycycline versus amoxicillin, cephalexin and enoxacin in bacterial infections in chronic bronchitis and asthma. Scand J Infect Dis 53(suppl):22–28, 1988.

70. Wolfson JS, Hooper DC: Fluoroquinolone antimicrobial agents. Clin Microbiol Rev 2:378–424, 1989.

71. Thys JP, Jacobs F, Byl B: Role of quinolones in the treatment of bronchopulmonary infections, particularly pneumococcal and community-acquired pneumonia. Eur J Clin Microbiol Infect Dis 10:304–315, 1991.

72. Arcieri G, Griffith E, Gruenwaldt G, et al: Ciprofloxacin: An update on clinical experience. Am J Med 82(suppl 4A):381–386, 1987.

73. Gleadhill IC, Ferguson WP, Lowry RC: Efficacy and safety of ciprofloxacin in patients with respiratory infections in comparison with amoxycillin. J Antimicrob Chemother 18(suppl D):133–138, 1986.

74. Schmidt EW, Zimmermann I, Ritzerfeld W, et al: Controlled prospective study of oral amoxicillin/clavulanate versus ciprofloxacin in acute exacerbations of chronic bronchitis. J Antimicrob Chemother 24(suppl B):185–193, 1989.

75. Kobayashi H, Takamura K, Takeda H, et al: Comparative clinical study of ciprofloxacin and cefaclor in the treatment of respiratory tract infections. Chemotherapy 34:1011–1037, 1986.

76. Gotfried MH, Ellison WT: Safety and efficacy of lomefloxacin versus cefaclor in the treatment of acute exacerbations of chronic bronchitis. Am J Med 92(suppl 4A):108S–113S, 1992.

77. Egede F, Kristensen I: A clinical comparative study of ofloxacin and pivampicillin in acute exacerbations of chronic bronchitis. J Antimicrob Chemother 22(suppl C):139–142, 1988.

78. Harazim H, Wimmer J, Mittermayer HP: An open randomized comparison of ofloxacin and doxycycline in lower respiratory tract infections. Drugs 34(suppl 1):71–73, 1987.

79. Rademaker CMA, Sips AP, Beumer HM, et al: A double-blind comparison of low-dose ofloxacin and amoxycillin-clavulanic acid in acute exacerbations of chronic bronchitis. J Antimicrob Chemother 26(suppl D):75–81, 1990.

80. Chodosh S, Tuck J, Pizzuto D, et al: Temafloxacin versus ciprofloxacin in acute bacterial exacerbations of chronic bronchitis. Presented at the 30th Annual Interscience Conference on Antimicrobial Agents and Chemotherapy, Atlanta, GA, October, 1990.

81. Aldons P, Carpentier P, Afarian J, et al: Safety and efficacy of temafloxacin in the treatment of COPD patients with acute bacterial infections. Presented at the 7th Mediterranean Congress of Chemotherapy, Barcelona, Spain, May, 1990.

82. Bachand RT: Comparative study of clarithromycin and ampicillin in

the treatment of patients with acute bacterial exacerbations of chronic bronchitis. J Antimicrob Chemother 27(suppl A):91–100, 1991.

83. Aldons PM: A comparison of clarithromycin with ampicillin in the treatment of outpatients with acute bacterial exacerbations of chronic bronchitis. J Antimicrob Chemother 27(suppl A):101–108, 1991.

84. Neu HC: The development of macrolides: Clarithromycin in perspective. J Antimicrob Chemother 27(suppl A):1–9, 1991.

85. Baldwin DR, Wise R, Andrews JM, et al: Azithromycin concentration at the sites of pulmonary infection. Eur Respir J 3:886–870, 1990.

86. Dark D: Multicenter evaluation of azithromycin and cefaclor in acute lower respiratory tract infections. Am J Med 91(suppl 3A):31S–35S, 1991.

87. Davies BI, Maesen FPV, van Noord JA: Clinical, bacteriological and pharmacokinetic results from an open trial of sultamicillin in patients with acute exacerbations of chronic bronchitis. J Antimicrob Chemother 13:161–170, 1984.

88. Vetter N, Feist H, Muhar F, et al: A comparative study of the efficacy of ceftazidime versus cefazolin and tobramycin in patients with acute exacerbations of chronic bronchitis. J Antimicrob Chemother 12(suppl A):35–39, 1983.

89. Wathen CG, Carbarns NJ, Jones PA, et al: Imipenem-cilastatin in the treatment of respiratory infections in patients with chronic airways obstruction. J Antimicrob Chemother 21:107–112, 1988.

90. Davies BI, Maesen FPV, Brouwers J: Cefoperazone in acute exacerbations of chronic bronchitis. J Antimicrob Chemother 9:149–155, 1982.

91. Maesen FPV, Davies BI, Drenth BMH, et al: Treatment of acute exacerbations of chronic bronchitis with cefotaxime: A controlled clinical trial. J Antimicrob Chemother 6(suppl A):187–192, 1980.

92. Maesen FPV, Davies BI, Brouwers J, et al: Latamoxef (moxalactam) in acute exacerbations of chronic bronchitis. J Antimicrob Chemother 11:115–123, 1983.

93. Maesen FPV, Davies BI, Brouwers J, et al: Is treatment of acute exacerbations of chronic bronchitis with intramuscular mezlocillin justifiable? J Antimicrob Chemother 12:169–173, 1983.

94. Maesen FPV, Davies BI, Teengs JP: Ceftriaxone in acute purulent exacerbations of chronic bronchitis. J Antimicrob Chemother 14:653–660, 1984.

95. Davies BI, Maesen FPV, Teengs JP: Aztreonam in patients with acute purulent exacerbations of chronic bronchitis: Failure to prevent emergence of pneumococcal infections. J Antimicrob Chemother 15:375–384, 1985.

96. Wiest PM, Flanigan T, Salata RA, et al: Serious infectious complications of corticosteroid therapy for COPD. Chest 95:1180–1184, 1989.

# INDEX

Note: Page numbers in *italics* refer to illustrations; page numbers followed by t refer to tables.

ISBN 0-7216-4347-7

90038